Solved Papers of
EMERGENCY MEDICINE
for Postgraduate Students

Solved Papers of
EMERGENCY MEDICINE
for Postgraduate Students

Editor

Devendra Richhariya
MBBS MD MBA Fellowship in Intensive Care Medicine
PG Diploma Medical Toxicology
Senior Emergency Physician
Gurugram, Haryana, India

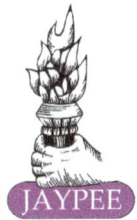

JAYPEE BROTHERS MEDICAL PUBLISHERS
The Health Sciences Publisher
New Delhi | London

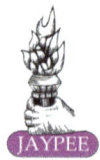
Jaypee Brothers Medical Publishers (P) Ltd

Headquarters
Jaypee Brothers Medical Publishers (P) Ltd
EMCA House, 23/23-B
Ansari Road, Daryaganj
New Delhi 110 002, India
Landline: +91-11-23272143, +91-11-23272703
+91-11-23282021, +91-11-23245672
Email: jaypee@jaypeebrothers.com

Overseas Office
JP Medical Ltd.
83, Victoria Street, London
SW1H 0HW (UK)
Phone: +44 20 3170 8910
Email: info@jpmedpub.com

Corporate Office
Jaypee Brothers Medical Publishers (P) Ltd
4838/24, Ansari Road, Daryaganj
New Delhi 110 002, India
Phone: +91-11-43574357
Fax: +91-11-43574314
Email: jaypee@jaypeebrothers.com

EU GPSR Authorised Representative
Logos Europe, 9 rue Nicolas Poussin
17000, La Rochelle, France
Phone: +33 (0) 6 67 93 73 78
E-mail: Contact@logoseurope.eu

Website: www.jaypeebrothers.com
Website: www.jaypeedigital.com

© 2024, Jaypee Brothers Medical Publishers

The views and opinions expressed in this book are solely those of the original contributor(s)/author(s) and do not necessarily represent those of editor(s) or publisher of the book.

All rights reserved. No part of this publication may be reproduced, stored or transmitted in any form or by any means, electronic, mechanical, photo copying, recording or otherwise, without the prior permission in writing of the publishers.

All brand names and product names used in this book are trade names, service marks, trademarks or registered trademarks of their respective owners. The publisher is not associated with any product or vendor mentioned in this book.

Medical knowledge and practice change constantly. This book is designed to provide accurate, authoritative information about the subject matter in question. However, readers are advised to check the most current information available on procedures included and check information from the manufacturer of each product to be administered, to verify the recommended dose, formula, method and duration of administration, adverse effects and contra indications. It is the responsibility of the practitioner to take all appropriate safety precautions. Neither the publisher nor the author(s)/editor(s) assume any liability for any injury and/or damage to persons or property arising from or related to use of material in this book.

This book is sold on the understanding that the publisher is not engaged in providing professional medical services. If such advice or services are required, the services of a competent medical professional should be sought.

Every effort has been made where necessary to contact holders of copyright to obtain permission to reproduce copyright material. If any have been inadvertently overlooked, the publisher will be pleased to make the necessary arrangements at the first opportunity.

Inquiries for bulk sales may be solicited at: jaypee@jaypeebrothers.com

Solved Papers of Emergency Medicine for Postgraduate Students

First Edition: **2024**

ISBN: 978-93-5696-218-7

Dedicated to

My parents

Contributors

Ajay Singh Thapa MD DM
Head (Emergency Medicine)
Department of Emergency Medicine
B & B Hospital
Kathmandu, Nepal

Anshul Jain MBBS MD MRCEM
Assistant Professor
Department of Emergency Medicine
Amrita Institute of Medical Sciences
Gurugram, Haryana, India

Aysegul Bayir MD
Professor Emergency Medicine
Faculty of Medicine
Department of Emergency Medicine
Selçuk University
Konya, Turkey

Bipin Karki MD DM
Resident (Critical Care Medicine)
Department of Emergency Medicine
Maharajgunj Medical Campus
Institute of Medicine
Tribhuvan University Teaching Hospital
Kathmandu, Nepal

Constatine AU
MBBS DPD PG Diploma SEM Diploma Clinical Toxicology PG Diploma Medical Toxicology (Cardiff) MSc in Infectious Diseases MRCS (Ed) FHKCEM FHKAM FRCEM
Medical Director
Department of Emergency Medicine
Emergency Care Training (HK) Rescue Products Limited
Hong Kong, China

Devisha Varma Jhunjhunwala
MBBS MEM
Clinical Associate
Emergency Department
PD Hinduja Hospital
Mumbai, Maharashtra, India

Devendra Richhariya
MBBS MD MBA Fellowship in Intensive Care Medicine PG Diploma Medical Toxicology
Senior Emergency Physician
Gurugram, Haryana, India

Egala VSSN Murthy MD IDCCM CIH CCEBDM
Emergency Physician and Intensivist
Department of Emergency Medicine
Maxcure Hospital
Hyderabad, Telangana, India

Jidhin Janardhanan MBBS DNB MRCEM
Head (Emergency Medicine)
Department of Emergency Medicine
Sree Narayana Institute of Medical Sciences (SNIMS)
Kochi, Kerala, India

Nandha Kumar Selvam
MBBS MEM (CCT-EM)
Registrar (Emergency Medicine)
Department of Emergency Medicine
Kovai Medical Center and Hospitals
Coimbatore, Tamil Nadu, India

Narendra Nath Jena
MBBS MEM MPH MBA
Director and Head
Accident and Emergency
Meenakshi Mission Hospital and Research Center
Madurai, Tamil Nadu, India

Noel Fernando
MBBS MD MRCEM FRCEM FFICM
Specialist in Emergency Medicine and Intensive Care
Department of Emergency Medicine
Queens Medical Centre
Nottingham, UK

Olita Shilpakar MD DM FRCP (Edinburgh)
Assistant Professor
Department of Emergency Medicine
Maharajgunj Medical Campus
Institute of Medicine
Tribhuvan University Teaching Hospital
Kathmandu, Nepal

Pradeep Kumar Botsa
MBBS CTCCM MEM PGCIH
Emergency Physician and Intensivist
Department of Emergency Medicine
Reliance Industries Limited
Vadodara, Gujarat, India

Rahul Solanki
MBBS MD FCCM
Director
Department of Emergency Medicine
Dewas Hospital and Research Centre
Dewas, Madhya Pradesh, India

Santosh Pandey
MBBS DNB FRCEM
Consultant
Department of Emergency Medicine
Maharaja Agrasen Hospital
New Delhi, India

Shweta Ashok
MBBS MEM FICM MBA (HHSM)
Consultant In-charge
Department of Emergency Medicine
Matsaya Clinics
Chennai, Tamil Nadu, India

Shweta Tyagi
MBBS FAEM MRCEM MBA
Head (Emergency Medicine)
Department of Emergency Medicine
Paras Health
Gurugram, Haryana, India

Sreekrishnan TP
MBBS MD
Consultant Emergency Medicine
Department of Emergency Medicine
Amrita Hospitals
Kochi, Kerala, India

Subbulakshmi Dhanabal
MBBS MEM
Associate Consultant
Emergency Department
Meenakshi Mission Hospital & Research Centre
Madurai, Tamil Nadu, India

Susmeet Mishra
DEM (RCGP, UK) MRCEM CCIDM (MUM)
Consultant and Head
Department of Emergency Medicine
SUM Ultimate Medicare
Bhubaneswar, Odisha, India

Preface

All power is within you; you can do anything and everything.

–Swami Vivekananda

Emergency medicine in India is no longer in a primitive phase; more and more expectations need to be fulfilled by the emergency physician toward quality patient care. Postgraduation program in emergency medicine is now the central part of academics in the emergency department and also in most of the medical schools in India. Emergency medicine postgraduate students are now acquiring and updating their knowledge through various platforms such as latest book and e-books articles simulation laboratory. This is our duty to provide them updated knowledge through various modes.

With this thought in mind, the 2nd edition of *Textbook of Emergency Medicine: Including Intensive Care & Trauma* was published which has been well appreciated by students and national and international faculties in view of its unique presentation of contents. *Textbook of Emergency Medicine: Including Intensive Care & Trauma,* 2nd edition, was published in two volumes consisting of 250 chapters and 22 sections with short answer questions (SAQs) after each chapter and multiple choice questions (MCQs) after each section.

In view of supporting the emergency medicine postgraduate students, we present solved questions from previous years' examination which enable them to prepare for exit examination in a short period of time, face the stressful period confidently, and clear the theory and practical examination. This book will be helpful for DNB (EM), MD (EM), MEM/CCT (EM), MRCEM, and FRCEM students.

Hopefully, all the postgraduate students will appreciate this effort as well. I extend my wishes to all the emergency medicine postgraduate students for their future endeavors.

Devendra Richhariya

Acknowledgments

I would like to thank all the authors for providing their chapters in spite of their busy schedules.

I would like to extend my special thanks to Shri Jitendar P Vij (Group Chairman), Mr Ankit Vij (Managing Director), Mr MS Mani (Group President), Ms Chetna Malhotra (Senior Director—Professional Publishing, Marketing, and Business Development), Ms Pooja Bhandari (Director—Production), and Mr Anand Kumar (Development Editor) of M/s Jaypee Brothers Medical Publishers (P) Ltd, New Delhi, India, for their invaluable contribution.

Contents

Emergency Medicine Paper 1 1
Devendra Richhariya

Emergency Medicine Paper 2 11
Devendra Richhariya

Emergency Medicine Paper 3 21
Devendra Richhariya

Emergency Medicine Paper 4 32
Devendra Richhariya

Emergency Medicine Paper 5 43
Santosh Pandey

Emergency Medicine Paper 6 51
Santosh Pandey

Emergency Medicine Paper 7 60
Anshul Jain

Emergency Medicine Paper 8 68
Anshul Jain

Emergency Medicine Paper 9 77
Olita Shilpakar, Bipin Karki

Emergency Medicine Paper 10 88
Bipin Karki, Olita Shilpakar

Emergency Medicine Paper 11 100
Devendra Richhariya

Emergency Medicine Paper 12 110
Devendra Richhariya

Emergency Medicine Paper 13 119
Aysegul Bayir

Emergency Medicine Paper 14 129
Aysegul Bayir

Emergency Medicine Paper 15 137
Shweta Ashok

Emergency Medicine Paper 16 151
Shweta Ashok

Emergency Medicine Paper 17 162
Devendra Richhariya

Emergency Medicine Paper 18 173
Devendra Richhariya

Emergency Medicine Paper 19 183
Rahul Solanki

Emergency Medicine Paper 20 195
Rahul Solanki

Emergency Medicine Paper 21 206
Pradeep Kumar Botsa

Emergency Medicine Paper 22 220
Ajay Singh Thapa

Emergency Medicine Paper 23 231
Ajay Singh Thapa

Emergency Medicine Paper 24 240
Devendra Richhariya

Emergency Medicine Paper 25 251
Devendra Richhariya

Emergency Medicine Paper 26 262
Devisha Varma Jhunjhunwala

Emergency Medicine Paper 27 273
Susmeet Mishra

Emergency Medicine Paper 28 289
Egala VSSN Murthy

Emergency Medicine Paper 29 299
Noel Fernando

Emergency Medicine Paper 30 324
Noel Fernando

Emergency Medicine Paper 31 341
Devendra Richhariya

Emergency Medicine Paper 32 351
Devendra Richhariya

Emergency Medicine Paper 33 360
Narendra Nath Jena, Subbulakshmi Dhanabal

Emergency Medicine Paper 34 373
Subbulakshmi Dhanabal, Narendra Nath Jena

Emergency Medicine Paper 35 382
Devendra Richhariya

Emergency Medicine Paper 36 393
Nandha Kumar Selvam

Emergency Medicine Paper 37 404
Devendra Richhariya

Emergency Medicine Paper 38 415
Devendra Richhariya

Emergency Medicine Paper 39 427
Devendra Richhariya

Emergency Medicine Paper 40 438
Constatine AU

Emergency Medicine Paper 41 447
Devendra Richhariya

Emergency Medicine Paper 42 455
Devendra Richhariya

Emergency Medicine Paper 43 466
Shweta Tyagi

Emergency Medicine Paper 44 478
Jidhin Janardhanan

Emergency Medicine Paper 45 486
Sreekrishnan TP

Emergency Medicine Paper 46 497
Sreekrishnan TP

Emergency Medicine Paper 47 506
Devendra Richhariya

Emergency Medicine Paper 48 516
Devendra Richhariya

Emergency Medicine Paper 49 525
Devendra Richhariya

Emergency Medicine Paper 50 541
Devendra Richhariya

Emergency Medicine Paper 51 553
Devendra Richhariya

Emergency Medicine Paper 52 569
Devendra Richhariya

Index 577

Emergency Medicine Paper 1

Devendra Richhariya

Question 1

1. Draw a labeled diagram of the conducting system of the heart.

Cardiac conducting system is made up of five elements (**Fig. 1**):
a. Sinoatrial (SA) node
b. Atrioventricular (AV) node
c. Bundle of His
d. Left and right bundle branches
e. Purkinje fibers.

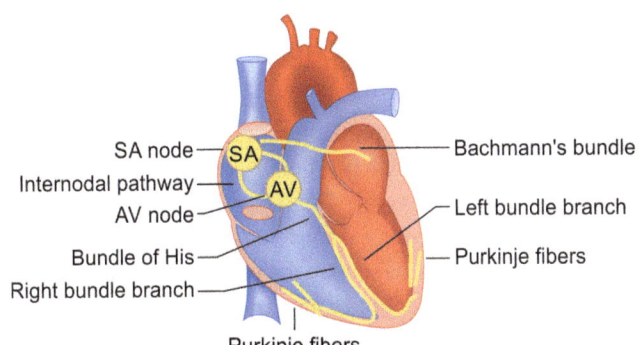

Fig. 1: Cardiac conducting system. (AV: atrioventricular; SA: sinoatrial)

2. What are the different mechanisms of the tachyarrhythmia?

Arrhythmogenic mechanisms with regard to the basic mechanisms of cardiac arrhythmia can be distinguished on two levels: cellular and tissue levels. Mechanisms acting at the cellular level comprise automaticity and triggered activity. The latter has been shown to be related to afterdepolarizations in the membrane potential. However, reentry-based arrhythmia is generated at the tissue level; it is observed most frequently and therefore, it represents the main topic of this study. Yet, as found in experiments, afterdepolarizations can be decisively involved in the reentry process (**Fig. 2**).

Automaticity: It is the ability to generate a spontaneous action potential. All cardiac cells can display this property, but, in a normal heart, most do not. Depending on the location within the heart, therefore, automaticity may be classified as either normal or abnormal. Cardiac cells with normal automaticity are called pacemaker cells. The dominant pacemaker of the heart is normally the sinus node, but there also exist cells capable of spontaneous diastolic depolarization, such as specialized fibers of the atria, AV junction, and the His-Purkinje system. These secondary pacemakers lie dormant (latent) until the sinus node activity is removed, allowing the latent pacemaker's rhythm to become visible.

Triggered rhythms: These are known to be caused by afterdepolarizations, which are oscillations in the membrane potential following an action potential. One mechanism by which triggered activity causes arrhythmia is observed when the afterdepolarization (of either type) is large enough to reach the threshold potential. The resulting action potential is called a triggered action potential. An arrhythmia is induced when impulse initiation shifts from the sinus node to the triggered focus. For this to happen, the rate of triggered impulses must be faster than the rate of the sinus node.

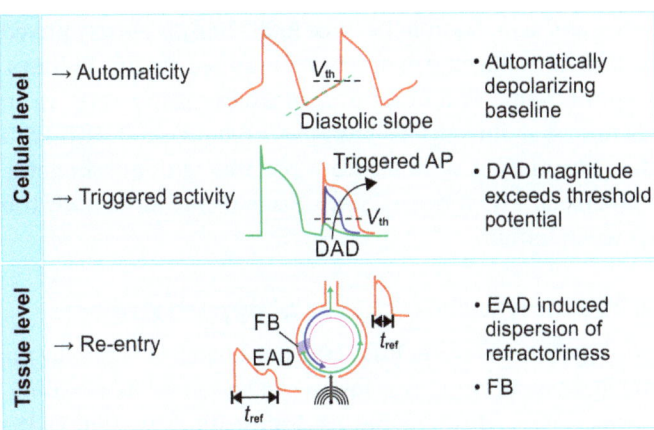

Fig. 2: Mechanisms of cardiac arrhythmia. (AP: action potential; DAD: delayed afterdepolarization; EAD: early afterdepolarization; FB: functional block; t_{ref}: reference travel; V_{th}: threshold potential)

3. Discuss the classification of anti-arrhythmic drugs.

Anti-arrhythmic drugs are classified in four groups as given in **Table 1**.

TABLE 1: Classification of anti-arrhythmic drugs.

Class I	IA	IB	IC
• Membrane stabilizing (Na channel blockers) • Class IA: Moderately prolong conduction • Class IB: Minimal effect on conduction • Class IC: Marked prolongation of conduction	• Quinidine • Procainamide • Disopyramide	• Lidocaine • Mexiletine	• Propafenone • Flecainide
Class II (blockade of β-adrenergic receptors)	• Propranolol • Esmolol • Sotalol (class III properties also)		
Class III (prolongation of repolarization)	• Amiodarone • Dronedarone • Dofetilide • Ibutilide		
Class IV (calcium channel blockers)	• Verapamil • Diltiazem		
Drugs for paroxysmal supraventricular tachycardia	• Adenosine • Digoxin		

Question 2

1. What is sodium homeostasis?

Sodium is an important electrolyte, mainly found in extracellular fluid, which helps to maintain fluid balance, blood pressure, nerve impulse conduction, and muscle contraction. The human body tightly maintains serum [Na^+] between 138 and 142 mEq/L despite what may be marked changes in daily intake depending on the person's diet. The sodium balance is the difference between the amount of Na absorbed by the gut and the amount excreted via urine, feces, and skin. Sodium balance in the body is closely linked to that of water and is finely maintained by the kidneys. Hyponatremia is a condition of excess water relative to Na^+ and is defined as a serum [Na^+] 100 mOsm/L H_2O with the exception of samples from patients with psychogenic polydipsia, which drives down urine osmolality below the typical minimum.

2. Mention various causes of hypernatremia.

Etiology: Serious water loss is the most common etiology for the hypernatremia. These losses can be caused by sweating, burns, losses through the gastrointestinal system (GIS) (vomiting, osmotic diarrhea, and loss of small intestine fluids), urinary losses, central diabetes insipidus (DI), nephrogenic DI, osmotic diuresis, diseases (adipsic DI) that affect the osmoreceptors in the hypothalamus, or the feeling of thirst. Intracellular water loss, excessive salt intake (intentional or unintentional increased oral intake of salt), iatrogenic (hypertonic saline infusion, sodium bicarbonate therapy, and intrauterine hypertonic saline administration for abortion induction), and some medications (lithium, phenytoin, and corticosteroids) can cause hypernatremia.

3. Discuss the pathophysiology of clinical effects of hypernatremia.

Pathophysiology: Extracellular and intracellular fluid osmolality are equal to each other. Water passes through the cell membrane comfortably. There are mainly sodium ions outside the cell and potassium ions inside the cell. Serum sodium concentration, as seen in the equation below, is closely related to the amount of potassium and water in the body.

Plasma osmolality: It is formulated as plasma osmolality: 2 (Na) mEq/L + [serum glucose (mg/dL)]/18 + [blood urea nitrogen (BUN) (mg/dL)]/2.8 and its normal limit is 275–290 mOsm/kg. Plasma sodium and plasma osmolality are kept in balance by water intake and excretion.

$$Na = Total\ body\ (Na + K)/total\ body\ water$$

Hypernatremia occurs due to either increased salt consumption, using hypertonic salt solutions, or loss of water from the body without electrolyte. When osmolality increases, arginine vasopressin (AVP) hormone and thirst are increased and a balance is achieved. Intracellular fluid is drawn into the intravascular area due to increased osmolality. Dehydration develops in the cells that work as an osmoreceptor or tonicity receptor in the brain. These cells work like a mechanoreceptor and provide AVP release and thirst. This regulatory system activates even when a large amount of salt is taken or fluid is lost and keeps serum sodium within normal limits. However, this physiological regulatory system may be insufficient for oral intake in people with impaired mental status, advanced elderly or care patients, critical care intensive care patients who are hospitalized, and children and infants.

Clinical findings: Advanced age, oral intake, impairment of consciousness, debility, physical disability, diuretic therapy, uncontrolled DI, hospitalization, and insufficient parent or nurse care at home are the risk factors for hypernatremia.

In physical examination, hemodynamic status should be evaluated first and vital parameters should be monitored. Clinical findings are based on volume deficiency, hypertonicity, and dehydration in the cells in the central nervous system. Neurological evaluation should be done very well. In patients with severe hypernatremia, brain hemorrhage due to tear may occur in the cerebral vessels. Hypotension, orthostatic hypotension, tachycardia, oliguria, dryness of the skin and mucous membranes, and turgor-tonus decrease occur due to hypovolemia. In addition, lethargy, irritability, cloudiness, confusion, widespread weakness, myoclonic jerks, seizures, and coma are the neurological signs and symptoms.

Question 3

1. Discuss the anatomy of wrist and hand as relevant to an emergency physician.

The human hand has 27 bones: the carpals or wrist accounts for eight, the metacarpals or palm contains five, the remaining 14 are digital bones (fingers and thumb). The palm has five bones known as the metacarpal bones, one to each of the five digits. These metacarpals have a head, a shaft, and a base. The joints of the hand include carpometacarpal joints found between the carpals and the metacarpals; the intermetacarpal joints among the metacarpals themselves; the metacarpophalangeal joints between the metacarpals and the proximal phalanges; and, finally, the interphalangeal joints found between the proximal phalanges **(Fig. 3)**.

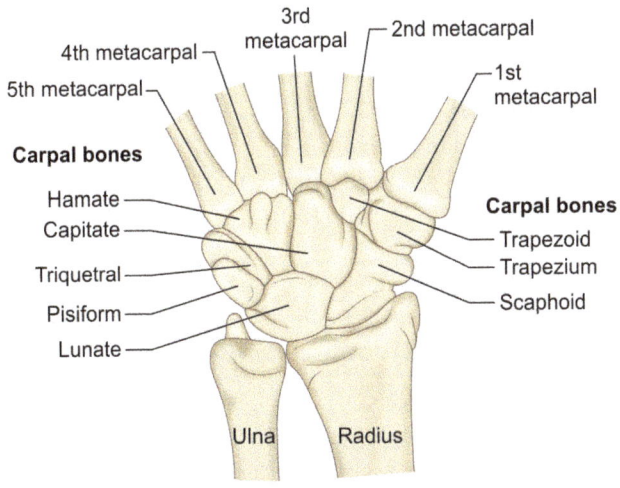

Fig. 3: Anatomy of wrist and hand.

2. Discuss the nerve supply of various muscles of the hand.

3. What are the actions of various muscles of hand?

The muscles of the hand are innervated by the radial, median, and ulnar nerves. The radial nerve innervates the finger extensors and the thumb abductor, i.e., the muscles that extend at the wrist and metacarpophalangeal joints (knuckles) and abduct and extend the thumb. The action of various muscles of hand and their innervation are given in **Table 2**.

TABLE 2: Intrinsic muscles of the hand and their innervation and actions.

Muscle	Action	Innervation
Thenar group		
Flexor pollicis brevis	Flexes thumb	Median nerve
Abductor pollicis brevis	Abducts thumb	
Opponens pollicis	Opposes thumb	
Hypothenar group		
Flexor digiti minimi	Flexes finger 5	Ulnar nerve
Abductor digiti minimi	Abducts finger 5	
Opponens digiti minimi	Opposition of finger 5	
Midpalmar group		
Lumbricals	Flexes 2nd–5th MP joints and extends 2nd–5th PIP and DIP joints	• Lateral 2 lumbricals: Median nerve • Medial 2 lumbricals: Ulnar nerve
Dorsal Interossei	Abducts fingers 2–5	Ulnar nerve
Palmar interossei	Adducts fingers 2–5	
Adductor pollicis	Adducts thumb	

(DIP: distal interphalangeal; MP: metacarpophalangeal; PIP: proximal interphalangeal)

Question 4

1. What is Kassirer–Bleich equation?

The *Henderson–Hasselbalch equation* shows that the pH is determined by the ratio of the serum bicarbonate (HCO_3) concentration and the partial pressure of carbon dioxide (PCO_2).

$pH = pK + \log (HCO_3)/(H_2CO_3)$ = Kidney/lung = [Metabolic/respiratory]

Kassirer-Bleich equation: $H^+ = 24 \times PCO_2/HCO_3$ (validity check) shows that pH is the function of ratio of bicarbonate to PCO_2.

2. How does the kidney regulate the acid–base balance?

The kidneys play a major role in the regulation of acid-base balance by reabsorbing bicarbonate filtered by the glomeruli and excreting titratable acids and ammonia into the urine **(Fig. 4)**.

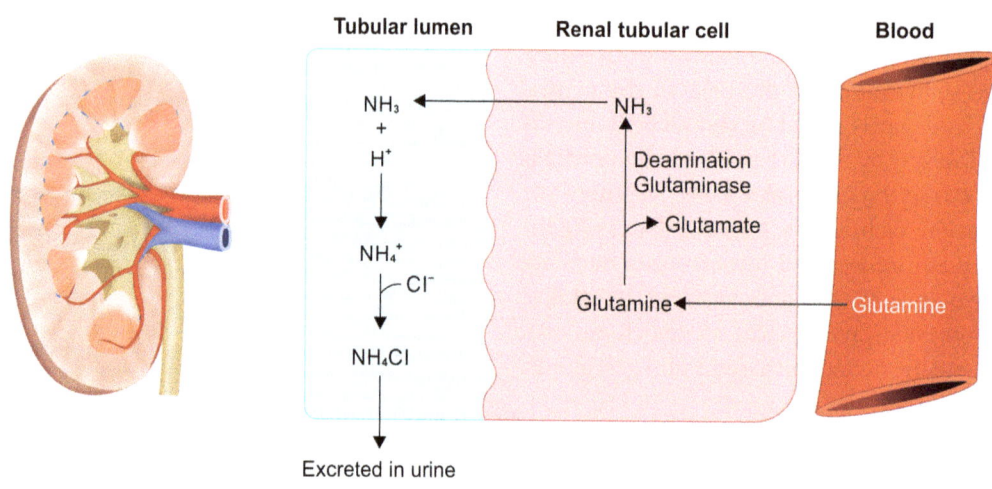

Fig. 4: Renal mechanism of acid–base balance.

3. Define anion gap and mention its clinical use.

Normal anion gap (AG) is 10 ± 2 mmol/L.

$$AG = Na^+ - (Cl^- + HCO_3^-)$$

The "normal" AG in patients with hypoalbuminemia is about 2.5 mEq/L lower for each 1 g/dL decrease in the plasma albumin concentration from normal.

Corrected AG = Calculated AG + 2.5 (albumin normal, i.e., 4 – albumin measured)

Raised AG acidosis: AG is raised in lactic acidosis (e.g., hypoxemia, ischemia, shock, sepsis), ketoacidosis (diabetes, starvation, and alcohol excess), renal failure (accumulation of sulfate, phosphate, and urate), poisoning (aspirin, methanol, and ethylene glycol), and massive rhabdomyolysis.

If the AG is raised, *calculate the osmolal gap* in case of compatible situations.
Osmolal gap = Measured osmolality – calculated osmolality
Serum osmolality = 2(Na) + BUN/2.8 + Glucose/18
Normal osmolal gap <15 mOsm/L
Osmolal gap may be increased in methanol poisoning, ethanol poisoning, hyperlipidemia chronic renal failure, and myeloma.

Normal AG (hyperchloremic) acidosis occurs predominantly due to loss of HCO_3^-

Non-anion gap (NAG) acidosis is seen in renal tubular acidosis (types 1, 2, and 4), diarrhea (HCO_3^- loss), adrenal insufficiency, ammonium chloride ingestion, urinary diversion (e.g., ureterosigmoidostomy), and drugs (e.g., acetazolamide).

4. Enumerate the causes of metabolic acidosis.

MUDPILERS is a mnemonic used to remember the causes of metabolic acidosis:
M—methanol
U—uremia
D—diabetic ketoacidosis (DKA)/alcoholic ketosis
P—paraldehyde
I—isoniazid
L—lactic acidosis
E—ethanol/ethylene glycol
R—rhabdomyolysis/renal failure
S—salicylates.

Question 5

1. Discuss noninvasive oxygen and carbon dioxide monitoring.

Pulse oximetry and capnography are widely used in clinical practice. They provide quick and noninvasive methods to estimate arterial oxygen saturation and carbon dioxide (CO_2)

tension in different situations including emergency departments (EDs), intensive care units, and during procedures. This chapter reviews the principles of surgery, accuracy, limitations, and clinical applications of these instruments.

2. What is the oxygen–hemoglobin dissociation curve?

Oxygen in blood depends on hemoglobin concentration and percentage saturation of hemoglobin with oxygen (SO_2). Partial pressure of oxygen (PO_2) is the driving force for oxygen molecule to bind with hemoglobin. So, the oxyhemoglobin dissociation curve shows SO_2 at any given PO_2 (generally we can say that the higher the PO_2, the higher the SO_2). But the curve is not linear; the *flat part of the curve* shows that PO_2 has little effect on SO_2 over this range. The *steep part of the curve* shows that even a small change in PO_2 makes a significant change in SO_2 over this range (**Fig. 5**).

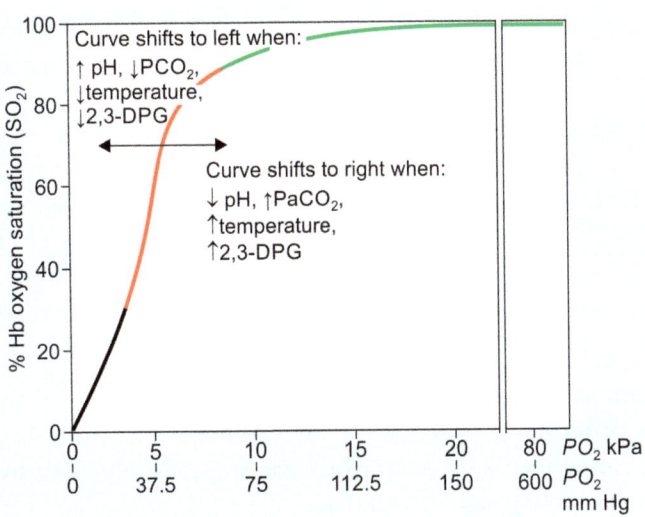

Fig. 5: Oxyhemoglobin dissociation curve. The curve defines the relationship between PO_2 and the SO_2. Note the sigmoid shape of the curve: it is relatively flat when PO_2 is >80 mm Hg (10.6 kPa) but steep when PO_2 falls below 60 mm Hg (8 kPa). (2,3-DPG: 2,3-diphosphoglyceric acid; PCO_2: partial pressure of carbon dioxide; $PaCO_2$: partial pressure of arterial carbon dioxide; PO_2: partial pressure of oxygen; SO_2: percentage saturation of hemoglobin with oxygen)

3. What is the utility of end-tidal CO_2 during cardiopulmonary resuscitation (CPR)?

The end-tidal CO_2 ($EtCO_2$) is the maximal partial pressure or concentration of CO_2 in the respiratory gases at the end of an exhaled breath. A capnometry monitor displays the $ETCO_2$ value alone, where as a capnography monitor displays the $ETCO_2$ value plus a continuous capnography waveform. Capnography is a mandatory tool in airway management in ED and ambulances. It is essential to confirm tube placement after intubation, monitoring of intubated patients in ED and also during medical transport. Capnometry is the continuous measurement of CO_2 in a sample of gas and is represented as a graphic form (time on X-axis and expired partial pressure of CO_2 on the Y-axis).

The capnography wave has four phases: Normal capnography wave morphology (**Fig. 6**).

Phase I (inspiratory phase): It represents the inspiratory phase, so no CO_2 is detected. The end of phase I represents the beginning of expiration, but because the initial gases expired originate from unventilated dead space, the capnography trace remains at zero.

Phase II (expiratory upstroke): It represents expiration of both dead space gas and alveolar gas from the respiratory bronchioles and alveoli.

Phase III (alveolar plateau): It represents the phase of expiration of alveolar gases. At the end of phase III, the maximal value of CO_2 measured is equivalent to the $EtCO_2$. Note that if all the alveoli contained exactly the same partial pressure of CO_2, phase III would be completely horizontal.

Phase IV (expiratory downstroke): It represents the beginning of the next breath, with the CO_2 content returning rapidly to zero. Healthy patients with normal respiratory function will produce a capnography trace with this form. Lung pathologies will change the appearance of the capnograph due to a number of different factors such as bronchoconstriction and obstruction to airflow, destruction of alveoli, an increase in the range of alveolar time constants (alveoli that empty at different rates), and an increase in lung ventilation (V)/perfusion (Q) spread (variation in the CO_2 content of each alveolus). As a result, the slope of phase III is often markedly increased in respiratory disease.

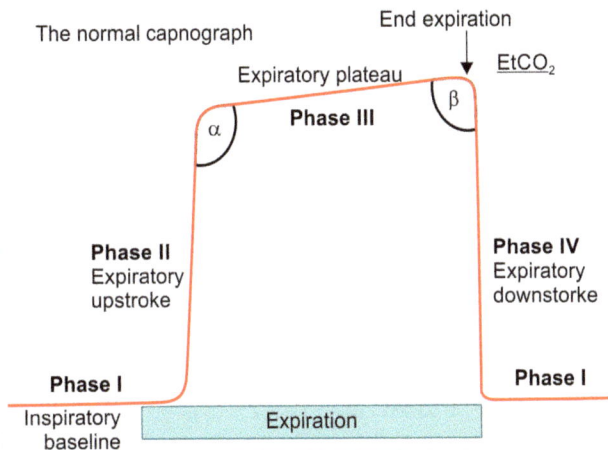

Fig. 6: Morphology of normal capnography wave. ($EtCO_2$: end tidal carbon dioxide)

Question 6

1. Name three low-molecular weight heparin (LMWH) along with their doses.

Prophylaxis for deep vein thrombosis and pulmonary embolism
a. *Dalteparin:* 2,500–5,000 IU SC once a day
b. *Enoxaparin:* 40 mg SC once daily in normal renal function, 30 mg SC twice daily for trauma patient
c. *Fondaparinux:* 2.5 mg SC once daily

Treatment for deep vein thrombosis and pulmonary embolism
a. *Enoxaparin:* 1 mg/kg SC every 12 hours or 1.5 mg/kg daily
b. *Dalteparin:* 200 units/kg SC once daily
c. *Tinzaparin:* 175 mg/kg once daily
d. *Fondaparinux:* <50 kg: 5 mg SC once daily, 50–100 kg: 7.5 mg SC once daily, >100 kg: 10 mg SC once daily.

2. Discuss the mechanism of action of unfractionated and LMWH.

Unfractionated heparin (UFH): It is a heterogenous mixture of polysaccharides. It has unpredictable anticoagulant effects, which are generally monitored by activated partial thromboplastin time (aPTT). UFH derivatives have no intrinsic anticoagulant activity; rather these agents bind to antithrombin and accelerate the rate at which it inhibits various coagulation proteases. Antithrombin inhibits activated coagulation factors, particularly thrombin and factor Xa, by serving as a "suicide substrate." Bleeding and heparin-induced thrombocytopenia (HIT) are major complications.

LMWH: They are polysaccharide chains with commercial preparations (enoxaparin, dalteparin, and tinzaparin). LMWH possesses many clinical advantages compared to UFH.

Fondaparinux: It is a synthetic pentasaccharide that binds to antithrombin and enhances its affinity for factor Xa, but not thrombin.

3. Discuss the methods to monitor anticoagulation therapy with UFH.

Monitoring anticoagulation therapy:

Target international randomized ratio (INR)
a. For prosthetic heart valve, INR 2.5–3.5
b. For all other conditions including deep vein thrombosis, pulmonary thromboembolism, and atrial fibrillation, INR 2–3
c. Higher INR is beneficial in patients with recurrent thromboembolic events while on anticoagulation.
d. Check INR four times per week initially in the first week of therapy and then two times per week for the next 2–3 weeks as fluctuations are more common.
e. If INR is stable, monitoring is done by doing INR once a week or once a fortnight.
f. In case of very stable INR, monitor once a month.
g. If any sign of external or internal bleeding such as bruising, epistaxis, hematuria, hemoptysis, hematemesis, or melena is observed, or if any patient is involved in a major trauma or suffers profuse or prolonged bleeding (more than 15 minutes), they should report to the ED.
h. If a patient develops the following symptoms, they should report to the ED:
  i. New-onset shortness of breath post valve surgery may be suggestive of valve thrombosis.
  ii. Stroke, sharp pain in limbs, or cold limbs. If the clot reaches to brain, it produces strokes; if it reaches to limb, it produces severe pain.
  iii. Fever and anemia after valve replacement may indicate infection.
  iv. Blood tests used in the ED to monitor anticoagulants:
    - Warfarin by getting prothrombin time (PT) and INR
    - Heparin—by getting partial thromboplastin time (PTT) and aPTT

Management of overanticoagulation:
a. Vitamin K is used as an antidote to coumarins anticoagulants (warfarin)—for stopping bleeding by correcting high PT and INR.
b. In case of overanticoagulation, INR > 4 without bleeding, skipping one or more dose is sufficient to achieve the therapeutic range. Oral 1 or 0.5 mg intravenous vitamin K can be added for faster correction and reduces the risk of minor hemorrhage. Avoid subcutaneous injection of vitamin K due to variable absorption.
c. In case of overanticoagulation with major bleeding, hospitalize the patient. Vitamin K alone is not sufficient, because its full effect occurs after 12–24 hours. Infusion of fresh frozen plasma (FFP) or coagulation factor concentrate is also required. Recheck INR after 6–8 hours and then daily for the next 3 days.
d. In case of a bleeding patient with normal INR, suspecting any other pathology may require temporary lowering of INR.
e. Protamine is used as an antidote to heparin—correct deranged aPTT.

Question 7

1. Classify various antimicrobial agents.
2. What is the mechanism of action of penicillin?
3. What are the adverse effects of penicillin?
4. What are the adverse effects of aminoglycosides?

Antimicrobials are antibiotics, antifungal, antiviral, antiparasitic, and antiprotozoal **(Flowchart 1)**.

Classification of antimicrobial agents on the basis of mechanism of action:
a. *Cell wall synthesis inhibitors:* Beta-lactamase (penicillin, cephalosporins, aztreonam, and imipenem) and polypeptides (vancomycin and bacitracin)
b. *Affect cell membrane functions:* Amphotericin B, nystatin, polymyxin B, and miconazole
c. *Protein synthesis inhibitors:* Aminoglycosides, chloramphenicol, erythromycin, tetracycline, clindamycin, and macrolides
d. *Inhibitors of essential metabolites (folate):* Sulfonamides and trimethoprim
e. *Inhibition of nucleic acid replications and transcriptions:* Quinolones and rifampin.

Mechanism of action of penicillin: Penicillin kills susceptible bacteria by specifically inhibiting the transpeptidase that catalyzes the final step in cell wall biosynthesis, the cross-linking of peptidoglycan.

Adverse effects of penicillin: Penicillin V and G can have adverse effects, including nausea, vomiting, diarrhea, rash, abdominal pain, and urticaria. In addition, penicillin G can have other adverse reactions, including muscle spasms, fever, chills, muscle pain, headache, tachycardia, flushing, tachypnea, and hypotension.

Adverse effects of aminoglycosides: Regular courses of aminoglycoside antibiotics may cause subclinical kidney damage leading to chronic kidney disease (CKD). This can manifest at the level of the glomerulus [causing decreased glomerular filtration rate (GFR)] and the tubules (causing altered excretion of electrolytes). Aminoglycosides appear to generate free radicals within the inner ear, with subsequent permanent damage to the sensory cells and neurons, resulting in permanent hearing loss. Two mutations in the mitochondrial 12S ribosomal ribonucleic acid (RNA) gene have been previously reported to predispose carriers to aminoglycoside-induced ototoxicity.

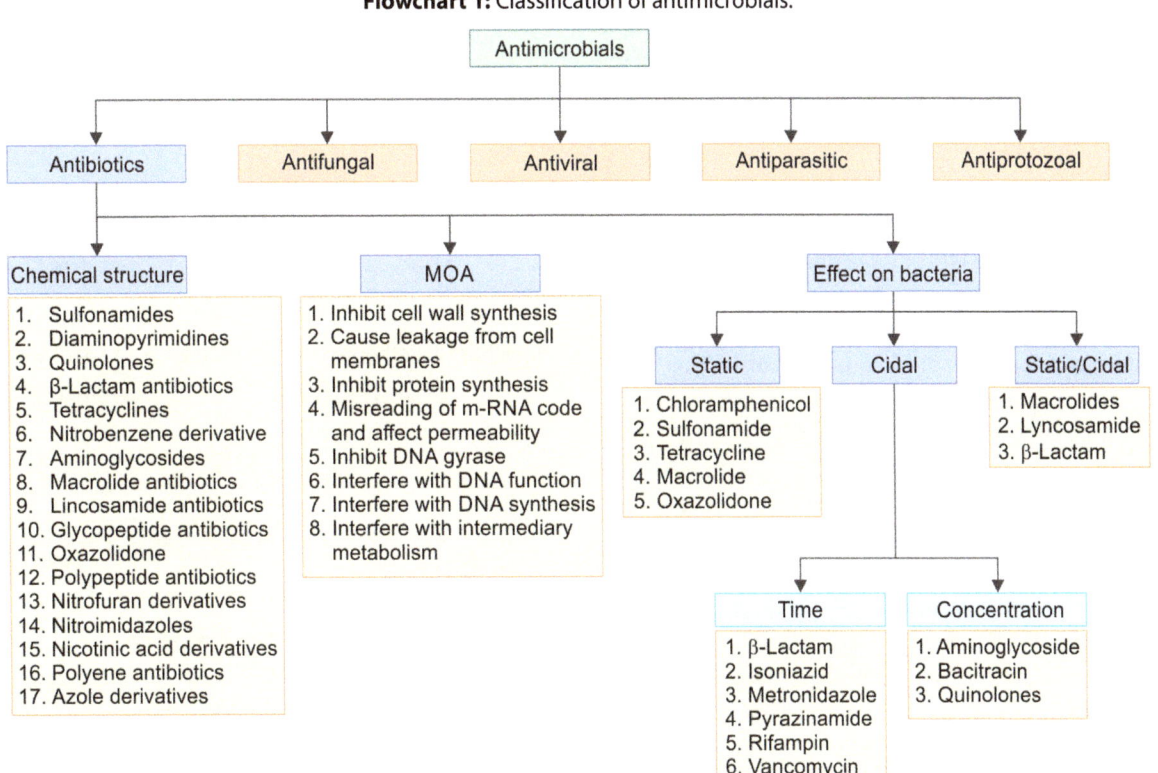

Flowchart 1: Classification of antimicrobials.

(DNA: deoxyribonucleic acid; MOA: mechanism of action; m-RNA: messenger ribonucleic acid)

Question 8

1. What are the diseases produced by various species of the *Clostridium*?

Clostridia are the most widely studied anaerobes, which are involved in a variety of human diseases, the most important of which are gas gangrene, tetanus, botulism, and pseudomembranous colitis and food poisoning.

2. Discuss the pathogenesis of tetanus.

Tetanus toxins act by a similar mechanism to botulinum toxin; tetanus toxin is taken up into nerve terminals of lower motor neurons, the nerve cells that activate the voluntary muscles. Tetanus toxin is a zinc-dependent metalloproteinase that targets a protein [synaptobrevin/vesicle-associated membrane protein (VAMP)] that is necessary for the release of neurotransmitter from nerve endings through fusion of synaptic vesicles with the neuronal plasma membrane. Flaccid paralysis may be the initial symptom of local tetanus infection, caused by interference with vesicular release of acetylcholine at the neuromuscular junction, as occurs with botulinum toxin. Extensive retrograde transport of tetanus toxin occurs in the axons of lower motor neurons and tetanus toxin reaches the spinal cord or brainstem. It crosses the synapses and is taken up by the nerve endings of inhibitory GABAergic and/or glycinergic neurons that control the activity of the lower motor neurons. Once the tetanus toxin reaches inside the inhibitory nerve terminals, it cleaves VAMP, thereby inhibiting the release of GABA and glycine, resulting in functional denervation of the lower motor neurons, which leads to rigidity and spasms due to hyperactivity and to increased muscle activity.

3. Discuss tetanus prophylaxis following an injury.

Tetanus toxoid: Tetanus immunization must be done, especially in patients who either have never been vaccinated (250 U of intramuscular human tetanus immune globulin) or did not have tetanus shots in the last 10 years [intramuscular or subcutaneous tetanus toxoid (0.5 mL)] **(Table 3)**.

TABLE 3: Tetanus prophylaxis in routine wound management (>18 years).

Tetanus immunization	Clean minor wound		All other wound*	
	Td	TIG	Td	TIG
<3 dose or uncertain	Yes	No	Yes	Yes
>3 dose				
Last dose within 5 years	No	No	No	No
Last dose within 5–10 years	No	No	Yes	No
Last dose >10 years	Yes	No	Yes	No

*All other wounds—contaminated wounds (feces, dirt, saliva, soil), puncture wounds, avulsions, burns, crush injuries, and frostbite.
(Td: tetanus-diphtheria toxoid; TIG: tetanus immune globulin)

Question 9

1. Discuss the common causes and pathophysiology of anaphylaxis.

Anaphylaxis is a severe systemic hypersensitivity reaction that is rapid in onset; characterized by life-threatening airway, breathing, and/or circulatory problems; and is usually associated with skin and mucosal changes. Because it can be triggered in some people by minute amounts of antigen (e.g., certain foods or single insect stings), anaphylaxis can be considered the most aberrant example of an imbalance between the cost and benefit of an immune response. The current understanding of the immunopathogenesis and pathophysiology of anaphylaxis **(Flowcharts 2 and 3)**, focusing on the roles of immunoglobulin E (IgE) and IgG antibodies, immune effector cells, and mediators, is thought to contribute to examples of the disorder. Anaphylaxis causes the immune system to release a flood of chemicals **(Table 4)** that can cause you to go into shock—blood pressure drops suddenly and the airways narrow, blocking breathing. Signs and symptoms include a rapid, weak pulse, skin rash, and nausea and vomiting.

Flowchart 2: Immunopathogenesis of anaphylactic shock.

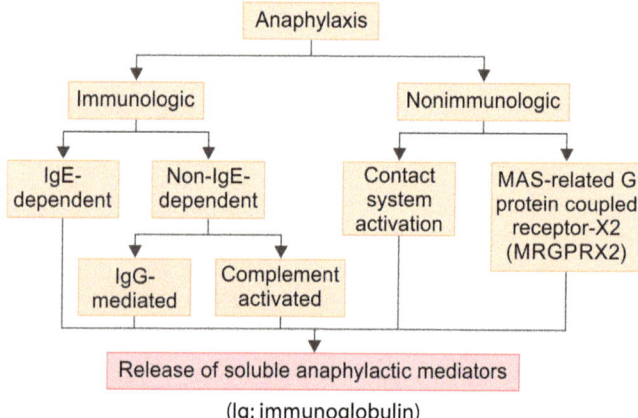

(Ig: immunoglobulin)

Flowchart 3: Pathophysiologic mechanism of anaphylactic shock.

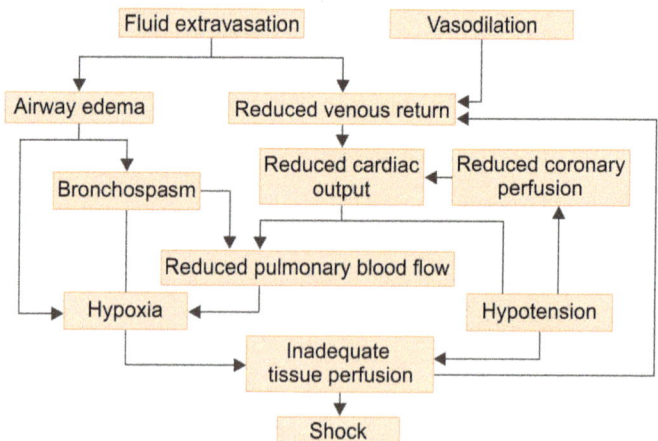

TABLE 4: Release of chemical mediators by activation of the immune system.

	Chemical mediator	Action
Arachidonic acid metabolites	• Cysteinyl • Leukotrienes • Prostaglandins • Platelet activating factor	Bronchoconstriction, coronary vasoconstriction, increased vascular permeability, mucus hypersecretion, and eosinophil activation and recruitment
Chemokines	• IL-8 • MIP-1α • Eosinophil • Chemotactic factors	Neutrophil and eosinophil chemotaxis, inflammatory cell recruitment, activation of NADPH oxidase
Cytokines	• GM-CSF • IL-3, -4, -5, -6, -10, and -13 • TNF-α	Eosinophil chemotaxis and activation, inflammatory cell activation and recruitment, induction of IgE-receptor expression, induction of apoptosis
Proteases	• Chymase • Tryptase • Carboxypeptidase A	Cleavage of complement proteins and neuropeptides, inflammatory-cell chemoattractant, conversion of angiotensin I to angiotensin II, activation of protease-activated receptor-2
Proteoglycans	• Chondroitin sulfate • Heparin	Anticoagulation, complement inhibition, eosinophil chemoattractant, kinin activation
Others	• Histamine • Nitric oxide	Vasodilation, bronchial and gastrointestinal smooth muscle contraction, mucus hypersecretion, vasodilation, increased vascular permeability

(GM-CSF: granulocyte-macrophage colony-stimulating factor; Ig: immunoglobulin; IL: interleukin; MIP-1α: macrophage inflammatory protein-1 alpha; NADPH: nicotinamide adenine dinucleotide phosphate; TNF-α: tumor necrosis factor alpha)

2. What are the clinical criteria for anaphylaxis diagnosis?

The Australasian Society of Clinical Immunology and Allergy defines anaphylaxis as any acute-onset illness with typical skin features (urticarial rash or erythema/flushing and/or angioedema), plus involvement of respiratory and/or cardiovascular and/or persistent severe gastrointestinal symptoms, or any acute onset of hypotension, bronchospasm, or upper airway obstruction where anaphylaxis is considered possible, even if typical skin features are not present. *Anaphylaxis is highly likely when any one of the following two criteria are fulfilled:*

Criteria 1: Acute onset of an illness (minutes to several hours) with simultaneous involvement of the skin, mucosal tissue, or both (e.g., generalized hives, pruritus or flushing, swollen lips–tongue–uvula), and at least one of the following:
a. Respiratory compromise (e.g., dyspnea, wheeze-bronchospasm, stridor, reduced peak expiratory flow, hypoxemia)
b. Reduced blood pressure or associated symptoms of end-organ dysfunction [e.g., hypotonia (collapse), syncope, incontinence]
c. Severe gastrointestinal symptoms (e.g., severe crampy abdominal pain, repetitive vomiting), especially after exposure to nonfood allergens

Criteria 2: Acute onset of hypotension or bronchospasm or laryngeal involvement after exposure to a known or highly probable allergen for that patient (minutes to several hours), even in the absence of typical skin involvement.

3. Write about two drugs used as first-line therapy of anaphylaxis.

Treatment of anaphylaxis
a. *Oxygenation:* It is done through face mask or endotracheal intubation, if needed. Mechanical ventilation is indicated for severe bronchospasm, apnea, or cardiac arrest.
b. *Epinephrine:* It is a universally recommended drug. Intramuscular dose is 0.3–1 mL
c. Intravenous dose 3–5 mL of 1:10,000 dilutions. *Mechanism of action:* It increases intracellular cyclic adenosine monophosphate (cAMP) levels in leukocytes and mast cells which inhibit the histamine release. It has beneficial effects on myocardial contractility, peripheral vascular tone, and bronchial smooth muscle.
d. *IV fluids and inotropes* comprise the treatment of choice. Norepinephrine infusion, methoxamine, phenylephrine, vasopressin, and methylene blue are tried in refractory cases.
e. *Nebulization:* With salbutamol in cases where bronchospasm is seen, aminophylline 5–6 mg/kg IV is given over 30 minutes. Ketamine and magnesium sulfate also can be used in severe cases of asthma.

Question 10

1. Discuss the pathophysiology and diagnostic criteria of diabetic ketoacidosis.

2. Mention important laboratory tests to be done in a case of suspected diabetic ketoacidosis.

Pathophysiology: Relative or absolute insulin deficiency in the presence of catabolic counter-regulatory hormones (glucagon, catecholamines, growth hormones, and cortisol) is the basic underlying mechanism. This leads to hepatic overproduction of glucose, unrestrained hepatic fatty acid oxidation, release of free fatty acids into the circulation from adipose tissue (lipolysis), and production of ketone bodies [β-hydroxybutyrate (β-OHB) and acetoacetate], resulting in ketonemia and metabolic acidosis. Hyperglycemia results in osmotic diuresis leading to dehydration and loss of electrolytes. Sodium depletion is worsened as insulin deficiency further diminishes renal sodium reabsorption. Metabolic acidosis leads to loss of intracellular potassium in exchange for hydrogen ions, and insulin deficiency also causes potassium loss from cells. Thus, there is high circulating plasma potassium. Based on the biochemical and clinical characteristics, diabetic ketoacidosis can be arbitrarily divided into mild, moderate, and severe types **(Table 5)**.

TABLE 5: Diagnostic criteria for diabetic ketoacidosis.

	Mild	Moderate	Severe
Plasma glucose (mg/dL)	>250	>250	>250
Arterial pH	7.25–7.30	7.00–7.24	<7.00
Serum bicarbonate (mEq/L)	15–18	10–15	<10
Urine ketones*	Positive	Positive	Positive
Serum ketones*	Positive	Positive	Positive
Effective serum osmolality (mOsm/kg)†	Variable	Variable	Variable
Anion gap‡	>10	>12	>12
Alteration in sensoria or mental obtundation	Alert	Alert/drowsy	Stupor/coma

*Nitroprusside reaction method.
†Calculation: 2 [measured Na⁺ (mEq/L)] + glucose (mg/dL)/18.
‡Calculation: (Na⁺) (Cl⁻ + HCO₃⁻) (mEq/L).

SUGGESTED READING

1. Australasian Society of Clinical Immunology and Allergy. [online] Available from: https://www.allergy.org.au/hp/papers/acute-management-of-anaphylaxis-guidelines. [Last accessed June, 2023]. (Question 9).
2. Erwin J, Varacallo M. Anatomy, Shoulder and Upper Limb, Wrist Joint. In: StatPearls [Internet]. Treasure Island, FL: StatPearls Publishing; 2023. (Question 3).
3. Richhariya D, Sharma B. Textbook of Emergency Medicine including Intensive Care and Trauma, 2nd edition. New Delhi: Jaypee Brothers Medical Publishers (P) Ltd; 2022. pp. 1314-6, 1657. (Question 8).
4. Richhariya D, Sharma B. Textbook of Emergency Medicine including Intensive Care and Trauma, 2nd edition. New Delhi: Jaypee Brothers Medical Publishers (P) Ltd; 2022. pp. 323-7. (Question 7).
5. Richhariya D, Sharma B. Textbook of Emergency Medicine including Intensive Care and Trauma, 2nd edition. New Delhi: Jaypee Brothers Medical Publishers (P) Ltd; 2022. pp. 473-80. (Question 1, 2, 4, and 5).
6. Richhariya D, Sharma B. Textbook of Emergency Medicine including Intensive Care and Trauma, 2nd edition. New Delhi: Jaypee Brothers Medical Publishers (P) Ltd; 2022. pp. 536-40. (Question 6).
7. Richhariya D, Sharma B. Textbook of Emergency Medicine including Intensive Care and Trauma, 2nd edition. New Delhi: Jaypee Brothers Medical Publishers (P) Ltd; 2022. pp. 871-6. (Question 10).
8. Richhariya D. Textbook of Emergency and Trauma Care, 1st edition. New Delhi: Jaypee Brothers Medical Publishers (P) Ltd; 2022. pp. 266-8. (Question 6).
9. Whyte AF, Soar J, Dodd A, Hughes A, Sargant N, Turner PJ. Emergency treatment of anaphylaxis: concise clinical guidance. Clin Med (Lond). 2022;22(4):332-9. (Question 9).

Emergency Medicine Paper 2

Devendra Richhariya

Question 1

1. Mention three anatomical and three physiological changes in pregnancy.
2. What is the importance of these changes in trauma management?

Knowledge of physiologic and anatomic changes in pregnancy and their clinical impact on symptoms and manifestation of traumatic injuries are important in management **(Table 1)**.

TABLE 1: Anatomic and physiologic changes in pregnancy.

Anatomic changes	Clinical relevance	Physiological changes	Clinical relevance
Edematous and friable airway	Difficult airway, may require smaller ETT	Increase in oxygen consumption	Require high flow oxygen
Uterus extent beyond bony pelvis after 12 weeks, gravid uterus after 20 weeks	• Direct injury to uterus • Supine hypotension due to compression of inferior vena cava	• Increase in plasma volume • Increase heart rate/low blood pressure	• Delay in identification of shock • Poor marker of hemodynamic stability
Bladder moves superiorly	Direct bladder injury	Increase in bladder and uterine blood flow	Increase in bleeding risk with direct injury
Diaphragm moves upward 4 cm	Pneumothorax, tension pneumothorax, tube placement 2–3 space upward	• Increase in renal plasma blood flow and GFR • Increase bicarbonate excretion	• Precaution with drugs which excrete through renal system • Susceptible to acidosis
Small bowel moves up	Direct blunt/penetrating bowel injury	Decrease in platelets, PT, PTT increase in fibrinogen and D-dimer	Precipitates disseminated intravascular coagulation (DIC) early
Peritoneum-abdominal wall stretches with progression of pregnancy	Poor assessment of organ injury intra-abdominal bleeding	Other hematopoietic changes in pregnancy are decrease in hemoglobin, hematocrit, and platelets, increase in white blood cell count fibrinogens factor VIII and X	Awareness about these changes helps in resuscitation and anticipation of various complications

(ETT: endotracheal tube; GFR: glomerular filtration rate; PT: prothrombin time; PTT: partial thromboplastin time)

3. What is supine hypotension syndrome and how do you correct it?

Cardiac output increases due to increased plasma volume, decreased vascular resistance, and increased maternal heart rate (an additional 10–15 beats/min). The supine positioning of pregnant trauma patients increases the risks of inferior vena cava compression and 20–30% reduction in cardiac output, due to gravid uterus (particularly during the 2nd and 3rd trimesters) **(Figs. 1A and B)**. Blood pressure is lower than normal (5–15 mm Hg less than usual) in the 2nd trimester, which causes difficulty in diagnosing hypovolemia secondary to bleeding, but returns to near normal levels at term.

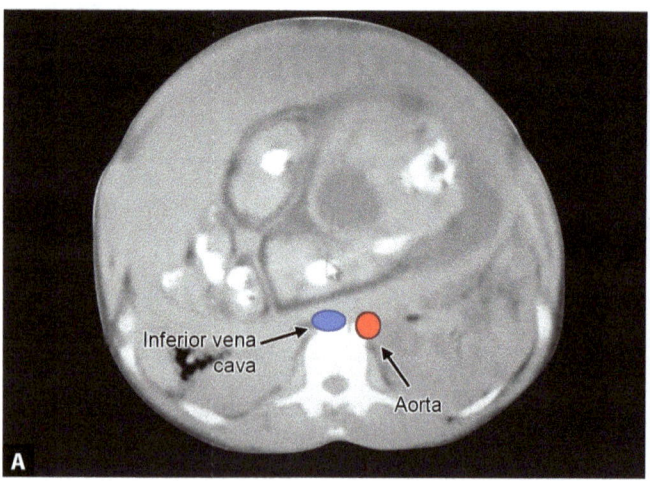
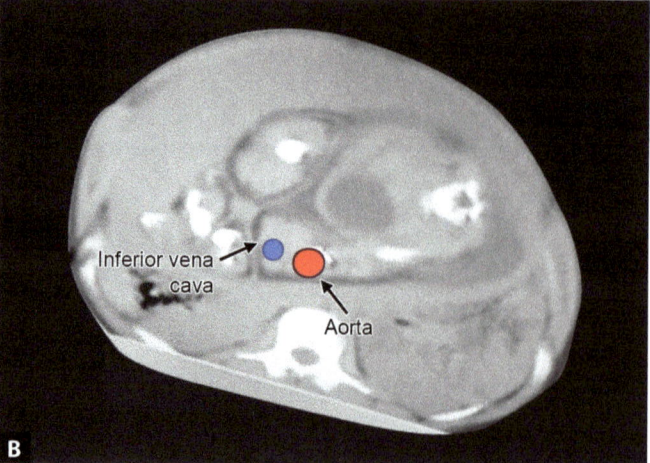

Figs. 1A and B: (A) Compression of the vena cava inferior in the supine position of the pregnant patient; (B) Disappearance of the compression with a tilt of about 15–30° on the right side.

Question 2

A 35-year-old multiparous woman presents with severe vaginal bleeding following vaginal delivery at 36 weeks.

1. Define postpartum hemorrhage.
2. What are the possible causes of severe bleeding in this patient?

Postpartum hemorrhage (also called PPH) occurs due to heavy bleeding after giving birth. It is a serious condition. It usually happens within 1 day of giving birth, but it can happen up to 12 weeks after having a baby. The causes of postpartum hemorrhage are called the four Ts (tone, trauma, tissue, and thrombin) **(Table 2)**. The conditions that may increase the risk for postpartum hemorrhage include the following:

- Placental abruption—the early detachment of the placenta from the uterus
- Placenta previa
- Overdistended uterus
- Multiple pregnancies
- Gestational hypertension or pre-eclampsia
- Having many previous births
- Prolonged labor
- Infection.

TABLE 2: Causes of postpartum hemorrhage.

Primary postpartum hemorrhage	Secondary postpartum hemorrhage
• Uterine atony • Retained placental fragments • Lower genital tract laceration • Uterine rupture • Uterine inversion • Hereditary coagulopathy	• Failure of uterine lining to sub involute • Retained placental tissue • Genital tract wounds • Uterogenital infections

3. Discuss initial management in the emergency department.
4. Explain the definitive management in case of continued bleeding.

- *Investigations:* Complete blood count (hemoglobin and hematocrit), coagulation profile, blood grouping and typing, urine analysis, blood culture, and ultrasound for viewing uterus.
- *Management:* The initial resuscitative steps include aggressive fluid and blood resuscitation while identifying and treating the underlying cause.
- *Tone:* Perform bimanual uterine massage. Drugs to improve uterine tone are—oxytocin 20 units in 1 L NS (or 10 units IM), misoprostol 1,000 µg PR/PO once methylergonovine 0.2 mg IM/IV/PO, carboprost 250 µg IM every 15–90 minutes.
- *Trauma:* Examine for cervical, vaginal or perineal laceration or hematoma. Repair laceration. Incise, drain and appropriately ligate bleeding vessel causing a hematoma. Correct uterine inversion with manual replacement. Uterine rupture requires surgery.
- *Tissue:* Inspect the placenta for missing fragments, if a portion is absent, manually evacuate the uterine cavity. Invasive placentation may require hysterectomy. Consider a balloon tamponade with either uterine-specific balloon device (Bakri or Rusch) or an adaptation of Foley catheter or condom as a temporizing measure.
- *Thrombin:* Consider DIC in the setting of severe pre-eclampsia, sepsis, placental abruption, shock or intrauterine fetal demise. Replace coagulation factors.

Question 3

1. Discuss clinical features of anterior cord syndrome.
2. Describe the features of posterior cord syndrome.

Anterior cord syndrome causes complete loss of movement, and pain and temperature loss, but it preserves light touch sensations. *Posterior cord syndrome* produces the opposite effect: It causes loss of light touch sensation, but it preserves movement, and pain and temperature sensation. Posterior cord syndrome is a rare type of incomplete spinal cord injury that affects the dorsal columns of the spinal cord (found in the posterior—or backside—region of the spinal cord), responsible for the perception of fine-touch, vibration, sense of self-movement, and body positioning (proprioception).

Incomplete spinal cord syndrome (ISCS) occurs when lesions involve specific structural and/or functional anatomic regions of the cord, with some preservation of sensory and/or motor function below the lesion. The clinical presentation of the incomplete spinal cord syndromes is largely determined by the involvement of the three tracts 1. corticospinal tract, 2. spinothalamic tract, and 3. posterior column of the spinal cord. There are eight types of incomplete spinal cord syndromes based on clinical presentations: *1. Central cord syndrome, 2. Brown–Séquard syndrome (unilateral cord syndrome), 3. Anterior cord syndrome, 4. Posterior syndrome, 5. Caudal equine syndrome, 6. Conus medullaris syndrome, 7. Subacute combined degeneration myelopathy, and 8. Cruciate paralysis—central cord syndrome due to syringomyelia, anterior cord syndrome due to anterior spinal artery occlusion, posterior cord syndrome due to posterior spinal artery occlusion.*

3. Differentiate spinal shock and neurogenic shock.

Neurogenic shock and spinal shock: In spinal cord injury (SCI) there are two conditions, *viz.,* (1) neurogenic shock and (2) spinal shock **(Table 3)**. Neurogenic shock is a cardiovascular event. It occurs when there is a cord injury above T6 level. The sympathetic nerve gets affected and due to peripheral vasodilatation, there is hypotension. Patient cannot develop tachycardia as the sympathetic nerve to the heart is affected. This is treated with fluids followed by vasopressors if necessary. *Spinal shock* is the state of complete paralysis due to spinal cord injury. There is flaccid paralysis with loss of reflexes including anal wink and bulbocavernosus reflex. This will recover as the neurological condition improves. SCI is often overlooked in (a) Head injury, (b) Intoxication, and (c) Polytrauma.

TABLE 3: Differentiating features of spinal shock and neurogenic shock.

	Spinal shock	**Neurogenic shock**
Definition	Immediate temporary loss of total power sensation and reflexes below the level of injury	Sudden loss of sympathetic nervous system
BP	Hypotension	Hypotension
Pulse	Bradycardia	Bradycardia
Bulbocavernosus reflex	Absent	Variable
Motor	Flaccid paralysis	Variable
Time	48–72 hours immediate after SCI	
Mechanism	Peripheral neurons become temporary unresponsive to brain stimuli	Disruption of autonomic pathway → loss of sympathetic tone and vasodilation
Management	• Immobilized at the scene and during transport • Rigid cervical collar and supportive blocks on a backboard with straps	• Airway support • Fluid management • Vasopressors • Atropine/temporary pacing

4. How will you manage neurogenic shock?

Maintaining mean arterial pressure (MAP) at 85–90 mm Hg for 7 days has been found to improve outcomes. The presence of bradycardia with hypotension can be due to neurogenic shock while head injury produces hypertension and bradycardia.

Use of steroids: The 2016 Cochrane review recommends against the use of steroids. But the AO Spine 2017 guidelines recommend steroids, i.e., methylprednisolone intravenously within 8 hours of cervical spine injury and continued for 24 hours. The dose of steroid should be 30 mg/kg bolus followed by 5.4 mg/kg/h for 23 hours. An increased risk of sepsis (pneumonia, septicemia) was noted with 48-hour steroid administration.

Question 4

1. Classify facial fractures.

Facial fractures are classified as below **(Fig. 2)**:

Le Fort I: Body of maxilla separated from pterygoid plate and nasal septum. Teeth and hard palate move.

Le Fort II: Pyramidal fracture across central maxilla and hard palate.

Le Fort III: Entire face is separated from skull from fractures of zygomatic suture line, across orbits and base of nose and ethmoids.

Le Fort IV: Includes Le Forte III and frontal bone.

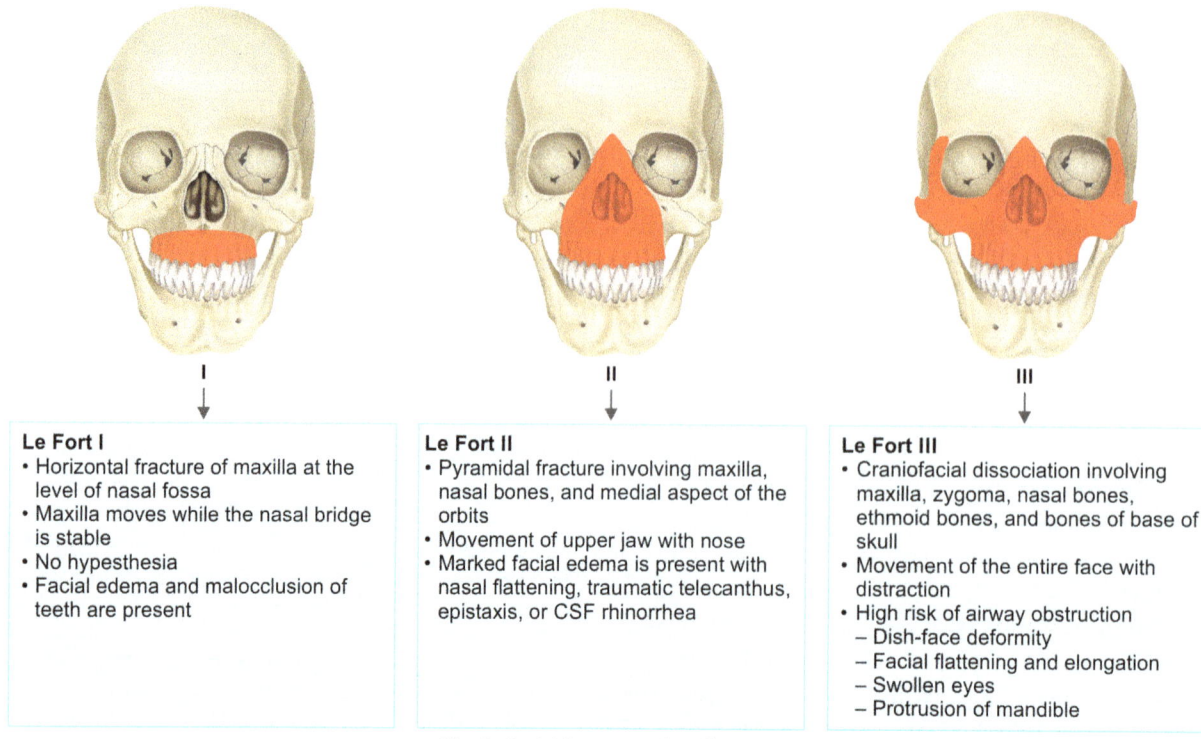

Fig. 2: Facial fractures classification.

2. Discuss airway management in a patient with facial injury.

3. Explain hemorrhage control in such a patient.

Management: To protect airway from hemorrhage and mechanical obstruction **(Flowchart 1)**.

Remove avulsed teeth or foreign bodies. Bag mask ventilation requires two people due to loss of normal structure. Always plan for difficult airway and to prevent administer of paralytics unless patient can be bagged effectively or alternate airway devices kept in place.

Keeping cricothyrotomy kept as a backup if other airway securing methods fail.

Hemorrhage: Control posterior nasal epistaxis early with nasal tampon, dual balloon device or Foley's catheter placement. After intubation, oral packing might be needed with severe facial bleeding.

Flowchart 1: Management of maxillofacial injuries.

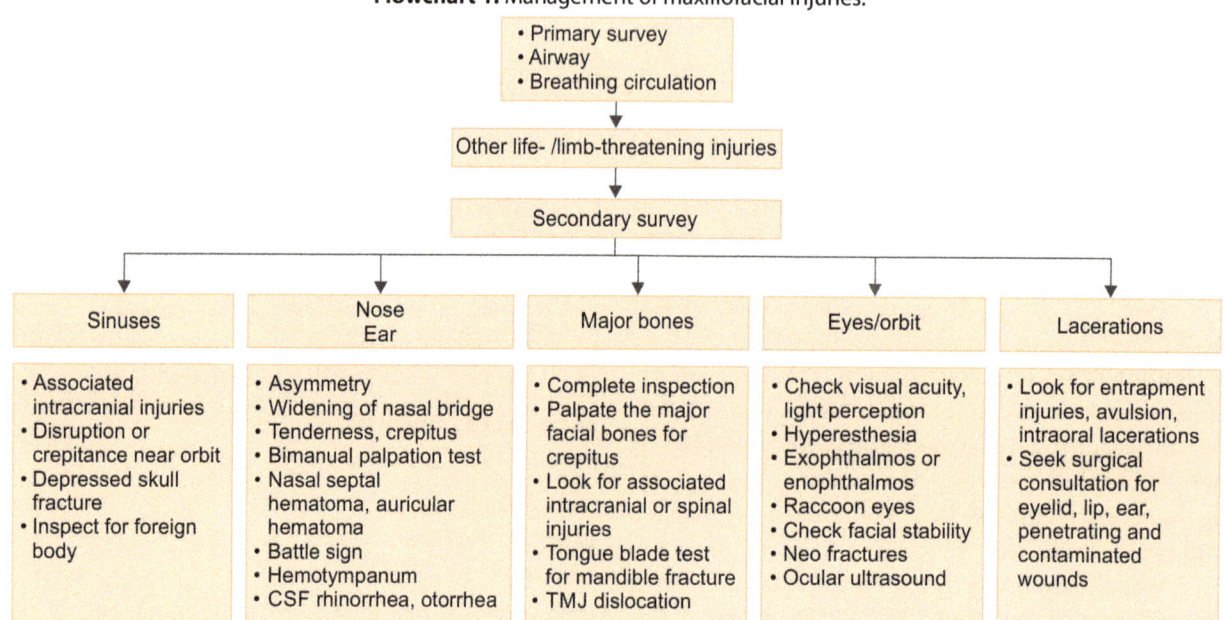

Question 5

A 60-year-old male patient comes to the emergency department with severe acute abdominal pain.

1. Enumerate your differential diagnoses.
2. How will you evaluate the patient clinically?
3. How will you investigate the patient?

Causes of acute lower abdominal pain are as follows:
- Aortic aneurysm
- Appendicitis
- Crohn's disease
- Diverticulitis
- Epiploic appendages
- Herpes zoster
- Inguinal hernia
- Meckel's diverticulum
- Psoas abscess

Differential diagnosis associated with diseases is given in **Table 4**.

TABLE 4: Differential diagnosis of abdominal pain.

Pain vomiting (+/– rigidity)	• Acute pancreatitis • Diabetic gastric paresis • Diabetic ketoacidosis • Incarcerated hernia
Pain/Vomiting/Distension	• Bowel obstruction • Cecal volvulus
Pain (+/–Vomiting)	• Acute diverticulitis • Adnexal torsion • Mesenteric ischemia • Myocardial ischemia • Testicular torsion
Pain/shock	• Abdominal sepsis • Aortic dissection • Hemorrhagic pancreatitis • Leaking/ruptured abdominal aortic aneurysm • Mesenteric ischemia • Myocardial ischemia • Ruptured ectopic
Pain shock rigidity	• Perforated appendix • Perforated diverticulum • Perforated ulcer • Ruptured esophagus • Splenic rupture
Distension (+/– Pain)	Elderly with bowel obstruction/volvulus

Evaluation: Start with a thorough history and physical examination including inspection, palpation, percussion, and auscultation of bowel sounds. Diagnoses testing such as plain radiographs, ultrasound, POCUS, and abdominal pelvic CT scan are used to further investigate the disease. Laboratory studies that may be appropriate in the evaluation of acute abdominal pain on the basis of clinical suspicion **(Table 5)**.

TABLE 5: Suggested investigations and conditions acute severe abdominal pain.

Laboratory test	Clinical suspicion
Amylase and lipase	Pancreatitis
• β-human chorionic gonadotrophin (β-hCG) • Serum/Urine • Qualitative/Quantitative	• Pregnancy • Ectopic or molar pregnancy
• Hemoglobin • Platelets • Coagulation studies • Liver function test	• GI bleed • End stage liver disease • Coagulopathy
Lactate	• Sepsis • Mesenteric ischemia
Liver function test	• Cholecystitis • Cholelithiasis • Hepatitis
Renal function test	• Dehydration • Renal insufficiency • Acute renal failure
Urine analysis	• Urinary tract infection • Pyelonephritis • Nephrolithiasis
ECG	Myocardial ischemia or infarction
Gonococcal/Chlamydial testing	• Cervicitis • Urethritis • Pelvic inflammatory disease

Question 6

1. Discuss hypotensive resuscitation in hemorrhagic shock.

Permissive hypotension implies accepting an adequate, not normal, blood pressure. It is employed in the actively bleeding patient until hemostasis is obtained, after which point definitive resuscitation begins. During resuscitation of hemorrhagic shock, volume infusion in the face of continued blood loss results in dilutional coagulopathy and hypothermia, while the transient elevation in blood pressure contributes to further bleeding from wounds and vessels. This approach may be associated with organ dysfunction, abdominal compartment syndrome, and death in major trauma patients. Permissive hypotension, therefore, can facilitate an environment that optimizes coagulation, albeit at the potential expense of optimal tissue perfusion pressure, until repair restores the integrity of the system.

Permissive hypotension is the act of maintaining a blood pressure lower than physiologic levels in a patient that has suffered from hemorrhagic blood loss. The practice is employed in order to maintain adequate vasoconstriction, organ perfusion, and prevent an undesired coagulopathy during initial fluid resuscitation. Permissive hypotension is contraindicated in patients with traumatic brain injury, because reduced perfusion pressure and oxygenation can lead to secondary brain injury. In such situations, a mean arterial pressure (MAP) of >80 mm Hg (a cerebral perfusion pressure of approximately 60 mm Hg), is required in order to maintain cerebral perfusion pressure.

2. Compare crystalloids and colloids for resuscitation.

Intravenous fluids are administered to virtually all acutely ill patients. The choice of the fluid should be individualized based on ongoing disease process, acid–base status, and electrolyte requirement. Thorough knowledge about intravenous fluids and their judicious use in the emergency department can improve patient outcomes.

Crystalloids are the oldest forms of intravenous fluids. They are basically simple solutions of electrolytes and/or sugars in water. They include isotonic solutions primarily used in resuscitation and hypotonic solutions used as maintenance fluid therapy. The most popular crystalloid in clinical practice, 0.9% saline, contains 154 mmol/L of sodium and chloride each. Thus, concentration of both sodium (plasma sodium ~140 mmol/L) and chloride (plasma chloride ~100 mmol/L) is much higher than in plasma, resulting in a strong ion difference (SID) of 0. SID is the difference between the predominantly positive charge (sodium) and negative charge (chloride) in plasma. Normal SID of plasma is about 40. Any decrease in SID produces acidosis and conversely any increase produces alkalosis. Infusion of large volumes of 0.9% saline leads to higher chloride concentrations in plasma and a decrease in SID. This decrease in SID (and hence bicarbonate) leads to hyperchloremic acidosis.

Balanced crystalloid, which is also known as *"physiological solutions",* have a chemical composition approximating that of extracellular fluid. These solutions employ metabolizable anions such as lactate, acetate, gluconate or maleate to maintain electroneutrality, as bicarbonate is unstable in plastic. They have concentrations of chloride similar to plasma and hence devoid of harmful hyperchloremic metabolic acidosis.

Colloids unlike crystalloids consist of large molecules and are believed to stay in the intravascular space for longer duration before leaking into the interstitium. They are used as resuscitation fluids in emergency department, critically ill, and during surgery. In the past it was thought that colloids are 3 to 4 times more effective than crystalloids in restoring the intravascular volume. This, however, was not substantiated in several recent trials, which suggested that only marginally lesser volume of colloids is required to produce similar hemodynamic effect when compared to crystalloids.

3. What is massive transfusion protocol (MTP)?

Massive transfusion protocol should be in place in every hospital and this protocol should be activated as soon as the emergency team recognizes the presence or likelihood of severe, ongoing hemorrhage. One example of MTP followed at authors' institute adapted from publication in journal of American College of Surgeons is shown below:

If the bleeding in trauma patients is unlikely or difficult to be controlled quickly, immediate transfusion of blood components in a 1:1:1 ratio of RBC, fresh frozen plasma (FFP), and platelets should be considered. In simple terms, if the emergency team recognizes that the patient will require four or more units of RBCs in 1 hour (or >10 units in 12–24 hours), they should start transfusing four units of RBCs, four units of FFP, and six units of random donor platelets [or one unit of single donor apheresis platelets (SDP) as one unit of SDP (also called apheresis platelets) is equivalent to six units of random donor platelets (RDP)]. Hypothermia must be controlled during transfusions with the help of inline warmers.

The Assessment of Blood Consumption (ABC) score in trauma was developed to assist clinicians in discerning when massive transfusion would be required to resuscitate trauma patients. Hemorrhage is the most common cause of early death in trauma patients. MTPs have been designed to accelerate the release of blood products but can result in waste if activated inappropriately. The ABC score **(Table 6)** has become a widely accepted score for MTP activation.

TABLE 6: ABC SCORE—massive blood transfusion protocol initiation ABC score ≥2.	
Components	Points
Penetrating injury	1
FAST positive	1
Heart rate	1
Systolic BP	1

Question 7

1. Enumerate causes of compartment syndrome.

- Trauma
- Crush injury

- Fracture (open/closed), fracture tibia, high energy fracture shaft femur, forearm
- Bleeding
- Prolonged vascular occlusion
- Burns
- Venomous bite
- Intraosseous fluid replacement
- IV fluid extravasation
- Tight bandage
- Postsurgery.

2. Explain the clinical features and diagnosis of compartment syndrome.

Compartment syndrome is a painful condition that occurs when pressure within the muscles builds to dangerous levels. This pressure can decrease blood flow, which prevents nourishment and oxygen from reaching nerve and muscle cells. Compartment syndrome results when injured muscle cells increase in size with intracellular fluid uptake while total space remains constant. This swelling results in increases in intracompartmental pressures. As pressure increases, blood flow to the damaged tissue decreases resulting in tissue ischemia and eventual necrosis. It is classically taught that increased pressures resulting in tissue ischemia for >6–8 hours result in permanent damage.

Compartment syndrome—clinical diagnosis:
- Pain out of proportion
- Palpable tense compartment
- Pain with passive stretch
- Paresthesia/Hypoesthesia
- Paralysis
- Pulselessness or pallor.

3. How will you manage it in the emergency department?

The treatment for compartment syndrome is fasciotomy **(Flowchart 2)**. This procedure allows the swelling muscle to expand outside of its compartment, thereby preserving afferent blood flow. Fasciotomy continues to be a controversial subject in the realm of crush syndrome management. Some authors argue that this is a lifesaving intervention that also decreases the risk for complications related to crush syndrome. Other studies have not shown such profound benefits with fasciotomy. The benefits of fasciotomy must be compared with the outcomes related to localized wound infection, sepsis, subsequent amputations, and increased mortality.

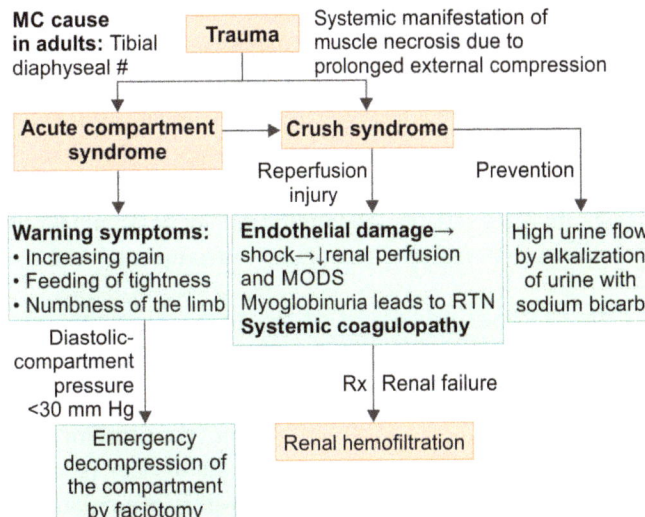

Flowchart 2: Treatment approach for compartment syndrome.

4. Enumerate the complications of compartment syndrome.

- Acidosis
- Hypercapnia
- Acute respiratory distress syndrome
- Sepsis
- Disseminated intravascular coagulation
- Rhabdomyolysis
- Multiorgan failure
- Disabling joint contracture
- Long standing muscle weakness
- Ulceration
- Loss of limb
- Death

Question 8

1. What is the classic triad of ruptured abdominal aortic aneurysm?

2. What are the external signs of acute aortic rupture?

The aorta is the most common site of an aneurysm in the abdominal cavity and anteroposterior diameter of >3.0 cm is classified as an aneurysm. Most abdominal aortic aneurysms (AAAs) occur in the infrarenal region. Most aneurysms are fusiform (not saccular), entire circumference and all layers of the vessel are involved. The mean diameter of the infrarenal aorta is 1.66–2.16 cm in older women and 1.99–2.39 cm in older men. The most important complication of AAA is rupture, which occurs almost exclusively in aneurysms >4 cm. The most important risk factors are smoking, family history of AAA, increasing age, and history of atherosclerotic disease. Most AAAs rupture into the retroperitoneal cavity, which results in the classical triad of pain, hypotension, and a *pulsatile mass*. Any older patient presenting to the ED with the clinical findings, of *abdominal pain, back pain, and shock*, ruptured or leaking AAA should be suspected, but these symptoms and signs presentation are variable. Abdominal pain or back pain is one of the prominent features in patients with a ruptured AAA.

3. Discuss management of acute aortic rupture.

- The early management of patients with suspected unstable AAA, either leaking or ruptured, should focus on rapid diagnosis and early definitive treatment. The presence of known risk factors for the disease (such as male gender, advanced age, and a history of smoking) in association with acute abdominal or back pain should raise the suspicion for an unstable AAA. Pulsatile mass on abdominal palpation has sensitivity ranging from 44–97%.
- Most useful tool in the diagnostic evaluation of AAA in emergency department is bedside ultrasonography. Ultrasound is a highly accurate test, with a sensitivity and specificity approaching 100% in detecting AAA for emergency physicians.
- CT is useful imaging modality for newly diagnosed AAA asymptomatic patients to define the anatomic details of the aneurysm; it should not be considered as the initial test of choice for patients with suspected ruptured AAA and instable patient.
- For those with a suspected ruptured AAA, aggressive resuscitation is priority, along with diagnostic measures, and consultation with vascular surgeon should occur simultaneously. Judicious fluid and blood replacement should begin for patients in shock, with large-bore, intravenous lines in place—once underlying disorder is an arterial rupture and hemorrhage is confirmed, vascular surgeon should be involved for surgical repair. For patients with an aneurysm >5.4 cm, referral should be made to vascular surgery. For those between 4.0 and 5.4 cm, surveillance with ultrasound is recommended every 6–12 month and, for those <4.0 cm, every 2–3 years is probably sufficient.

Question 9

1. Discuss differential diagnosis of acute scrotal pain.

The presentation of an acute scrotum can be broken down into four subcategories: (1) *the painful swollen testicle*, (2) *the painless swollen testicle*, (3) *the erythematous testicle*, and (4) *the traumatic testicle*. Within each of these groups, there is a diagnosis that cannot be missed. However, not all scrotal emergencies present with pain in the genital area. It is important to rule out scrotal emergencies in patients presenting with lower abdominal pain **(Table 7)**.

TABLE 7: Differential diagnoses for acute scrotal pain.

Ischemic	Testicular torsion, torsion of the testicular appendage
Infectious	Epididymitis, epididymo-orchitis, orchitis, scrotal cellulitis, scrotal abscess, Fournier gangrene, Hansen disease, filariasis
Traumatic	*Blunt:* Testicular contusion, testicular rupture, penetrating testicular rupture, hematocele, scrotal degloving
Inflammatory	Henoch–Schönlein purpura
Idiopathic	Idiopathic scrotal swelling
Oncologic	Testicular tumors
Other	Strangulated/incarcerated inguinal hernia, referred pain from abdominal pathology, e.g., ruptured abdominal aortic aneurysm or nephrolithiasis

2. What is Prehn's sign?

On normal physical examination, the epididymis is found at the posterior-lateral aspect of the testicle. When palpated it feels soft and fleshy, similar to an earlobe. *In epididymitis*, the epididymis may be tender on palpation. Patients may not have testicular tenderness. The provider should also check for *Prehn's sign*, which is relief of pain in the lateral recumbent position or with scrotal elevation. *If orchitis is present*, patients will have more testicular involvement, with increased testicular swelling and tenderness.

3. How will you diagnose torsion testis?

Testicular torsion occurs when the spermatic cord twists causing venous congestion, decreased arterial blood flow and eventually ischemia of the testicle. There are two features of the clinical history that have been shown to increase the likelihood of diagnosis. Presence of nausea and/or vomiting and <24 hours since the onset of pain has both been proven to be associated with testicular torsion **(Table 8)**.

TABLE 8: TWIST score (testicular workup for ischemia and suspected torsion).

History and physical presentation	Points
Testicular swelling	2
Hard testicle	2
Absent cremasteric reflex	1
Nausea or vomiting	1
High-riding testicle	1
High risk–7 points. 100% sensitive and specific for testicular torsion.	

In general, ultrasonography is performed by a radiologist or ultrasonography technician; however, bedside ultrasonography by an emergency physician can also aid in diagnosis. Emergency physicians can accurately diagnose patients presenting with acute scrotal pain using bedside ultrasonography. Ultrasonography is the diagnostic modality of choice when evaluating a painful scrotum. In general, laboratory work and urinalysis are not helpful in the diagnosis of testicular torsion but may help with ruling in epididymitis. Ultrasonography findings consistent with testicular torsion include absent or diminished intra-testicular blood flow in the symptomatic testicle when compared with the asymptomatic testicle, or evidence of spermatic cord torsion with a *"whirlpool or snail sign"*. Comparison of flow between both testicles is an important step in assessing for torsion. Imaging the spermatic cord to find a kink in the cord is more sensitive than color Doppler alone in adults and children.

4. How you will perform detorsion of the testis?

- Testicular torsion is time sensitive emergency. Manual detorsion can be attempted before surgical intervention but should not delay surgical intervention. *Trials of manual detorsion* have been found to decrease ischemia time. Even if the testicle is manually detorsed, surgery is still required. Surgical exploration is the definitive management for testicular torsion. Before performing manual detorsion, it must be explained that the procedure is painful but, if successful, it will alleviate the pain. Analgesic medication, local analgesia injection (i.e., local lidocaine), or procedural sedation should be administered.
- Stand at the foot of the bed or to the right of the patient. Holding the testicle between the thumb and index finger, rotate it in an outward direction (like opening a book) from medial to lateral. The initial attempt should be with one and a half full rotations (540°). Relief of pain is a positive end point. You can also reassess with bedside ultrasonography. If the pain worsens with detorsion in the medial to lateral rotation, detorse in the lateral to medial direction, because a third of testicular torsions occurs with medial to lateral rotation.

Question 10

1. Mention the six killers in thoracic trauma.

The Lethal Six (airway obstruction, tension pneumothorax, cardiac tamponade, open pneumothorax, massive hemothorax, and flail chest) are immediate, life-threatening injuries that require evaluation and treatment during primary survey.

2. Explain the clinical features of tension pneumothorax.

Tension pneumothorax is a life-threatening chest wound leading to a one-way valve, drawing more and more air into the chest without an escape, leading to lung collapse and contralateral compression of the lung, great vessels, and veno-caval structures. This leads to shock, hypoxia, decreased cardiac output, and death.

3. Discuss procedure for needle decompression.

- *Emergent needle thoracocentesis:* It must be decompressed with needle thoracostomy or at least a 5-cm 14G angiographic catheter, common site of insertion is in the 2nd intercostal space at the midclavicular line or the lateral chest 4–5th interspace anterior axillary line.
- Chest tube must be performed immediately after needle decompression. Insert over the top of the 5th rib in mid-axillary line. The most common cause of serious injury as a result of chest drain is incorrect site of placement. Confirm that the drain lies within the chest wall cavity by looking for fogging of the tube and swinging of the chest drain with respiration.
- Do not clamp the chest drain or apply suction. The underwater seal needs to remain below the insertion site at all times. Gross surgical emphysema with pneumomediastinum and a chest drain that continues to bubble, suggest tracheobronchial injury. Cardiac tamponade can give similar signs clinically, shock with distended veins. With FAST and CXR along with mechanism of injury can help to differentiate between the two.

4. Explain the procedure for intercostal drain insertion.

- Intercostal chest drains are inserted into the pleural or mediastinal spaces to remove abnormal collections of air, blood, pus or fluid and in many acute and chronic conditions especially when respiratory function is compromised.
- The procedure is usually performed by surgeons and chest physicians, but every emergency physician should be well versed with the technique of insertion of chest drain. Insertion of an intercostal chest drain is indicated for appropriate lung re-expansion in pneumothoraces, complicated parapneumonic effusions or empyema,

hemothoraces, bedside pleurodesis, and following cardiothoracic surgery or thoracoscopic procedures.
- Small-bore chest tube (SBCT 14F or less) or medium-bore chest tubes (MBCT) are typically placed using the Seldinger technique, whereas LBCT (>24F) can be inserted by blunt dissection or the trocar technique.
- Chest drains are usually inserted in the triangle of safety, which is defined anteriorly by the fold of pectoralis major, posteriorly fold of latissimus dorsi, and inferiorly by a line drawn downward from nipple, which usually corresponds to 5th or 6th intercostal space in the mid-axillary line.

SUGGESTED READING

1. Richhariya D, Sharma B. Textbook of Emergency Medicine including Intensive Care and Trauma, 2nd edition. New Delhi: Jaypee Brothers Medical Publishers (P) Ltd; 2022. pp. 1646-51. (Question 1).
2. Richhariya D, Sharma B. Textbook of Emergency Medicine including Intensive Care and Trauma, 2nd edition. New Delhi: Jaypee Brothers Medical Publishers (P) Ltd; 2022. pp. 1112-3. (Question 2).
3. Richhariya D, Sharma B. Textbook of Emergency Medicine including Intensive Care and Trauma, 2nd edition. New Delhi: Jaypee Brothers Medical Publishers (P) Ltd; 2022. pp. 1570-2. (Question 3).
4. Richhariya D, Sharma B. Textbook of Emergency Medicine including Intensive Care and Trauma, 2nd edition. New Delhi: Jaypee Brothers Medical Publishers (P) Ltd; 2022. pp. 1551-5. (Question 4).
5. Richhariya D, Sharma B. Textbook of Emergency Medicine including Intensive Care and Trauma, 2nd edition. New Delhi: Jaypee Brothers Medical Publishers (P) Ltd; 2022. pp. 633-9. (Question 5).
6. Richhariya D, Sharma B. Textbook of Emergency Medicine including Intensive Care and Trauma, 2nd edition. New Delhi: Jaypee Brothers Medical Publishers (P) Ltd; 2022. pp. 291-4, 986-92, 1537-38. (Question 6).
7. Richhariya D, Sharma B. Textbook of Emergency Medicine including Intensive Care and Trauma, 2nd edition. New Delhi: Jaypee Brothers Medical Publishers (P) Ltd; 2022. pp. 1671-3. (Question 7).
8. Richhariya D, Sharma B. Textbook of Emergency Medicine including Intensive Care and Trauma, 2nd edition. New Delhi: Jaypee Brothers Medical Publishers (P) Ltd; 2022. pp. 720-2. (Question 8).
9. Richhariya D, Sharma B. Textbook of Emergency Medicine including Intensive Care and Trauma, 2nd edition. New Delhi: Jaypee Brothers Medical Publishers (P) Ltd; 2022. pp. 784-790. (Question 9).
10. Richhariya D, Sharma B. Textbook of Emergency Medicine including Intensive Care and Trauma, 2nd edition. New Delhi: Jaypee Brothers Medical Publishers (P) Ltd; 2022. pp. 605-12, 1582-3. (Question 10).

Emergency Medicine Paper 3

Devendra Richhariya

Question 1

1. Enumerate stroke mimics.

2. What are the inclusion and exclusion criteria for thrombolysis in acute stroke?

Cerebral stroke mimics are given in **Table 1**.

TABLE 1: Stroke mimics.

Toxic-metabolic	• Hypoglycemia or hyperglycemia • Hyponatremia or hypernatremia • Ingestion or overdose • Drug toxicity • Intoxication (alcohol, illicit drugs) • Hepatic encephalopathy
Intracranial hemorrhage	Intracerebral hemorrhage, subarachnoid hemorrhage, subdural hematoma
Infectious	• Sepsis • Encephalitis • Meningitis
Structural lesions	• Brain mass or tumor • Spinal cord lesion
Others	• Demyelinating disease (i.e., multiple sclerosis), seizure or Todd paralysis • Migraine • Idiopathic intracranial hypertension • Reversible cerebral vasoconstrictive syndrome • Central nervous system vasculitis • Vestibular dysfunction • Hypertensive encephalopathy • Peripheral neuropathy • Dementia • Conversion disorder

Inclusion and exclusion criteria for ischemic stroke thrombolysis are given in **Box 1**.

3. Discuss standard method of thrombolysis in ischemic stroke.

Dose of tPA: As per the guidelines infuse 0.9 mg/kg (maximum dose 90 mg) over 60 minutes, with 10% of the dose given as a bolus over 1 minute.

For treatment within 3 hours of stroke onset, alteplase led to a good outcome for 33%, versus 23% for control [odds ratio (OR) 1.75, 95% CI 1.35–2.27]. The number needed to treat (NNT) for one additional patient to achieve a good outcome was 10.

BOX 1: Inclusion and exclusion criteria for intravenous tPA infusion.

Inclusion criteria:
- Diagnosis of ischemic stroke causing measurable neurological deficit
- Onset of symptoms <3 hours before beginning treatment
- Aged ≥18 years
- Exclusion criteria
- Significant head trauma or prior stroke in previous 3 months
- Symptoms suggest subarachnoid hemorrhage
- Arterial puncture at noncompressible site in previous 7 days
- History of previous intracranial hemorrhage
- Intracranial neoplasm, arteriovenous malformation, or aneurysm
- Recent intracranial or intraspinal surgery
- Elevated blood pressure (systolic >185 mm Hg or diastolic >110 mm Hg)
- Active internal bleeding
- Acute bleeding diathesis
- Platelet count <100,000/mm^3
- Heparin received within 48 hours, resulting in abnormally elevated aPTT greater than the upper limit of normal
- Current use of anticoagulant with INR >1.7 or PT >15 seconds
- Current use of direct thrombin inhibitors or direct factor Xa inhibitors with elevated sensitive laboratory tests (such as aPTT, INR, platelet count, and ECT; TT; or appropriate factor Xa activity assays)
- Blood glucose concentration <50 mg/dL (2.7 mmol/L)
- CT demonstrates multilobar infarction (hypodensity >1/3 cerebral hemisphere)

Relative exclusion criteria:
- Recent experience suggests that under some circumstances—with careful consideration and weighting of risk to benefit—patients may receive fibrinolytic therapy despite 1 or more relative contraindications. Consider risk to benefit of IV rtPA administration carefully if any of these relative contraindications are present:
  – Only minor or rapidly improving stroke symptoms (clearing spontaneously)
  – Pregnancy
  – Seizure at onset with postictal residual neurological impairments
  – Major surgery or serious trauma within previous 14 days
  – Recent gastrointestinal or urinary tract hemorrhage (within previous 21 days)
  – Recent acute myocardial infarction (within previous 3 months)

(aPTT: activated partial thromboplastin clotting time; INR: international normalized ratio; tPA: tissue plasminogen activator)

For treatment from 3 to 4.5 hours, the proportion with a good outcome in the alteplase and control groups was 35 and 30% (OR 1.26, 95% CI 1.05–1.51, NNT 20).

The benefit of intravenous (IV) defibrinogenating agents and of IV fibrinolytic agents other than alteplase and tenecteplase is unproven; therefore, their administration is not recommended outside a clinical trial. Tenecteplase administered as a 0.4 mg/kg single IV bolus has not been proven to be superior or noninferior to alteplase but might be considered as an alternative to alteplase in patients with minor neurological impairment and no major intracranial occlusion.

Question 2

1. What are the causes of acute onset of dyspnea with wheezing?

Breathing difficulty (acute dyspnea) is the most common manifestation with which the patients come to emergency department (ED). It requires several steps for differentiation and the risk stratification of patients presenting with SOB, i.e., shortness of breath **(Table 2)**. There should be methodological approach by the doctors present in ED.

TABLE 2: The differential diagnosis for acute dyspnea.

Head and neck	Cardiac	Miscellaneous
Angioedema	ACS	Hyperventilation
Anaphylaxis	Decompensated heart failure	Anxiety
Pharyngeal infection	Pulmonary edema (flash)	Pneumomediastinum
Deep neck infection	High output failure	Lung tumor
Foreign body	Cardiomyopathy	Massive pleural effusion
Neck trauma	Arrhythmia	Intra-abdominal process
Pulmonary	Valvular dysfunction	Ascites
COPD exacerbation	Cardiac tamponade	Pregnancy
BA exacerbation	**Toxic/metabolic**	Massive obesity
Pulmonary embolism	Organophosphate	**Neurological**
Pneumothorax	Salicylate	Stroke
Pneumonia	CO poisoning	Neuromuscular disease
ARDS	Toxic ingestion	**Chest wall**
Lung contusion or injury	DKA	Rib fracture
Hemorrhage	Sepsis	Flail chest
	Anemia	

(ARDS: acute respiratory distress syndrome; COPD: chronic obstructive pulmonary disease; DKA: diabetic ketoacidosis)

2. What is grading of acute severe asthma?

Severity of asthma: The assessment of severity can be done based on GINA guidelines. On physical examination, cyanosis, nasal flaring, use of accessory muscles of respiration leading to intercostal or supraclavicular indrawing, tachycardia, tachypnea, hypotension, and altered level of consciousness are at higher risk of fatal asthma and need special attention. On auscultation bilateral rhonchi can be present silent chest without wheezing indicated severe airflow obstruction. Symptoms and finding do not correlate well with severity of symptoms so forced expiratory volume in 1 second and peak expiratory flow rate (PEFR) are important parameters in categorizing the severity of acute asthma. The other parameters to classify severity of asthma are summarized in **Flowchart 1**.

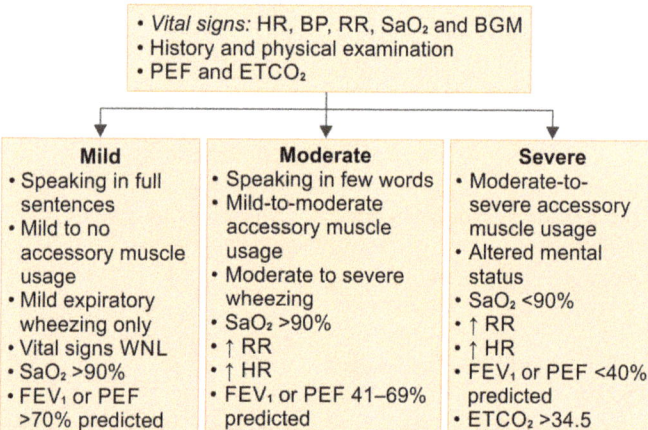

Flowchart 1: Severity of asthma.

(BGM: blood glucose meter; BP: blood pressure; $ETCO_2$: end-tidal carbon dioxide; FEV1: forced expiratory volume in 1 second; HR: heart rate; PEF: peak expiratory flow; RR: respiratory rate; SaO_2: oxygen saturation; WNL: within normal limit)

3. Discuss the modes of noninvasive ventilation, indications, and contraindications.

There are two modes of NIV—continuous positive airway pressure (CPAP) and bilevel positive airway pressure (BiPAP). In CPAP same pressure is applied/set during inspiratory and expiratory phase of respiratory cycle. CPAP is comparable to positive end expiratory pressure (PEEP) used in invasive mechanical ventilation. CPAP is most useful in hypoxic respiratory failure. In BiPAP different pressure applied/set in inspiratory and expiratory phase of respiratory cycle, these pressures known as IPAP (inspiratory positive airway pressure) and EPAP (expiratory positive airway pressure). EPAP is the pressure which is comparable to the pressure of CPAP. BiPAP is useful in both hypercapnic as well as hypoxic respiratory failure. High flow nasal cannula (HFNC) is a recent method of delivering NIV through nasal cannula instead of tight-fitting face mask.

Continuous positive airway pressure: This mode can be used in patients, who are breathing spontaneously (a must). At end expiration, pressure in airways equals to pressure at mouth and both equate with normal atmospheric pressure. Surfactant prevents collapse of the alveoli which would have otherwise collapsed at this low end-expiratory pressure.

Bilevel positive airway pressure: CPAP does not provide support during inspiration as it only maintains positive pressure in airways. So, PSV was added to provide pressure support during inspiration in patients with poor respiratory effort. This resulted in creation of a new mode called BiPAP. So BiPAP has two components providing pressures at two levels, i.e., inspiratory and expiratory level; (1) PSV—which provides inspiratory pressure, and (2) PEEP—which provides expiratory pressure. BiPAP and CPAP both have disadvantage of propensity toward hyperinflation of lung. Further indications and contraindications are discussed in **Table 3**.

TABLE 3: Indications and contraindications of noninvasive ventilation (NIV).

Indications	Contraindications
• Acute exacerbation of chronic obstructive pulmonary disease where PaCO$_2$ >45 mm Hg or pH <7.30 • Cardiogenic pulmonary edema • Acute hypoxemic respiratory failure • Obstructive sleep apnea-hypopnea syndrome • Congestive heart failure • Obesity hypoventilation syndrome • Immunocompromised host with acute respiratory failure • Postextubation and respiratory failure after extubation • Facilitate weaning • Asthma and status asthmaticus	• Patients having no spontaneous breathing • Unconscious patient • Severe hemodynamic instability of the patient • Upper airway obstruction • Facial trauma in a patient • Pneumothorax • Inability to cooperate, protect the airway, or clear secretions • High aspiration risk • Prologed duration of mechanical ventilation anticipated • Recent esophageal anastomosis

Question 3

1. What are toxidromes?

2. Enumerate toxidromes.

3. Discuss the features of various toxidromes.

Toxic syndrome: Toxidromes—the word "toxidrome" is used when a specific class of toxin/chemical/poison produces a group of signs and symptoms. Toxidromes are helpful in identifying the particular toxins and narrow down the differential diagnosis when history is uncertain or inadequate. On the basis of these toxidromes (group of signs and symptoms specific to toxins) physician incorporates appropriate diagnostic tests and treatment into their management plan. But confusing mixed syndrome picture appears in cases of polydrug overdoses. Common toxidromes are anticholinergic syndrome, sympathomimetic syndrome, opioid/sedative/ethanol syndrome, cholinergic syndrome, and serotonin syndrome. The salient features of common toxidromes are listed in **Table 4**.

TABLE 4: Toxidromes—common toxic syndrome

Drugs	Common syndromic features
Cholinergic: (Organophosphorus, carbamates insecticides physostigmine, edrophonium, some mushroom)	Confusion, CNS depression, weakness, salivation lacrimation, urinary/fecal incontinence, abdominal cramps, vomiting, muscle fasciculation, pulmonary edema, miosis, bradycardia/tachycardia, seizure
Anticholinergics: Antihistamine antiparkinsonians, atropine scopolamine, amantadine, antipsychotics, antidepressants antispasmodics, muscle relaxants	Delirium tachycardia dry flushed skin, dilated pupil myoclonus, temperature, urinary retention, diminished bowel sound, seizure
Sympathomimetics: Cocaine amphetamines, methamphetamines, decongestant in cough syrup (phenylpropanolamine, ephedrine, pseudoephedrine)	Delusion, paranoia, tachycardia, hypertension, hyperpyrexia, diaphoresis mydriasis, hyperreflexia, seizure, hypotension, arrhythmias
Opioid/sedative/ethanol: Narcotics, barbiturates, benzodiazepines, ethchlorvynol, glutethimide, ethanol clonidine meprobamate	Respiratory depression, hypotension, miosis, bradycardia, hypothermic, pulmonary edema, diminished bowel sound, hyporeflexia, seizure, coma
Salicylates	Fever, metabolic acidosis, respiratory alkalosis, tinnitus, and altered sensorium
Serotonins: SSRI, TCA, and MAOI	Hyperreflexia, clonus, sweating, tremor, flushing, and hypertension

(CNS: central nervous system; MAOI: monoamine oxidase inhibitors; SSRI: selective serotonin reuptake inhibitors; TCA: tricyclic antidepressants)

Question 4

1. Define and classify acute coronary syndrome (ACS).

Acute coronary syndrome refers to the clinical spectrum of coronary artery diseases (CADs) that include ST-segment elevation myocardial infarction (STEMI) and non-ST elevation ACS (NSTE-ACS). The NSTE-ACS encompasses non-ST-segment elevation myocardial infarction (NSTEMI) and unstable angina (UA). Acute myocardial infarction (AMI) is any ACS with clinical evidence of 1) myocardial injury with serial elevated cardiac troponin (cTn) levels and at least one cTn value above the 99th percentile of upper reference limit (URL) and 2) cardiac tissue necrosis consistent with myocardial ischemia **(Table 5)**.

TABLE 5: Types of acute coronary syndrome presentation.

Types	Clinical setting	Etiology/findings
Type 1	Spontaneous MI	• Rupture, ulceration, fissuring, erosion or dissection of atherosclerotic plaque *OR* • Distal platelet emboli with resultant myocyte necrosis
Type 2	MI secondary to ischemic imbalance	Non-CAD related condition such as arrhythmia, coronary embolus, coronary endothelial dysfunction, coronary artery spasm, anemia, tachycardia, respiratory failure, pulmonary embolism, severe aortic stenosis, hypotension, hypertension, sepsis, use of cardiotoxic drugs, stress, cocaine and tobacco use
Type 3	MI resulting in death when biomarker values are unavailable	• Death due to cardiac arrest before blood samples could be obtained or before cardiac biomarkers could rise • ECG shows new ischemic changes or new LBBB
Type 4a	MI related to PCI (recurrent MI)	cTn elevation to >5 times the 99th percentile of URL or >20% in patients with normal pre-PCI values *AND* one of the following: • Angina • *ECG:* New ischemic changes • *Angiography:* Either reduced blood flow or blockage • *Imaging studies:* New regional wall motion abnormality
Type 4b	MI related to stent thrombosis (recurrent MI)	Stent thrombosis on angiography or autopsy *AND* Rise and/or fall in cardiac biomarker levels
Type 5	MI related to CABG (recurrent MI)	Cardiac biomarkers values >10 times with 99th percentile of URL in patients with normal pre-CABG values *AND* one of the following: • *ECG:* New pathological Q waves or LBBB • *Angiography:* Occlusion of a new graft or native coronary artery • *Imaging:* New regional wall motion abnormality

(CABG: coronary artery bypass surgery; CAD: coronary artery disease; cTn: cardiac troponin; ECG: electrocardiogram; LBBB: left bundle branch block; MI: myocardial infarction; PCI: percutaneous coronary intervention; URL: upper reference level)

2. What is the use of cardiac enzymes in diagnosis of acute myocardial infarction?

Cardiac markers for diagnosis and risk stratification: Timing of cardiac markers—in patients with symptoms consistent with ACS:

- Immediately send blood samples for cardiac troponin I (cTnI) or cardiac troponin T (cTnT)
- Reassess cTnI or cTnT 3–6 hours after symptom onset
- *After 6 hours:* If initial and serial cTn values are normal, and/or patient has ECG changes, and/or patient is in immediate/high risk category
- *Day 3 or 4:* In patients with MI to assess infarct size

An increased cTn suggests myocardial cell injury but does not throw light on cause of the injury as cTn values increase in many other cardiac/noncardiac causes. Imaging techniques such as angiography are used to find the cause and actual site of injury.

Role of other cardiac markers in ACS diagnosis: Other cardiac markers include creatinine kinase (CK), myoglobin, and B-type natriuretic peptide (BNP). The sensitivity and specificity of CK levels for cardiac damage are lower compared to other markers as raised CK levels are usually associated with many noncardiac conditions as well. CK myocardial isoenzyme (CK-MB) is useful for early diagnosis of acute MI. Unlike CK level, CK-MB is more specific to cardiac injury but it cannot help in ascertaining infarct size; however, it is useful in detecting early reinfarction. CK-MB and myoglobin are not required if contemporary troponin assays are being performed as they do not add any additional diagnostic value. BNP or N-terminal (NT)-pro hormone BNP (NT–pro-BNP) is sometimes done in patients with suspected ACS to assess risk and as a prognostic marker.

3. Explain TIMI risk scoring.

Initial evaluation at ED/when first seen: Initial evaluation is aimed at establishing diagnosis of ACS, assessing risk and differentiating into STEMI, NSTEMI, and UA (unstable angina) for further management. Physicians initially make a working diagnosis of ACS based on the symptoms, medical history (including assessing risk factors for CAD), and physical evaluation, which is further confirmed by serial electrocardiograms (ECG) and serial serologic cardiac markers. Further management is based on risk prognosis assessed by two commonly used risk assessment tools: (1) Thrombolysis in Myocardial Infarction (TIMI) risk score and (2) the Global Registry of Acute Coronary Events (GRACE) risk score **(Table 6)**. After initial evaluation and risk stratification, treatment depends on whether patient has STEMI, NSTEMI or unstable angina (UA). The primary aim of the treatment for ACS is to relieve distress, reduce cardiac workload, reverse ischemia, interrupt thrombosis, and prevent complications. Patients having confirmed STEMI require more intensive management and monitoring than NSTE-ACS.

TABLE 6: Risk scores for risk stratification of acute coronary syndrome.

TIMI risk score for STEMI	TIMI risk score for NSTE-ACS	GRACE risk score for entire spectrum of ACS
Score: 0–14 (scores ≥3–high risk)	Score: 0–7 (scores ≥3–high risk)	Range: 1–372 Low risk: <109 Intermediate risk: 109–140 High risk: >141
Based on 8 variables at admission: 1. ≥65 years 2. Risk factors: Diabetes mellitus, angina, hypertension 3. SBP <100 4. Heart rate >100 5. Weight <67 kg 6. Anterior STE or LBBB 7. Treatment start >4 hours 8. Killip class II–IV	Based on one point each for 7 variables at admission: 1. ≥65 years of age 2. ≥3 risk factors for CAD 3. Prior ≥50% coronary stenosis 4. ST deviation on ECG 5. ≥2 anginal events in prior 24 hours 6. Aspirin use in prior 7 days 7. Elevated cardiac biomarkers	Based on 8 variables at admission: 1. Age 2. Heart rate 3. SBP 4. Serum creatinine 5. Killip class 6. Cardiac arrest 7. ST-segment deviation on ECG 8. Elevated cardiac enzymes/markers

(ACS: acute coronary syndrome; ECG: electrocardiogram; LBBB: left bundle branch block; NSTE-ACS: non-ST elevation ACS; SBP: systolic blood pressure; STE: ST-segment elevation; STEMI: ST-segment elevation myocardial infarction)

4. Discuss percutaneous coronary intervention versus thrombolysis in ST elevation MI.

Reperfusion is indicated for all patients with ≤12 hour duration of symptoms and persistent ST-segment elevation. Fibrinolysis with tenecteplase, alteplase, or reteplase is recommended if revascularization is expected to be delayed beyond 2 hours **(Table 7)**. Primary percutaneous coronary intervention (PCI), when performed in a timely manner, is preferred to fibrinolytic therapy for reperfusion therapy during ST-segment–elevation myocardial infarction (STEMI).

Percutaneous coronary intervention is preferred if the medical contact-to-balloon time is less than 90 minutes, or if there are other reasons [e.g., contraindications to thrombolysis, symptom onset of >3 hours or high-risk STEMI (cardiogenic shock, or Killip class 3 or greater)].

TABLE 7: Fibrinolytic agents and doses.

Streptokinase	• 1.5 million IU • Infused over 1 hour in 45 mL NaCl
Alteplase	15 mg loading dose followed by 50 mg over 30 minutes and 35 mg over next 1 hour (Total duration of infusion 90 minutes) and concurrent use of heparin (0.75 mg/kg not to exceed 50 mg over 30 minutes and 0.50 mg/kg and not to exceed 35 mg over next 1 hour)
Reteplase	• Given as double bolus by 10 U+10 U (no infusion) • 10 U bolus over 2 minutes wait for 30 minutes and repeat 10 U over 2 minutes and concurrent use of heparin
Tenecteplase	30–50 mg single weight-based bolus over 5–10 seconds and concurrent use of heparin

Question 5

1. Define upper gastrointestinal (GI) bleeding.

The GI bleed is defined as bleeding in the GI tract from mouth to anus. It is further divided into upper GI bleed (bleed that occurs from source in esophagus to ligament of Treitz in duodenum) and lower GI bleed (bleed that occurs from source distal to ligament of Treitz).

2. Enumerate the causes of massive upper GI bleeding.

The commonest causes of upper GI bleed are peptic ulcer, varices (esophageal or gastric), Mallory-Weiss tear, and neoplasms. Other common causes of upper GI bleed include esophagitis, erosive gastritis, vascular malformations, and Dieulafoy's lesions.

3. Explain the ED management of massive upper GI bleeding.

The emergent treatment of the patient presenting with GI bleed is very important. Initial rapid resuscitative measures should be promptly started in emergency which includes putting two large bore IV cannula and fluid resuscitation. Blood samples should be collected for complete blood counts, liver and renal function tests, coagulation profile and blood grouping/crossmatching. Patients with massive upper GI bleed may need endotracheal intubation for airway protection **(Flowchart 2)**.

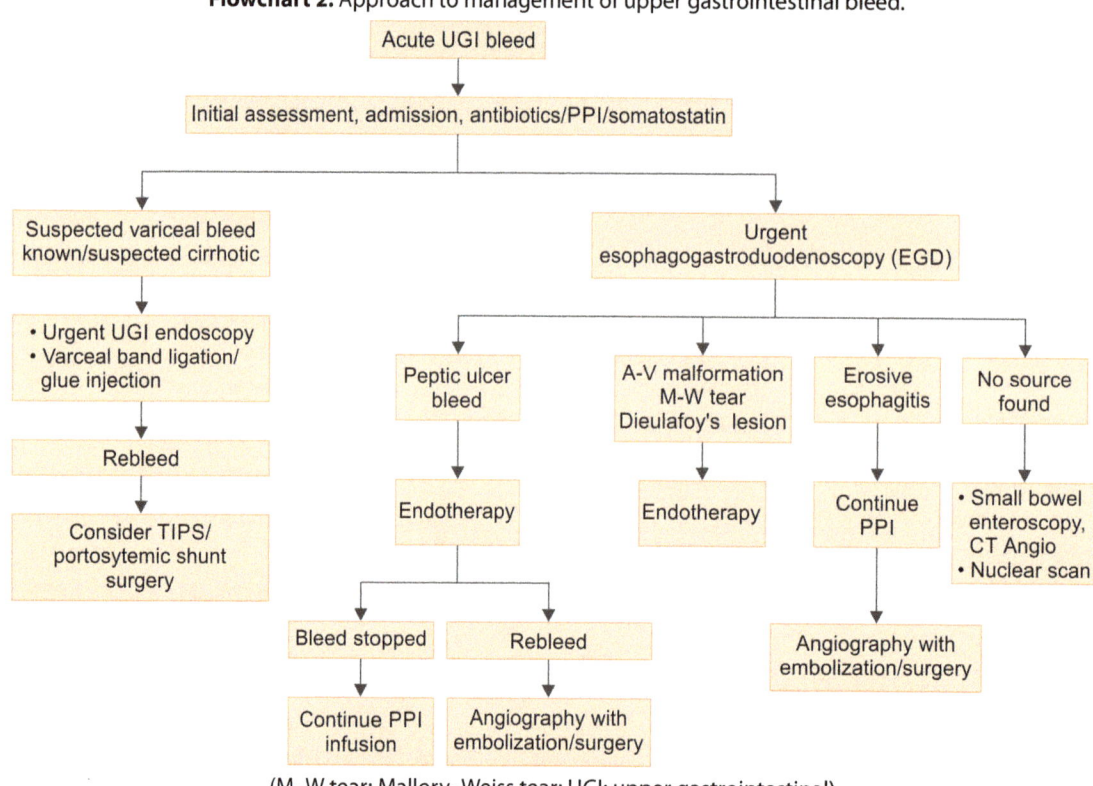

Flowchart 2: Approach to management of upper gastrointestinal bleed.

(M–W tear: Mallory–Weiss tear; UGI: upper gastrointestinal)

4. Discuss the pros and cons of different modalities of treatment.

Upper endoscopy and colonoscopy are the mainstay of initial investigations. Angiography and radionuclide imaging are best suited for acute overt gastrointestinal (GI) bleeding. Capsule endoscopy and deep enteroscopy play significant roles in the diagnosis of obscure GI bleeding, usually from the small bowel.

Antibiotics: Every patient should be started with antibiotics to prevent sepsis caused by bacterial translocation from the gut, particularly in cirrhotic. The risk of rebleed is more in patient who develop bacterial infections.

Packed RBC transfusion: Patients presenting with massive GI bleed should be given packed RBC in the ED only as rapid blood loss can result in vital organ hypoperfusion leading to multiorgan dysfunction. In euvolemic patients with upper GI hemorrhage, the PRBC transfusion should be planned to *target hemoglobin level of 7 g*. Overzealous PRBC transfusion should be avoided.

Nasogastric tube placement: There is a controversial role of nasogastric tube placement in all GI bleeds, can be useful in upper GI bleed.

Proton-pump inhibitors (PPI): Intravenous PPI is recommended in all patients presenting with acute upper GI bleed. Emergency physician should consider intravenous PPI in all patients with upper GI hemorrhage before the endoscopic therapy.

Anticoagulation reversal: Patients with acute GI bleed who are on anticoagulants, efforts should be made by emergency physician to reverse the effect of anticoagulant. Patients on warfarin or dicoumarin (vitamin K antagonists) should be given *intravenous dose of Vitamin K*.

Somatostatin and its long-acting analog, octreotide, cause selective splanchnic vasoconstriction thus cause reduction in portal pressure.

Terlipressin causes vasoconstriction and therefore reduces portal blood flow and also increases the resistance to variceal blood. This drug is widely used and recommended for variceal bleed.

Question 6

1. Discuss the clinical features of organophosphorus (OP) poisoning.

Patients with massive ingestions can become symptomatic very quickly, sometimes within 5 minutes following ingestion, and deaths have occurred within 15 minutes of ingestion. Most victims, however, become symptomatic in about 8 hours of exposure, and virtually all within 24 hours.

I. *Muscarinic effects (hollow organ parasympathetic manifestations):* Common manifestations include bronchoconstriction with wheezing and dyspnea, cough, pulmonary edema, vomiting, diarrhea, abdominal cramps, increased salivation, lacrimation, and sweating, bradycardia, hypotension, miosis, and urinary incontinence. Excessive salivation, nausea, vomiting, abdominal cramps, and diarrhea are common muscarinic effects, and have been reported even following the cutaneous absorption of organophosphate. Bradycardia and hypotension occur following moderate to severe poisoning. Bronchorrhea can be so profuse that it mimics pulmonary edema even when the lungs are not edematous.

II. *Nicotinic effects* (autonomic ganglionic and somatic motor effects due to stimulation of nicotinic adrenal receptors and postganglionic sympathetic fibers): Fasciculations, weakness, hypertension, tachycardia, and paralysis. Mydriasis has been reported in as many as 13% of cases, presumably from nicotinic stimulation of sympathetic receptors. Muscle weakness, fatiguability, and fasciculations are very common.

2. Outline OP poisoning management in the ED.

The initial treatment for a patient exposed to OP compounds must be directed at ensuring an adequate airway and ventilation, and at reversing excessive muscarinic effects. Seizures must be treated with standard anticonvulsants such as benzodiazepines or barbiturates.

Decontamination: Procedure—
- Shower is preferable. Make the patient stand (if he/she is able to) under the shower, or seated in a chair.
- Wash with cold water for 5 minutes from head to toe using nongermicidal soap. Rinse hair well.
- Repeat the wash and rinse procedure with warm water.
- Repeat the wash and rinse procedure with hot water.

Treating personnel should protect themselves with water-impermeable gowns, masks with eye shields, and shoe covers

Atropine: A competitive antagonist of acetylcholine at the muscarinic postsynaptic membrane and in the CNS; will block the muscarinic manifestations of organophosphate poisoning.

Pralidoxime: This is a nucleophilic oxime which helps to regenerate acetylcholinesterase at muscarinic, nicotinic, and CNS sites.

Supportive measures: Maintain airway patency and oxygenation. Suction secretions. Endotracheal intubation and mechanical ventilation may be necessary. Monitor pulse oximetry or arterial blood gases to determine need for supplemental oxygen.

Prevention of further exposure: After the patient has recovered, he/she should not be re-exposed to organophosphates.

3. Give a differential diagnosis of acute flaccid paralysis (AFP).

Acute flaccid paralysis is a complex clinical syndrome characterized by rapid onset of weakness of limbs which may include muscles of respiration and swallowing, rapidly progressing to maximum severity within few days. The term "flaccid" indicates decreased tone of affected muscles. It includes broad spectrum of diseases which may vary with age and region. Poliomyelitis was one of the most common causes of acute flaccid paralysis. However, because of global polio eradication initiative by WHO, poliomyelitis has reached near eradication in world. Hence, other causes of AFP must be sought and evaluated. Early diagnosis in ED significantly improves the outcome of the patient **(Table 8)**.

TABLE 8: Etiology of acute flaccid paralysis.	
Metabolic causes	- Hypokalemia - Hyperkalemia - Hypophosphatemia - Thiamine deficiency
Muscle disorders	- Infection—viral myositis - Inflammatory myopathy—polymyositis, dermatomyositis
Disorder of neuromuscular junction	- Myasthenia gravis crisis - Lambert–Eaton syndrome - Botulism - Tick paralysis - Snake bite - Organophosphate poisoning
Neuropathy	- Guillain–Barré syndrome - Porphyria - Diphtheria - Vasculitis
Anterior horn cell disease	- Poliomyelitis - Paraneoplastic
Spinal cord diseases	- Trauma - Transverse myelitis - Anterior spinal artery syndrome

Question 7

1. State the RIFLE criteria for classification of acute kidney injury.

The acronym RIFLE defines three grades of increasing severity of acute kidney injury (risk, injury, and failure, respectively, R, I, and F) and two outcome variables (loss and end-stage kidney disease, respectively, L and E) **(Table 9)**.

TABLE 9: RIFLE criteria for acute kidney injury.

Category	Criteria
Risk (R)	Increased serum creatinine level by 1.5 times or GFR decrease by >25%
Injury (I)	Increased serum creatinine level by 2.0 times or GFR decrease by >50%
Failure (F)	Increased serum creatinine level by 3.0 times, GFR decease by >75% or serum creatinine level ≥354 µmol/L
Loss (L)	Persistent acute renal failure or compete loss of function for >4 weeks
End stage kidney disease (E)	End-stage kidney disease for >3 months

(GFR: glomerular filtration rate)

2. Discuss ECG changes of hyperkalemia.

The most common ECG changes of hyperkalemia findings are tall, peaked T waves with shortened QT interval, lengthening of PR interval and QRS duration, absence of P waves, and ultimately sine wave pattern as the QRS progresses in duration. Various ECG changes seen as potassium level increases are shown in **Table 10**.

TABLE 10: Electrocardiogram changes in hyperkalemia.

Potassium level (mmol/L)	Mechanism	ECG changes
5.5–6.5	Repolarization abnormalities	Peaked T waves
6.5–7.0	Progressive atrial paralysis	• P wave widening/flattening • PR prolongation • P waves eventuality disappear
7.0–9.0	Conduction abnormalities	*Bradyarrhythmias:* Sinus bradycardia; high-grade AV block with slow junctional and ventricular escape rhythms; slow AF conduction blocks (bundle branch block, fasciculate blocks); prolonged QRS interval with bizarre QRS morphology
>9.0	All of the above	• Development of sine wave appearance (preterminal rhythm), asystole ventricular fibrillation • PEA with bizarre, wide complex rhythm

3. Discuss the management of hyperkalemia in the ED.

Clinical manifestations of hyperkalemia which occurs at potassium levels >7.0 mEq/L include muscle weakness/paralysis and cardiac arrhythmias secondary to conduction abnormalities. Hyperkalemia causing conduction abnormalities is detected on electrocardiograms (ECG). In patients with hyperkalemia and ECG changes, administration of calcium gluconate or calcium carbonate (1 g IV over minutes, repeat as needed) is recommended to stabilize the cardiac membrane. Then use drugs which promote potassium ions to shift intracellularly are regular insulin (10 U IV or weight-based and administered with glucose), β_2-adrenergic agonists (nebulized albuterol), or sodium bicarbonate (50 mEq/50 mL IV). After this if the patient's volume status has been assessed and determined to be hypervolemic or euvolemic with appropriate supportive fluids one can use loop diuretics (furosemide, 40–60 mg IV) or cation resins (sodium polystyrene sulfonate, 15 g orally) to eliminate potassium in the urine and stool **(Table 11)**. There is limited evidence regarding use of cation resins, such as sodium polystyrene sulfonate (Kayexalate), there are some potential untoward effects and that may outweigh benefits. Newer binding agents, such as patiromer and sodium zirconium cyclosilicate (ZS-9) are studied recently. Patiromer is a synthetic polymer of nonabsorbable beads that exchanges calcium for potassium excretion in the stool in the distal colon. A recent meta-analysis investigating patiromer and ZS-9 found that these agents were more efficacious compared with Kayexalate, although further studies are warranted to test side effects, use in specific patient populations, and medication interactions.

4. What are the indications for emergent dialysis?

Indications for emergent dialysis **(Table 12)** are: (1) Acidosis (pH 6.5 refractory to treatment), (2) Ingestions of dialyzable drugs (salicylates, lithium, toxic alcohols), (3) Overload (especially with hypertension, increasing oxygen requirements), and (4) Uremia (bleeding, pericarditis, encephalopathy).

TABLE 11: Drugs to treat hyperkalemia—dose onset duration

Effect	Treatment	Dose	Onset	Duration
Stabilize membrane	Calcium gluconate and Calcium carbonate	10 mL IV over 10 minutes	Immediate	30–60 minutes
Shifters	• Albuterol • Insulin • Sodium bicarbonate	• 10–20 mg nebulization • 10 units IV with dextrose 25–50 g • 150 mmol IV	• 30 minutes • 20 minutes • Hours	• 2 hours • 4–6 hours • Hours
Excretors	• Furosemide • Sodium polystyrene	• 40–80 mg IV • 15–30 g in 15–30 mL	• 15 minutes • Hours	2–3 hours 4–6 hours
Definitive	Hemodialysis		Immediate	3 hours

TABLE 12: Mnemonic for emergent hemodialysis indications.

A	*Acidemia:* Severe metabolic acidosis despite adequate medical optimization (pH <7.1)
E	*Electrolytes:* Particularly hyperkalemia refractory to medical therapy
I	*Ingestion:* Poisoning by drugs that are able to be eliminated with RRT
O	*Overload:* Volume overload resulting in hypoxic respiratory failure necessitating mechanical ventilation
U	*Uremia:* Complications secondary to increased BUN (bleeding, pericarditis, encephalopathy)

(BUN: blood urea nitrogen)
Source: Data adapted from Nee P, Bailey D, Todd V, Lewington AJ, Wootten AE, Sim KJ. Critical care in the emergency department: acute kidney injury. Emerg Med J. 2016;33:361-5.

Question 8

1. Discuss the pathogenesis and clinical features of staphylococcal toxic shock syndrome.

Staphylococcal scalded skin syndrome, also known as Ritter disease is a disease characterized by denudation of the skin caused by exotoxin producing strains of the *Staphylococcus* species, typically from a distant site. It usually presents 48 hours after birth and is rare in children >6 years.

Commonly seen in infants and children due to exotoxin released by *Staphylococcus aureus* group 2 phage 71. Exotoxin is an epidermolytic toxin also called exfoliating toxin or epidermolysin.

Clinically, intense erythematous cutaneous eruptions occur following an upper respiratory tract infection or purulent conjunctivitis. Painful erosions appear when erythematous sheets of skin are shed which is referred to as potato chip desquamation. Patient should be admitted and treated promptly with antibiotics covering *Staphylococcus aureus*.

2. What are the diagnostic criteria of staphylococcal toxic shock syndrome?

Staphylococcal scalded skin syndrome tends to appear abruptly with diffuse erythema and fever. The diagnosis can be confirmed by a *skin biopsy*, which can be expedited by frozen section processing, as staphylococcal scalded skin syndrome should be distinguished from life-threatening toxic epidermal necrolysis.

Question 9

1. Explain the precipitating factors for thyroid storm.

Thyroid storm is unrecognized, undertreated, life-threatening form of severe thyrotoxicosis. Thyroid storm is rare and mostly acute reaction to thyroid and nonthyroid surgery, trauma infections contrast media, amiodarone, after delivery in preexisting hyperthyroidism. Other risk factors are acute coronary syndrome, pulmonary embolism, and diabetic ketoacidosis.

2. What are the diagnostic criteria for thyroid storm?

Prompt recognitions and treatment is warranted as mortality is almost 100%. The causes of mortality in patient of thyroid storm: Sepsis, multiorgan failure, congestive heart failure arrhythmias, disseminated intravascular, and coagulation. Clinical features of thyroid storm are typical—include hyperpyrexia, out of proportion tachycardia, altered mental status (agitation, delirium coma) along with clinical picture of hyperthyroidism. Classic features of thyroid storm include fever, marked tachycardia, heart failure, tremor, nausea and vomiting, diarrhea, dehydration, restlessness, extreme agitation, delirium or coma. Fever is typical and may be >105.8°F (41°C).

3. Discuss the investigations you will do in such a case.

Thyroid function test: Usual findings include elevated triiodothyronine (T3), thyroxine (T4), and free T4 levels; increased T3 resin uptake; suppressed thyroid-stimulating hormone (TSH) levels; and an elevated 24-hour iodine uptake.

4. Explain the ED management of thyroid storm.

The management of thyroid storm is summarized in **Table 13**.

TABLE 13: Management of thyroid storm.

Beta-adrenergic blockers	• Propranolol 60–80 mg orally every 4 hours (IV 0.5–1.0 mg as test dose then repeat 1–2 mg every 15 minutes till desired effect then 1–2 mg every 3 hours) or • Metoprolol 25–50 mg orally every 6 hours or • Esmolol 50–100 µg/kg/min infusion
Inhibition of thyroid hormone synthesis	Propylthiouracil 500–1,000 mg loading then 250 mg every 4 hours or Methimazole 60–80 mg/day
Inhibition of thyroid hormone release	• Saturated potassium iodide solution (50 mg/drop) 1–2 drops orally or per rectally or • Lugol's solution 5–7 drops
Corticosteroid	Hydrocortisone 300 mg IV then 100 mg every 8 hours
Treatment of underlying precipitant	Empirical antibiotics
Supportive measures	Volume resuscitation cooling blankets, fan ice packs/lavage
Others	Lorazepam, diazepam

Question 10

1. Enumerate heat emergencies.
2. Discuss clinical presentation of heat stroke.
3. Explain the management of heat stroke in the ED.

Heat emergencies/illness is a spectrum of disorders due to environmental exposure to heat. It ranges from minor conditions such as heat cramps, heat syncope, and heat exhaustion to the more severe condition known as heat stroke. A number of heat illnesses exist across a broad spectrum of presentations **(Table 14)**.

TABLE 14: Classification of heat Illness.	
Types	Characteristic feature
Heat cramps	Muscular pain which happens after exercise in hot conditions
Heat edema	Cutaneous condition characterized by dependent edema from vasodilatory pooling
Heat rash	Irritation of the skin that results from excessive sweating during hot and humid weather
Heat tetany	A result of short periods of stress in intense heat. Symptoms may include hyperventilation, respiratory problems, numbness or tingling, or muscle spasms
Heat syncope	Dizziness as a result of excess heat
Heat exhaustion	A precursor of a heatstroke which includes heavy sweating, rapid breathing, and a fast, weak pulse
Heat stroke	A core body temperature of >40°C (104°F) due to environmental heat exposure with either a lack or dysfunction of the central and peripheral thermoregulation center. Symptoms include dry skin, rapid, strong pulse, and dizziness

Investigations: Important recommended investigations are: Complete blood count (CBC), liver function tests (LFTs), urea and electrolytes (U&E) glucose urate—maybe a predictor of acute kidney injury creatine kinase; maybe a predictor of rhabdomyolysis. Coagulation studies, arterial blood gases, and urinalysis may show myoglobinuria and impending acute kidney injury; and ECG, chest X-ray (CXR)— to check for aspiration/pulmonary edema.

Treatment

- Maintain airway breathing and circulation, cardiac monitoring. Monitor core body temperature regularly.
- Treatment of heat stroke involves rapid mechanical cooling along with resuscitation measures. The body temperature must be lowered quickly.
- The patient should be moved to a cool area which is either indoor or in a shade and clothing may need to be removed to promote passive clothing.
- Active cooling methods include immersion in cold water, or a hyperthermia vest can be applied. Cold compresses to the torso, head, neck, and groin will help in bringing the body core temperature down. A fan or dehumidifying air-conditioning unit may be used to aid in evaporation of the water.
- Immersion should be avoided for an unconscious person, but if there is no alternative, the patients' head must be held above water.
- Dantrolene, a direct-acting paralytic which abolishes shuddering and is effective in many other forms of hyperthermia has no individual or additive effects to cooling in the context of heat stroke, showing a lack of endogenous thermogenic response to cold water immersion. Aggressive ice-water immersion is the gold standard for life-threatening heat stroke.
- Adequate hydration is essential adjunct to cool the temperature. In mild cases of dehydration, adequate hydration can be achieved by drinking water, or isotonic sport drinks. In exercise- or heat-induced dehydration, an imbalance of electrolytes can occur and is exacerbated by over consumption of water.
- Hyponatremia can be corrected by intake of hypertonic fluids. Absorption is rapid and complete in most people but in the event of confusion, impaired conscious level or if the patient is unable to tolerate oral fluid, then an IV rehydration and electrolyte replacement may be required. The person's condition should be reassessed at regular intervals including the vital signs to ensure stability.

SUGGESTED READING

1. Richhariya D, Sharma B. Textbook of Emergency Medicine including Intensive Care and Trauma, 2nd edition. New Delhi: Jaypee Brothers Medical Publishers (P) Ltd; 2022. pp. 820-7. (Question 1).
2. Richhariya D, Sharma B. Textbook of Emergency Medicine including Intensive Care and Trauma, 2nd edition. New Delhi: Jaypee Brothers Medical Publishers (P) Ltd; 2022. pp. 255, 575-81. (Question 2).

3. Richhariya D, Sharma B. Textbook of Emergency Medicine including Intensive Care and Trauma, 2nd edition. New Delhi: Jaypee Brothers Medical Publishers (P) Ltd; 2022. p. 1395. (Question 3).
4. Richhariya D, Sharma B. Textbook of Emergency Medicine including Intensive Care and Trauma, 2nd edition. New Delhi: Jaypee Brothers Medical Publishers (P) Ltd; 2022. pp. 452-9. (Question 4).
5. Richhariya D, Sharma B. Textbook of Emergency Medicine including Intensive Care and Trauma, 2nd edition. New Delhi: Jaypee Brothers Medical Publishers (P) Ltd; 2022. pp. 656-60. (Question 5).
6. Richhariya D, Sharma B. Textbook of Emergency Medicine including Intensive Care and Trauma, 2nd edition. New Delhi: Jaypee Brothers Medical Publishers (P) Ltd; 2022. pp. 838-40, 1405-16. (Question 6).
7. Richhariya D, Sharma B. Textbook of Emergency Medicine including Intensive Care and Trauma, 2nd edition. New Delhi: Jaypee Brothers Medical Publishers (P) Ltd; 2022. pp. 743-52. (Question 7).
8. Richhariya D, Sharma B. Textbook of Emergency Medicine including Intensive Care and Trauma, 2nd edition. New Delhi: Jaypee Brothers Medical Publishers (P) Ltd; 2022. p. 1027. (Question 8).
9. Richhariya D, Sharma B. Textbook of Emergency Medicine including Intensive Care and Trauma, 2nd edition. New Delhi: Jaypee Brothers Medical Publishers (P) Ltd; 2022. p. 891. (Question 9).
10. Richhariya D, Sharma B. Textbook of Emergency Medicine including Intensive Care and Trauma, 2nd edition. New Delhi: Jaypee Brothers Medical Publishers (P) Ltd; 2022. pp. 1692-6. (Question 10).

Emergency Medicine Paper 4

Devendra Richhariya

Question 1

1. List six common signs and symptoms of increased intracranial pressure (ICP) in infants.

Common signs and symptoms of idiopathic intracranial hypertension (IIH) in the young include headache, vomiting, blurred vision, and diplopia. Headaches are intermittent, diffuse, and worse at night; they may awaken the child and are often aggravated by sudden movement.

Infants: Tense/bulging fontanel separated cranial sutures, irritable high pitch cry, increased occipital circumference, distended scalp vein changes in feeding, setting-Sun sign **(Fig. 1)**.

Children: Headache, nausea, vomiting, diplopia, blurred vision, seizures.

2. What is an impact seizure?

Early and late post-traumatic seizures frequently indicate structural brain damage and transition to chronic, post-traumatic epilepsy. Some authors suggest that most impact seizures are nonepileptic in origin and hence coined the term "concussive convulsions" for benign impact seizures.

3. Discuss setting-Sun sign.

The setting-Sun phenomenon is an ophthalmologic sign in young children resulting from upward-gaze paresis.

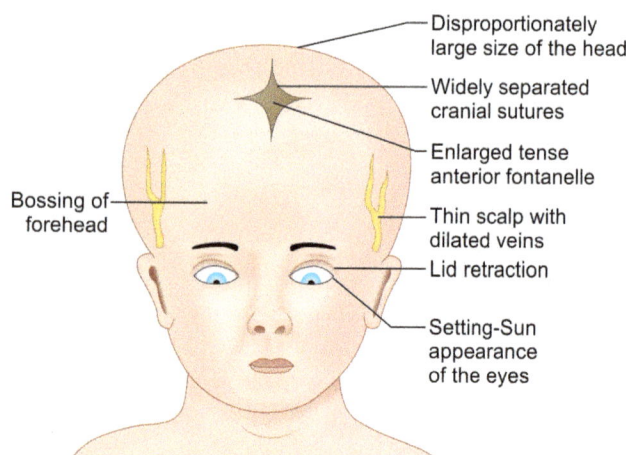

Fig. 1: Signs and symptoms of increased intracranial pressure in infants.

In this condition, the eyes appear driven downward, the sclera may be seen between the upper eyelid and the iris, and part of the lower pupil may be covered by the lower eyelid. Setting-Sun eyes are most often associated with neurological conditions that cause an increase in ICP and affect the part of the brain that controls eye movement. One such condition is hydrocephalus.

4. Outline the management of hydrocephalus in infants.

Management of hydrocephalus directed toward:
- Reducing ICP
- Prevention and management of complications
- Medical management includes use of diuretics which provide temporary relief
- Surgical management includes insertion of shunt **(Fig. 2)**

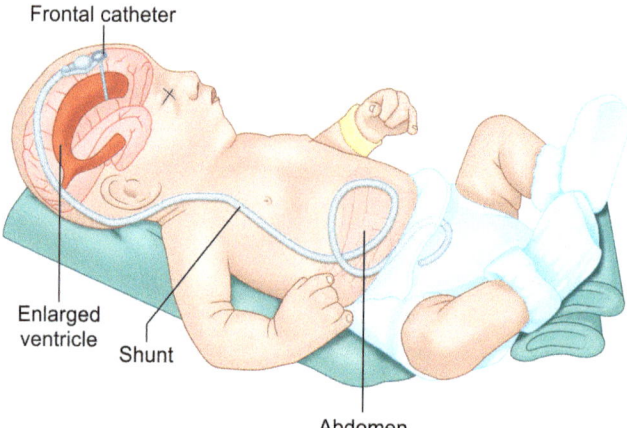

Fig. 2: Insertion of shunt to manage hydrocephalus.

Question 2

1. What are the indications for intraosseous (IO) access?

The following clinical situations represent patient groups in whom vascular access is notably difficult or who need access repeatedly but characteristically have limited vascular access.

Intraosseous access can be considered clinically appropriate on the basis of a short-term need for patients:

- With chronic disease who have been admitted to the hospital for treatment of a medical event, e.g., the deteriorating patient with chronic obstructive pulmonary disease.
- With limited vascular access due to aggressive treatment modalities, e.g., fistulas, grafts, shunts, mastectomies, or multiple central line placements.
- For whom rapid response teams are called to prevent an emergent situation and in whom obtaining peripheral or central intravenous (IV) access is difficult.
- Who experience an unexpected medical event that causes their peripheral or central IV device to become nonfunctional, e.g., infiltration or occlusion, and difficult to reestablish.
- Who have limited peripheral access due to morbid obesity.
- Who experience intractable pain.
- Who are in the early stages of sepsis.
- Who are receiving palliative or hospice care.
- Who are undergoing anesthesia and experience prolonged, difficult, or failed IV access.

2. Discuss different sites available for it and outline its procedure.

Sternum, clavicle, humeral head, iliac crest, distal femur, proximal tibia, distal tibia, and calcaneus are all potential sites for IO access.

3. What are the complications?

Complications are reported in connection with IO access. Most are avoidable with proper education and training. Complications associated with IO access include extravasation from dislodgement, iatrogenic fracture, growth plate injury, infection, fat emboli, compartment syndrome, and osteomyelitis.

Intraosseous access should be avoided in the following situations:
- Fractures in the same extremity as the targeted bone
- Previous surgery involving hardware in the bone targeted for IO access
- Infection at the insertion site or within the targeted bone
- Local vascular compromise
- Previous failed IO insertion within 24 hours in the targeted bone
- Inability to locate the landmarks.

4. What drugs can be given through IO route?

Intraosseous access is a fast, easy, and completely acceptable alternative. IO access uses the medullary cavity within bones as a noncollapsible vein. These cavities drain into venous channels that exit the bone into the systemic circulation, much like peripheral veins. While all resuscitation drugs can be given by the IO route, key drugs and fluids usable by IO access:

Adenosine, amiodarone, atropine, dobutamine, dopamine, epinephrine, etomidate, heparin, insulin, lidocaine, morphine, norepinephrine, propofol, blood products—red blood cells/platelet/fresh frozen plasma, resuscitative fluids: crystalloids/colloid/Ringer's lactate, contrast products.

Question 3

1. What are the recent clinical trials done on management of hypertensive intracerebral hemorrhage (ICH)?
2. Discuss briefly the trials.

Antihypertensive Treatment of Acute Cerebral Hemorrhage (ATACH-2) trial: Recent clinical trials have focused on determining the clinical efficacy of early intensive systolic blood pressure (SBP) reduction in ICH patients. The ATACH-2 trial was the latest phase 3 randomized controlled multicenter clinical trial aimed to study the efficacy of early intensive reduction of SBP in ICH patients.

Intensive Blood Pressure Reduction in Acute Cerebral Hemorrhage Trial (INTERACT II): The INTERACT II randomized 2,839 patients with ICH within 6 hours of symptom onset to intensive SBP reduction, with a target of <140 mm Hg within 1 hour, or guideline-recommended SBP reduction, with a target of <180 mm Hg using a variety of antihypertensive medications **(Table 1)**.

TABLE 1: Differences between INTERACT II and ATACH II.

Trial design issues	INTERACT II design	ATACH II design
Frequent transient or moderate elevation in SBP in subjects with ICH	Inclusion of patients with initial SBP of 150 mm Hg or greater	Inclusion of patients with initial SBP of 180 mm Hg or greater; exclusion of patients with spontaneous reduction in SBP prior to randomization
Short time window for preventing hematoma expansion	Inclusion and treatment of patients with symptom onset of 6 hours or less	Inclusion and treatment of patients with symptom onset of 4.5 hours or less

Contd...

Contd...

Trial design issues	INTERACT II design	ATACH II design
Very high likelihood of death within 24 hours in patients with high severity	Investigator judgment	Exclusion of patients with parenchymal hematoma volume <60 cc, large amount of IVH, or pontine ICHs
Surgical evacuation of ICH may confound the effect of trial intervention	Investigator judgment	Exclusion of cerebellar hemorrhages and those in whom surgery is indicated at time of randomization
High rate of hematoma expansion associated with anticoagulant-related ICHs	Included with INR correction based on investigator discretion	Included but require INR correction to value <1.5 prior to randomization using prothrombin complex concentrate
Imbalance between treatment groups for known factors that influence prognosis or treatment responsiveness	Large sample size; sensitivity analyses after adjusting for potential confounders	Postrandomization adjusted analyses (adjusted for GCS score, IVH, and hematoma volume)
Heterogeneity of IV antihypertensive treatment can reduce effectiveness of SBP lowering and effect ICP	Several BP-lowering protocols using urapidil, labetalol, hydralazine, metoprolol, and nicardipine	Single agent—IV nicardipine, in all patients
Effect of intensive SBP reduction post-24 hours independent of hematoma expansion	A SBP level of <140 mm maintained for the next 7 days in intensive SBP reduction group	The SBP goals after first 24 hours same in both treatment groups
Time to achieve therapeutic goals important for benefit	33% reaching therapeutic goals within 1 hour in those allocated to intensive SBP reduction	ATACH I suggested that 90% of subjects can reach therapeutic goals within 2 hours. Interim monitoring in ATACH II demonstrates similar observation
Heterogeneity in intensity of medical care in subjects between sites can affect the rates of death and disability	Not addressed	Review of patient care profile at each site by IOC
Definition of primary outcome easy to interpret with direct clinical relevance	A dichotomous outcome mRS score of 0–2 vs. 3–6	A dichotomous outcome mRS score of 0–3 vs. 4–6
Ascertainment of safety or adverse events with determination of causal effect of trial intervention	Investigator judgment	Review by IOC regarding relationship to treatment intervention and intensity of medical care
Large magnitude of benefit of trial intervention required to change clinical practices	Absolute risk reduction anticipated ≥7%; actual 3.6%	Absolute risk reduction anticipated ≥10%

(ATACH: Antihypertensive treatment of acute cerebral hemorrhage; GCS: Glasgow Coma Scale; ICP: intracranial pressure; ICH: intracerebral hemorrhage; INR: international normalized ratio; INTERACT II: Intensive Blood Pressure Reduction in Acute Cerebral Hemorrhage Trial; IOC: independent oversight committee; IV: intravenous; IVH: intraventricular hemorrhage; mRS: modified Rankin scale; SBP: systolic blood pressure)

3. What are the latest guidelines for the management of hypertensive ICH?

The latest recommendation for the target point is SBP <140 mm Hg in ICH that should be achieved during the first hour using titratable agents to prevent the expansion of present hematoma. However, if elevated ICP presents based on signs, symptoms, and radiologic findings; the physician should decrease blood pressure to the point that cerebral perfusion pressure (CPP) remains in the range of 60–80 mm Hg. IV labetalol and nicardipine are the first-line agents. Angiotensin-converting enzyme inhibitors (ACEIs) such as enalapril could be administered as the second-line option. It seems that nitroprusside and nitroglycerine may increase ICP, so they should be avoided.

In subarachnoid hemorrhage (SAH) the target point is SBP <160 mm Hg that could be achieved by various titratable agents such as nicardipine or labetalol to prevent stroke and re-bleeding, and also maintaining proper CPP. As mentioned in case of ICH, nitroprusside should be also avoided in SAH. Oral nimodipine improves neurological outcomes and should be administered to all patients with SAH.

Question 4

1. Mention the changes in the American Heart Association (AHA) guidelines of cardiopulmonary resuscitation (CPR) in an adult with cardiac arrest.

The American Heart Association guidelines for adult, pediatric, neonatal, resuscitation are revised in year 2020. These guidelines are helpful for the resuscitation providers and instructors during cardiac arrest resuscitation and also result in changes in resuscitation training and practice. The changes in the 2020 AHA guidelines for CPR are summarized here:

- Easy to remember resuscitation scenarios, algorithms, and visual aids guidance for basic life support (BLS) and advanced cardiac life support (ACLS) are developed.
- Re-emphasis is given on the importance of early initiation of CPR by lay rescuers.
- Early epinephrine administration has been reaffirmed, with emphasis like previous guidelines.
- Use of real-time audio-visual feedback is suggested as a means to maintain CPR quality.
- To improve CPR quality, continuous measure of arterial blood pressure and end tidal carbon dioxide ($ETCO_2$) during ACLS resuscitation is emphasized.
- Routine use of double sequential defibrillation is not recommended as per recent evidences.
- For medication administration during ACLS resuscitation, IV access is the preferred route but IO access is acceptable if IV access is not available.
- After return of spontaneous circulation (ROSC), patient care requires close attention to oxygenation, blood pressure control, evaluation for percutaneous coronary intervention, targeted temperature management (TTM), and multimodal neuroprognostication.
- Postcardiac arrest recovery is long and continues process after the initial hospitalization, patients should have formal assessment and support for their physical, cognitive, and psychosocial needs.
- Debriefing after resuscitation for lay rescuers, emergency medical services (EMS) providers, and hospital-based healthcare workers is beneficial to support their mental health and well-being.
- Management of cardiac arrest in pregnancy focuses on maternal resuscitation, improve the chances of successful resuscitation of the mother with preparation for early perimortem cesarean delivery if necessary to save the infant.

The changes in algorithms and other performance aids are:

- A sixth link, *recovery,* is added to the resuscitation— chains of survival **(Fig. 3)**.
- The emphasis is given on the role of early epinephrine administration for patients with non-shockable rhythms in the Universal Adult Cardiac Arrest Algorithm (modified now).
- Two new algorithms for opioid-associated emergency have been added for lay rescuers and trained rescuers.
- The postcardiac arrest care algorithm was updated to emphasize the need to prevent hyperoxia, hypoxemia, and hypotension.
- In postcardiac arrest care section new diagram is added to guide and inform neuroprognostication.
- A new algorithm has been added to address cardiac arrest in pregnancy.

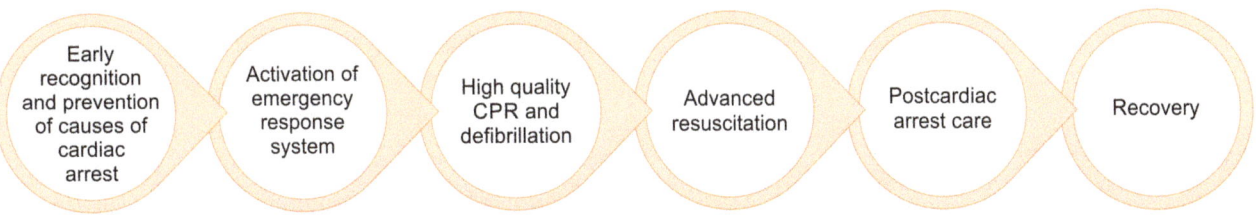

Fig. 3: Resuscitation—updated chain of survival. (CPR: cardiopulmonary resuscitation)

2. What are H's and T's?

The **H's and T's** are the reversible conditions of cardiac arrest **(Table 2)**.

TABLE 2: Causes of cardiac arrest (H's and T's).

H	T
• Hypovolemia	• Toxins/tablets
• Hypoxia	• Tamponade
• Hydrogen ion (acidosis)	• Tension pneumothorax
• Hyperkalemia, hypokalemia	• Thrombosis
• Hypothermia	• Thromboembolism
• Hypoglycemia	• Trauma

3. What is high quality CPR?

Five main components of high-performance CPR have been identified—*chest compression fraction (CCF), chest compression rate, chest compression depth, chest recoil (residual leaning), and ventilation.* CCF >80%, compression rate of 100–120/min, compression depth of at least 50 mm (2 inches) in adults and at least 1/3 the AP dimension of the chest in infants and children. These CPR components were identified because of their contribution to blood flow and outcome.

Question 5

A 2-year-old child is brought with drooling and noisy breathing.

1. Mention the differential diagnosis.

Noisy breathing/stridor in infants and children can have several different causes, including:

- *Croup:* This is a viral infection that causes inflammation of the upper airway, which can result in a barking cough, hoarseness, and stridor.
- *Epiglottitis:* This is a bacterial infection that causes inflammation and swelling of the epiglottis, which can lead to difficulty breathing and stridor.
- *Foreign body aspiration:* This occurs when a child inhales a foreign object, such as a toy or food, which can cause obstruction of the airway and stridor.
- *Anaphylaxis:* This is a severe allergic reaction that can cause swelling of the throat and airway, leading to difficulty breathing and stridor.
- *Trauma to the neck or airway:* This can occur as a result of a fall, car accident, or other injury, and can lead to obstruction of the airway and stridor.
- *Vocal cord dysfunction:* This occurs when the vocal cords do not function properly, causing difficulty breathing and stridor.
- *Tonsillitis:* Inflammation of the tonsils can cause difficulty breathing and stridor.
- *Congenital abnormalities:* Infants may be born with structural abnormalities in the airway that can cause stridor, such as laryngomalacia or tracheomalacia.

2. How will you prepare to secure the airway if needed?

The Pediatric Advanced Life Support (PALS) guidelines recommend assessing the unresponsive pediatric patient by first checking for normal breathing and a pulse. Breathing is ideally assessed by observation for any chest rise for a maximum of 10 seconds while simultaneously palpating for a pulse over the region of the brachial artery for infants and the carotid or femoral artery for children.

Respiratory arrest: If breathing is absent or abnormal (e.g., gasping), but a pulse is present, management consists of providing 12–20 adequate "rescue breaths" per minute (approximately 1 breath every 3–5 seconds) over 1 second with visible chest rise. Continue this with a pulse check every 2 minutes to check for progression to cardiac arrest.

An advanced airway, such as an endotracheal tube, allows for decreased subsequent interruptions during chest compressions. However, a systematic review from 2019 focused on comparing bag-valve-mask ventilation (BMV) versus endotracheal intubation use for out-of-hospital cardiac arrest (OHCA) showed no significant difference in good neurological outcome or survival to hospital discharge between both groups. Therefore, it is reasonable to continue with BMV, at least during OHCA, rather than expedite the establishment of an advanced airway.

3. Discuss the drug treatment of this child.

Croup (viral laryngotracheobronchitis) is the most common cause of stridor outside the neonatal period, commonly affecting children 6 months to 3 years old. It is caused by a viral infection that inflames the upper airways, including the larynx, trachea, and bronchi. The most common causes are: Parainfluenza virus and rhinovirus. *Other causes are:* Influenza respiratory syncytial virus (RSV), metapneumovirus, enterovirus, and coronavirus. The treatment of croup depends on the severity of the symptoms. In most cases, croup is a self-limited illness that improves on its own within a few days.

The following treatments may be recommended to help alleviate symptoms and improve the child's comfort:

Humidifier: Using a cool-mist humidifier in the child's bedroom can help to relieve cough and ease breathing. Alternatively, taking the child into a steamy bathroom for a few minutes can also be effective.

Rest: Encouraging the child to rest and limiting physical activity can help to reduce the strain on the respiratory system and promote healing.

Fluids: Making sure the child drinks plenty of fluids can help to prevent dehydration, thin out mucus secretions, and make coughing more productive.

Medications: Over-the-counter pain relievers, such as acetaminophen or ibuprofen, can be given to help reduce fever and relieve pain. Oral steroids may be prescribed to help reduce inflammation in the airways and improve breathing, hence, reducing the duration of the disease. Recommended is dexamethasone single dose of 0.6 mg/kg per oral.

Emergency care: In rare cases of severe croup, where the child is struggling to breathe, hospitalization may be necessary. In the hospital, the child may receive supplemental oxygen, nebulized medications, and other treatments to help alleviate symptoms and improve breathing.

For severe croup with persistent respiratory failure despite medical therapy, endotracheal intubation may be necessary. There is insufficient evidence to determine whether nebulized beta agonists are beneficial with croup, as it causes vasodilation, which may worsen upper airway edema. Hence, β-agonists are not recommended in croup.

Question 6

1. Name newer antiepileptic drugs.

Newer antiepileptic drugs are:
- *Levetiracetam*
- *Lamotrigine*
- *Oxcarbazepine*
- *Eslicarbazepine acetate*
- *Zonisamide*
- *Topiramate*
- *Gabapentin*
- *Pregabalin.*

2. Discuss dose and advantages of levetiracetam.

Dose

Levetiracetam—status epilepticus—60 mg/kg (up to maximum 4,500 mg) infused over 10 minutes. If patient weight is >75 kg then dose is 4.5 g.

Advantages of levetiracetam.
- Nonenzyme induces antiepileptic drug
- No serum level monitoring
- Not induce drug fever or cutaneous hypersensitivity reaction
- Less adverse drug reaction
- Less drug-drug interaction
- Intravenous: Oral = 1:1.

3. Give algorithm for management of status epilepticus.

Primary management should aim at stabilization of airway, breathing, circulation and administration of medications to terminate the clinical and electrical seizure. Airway, breathing and circulation management is as described before. After stabilization of airway, breathing and circulation arterial blood gas analysis may be performed. Initial hyperpyrexia, acidosis, and hypertension may not be immediately treated as it usually subsides without any corrective measures. All the patients should get a blood glucose level—serum calcium, magnesium, sodium, and potassium levels. If the patient is known epileptic on medication, then blood levels of antiepileptic medications must be performed. Based on history and clinical findings other investigations such as CT scan, lumbar puncture, blood toxicology panel may be performed **(Table 3)**.

TABLE 3: Treatment summary for status epilepticus.

Immediate treatment (first 5–10 minutes)	
Monitoring of vitals	Airway, oxygen, cardiac monitor
Securing intravenous (IV) lines	Two lines for blood samples and starting treatment
To start IV fluids	• Fluid of choice is normal saline • To give 100 mg IV thiamine and 50 mL of 50% dextrose in patients with history of alcoholism
First antiepileptic	• To give lorazepam/midazolam/diazepam IV • 0.1 mg/kg bolus dose of IV lorazepam in equal volume of diluent by slow IV push at ~2 mg/min
Repeat dose if seizure persists	Repeat another half of the bolus dose if seizures are not controlled
Early treatment for next 10–60 minutes	
Loading antiepileptic 2nd line IV agent	• *Phenytoin:* IV infusion 15 mg/kg @ 50 mg/min (*Fosphenytoin:* IV infusion 15 mg PE/kg @ 100 mg PE/min) • *Valproate:* IV infusion 25 mg/kg at 3–6 mg/kg/min • *Phenobarbital:* IV infusion 10 mg/kg at a maximum rate of 100 mg/min • *Levetiracetam:* 20 mg/kg bolus of over 15 minutes
If seizure persists then two options	• Repeat half dose of any of the above-mentioned antiepileptic drugs • To load with any of the other antiepileptic drugs
Refractory status epilepticus (>60 minutes on going convulsions)	
Midazolam infusion (possible to avoid ventilator support)	• *Loading:* 0.2 mg/kg by slow IV bolus • *Maintenance IV dose:* 0.1–0.4 mg/kg/h • *Maximum IV dose:* 2.0–3.0 mg/kg/h
Thiopental sodium	• Loading 3–5 mg/kg at 0.2–0.4 mg/kg/min • Maintenance IV dose: 3.0–5.0 mg/kg/h • Maximum IV dose: 5.0 mg/kg/h
Propofol infusion	• *Loading dose:* 1–2 mg/kg at 10 mg/min • *Maintenance IV dose:* 2–10 mg/kg/h • *Maximum IV dose:* 15 mg/kg/h
Malignant/super-refractory status epilepticus (seizures >24 h)	
Magnesium infusion	• *Loading:* 2–6 g/h • Maintenance 3.5 mmol/L
Hypothermia	• 32–35°C for <48 hours • Endovascular cooling vs. external cooling
Immunotherapy	• IV methylprednisolone 1 g/day × 5 days • IV immunoglobulins 0.4 g/kg/day × 5 days • Plasma exchange
Ketogenic diet	• 1:1 or 1:4 ketogenic diet • To avoid glucose containing fluids
Epilepsy surgery	Consider surgery in special circumstances with documented brain lesions responsible for status

(PE: Phenytoin sodium equivalent)

Question 7

1. What is TTM?

Studies suggest that after achieving ROSC (period of global cerebral hypoxia-ischemia), mild-induced hypothermia is used as a neuroprotective and outcome improving measures. Mild-induced hypothermia suppresses the many pathological process leading to delayed cell death, including apoptosis (programmed cell death). Hypothermia reduces the release of excitatory amino acids, free radicals and decreases the cerebral metabolic rate for oxygen ($CMRO_2$) by about 6% for each 1°C reduction in core temperature. Hypothermia reduces the inflammatory response associated with the postcardiac arrest syndrome. The previous term "therapeutic hypothermia" is replaced by new term "targeted temperature management". Several treatment recommendations on TTM by "The Advanced Life Support Task Force of the International Liaison Committee on Resuscitation" (ILCOR):

Targeted temperature management is indicated for adults after OHCA with an initial shockable/nonshockable rhythm or any other initial rhythm who remain unresponsive after ROSC. Temperature is maintained between 32° and 36°C with temperature control monitoring system. Minimum duration of TTM should be at least 24 hours. Following the TTM trial, many intensive care clinicians elected to use 36°C as the target temperature for postcardiac arrest temperature control. This has several advantages of selecting temperature of 36°C compared with a target temperature of 33°C: Vasopressor support is reduced to minimum with lower lactate levels. The rewarming phase is shorter and chances of rebound hyperthermia after rewarming are less.

2. Discuss the methods of lowering temperature in the post-return of spontaneous circulation patient.

Methods of inducing and/or maintaining TTM include:
- The first inexpensive method is by simple ice packs and/or wet towels. For nursing staff this method is time-consuming, also temperature fluctuations will be more, and controlled rewarming is not possible.
- Cooling blankets or pads.
- Water or air circulating blankets.
- Water circulating gel-coated pads.
- Trans-nasal evaporative cooling—large multicenter randomized controlled trials are needed.
- Intravascular heat exchanger, placed usually in the femoral or subclavian veins.
- Extracorporeal circulation [e.g., cardiopulmonary bypass, extracorporeal membrane oxygenation (ECMO)].

3. Mention trials done on TTM.

The Targeted Temperature Management-2 (TTM2) trial was the largest trial conducted to date, across 14 countries with >1,800 subjects, and published in 2021. It compared the effect of targeted hypothermia at 33°C to targeted normothermia at 37.5°C.

Question 8

1. Define multiple casualty and mass casualty.

Disaster is defined as per Disaster Management ACT, 2005, "A catastrophe, mishap, calamity or grave occurrence in any area, arising from natural or man-made causes, or by accident or negligence which results in substantial loss of life or human suffering or damage to, and destruction of property, or damage to, or degradation of environment and is of such a nature or magnitude as to be beyond the coping capacity of the community of the affected area."

2. How would you develop a hospital disaster plan?

Establishing the emergency operation center (EOC): It serves as central command post during a disaster, generally established outside the emergency department should be large enough for key people and support staff. It should be located in a safe area.

How to activate and when to activate incident command center (ICS)? **(Table 4)**

TABLE 4: Overall responsibilities of head of incident command center.			
Logistic (Provide support)	*Planning (Prepare action plan)*	*Finance (Cost accounting and procurement)*	*Operations (Direct tactical action)*
• Responsible for acquisition and maintenance of facilities, services • Personnel equipment materials	• Collect, analyze, display information • Prepare incident action plan • Maintain situation and resource status • Maintain incident documentation • Prepare demobilization • Promote continuity of operations	• Monitors incident costs • Maintains financial records • Administers procurement contracts	Carry out the medical objective to the best of their ability
Other important command staff			
Public information officer	*Safety officer*		*Liaison officer*
Provide information to the news media, serves as the one central point for information dissemination	Monitors the facility and anticipates, detects, and corrects unsafe situations		Function as incident contact person for representatives from other assisting and cooperating agencies

- Determine who will activate the ICS
- Notification to hospital personnel
- Briefing to all core members regarding assignments and clear immediate direction.
- Activation of ICS should be announced using standardized codes, such as "disaster code".

3. Explain triaging during mass casualty.

In mass casualty situation number of patients and their severity are much more than the existing capability for management. Triage is most important part of any disaster response. The main objective of mass casualty/disaster triage is to do the maximum help to maximum number of people. Major incident which causes the mass casualties are road traffic accident, building collapse, earthquake, flood, major fire, train derailment, explosion, air crash, terrorist attack, hazardous material release. Main objectives of triaging in disaster and mass casualty are—to decompress the disaster area, most critical casualty should get best care and special care for burn and crush injuries. In this critical situation simple triaging format (START **Flowchart 1** and SALT **Flowchart 2**) should be used. *Use START/SALT triaging methods in adult age group mass casualty.*

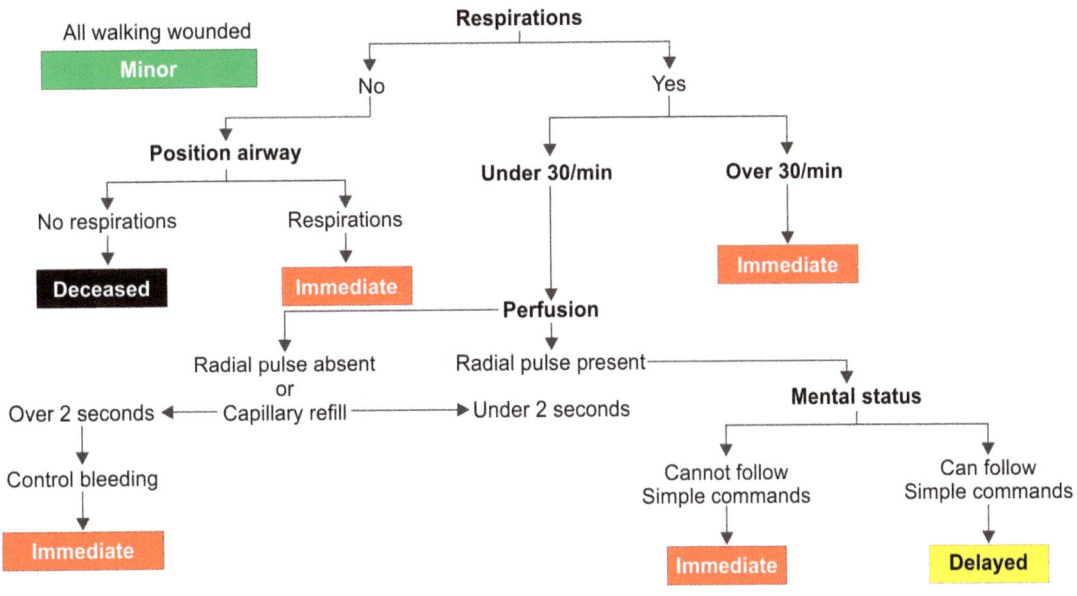

Flowchart 1: START triaging (based on respiration, perfusion, and mental status assessment).

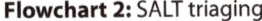

Flowchart 2: SALT triaging.

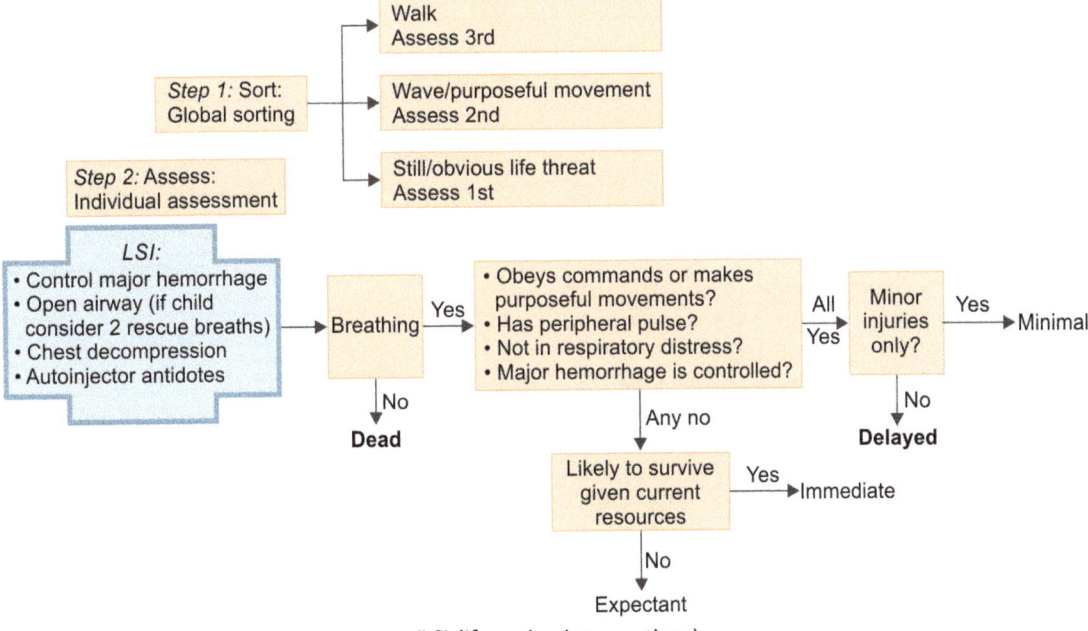

(LSI: life-saving interventions)

Triaging in pediatric age group: Children are usually uncooperative during examination and give poor history therefore it is very important to recognize markers of serious illness. Useful signs are drowsiness, hypotonia, respiratory grunt, wheeze, crepitation, stridor tachypnea, pallor, fever, signs of dehydration, abnormal posture, cold periphery, vomit or less urination, convulsion, and tender abdomen. *Use JumpSTART* **(Flowchart 3)** *triaging methods in pediatric age group mass casualty.*

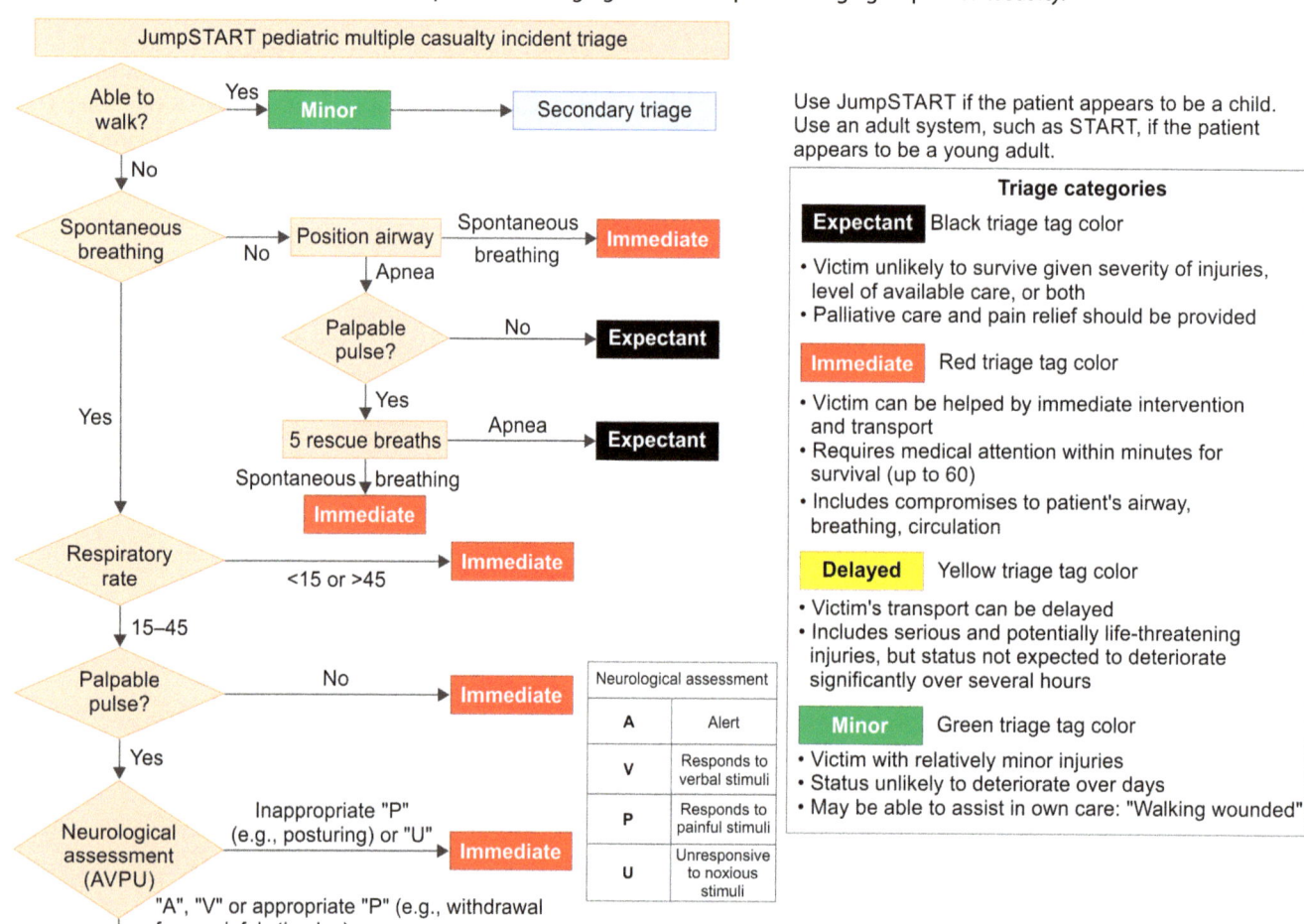

Flowchart 3: JumpSTART 2C triaging methods in pediatric age group mass casualty.

Question 9

1. Discuss the recent definitions for sepsis and septic shock.

The Sepsis-3 (2016) defines sepsis as *"A life-threatening organ dysfunction caused by dysregulated host response to infection"*; whereas septic shock is recognized as *"A subset of sepsis in which underlying circulatory and cellular metabolism abnormalities are profound enough to substantially increase mortality."*

Sepsis-3 definition suggests clinical criteria to operationalize and rapidly categorize patients according to new definition. A qSOFA score of ≥2 points **(Table 5)** or a worsening SOFA score of ≥ 2 point is taken as marker of organ dysfunction and in event of suspected infection qualifies for sepsis.

TABLE 5: qSOFA score.

H	**H**ypotension: SBP less than or equal to 100 mm Hg
A	**A**ltered mental status (any GCS <15)
T	**T**achypnea: Respiratory rate greater than or equal to 22/min

2. What is the role of different vasopressors in septic shock?

Septic shock management starts with source control, volume assessment correction of hypovolemia timely and appropriate antibiotics; vasopressors are also required to maintain perfusion. Norepinephrine is the drug of choice in shock related to sepsis. Perfusion markers should be assessed regularly such as urine output, mental status, skin perfusion, serum lactate levels. If resuscitation goals are not met then vasopressin should be started in low dose (0.04 U/min) is safe and effective. If patient has myocardial dysfunction (elevated cardiac filling pressor, low cardiac output and signs of low perfusion in spite of fluid and vasopressor therapy) then dobutamine can be added. Dopamine can only be added in patient with low risk for arrhythmias **(Fig. 4)**.

3. What are the goals in first 6 hours of its management?

The 1-hour bundle is composed of the following five elements—measuring the lactate level, obtaining blood culture prior to administration of antibiotics, administering broad-spectrum antibiotics, beginning rapid administration of 30 mL/kg crystalloid fluid for hypotension or lactate ≥4 mmol/L **(Table 6)**.

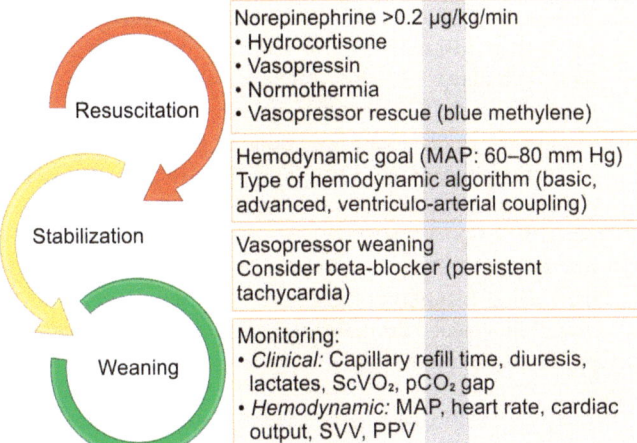

Fig. 4: Vasopressor therapy principles. (MAP: mean arterial pressure; PPV: pulse pressure variation; SVV: stroke volume variation)

TABLE 6: Surviving sepsis guidelines.

Hour-1 bundle of surviving sepsis campaign	
Bundle elements to be completed within 1st hour	• Measure lactate level. Remeasure if initial lactate is >2 mmol/L • Obtain blood cultures prior to administration of antibiotics best practice statement • Administer broad-spectrum antibiotics strong recommendation • Rapidly administer 30 mL/kg crystalloid for hypotension or lactate ≥4 mmol/L • Apply vasopressors if patient is hypotensive during or after fluid resuscitation to maintain MAP ≥65 mm Hg
"Time zero" or "time of presentation"	Time of triage at the first point of contact or, if patient is referred from another care location, represent the time when sepsis is first identified through chart review
Hour 6 bundle	
• Repeat lactic acid if initial lactic acid >2 • Vasopressors if hypotensive • Repeat physical examination (MAP: mean arterial pressure)	

Question 10

1. Define randomized clinical trial (RCT).

Randomization is a scientific method of allocation of subjects between the treatment and control groups. This method ensures that there is no bias or preference in selecting specific treatment for any subjects. Further, randomization provides equal chance/probability to subjects for allocation into different groups. Importantly a prerequisite all statistical tests of significance assume that the sample drawn is random, which is met through randomization.

Randomization techniques used in RCTs are simple randomization or stratified randomization. In simple randomization, subjects are allocated to different groups without any matching. On the other hand, in stratified randomization technique, subjects are classified in groups, i.e., strata and then within a group they are randomized to various treatment groups. This ensures matching of subjects for confounding factors that might influence the outcome and thus helps in drawing the valid conclusions netting out the effects of confounders. For allocation of subjects in different groups, the random numbers are generated through computer using appropriate mathematical algorithms. In case of two groups generally, odd numbers correspond to group I and even numbers for group II.

As an example, in case of two groups with sample size of 30 each, a sequence of 60 two digit random numbers are generated of which 30 are odd and 30 even. The sequence of random numbers will be kept in the opaque sealed envelopes. In this the serial numbers will be written on the envelopes and the group to which the subject at that serial number to be allocated will be kept inside the envelope. After recruitment of the subjects and taking their consents, the allocation of the subjects to two groups will be based on the sequence of random number kept in opaque envelopes. The envelops will be kept with biostatistician and will be opened after recruitment of the subjects and obtaining the consent.

2. Compare prospective and retrospective studies.

In prospective studies, individuals are followed over time and data about them are collected as their characteristics or circumstances change. Birth cohort studies are a good example of prospective studies. In retrospective studies, individuals are sampled and information is collected about their past. For example, a medical researcher is investigating the causes of human immunodeficiency virus (HIV) in humans. A retrospective approach will recruit subjects who are HIV positive, while a prospective approach will recruit people who are HIV negative but are at risk of contracting the disease.

3. Which common statistical methods are employed for categorical variables? Discuss any one of them.

Examples of categorical variables are *race, sex, age group, and educational level*. While the latter two variables may also be considered in a numerical manner by using exact values for age and highest grade completed, it is often more informative to categorize such variables into a relatively small number of groups. Categorical variables, including nominal and ordinal variables, are described by tabulating their frequencies or probability. If two variables are associated, the probability of one will depend on the probability of the other.

◼ SUGGESTED READING

1. Richhariya D, Sharma B. Textbook of Emergency Medicine including Intensive Care and Trauma, 2nd edition. New Delhi: Jaypee Brothers Medical Publishers (P) Ltd; 2022. pp. 1142-6. (Question 1).
2. Richhariya D, Sharma B. Textbook of Emergency Medicine including Intensive Care and Trauma, 2nd edition. New Delhi: Jaypee Brothers Medical Publishers (P) Ltd; 2022. pp. 281-90. (Question 2).
3. Richhariya D, Sharma B. Textbook of Emergency Medicine including Intensive Care and Trauma, 2nd edition. New Delhi: Jaypee Brothers Medical Publishers (P) Ltd; 2022. pp. 829-31. (Question 3).
4. Richhariya D, Sharma B. Textbook of Emergency Medicine including Intensive Care and Trauma, 2nd edition. New Delhi: Jaypee Brothers Medical Publishers (P) Ltd; 2022. pp. 220-8. (Question 4).
5. Richhariya D, Sharma B. Textbook of Emergency Medicine including Intensive Care and Trauma, 2nd edition. New Delhi: Jaypee Brothers Medical Publishers (P) Ltd; 2022. pp. 1129, 1187-9. (Question 5).
6. Richhariya D, Sharma B. Textbook of Emergency Medicine including Intensive Care and Trauma, 2nd edition. New Delhi: Jaypee Brothers Medical Publishers (P) Ltd; 2022. p. 836. (Question 6).
7. Richhariya D, Sharma B. Textbook of Emergency Medicine including Intensive Care and Trauma, 2nd edition. New Delhi: Jaypee Brothers Medical Publishers (P) Ltd; 2022. p. 237. (Question 7).
8. Richhariya D, Sharma B. Textbook of Emergency Medicine including Intensive Care and Trauma, 2nd edition. New Delhi: Jaypee Brothers Medical Publishers (P) Ltd; 2022. pp. 42-3, 172-9. (Question 8).
9. Richhariya D, Sharma B. Textbook of Emergency Medicine including Intensive Care and Trauma, 2nd edition. New Delhi: Jaypee Brothers Medical Publishers (P) Ltd; 2022. pp. 319-27. (Question 9).
10. Richhariya D, Sharma B. Textbook of Emergency Medicine including Intensive Care and Trauma, 2nd edition. New Delhi: Jaypee Brothers Medical Publishers (P) Ltd; 2022. pp. 80-90. (Question 10).

Emergency Medicine Paper 5

Santosh Pandey

Question 1

1. Discuss sodium homeostasis.

Sodium is an important electrolyte mainly found in extracellular fluid, which helps maintain fluid balance, blood pressure, nerve impulse conduction, and muscle contraction. The human body tightly maintains serum [Na^+] between 138 and 142 mEq/L despite what may be marked changes in daily intake depending on the person's diet. The sodium balance is the difference between the amount of Na absorbed by the gut and the amount excreted via urine, feces, and skin. Sodium balance in the body is closely linked to that of water and is finely maintained by the kidneys. Hyponatremia is a condition of excess water relative to Na^+ and is defined as a serum [Na^+] 100 mOsm/L H_2O with the exception of samples from patients with psychogenic polydipsia, which drives down urine osmolality below the typical minimum.

2. Mention various causes of hyponatremia.

Causes of hyponatremia are as follows:
a. Diarrhea and vomiting
b. Diuretics (most common thiazides)
c. Chronic heart failure and cirrhosis
d. Nephrotic syndrome
e. Acute or chronic kidney disease
f. Syndrome of inappropriate antidiuretic hormone secretion (SIADH)
g. Hypothyroidism
h. Glucocorticoid deficiency
i. Mineralocorticoid deficiency
j. Salt-losing nephropathies
k. Cerebral-salt-wasting

3. Explain the pathophysiology of clinical effects of hyponatremia.

The most important symptoms of hyponatremia are due to its effects on the brain; symptoms can be divided into moderately severe and severe, according to a European clinical practice guideline.

Moderately severe symptoms often start when a plasma [Na] is <130 mEq/L and consist of headache, nausea, disorientation, confusion, agitation, ataxia, and areflexia. When [Na^+] reach levels <120 mEq/L, **severe** symptoms may develop including intractable vomiting, seizures, coma, and ultimately respiratory arrest due to brainstem herniation. Brain injury may become irreversible.

The symptoms of hyponatremia can be due to **many other conditions**. The presence of hyponatremia-related symptoms is directly related to the rapidity of onset. After a certain period, brain cells begin to adapt to hyponatremia. Initially the hypo-osmolality drives water into the brain cells yielding swelling. Due to the rigid skull, intracranial hypertension occurs and the described symptoms begin. After 48 hours, the brain cells start to adapt by extruding Na^+, K^+, Cl^-, and organic osmolytes such as glycine and taurine from the cells, reducing cell osmolality, and preventing further water uptake. In several clinical or physiologic conditions, this adaptation mechanism is impaired, as in the syndrome of inappropriate antidiuretic hormone (ADH) secretion, in children, in menstruating women, and in hypoxia. In such cases, symptoms are more severe and persistent.

Question 2

1. Draw a labeled diagram of portal venous system.

Portal venous system (PVS) drains blood from the gastrointestinal tract (apart from the lower section of rectum), spleen, pancreas, and gallbladder to the liver (**Fig. 1**).

2. Enumerate causes of portal hypertension.

Various causes of portal hypertension are as in **Table 1**.

3. Explain the pathophysiology of ascites in cirrhosis of liver.

Ascites formation in cirrhosis can be due to the following:
a. Hypoalbuminemia
b. Decrease the plasma oncotic pressure

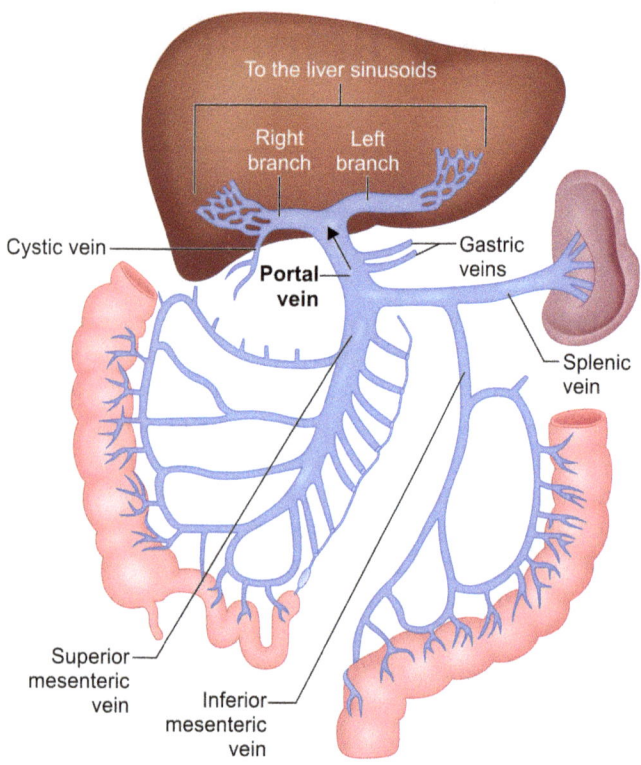

Fig. 1: Portal venous system.

TABLE 1: Causes of portal hypertension.		
Prehepatic	**Intrahepatic**	**Posthepatic**
Portal or splenic vein thrombosis	Primary biliary cirrhosis	Budd–Chiari syndrome
Congenital portal vein stenosis	Cirrhosis, Wilson disease Autoimmune hepatitis	IVC thrombosis
Arteriovenous fistula	Infiltrative liver disease	Congestive heart disease
Superior vena cava occlusion	Idiopathic portal hypertension	Constrictive pericarditis
	Congenital hepatic fibrosis	Tricuspid value disease
	Nodular regenerative hyperplasia	
	Veno-occlusive disease	

(IVC: inferior vena cava)

c. Portal hypertension (only localizes the fluid in the peritoneal cavity)
d. Increased oozing of "hepatic lymph" from the surface of liver (weeping liver)
e. Secondary hyperaldosteronism
f. Increased level of ADH
g. Decreased appetite (decreased intake of protein)

Question 3

1. Explain Bayes' theorem.

Bayes' theorem describes the probability of occurrence of an event related to any condition. It is also considered for the case of conditional probability. Bayes' theorem is also known as formula for the probability of "causes". For example, if we have to calculate the probability of taking a blue ball from the second bag out of the three different bags of ball, where each bag contains three different color balls viz., red, blue, black. In this case probability of occurrence of an event is calculated depending on other conditions is known as conditional probability.

Conditional probability: Bayes' Theorem

$$P(A|B) = \frac{P(B|A)\, P(A)}{P(B)}$$

2. What are the measures of diagnostic test accuracy?

Diagnostic accuracy of any diagnostic procedure or a test gives us an answer to the following question: How well this test discriminates between certain two conditions of interest? This discriminative ability can be quantified by the measures of diagnostic accuracy:
a. Sensitivity and specificity
b. Positive and negative predicative values (PPV, NPV)
c. Likelihood ratio
d. The area under the receiver operating characteristic (ROC) curve
e. Youden's index
f. Diagnostic odds ratio (DOR)

3. Discuss receiver operating characteristic curve.

There is a pair of diagnostic sensitivity and specificity values for every individual cut-off. To construct a ROC graph **(Fig. 2)**, we plot these pairs of values on the graph with the 1-specificity on the x-axis and sensitivity on the y-axis. The shape of ROC curve and the area under the curve (AUC) help us estimate how high the discriminative power of a test is. The AUC can have any value between 0 and 1 and it is a good indicator of the goodness of the test. The perfect diagnostic test has an AUC 1.0, whereas a non-discriminating test has an area 0.5.

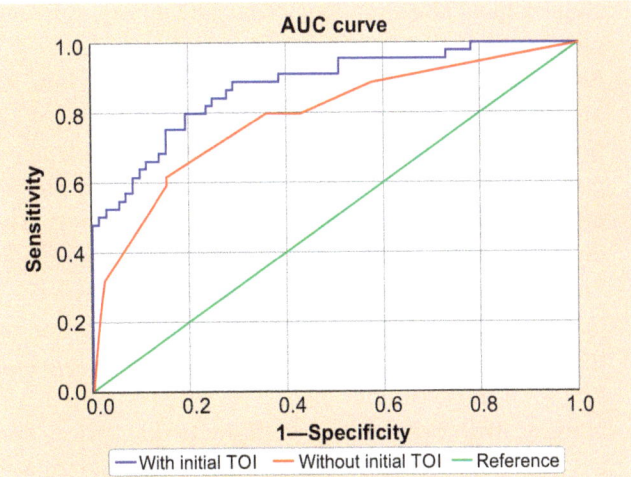

Fig. 2: Receiver operating characteristic (ROC) curve.

Question 4

1. Discuss bioavailability of a drug.

Bioavailability refers to the rate and extent of absorption of a drug from a dosage form administered by any route, as determined by its concentration-time curve in blood or by its excretion in urine. It is a measure of fraction of administered dose of a drug that reaches the systemic circulation in the unchanged form. Bioavailability of drug injected intravenous (IV) is 100%, but is frequently lower after oral ingestion because drug may be incompletely absorbed. The absorbed drug may undergo first pass metabolism in the intestinal wall/liver or be excretion in bile. Incomplete bioavailability after subcutaneous or intramuscular injection is less common but may occur due to local binding of the drug. Bioavailability variation assumes practical significance for drugs with low safety margin (digoxin) or where dosage needs precise control (oral hypoglycemics, oral anticoagulants). It may be responsible for success or failure of an antimicrobial regimen.

2. Elaborate "first pass effect" of a drug.

First pass metabolism of a drug during its passage from the site of absorption into the systemic circulation. All orally administered drugs are exposed to drug metabolizing enzymes in the intestinal wall and liver (where they first reach through portal vein). Presystemic metabolism in the gut and liver can be avoided by administering the drug through sublingual, transdermal or parenteral routes. However, limited presystemic metabolism can occur in the skin (transdermally administered drug) and in the lungs (for drug reaching venous blood through any route). The extent of first pass metabolism differs for different drugs and is an important determinant of oral bioavailability.

3. Explain the clinical implications of half-life measurement of a drug.

The plasma half-life ($t1/2$) of a drug is the time taken for its plasma concentration to be reduced to half of its original value. Understanding the concept of half-life is useful for determining excretion rates as well as steady-state concentrations for any specific drug. Different drugs have different half-lives, however they all follow this rule—after one half-life has passed, 50% of the initial drug amount is removed from the body. The characteristic decrease of drugs overtime has long been studied in a field known as pharmacokinetics and is depicted by different equations. Most clinically drugs tend to follow first pass first-order pharmacokinetics, i.e., their drug elimination rates are proportional to plasma concentrations. In contrast, a few drugs follow zero-order elimination in which the drug is amount decreases by a constant amount over time regardless of the initial concentration of ethanol.

Question 5

1. What are baroreceptors?

The baroreceptors are stretch receptors in the walls of the heart and blood vessels. They are a type of mechano-receptors allowing for relaying information derived from blood pressure within the autonomic nervous.

2. Discuss common locations of baroreceptors in body.

Common locations of baroreceptors in the body are explained here:
a. The carotid sinus and aortic arch receptors monitor the arterial circulation. The carotid sinus is a small dilation of the internal carotid artery just above the bifurcation of the common carotid into external and internal carotid branches.
b. Receptors are also located in the walls of the right and left atria at the entrance of the superior and inferior vena cava and the pulmonary veins, as well as in the pulmonary circulation.

3. What is baroreflex?

Baroreflex has a pivotal role in blood pressure regulation. Changes in blood pressure elicit changes in stretch of carotid and aortic baroreceptors. The altered baro-receptors stretch is conveyed to medullary brain stem nuclei via the glossopharyngeal and vagus nerves **Flowchart 1**.

Flowchart 1: Baroreflex.

```
Blood pressure increases → Increased baroreceptor activity → Increase in number of afferent impulses toward the cardiovascular center → Increased PSNS activity / Decreased SNS activity → Decrease in cardiac output and vasodilation to reduce blood pressure

Blood pressure decreases → Decreased baroreceptor activity → Decrease in number of afferent impulses toward the cardiovascular center → Increased SNS activity / Decreased PSNS activity → Increase in cardiac output and vasoconstriction to increase blood pressure
```

(PSNS: parasympathetic nervous system; SNS: sympathetic nervous system)

4. Discuss management of orthostatic hypotension.

Orthostatic hypotension is fall in systolic blood pressure by 20 mm Hg in standing as compared to supine, within 2–3 minutes of standing. Treatment of orthostatic hypotension is directed at the cause rather than the low blood pressure itself. No specific treatment is currently available that achieves all the goals. Hydration plays key role if dehydration causes orthostatic hypotension. If a medication, e.g., diuretic alpha-blocker, etc., causes low blood pressure when standing, treatment may involve changing the dose or stopping the drug. Therapies primarily consist of a combination of vasoconstrictors drugs, volume expansion, compression garments, and postural adjustments. Education about orthostatic stressors and warnings symptoms empowers the patient to adopt easy lifestyle changes to minimize and handle orthostatic stress.

Question 6

1. How do lungs regulate acid base balance?

Lungs play important role in regulating acid-base balance by controlling CO_2 to maintain pH. As CO_2 accumulates in the blood, the pH of the blood decreases. The brain regulates the amount of CO_2 that is exhaled by controlling the speed and depth of respiration. When pH decreases leads to hyperventilation and eliminates CO_2. When pH increases leads to hypoventilation and increases CO_2 in body.

2. Enumerate the pathophysiology of metabolic alkalosis.

a. Metabolic alkalosis results from gain of bicarbonate or loss of acid.
b. Neurological abnormalities especially tetany, seizures, neuromuscular instability are common.
c. Reduction in H^+ results in decreased ionized calcium, K^+, Mg, and PO_4 levels.
d. Alkalemia particularly concerned in chronic obstructive pulmonary disease (COPD) patients in which further decreases respiration. Many patients with COPD take diuretics, leading to a contraction alkalosis.
e. Bicarbonate and chloride homeostasis is intertwined.
f. Condition that results in chloride loss such as vomiting tends to reduce serum chloride concentration and extracellular volume, leads to mineralocorticoid activity, which enhances sodium reabsorption and K^+, H^+ secretion in distal tubule, which increases bicarbonate production, leads to urine alkaline and largely free of chloride (<10 mEq/L), results in hypokalemia, hypochloremia alkalosis that responds to normal saline.
g. Other diseases that cause metabolic alkalosis are associated with normovolemic or hypervolemia and often included hypertension.
h. These diseases cause excess mineralocorticoid activity not associated with hypovolemia, so urine chloride is normal or elevated (>10 mEq/L) and alkalosis cannot be reversed with normal saline.
i. The compensation for metabolic alkalosis involves reduction in alveolar ventilation.
j. PCO_2 in patients with significant metabolic alkalosis should rise by 0.7 mm Hg for each milliequivalent increase in HCO_3.
k. PCO_2 rarely rises by above 55 mm Hg in compensation for metabolic alkalosis.

3. What are the common causes of metabolic alkalosis?

Metabolic alkalosis, **a disorder that elevates the serum bicarbonate**, can result from several mechanisms (Table 2)—intracellular shift of hydrogen ions; gastrointestinal loss of hydrogen ions; excessive renal hydrogen ion loss; administration and retention of bicarbonate ions; or volume contraction.

TABLE 2: Common causes of metabolic alkalosis.

Chloride responsive	Chloride unresponsive
• Vomiting	• Renal artery stenosis
• Diarrhea	• Renin secreting tumors
• Diuretic therapy	• Adrenaline hyperplasia
• Cystic fibrosis	• Hyperaldosteronism
• Chloride wasting enteropathy	• Cushing syndrome
	• Exogenous mineralocorticosteroids

Question 7

1. Discuss anatomy of lower motor neurons with a suitable diagram.

The lower motor neuron is responsible for transmitting the signal from the upper motor neuron to the effector muscle to perform a movement **(Fig. 3)**. There are three broad types of lower motor neurons—somatic motor neurons, special visceral efferent (branchial) motor neurons, and general visceral motor neurons.

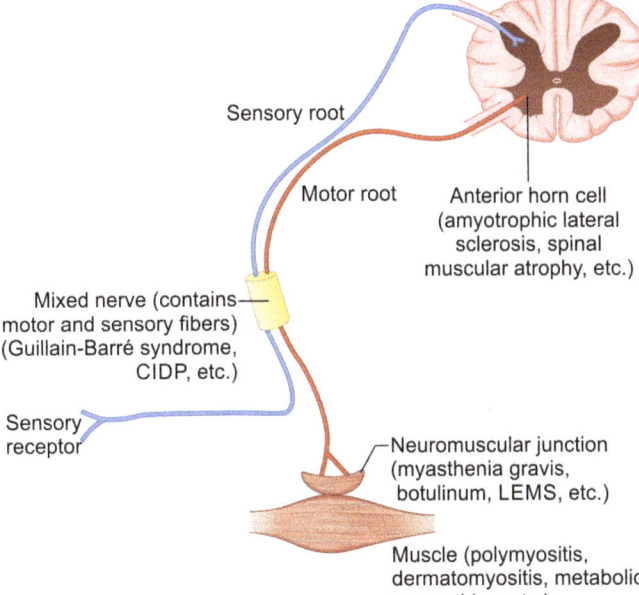

Fig. 3: Anatomical stations underlying Lower motor neuron weakness. (CIDP: chronic inflammatory demyelinating polyneuropathy; LEMS: Lambert–Eaton myasthenic syndrome)

2. Explain the clinical signs characteristics of lower motor neuron disease.

The anterior horn cells and its dendrite up to the motor end plate, and the cranial nerve nuclei with the cranial nerves constitute lower motor neurons. The features of lower motor neuron palsy are as follows:
a. Paralysis of the individual muscle supplied by the segment or nerve
b. Atrophy and wasting are cardinal features
c. Flaccidity (hypotonia)
d. Fasciculations may be present
e. Power is very much affected (may be power zero) as compared to upper motor neuron lesions (UML) lesions
f. Superficial reflexes—lost
g. Deep reflexes—lost or diminished
h. Clonus-absent
i. Tropical changes in skin—common
j. Planter response—flexor or no response

3. Enumerate the causes of episodic generalized weakness.

The causes of episodic generalized weakness are as follows:
a. Familial Hyperkalemic periodic paralysis
b. Hypokalemic periodic paralysis type-1
c. Hypokalemic periodic paralysis type-2
d. Metabolic myopathies—glycogen storage disease, fatty acid oxidation defects
e. Mitochondrial myopathies
f. Acute intermittent porphyria
g. Drugs/toxins—statins, alcohol, amphetamine, cocaine, heroin, etc.

Question 8

1. Define "ataxia".

Ataxia is an uncoordinated movement. A gait disorder is an abnormal pattern or style of walking. Ataxia is a term for a group of disorders that affect coordination, balance, and speech. Any part of the body can be affected, but people with ataxia often have difficulties with balance and walking, speaking and swallowing.

2. What are various features of cerebellar disease?

Clinical manifestations of cerebellar disease include the following:
a. Detailed history with onset of symptoms and its progression.
b. Ataxia, tremors, as well as nystagmus and cognitive dysfunction. Other signs are slowing of saccadic movements, ophthalmoplegia, optic neuritis, seizures, pyramidal signs, and dysautonomia. General physical examination of the patient with ataxia or gait disorder should include examination of orthostatic vital signs. The testing of cranial nerves, mental status, sensation, and the motor system is necessary. Gait testing is one of the aspects of directed neurological examination. Observe the patient sitting upright in the stretcher, and then tell patient to rise, stand, and walk and turn around. Tandem gait is toe-to-toe walking and also tests many elements of nervous system. Cerebellar functions are tested by asking the patient to perform smooth voluntary movements and rapidly alternating movements.

3. How do you differentiate between cerebellar ataxia and sensory state?

Various tests are available to differentiate between ataxia and sensory ataxia. Following are the few discussed here:

a. **Dyssynergia** (breakdown of movements into parts), **dysmetria** (inaccurate fine movements), or **dysdiadochokinesia** (clumsy rapid movements) may indicate a lateral cerebellar lesion. The rapid thigh-slapping test particularly examines rapidly alternating movements. This is correctly performed by asking the patient to pat the thigh with the palm then the back of the same hand in alternating fashion, making a sound with each rapid slap. The maneuver is performed with each hand in turn.
b. The **finger-to-nose test** may be helpful in distinguishing between cerebellar and posterior column (proprioceptive) lesions. Performing this test with the eyes closed tests proprioception in the upper extremity.
c. A test for cerebellar function that emphasizes the lower extremities is the **heel-toe-shin test**. In cerebellar disease, the heel may initially overshoot the other shin or knee, and the action is done with a series of jerky movements. In posterior column disease, there may be difficulty locating the knee, and the movement down the shin typically weaves from side to side or falls off.
d. Another test commonly used for cerebellar function is the **Stewart–Holmes rebound sign** (with sudden release of the flexed forearm, the individual fails to check the movement). Another example of rebound phenomena is when a tapped outstretched arm oscillates back and forth for several cycles.
e. The **Romberg test** is primarily a test of sensation, and if positive may distinguish sensory from motor ataxia. While standing with arms outstretched and eyes open, observe the patient for signs of unsteadiness. The feet should be narrowly spaced, and the posture should be easily maintained. The inability to maintain a steady standing posture (or, in extreme cases, a seated position) confirms that an ataxia is present but does not yet give any information about the type of ataxia. Then ask the patient to close the eyes to eliminate visually orienting information. If the ataxia worsens with the loss of visual input, then the Romberg sign is present or positive, suggesting sensory ataxia with a problem of proprioceptive input (posterior column, vestibular dysfunction), or a peripheral neuropathy. Further neurologic examination is indicated to confirm the suspicion of sensory ataxia. In patients who show little or no change in unsteadiness with eye closure (Romberg test–negative), a motor ataxia is suggested with possible localization of that problem to the cerebellum.

Note that many normal individuals will have some small increase in unsteadiness with eye closure.

Question 9

1. Discuss pathophysiology of hyperosmolar hyperglycemic syndrome/state.

The development of hyperosmolar hyperglycemic syndrome/state (HHS) is attributed to three main factors: (1) insulin resistance and/or deficiency; (2) an inflammatory state with marked elevation in proinflammatory cytokines (C-reactive protein, interleukins, tumor necrosis factors) and counterregulatory hormones (growth hormone, cortisol) that cause increased hepatic gluconeogenesis and glycogenolysis; and (3) osmotic diuresis followed by impaired renal excretion of glucose.

In a patient with type 2 diabetes, physiologic stresses combined with inadequate water intake in an environment of insulin resistance or deficiency lead to HHS. As serum glucose concentration increases, an osmotic gradient develops, attracting water from the intracellular space into the intravascular compartment, causing cellular dehydration. The initial increase in intravascular volume is accompanied by a temporary increase in the glomerular filtration rate. As serum glucose concentration increases, the capacity of the kidneys to reabsorb glucose is exceeded, and glucosuria and osmotic diuresis occur. During osmotic diuresis, significant urinary loss of sodium and potassium, as well as more modest losses of calcium, phosphate, and magnesium may occur. As volume depletion progresses, renal perfusion decreases, and the glomerular filtration rate is reduced. Renal tubular excretion of glucose is impaired, which further worsens hyperglycemia. A sustained osmotic diuresis may result in total body water losses that often exceed 20–25% of total body weight, or approximately 8–12 L in a 70-kg patient. The relative lack of severe ketoacidosis in HHS is poorly understood and has been attributed to three possible mechanisms: (1) higher levels of endogenous insulin than are seen in diabetic ketoacidosis, which inhibits lipolysis; (2) lower levels of counterregulatory "stress" hormones; (3) inhibition of lipolysis by the hyperosmolar state itself. Evidence of significant ketoacidosis in a patient thought to have type 2 diabetes should bring into question the possibility of variants of type 1 diabetes, such as latent autoimmune diabetes in adults.

2. Explain the diagnostic criteria of hyperosmolar hyperglycemic state.

Hyperosmolar hyperglycemic state is defined by the following:

a. Severe hyperglycemic with serum glucose usually >600 mg/dL
b. Arterial pH >7.3
c. Elevated calculated plasma osmolality
d. Serum bicarbonate >15 mEq/L
e. Serum ketones negative or slightly positive.

3. How do you differentiate between hyperosmolar hyperglycemic state and diabetic ketoacidosis?

Differentiating features are as given in **Table 3**.

TABLE 3: Differentiating features of HHS and DKA.

	Hyperosmolar hyperglycemic state	Diabetic ketoacidosis
Plasma glucose	>600 mg/dL	>250 mg/dL
pH	>7.30	<7.30
Serum bicarbonate	>15 mEq/L	<18 mEq/L
Urine acetoacetate	– or small	+
Serum ketones	– or small	+
Serum osmolality	>320 mOsm/kg	Variable
Anion gap	<12 mEq/L	>12 mmol/L

(DKA: diabetes-related ketoacidosis; HHS: hyperosmolar hyperglycemic syndrome/state)

Question 10

1. Draw a labeled diagram of middle ear.

The middle ear includes three small bones— (1) the hammer (malleus), (2) anvil (incus), and (3) stirrup (stapes) **(Fig. 4)**. The middle ear is separated from your external ear by the eardrum and connected to the back of your nose and throat by a narrow passageway called the Eustachian tube.

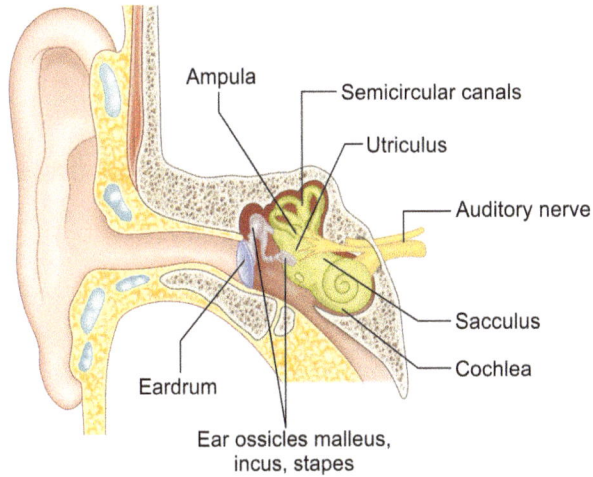

Fig. 4: Sagittal section of the middle ear and related structures.

2. What are the causes of "otitis externa"?

External otitis is an inflammation of the external auditory canal. The protective lipid layer may be disrupted by high humidity, increased temperature, and maceration of the skin after prolonged exposure to moisture and local trauma that ultimately results in introduction of bacteria. Otitis externa is usually caused by *Pseudomonas aeruginosa* and *Staphylococcus aureus*, but can also be polymicrobial. Occurring most common in summer and tropical climate it is known as swimmer's ear.

3. How do you differentiate between sensorineural deafness and conductive deafness?

The outer and middle ears mediate conductive hearing. The inner ear mediates sensorineural hearing.

Weber test: This test has been mainly used to establish a diagnosis in patients with unilateral hearing loss to distinguish between conductive and sensorineural hearing loss. In conductive hearing loss, the sound should lateralize to the affected side, however in patients with sensorineural hearing loss, the sound lateralizes to the contralateral side. Weber test is often combined with the Rinne test to detect the location and nature of hearing loss.

■ SUGGESTED READING

1. Richhariya D, Sharma B. Textbook of Emergency Medicine including Intensive Care and Trauma, 2nd edition. New Delhi: Jaypee Brothers Medical Publishers (P) Ltd; 2022. pp. 311-13. (Question 1).
2. Richhariya D, Sharma B. Textbook of Emergency Medicine including Intensive Care and Trauma, 2nd edition. New Delhi: Jaypee Brothers Medical Publishers (P) Ltd; 2022. p. 687. (Question 2).
3. Richhariya D, Sharma B. Textbook of Emergency Medicine including Intensive Care and Trauma, 2nd edition. New Delhi: Jaypee Brothers Medical Publishers (P) Ltd; 2022. pp. 80-90. (Question 3).
4. Researchgate.net. (2016). Study of regulatory requirements for the conduct of bioequivalence studies in US, Europe, Canada, India, ASEAN and SADC countries: Impact on generic drug substitution. [online] Available from: https://www.researchgate.net/figure/Factors-affecting-bioavailability-of-drugs_fig2_301787198 [Last accessed April, 2023]. (Question 4).
5. Richhariya D, Sharma B. Textbook of Emergency Medicine including Intensive Care and Trauma, 2nd edition. New Delhi: Jaypee Brothers Medical Publishers (P) Ltd; 2022. pp. 415-18. (Question 5).
6. Richhariya D, Sharma B. Textbook of Emergency Medicine including Intensive Care and Trauma, 2nd edition. New Delhi: Jaypee Brothers Medical Publishers (P) Ltd; 2022. pp. 303-10. (Question 6).

7. Richhariya D, Sharma B. Textbook of Emergency Medicine including Intensive Care and Trauma, 2nd edition. New Delhi: Jaypee Brothers Medical Publishers (P) Ltd; 2022. pp. 838-843. (Question 7).
8. Richhariya D, Sharma B. Textbook of Emergency Medicine including Intensive Care and Trauma, 2nd edition. New Delhi: Jaypee Brothers Medical Publishers (P) Ltd; 2022. pp. 801-13. (Question 8).
9. Richhariya D, Sharma B. Textbook of Emergency Medicine including Intensive Care and Trauma, 2nd edition. New Delhi: Jaypee Brothers Medical Publishers (P) Ltd; 2022. pp. 877-81. (Question 9).
10. Richhariya D, Sharma B. Textbook of Emergency Medicine including Intensive Care and Trauma, 2nd edition. New Delhi: Jaypee Brothers Medical Publishers (P) Ltd; 2022. pp. 907-14. (Question 10).

Emergency Medicine Paper 6

Santosh Pandey

Question 1

1. Discuss the classification of thermal burns based on depth.

Superficial or epidermal burns involve only the epidermal layer of skin. Partial-thickness burns involve the epidermis and portions of the dermis. Full-thickness burns extend through and destroy all layers of the dermis **(Table 1)**.

TABLE 1: Classification of thermal burn based on depth.

Burn depth	Histology/Anatomy	Example	Healing
Superficial (1 degree)	• Epidermis • No blisters, painful	Sunburn	7 days
Superficial partial thickness (2nd degree)	• Epidermis and superficial dermis • Blisters and very painful	Hot water scald	14–21 days, no scar
Deep partial thickness (Deep 2nd degree)	• Epidermis, and deep dermis, sweat glands, hair follicle • Blister and very painful	Hot liquid steam, flame	3–8 weeks, permanent scar
Full thickness (3rd degree)	Entire epidermis and dermis charred, pale, leathery, no pain	Flame	Months, severe scarring
Fourth degree	Entire epidermis and dermis, as well as bone, fat	Flame	Months

2. Enumerate the rule of nine in adults.

It is used for estimation of adult burn size. The front and back of each arm and hand equal 9% of the body's surface area. The chest equals 9% and the stomach equals 9% of the body's surface area. The upper back equals 9% and the lower back equals 9% of the body's surface area. The front and back of each leg and foot equal 18% of the body's surface area **(Fig. 1)**.

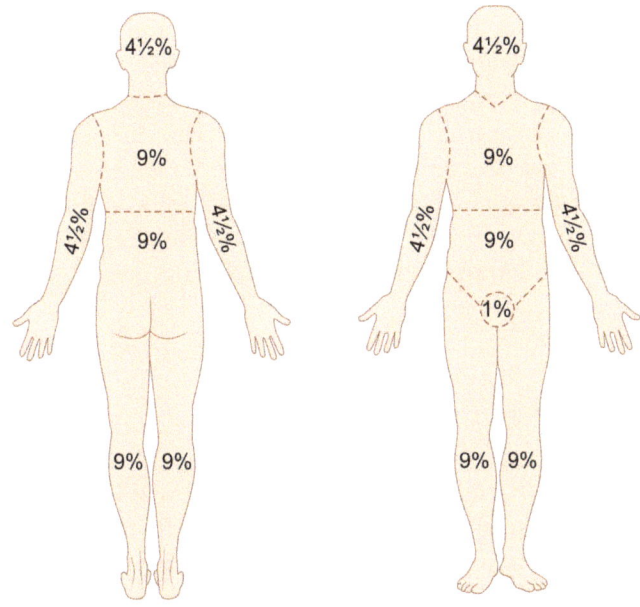

Fig. 1: Rule of nine—estimation of adult burn.

3. Discuss fluid requirement in an adult weighing 60 kg with 30% burns.

Adult weight—60 kg, 30% burns
Fluid requirement, according to Parkland formula:
  4 mL × weight (kg) × % burn
  4 mL × 60 × 30 = 7,200 mL over 24 hours
  3,600 mL over first 8 hours from time of burn
  Next 3,600 mL over 16 hours

Question 2

1. List the common causes of hemorrhagic shock in a male patient.

Causes of hemorrhagic shock in males
a. *Traumatic:* (i) long bone fractures (ii) hemothorax (iii) hemoperitoneum (iv) large vessel injury
b. *Gastrointestinal:* (i) esophageal varices (ii) gastric and duodenal ulcer (iii) Mallory-Weiss tear (iv) colon cancers and ulcerations
c. Ruptured aneurysm
d. Coagulopathy

2. Explain the role of tranexamic acid in a patient with trauma.

Role of tranexamic acid: Tranexamic acid is an antifibrinolytic agent that reduces blood loss after surgery and may reduce blood loss after traumatic injury. It prevents cleavage of plasmin and degradation of fibrin. As early as possible after injury, with administration of tranexamic acid, within 1 hour of injury decreases relative risk from bleeding by 32% and within 1–3 hours by 21%. Administration of tranexamic acid >3 hours after injury is less effective and potentially harmful. Tranexamic acid must be given before transfer/arrival to a trauma center in order to meet the time requirement of early administration. The dose is 1 gm intravenous (IV) bolus over 10 minutes, followed by 1 gm IV over 8 hours. According to CRASH-3 trial, tranexamic acid is safe in patients with traumatic brain injury and that treatment within 3 hours of injury reduces head injury-related death.

3. Discuss the complications of "massive transfusion" in trauma.

Complications of massive blood transfusion: Administration of at least 10 units of red blood cells (RBCs) in 24 hours.
a. Hypothermia is common in these patients and can reduce clotting factor activity
b. Hypocalcemia
c. Hypomagnesemia
d. Hypo/hyperkalemia
e. Acidosis is common finding in massive transfusions
f. Alkalosis is seen sometimes due to citrate toxicity
g. Coagulopathy and thrombocytopenia.

Question 3

A 20-year-old unmarried female patient comes to an emergency department with acute severe lower abdominal pain.

1. Enumerate causes of pain in the patient.

Causes of acute lower abdominal pain are as follows:
a. Aortic aneurysm
b. Appendicitis
c. Crohn's disease
d. Diverticulitis
e. Ectopic pregnancy
f. Endometriosis
g. Epiploic appendages
h. Herpes zoster
i. Inguinal hernia
j. Meckel's diverticulum
k. Ovarian cyst
l. Ovarian torsion
m. Pelvic inflammatory disease
n. Psoas abscess

2. Explain the helpful clinical findings in differential diagnosis.

Clinical findings associated with diseases **(Table 2)**:

TABLE 2: Differential diagnosis of abdominal pain.

Pain/vomiting (± rigidity)	Pain/vomiting/ distention	Pain (± vomiting)
Acute pancreatitis	Bowel obstruction	Acute diverticulitis
Diabetic gastric paresis	Cecal volvulus	Adnexal torsion
Diabetic ketoacidosis		Mesenteric ischemia
Incarcerated hernia		• Myocardial ischemia • Testicular torsion
Pain/shock	**Pain/shock/rigidity**	**Distention (± pain)**
Abdominal sepsis	Perforated appendix	Elderly with bowel obstruction/volvulus
Aortic dissection	Perforated diverticulum	
Hemorrhagic pancreatitis	Perforated ulcer	
Leaking/ruptured abdominal aortic aneurysm	Ruptured esophagus	
	Splenic rupture	
Mesenteric ischemia (late)		
Myocardial ischemia		
Ruptured ectopic pregnancy		

3. How will you investigate the patient?

Start with a thorough history and physical examination including inspection, palpation, percussion, and auscultation of bowel sounds. Diagnoses testing such as plain radiographs, ultrasound, point of care ultrasonography (POCUS), abdominal pelvic computed tomography (CT) scan are used to further investigate the disease. Laboratory studies those may be appropriate in the evaluation of acute abdominal pain on the basis of clinical suspicion **(Table 3)**.

TABLE 3: Suggested laboratory test in abdominal pain evaluation.	
Laboratory test	**Clinical suspicion**
Amylase (if lipase not available)	Pancreatitis
Lipase	Pancreatitis
β-Human chorionic gonadotropin serum or urine Qualitative or quantitative	• Pregnancy • Ectopic or molar pregnancy
Coagulation studies (prothrombin time/partial thromboplastin time)	• GI bleeding • End-stage liver disease coagulopathy
Electrolytes	• Dehydration • Endocrine or metabolic disorder
Glucose	Diabetic ketoacidosis pancreatitis
Gonococcal/chlamydia testing	• Cervicitis/urethritis • Pelvic inflammatory disease
Hemoglobin	GI bleeding
Lactate	Mesenteric ischemia sepsis
Liver function tests	Cholecystitis cholecystitis hepatitis
Platelets	GI bleeding
Renal function tests	Dehydration renal insufficiency acute renal failure
Urinalysis	• Urinary tract infection • Pyelonephritis • Nephrolithiasis
ECG	Myocardial ischemia or infarction

(ECG: electrocardiogram; GI: gastrointestinal)

4. Outline the management of acute severe lower abdominal pain in the emergency department.

Symptomatic treatment is to be given in the emergency department. Nonsteroidal anti-inflammatory drugs (NSAIDs) and opioids are the choice of analgesia. Administer antiemetics—dosage of IV ondansetron is 4 or 8 mg to a maximum of 32 mg daily. Dosage of IV metoclopramide is 10 mg. Consider placements of nasogastric tubes and catheters. Algorithm for management of abdominal pain in the emergency department is shown in **Flowchart 1**.

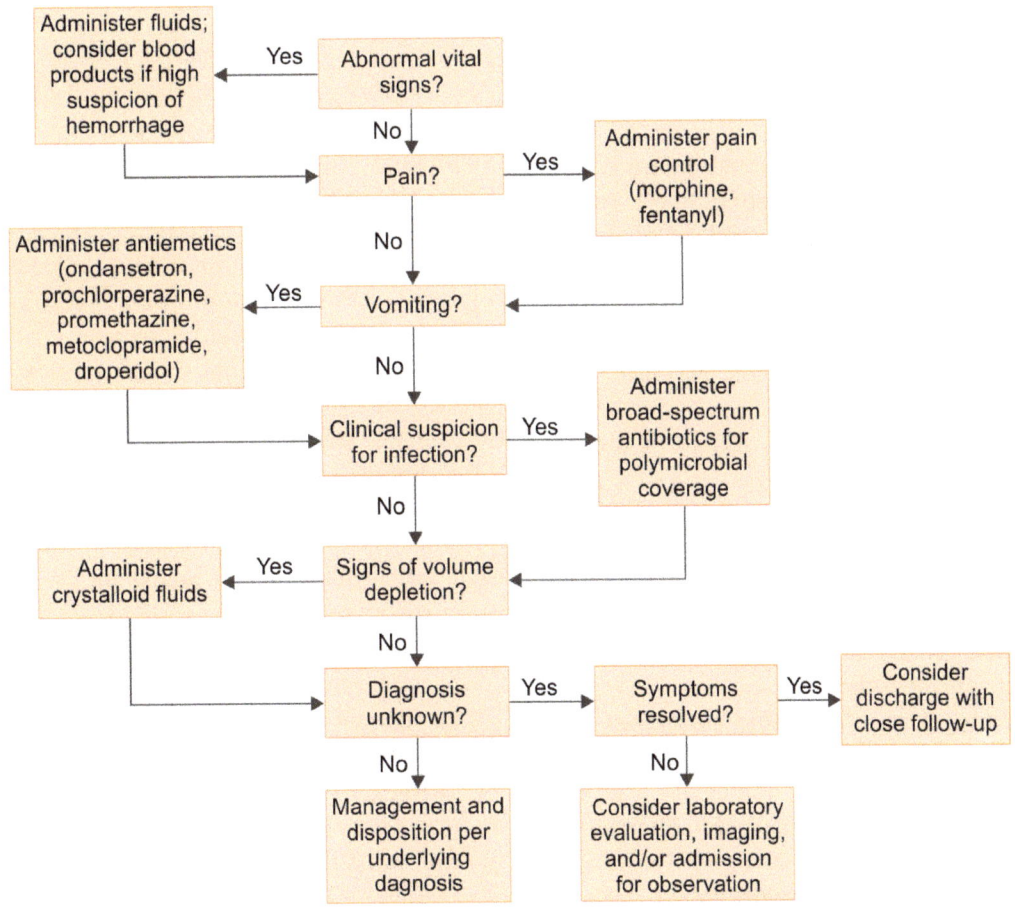

Flowchart 1: Approach to management of abdominal pain.

Question 4

1. Classify fracture of femur.

Fracture of femur are classified as proximal femur fracture and femoral shaft fracture. Further proximal femur fractures are as mentioned here.

a. Femoral head—intracapsular
b. Femoral neck—intracapsular
c. Greater trochanter—extracapsular
d. Lesser trochanter—extracapsular
e. Intertrochanteric—extracapsular
f. Subtrochanteric—extracapsular

2. How will you diagnose fracture neck of femur?

Femoral neck fractures present with the history of fall especially in older adults and more frequently in females with mild pain in groin or inner thigh, to severe pain with subtle movement. Those with displaced fractures are unable to bear weight. On physical examination the affected limb appears as shortened, abducted, and externally rotated. X-ray pelvis anteroposterior (AP) view and X-ray hip AP and lateral should be obtained on which disruption of bony cortex and trabecular lines can be seen.

3. How will you manage a patient with femoral shaft fracture in the emergency department?

Patients with femoral pathology need hemodynamic stabilization and hence crystalloids should be started for resuscitation. A Foley's catheter should be placed and patient should be restricted to take nothing by mouth [*nil per os* (NPO)] until an orthopedic surgeon sees the patient. Blood group crossmatching should be done. For pain management NSAIDs or parenteral opioid-based analgesics should be used.

X-ray femur AP and lateral views should be obtained along with X-ray pelvis, hips, and knee.

For open fractures prophylactic broad spectrum antibiotics (usually first generation cephalosporin along with gentamycin) and tetanus toxoid should be given along with irrigation. Cover the open wound or exposed wound with saline-soaked gauze which further requires operative washout and debridement.

Reduce fracture to near anatomic alignment using in-line traction, which reduces pain and helps prevent hematoma. Hold reduction by a traction device (e.g., Hare, Buck). Traction splints are contraindicated in open fracture or suspected nerve, knee, vascular injury. Neovascular examination with focus on sciatic nerve is done.

4. What are complications of various types of femur fractures?

Complications of various fractures are as follows:
a. Head of femur fracture—avascular necrosis, post-traumatic arthritis, sciatic nerve injury, heterotopic ossification.
b. Femoral neck fractures—avascular necrosis, infection, deep vein thrombosis (DVT) and/or pulmonary embolism.
c. Greater trochanteric—nonunion.
d. Lesser trochanteric—nonunion.
e. Intertrochanteric—DVT and/or pulmonary embolism, infection.
f. Subtrochanteric—DVT and/or pulmonary embolism, infection, malunion (shortened limb), nonunion.
g. Shaft of femur fracture—hemorrhagic shock, neovascular injury, infection.

Question 5

A 35-year-old male presents to the emergency department after a road traffic accident. The pre-hospital emergency technician noted a blood pressure of 70 mm Hg systolic.

1. How will you manage his airway?

Airway management: Clinicians must quickly and accurately assess patient's airway patency and adequacy of ventilation. Pulse oximetry and end-tidal carbon dioxide (CO_2) measurements are essential. If problems identified take immediate action to improve oxygenation and reduce risk of further ventilation compromise. These measures include airway maintenance techniques, definitive airway, and supplemental oxygen. Because all these actions potentially require neck motion, restrictions of cervical motion is necessary in all trauma patients at risk for spinal injury until it has been excluded by appropriate radiographs adjuncts and clinical evaluation. In drug-assisted intubation, use of etomidate does not affect blood pressure/intracranial pressure. It provides adequate sedation, which is advantageous for this patient, then use succinylcholine.

1. *Be prepared:* Suction, oxygen, oropharyngeal, and nasopharyngeal airways bag mask, gum elastic bougie, extraglottic devices, surgical needle, cricothyrotomy kit, endotracheal tube, pulse oximeter, CO_2 detection device drugs.
2. *Preoxygenate:* Oxygen/bag mask/nasal airways
3. *Not able to oxygenate:* Definitive airway/surgical airways

4. *Able to oxygenate:* If yes—assess airway anatomy for ease of intubation [Look-Evaluate-Mallampati-Obstruction-Neck (LEMON)]. If easy—perform drug-assisted intubation. If unsuccessful—consider adjunct [laryngeal mask airway (LMA)] and definitive airway and surgical airways.

2. How will you evaluate his breathing during primary view?

Ventilation requires adequate function of lungs, chest wall, and diaphragm; therefore clinicians must rapidly examine and evaluate each component. To adequately assess jugular venous distension, position of trachea, and chest wall excursion, expose patient's chest and neck. Perform auscultation, ensure gas flow in lungs. Visual inspection and palpation can detect injuries to chest wall.

Percussion also identifies abnormalities. Injuries that significantly impair ventilation in short-term include:
a. Tension pneumothorax
b. Massive hemothorax
c. Open pneumothorax
d. Tracheal/bronchial injury

Because tension pneumothorax compromises ventilation and circulation dramatically, so chest decompression follows immediately.

3. In a patient who is hypotensive due to trauma, what are the probable findings on sonography?

Sonographic findings: Right upper quadrant view—the perihepatic area and the potential space between the liver and kidney, otherwise known as Morrison's pouch, it is more sensitive area to detect intraperitoneal fluid indicate blunt abdominal trauma and liver injury.

Left upper quadrant view—free fluid in perisplenic view indicates blunt abdominal trauma and splenic injury.

Pelvic view: In reverse Trendelenburg position free fluid presence will enhance and indicate blunt abdominal trauma and any bladder injury.

Cardiac view: Presence of free fluid around pericardial space indicates pericardial effusion and cardiac tamponade.

Chest view: Presence of fluid in around lungs indicates hemothorax; barcode sign positive and lung point—tension pneumothorax.

Question 6

1. Discuss various etiological agents producing gas gangrene.

The most common etiological agent of gas gangrene is clostridium perfringens.

Other common clostridial species that can cause gas gangrene are clostridium bifermentans, clostridium septicum, clostridium sporogeneses, clostridium novyi, clostridium fallax, clostridium histolyticum, clostridium tertium. Some aerobic gram-negative bacteria can also cause gas gangrene such as *Escherichia coli* (*E. coli*), *Proteus* species, *Pseudomonas aeruginosa* and *Klebsiella pneumoniae*.

2. Explain the pathogenesis of gas gangrene.

The induction of gas gangrene involves contamination with clostridial spores in post-traumatic or postoperative lesions. Disrupted or necrotic tissue provides the necessary enzymes and low oxidation/reduction potential, allowing for spore germination. The pathogenesis of gas gangrene typically involves the exotoxin of clostridium, of which >20 have been identified. Alpha toxin is the most prevalent and causes platelet and leucocyte destruction, widespread capillary damage, hemolysis, tissue necrosis, and often death. Local effects include necrosis of muscle, subcutaneous fat, and thrombosis of blood vessels. Marked edema can further compromise blood supply. Fermentation of glucose is the main mechanism of gas gangrene which is nitrogen (74.5%), oxygen (16.1%), hydrogen (5.9%), carbon dioxide (3.4%). Systemically hemolysis results in hypotension, acute tubular necrosis, and renal failure.

3. How will you manage gas gangrene in emergency?

The treatment of gas gangrene involves three-pronged approach, i.e.,
a. Antibiotics
b. Surgery
c. Hyperbaric oxygen therapy

A combination of penicillin along with clindamycin should be used.

Fasciotomy for compartment syndrome can be done. Copious irrigation with normal saline (NS) solutions or 3% liquid hydrogen peroxide should be performed. Debridement of wound should be done as soon as possible. The hyperbaric oxygen therapy protocol for gas gangrene is 3.0 ATA (atmospheric absolute of pressure) for 90 minutes three times a day in the first 24 hours and then twice daily for the next 2–5 days.

4. Discuss the systemic complications related to necrotizing soft tissues infections.

Necrotizing soft tissue infections including necrotizing fasciitis, Fournier's gangrene are rapidly spreading, deep, typically mixed infections that result in profound morbidity and mortality.

The rapid necrotizing process begins with direct invasion of subcutaneous tissue from external trauma or direct spread from a perforated viscus. Bacteria proliferate and release exotoxins leading to tissue ischemia, liquefaction necrosis, and systemic toxicity. Systemic manifestations include a low-grade fever with tachycardia out of proportion to the fever. In fulminant necrotizing infections, particularly from *Vibrio vulnificus* (*V. vulnificus*), patients may have cardiovascular collapse due to release of bacterial toxins and release of cytokines, and they may be confused, irritable, or have a rapid deterioration of mental status.

Question 7

1. Enumerate anatomy of rotator cuff around shoulder.

Rotator cuff muscles surround the proximal humerus and help to move the arm in different directions.

Four muscles form the rotator cuff **(Fig. 2)**:
1. *Supraspinatus muscle*—arises from supraspinatus fossa on dorsal scapula/attaches to superior facet on greater tuberosity of humerus/abducts the arm.
2. *Infraspinatus muscle*—arises from infraspinous fossa on dorsal aspect of scapula/attaches to middle facet of greater tuberosity of humerus/externally rotates the arm.
3. *Teres minor*—arises from superior part of lateral border of scapula/attaches to inferior facet of greater tuberosity of humerus/externally rotating of arm.
4. *Subscapularis*—arises from ventral surface of scapula/attaches to lesser tuberosity of humerus/internally rotates the arm.

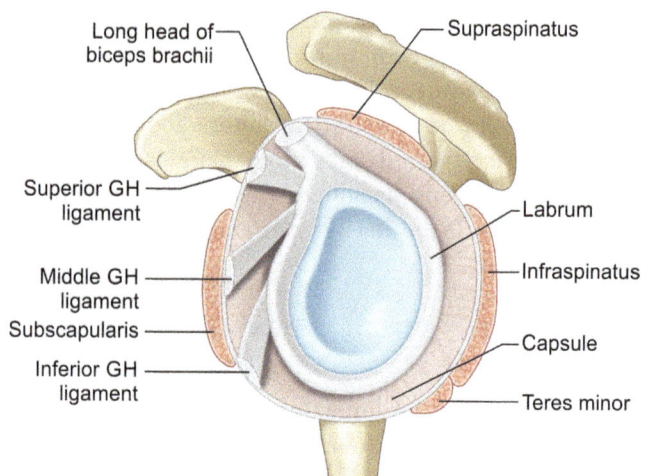

Fig. 2: Anatomy of rotator cuff around shoulder. (GH: glenohumeral)

2. Examine the findings in rotator cuff injuries.

Drop arm test (supraspinatus muscle): Ask the patient to lower the arm slowly from abduction. Positive test result—immediate drop of the arm accompanied by pain.

External rotation lag test (infraspinatus and supraspinatus): Examiner passively rotates the patient's arm in external rotation.

Positive test result—patient unable to maintain a position of full external rotation.

Internal rotation lag test (subscapularis): Hand of the patient's affected arm is lifted off of back by the examiner, and ask to maintain position. Positive result—unable to maintain position.

3. How will you investigate a patient with suspected rotator cuff injury?

X-ray: It does not show rotator cuff tear but to visualize the bone spurs or other potential cause of pain like arthritis.
Ultrasound: This test helps to produce images of structures particularly soft tissue such as muscle and tendons. It helps to assess the structure during movement.
Magnetic resonance imaging (MRI): It helps in displaying all structures in great detail.

Question 8

A 55-year-old smoker with type 2 diabetes presents to the emergency with pain in left leg and discomfort and discoloration of big toe.

1. Enumerate the causes and differential of this presentation.

The differentials and causes for acute limb ischemia include:
a. Atherosclerosis
b. Cardiac source—atrial fibrillation, rheumatic heart disease (RHD), mechanical valves, postmyocardial infarction thrombus, atrial myxomas, endocarditis
c. Cholesterol emboli
d. Vasculitis, rheumatoid arthritis, lupus, polyarteritis nodosa
e. Raynaud's disease
f. Takayasu arteritis
g. Thromboangiitis proliferans (Buerger's disease)
h. Human immunodeficiency virus (HIV) arteritis
i. Hypothenar hammer syndrome
j. Popliteal artery entrapment
k. External iliac artery thrombosis

l. Local arterial trauma
m. Shock related
n. Thoracic aortic dissection.

2. How will you evaluate this patient in emergency?

Obtain an adequate history, focusing on timing and acuity of symptom onset, pattern of claudication, any previous revascularization or diagnosing of ischemia, and assessment of risk factors. On physical examination look at skin and palpate peripheral pulses of both extremities.

Listen to the heart and abdomen, seeking bruits and murmurs. POCUS helps to detect an abnormal aortic aneurysm. Doppler examination is done to assess ankle brachial index. Patients with chronic peripheral arterial disease have an ankle brachial index of <0.9, while values of <0.4 suggest severe disease. Laboratory evaluation includes creatinine kinase, myoglobin, serum lactate, serum electrolytes and glucose, renal function [blood urea nitrogen (BUN) and creatinine], complete blood count (CBC), and coagulation profile.

3. How will you perform the medical management of this patient?

The medical management of acute limb ischemia in emergency department involves: Stratifying the patients with **Rutherford criteria** in conjunction with early surgical consultation guides initial care.

Rutherford criteria for acute limb ischemia: Patients with stage 1 and 2 a limb ischemia may undergo diagnostic imaging workup before definitive treatment. Patients with stage 2b ischemia often require immediate revascularization. Patients with stage 3 have irreversible damage and require amputation.

Question 9

A 70-year-old patient presents with dysphagia to solids.

1. Enumerate the causes of dysphagia at this age.

The causes for dysphagia are as follows:
a. Neuromuscular vascular
b. Cerebrovascular accident
c. *Immunologic:* Dermatomyositis, multiple sclerosis, myasthenia gravis, polymyositis scleroderma
d. *Infectious:* Botulism, diphtheria, poliomyelitis, rabies, Sydenham chorea, tetanus
e. *Metabolic:* Lead poisoning, magnesium deficiency
f. Alzheimer's disease, amyotrophic lateral sclerosis, brain tumor, depression, diabetic neuropathy, familial dysautonomia, metabolic myopathies (e.g., thyrotoxicosis), muscular dystrophies, Parkinson's disease
g. *Obstructive:* Aortic aneurysm, esophageal motility disorder (e.g., achalasia, diffuse esophageal spasm, nutcracker esophagus), esophageal rings, esophageal stricture, esophageal webs, esophagitis, foreign bodies, hypertrophic cervical spurs, inflammatory lesions, left atrial enlargement, mediastinal mass, neoplasm, thyroid enlargement, vascular anomalies (e.g., enlarged aorta, aberrant subclavian artery), Zenker diverticulum
h. *Other:* Alcoholism, decreased saliva production (Sjögren's syndrome, postirradiation), diabetes, functional, gastro-esophageal reflux disease.

2. How would you evaluate this patient?

A thorough history and physical examination should be done. The diagnosis of underlying pathology can be done by upper endoscopy, video esophagography, barium swallow, or esophageal manometry. If neoplasm is suspected CT imaging of neck and chest may be indicated in the emergency department.

3. Discuss the management of acute dysphagia in elderly.

Achalasia is the only motility disorder for which reasonably reliable studies support specific treatment. Previously, pharmacologic therapies such as nitrates and calcium channel blockers have been used with the goal of decreasing tone of the lower esophageal sphincter (LES). More recently, surgical interventions such as peroral endoscopic myotomy (POEM) have been used as first-line therapy in patients with achalasia who are able to tolerate surgical intervention. Pharmacologic therapy remains available as a bridge to more definitive intervention or in patients who are unable to tolerate an invasive procedure.

Endoscopic botulinum toxin injection remains available as an acceptable treatment option in patients; although as with other medical therapies are commonly reserved for patients unable to tolerate more invasive procedures. Medical therapy for esophageal motility disorders is limited, and clinical impacts are typically minimal. Anticholinergic drugs such as hyoscyamine sulfate or dicyclomine have been used because they decrease the amplitude of esophageal peristalsis and LES pressure. However, because these drugs delay gastric emptying and decrease esophageal peristalsis, they may exacerbate reflux symptoms. Other therapies include the use of calcium channel blockers, which decrease LES pressure and the amplitude of esophageal contractions.

Question 10

A 60-year-old hypertensive patient presents with severe headache for 3 hours.

1. List different causes of acute headache.

Causes of acute headache are:
a. *Due to hemorrhage*—intracranial hemorrhage "Sentinel" aneurysmal headache spontaneous subarachnoid and intracerebral hemorrhage
b. *Due to vascular causes*—carotid or vertebrobasilar dissection, reversible cerebral vasoconstriction syndrome, cerebral venous thrombosis, posterior reversible encephalopathy
c. *Other causes*—coital headache, Valsalva-associated headache, spontaneous intracranial hypotension, acute hydrocephalus, pituitary apoplexy, acute angle closure glaucoma, primary headache syndromes (migraine, cluster headache).

2. How will you investigate a patient with suspicion of subarachnoid hemorrhage?

Subarachnoid hemorrhage can be ruled out with 100% sensitivity by applying Ottawa subarachnoid hemorrhagic rule for headache evaluation, i.e.,
a. Age >40 years
b. Neck pain or stiffness
c. Loss of consciousness
d. Onset during exertion
e. Thunderclap headache
f. Limited neck flexion on examination

The initial diagnostic modality in suspected subarachnoid hemorrhage (SAH) patients is noncontrast CT scan of head. CT angiography and MRI are done after a negative CT head. Cerebrospinal fluid (CSF) analysis through lumbar puncture is done after normal CT head to rule out infections. **Table 4** shows grading scale of subarachnoid hemorrhage (Hunt and Hess scale).

TABLE 4: Grading scales for subarachnoid hemorrhage.

Grade	Hunt and Hess scale	World Federation of Neurosurgical Societies scale
1	Mild headache, normal mental status, no cranial nerve or motor findings	GCS of 15, no motor deficits
2	Severe headache, normal mental status, may have cranial nerve deficits	GCS of 13 or 14, no motor deficits
3	Somnolent, confused, may have cranial nerve or mild motor deficit	GCS of 13 or 14, with motor deficits
4	Stupor, moderate to severe motor deficit, may have intermittent reflex posturing	GCS of 7–12, with or without motor deficits
5	Coma, reflex posturing or flaccid	GCS of 3–6, with or without motor deficits

(GCS: Glasgow Coma Scale)

3. How will you manage a patient with subarachnoid hemorrhage in emergency department?

Management of SAH in emergency department: Subarachnoid hemorrhage is a life-threatening condition. The prevention of complications such as vasospasm, hydrocephalus, and permanent brain damage is priority. Reassess the Glasgow coma scale and pupillary responses regularly. Control blood pressure (BP) with agent such as labetalol and nicardipine to balance the risk of stroke, rebleeding, and maintenance of cerebral perfusion pressure. A decrease in systolic blood pressure to a range of 120-160 mm hg is recommended. Antifibrinolytics such as tranexamic acid or aminocaproic acid can be used to prevent aneurysmal rebleeding. Vasospasm is most common 2 days-3 weeks after SAH therefore nimodipine 60 mg PO (*per os*—orally) every 4 hours is indicated and should be initiated within 96 hours of symptom onset. Initiating hypertension, hypervolemia, and hemodilution therapy (**HHH therapy**) to prevent vasospasm in SAH patients, i.e.,
a. *Hemodilution:* Hemodilution goes hand-in-hand with hypervolemia to decrease viscosity and facilitate blood flow through the cerebral vasculature.
b. *Hypervolemia:* Fluid volume should be optimal with central venous pressure (CVP) 8-12 mm Hg (higher if vented due to the artificial elevation in pressure due to mechanical ventilation)
c. *Hypertension:* As mentioned above.

SUGGESTED READING

1. Richhariya D, Sharma B. Textbook of Emergency Medicine including Intensive Care and Trauma, 2nd edition. New Delhi: Jaypee Brothers Medical Publishers (P) Ltd; 2022. pp. 1675-85. (Question 1).
2. Richhariya D, Sharma B. Textbook of Emergency Medicine including Intensive Care and Trauma, 2nd edition. New Delhi: Jaypee Brothers Medical Publishers (P) Ltd; 2022. pp. 1537. (Question 2).

3. Richhariya D, Sharma B. Textbook of Emergency Medicine including Intensive Care and Trauma, 2nd edition. New Delhi: Jaypee Brothers Medical Publishers (P) Ltd; 2022. pp. 633-9. (Question 3).
4. Richhariya D, Sharma B. Textbook of Emergency Medicine including Intensive Care and Trauma, 2nd edition. New Delhi: Jaypee Brothers Medical Publishers (P) Ltd; 2022. pp. 1615-9. (Question 4).
5. Richhariya D, Sharma B. Textbook of Emergency Medicine including Intensive Care and Trauma, 2nd edition. New Delhi: Jaypee Brothers Medical Publishers (P) Ltd; 2022. pp. 1524-2. (Question 5).
6. Richhariya D, Sharma B. Textbook of Emergency Medicine including Intensive Care and Trauma, 2nd edition. New Delhi: Jaypee Brothers Medical Publishers (P) Ltd; 2022. pp. 1353. (Question 6).
7. Richhariya D, Sharma B. Textbook of Emergency Medicine including Intensive Care and Trauma, 2nd edition. New Delhi: Jaypee Brothers Medical Publishers (P) Ltd; 2022. pp. 1603-10. (Question 7).
8. Richhariya D, Sharma B. Textbook of Emergency Medicine including Intensive Care and Trauma, 2nd edition. New Delhi: Jaypee Brothers Medical Publishers (P) Ltd; 2022. pp. 547-50. (Question 8).
9. Richhariya D, Sharma B. Textbook of Emergency Medicine including Intensive Care and Trauma, 2nd edition. New Delhi: Jaypee Brothers Medical Publishers (P) Ltd; 2022. pp. 662-3. (Question 9).
10. Richhariya D, Sharma B. Textbook of Emergency Medicine including Intensive Care and Trauma, 2nd edition. New Delhi: Jaypee Brothers Medical Publishers (P) Ltd; 2022. pp. 796-800; 828-31. (Question 10).

Emergency Medicine Paper 7

Anshul Jain

Question 1

A young pregnant lady presents to an emergency department with headache and her blood pressure is 200/110 mm of Hg.

1. Discuss differential diagnosis.

a. *Chronic hypertension in pregnancy:* Systolic blood pressure (BP) ≥140 mm Hg and Diastolic BP ≥90 mm Hg without any evidence of proteinuria or any organ dysfunction.
b. *Preeclampsia:* Presence of hypertension (>140 mm Hg systolic or >90 mm Hg diastolic) after 20 weeks of gestation combined with proteinuria or other maternal organ dysfunction (renal/liver/neurological).
c. *Hemolysis, elevated liver enzymes, and low platelets (HELLP) syndrome:* Severe form of preeclampsia, characterized by hemolysis, elevated liver enzymes [alanine transaminase (ALT) and aspartate transaminase (AST) levels >100], and low platelet counts (<1 lakh/mL).
d. *Eclampsia:* Development of new onset seizures superimposed upon preeclampsia, between 20 weeks of gestation and 4 weeks postpartum.

2. How will you evaluate this patient?

Patient needs to be evaluated for preeclampsia.

The severe features of preeclampsia are:
a. Systolic BP of ≥160 mm Hg and diastolic of ≥90 mm Hg on two separate occasions at least 4 hours apart when the patient is on bed.
b. Proteinuria ≥300 mg in 24 hours.
c. Evidence of maternal end organ dysfunction (headache or visual disturbances, thrombocytopenia <1 lakh/mL, impaired liver functions or persistent right upper quadrant or epigastric pain unresponsive to medications, progressive renal insufficiency, and signs of pulmonary edema).

Lab investigations recommended (**Table 1**) are as following:

TABLE 1: Lab investigations recommended.

Test	Comments
CBC with differentials	Hemoconcentration or decreasing hematocrit, low platelets may indicate severe disease
Creatinine	Elevation suggests severe disease
ALT and AST levels	Elevation suggests severe disease
Lactate dehydrogenase	Elevation suggests microangiopathic hemolysis
Protein in urine	≥1 + proteinuria, >5 g/24 hours suggest severe disease
Protein/creatinine ratio	0.1–0.3 indicate need for 24-hour collection
Uric acid levels	Level ≥5.5 mg/dL suggests superimposed preeclampsia on chronic hypertension

(CBC: complete blood count; ALT: alanine transaminase; AST: aspartate transaminase)

3. How will you manage this patient in emergency department?

Management of this patient in emergency: As patient is having signs of severe preeclampsia, primary goal of the management will be to reduce her BP and definitive treatment will be delivery of the fetus.

Management of eclampsia and severe preeclampsia:
a. Control seizures with magnesium sulfate intravenous (IV) 4-6 g in 100 mL saline over 20-30 minutes followed by infusion of magnesium sulfate 2 g/h for at least 24 hours. Watch for the signs of magnesium toxicity such as diminished patellar reflexes and slow respiratory rate.
b. Control BP after seizure control.
c. Obtain lab investigations to assess the organ damage.
d. Monitor urine output, maintain at <25 mL/h.
e. Limit the use of intravenous fluids unless indicated.
f. Avoid diuretics and hyperosmolar agents.
g. Perform a computed tomography (CT) head if decreased consciousness.
h. Initiate the steps to delivery.

Antihypertensives which can be safely used to treat severe preeclampsia are:
a. Labetalol—selective alpha and nonselective beta antagonist, 20 mg IV then 40–80 mg IV every 10 minutes as needed (maximum 300 mg), infusion @1–2 mg/min.
b. Hydralazine—arterial vasodilator, 5 mg IV or 10 mg intramuscular (IM), to be repeated after 20 minutes interval if BP does not reduce.
c. Nifedipine—calcium channel antagonist, 10 mg PO to be repeated after 30 minutes.

Question 2

1. Define delirium.

Delirium is defined as abrupt disorder characterized by impairment of attention and cognition.

2. List types of delirium.

Types of delirium:
a. *Hyperactive delirium:* Restlessness, agitation, rapid mood swings or hallucinations.
b. *Hypoactive delirium:* Inactivity, sluggishness or abnormal drowsiness.
c. *Mixed delirium:* It includes both the symptoms of hyperactive and hypoactive delirium.

3. Enumerate causes of delirium in elderly.

The causes of delirium in elderly **(Table 2)** are as follows:

TABLE 2: Causes of delirium in elderly.

Infectious	• Urinary tract infection • Sepsis • Meningitis • Pneumonia
Metabolic/toxic	• Hypoglycemia • Alcohol ingestion • Electrolyte abnormalities • Hepatic encephalopathy • Alcohol withdrawal
Neurological	• Stroke or transient Ischemic attack • Seizure • Subarachnoid hemorrhage • Intracranial hemorrhage • CNS mass lesion • Subdural hematoma
Cardiopulmonary	• Myocardial infarction • Congestive cardiac failure
Drug related	• Alcohol withdrawal • Sedatives or hypnotics • Narcotic analgesics

3. How will you manage a delirious patient?

Management of a patient in delirium

Diagnosis: Delirium is a clinical diagnosis, so thorough history and physical examination is a must for the diagnosis. Compared to the patient's baseline, acute onset of attention deficits and cognitive abnormalities, fluctuating in course is virtually diagnostic of delirium.

Screening tools: Delirium Triage Screen (incorporates the Richmond Agitation-Sedation Scale) and highly specific *Brief Confusion Assessment Method.*

The treatment procedure is shown in **Flowchart 1**.

Flowchart 1: Treatment of a patient in delirium.

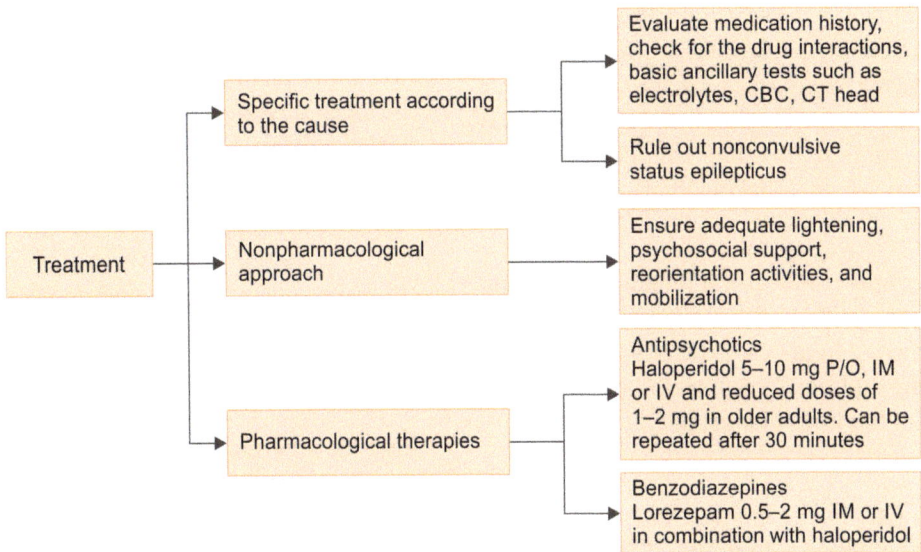

(CBC: complete blood count; CT: computed tomography; IM: intramuscular; IV: intravenous)

Question 3

1. Enumerate the causes of chest pain in emergency.

The causes of acute chest pain in emergency **(Table 3)** are as follows:

TABLE 3: Causes of acute chest pain in emergency.

Visceral pain	Pleuritic pain	Chest wall pain
Unstable angina	Pulmonary embolism	Costochondritis (Tietze's syndrome)
Aortic dissection	Pneumonia	Fibromyalgia
Myocardial infarction	Pericarditis	Intercostal nerve syndromes
Esophageal reflux	Pleurisy	
Esophageal rupture	Spontaneous pneumothorax	

2. Discuss the role of biomarkers in evaluation of chest pain in emergency.

Role of cardiac biomarkers

Indication: Cardiac markers are very useful in cases where electrocardiograms (ECGs) are non-diagnostic and risk stratification needs to be done in patients with ST-elevation myocardial infarction (STEMI), non-ST-elevation myocardial infarction (NSTEMI), and unstable angina.

Troponins: Because of the superior sensitivity and specificity as compared to other markers, cardiac troponins are the best to identify any myocardial cell injury. Serial measurements, particularly performed at least 6 hours of the symptom onset markedly improve the sensitivity of cardiac troponins to diagnose acute MI. Troponins may also be elevated in some noncardiac conditions such as pulmonary embolism, sepsis, renal insufficiency, and even in physical exertion.

Creatinine phosphokinase (CPK-MB): It remains the second best alternative to troponins in the setting of acute MI. It is detectable as early as 3 hours after the onset of necrosis, peaks at 20–24 hours and becomes normal after 2–3 days of injury. Because of the lack of specificity, their role has decreased in recent years.

Myoglobin: Its level rises in 1–2 hours, peaks in 5–7 hours, and returns to the baseline in 24 hours. It is the earliest indicator of myocardial injury, but due to extreme lack of specificity not used nowadays.

3. Discuss the management of saddle thrombus in pulmonary artery.

Saddle thromboembolism is a rare type of acute pulmonary embolism in which thrombus is present at the bifurcation of the main pulmonary artery and presents with significant hemodynamic instability.

Management options are given as below:

Anticoagulation: Two options are available—unfractionated heparin and LMWH (low molecular weight heparin).

1. Unfractionated heparin dose—80 units/kg bolus then 18 units/kg/h infusion.
   LMWH—1 mg/kg subcutaneously every 12 hourly.
   Factor Xa Inhibitors—fondaparinux.
   Target specific anticoagulants—dabigatran (150 mg P/O BD), rivaroxaban, and apixaban.
2. *Systemic thrombolysis:* Consider this step in those with no contraindications of thrombolysis and patients with significant hypotension with shock.
   Alteplase—10 mg IV bolus, then 90 mg IV infused over 2 hours.
3. *Catheter-directed thrombolysis:* Indicated in older patients with embolism in which risk of intracranial bleed is high. Dose required is quite less—10 mg alteplase.
4. *Surgical embolectomy:* Particularly for young patients with proximal embolus and hypotension.

Question 4

1. Discuss the role of gastric lavage in poisoning.

a. For clearing the stomach contents and to prevent the further spread of the poison.
b. In case of medicolegal issues, appropriate samples can be taken through gastric lavage and sent to the forensics for identification of an unknown poison.

2. How does multiple dose-activated charcoal (MDAC) help in patient of acute poisoning?

a. Unlike single dose-activated charcoal, which prevents the absorption of a drug, MDAC also facilitates the removal of the toxin which has already been absorbed.
b. It decreases xenobiotic absorption and elimination half-life when large amount of toxins are ingested and dissolution is delayed.
c. It also creates a hemoperfusion substrate for the gut wall microcirculation to permit "gastrointestinal dialysis" which creates a concentration gradient into the stools, which are then eliminated by defecation.

d. It interferes with the enterohepatic circulation of certain drugs, thereby affecting the reabsorption of these drugs.

3. How will you perform whole bowel irrigation in patient of acute poisoning?

a. Indicated in certain ingestions such as extended-release preparations, illicit drug packets and metals (iron and lead).
b. It is performed with a balanced polyethylene glycol solution that does not participate in the fluid exchange nor become absorbed into the body.
c. To be effective, it requires a rate of 2 L/h in an adult, consequently this will require placement of a nasogastric tube.
d. It is contraindicated in conditions causing hypoperfusion of gut or obstruction of bowel, where there can be increased chances of morbidity and mortality.

Question 5

1. Write staging of chronic kidney disease.

Stages of chronic kidney disease are depicted in **Table 4**.

TABLE 4: Stages of chronic kidney disease.

Stage	GFR	Comments
Stage 1	GFR ≥90 mL/min/1.73 m²	Non-GFR evidence of kidney damage present
Stage 2	GFR 60–89 mL/min/1.73 m²	Mild disease
Stage 3	GFR 30–59 mL/min/1.73 m²	Mild to moderate disease
Stage 4	GFR 15–29 mL/min/1.73 m²	Moderate to severe disease
Stage 5	GFR <15 mL/min/1.73 m²	Dialysis or transplant needed

(GFR: glomerular filtration rate)

2. Enumerate emergency complications of end stage chronic kidney disease (CKD).

a. Uncontrolled hyperkalemia (Serum K⁺ >6.5 mmol/L or rising)
b. Refractory fluid overload in association of persistent hypoxia or lack of response to the conservative measures.
c. Uremic pericarditis.
d. Persistent uremia/metabolic encephalopathy, asterixis or seizures.
e. Serum sodium level of <115 or >165 mEq/L.
f. Severe metabolic acidosis with concomitant acute kidney injury.
g. Bleeding dyscrasia secondary to uremia.

3. Write the emergency complications of hemodialysis.

Following are the emergency complications of hemodialysis (**Box 1**):

BOX 1: Emergency complications of hemodialysis.

Vascular access-related complications:
- Bleeding from the dialysis puncture site
- Infection of the vascular access due to recurrent bacteremia

Nonvascular access-related complications:
- *Significant hypotension:* It may occur as a result of acute reduction in the circulating intravascular volume and failure of the patient's hemostatic mechanisms to compensate for it; need to rule out other life-threatening causes such acute pericardial tamponade and pulmonary embolism.
- *Acute onset shortness of breath:* May be due to sudden cardiac failure, pericardial tamponade, pleural effusion or pleural hemorrhage.
- *Chest pain:* Most episodes of chest pain are likely to be ischemic in origin, as chronic kidney disease itself is a disease with high risk of coronary artery disease. Among nonischemic causes, most common is pericarditis which has to be ruled out—history of fever, friction rub on auscultation, and atrial dysarrhymias.
- *Neurologic dysfunction:* Most common is disequilirium syndrome (a constellation of symptoms and signs from the rapid changes of body fluid composition and serum osmolality). Other causes may be uremic encephalopathy or meningitis.

Question 6

A young male patient presents in emergency with fever and purpuric rash.

1. Enumerate causes.

Following are the infectious and noninfectious causes (**Box 2**):

BOX 2: Infectious and noninfectious causes.

Infectious causes
- *Bacterial:* Rickettsia, erysipelas, toxic shock syndrome, typhoid fever, leptospirosis
- *Viral:* Dengue fever, chikungunia, measles, rubella, infectious mononucleosis, chicken pox

Noninfectious causes
- Drug reactions
- Connective tissue disorders
- Others—small vessel vasculitis, Urticaria, Erthyema Nodosum

2. Enumerate "warning signs" in dengue fever.

a. Abdominal pain or tenderness.
b. Persistent vomiting.
c. Clinical fluid accumulation (ascites, pleural effusion).

d. Mucosal bleeding.
e. Lethargy or restlessness.
f. Hepatomegaly >2 cm.
g. Increase in the hematocrit concurrent with rapid decrease in the platelet count.

3. How will you treat a dengue shock syndrome Grade IV or severe dengue shock?

Following are the steps to treat a dengue shock syndrome Grade IV or severe dengue shock (**Flowchart 2**):

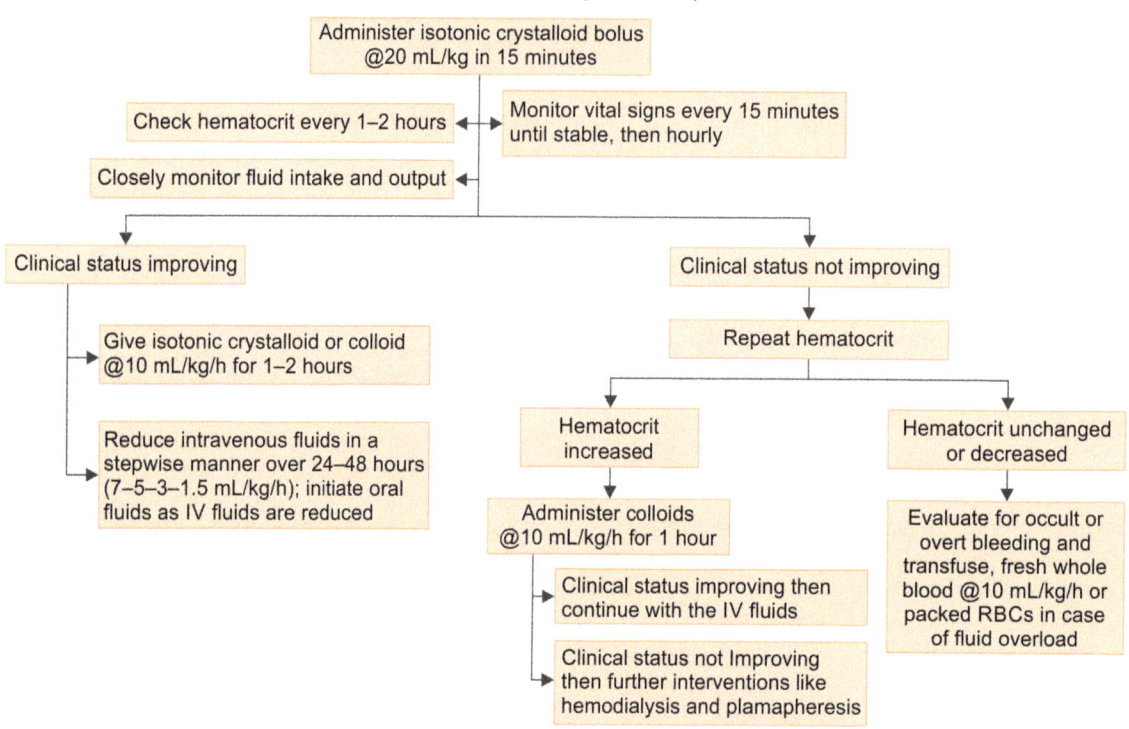

Flowchart 2: Steps to treat a dengue shock syndrome Grade IV.

(IV: intravenous; RBCs: red blood cells)

Question 7

1. Enumerate precipitating factors for Addisonian crisis.

a. *Drug-induced adrenal enzyme inhibitors:* Etomidate, aminoglutethimide, mitotane, and ketoconazole.
b. *Infections:*
   i. Tuberculosis (most common cause of adrenal insufficiency).
   ii. Fungal or bacterial sepsis.
   iii. Acquired immunodeficiency syndrome involving adrenal gland.
c. *Infiltrative disorders:* Sarcoidosis, hemochromatosis, amyloidosis, lymphoma, and metastatic cancer.
d. *Surgery:* Bilateral adrenalectomy and bariatric surgery.
e. *Hereditary:* Congenital adrenal hyperplasia, familial glucocorticoid deficiency, and adrenal hypoplasia.
f. Autoimmune causes.
g. *Adrenal hemorrhage:* Meningococcal sepsis, anticoagulants or trauma.

2. Enumerate clinical features of Addisonian crisis:

a. Refractory hypotension and dehydration not responding to fluids and pressors.
b. Recurrent hypoglycemia
c. Electrolyte imbalances (hyponatremia, hyperkalemia)
d. Hyperpigmentation
e. Generalized weakness or fatigue
f. Weight loss
g. Orthostasis, syncope
h. Vitiligo

3. Outline management of Addisonian crisis.

Management of Addisonian crisis is summarized in **Figure 1**.
a. Bedside glucose determination to identify hypoglycemia.
b. Complete blood count, serum electrolytes, calcium levels, hepatic function tests, ECG, and urinalysis.
c. Additional tests such as chest X-ray to rule out tuberculosis and abdominal CT to rule out adrenal hemorrhage can be carried out.

Treatment of Addisonian crisis

Administer IV fluids for hypotension
- Use dextrose containing saline if hypoglycemia (begin with D5/NS)

Give steroids
- Hydrocortisone 100 mg IV bolus (drug of choice for adrenal insufficiency), if no IV access, then give 100 mg IM, then start infusion @200 mg/24 hours or 100 mg 6 hourly or
- Dexamethasone—4 mg IV bolus, add fludrocortisone 100 μg/day as dexamethasone does not have mineralocorticoid

Supportive care
- Maintain airway breathing and circulation
- Consider giving bolus glucose, thiamine, or naloxone if altered sensorium
- Correct sodium potassium or calcium if abnormal

Vasopressors
- Consider giving vasopressors if not responding to IV fluids and persistent hypotension

Determine the underlying cause
- Investigate for sepsis, adrenal hemorrhage or any CNS abnormality

Optimization of steroids
- Patients may require lifelong administration of steroids + androgen supplementation; increase the doses in stress situations upto three times the normal to satisfy the daily requirement of cortisol

Fig. 1: Treatment of Addisonian crisis. (CNS: central nervous system; IM: intramuscular; IV: intravenous)

Question 8

1. Enumerate causes of acute flaccid paralysis.

a. Neuroparalytic snake envenomation
b. Guillain–Barré syndrome
c. Hypokalemic paralysis
d. Acute intermittent porphyria
e. Viral meningoencephalitis
f. Acute transverse myelitis
g. Myasthenic crisis
h. Poliomyelitis
i. Botulism.

2. How will you manage a patient of "krait bite"?

a. *General management:*
   i. *Protection of airway:* Oxygen support @ 15 L/min via nonrebreather mask (NRBM), mechanical ventilation may be required if airway is compromised.
   ii. *Breathing:* Maintain oxygen saturation and respiratory rate.
   iii. *Circulation:* Insert two large-bore IV cannulas and start IV crystalloids if the patient is in shock.
b. *Anti-snake venom (ASV):*
   i. Start ASV intravenous 10 vials mixed with 500 mL saline to be given over 30–60 minutes.
   ii. Repeat 10 vials ASV if neurological symptoms do not resolve after 1 hour.
   iii. Watch for any anaphylactic reactions.
c. Krait venom affects the presynaptic fibers where calcium ion acts as a neurotransmitter. So, inject calcium gluconate 10 mL IV slowly over 5–10 minutes every 6 hourly and continue till neuroparalysis recovers which may last for 5–7 days.

3. Write complications associated with of anti-snake venom administration.

a. Rarely patients may have life-threatening anaphylactic reactions such as hypotension, bronchospasm, and angioedema.
b. *Early anaphylactic reactions* occur about 10–180 minutes of the start of the therapy and are characterized by itching, urticaria, dry cough, diarrhea, nausea and vomiting, abdominal pain, and fever.
c. *Pyrogenic reactions* usually develop 1–2 hours after treatment. Symptoms include chills and rigors, fever, and hypotension. These reactions are caused by contamination of the ASV with pyrogens during the manufacturing process.
d. Any new sign or symptom after starting the ASV in drip should be suspected as a reaction to ASV.
e. *Late (serum sickness type) reactions* develop 1–12 (mean 7) days after treatment. Clinical features include fever, nausea, vomiting, diarrhea, itching, recurrent urticaria, arthralgia, myalgia, lymphadenopathy, immune complex nephritis, and rarely, encephalopathy.

Question 9

1. Write causes of vesiculobullous skin lesions.

a. Bullous pemphigoid
b. Pemphigus vulgaris
c. Dermatitis herpetiformis
d. Darier's disease
e. Pemphigus foliaceous
f. Epidermolysis bullosa
g. Drug reactions.

2. Enumerate clinical features of pemphigus vulgaris.

a. *Mucosal involvement:* Oral cavity is the most common site of mucosal lesions; other sites may also be present such as conjunctiva, nose, esophagus, cervix, vagina, and anus.
b. Painful blisters that rupture easily.
c. *Nikolsky sign:* Induction of blistering via mechanical pressure at the edge of the blister or on normal skin.

3. Write treatment of pemphigus vulgaris.

a. *Attaining disease control:* This is the first priority which is achieved through administration of systemic glucocorticoids (prednisolone 0.5-1 mg/kg/day) or a combination of steroids with rituximab.
b. *Incorporating adjuvant immunosuppressive therapy:* Adjuvant immunosuppressants such mycophenolate mofetil or azathioprine are typically advised at the start of the therapy to reduce the dependence on systemic glucocorticoids.
c. *Tapering and cessation of therapy following achievement of disease control:* Therapy is reduced to lowest dose possible so as to prevent the appearance of new lesions.
d. *Symptom management:* Measures are aimed at managing oral pain and cutaneous wounds are additional.

Question 10

1. Enumerate "cold-related emergencies".

a. *Frostbite:*
   i. Frostbite involves tissue freezing with the formation of ice crystals in the tissues.
   ii. Tissue injury occurs due to the structural damage to the cells due to ice crystal formation and to microvascular thrombosis and stasis.
   iii. The term "frostnip" refers to the superficial freezing injury manifested by transient numbness and tingling that resolves after rewarming.
b. *Non-freezing cold injuries:*
   i. *Immersion injuries (trench foot):* It is produced by prolonged exposure to wet cold at temperatures above freezing. It develops slowly over several days resulting in the neurological damage. Most patients of immersion injury are military personnel who have worn boots continuously for several days or weeks.
   ii. *Chilblains or pernio:* Mild form of cold injury which often follows repetitive exposure in susceptible individuals. It appears within 24 hours of the exposure and most commonly affects the face, dorsa of the feet and hands, and pretibial areas. Young females with Raynaud's phenomenon, SLE (systemic lupus erythematosus) or antiphospholipid antibodies are at increased risk. Plaques, blue nodules, or ulceration may develop. These painful lesions last for 1-2 weeks.
   iii. *Panniculitis:* It is characterized by mild degrees of necrosis of subcutaneous fat tissues that develops during prolonged exposure to temperatures above freezing.
   iv. *Cold urticaria:* Hypersensitivity to cold air or water which in rare case can lead to anaphylaxis.

2. Write clinical presentation of hypothermia.

SWISS system classification: This system of classification correlates clinical signs with the standard core temperature ranges of mild, moderate, and severe hypothermia as well as two additional stages—profound hypothermia and death due to hypothermia.

Stages of hypothermia (HT) are:

HT I: Clear consciousness with shivering: 35°-32°C

HT II: Impaired consciousness without shivering: 32°-24°C

HT III: Unconsciousness: 28°-24°C

HT IV: Apparent death: 24°-13.7°C

HT V: Death due to irreversible hypothermia: <13.7°C.

Patients having moderate hypothermia (HT II) **(Table 5)** are likely to be shivering if the core temperature is above 30°-31°C. Rescuers are advised to focus on the level of consciousness rather than the presence or absence of shivering. Trauma and other medical conditions that cause decreased level of consciousness or abnormal vital signs can lead to confusion while classifying the patients. As these conditions may also suppress or abolish shivering the rescuers may rewarm more aggressively at a given core temperature than would otherwise be necessary.

TABLE 5: Signs and symptoms of hypothermia.

System	Features		
	Mild (35°–32°C)	Moderate (32°–28°C)	Severe (<28°C)
CNS	Amnesia, dysarthria, impaired judgement	Drowsiness, mydriasis, paradoxical undressing, hallucinations	Coma, loss of ocular reflexes
CVS	Tachycardia progressing to bradycardia, raised BP	Atrial and ventricular arrhythmias, lowered BP, J wave on ECG	Severe hypotension, bradycardia, asystole
Respiratory system	Tachypnea followed by decrease in minute volume, bronchospasm	Hypoventilation	Pulmonary edema, apnea
Renal and endocrine systems	Cold diuresis, shivering	Increased renal blood flow	Decreased renal blood flow, oliguria, poikilothermic
Musculoskeletal system	Increased muscle tone followed by fatiguing, anoxia	Hyporeflexia, rigidity	No motion, peripheral areflexia

(BP: blood pressure; CNS: central nervous system; CVS: cyclic vomiting syndrome; ECG: electrocardiogram)

3. Write management of accidental hypothermia.

Initiate management of accidental hypothermia as described in **Table 6**.

TABLE 6: Staging and management of accidental hypothermia.

Stage	Clinical symptoms	Typical core temperature	Treatment
HT I	Conscious, shivering	35°–32°C	Warm environment and clothing, warm sweet drinks, and active movement (if possible)
HT II	Impaired consciousness, not shivering	<32°–28°C	Cardiac monitoring, minimal and cautious movements to avoid arrhythmias, horizontal position and immobilization, full-body insulation, active external and minimally invasive rewarming techniques (warm environment; chemical, electrical, or forced-air heating packs or blankets; warm parenteral fluids)
HT III	Unconscious, not shivering vital signs present	<28°–24°C	HT II management plus airway management as required; ECMO or CPB in cases with cardiac instability that is refractory to medical management
HT IV	No vital signs	<24°C	HT II and III management plus CPR and up to three doses of epinephrine (at an intravenous or intraosseous dose of 1 mg) and defibrillation, with further dosing guided by clinical response; rewarming with ECMO or CPB (if available) or CPR with active external and alternative internal rewarming

Hypothermia may be determined clinically on the basis of vital signs with the use of the Swiss staging system. CPB denotes cardiopulmonary bypass, CPR—cardiopulmonary resuscitation, and ECMO—extracorporeal membrane oxygenation.
Measurement of body core temperature is helpful but not mandatory. The risk of cardiac arrest increases as the core temperature drops below 32°C and increases substantially if the temperature is <28°C. To convert values for temperature to degrees Fahrenheit, multiply by 9/5 and add 32.

SUGGESTED READING

1. Richhariya D, Sharma B. Textbook of Emergency Medicine including Intensive Care and Trauma, 2nd edition. New Delhi: Jaypee Brothers Medical Publishers (P) Ltd; 2022. pp. 1086-94. (Question 1).
2. Richhariya D. Sharma B. Textbook of Emergency Medicine including Intensive Care and Trauma, 2nd edition. New Delhi: Jaypee Brothers Medical Publishers (P) Ltd; 2022. pp. 814-9. (Question 2).
3. Richhariya D, Sharma B. Textbook of Emergency Medicine including Intensive Care and Trauma, 2nd edition. New Delhi: Jaypee Brothers Medical Publishers (P) Ltd; 2022. pp. 405, 523, 534. (Question 3).
4. Richhariya D, Sharma B. Textbook of Emergency Medicine including Intensive Care and Trauma, 2nd edition. New Delhi: Jaypee Brothers Medical Publishers (P) Ltd; 2022. p. 1394. (Question 4).
5. Richhariya D, Sharma B. Textbook of Emergency Medicine including Intensive Care and Trauma, 2nd edition. New Delhi: Jaypee Brothers Medical Publishers (P) Ltd; 2022. pp. 753-60. (Question 5).
6. Richhariya D, Sharma B. Textbook of Emergency Medicine including Intensive Care and Trauma, 2nd edition. New Delhi: Jaypee Brothers Medical Publishers (P) Ltd; 2022. pp. 1317-27. (Question 6).
7. Richhariya D, Sharma B. Textbook of Emergency Medicine including Intensive Care and Trauma, 2nd edition. New Delhi: Jaypee Brothers Medical Publishers (P) Ltd; 2022. pp. 894-8. (Question 7).
8. Richhariya D, Sharma B. Textbook of Emergency Medicine including Intensive Care and Trauma, 2nd edition. New Delhi: Jaypee Brothers Medical Publishers (P) Ltd; 2022. pp. 838, 1725. (Question 8).
9. Richhariya D, Sharma B. Textbook of Emergency Medicine including Intensive Care and Trauma, 2nd edition. New Delhi: Jaypee Brothers Medical Publishers (P) Ltd; 2022. pp. 1021-2. (Question 9).
10. Richhariya D, Sharma B. Textbook of Emergency Medicine including Intensive Care and Trauma, 2nd edition. New Delhi: Jaypee Brothers Medical Publishers (P) Ltd; 2022. pp. 1686-91. (Question 10).

Emergency Medicine Paper 8

Anshul Jain

Question 1

1. Tabulate differences in single rescuer cardiopulmonary resuscitation (CPR) in a neonate, infant, and child in cardiac arrest (Table 1).

TABLE 1: Cardiopulmonary resuscitation in neonate, infant, and child.

Components	Neonate	Infant	Child
CPR hand placement	Two-finger technique	One hand on the forehead and two fingers on the center of chest in the lower half of the sternum just below the nipple line	One hand in the center of the chest just below the sternum and the other hand above it
CPR compression depths	At least 1.5 inches	At least 1.5 inches	At least 2 inches
Rapid assessment	• Term gestation? • Crying? • Good muscle tone?	Check for respiration and brachial pulse	Check for the carotid pulse
CPR compressions per minute	30:2 (single rescuer)	30:2 (single rescuer)	30:2 (single rescuer)

(CPR: cardiopulmonary resuscitation)

2. What is the role of vasopressin in adult CPR?

a. Vasopressin is a nonadrenergic peripheral vasoconstrictor that causes coronary and renal vasoconstriction.
b. Vasopressin was removed from the American Heart Association Adult Cardiac Arrest Algorithm in 2015 when initial trials failed to demonstrate any significant benefit when compared with or combined with epinephrine.
c. As per the updated advanced cardiac life support (ACLS) 2019 guidelines, vasopressin may be considered during cardiac arrest in combination with epinephrine but provides no added advantage when used as a substitute for epinephrine (Level of Evidence C-LD).

3. What is the role of coronary angiography in an adult in postcardiac arrest phase?

a. The COACT (Coronary Angiography After Cardiac Arrest) trial showed that immediate angiography with an intent to revascularize is not superior to delayed angiography among patients presenting with out-of-hospital cardiac arrest secondary to a shockable rhythm and with no echocardiography (ECG) evidence of ST-segment elevations post-return of spontaneous circulation (ROSC).

Question 2

A 1-year-old child weighing 7 kg presents with diarrhea for 2 days.

1. How do you evaluate the degree of dehydration?

A child with diarrhea should be assessed for (a) dehydration, (b) blood in diarrhea, (c) coexisting malnutrition, and (d) serious nonintestinal infections. **Table 2** and by child dehydration scale **Table 3**.

TABLE 2: Severity of dehydration in a child.

Signs and symptoms	Mild dehydration (3–5%)	Moderate dehydration (5–10%)	Severe dehydration (> 10%)
Dry mucous membrane	±	+	+
Reduced skin turgor	–	±	+
Depressed anterior fontanelle	–	+	+
Mental status	Alert	Irritable	Lethargic
Sunken eyeballs	–	+	+
Hypotension	–	±	+
Capillary refill time	<2 seconds	>2 seconds	>2 seconds

TABLE 3: Clinical dehydration scale.

Symptoms	0 (no dehydration) <3%	1 (some dehydration) 3–6%	2 (moderate dehydration) >6%
General appearance	Normal	Thirsty, restless, or lethargic	Drowsy, sweaty, or comatose
Eyes	Normal	Slightly sunken	Very much sunken
Mucous membranes	Moist	Sticky	Dry
Tears	Present	Decreased	absent

2. What is the complication of oral rehydration solution?

a. Electrolyte imbalances
b. Upper gastrointestinal hemorrhage
c. Restlessness
d. Irritability
e. Swelling of ankles
f. Seizures.

3. Discuss the management of the above-mentioned child if he has severe dehydration.

a. *Monitoring airway:* Start oxygen and attach monitors.
b. *IV rehydration*: Take two large-bore IV cannulas and give 140 mL of 0.9% normal saline (NS) bolus over 5 minutes and then repeat if the patient is hemodynamically unstable.
c. *Replacement of ongoing losses after initial rehydration:* 5–10 mL of 0.9% NS (70 mL) or 5% dextrose in 0.9% NS to be given after every watery stool and 2 mL/kg (14 mL) 0.9% NS or 5% dextrose in 0.9% NS to be given after every emesis.
d. *Maintenance fluids:* @ 28 mL/h isotonic fluids to be given as maintenance.
e. *Investigations to be done:* Electrolytes, blood urea nitrogen (BUN), creatinine, calcium, and glucose levels, and urinalysis.

Question 3

1. What is rapid-sequence intubation (RSI)?

Seven Ps of RSI are:
1. *Preparation:* In the initial phase, the patient is assessed for intubation difficulty, unless this has already been done, and the intubation is planned, including determining dosages and sequence of drugs, tube size, and laryngoscope type, blade, and size. Drugs are drawn up and labeled. All patients require continuous cardiac and pulse oximetry monitoring.
2. *Preoxygenation:* Administration of 100% oxygen for 3 minutes of normal tidal volume breathing in a normal healthy adult establishes an adequate oxygen reservoir to permit 6–8 minutes of safe apnea before oxygen desaturation to < 90% occurs.
3. *Pretreatment:* During this phase, drugs are administered 3 minutes before the administration of a paralytic agent and an induction agent to mitigate the adverse physiologic effects of laryngoscopy and intubation on the patient's presenting condition.
4. *Paralysis with induction:* In this phase, a potent sedative agent is administered by rapid IV push in a dose capable of producing unconsciousness rapidly. This is immediately followed by rapid administration of an intubating dose of a neuromuscular blocking agent (NMBA), either succinylcholine at a dose of 1.5 mg/kg IV or rocuronium at a dose of 1 mg/kg.
5. *Positioning:* The patient should be positioned for intubation as consciousness is lost. Usually, positioning involves head extension, often with flexion of the neck on the body.
6. *Placement of the tube:* Approximately 45–60 seconds after administration of the NMBA, the patient is relaxed sufficiently to permit laryngoscopy. This is assessed most easily by moving the mandible to test for mobility and absence of muscle tone.
7. *Postintubation management:* After confirmation of tube placement by end-tidal carbon dioxide ($ETCO_2$), obtain a chest radiograph to confirm that mainstem intubation has not occurred and to assess the lungs. If available, place the patient on continuous capnography.

2. What are the preferred induction agents in RSI?

a. *Ketamine:* Dose: 1.5 mg/kg IV; Onset: 60–90 seconds; Duration: 10–20 minutes; Use: Any RSI, especially if hemodynamically unstable [OK in traumatic brain injury (TBI), does not increase intracranial pressure (ICP)] despite traditional dogma] or if reactive airways disease (causes bronchodilation)
b. *Propofol:* Dose: 1–2.5 mg/kg; Onset: 15–45 seconds; Duration: 5–10 minutes; Use: Hemodynamically stable patients, reactive airways disease, status epilepticus
c. *Fentanyl:* Dose: 2–10 µg/kg; Onset: <60 seconds; Duration: Dose dependent (30 minutes for 1–2 µg/kg, 6 hours for 100 µg/kg); Use: May be used in a low dose as a sympatholytic premedication
d. *Midazolam:* Dose: 0.3 mg/kg; Onset: 60–90 seconds; Duration: 15–30 minutes not usually recommended for RSI

e. *Etomidate:* Dose: 0.3 mg/kg IV Onset: 10–15 seconds; Use: Suitable for most situations including hemodynamically unstable situations, other than sepsis or seizures.

3. What are the contraindications for using succinylcholine in RSI?

a. Burns >10% body surface area
b. Crush injuries can lead to rhabdomyolysis and hyperkalemia.
c. Denervation (stroke/spinal cord injuries)
d. Neuromuscular disorders (amyotrophic lateral sclerosis, muscular dystrophy, and multiple sclerosis)
e. Intra-abdominal sepsis

Question 4

1. Discuss the revised Geneva score for diagnosis of pulmonary embolism (PE).

Three scoring systems have been prospectively tested and validated in large clinical trials: Wells score, Geneva score **(Table 4)**, and Pisa score. The Pisa score is more appropriately used for hospitalized patients, whereas the Wells and Geneva scores were developed for use in the emergency department (ED).

2. Name newer anticoagulants in treatment of venous thromboembolism (VTE).

Systemic anticoagulation is the mainstay of the treatment for VTE **(Table 5)**.

TABLE 4: Revised Geneva score for assessing probability of pulmonary embolism.

Clinical variables	Points
>65 years of age	1
History of venous thromboembolism	1
Lower limb fracture (in previous month) or surgery requiring anesthesia	1
Malignancy (active)	1
Leg pain (unilateral)	1
Hemoptysis	1
Unilateral limb edema or pain	1
Heart rate >95 bpm	1

Note: Interpretation of score: 0–3 indicates low probability, 4–10 indicates moderate probability, and >10 indicates high probability of pulmonary embolism.

TABLE 5: Treatment for deep vein thrombosis and pulmonary embolism.

Unfractionated heparin	80 units/kg IV bolus followed by 18 units/kg/h continuous infusion, with aPTT checked after 6 hours and infusion adjusted to maintain aPTT 1.5–2.5 times the standard
Enoxaparin	1 mg/kg SC every 12 hours or 1.5 mg/kg daily
Dalteparin	200 units/kg SC once daily
Tinzaparin	175 mg/kg once daily
Fondaparinux	<50 kg: 5 mg SC once daily, 50–100 kg: 7.5 mg SC once daily, and >100 kg: 10 mg SC once daily
Warfarin	2–5 mg/day for 2–4 days, followed by 1–10 mg/day as indicated by INR
Dabigatran	150 mg PO twice daily (after 5–10 days of parenteral anticoagulation)
Apixaban	10 mg PO twice daily for 7 days and then 5 mg twice daily
Rivaroxaban	15 mg PO twice daily for 21 days and then 20 mg once daily
Streptokinase	2,50,000 unit IV bolus followed by 1,00,000 unit/h continuous infusion for 1–3 days or alteplase 100 mg IV infused over 2 hours or tenecteplase weight-tiered single IV bolus (<60 kg: 30 mg), (60–70 kg: 35 mg), (70–80 kg: 40 mg), (80–90 kg: 45 mg), and (>90 kg: 50 mg)

(aPTT: activated partial thromboplastin time; INR: international normalized ratio; IV: intravenous)

3. Discuss the treatment of subsegmental PE.

a. Isolated subsegmental PE is a filling defect seen in one small pulmonary artery, usually <3 mm in diameter.
b. Patients with only subsegmental PE without any risk factors should be started on oral anticoagulants (apixaban 10 mg BD or rivaroxaban 15 mg BD) for 1 month.
c. Check for the D-dimer levels after 1 month.
d. If the levels are normal, then stop the anticoagulation and assess for the risk factors.

Question 5

A young child is admitted in the emergency with upper respiratory infection (URI) and respiratory distress. You notice a "whoop".

1. What are the clinical features of this disease in adults?

The disease is characterized by three clinical stages—catarrhal stage, paroxysmal stage, and convalescent stage. Pertussis begins with mild upper respiratory tract symptoms and cough; this catarrhal stage usually lasts 1–2 weeks. The disease progresses to severe paroxysms of a staccato cough, followed by post-tussive emesis, and may be accompanied by periods of cyanosis. The paroxysmal stage lasts 2–4 weeks and is followed by a convalescent stage, during which symptoms gradually wane. Adults generally do not have a classical presentation of pertussis. They have a milder but a prolonged phase of illness. Adults are considered to be the reservoir of the disease.

2. Discuss the treatment of *Bordetella pertussis* infection.

a. Monitoring of airway, breathing, and circulation
b. Supportive care
c. Drug of choice is azithromycin
d. Other drugs can also be given such as erythromycin and trimethoprim–sulfamethoxazole
e. Erythromycin has a risk of causing infantile hypertrophic pyloric stenosis, so azithromycin is the preferred drug
f. Antimicrobials have no effect on disease progression after the progression to paroxysmal stage but limit the spread of organisms.

3. What is the role of vaccination?

There are two vaccines that include protection against whooping cough: The DTaP vaccine protects young children from diphtheria, tetanus, and whooping cough. The TDaP vaccine protects preteens, teens, and adults from tetanus, diphtheria, and whooping cough. The Centers for Disease Control and Prevention (CDC) routinely recommends DTaP at 2, 4, and 6 months, at 15–18 months, and at 4–6 years. The CDC routinely recommends TDaP for children of age 7–10 years who are not fully vaccinated against pertussis: Single dose of TDaP for those who are not fully vaccinated.

Question 6

Surviving Sepsis Campaign: International Guidelines for management of severe sepsis were revised in 2016. As per the guidelines, discuss the following.

1. Initial resuscitation of septic shock.

Intravenous crystalloids and hemodynamic monitoring are recommended, as given in **Table 6**.

TABLE 6: Initial resuscitation of septic shock.

Points	Weak Recommendation	Strong Recommendation
For the patients with sepsis-induced hypoperfusion/septic shock, start IV crystalloids at least @ 30 mL/kg within 3 hours of identification of shock	Yes	–
Dynamic measures to be used to guide fluid resuscitation instead of physical examination or static parameters alone	Yes	–
Guidelines suggest to use subsequent decreasing levels of lactates as a sign of improvement	Yes	–
Capillary refill time to be used as an adjunct to guide the resuscitation to other parameters	Yes	–
Antimicrobials to be given immediately or within 1 hour of recognition of septic shock	–	Yes

2. Use of antibiotics.

a. Early administration of appropriate antimicrobials is one of the most effective interventions to reduce mortality in patients with sepsis.
b. Surviving Sepsis Guidelines 2021 suggest initiating antibiotics in patients with possible sepsis without shock as soon as sepsis appears to be the most likely diagnosis, and no later than 3 hours after sepsis was first suspected if concern for sepsis still persists at that time.
c. Overall, given the high risk of death with septic shock and the strong association of antimicrobial timing and mortality, the panel issued a strong recommendation to administer antimicrobials immediately, and within 1 hour, in all patients with potential septic shock.
d. For patients with possible sepsis without shock, the panel recommended a rapid assessment of infectious and noninfectious etiologies of illness be undertaken to determine, within 3 hours, whether antibiotics should be administered or whether antibiotics should be deferred while continuing to monitor the patient closely.

3. Use of vasoactive medications.

a. For adults with septic shock, the panel *recommends* using norepinephrine as the first-line agent over other vasopressors.
b. For adults with septic shock on norepinephrine with inadequate mean arterial pressure (MAP) levels, the panel *suggests* adding vasopressin instead of escalating the dose of norepinephrine.

c. For adults with septic shock and inadequate MAP levels despite norepinephrine and vasopressin, the panel *suggests* adding epinephrine.

Question 7

1. Discuss the principles of managing serious traumatic brain injury in children.

a. Management of traumatic brain injury in children involves the rapid, early assessment and management of the airway, breathing, circulation, disability, exposures (ABCDEs), as well as appropriate neurosurgical involvement from the beginning of treatment.
b. Focus is on preventing secondary brain injuries—hypoxia and hypoperfusion.
c. Differences in the anatomy of adult head and pediatric head:
   i. The cranial vault of a child is larger and heavier in proportion to the total body mass. This predisposes young children to high degrees of torque that are generated by forces along the cervical spine axis.
   ii. Sutures within the pediatric skull are both protective and detrimental to the outcome of head injury. Although the cranium may be more pliable relative to traumatic insult, forces are generated internally that predispose the pediatric patient to parenchymal injury in the absence of skull fractures.
   iii. The pediatric brain is less myelinated, with higher water content, predisposing it to shearing forces, further injury, and posttraumatic seizures.
   iv. For performing head CT in pediatric age group, Pediatric Emergency Care Applied Research Network (PECARN) criteria are used **(Flowchart 1)**.
   v. Early and controlled intubation is recommended in pediatric traumatic brain injury with deteriorating Glasgow Coma Score (GCS).
   vi. The use of anticonvulsants after moderate-to-severe head injury in children is controversial. Early prophylaxis does not decrease the incidence of late seizures and is not recommended for this purpose. However, because early seizures after trauma are discordant with the management principles of acute brain injury, some guidelines suggest the use of prophylactic anticonvulsants (most often phenytoin or levetiracetam).
   vii. Herniation syndromes in children are similar to those in adults. Management of suspected acute herniation begins with immediate controlled hyperventilation.

Flowchart 1: PECARN criteria suggested CT algorithm for children (A) younger than 2 years and (B) for those aged 2 years or older with GCS of 14–15 after head trauma.

(A)
- GCS = 14 or other signs of altered mental status, or palpable skull fracture
  - Yes (13.9% of population, 4.4% risk of ciTBI) → CT recommended
  - No ↓
- Occipital or parietal or temporal scalp hematoma, or history of LOC ≥5 seconds, or severe mechanism of injury, or not acting normally per parent
  - Yes (32.6% of population, 0.9% risk of ciTBI) → Observation versus CT on the basis of other clinical factors including:
    - Physician experience
    - Multiple versus isolated findings
    - Worsening symptoms or signs after emergency department observation
    - Age <3 months
    - Parental preference
  - No (53.5 of population, <0.02% risk of ciTBI) → CT not recommended

(B)
- GCS = 14 or other signs of altered mental status, or signs of basilar skull fracture
  - Yes (14.0% of population, 4.3% risk of ciTBI) → CT recommended
  - No ↓
- History of LOC, or history of vomiting, or severe mechanism of injury, or severe headache
  - Yes (27.7% of population, 0.9% risk of ciTBI) → Observation versus CT on the basis of other clinical factors including:
    - Physician experience
    - Multiple versus isolated findings
    - Worsening symptoms or signs after emergency department observation
    - Parental preference
  - No (58.3 of population, <0.05% risk of ciTBI) → CT not recommended

(GCS: Glasgow Coma Scale; LOC: loss of consciousness; ciTBI: clinically important traumatic brain injury)

2. What is revised trauma score?

Revised trauma score is a physiological scoring system used in trauma patients based on initial vital signs of the patient. The lower the score, the higher the degree of injury. Score ranges from 0 to 12 **(Table 7)**.

TABLE 7: Revised trauma scale.

RTS	GCS	Systolic BP (mm Hg)	Respiratory rate
4	13–15	>89	10–29
3	9–12	76–89	>29
2	6–8	50–75	6–9
1	4–5	1–49	1–5
0	3	0	0

(BP: blood pressure; GCS: Glasgow coma scale; RTS: revised trauma scale)

Question 8

1. What are the indications for "procedural sedation" in a child?

Procedural sedation is indicated any time a pediatric patient requires a procedure that requires anxiolysis for the proper technique or intervention that will cause significant discomfort. The level of sedation is tailored to the amount of sedation needed depending on the amount of pain or anxiety that will be caused by the procedure or the necessity to keep the patient still. For instance, a child may require anxiolysis in order to obtain CT or MRI imaging or need deeper sedation for more painful procedures such as fracture reduction or complex lacerations.

The patient's vital signs and overall stability must be taken into account in unscheduled procedures, along with consideration of the patient's history of chronic disease or genetic abnormalities (e.g., cardiovascular or respiratory disease, Down syndrome, cerebral palsy), medication history, and allergies. The physical status evaluation of the airway is based on the American Society of Anesthesiologists (ASA) classification system:

- *ASA class I:* Healthy patient with no acute or chronic disease and normal body mass index (BMI) percentile for age
- *ASA class II:* Patient with mild systemic disease without acute worsening or exacerbation. Examples include asymptomatic congenital heart disease, well-controlled dysrhythmia, well-controlled epilepsy, and asthma without exacerbation.
- *ASA class III:* Patient with severe systemic disease without immediate danger of death, including uncorrected stable congenital cardiac abnormality, poorly controlled epilepsy, cystic fibrosis, morbid obesity, metabolic disease, and history of organ transplantation.
- *ASA class IV:* Patient with severe systemic disease that represents a constant threat to life, such as symptomatic congenital cardiac abnormality, severe trauma, sepsis, severe respiratory distress, congestive heart failure, and acute hypoxic–ischemic encephalopathy.
- *ASA class V:* Moribund patients not expected to survive without operation, including massive trauma, a patient requiring extracorporeal membrane oxygenation (ECMO), intracranial hemorrhage with mass effect, respiratory failure or arrest, and multiple organ system dysfunction.
- *ASA class VI:* Patient declared brain dead whose organs are being harvested for donor purposes.

2. List the preferred agents for procedural sedation in children.

The ED is the place where sedation and analgesia are provided for unscheduled procedures. In procedural sedation and analgesia (PSA) processes, various anxiolytics, sedatives, hypnotics, and/or dissociative medication are being used. These agents provide amnesia, decrease awareness, and increase a patient's comfort and safety during diagnostic and therapeutic procedures in the ED **(Table 8)**.

TABLE 8: Drugs for procedural sedation.

Drugs	Dose	Onset of action	Effectiveness	Comments
Propofol	• 0.5–1 mg/kg • Repeat dose 0.25–0.5 mg/kg • In elderly 0.25–0.5 mg/kg	<1 minute	<10 minutes	• Good for orthopedic reduction as rapid onset and short duration of action • Respiratory depression may occur • Do not provide analgesia
Ketamine	• 1–1.5 mg/kg over 1 minute • Repeat dose 0.5–1 mg/kg • For only analgesia 0.1–0.3 mg/kg	<1 minute	10 minutes	• Acts as both sedative and analgesia safer in comorbid conditions • Provides cardiorespiratory stability. • To be avoided in psychiatric illness
Etomidate	• 0.1–0.2 mg/kg • Repeat dose 0.05 mg /kg	Less than a minute	<5 minutes	• Useful for short procedure and cardioversion • Minimum cardiac and respiratory depression

Contd...

Contd...

Drugs	Dose	Onset of action	Effectiveness	Comments
Ketamine + Propofol (ketofol-single syringe)	0.5 mg + 0.5 mg	<1 minute	<10 minutes	• Ketamine adds analgesic properties. Blunt propofol induces hypotension, good for prolonged procedure • Longer time for recovery if ratio increases
Midazolam	• 1–2.5 mg • Repeat dose 0.5–2.5 mg • Repeat dose in every 3 minutes • For elderly dose 0.05 mg/kg	<5 minutes	30–60 minutes	• Useful for longer procedures • Does not provide analgesia, so combined with analgesic • Cardiovascular and respiratory depression
Fentanyl	• 0.5–1.5 µg/kg • Repeat dose is the same every 2–3 minutes • In elderly, dose is 0.25 µg/kg	<2 minutes	30–60 minutes	• Monotherapy used for minimal sedation • Respiratory depression may occur
Alfentanil	• 10 µg/kg • Repeat dose also same • Reduced dose is used in elderly	Less than a minute	<10 minutes	• Fast onset and short duration of action • Increased risk of apnea
Remifentanil	• 0.16 µg/kg/min infusion or 1 µg/kg bolus • Less doses in elderly	Immediate	10 minutes	• Fast onset and short duration of action • Increased risk of apnea

3. What precautions/monitoring you would follow in a sedated child after procedural sedation?

a. After the procedure, monitoring in the ED is necessary until recovery is complete and the child has resumed the presedation level of consciousness.
b. Monitoring should include obtaining vital signs at regular intervals (every 5 minutes while sedated and less frequently once awake) and continuous display of heart rate and oxygen saturation if not fully alert.
c. There is an increased risk of respiratory depression during the procedure. For this reason, patients should be monitored in a recovery area that is equipped with a suction device, the ability to deliver >90% oxygen, positive-pressure ventilation using a bag-valve mask, and rescue equipment for airway and ventilatory support.
d. If sedation was performed using ketamine, even with the preadministration of ondansetron, nausea and vomiting may occur and should be anticipated.
e. Parents should review and understand written postsedation discharge instructions, which advise them to closely observe their child for abnormal somnolence and to restrict activities that require coordination until all medication effects have worn off.
f. Parents should also be warned that delayed sequelae of sedation, including vivid dreams, sleep disturbance, and behavioral dysregulation, may occur up to 24 hours after sedation.
g. Parents should be advised to protect the child from falls due to incoordination for several hours after discharge.

Question 9

A young boy presents to the emergency with painful red eye with photophobia.

1. List the causes.

a. Conjunctivitis
b. Corneal abrasions
c. Foreign bodies
d. Ocular burns
e. Corneal ulcers
f. Keratitis
g. Acute angle closure glaucoma
h. Anterior uveitis (iritis)
i. Scleritis/episcleritis
j. Cellulitis (preorbital and orbital)
k. Subconjunctival hemorrhage.

2. How will you evaluate a child for corneal abrasion?

a. A thorough eye examination should be performed.
b. The upper lid should be everted, looking for subtarsal foreign bodies. Fluorescein should be instilled to assess for a corneal abrasion or a corneal foreign body.
c. A penetrating injury can be very subtle and the eye should be carefully inspected with a slit lamp for a corneoscleral wound.
d. Other signs include reduced visual acuity, pupil irregularity, hyphema (bleeding into the anterior chamber), and/or vitreous hemorrhage.

Management of corneal trauma: Nonpenetrating trauma
a. *Foreign body removal:* Local anesthetic drops should be instilled and the foreign body removed with a cotton bud. If this is unsuccessful, a 23 G needle can be used, with a slit lamp.
b. If removal is incomplete, referral to ophthalmology is required.
c. Topical antibiotics
d. Dilation of the pupil with cyclopentolate can ease the pain from iris spasm.
e. Oral analgesics
f. Eye pad (only required for patient comfort)

Management of corneal trauma: Penetrating trauma
a. Orbital X-ray (eyes up, eyes down) to look for a radio-opaque foreign body
b. Apply an eye shield (an eye pad should not be used because the pressure on the eye may exacerbate the injury).
c. Analgesia
d. Ensure adequate tetanus prophylaxis.
e. Urgent ophthalmology referral

3. Treatment of a child with chemical injury in the eye.

a. Irrigation should begin at the scene and continue in the ED with 1–2 L of NS.
b. Instil a topical anesthetic and continue irrigation for at least 30 minutes. Then check pH by touching a strip of litmus paper to the inferior conjunctival fornix. *If the pH is >7.4, continue irrigation until the pH remains neutral 30 minutes after the last irrigation.*
c. After irrigation and maintenance of ocular pH >7.4, perform the eye examination. Inspect the facial skin and eyelids for burns. Evert the eyelids and remove any particulate matter with a cotton applicator.
d. Document visual acuity and measure intraocular pressure. Intraocular pressure may be increased if the trabecular meshwork has been damaged.
e. Use the slit lamp to evaluate corneal injury and to detect for cells and flare in the anterior chamber. Injury to the cornea may range from punctate defects to complete loss of epithelium. The cornea may become cloudy with severe burns.
f. Urgent pediatric ophthalmology consult is a must.
g. A topical cycloplegic agent (cyclopentolate 1%, one drop) should be used three times daily for pain reduction if an epithelial defect is present.

Question 10

A young child is brought to the emergency with multiple bruises.

1. When would you suspect child abuse based on the presence of multiple bruises?

a. Injuries inconsistent with the history given
b. Injuries inappropriate for the developmental age
c. Changing history either between parents/carers/child or alterations over time
d. Vague history or lacking details
e. Delay in seeking medical attention with no adequate explanation
f. Abnormal parental attitudes (e.g., lack of parental concern)
g. *Frequent ED attendances:* Children with three or more attendances for different conditions in the past year.

2. What are the other injuries noted in abused children?

a. *Bruising:* Especially in areas that are not usually injured (e.g., not on a bony prominence) and if in the pattern of a hand, ligature, stick, teeth marks, grip, or implement
b. *Lacerations, abrasions, and scars:* For which there is inadequate explanation
c. *Bite marks*
d. *Burns and scalds:* Especially on areas that would not be expected to come into contact with a hot object in an accident (e.g., back of hands, soles, buttocks), or in the shape of an implement (e.g., cigarette, iron), or suggesting immersion
e. *Fractures:* That are multiple and/or of different ages without adequate explanation (i.e., no medical condition that predisposes to fragile bones, e.g., osteogenesis imperfecta, osteopenia, prematurity). These include fractures of ribs or the spine.
f. *Intracranial injuries:* In the absence of major confirmed accidental trauma or known medical cause
g. Eye trauma (e.g., retinal hemorrhages or eye injuries in the absence of confirmed major trauma or medical explanation)
h. Oral injury such as a torn frenulum, without adequate explanation

3. How would you investigate and treat an abused child?

a. The immediate management should involve ensuring that the child is pain free and treating any injuries or illness appropriately.
b. Meticulous documentation is essential. Notes should be factual (e.g., 4 × 1 cm round bruises found on the medial aspect of the left upper arm) and not attribute blame or causation (e.g., finger imprints found on the medial

aspect of the left upper arm). Documenting injuries in a diagram is a useful way to capture information.
c. If sexual assault is suspected, a genital examination should not be pursued in the ED. This should be performed only once, by a senior clinician in child protection, in collaboration with a police surgeon (clinical forensic physician).
d. Further information should be gathered about the child, e.g., checking whether the child or any siblings are known to social services or whether they are subject of a child protection plan, looking up previous ED attendances, contacting the child's previous doctor to gain past medical history of the child and family (parental–maternal health and substance abuse issues).

SUGGESTED READING

1. Richhariya D, Sharma B. Textbook of Emergency Medicine including Intensive Care and Trauma, 2nd edition. New Delhi: Jaypee Brothers Medical Publishers (P) Ltd; 2022. pp. 1124-35. (Question 1).
2. Richhariya D, Sharma B. Textbook of Emergency Medicine including Intensive Care and Trauma, 2nd edition. New Delhi: Jaypee Brothers Medical Publishers (P) Ltd; 2022. pp. 1177-80. (Question 2).
3. Richhariya D, Sharma B. Textbook of Emergency Medicine including Intensive Care and Trauma, 2nd edition. New Delhi: Jaypee Brothers Medical Publishers (P) Ltd; 2022. pp. 208-18. (Question 3).
4. Richhariya D, Sharma B. Textbook of Emergency Medicine including Intensive Care and Trauma, 2nd edition. New Delhi: Jaypee Brothers Medical Publishers (P) Ltd; 2022. pp. 521-8. (Question 4).
5. Richhariya D, Sharma B. Textbook of Emergency Medicine including Intensive Care and Trauma, 2nd edition. New Delhi: Jaypee Brothers Medical Publishers (P) Ltd; 2022. pp. 1185-9. (Question 5).
6. Richhariya D, Sharma B. Textbook of Emergency Medicine including Intensive Care and Trauma, 2nd edition. New Delhi: Jaypee Brothers Medical Publishers (P) Ltd; 2022. pp. 319-27. (Question 6).
7. Richhariya D, Sharma B. Textbook of Emergency Medicine including Intensive Care and Trauma, 2nd edition. New Delhi: Jaypee Brothers Medical Publishers (P) Ltd; 2022. pp. 1641-5. (Question 7).
8. Richhariya D, Sharma B. Textbook of Emergency Medicine including intensive care & Trauma, 2nd edition. New Delhi: Jaypee Brothers Medical Publishers (P) Ltd; 2022. pp. 350-4. (Question 8).
9. Richhariya D, Sharma B. Textbook of Emergency Medicine including intensive care & Trauma, 2nd edition. New Delhi: Jaypee Brothers Medical Publishers (P) Ltd; 2022. pp. 900-6. (Question 9).
10. Richhariya D, Sharma B. Textbook of Emergency Medicine including intensive care & Trauma, 2nd edition. New Delhi: Jaypee Brothers Medical Publishers (P) Ltd; 2022. pp. 1641-5. (Question 10).

Emergency Medicine Paper 9

Olita Shilpakar, Bipin Karki

Question 1

1. How do you predict difficult airway by LEMON and MOANS method?

The LEMON method is a tool developed to determine any airway management difficulties. It is a fast and easy technique to evaluate a patient's airways in the emergency situation. It has shown to have reasonable sensitivity and high negative predictive value.

It consists of the following assessments:
a. L—Look externally (facial trauma, large incisors, beard or moustache, and large tongue)
b. E—Evaluate the 3-3-2 rule (incisor distance <3 finger-breadths, hyoid/mental distance <3 finger-breadths, thyroid-to-mouth distance <2 finger-breadths)
c. M—Mallampati (Mallampati score ≥3)
d. O—Obstruction (presence of any condition that could cause an obstructed airway)
e. N—Neck mobility (limited neck mobility).

The predictors of difficult bag-mask ventilation are described by the mnemonic "MOANS." It is also a reliable and instant technique to assess the airway in emergency conditions.

It stands for:
a. M—Suboptimal mask seal
b. O—Obstruction or obesity
c. A—Advanced age (>55 years old)
d. N—No teeth
e. S—Stiffness of the lungs

2. Explain the role of rapid-sequence intubation in unstable cervical spine.

Unstable cervical spine is an indication for rapid-sequence intubation (RSI).

Patients with suspected cervical spine injury are mostly intubated via direct laryngoscopy (DL) with in-line cervical spine immobilization. With this approach, excessive lifting force may be required since the glottis view can be inadequate. In case of an unstable cervical spine, a flexible bronchoscope is used to minimize cervical spine motion. However, in the emergency setting, a videolaryngoscope should be used if available. A videolaryngoscope with a hyperangulated blade shape provides superior laryngeal views without excessive cervical spine movement. It also has higher intubation success rates as compared to the conventional DL. The intubating laryngeal mask airway (I-LMA) is another device which helps to minimize cervical spine movement during intubation than DL. However, in cases where these devices are not available, the traditional in-line cervical spine immobilization is the key to perform RSI in an unstable cervical spine.

3. What are supraglottic airways?

Supraglottic airways (SGAs) are devices placed in the oropharynx, allowing for oxygenation and ventilation without the visualized or surgical insertion of a tube into the trachea. These devices bridge to endotracheal intubation or a rescue device after unsuccessful intubation efforts. They provide some aspiration protection but do not fully secure the airway and can only withstand a small amount of positive-pressure ventilation so they are not used for prolonged ventilation. They are mostly used in apneic, unconscious patients since their large cuffs can cause gagging and discomfort in awake patients. In the out-of-hospital setting, these devices improve survival after cardiac arrest compared to endotracheal intubation.

After inserting the SGA, confirmation of proper position is done with end-tidal carbon dioxide and is secured with a tape. Different types of SGAs are commercially available. Some of the important ones are described below:

I-gel: The i-gel has a soft, gel-like cuff that seals the perilaryngeal structures without inflation which limits tissue compression caused by large cuffed devices. Lubricate the gel-like cuff prior to insertion and advance the device into the posterior pharynx until resistance is met and the lips align with the lip line on the i-gel. Complications of i-gel include laryngospasm and sore throat and rarely vasovagal asystole and glottic hematoma. The i-gel is available in various sizes for patients from 2 to >90 kg.

King laryngeal tube (King LT): It is a single-lumen tube with a proximal cuff that seals the posterior oropharynx, while a distal cuff occludes the esophagus. It is placed blindly into the oropharynx until the lip aligns with the device lip line. The balloon is then inflated to a pressure of 60 cmH$_2$O. Tongue engorgement is a complication of this tube since the proximal balloon can impair venous drainage of the tongue which can be overcome by removing the tube. It is available in several sizes depending on the patient's height: 4–5 feet, size 3 (yellow); 5–6 feet, size 4 (red); and >6 feet, size 5 (purple).

LMA: It is an SGA placed blindly through the mouth by occluding the structures around the larynx. It consists of a single cuff inflated with 20–30 mL of air. To insert the LMA, place a gloved index finger into the oropharynx to guide the device into the oropharynx and position the cuff around the larynx. It is useful when the vocal cords cannot be visualized during intubation attempts. There are various models, including an I-LMA, that allow an endotracheal tube to be passed through the lumen. Complications of the LMA include partial or complete airway obstruction and aspiration of gastric contents. LMA is available in several sizes based on the patient's estimated body weight: 50–70 kg, size 4; 70–100 kg, size 5; and >100 kg, size 6.

Question 2

1. Show a diagram depicting anatomy of subclavian vein relevant to its venous access.

Anatomy of subclavian vein is shown in **Figures 1A and B**.

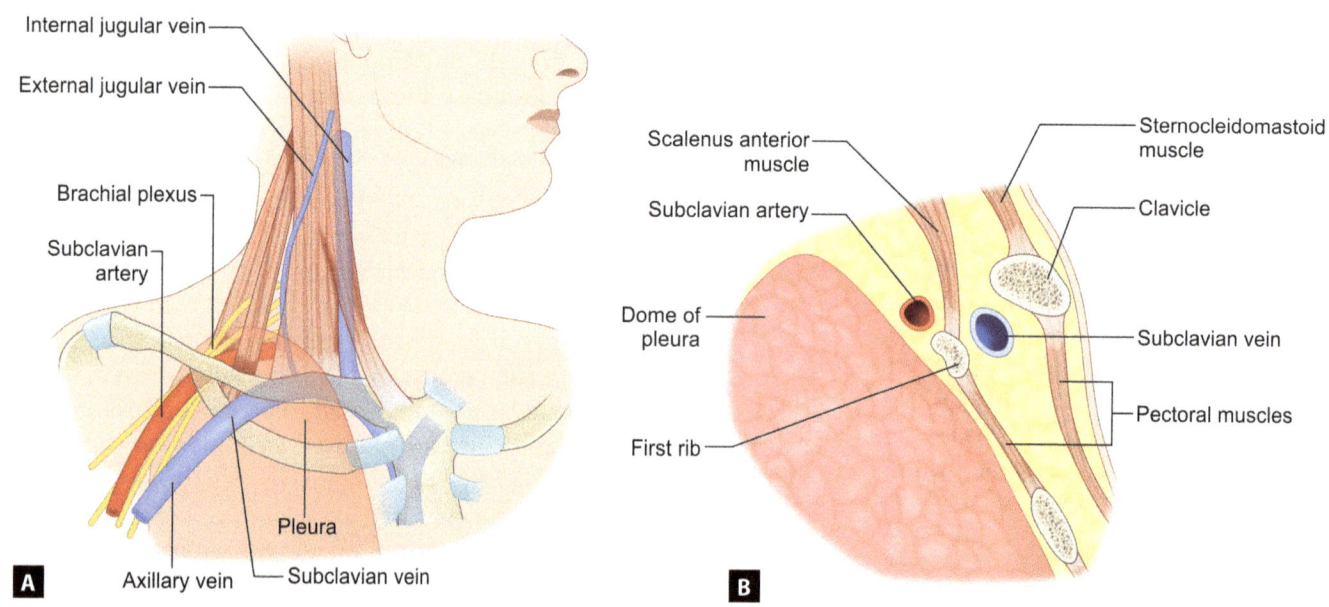

Figs. 1A and B: (A) Anatomy of subclavian vein; (B) Cross-section showing relation to clavicle.

2. What are the indications of central venous catheterization in the emergency department?

a. Inability to obtain peripheral access
b. Central circulation access needed for procedures such as urgent hemodialysis, pulmonary artery catheter placement, and transvenous pacemaker placement
c. Measurement of central venous pressure in conditions such as sepsis, congestive heart failure, and pericardial effusion
d. Administration of medications, e.g., vasopressors, concentrated ionic solutions, or cytotoxic chemotherapeutic agents.

3. List the complications of central venous catheterization.

a. Pneumothorax
b. Arterial puncture
c. Mispositioning
d. Catheter-associated infection
e. Thrombosis
f. Chylothorax (injury to the thoracic duct on left-sided attempts)
g. Hydrothorax/hydromediastinum (infusion into the pleural space)
h. Air embolism

i. Great vessel or right atrial perforation (hemothorax, tamponade)
j. Airway compromise (tracheal injury, hematoma with airway compression).

4. List the complications of peripheral venous access.

a. Hematoma formation
b. Pain at the site of access
c. Extravasation of fluids
d. Phlebitis
e. Cellulitis
f. Neurovascular injury
g. Bacteremia
h. Sepsis
i. Deep vein thrombosis (DVT)
j. Tissue necrosis.

Question 3

1. Explain the conduction system of the heart.

The cardiac conduction system contains specialized cells and nodes that control the heart **(Fig. 2)**. These are the sinoatrial (SA) node, atrioventricular (AV) node, bundle of His (atrioventricular bundle), and Purkinje fibers.

SA node: It is called the heart's natural pacemaker. It sends the electrical impulses that start the heartbeat. It is at the edge of the right atrium near the superior vena cava. The autonomic nervous system controls how fast or slow the SA node sends electrical signals. The autonomic nervous system includes:
a. Sympathetic nervous system (fight or flight response) makes the SA node work faster, which increases the heart rate.
b. Parasympathetic nervous system (rest and digest response) makes the SA node work slower, which decreases the heart rate.

AV node: It is located in an area known as the triangle of Koch (located between the septal leaflet of the tricuspid valve, the coronary sinus, and the membranous portion of the interatrial septum). The AV node delays the SA node's electrical signal by a fraction of a second each time. The delay ensures that the atria are empty of blood before the contraction stops. The atria are the heart's upper chambers which receive blood from the body and empty it into the ventricles.

Bundle of His: It is also called the AV bundle. It is a branch of fibers (nerve cells) that extends from the AV node. This fiber bundle receives the electrical signal from the AV node and carries it to the Purkinje fibers.

The bundle of His runs down the length of the interventricular septum, the structure that separates the right and left ventricles. The bundle of His has two branches:
a. Left bundle branch sends electrical signals through the Purkinje fibers to the left ventricle.
b. Right bundle branch sends electrical signals through the Purkinje fibers to the right ventricle.

Purkinje fibers: These fibers are branches of specialized nerve cells. They send electrical signals very quickly to the right and left heart ventricles. Purkinje fibers in the subendocardial surface of the ventricle walls. The subendocardial surface is part of the endocardium, the inner layer of tissue that lines the heart's chambers. When the Purkinje fibers deliver electrical signals to the ventricles, the ventricles contract. As they contract, blood flows from the right ventricle to the *pulmonary arteries* and from the left ventricle to the *aorta*. The aorta is the body's largest artery. It sends blood from the heart to the rest of the body.

2. Discuss normal electrocardiogram (ECG) waves and intervals.

The normal ECG waves and intervals are as follows **(Fig. 3)**:

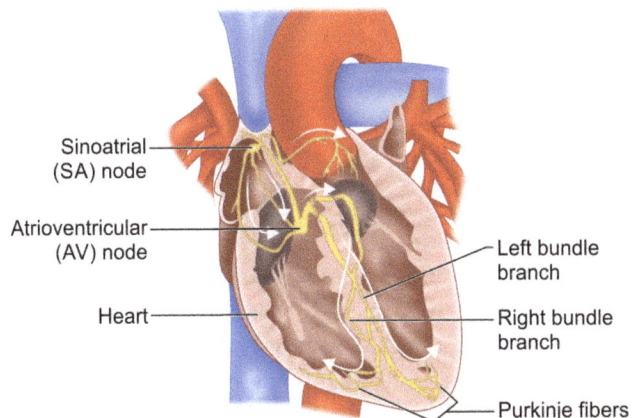

Fig. 2: Conduction system of the heart.

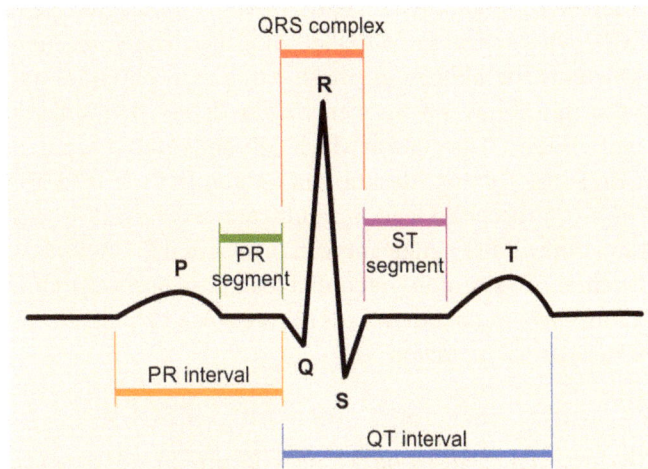

Fig. 3: Normal ECG intervals.

P wave (atrial depolarization): It is the first positive deflection with a height of 2.5 mm. If the height is >2.5 mm, it is known as "p" pulmonale/right atrial enlargement. It has a width of 3 mm; a width of >3 mm width is known as "P" mitrale/left atrial enlargement. P wave is absent in atrial fibrillation and supraventricular tachycardia and is deformed in atrial flutter (saw tooth).

Q wave: It is the first negative deflection. Q wave in lead III can be ignored. It is one-fourth of R wave and is seen in irreversible ischemia or infarction. It is significant if it has a width of 0.04 second and a depth of 4 mm/0.4 mV.

QRS complex (ventricular depolarization): The normal QRS duration is 60–100 ms. Narrow complexes (QRS <100 ms) are supraventricular in origin. Broad complexes (QRS >100 ms) are ventricular in origin or due to bundle branch block, hyperkalemia, or sodium channel blockade.

T wave (ventricular repolarization): It shows a positive deflection after QRS complex, slightly asymmetrical (symmetrical T wave should be consider pathological until proven otherwise), and negative deflection in aVR and V1. Normally, it is <5 mm/5 SS in limb lead and <10 mm/10 SS in precordial lead. Tall, flat, and inverted T waves are pathological.

PR interval: It extends from the beginning of P wave to the beginning of QRS complex. It denotes the conduction of action potential from atria to ventricles. A long PR interval is seen in heart block, whereas a short PR interval is seen in Wolff—Parkinson—White (WPW) syndrome (delta wave). The normal PR interval is 0.12–0.2 second (3–5 SS).

QT interval: It extends from the beginning of Q wave to the end of T wave with a normal duration of 0.35–0.44 second (9–11 SS). It is shortened in hypercalcemia, hyperthermia, digitalis therapy, and vagal stimulation and is prolonged in hypocalcemia, quinidine, procainamide, and central nervous system (CNS) insult.

ST segment: It denotes the end of QRS to the beginning of T wave. These segments are isoelectric lines. The ST segment represents the plateau or phase 2 of action potential and is the time between the ventricular depolarization and repolarization. The point at which QRS ends and ST segment begin is the J point. Elevation of >1 mm in limb lead and 2 mm in precordial lead is significant. ST elevation with convex upward is significant with myocardial infarction. An elevation of >2 mm in precordial lead (2 consecutive) and >1 mm elevation in other leads (2 consecutive) is significant for myocardial infarction.

3. List the causes of QT interval prolongation.

The important causes of QT interval prolongation are as follows:

- Hypokalemia, hypomagnesemia, hypocalcemia, hypothermia, myocardial ischemia, return of spontaneous circulation (ROSC) postcardiac arrest, raised intracranial pressure, and congenital long QT syndrome.
- *Medications/drugs:* Antifungals, antibiotics, and anti-arrhythmics

Question 4

1. Explain a normal oxygen dissociation curve.

A normal oxygen dissociation curve demonstrates the relationship of the partial pressure of oxygen (PO_2) in the plasma to the saturation of hemoglobin molecules with oxygen (O_2). P_{50} is the PO_2 at which hemoglobin is 50% saturated and correlates with PO_2 of 27 mm Hg normally. Normal mixed venous blood has an oxygen partial pressure ($PmvO_2$) of 40 mm Hg and an oxyhemoglobin saturation of 75%. A partial pressure of arterial oxygen (PaO_2) of 60 mm Hg normally results in approximately 90% saturation of hemoglobin **(Fig. 4)**.

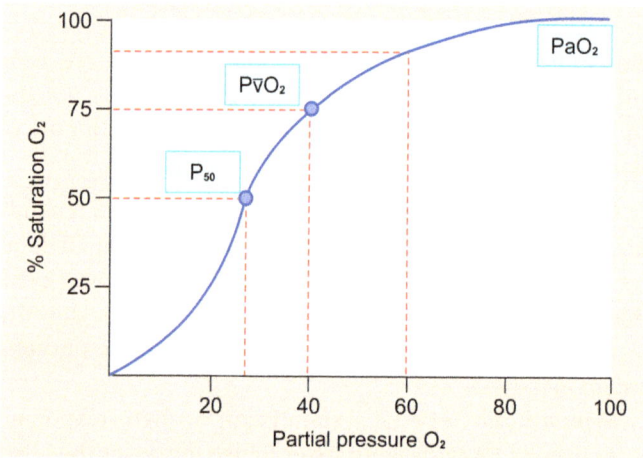

Fig. 4: Oxyhemoglobin dissociation curve.

2. What are the factors causing shifts in oxygen dissociation curve?

There are several important factors that affect the oxygen–hemoglobin dissociation curve. These factors include the following:
a. pH
b. Temperature
c. Carbon dioxide
d. 2,3-bisphosphoglycerate (BPG)
e. Carbon monoxide (CO)

By increasing the hydrogen ion concentration (and therefore the pH), the temperature, the carbon dioxide concentration, or the amount of 2,3-BPG present in the red blood cell, there is a decrease in the affinity of hemoglobin to oxygen and therefore curve shifts to the right side which allows to unload more oxygen to the tissues. By increasing the concentration of

CO, there is increase in the affinity of hemoglobin for oxygen and therefore the curve shifts to the left side. This means that less oxygen will be delivered to the tissues.

3. What are the clinical applications of central venous oxygen saturation?

Venous oxygen saturation (SvO_2) is a measure of the oxygen content of the blood returning to the right side of the heart after perfusing the entire body. When the oxygen supply is insufficient to meet the metabolic demands of the tissues, an abnormal SvO_2 ensues and reflects an inadequacy in the systemic oxygenation. SvO_2 is, therefore, dependent on oxygen delivery and oxygen extraction.

Venous oximetry is used in certain clinical settings of hemodynamic instability, such as in critical illnesses, perioperative periods of major surgeries, heart failure, and sepsis. A less invasive method of measuring SvO_2 is via a central venous catheter positioned in the superior vena cava and is called the central venous oxygen saturation ($ScvO_2$).

a. It provides an understanding of the patient's oxygen delivery, oxygen consumption, and cardiac output. It acts as a surrogate for SvO_2 and thus provides a surrogate measure of oxygen flux, reflecting the balance between oxygen delivery (DO_2) and consumption (VO_2).
b. It is advocated by the Surviving Sepsis Guidelines as part of early goal-directed therapy for septic shock (target $ScvO_2$ >70%) The optimization of low $ScvO_2$ (70%) has been successfully used in a protocolized approach to septic shock. Normal or high values are less indicative of the degree of shock.
c. It may have a role in the management of postoperative patients.

Question 5

1. Discuss the regulation of acid–base balance by kidneys.

Plasma [H⁺] is influenced by the rate of endogenous production, the rate of excretion, exogenous addition, and the buffering capacity of the body. Buffers mitigate the impact of large changes in available hydrogen ion on plasma pH. Buffer systems that are effective at physiologic pH include hemoglobin, phosphate, and proteins such as albumin and bicarbonate. The [H⁺] is the result of all physiologic buffers acting on the common pool of hydrogen ions.

The quantity of [HCO_3^-] in relation to carbonic acid buffer in the system is not fixed but varies according to physiologic need. This flexibility is largely provided by pulmonary exhalation of carbon dioxide (CO_2), which can vary significantly and change rapidly as required by alterations in the underlying acid–base status. The kidney regulates HCO_3^- excretion and the formation of new HCO_3^-. The rate of these processes is dependent on the underlying acid–base status. The renal response to pulmonary acid–base disturbances begins within 30 minutes of onset but requires hours to days to achieve equilibrium.

Any condition that acts to increase [H⁺]—whether through endogenous production, decreased buffering capacity, decreased excretion, or exogenous addition—is known as acidosis. Similarly, any condition that acts to decrease [H⁺] is termed alkalosis. The terms acidemia and alkalemia refer to the net imbalance of [H⁺] in the blood.

2. What is normal anion gap metabolic acidosis?

The non-anion gap (AG) type of acidosis is often referred to as "normal" AG acidosis. Some texts refer to this as hyperchloremic metabolic acidosis, but not all cases of normal AG acidosis are associated with hyperchloremia.

Causes of normal AG metabolic acidosis are as follows:

With a tendency to hyperkalemia:
a. Subsiding diabetic ketoacidosis
b. Early uremic acidosis
c. Early obstructive uropathy
d. Renal tubular acidosis, type IV
e. Hypoaldosteronism (Addison's disease)
f. Infusion or ingestion of HCl, NH_4Cl, lysine-HCl, or arginine-HCl
g. Potassium-sparing diuretics.

With a tendency to hypokalemia:
a. Renal tubular acidosis, type I (classical distal acidosis)
b. Renal tubular acidosis, type II (proximal acidosis)
c. Acetazolamide; carbonic anhydrase inhibitor, causing functional renal tubular acidosis
d. Acute diarrhea with losses of HCO_3^- and K⁺
e. Ureterosigmoidostomy with increased resorption of [H⁺] and [Cl⁻] and losses of HCO_3^- and K⁺
f. Obstruction of artificial ileal bladder
g. Fluid resuscitation with unbalanced, high chloride content crystalloids (dilution acidosis)

3. What is high anion gap metabolic acidosis?

High AG metabolic acidosis is a form of metabolic acidosis characterized by a high anion gap.

The etiology of high AG metabolic acidosis is as follows **(Table 1)**.

Renal failure (uremia), diabetic ketoacidosis, alcoholic starvation, lactic-acidosis, sepsis, cardiac arrest, and liver failure drugs like iron, metformin, cyanide, salicylate, isoniazid cyanide, CO, thiamine deficiency exogenous poisoning methanol ethylene glycol.

TABLE 1: GOLDMARK mnemonic for the high anion gap metabolic acidosis.

Letter	Parameter	Potential causes
G	Glycols	Ingestion/infusion of ethylene, propylene, or diethylene glycol; metabolism generates glyoxylic, oxalic, D- and L-lactic acid
O	5-oxoproline	Chronic acetaminophen use can generate 5-oxoproline (a strong acid that is also called pyroglutamic acid)
L	L-Lactic acidosis	Multiple etiologies of types A and B lactic acidosis
D	D-Lactic acidosis	Carbohydrate loading in patients with short gut syndromes
M	Methanol	Metabolism generates formic acid
A	Aspirin	Toxic levels generate multiple organic acids including keto acids
R	Renal failure	Accumulation of multiple inorganic and organic acids including sulfuric and phosphoric acid
K	Ketoacidosis	B-OH butyric and acetoacetic acid

Question 6

1. Enumerate sedation agents for procedural sedation.

The agents for procedural sedation are propofol, ketamine, etomidate, midazolam, fentanyl, alfentanil, remifentanil, dexmedetomidine, nitrous oxide, and methohexital.

2. Discuss any three sedation agents.

a. *Propofol:*
Recommended IV dose: 0.5–1.0 mg/kg (elderly: 0.25–0.5 mg/kg)

Repeat dosing: 0.25–0.5 mg/kg; Onset of action: 10–50 seconds

Average effective action: <10 minutes

Advantages: Rapid onset, short duration of action, good agent for orthopedic reductions

Side effects/disadvantages: Does not provide analgesia, may cause respiratory depression (increased risk in elderly patients), may burn on injection; lidocaine added to syringe can decrease pain.

b. *Fentanyl:*
Recommended IV dose: 0.5–1.5 µg/kg; start with 0.25 µg/kg in elderly

Repeat dose: 0.5–1.5 µg/kg, can repeat every 1–3 minutes (longer between-dose intervals are recommended if larger initial doses are given)

Onset of action: Effect in 1–2 minutes

Average effective action: 30–60 minutes

Advantages: Given in combination with sedatives that lack analgesic properties; monotherapy may be used for minimal sedation

Side effects/disadvantages: Monotherapy for moderate or deep sedation will not provide adequate sedation/amnestic effects, or respiratory depression.

c. *Ketamine:*
Recommended IV dose: 1.0–1.5 mg/kg (give over 30–60 seconds)

Repeat dosing: 0.5–1.0 mg/kg, for analgesia only (subdissociative dose): 0.1–0.3 mg/kg

Onset of action: <1 minute

Average effective action: <10 minutes

Advantages: Ketamine adds analgesia without opioids; ketamine component blunts propofol-induced hypotension, combination good for prolonged procedures

Side effects/disadvantages: Higher *ketamine:propofol ratios* lead to longer recovery; do not reduce clinically important adverse events; while not harmful, objective benefits have mixed evidence.

3. What are the requirements for monitoring a patient during procedural sedation?

Procedural sedation requires both interactive and physiologic monitoring. Interactive monitoring includes direct visualization of the patient's airway and chest wall motion, chest auscultation, monitoring patient responsiveness, and providing appropriate maneuvers to maintain the patient's airway and ventilation. Physiologic monitoring includes continual tracking of arterial oxygenation, ventilation, blood pressure, and cardiac rate/rhythm. Cardiac monitoring is recommended for patients with preexisting cardiac disease or dysrhythmias or during procedures such as cardioversion. Monitor arterial oxygen saturation with pulse oximetry. However, pulse oximetry is not a substitute for monitoring ventilation because hypoventilation or apnea develops before oxygen saturation decreases, especially in patients who receive supplemental oxygen. The recommended extent of monitoring is determined by the level of sedation as shown in **Table 2**. A structured assessment, such as the *Aldrete score* **(Table 3)**, can be used to assess the patient's recovery and safety for discharge.

TABLE 2: Parameters of monitoring a patient during procedural sedation.

Target level of sedation	Level of consciousness	Heart rate	Respiratory rate	Blood pressure	Oxygen saturation	Capnography end-tidal CO_2
Minimal	Observe frequently	Record every 15 minutes	Record every 15 minutes	Record every 15 minutes and after sedative boluses	Monitor continuously	No recommendation
Dissociative	Observe constantly	Monitor continuously	Continuous direct observation	Record at initiation, frequent monitoring generally unnecessary	Monitor continuously	Recommend continuous monitoring
Moderate	Observe constantly	Monitor continuously	Continuous direct observation	Record every 5 minutes and after sedative boluses	Monitor continuously	Recommend continuous monitoring
Deep	Observe constantly	Monitor continuously	Continuous direct observation	Record every 5 minutes and after sedative boluses	Monitor continuously	Recommend continuous monitoring

TABLE 3: Aldrete score: Assessment of the patient recovery and safety for discharge.

Activity	Respiration	Circulation	Consciousness	Oxygen saturation
Score 2: Moves all extremities voluntarily/on command	*Score 2:* Breathes deeply and coughs freely	*Score 2:* BP + 20 mm Hg of preanesthetic level	*Score 2:* Fully awake	*Score 2:* SpO_2 >92% on room air
Score 1: Moves 2 extremities	*Score 1:* Dyspneic, shallow or limited breathing	*Score 1:* BP + 20–50 mm Hg of preanesthetic levels	*Score 1:* Arousable on calling	*Score 1:* Supplemental O_2 required to maintain SpO_2 >92%
Score 0: Unable to move extremities	*Score 0:* Apneic	*Score 0:* BP + 50 mm Hg of preanesthetic levels	*Score 0:* Not responding	*Score 0:* SpO_2 <92% with supplemental O_2

(BP: blood pressure; SpO_2: oxygen saturation)
Note: Aldrete score: A score of ≥9 is appropriate for safe discharge.

Question 7

1. Describe various volumes given by a spirometer.

Spirometers can measure three of the four lung volumes: (1) inspiratory reserve volume (IRV), (2) tidal volume (TV), and (3) expiratory reserve volume (ERV), but cannot measure residual volume. Four lung capacities are also important: (1) inspiratory capacity, (2) vital capacity, (3) functional residual capacity, and (4) total lung capacity. Pulmonary ventilation is the product of TV and respiratory frequency. The maximum voluntary ventilation is the maximum air that can be moved per minute.

The spirometer helps in identifying several useful lung volumes.

These are:
a. *TV* is the amount of air breathed in and out during normal, restful breathing. Its typical value is about 500 mL = 0.5 L. The magnitude of the TV depends on the size of the individual and their metabolic state. TV usually varies from breath to breath.
b. *IRV* is the additional volume of air that can be inspired at the end of a normal or tidal inspiration. The typical value for a young adult male of normal size is about 3,000 mL.
c. *ERV* is the additional volume of air that can be expired after a normal or tidal expiration. The typical value of ERV is about 1,100 mL for a young adult male.

2. Define anatomic, physiologic, and mechanical dead spaces.

Dead space represents the volume of ventilated air that does not participate in gas exchange.

Anatomical dead space is represented by the volume of air that fills the conducting zone of respiration made up by the nose, trachea, and bronchi. This volume is considered to be 30% of normal TV (500 mL); therefore, the value of anatomic dead space is 150 mL.

Physiologic or total dead space is equal to anatomic plus alveolar dead space which is the volume of air in the respiratory zone that does not take part in gas exchange. The respiratory zone is comprised of respiratory bronchioles, alveolar duct, alveolar sac, and alveoli. In a healthy adult, alveolar dead space can be considered negligible. Therefore, physiologic dead space is equivalent to anatomic dead space. One can see an increase in the value of physiologic dead space in lung disease states where the diffusion membrane of alveoli does not function properly or when there are ventilation/perfusion mismatch defects.

Mechanical dead space is dead space in an apparatus in which the breathing gas must flow in both directions as the user breathes in and out, increasing the necessary respiratory effort to get the same amount of usable air or breathing gas, and risking accumulation of carbon dioxide from shallow breaths.

3. Discuss the clinical importance of various dead spaces during invasive ventilation.

Dead space measurements have been shown to provide useful information in patients with severe respiratory failure both for management and for prognosis. The concept of dead space was originally described by Bohr. Dead space is divided into the normal anatomic dead space, which exists in the large and small airways and normally do not participate in gas exchange and the alveolar dead space, when there is reduced or no blood flow to a given area of lung that is still receiving ventilation. The sum of anatomical V_D and alveolar V_D is referred to as the physiologic dead space. Traditionally, dead space is expressed as a fraction of the tidal volume (V_T), i.e., physiologic V_D/V_T, but it may also be expressed as anatomical V_D/V_T or alveolar V_D/V_T.

An invasive technique for measuring dead space was described by Enghoff as a modification of the Bohr equation. This has become the standard technique for measurement of dead space. In contrast, the original Bohr equation utilizes the alveolar P rather than the arterial P.

The Enghoff calculation of dead space is affected by the level of shunt. V_D/V_T measured according to either technique was significantly elevated at all levels of positive end expiratory pressure (PEEP). However, the alveolar V_D measured with the Bohr technique was not significantly increased at PEEP levels up to +15 cmH$_2$O, after which it increased at higher PEEP levels up to +30 cmH$_2$O. In contrast, the alveolar V_D calculated with the Enghoff technique was significantly elevated at all levels of PEEP, although there was a slight decrease at levels of +15 cmH$_2$O or higher. They attribute the changes in Bohr dead space to "stress" on the lungs, whereas the changes in the Enghoff dead space are attributed to the shunt effect.

Question 8

1. Explain noninvasive arterial blood pressure monitoring.

The systolic pressure is the maximum pressure during ventricular ejection, and the diastolic pressure is the lowest pressure in the blood vessels between heartbeats during ventricular filling. The difference between systolic and diastolic pressures is the pulse pressure. Because the vascular circuit is elastic, both systolic and diastolic pressures vary throughout the vascular system. Systolic pressure can increase by up to 20 mm Hg, whereas the diastolic pressure similarly decreases as the pressure wave moves peripherally from the aorta. However, mean arterial pressure (MAP) varies by only 1–2 mm Hg, whether measured centrally or peripherally; in practice, estimate MAP using the sum of the diastolic pressure and one third of the pulse pressure.

MAP = Diastolic blood pressure + [Pulse pressure/3]

The different ways of noninvasive arterial blood pressure monitoring are as follows:

Palpation: Traditional teaching is that the ability to palpate the radial, femoral, or carotid pulse represents a minimum systolic pressure of 80, 70, or 60 mm Hg, respectively. However, two small studies showed that these values generally overestimate the patient's systolic blood pressure and are not included in the ninth edition of the Advanced Trauma Life Support guidelines.

Sphygmomanometry: This method uses a sphygmomanometer. The cuff is placed around the upper arm, and the bell is held over the brachial artery as the cuff is gradually inflated to at least 30 mm Hg above the point where the radial artery sound disappears. During cuff deflation, the first tapping sound (Korotkoff sound) corresponds to the systolic pressure, while the disappearance of these sounds corresponds to the diastolic pressure. An inappropriately small cuff results in falsely elevated blood pressure measurements, and an inappropriately large cuff results in falsely low measurements.

Sphygmomanometric measurements of blood pressure often report slightly higher systolic pressure and lower diastolic pressure than those reported from simultaneous direct measurement using an intra-arterial catheter. This is because the reflected pressure waves summate with cuff inflation and increase systolic pressure, whereas the ischemic vasodilation downstream from the occluded cuff decreases cuff opening diastolic pressure. In normotensive patients, use the arm or leg for noninvasive blood pressure measurements; in critically ill and hypotensive patients, noninvasive arm measurements are usually temporizing while establishing arterial line access.

Oscillometry: Most automated blood pressure monitors use oscillometry. The device analyzes the amplitude of the fluctuations (or oscillations) in blood pressure in a sphygmomanometer cuff and converts it to a pressure measurement without the need for auscultation. With gradual deflation of the cuff, oscillations begin above systolic pressure. The point of maximum oscillation corresponds to MAP. Noninvasive measurements overestimate the systolic blood pressure compared to invasive arterial monitoring, but the calculated MAP shows better correlation and thus is more reliable in the critically ill patient.

2. Explain invasive arterial blood pressure monitoring.

The arterial catheter measures MAP and pulse pressure, estimates CO, and enables repeated blood sampling. The International Consensus Conference for Hemodynamic Monitoring in Shock recommends invasive blood pressure monitoring for patients with refractory shock receiving vasoactive agents.

Placement of an intra-arterial catheter requires knowledge of the anatomic landmarks of the selected site. US guidance aids placement. The catheter insertion is either directly over a needle or over a guidewire (called the Seldinger technique). The Allen test, compression of both the ulnar and radial arteries with subsequent release of the ulnar artery pressure to see if "pink" returns, confirms collateral blood flow before radial artery catheterization. After successful arterial catheterization, connect the catheter to the pressure transducer and look for an arterial waveform. The square wave flush test is applied to determine if artifacts in the tubing and recording system are damping the pressure measurements. An overdamped system suggests that air bubbles in the tubing falsely lower pressure measurements. An underdamped system will overestimate systolic pressure and underestimate diastolic pressure. Flushing the system should remove the air bubbles. If this does not fix the problem, replace the tubing.

3. Explain noninvasive cardiac output monitoring.

Minimally invasive or noninvasive hemodynamic monitoring techniques to measure CO in the emergency department setting includes transthoracic echocardiography and pulse contour waveform analysis.

Transthoracic echocardiography: It is an accurate tool to estimate CO in the critically ill patient recommended by the American Society of Echocardiography. Using the parasternal long axis to measure the left ventricular outflow tract diameter and pulse wave Doppler in the apical four-chamber view to measure stroke volume from the left ventricular outflow tract, one can reliably estimate CO.

Pulse contour analysis: Devices using pulse contour analysis quantify CO, stroke volume, and stroke volume or pulse pressure variation to help guide resuscitation. The devices require placement of an indwelling arterial catheter and a central venous catheter to obtain central venous pressure measurement and derive systemic vascular resistance. These devices require a mechanically ventilated patient with a set tidal volume of 8 mL/kg. Also, because these devices rely on pulse contour analysis as the primary means of CO measurement, they cannot be used in the presence of cardiac dysrhythmias (e.g., atrial fibrillation) or mechanical circulatory devices.

Question 9

1. Explain the anatomic changes in pregnancy affecting airway management during pregnancy.

There are significant anatomic changes during pregnancy which may cause difficulty in airway management. There is fluid retention which causes edema within the structures of the upper airway. Important landmarks of airway can be distorted due to weight gain with adipose deposition. There can thus be difficulty with mask ventilation, laryngoscopy, glottic visualization, and endotracheal intubation. Desaturation can also occur quickly due to maternal increased oxygen consumption and decreased functional residual capacity. Moreover, the incidence of Mallampati class III airways also increases which makes the intubation more difficult. There is likelihood of airway bleeding and swelling due to mucosal engorgement and increased capillary friability. Pregnant obese women may also have redundant pharyngeal and palatal folds in the airways which may hinder the intubation process. Decreased lower esophageal tone, increased intra-abdominal pressure, decreased gastric emptying, and a full stomach increase the likelihood of gastric aspiration making airway management difficult.

2. Explain the physiological changes in pregnancy relevant to resuscitation.

Physiologic changes in pregnancy that may affect the resuscitation are given in **Table 4**.

TABLE 4: Physiologic changes in pregnancy affecting resuscitation.

System	Parameters	Comment
Cardiovascular	Cardiac output	Increases 30–50%
	Peripheral resistance	Decreases 20%
	Blood pressure	Decreases 10–15 mm Hg systolic in the first half of pregnancy; then back to baseline
	Blood volume	100 mL/kg or 6–7 L
	Central venous pressure	May be increased up to 10 mm Hg
	Central venous oxygen saturation	Increases as high as 80%
	Plasma volume	Increases 30–50%
Hematologic	Fibrinogen, factors V, VII, VIII, X, von Willebrand factor	Increase, with heightened risk for venous thromboembolism in the second half of pregnancy
Respiratory and pulmonary	Upper airway edema, hyperemia, and friability	Estrogen and volume effects; can result in difficult airway
	Diaphragm elevation	Higher thoracostomy tube insertion site during pregnancy
	Hemoglobin F has greater affinity for oxygen than maternal hemoglobin	Fetal oxygen maintained at expense of maternal oxygenation; maintain maternal oxygen saturation >95%
	Respiratory rate	No change
	Tidal volume, minute ventilation	Increase
Renal and urinary	Progesterone dilates renal collecting system; ureteral peristalsis decreases	Renal US may show mild hydronephrosis; increased risk for ascending infection
Gastrointestinal	Alkaline phosphatase rises from placental production; bile is more lithogenic	Increased risk of cholecystitis/cholelithiasis
	Decreased lower esophageal tone; decreased gastric emptying	Increased likelihood of aspiration of gastric contents
Uteroplacental unit	25% of blood flow directed to uteroplacental unit; no autoregulation of blood flow; enlarging uterus can compress vena cava and vessels below the diaphragm; supine hypotension syndrome can occur after 30 minutes of supine position	Place patient in left lateral tilt position during the third trimester; replace volume adequately to account for increased blood and plasma volume in pregnancy; avoid femoral and lower extremity site for blood and volume delivery in the second half of pregnancy

3. Discuss briefly special steps of cardiopulmonary resuscitation during pregnancy.

Special steps of cardiopulmonary resuscitation during pregnancy are shown in **Flowchart 1**.

Question 10

1. What is Vaughan-William's classification of anti-arrhythmic agents?

Anti-arrhythmic drug classification is given in **Table 5**.

TABLE 5: Anti-arrhythmic drug classification.

Action	Class and medications
Sodium channel blockers	*Class Ia:* Procainamide *Class Ib:* Lidocaine *Class Ic:* Flecainide, propafenone
β-Blockers	*Class II:* Esmolol, labetalol, metoprolol, propranolol
Potassium channel blockers	*Class III:* Amiodarone, dronedarone, dofetilide, ibutilide, sotalol
Calcium channel blockers	*Class IV:* Diltiazem, verapamil, nicardipine

2. Discuss briefly about class I anti-arrhythmic agents.

Class I agents block fast sodium channels and are further categorized based on their degree of blockade into classes Ia (moderate blockade), Ib (weak blockade), and Ic (strong blockade). They increase the excitability threshold, requiring more sodium channels to open in order to overcome the potassium current and generate an action potential. This effect increases the refractory period and can be useful in terminating reentry currents. In addition, some class I agents block potassium channels and exhibit antimuscarinic effects. The examples of class I anti-arrhythmic agents are as follows:

Class Ia: Procainamide

Class Ib: Lidocaine

Class Ic: Flecainide, propafenone

3. Discuss briefly about class III anti-arrhythmic agents.

Class III anti-arrhythmic medications inhibit inward potassium currents leading to a significantly longer refractory period.

Flowchart 1: Cardiac arrest in pregnancy in-hospital ACLS algorithm.

```
┌─────────────────────────────────┐           ┌──────────────────────────────────────────────────────────┐
│ Continue BLS/ACLS               │           │                  Maternal cardiac arrest                 │
│ • High-quality CPR              │           ├──────────────────────────────────────────────────────────┤
│ • Defibrillation when indicated │           │ • Team planning should be done in collaboration with the │
│ • Other ACLS interventions      │           │   obstetric, neonatal, emergency, anesthesiology,        │
│   (e.g., epinephrine)           │           │   intensive care, and cardiac arrest services            │
└─────────────┬───────────────────┘           │ • Priorities for pregnant women in cardiac arrest should │
              ▼                               │   include provision of high-quality CPR and relief of    │
   Assemble maternal cardiac arrest team      │   aortocaval compression with lateral uterine            │
              │                               │   displacement                                           │
              ▼                               │ • The goal of perimortem cesarean delivery is to improve │
        Consider etiology                     │   maternal and fetal outcomes                            │
           of arrest                          │ • Ideally, perform perimortem cesarean delivery in 5     │
       ┌──────┴──────┐                        │   minutes, depending on provider resources and skill sets│
       ▼             ▼                        ├──────────────────────────────────────────────────────────┤
```

Perform maternal interventions
- Perform airway management
- Administer 100% O₂, avoid excess ventilation
- Place IV above diaphragm
- If receiving IV magnesium, stop and give calcium chloride or gluconate

Perform obstetric interventions
- Provide continuous lateral uterine displacement
- Detach fetal monitors
- Prepare for perimortem cesarean delivery

Continue BLS/ACLS
- High-quality CPR
- Defibrillation when indicated
- Other ACLS interventions (e.g., epinephrine)

Perform perimortem cesarean delivery
- If no ROSC in 5 minutes, consider immediate perimortem cesarean delivery

Neonatal team to receive neonate

Advanced airway
- In pregnancy, a difficult airway is common. Use the most experienced provider
- Provide endotracheal intubation or supraglottic advanced airway
- Perform waveform capnography or capnometry to confirm and monitor ET tube placement
- Once advanced airway is in place, give 1 breath every 6 seconds (10 breaths/min) with continuous chest compressions

Potential etiology of maternal cardiac arrest

A Anesthetic complications
B Bleeding
C Cardiovascular
D Drugs
E Embolic
F Fever
G General nonobstetric causes of cardiac arrest (H's and T's)
H Hypertension

(ACLS: advanced cardiac life support; BLS: basic life support; CPR: cardiopulmonary resuscitation; ROSC: return of spontaneous circulation)

Myocardial tissue in a refractory state is resistant to reentrant conduction circuits that may produce arrhythmia. These agents prolong the QT interval, which is associated with significant risk for torsades de pointes. The class III anti-arrhythmic agents are amiodarone, dronedarone, dofetilide, ibutilide, and sotalol.

SUGGESTED READING

1. Richhariya D, Sharma B. Textbook of Emergency Medicine including Intensive Care and Trauma, 2nd edition. New Delhi: Jaypee Brothers Medical Publishers (P) Ltd; 2022. pp. 205 and 210. (Question 1).
2. Richhariya D, Sharma B. Textbook of Emergency Medicine including Intensive Care and Trauma, 2nd edition. New Delhi: Jaypee Brothers Medical Publishers (P) Ltd; 2022. p. 284. (Question 2).
3. Richhariya D, Sharma B. Textbook of Emergency Medicine including Intensive Care and Trauma, 2nd edition. New Delhi: Jaypee Brothers Medical Publishers (P) Ltd; 2022. pp. 421-33. (Question 3).
4. Richhariya D, Sharma B. Textbook of Emergency Medicine including Intensive Care and Trauma, 2nd edition. New Delhi: Jaypee Brothers Medical Publishers (P) Ltd; 2022. p. 304. (Question 4).
5. Richhariya D, Sharma B. Textbook of Emergency Medicine including Intensive Care and Trauma, 2nd edition. New Delhi: Jaypee Brothers Medical Publishers (P) Ltd; 2022. pp. 303-9. (Question 5).
6. Richhariya D, Sharma B. Textbook of Emergency Medicine including Intensive Care and Trauma, 2nd edition. New Delhi: Jaypee Brothers Medical Publishers (P) Ltd; 2022. pp. 350-4. (Question 6).
7. Richhariya D, Sharma B. Textbook of Emergency Medicine including Intensive Care and Trauma, 2nd edition. New Delhi: Jaypee Brothers Medical Publishers (P) Ltd; 2022. p. 580. (Question 7).
8. Richhariya D, Sharma B. Textbook of Emergency Medicine including Intensive Care and Trauma, 2nd edition. New Delhi: Jaypee Brothers Medical Publishers (P) Ltd; 2022. p. 298. (Question 8).
9. Richhariya D, Sharma B. Textbook of Emergency Medicine including Intensive Care and Trauma, 2nd edition. New Delhi: Jaypee Brothers Medical Publishers (P) Ltd; 2022. p. 1116. (Question 9).
10. Richhariya D, Sharma D. Textbook of Emergency Medicine including Intensive Care and Trauma, 2nd edition. New Delhi: Jaypee Brothers Medical Publishers (P) Ltd; 2022. p. 478. (Question 10).

Emergency Medicine Paper 10

Bipin Karki, Olita Shilpakar

Question 1

A 32-year-old is brought to the emergency department (ED) 1 hour after an accident. On arrival, he is talking in incomprehensible words. His vitals are: Respiratory rate (RR) 32 breaths/min, oxygen saturation (SpO₂) 92% on room air, pulse rate (PR) 118 beats/min, and blood pressure (BP) 88/60 mm Hg. He is opening his eyes to painful stimulus. He withdraws right upper and lower extremities on painful stimulus with no movement of the left side. The right pupil is fixed and dilated.

1. What is his Glasgow Coma Score (GCS)?

His GCS is 9. GCS of this given patient is 9 (E2V3M4)

2. Describe a stepwise approach to the patient in the ED.

Resuscitation and initial stabilization is the key to management in any patient coming to the ED. Primary survey is done by following the ABCDE (airway, breathing, circulation, disability, and exposure) approach.

a. *Airway:* Maintain airway. Take spinal precautions by applying a cervical collar. If severe injury with a GCS of <8, the patient requires intubation. Use of short-acting induction agents that have limited effect on BP or intracranial pressure (ICP) is recommended. Maintain in-line cervical spine stabilization during intubation.
b. *Breathing:* Maintain oxygenation and use capnometry to control partial pressure of carbon dioxide (PCO_2) and avoid hyperventilation. Prolonged (>6 hours) hypocapnia causes cerebral vasoconstriction and worsens cerebral ischemia. Keep SpO_2 >90%, partial pressure of oxygen (PaO_2) >60 mm Hg, and PCO_2 at 35–45 mm Hg.
c. *Circulation:* Provide aggressive fluid resuscitation to prevent hypotension and secondary brain injury. Normal saline is recommended for volume resuscitation. Maintain systolic blood pressure (SBP) at ≥110 mm Hg for patients 15–49 years old. A BP within "normal" range may be inadequate to maintain adequate flow and cerebral perfusion pressure (CPP) if ICP is increased. Permissive hypotension worsens outcome in patients with brain injury.
d. *Disability:* Check GCS for changes and for signs of impending herniation/deterioration. Change of >2 points should prompt further workup. Check glucose levels. Treat hypoglycemia and hyperglycemia.
e. *Exposure and temperature control:* All clothes of the patient should be removed, so that no injuries are missed. Maintain the temperature between 36 and 38.3°C. This is then followed by the secondary survey which includes head to toe examination and log roll. AMPLE (allergies, medications, past medical history, last meal taken and events) history is taken and reassessment of the primary survey is done and managed accordingly.

3. How will you prevent further deterioration in brain injury?

Apart from maintaining the ABCDE and initiating management accordingly, in order to prevent further deterioration in brain injury, the following points need to be considered:

a. *Patient positioning:* Keep the head of the bed at 30°. Raising the head of the bed may improve cerebral blood flow by lowering ICP.
b. *Identify and treat raised ICP:* Indicators of rising ICP include severe headache, visual changes, numbness, focal weakness, nausea, vomiting, seizure, change in mental status, lethargy, hypertension, coma, bradycardia, and agonal respirations. Signs of impending transtentorial herniation include unilateral or bilateral pupillary dilation, hemiparesis, motor posturing, and/or progressive neurologic deterioration. Measure neurologic deterioration by comparing sequential GCS scores. In a patient with a rapidly deteriorating GCS, if time permits, obtain a repeat head computed tomography (CT) to identify an expanding intracranial hematoma. CT signs of intracranial hypertension are loss of symmetry, attenuation of the visibility of sulci and gyri, compressed lateral ventricles, and poor gray/white matter distinction. Papilledema is a sign of increased ICP. Manage with inj. Mannitol 1 g/kg IV bolus. Mannitol is an osmotic agent

that can reduce ICP and improve cerebral blood flow, CPP, and brain metabolism. It has an effect within 30 minutes and expands plasma volume and can improve oxygen-carrying capacity. Administer mannitol by repetitive bolus (0.25–1 g/kg). Consider adding hypertonic saline (3% NaCl 250 mL/30 min) for refractory elevations in ICP.

c. *Glucose control:* Hyperglycemia in traumatic brain injury (TBI) is associated with worse outcome. Tight hyperglycemic control is recommended in patients with moderate to severe TBI. Insulin drips may be required to achieve adequate control (glucose 100–180 mg/dL or 5.55–9.99 mmol/L).

d. *Temperature control:* Elevated temperature is associated with an increased metabolic demand and excessive glutamate release. Elevated temperature elevates ICP and worsens outcome in many neurologic critical care conditions including TBI. Treat fever with the goal of normothermia.

e. *Seizure treatment and prophylaxis:* Seizures after head injury can change the neurologic examination, alter oxygen delivery and cerebral blood flow, and increase ICP. Prolonged seizures can worsen secondary injury. Treat acute seizures with midazolam or lorazepam. Administer prophylactic phenytoin/fosphenytoin if the GCS is ≤10, if the patient has an abnormal head CT scan, or if the patient has had an acute seizure after the injury. The dose is 18 mg/kg IV at 25 mg/min. Prophylactic anticonvulsants reduce the occurrence of post-traumatic seizures within the first week. Phenytoin/fosphenytoin is the agent most studied. Levetiracetam can be used, but there are fewer data supporting its use.

Question 2

A 16-year-old boy presents to ED complaining of shortness of breath and pain on the right side of chest. He informs being beaten by hockey sticks in playground 30 minutes ago. His vitals are: RR 28 beats/min, SpO$_2$ 80% on room air, PR 110 beats/min, and BP 90/50 mm Hg. His GCS is 15/15 with normal pupils and no deficits.

1. What are the possible chest injuries in this patient?

The possible chest injuries in this patient could be:
a. Tension pneumothorax
b. Massive hemothorax
c. Pulmonary contusions
d. Pneumomediastinum
e. Pulmonary hematomas
f. Multiple rib fractures
g. Flail chest.

2. How will you detect various chest injuries in the ED?

Chest injuries can be detected in the ED by various means:
a. *Chest X-ray:* Plain chest radiographs are helpful to screen for abnormal mediastinal contours, hemothorax, pneumothorax, pulmonary contusions, diaphragmatic injury, and osseous trauma.
b. *Point-of-care ultrasound* (*POCUS*): It can quickly diagnose pneumothorax, hemothorax, and pericardial tamponade as part of the extended focused assessment with sonography in trauma (FAST) examination.
c. *CT:* It can detect major and occult injuries and identify the need for additional interventions but may demonstrate incidental findings that require follow-up and do not change acute care. CT is more sensitive for detecting pulmonary contusion and hemothorax than plain radiography.

3. How will you relieve him of his pain?

Effective analgesia prevents hypoventilation and enables deep breathing and adequate coughing with clearance of secretions. Initial analgesia with intravenous paracetamol and nonsteroidal anti-inflammatories (NSAIDs) if not contraindicated should be administered followed by opioids. Early use of serratus anterior plane block (SAPB) and erector spinae plane block (ESPB) for patients presenting with rib injuries as these are well known and safe alternatives to opioids. Regional anesthesia in the form of paravertebral block, SAPB, or ESPB can be considered depending on the location of fractures and expertise to administer. Thoracic epidurals can be considered for bilateral rib fractures in patients without contraindications.

4. The patient was intubated by an intern and put on ventilator. However, the boy suddenly collapses with unrecordable BP. Enumerate the probable causes of his deterioration.

The probable causes of deterioration in this case could be due to the following reasons:
a. Displaced endotracheal tube (ETT)
b. Obstruction anywhere in the circuit
c. Pneumothorax, pulmonary embolism, pulmonary edema
d. Equipment failure, e.g., ventilator malfunction or disconnect
e. Stacked breaths
f. Esophageal intubation.

Question 3

A 56-year-old male has been wheeled into your ED with deep second-degree burns involving both upper limbs. He had an unsuccessful attempt trying to save his wife from fire within a closed compartment having wool garments. He is highly agitated and coughing black sputum.

1. What are your initial concerns in managing this patient?

This is a case of second-degree burn with inhalational injury. Airway compromise in such patients is a major concern since inhalation injury damages endothelial cells, produces mucosal edema of the small airways, and decreases alveolar surfactant activity, resulting in bronchospasm, airflow obstruction, and atelectasis. Although lower airway edema may not be clinically evident for up to 24 hours, upper airway edema can occur rapidly. For this reason, airway protection is essential in this patient.

2. How will you manage the various inhalational injuries produced by smoke?

Treat suspected inhalation injury with humidified 100% oxygen, intubation and ventilation, bronchodilators, lung-protective vent settings, and aggressive pulmonary toilet. Hyperbaric oxygen may be necessary for severe carbon monoxide poisoning. Provide humidified oxygen (100%) by face mask. Obtain arterial blood gas concentrations, including carboxyhemoglobin levels. Control of the upper airway is achieved by prompt endotracheal intubation.

Indications for intubation include:
a. Full-thickness burns of the face or perioral region
b. Circumferential neck burns
c. Acute respiratory distress
d. Progressive hoarseness or air hunger
e. Respiratory depression or altered mental status
f. Supraglottic edema and inflammation on bronchoscopy.

3. Discuss Parkland's formula for fluid resuscitation of burn in adults.

Adults:
a. Lactated ringer's (LR) 4 mL × weight (kg) × % burned surface area (BSA) burned over the initial 24 hours
b. Half over the first 8 hours from the time of burn
c. Other half over the subsequent 16 hours
d. *Example:* 70 kg adult with 40% second- and third-degree burns: 4 mL × 70 kg × 40 = 11,200 mL over 24 hours.

Children:
a. LR 3 mL × weight (kg) × %BSA burned over initial 24 hours plus maintenance
b. Half over the first 8 hours from the time of burn
c. Other half over the subsequent 16 hours.

Question 4

1. Enumerate common causes of acute pancreatitis.

The causes of acute pancreatitis are shown in **Table 1**.

TABLE 1: Causes of pancreatitis.	
Common	• Gallstones (35–75%) • Alcohol (25–35%) • Idiopathic (10–20%) • Increases with age
Uncommon	• Hypertriglyceridemia (fasting triglycerides >1,000 mg/dL) (1–4%) • Endoscopic retrograde cholangiopancreatography • Drugs (1.4–2%)
More uncommon (total <8% of cases)	• Abdominal trauma • Postoperative complications, especially post-cardiopulmonary bypass • Hyperparathyroidism • Infection (bacterial, viral, or parasitic) • Autoimmune disease • Tumor (pancreatic, ampullary) • Hypercalcemia • Cystic fibrosis
Rare	• Ischemia • Posterior penetrating ulcer • Toxin exposure
Unknown	Congenital abnormalities

2. How do you assess the severity of acute pancreatitis in ED?

There are many different scoring systems to assess the severity of acute pancreatitis in the ED. They are:
a. Ranson's criteria
b. Acute physiology and chronic health examination-II
c. Modified GCS
d. Bedside index for severity in acute pancreatitis
e. Balthazar CT severity index.

Systemic inflammatory response syndrome at admission and persistent at 48 hours predicts severe acute pancreatitis more simply and as accurately as the various scoring systems. A number of other clinical findings at the initial assessment are associated with the severity of disease. These findings include the following:

a. Patient characteristics (age >55 years, obesity, altered mental status, comorbidities)
b. Laboratory findings [blood urea nitrogen (BUN) >20 mg/dL or rising; hematocrit >44% or rising; increased creatinine]
c. Radiologic findings (many or large extra pancreatic fluid collections, pleural effusions, and pulmonary infiltrates).

Overall, acute pancreatitis has a mortality rate of approximately 1%. Most patients with acute pancreatitis die from multiorgan failure. The sensitivity of systemic inflammatory response syndrome on admission for mortality is 100% with a specificity of 31%, whereas the sensitivity and specificity of systemic inflammatory response syndrome at 48 hours (persistent systemic inflammatory response syndrome) are 77–89% and 79–86%, respectively. Systemic inflammatory response syndrome at admission and 48 hours, combined with patient characteristics (age, comorbidities, and obesity) and response to treatment, helps predict outcome.

3. What are the criteria for diagnostic studies in a patient with suspected acute pancreatitis?

There are three criteria to be considered in acute pancreatitis; the diagnosis is based on at least two out of three of them:
a. Clinical presentation consistent with acute pancreatitis
b. A serum lipase or amylase value elevated above the upper limit of normal
c. Imaging findings characteristic of acute pancreatitis [IV contrast-enhanced CT, magnetic resonance imaging (MRI), or transabdominal ultrasound].

4. What are the local complications seen in acute pancreatitis?

Local complications of acute pancreatitis are acute peripancreatic fluid collections, pancreatic pseudocyst, acute pancreatic or peripancreatic necrosis, walled-off necrosis, gastric outlet dysfunction, splenic and portal vein thrombosis, and colonic inflammation/necrosis.

Question 5

A 25-year-old female presents with sudden loss of vision in her right eye.

1. Describe briefly various causes of painless loss of vision.

The different causes of painless loss of vision are:
a. Central retinal artery occlusion
b. Central retinal vein occlusion
c. Acute ischemic optic neuropathy
d. Vitreous hemorrhage
e. Amaurosis fugax
f. Transient ischemic attack
g. Retinal detachment.

Central retinal artery occlusion: Its causes include carotid or cardiac embolus, retinal artery thrombosis, giant cell arteritis, vasculitis (lupus, polyarteritis nodosa), sickle cell disease, trauma, vasospasm (migraine), elevated intraocular pressure (glaucoma), hypercoagulable states, and low retinal blood flow (carotid stenosis or hypotension). Sudden (occurring over seconds), profound, painless, monocular loss of vision is characteristic of a central retinal artery occlusion. The event is often preceded by episodes of amaurosis fugax. Physical examination will often reveal an afferent pupillary defect in addition to the pale retina and cherry red macula. Recent studies support IV tissue plasminogen activator within 4.5 hours of symptom onset; however, immediate consultation with an ophthalmologist and neurologist immediately when suspecting acute central retinal artery occlusion is recommended since irreversible loss of visual function occurs after 4 hours of ischemia.

Central retinal vein occlusion: Thrombosis of the central retinal vein causes retinal venous stasis, edema, and hemorrhage. Risk factors include diabetes, hypertension, cerebrovascular disease, cardiovascular disease, dyslipidemia, hypercoagulable states, vasculitis, glaucoma, compression of the vein in thyroid disease, and orbital tumors. Loss of vision is variable, ranging from vague blurring to rapid, painless, and monocular loss of vision. Funduscopic examination reveals optic disk edema and diffuse retinal hemorrhages in all quadrants ("blood-and-thunder fundus"), antivascular endothelial growth factor and laser-induced chorioretinal anastomosis show promise but immediate consultation with neurology and ophthalmology is recommended.

Retinal detachment/flashing lights and/or floaters: Complaints about new-onset flashing lights and/or floaters commonly cause patients to seek urgent medical attention. The first distinction to make is if the symptoms are monocular or binocular. Binocular complaints are almost always intracranial (i.e., ophthalmic migraines), whereas monocular complaints are almost always related to the symptomatic eye. Symptoms may include flashes of light, floaters, a dark veil or curtain in the field of vision, and decreased peripheral and/or central visual acuity. This is an emergent condition requiring a retina specialist to evaluate and treat the patient. Diagnosing a retinal detachment or tear or vitreous detachment requires a dilated indirect ophthalmoscopic evaluation by an ophthalmologist within 24 hours. Most tears occur in the peripheral retina, which is not visualized on the direct funduscopic examination. A large retinal detachment will appear as a pale billowing parachute on dilated funduscopic examination.

2. Describe briefly various causes of painful loss of vision.

The various causes of painful loss of vision are acute angle-closure glaucoma, optic neuritis, giant cell arteritis, and uveitis.

Acute angle-closure glaucoma: It is sudden in onset with severe eye pain and frontal or supraorbital headache and may result in severe visual impairment if not treated quickly. Patients might also complain of blurred vision, nausea, and vomiting. It may be misdiagnosed as migraine, temporal arteritis, subarachnoid hemorrhage, or intra-abdominal emergency. Examination reveals a fixed, midposition pupil, and a hazy (cloudy/steamy) cornea with conjunctival injection most prominent at the limbus. Normal intraocular pressure is 10–20 mm Hg; ocular pressure may exceed 60–80 mm Hg in an acute attack. The initial treatment combines the effects of a carbonic anhydrase inhibitor (IV, PO, or topical), a topical β-blocker, and a topical α-agonist. If the intraocular pressure does not drop significantly with resolution of associated symptoms in the first hour (usually below 40 mm Hg), IV mannitol should be given if there are no contraindications. Definitive treatment is peripheral laser iridotomy (iridectomy).

Optic neuritis: Acute optic neuritis may present without the complaint of pain, but patients frequently have mild-to-moderate pain with eye movement (19–92%). Visual acuity can range from mildly reduced to profound loss with no light perception. Reduction of vision occurs most commonly over days, but occasionally over hours. Visual loss is usually unilateral but can be bilateral. Color vision is affected more commonly than visual acuity, and there may be visual field deficits. Optic neuritis can be idiopathic or an initial presentation of multiple sclerosis. Other causes of optic neuritis include post childhood vaccination; viral infections such as measles, mumps, chickenpox, encephalitis, herpes zoster, and mononucleosis; inflammation of structures contiguous with the optic nerve such as the meninges, orbit, and sinuses; and other infections, including syphilis, tuberculosis, *Cryptococcus*, and sarcoidosis. Neurology and ophthalmology consultation is needed to establish a diagnosis. MRI results are important prognosticators for optic neuritis.

Question 6

1. List the incomplete spinal cord syndromes.

The incomplete spinal cord syndromes are as follows:
a. Anterior cord syndrome
b. Central cord syndrome
c. Brown-Séquard syndrome.

Anterior cord syndrome: It results from damage to the corticospinal and spinothalamic pathways, with preservation of posterior column function. This is manifested by loss of motor function, pain, and temperature sensation distal to the lesion. Only vibration, position, and tactile sensation are preserved. This syndrome may occur following direct injury to the anterior spinal cord. Flexion of the cervical spine may result in cord contusion or bone injury with secondary cord injury. Alternatively, thrombosis of the anterior spinal artery can cause ischemic injury to the anterior cord. Anterior cord injury can also be produced by an extrinsic mass that is amenable to surgical decompression. The overall prognosis for recovery of function is poor.

Central cord syndrome: It is usually seen in older patients with preexisting cervical spondylosis who sustain a hyperextension injury. As named, this injury preferentially involves the central portion of the cord more than the peripheral. The centrally located fibers of the corticospinal and spinothalamic tracts are affected. The neural tracts providing function to the upper extremities are most medial in position compared with the thoracic, lower extremity, and sacral fibers that have a more lateral distribution. Clinically, patients with a central cord syndrome present with decreased strength and, to a lesser degree, decreased pain and temperature sensation, more in the upper than in the lower extremities. Vibration and position sensation are usually preserved. Spastic paraparesis or spastic quadriparesis can also be seen. The majority will have bowel and bladder control, although this may be impaired in the more severe cases.

Brown-Séquard syndrome: It results from hemisection of the cord. It is manifested by ipsilateral loss of motor function, proprioception, and vibratory sensation, and contralateral loss of pain and temperature sensation. The most common cause of this syndrome is penetrating injury. It can also be caused by lateral cord compression secondary to disk protrusion, hematomas, spine fractures, infections, spinal cord infarctions, multiple sclerosis, or tumors.

2. Discuss the process of management of neurogenic shock.

Neurogenic shock is a type of distributive shock that can occur with central nervous system (CNS) or spinal cord injury.

Loss of peripheral sympathetic innervation results in extreme vasodilatation secondary to loss of sympathetic arterial tone. This causes blood pooling in the distal circulation with resultant hypotension. If the T1 through T4 cord levels are compromised, loss of sympathetic innervation to the heart leaves unopposed vagal parasympathetic cardiac innervation. This results in bradycardia or an absence of reflex tachycardia. Patients with neurogenic shock are warm, peripherally vasodilated, and hypotensive with a relative bradycardia. The diagnosis of neurogenic shock is one of exclusion. Management of neurogenic shock is as follows:

a. *Airway:* As a general rule, all patients with a complete cervical injury above C5 should be intubated as soon as possible.
   Absolute indications: Complete cervical spine injury above C5 level, respiratory distress, hypoxemia despite attempts at oxygenation, and severe respiratory acidosis.
   Relative indications: Complaint of shortness of breath, development of "quad breathing" or "belly breathing" (abdomen goes out sharply with inspiration), vital capacity (VC) of <10 mL/kg or decreasing VC. Requirement of patient transfer from ED (MRI, transfer to another facility).

b. *Breathing:* Supplemental oxygen is administered to maintain a SpO_2 >95%. Hypoxemia can be extremely detrimental to patients with neurological injury and can cause severe bradycardia in patients with high cervical injuries due to vagal stimulation.

c. *Circulation:* Fluid resuscitation *"filling the tank"* by infusion of IV crystalloids since the loss of sympathetic tone leads to vasodilation and the need for an increase in the circulating blood volume.

d. *Monitoring:* Pulmonary artery catheter to avoid excessive fluid replacement, with resultant heart failure and pulmonary edema. Mean arterial BP should be maintained at 85–90 mm Hg for the first 7 days after acute spine injury. Second line therapy: Inotropic support as per requirement.

3. Mention the mechanisms of injuries encountered in cervical spine trauma with an example in each category.

Mechanisms of cervical spine trauma with example are shown in **Table 2**.

TABLE 2: Mechanisms of cervical spine injury.

Mechanism of injury	Injury
Flexion	• Anterior subluxation (hyperflexion sprain) (usually stable, but depends on the integrity of posterior ligaments) • Atlantoaxial dislocation (unstable) • Bilateral interfacetal dislocation (unstable) • Simple wedge (compression) fracture (usually stable) • Spinous process avulsion fracture (stable) • Flexion teardrop fracture (highly unstable)
Flexion rotation	• Unilateral facet dislocation (stable unless associated with an articular mass fracture) • Fracture of lateral mass (can be unstable)
Vertical compression	• Jefferson burst fracture of atlas (potentially unstable) • Burst fracture (unstable)
Extension	• Hyperextension dislocation (unstable) • Hyperextension teardrop fracture or extension corner avulsion fracture (unstable in extension) • Fracture of posterior arch of atlas (stable) • Laminar fracture (usually stable) • Traumatic spondylolisthesis (Hangman's fracture) (unstable)
Injuries caused by a combination of mechanisms or poorly understood mechanisms	• Occipital condyle fractures (usually stable) • Atlanto-occipital dissociation (AOD) (highly unstable) • Odontoid (dens) fractures (types II and III are unstable)

Question 7

1. List the various causes of acute scrotal pain.

The various causes of acute scrotal pain are testicular torsion, epididymitis, and appendage torsion.

2. How do you differentiate clinically among them?

The differential diagnosis of acute scrotal pain is shown in **Table 3**.

TABLE 3: Differential diagnosis of acute scrotal pain.

	Testicular torsion	Epididymitis	Appendage torsion
Historical features			
Peak incidence	Neonates, adolescents	Adolescents, young adults	Prepubertal
Risk factors	Undescended testicle (neonate), rapid increase in testicular size (adolescent), failure of prior orchiopexy	Sexual activity/promiscuity, genitourinary (GU) anomalies, GU instrumentation	Presence of appendages
Pain onset	Sudden	Gradual, progressive	Variable
Nausea/vomiting	More likely	Less likely	Less likely
Dysuria	Less likely	More likely	Less likely
Physical findings			
Fever	Less likely	More likely, particularly in advanced disease (epididymoorchitis)	Less likely
Location of swelling/tenderness (early)	Testicle, progressing to diffuse hemiscrotal involvement	Epididymis, progressing to diffuse hemiscrotal involvement	Localized to head of affected testicle or epididymis
Cremasteric reflex	Testicular torsion less likely if present	May be present or absent	May be present or absent
Testicle position	High riding, transverse alignment	Normal position, vertical alignment	Normal position, vertical alignment

3. Discuss the treatment options for testicular torsion in ED.

Testicular torsion is a common condition that is encountered in the ED. Manual detorsion of the affected testis successfully, though a painful procedure, can be considered initially as an emergency. Most testes twist in a lateral to medial fashion (two thirds of cases) so detorsion initially should be done in a medial to lateral motion. Detorsion is typically done in a manner similar to opening a book. If one were to stand at the patient's feet, the patient's right testis would be rotated in a counterclockwise fashion and the patient's left testis in a clockwise fashion. The initial attempt should include one and one-half rotations (540°). Any relief of pain is a positive end point, and the success of the maneuver can be assessed with Doppler ultrasound, demonstrating restoration of blood flow. An occasional patient will require manipulation beyond the initial one and one-half rotations. A worsening of the patient's pain suggests that detorsion should then be done in the opposite direction (one third of cases). Final management of testicular torsion is surgical fixation by the urologist.

Question 8

1. Explain the anatomy of knee relevant to trauma.

The knee consists of two joints: (1) The tibiofemoral joint and (2) the patellofemoral joint **(Fig. 1)**. Within the tibiofemoral joint, the distal femur (comprised of the medial and lateral femoral condyles) articulates with the proximal tibia (comprised of the medial and lateral tibial condyles) **(Fig. 2)**.

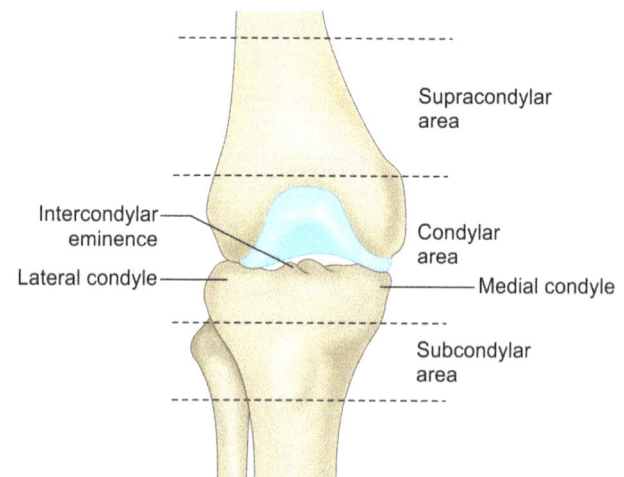

Fig. 1: The supracondylar and condylar areas of the femur, and the medial and subcondylar areas of the tibia.

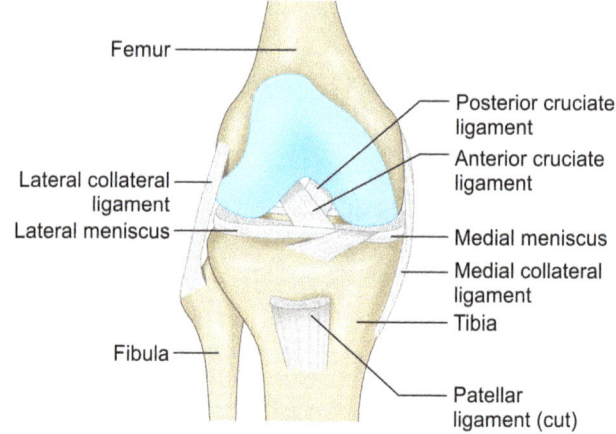

Fig. 2: Ligaments of the right knee joint. The articular capsule and the patella have been removed.

2. Discuss important neurovascular complications of injuries to knee.

Popliteal artery injury can occur from fractures about the knee, especially femoral condyle fractures or displaced tibial plateau fractures, and from ligamentous injuries such as isolated posterior cruciate ligament injuries, multiple ligamentous injuries, or knee dislocation. Popliteal artery circulation must be restored within 8 hours to avoid amputation, because collateral circulation is insufficient to maintain blood flow to the leg. Measure distal pulses on ED admission and after any manipulation and compare pulses to those in the noninjured leg. A diminished pulse raises concern for vascular injury and should not be interpreted as vascular spasm. It is important to remember that vascular injury can be present even in the presence of normal pulses. Ancillary studies include measurement of the ankle–brachial index and duplex ultrasound (reported to be 95% sensitive and 99% specific for arterial injury but can miss small intimal tears). Patients with normal pulses and an ankle–brachial index ≥0.9 can be observed. Vascular compromise is suspected in patients with abnormal palpable and Doppler pulses and/or ankle-brachial index <0.9 and warrants further vascular imaging and consultation. Vascular surgery consultation can aid in determining the need for CT angiogram versus on-table angiography and can help monitor for the development of compartment syndrome, venous injury, and arterial thrombosis.

Peroneal nerve injuries (stretch or, less often, transection) can result from severe ligamentous knee injuries or knee dislocations. Nearly half of the fibular head fractures or avulsions are associated with peroneal nerve injury. The deep peroneal nerve provides sensation to the first dorsal web space of the toes and allows dorsiflexion of the foot and extension of the toes. Injury results in foot drop and gait difficulty. Prognosis is variable, depending on the severity of injury.

3. Discuss meniscal and ligament injuries around knee joint.

The knee joint depends on ligaments and muscles for support and is frequently subjected to injuries from traumatic forces, including hyperextension, valgus and varus stresses, and anteroposterior displacement. The most common forces are valgus, which produce injuries to the medial side of the knee. Injuries to the lateral side of the knee are produced by varus stresses. Such forces may result in a strain or rupture of the medial or lateral collateral ligaments, the anterior or posterior cruciate ligaments, or the capsular structures, or a tear in the medial or lateral menisci.

a. *Medial collateral ligament and lateral collateral ligament injuries:* The medial stabilizers of the knee are tested by applying a valgus stress to the knee at 0° and in approximately 30° of flexion to determine the integrity of the medial capsular and ligamentous structures. The medial collateral ligament supplies the majority of restraint to valgus deformities of the knee in all stages of flexion. A varus force is then applied to the lateral aspect of the knee to ascertain the integrity of the lateral structures. The lateral collateral ligament, analogous to the medial collateral ligament, is the major restraint to varus laxity on the knee at all positions of flexion. Injuries to these ligaments can include a strain, partial tear, or complete rupture. If there is no demonstrated laxity but the valgus or varus test reproduces pain, a grade 1 strain has likely occurred. If there is a laxity demonstrated without a firm end point compared with the other knee, this is concerning for a complete tear of the medial or lateral collateral ligament. If there is laxity with the varus or valgus test performed with 30° of flexion, similar maneuvers should be applied with the leg in full extension, if possible. Laxity to valgus stress while in full extension indicates a significant lesion involving the entire medial collateral ligament complex and/or in association with a cruciate ligament and posterior capsule tear. Laxity to varus stress in full extension likewise indicates a significant injury that may involve the posterolateral corner of the knee as well as the cruciate ligaments. Peroneal nerve injuries may also occur in lateral injuries. Although these tests may aid in the diagnosis of medial collateral ligament and lateral collateral ligament injuries, there are no adequate published reports to allow comment on their sensitivity and specificity.

b. *Anterior cruciate ligament injuries:* The mechanism of injury to the anterior cruciate ligament is usually noncontact—a deceleration, hyperextension, or marked internal rotation of the tibia on the femur resulting in an injury to this ligament. Injury is often associated with a "pop," swelling that develops within hours, and a sense of instability. The pop is considered pathognomonic for anterior cruciate ligament injury. The history of this mechanism of injury combined with the presence of a traumatic effusion is very suggestive of an anterior cruciate ligament disruption. The diagnosis of an anterior cruciate ligament injury is made using the *Lachman test*, the anterior drawer sign, and the pivot shift. The Lachman test is the most sensitive and specific test (81% for both). For this test, the examiner places the knee in 30° of flexion and stabilizes the femur above the knee with his or her nondominant hand. The dominant hand is placed grasping the lower leg at the level of the tibial tubercle, and the examiner introduces an anterior force, attempting to displace the tibia anteriorly on the femur. If a displacement compared with the opposite knee is found, or if there is a soft end point, then a tear in the anterior cruciate ligament has occurred.

The *anterior drawer test* is only approximately 38% sensitive and 81% specific. This maneuver is performed with a 45° flexion at the hip and a 90° flexion at the knee. Then, an attempt is made to displace the tibia from the femur in an anterior direction. A displacement of >6 mm compared with the normal, opposite knee indicates an injury to the anterior cruciate ligament. False-negative findings may be associated with this maneuver. False-positive results may occur when there is a posterior cruciate ligament tear as the tibia will start out in a more posterior position, thus allowing for a perceived increase in translation when moved anteriorly. Although the Lachman test is more sensitive than the anterior drawer test and is able to identify partial tears in the anterior cruciate ligament, it can be difficult to perform on patients with large legs.

The *pivot shift* is the third maneuver by which the examiner can determine the integrity of the anterior cruciate ligament. It may be painful to the patient and is often most easily tested under anesthesia in the operating room. The pivot shift test without anesthesia was found to be only 28% sensitive but 81% specific. With the patient supine and relaxed, lift the heel of the foot to approximately 45° of hip flexion with the knee fully extended. The opposite hand grasps the knee with the thumb behind the fibular head. Then internally rotate the ankle and knee, apply a valgus force to the knee, and flex the knee. If an anterior subluxation of the tibia is present, a sudden visible, audible, and palpable reduction of the subluxation occurs at about 20–30° of flexion. This indicates a deficit in the anterior cruciate ligament, which is required to stabilize the knee in this position. Other tests are described in the literature to determine the integrity of the anterior cruciate ligament, including the jerk test and dynamic extension testing.

c. *Posterior cruciate ligament injuries:* The posterior cruciate ligament can be injured in isolation or in combination with other ligamentous structures of the knee. In contrast to anterior cruciate ligament injuries, isolated posterior cruciate ligament injuries are much less common. The posterior cruciate ligament provides initial resistance to posterior translation at all angles of flexion of the knee. The mechanism of injury then is usually an anterior-to-posterior force applied to the tibia or lower leg. Nearly all posterior cruciate ligament injuries diagnosed in the ED are seen in association with other ligamentous injuries. A deficit of this ligament is identified by the posterior drawer test and the sag sign. The posterior drawer test is performed with the knee and hip in flexion as described for the anterior drawer test. The physician applies a posterior force to the tibial tubercle. If there is displacement posteriorly, then the examiner can diagnose an injury to this ligament. One might also notice a sag sign, where there is a posterior sag or drop back of the tibial tubercle because of loss of integrity of the posterior cruciate ligament when observing the knee with 45° flexion at the hip and 90° flexion at the knee.

d. *Posterolateral injury:* This injury is difficult to detect and involves a tear of the popliteus–arcuate complex, which may occur in combination with lateral ligament injury and possible anterior cruciate ligament or posterior cruciate ligament injury. Isolated injuries to the popliteus–arcuate complex are rare and demonstrated by testing at 0–30° of flexion for maximal posterior translation and at 90° of flexion for maximal external rotation compared with that of the normal opposite knee.

e. *Meniscal injuries*: These injuries occur by themselves or in combination with ligamentous injuries. Anterior cruciate ligament injuries are commonly associated with meniscal injuries. Cutting, squatting, or twisting maneuvers may cause injury to the meniscus. The medial meniscus is approximately twice as likely as the lateral meniscus to be injured. Many of the tears involve the peripheral posterior aspect of the meniscus. The combination of a suggestive history and physical findings on examination should lead to the diagnosis of a meniscal tear. If the patient experiences painful locking of the knee joint on either flexion or extension limiting further activity, it points to the diagnosis of a torn meniscus. Other signs of a meniscal tear include effusions that occur after activity; a sensation of popping, clicking, or snapping; a feeling of instability in the joint, especially with activity; and tenderness in the anterior joint space after excessive activity. On examination, atrophy of the quadriceps muscle as a result of disuse and joint-line tenderness can be found. Definitive diagnosis can be made by MRI or arthroscopy. The definitive surgical treatment is usually partial meniscectomy or meniscal repair.

Question 9

1. List the regional nerve entrapment syndromes of the hip.

a. *Lateral femoral cutaneous nerve entrapment/meralgia paresthesia (anterolateral thigh pain):* This condition is the most common among the lower extremity nerve entrapment syndromes and is the compressive inflammation of the lateral femoral cutaneous nerve. The nerve enters the thigh under the inguinal ligament near the anterior superior iliac spine and is subjected to minor recurring traumatic events. Nerve irritation can also be triggered by tight clothing or heavy belts, seat belts, pregnancy, certain sitting positions, repetitive flexion/extension of the leg, trauma, surgical interventions such as appendectomy or hysterectomy, and obesity. Patients present with pain to the hip area, thigh, or groin along the proximal anterior lateral aspect of the leg, burning or tingling paresthesias, and hypersensitivity to light touch. Pain may be worsened during physical examination by tapping over the area of the anterior superior iliac spine. Management includes limiting the exacerbating activity, NSAIDs, local injections, weight loss, and rarely surgical excision of the nerve.

b. *Obturator nerve entrapment (medial thigh/groin pain):* It is a sequela of pelvic fractures or abdominal/pelvic surgery. Exercise-induced medial thigh is the predominant symptom and is aggravated by movement of the hip. Imaging studies are of limited value. Chronic denervation can be revealed by needle electromyography. Pain may be relieved by local injection of lidocaine into the area of the nerve.

c. *Ilioinguinal nerve entrapment (groin pain):* Hypertrophy of the abdominal wall musculature or pregnancy is the main cause of nerve entrapment. Hyperextension of the hip produces pain and hypoesthesia in the distribution of the nerve resulting in groin pain.

d. *Piriformis syndrome (buttock/posterior thigh pain):* Irritation of the sciatic nerve from the piriformis muscle causes pain in the buttocks and hamstring muscles. It is worsened by sitting, climbing stairs, or squatting and is exacerbated by hip flexion and passive internal rotation. The patient is managed conservatively.

2. List the bursal syndromes of the knee.

a. *Pes anserine bursitis (anterior medial knee pain):* The pes anserine (Latin for three-toed foot of the goose) bursa lies deep to the three tendons that insert on the medial aspect of the tibia below the knee joint—the gracilis, sartorius, and semitendinosus and above the medial collateral ligament and medial femoral condyle. Pes anserine bursitis is common in obese women with osteoarthritis of the knee, in runners, and with overuse syndromes. The patient complains of anterior medial pain below the joint line, focal swelling over the bursa, and increased tenderness to palpation.

b. *Prepatellar bursitis (pain anterior to the patella):* This is also known as *housemaid's knee, nun's knee,* or *carpet-layer's knee*. Inflammation of bursa through repetitive kneeling on hard surfaces presents with mild pain and a restricted range of motion from the swelling or as an effusion over the lower pole of the patella. This swelling is tender to palpation, and bursal margins are often palpable. The prepatellar bursa is also one of the more common sites for septic bursitis, especially in children.

3. List knee myofascial syndromes.

Knee myofascial syndromes are also known as overuse syndromes.

a. *Patellofemoral syndrome/runner's knee (anterior knee pain):* This syndrome is a major cause of anterior knee pain, with three typical causes: focal trauma (least common), overuse, and abnormal patellar tracking as it glides and rotates in the patellar groove. A major contributor to abnormal patellar tracking is weakness of the quadriceps muscle. The syndrome is more common in females due to the presence of an abnormal Q angle (>20°), resulting from a broader pelvis. The Q angle is measured at the junction of a line drawn from the anterior superior iliac spine to the central patella and a second line drawn from the central patella to the tibial tubercle. A normal angle is approximately 15°. An increased Q angle increases the risk for patellar subluxation. Because of this relationship, females have a 50–100% greater incidence of knee injuries compared with males in both athletes and nonathletes. The symptoms of anterior knee pain are gradual in onset, nonradiating, and typically unilateral. Pain is exacerbated by prolonged flexion of the knee, such as sitting in on-air flights or at the movie theater. Pain frequently occurs with activities of daily living, such as walking, and especially with stair-climbing. The presence of crepitus to palpation at the patellofemoral joint suggests degenerative changes but may be normal. The patellar grind test is accomplished by direct anterior to posterior pressure on the patella or the quadriceps tendon while asking the patient to contract the quadriceps muscles. A positive test evokes sudden patellar pain and relaxation of the muscle. The opposite test involves lifting the patella away from the knee joint while passively bending and straightening the knee. If this relieves pain, the patellofemoral joint is likely the source. Radiographic studies are of limited value but may detect arthritis. Treatment involves the usual conservative measures, with an emphasis on physical therapy and strengthening.

Brace support of the knee will also help correct the patellofemoral mechanism. Inflammatory pain to the knee may last for months to a few years following surgery or trauma and is based on a genetic predisposition to arthrofibrosis from these insults. Arthroscopy may cause the release of calcium pyrophosphate from tissue, resulting in a severe synovitis.

b. *Chondromalacia patellae (anterior knee pain):* It refers to the softening of the cartilage on the posterior surface of the patella, most commonly occurring with the patellofemoral syndrome. This diagnosis is made by direct arthroscopic visualization of a ragged appearance of the affected cartilage.

c. *Medial plica syndrome (anterior medial knee pain):* The plica syndrome is uncommon and is difficult to distinguish from other causes of patellofemoral pain. Plicae are abnormal, redundant folds in the connective tissue of the knee, persisting from embryologic septa that initially divide the knee into compartments, normally disappearing as the fetus matures. Plicae become symptomatic for unclear reasons. Recurring synovitis may result in a palpable, inelastic band that interferes with normal knee movement and pain. This band-like structure is best palpated parallel to the medial border of the patella and produces pain in the area of the medial femoral condyle that radiates anteriorly. Pain may be brought on with activity or may occur at rest. Patients may also report a snapping sensation as the plica moves over the femoral condyle with repeated flexion and extension. Arthroscopy or MRI findings confirm the diagnosis. Treatment is conservative, with strengthening and stretching exercises; some patients require arthroscopic resection of the band.

d. *Iliotibial band syndrome (lateral knee pain):* It is the most common in distance runners or cyclists. The iliotibial band inserts onto the lateral femoral and tibial condyles. The thickened fascia serves as a ligament and stabilizes the joint in extension. With overuse, the bursa underlying the band becomes irritated.

Question 10

1. What are the causes of chest pain during the third trimester of pregnancy?

Chest pain can be caused due to a number of reasons during pregnancy; most of the differential diagnoses are similar to nonpregnant women. The important causes are as follows:
a. Acute coronary syndrome
b. Aortic dissection
c. Cardiomyopathy
d. Spontaneous coronary artery dissection
e. Coronary vasospasm
f. Coronary embolus
g. Peripartum cardiomyopathy
h. Sympathetic crashing acute pulmonary edema

Aortic dissection, cardiomyopathy, and acute coronary syndrome are common in pregnancy. Acute coronary syndrome is three times more common in pregnancy when compared to nonpregnant women of the same age group. It is caused in pregnancy by spontaneous coronary artery dissection, coronary vasospasm, or coronary embolus.

Spontaneous coronary artery dissection is the most common cause of pregnancy-related acute myocardial infarction and is frequent in the third trimester of pregnancy or in the postpartum period. It is due to progesterone-related vessel wall changes and shear forces secondary to increased blood volume. It is frequently found in multiple vessels and is associated with an increased incidence of cardiogenic shock, life-threatening arrhythmias, and a high maternal and fetal mortality.

Coronary vasospasm is more common in patients with migraine headaches, whereas coronary emboli are seen commonly in pregnancy considering the fact that it is a hypercoagulable state. Treatment of acute coronary syndrome in pregnancy is complicated since many drugs in current acute coronary syndrome guidelines are not recommended in pregnancy or have limited human safety data. It is therefore recommended to resuscitate and stabilize the patient as for any nonpregnant patient and obtain emergent cardiology consultation for further management.

2. Define severe preeclampsia.

Preeclampsia is defined as the presence of de novo hypertension (>140 mm Hg systolic or >90 mm Hg diastolic) after 20 weeks of gestation combined with proteinuria or other maternal organ dysfunction (renal, liver, neurologic).

Severe preeclampsia is the condition which includes the following features:
a. Systolic blood pressure is ≥160 mm Hg or diastolic BP is ≥110 mm Hg on two occasions at least 4 hours apart while the patient is on bed rest.
b. Thrombocytopenia (<100,000 platelets/mL)
c. Impaired liver function (liver enzyme levels increased to twice normal) or persistent right upper quadrant/epigastric pain unresponsive to medication and not accounted for by a different diagnosis)
d. Progressive renal insufficiency (serum creatinine >1.1 mg/dL or doubling of creatinine level without other renal disease)
e. Pulmonary edema
f. Cerebral or visual disturbances

3. Discuss abruptio placentae.

Abruptio placentae is the premature separation of a normally implanted placenta from the uterine lining. The incidence of spontaneous abruption is highest between 24 and 32 weeks of gestation. Placental abruption is an obstetric emergency which increases the risk of maternal morbidity or mortality and may also have a detrimental effect on the fetus. Abruption can cause uteroplacental insufficiency and fetal distress or demise. Risk factors for abruption include abdominal trauma, oligohydramnios, chorioamnionitis, advanced maternal age or parity, chronic or pregnancy induced hypertension, vasculitis, and cocaine or tobacco use. Maternal complications include coagulopathy, hemorrhagic shock, uterine rupture, and multiple organ failure. Diagnosis is done clinically. Electronic fetal monitoring (cardiotocodynamometry) and transvaginal ultrasound also help in the diagnosis of placental abruption. Initial management consists of maternal stabilization; cardiotocographic monitoring to detect fetal distress followed by immediate delivery is indicated for severe abruption.

■ SUGGESTED READING

1. Richhariya D, Sharma B. Textbook of Emergency Medicine including Intensive Care and Trauma, 2nd edition. New Delhi: Jaypee Brothers Medical Publishers (P) Ltd; 2022. pp. 1557-63. (Question 1).
2. Richhariya D, Sharma B. Textbook of Emergency Medicine including Intensive Care and Trauma, 2nd edition. New Delhi: Jaypee Brothers Medical Publishers (P) Ltd; 2022. pp. 1579-88. (Question 2).
3. Richhariya D, Sharma B. Textbook of Emergency Medicine including Intensive Care and Trauma, 2nd edition. New Delhi: Jaypee Brothers Medical Publishers (P) Ltd; 2022. pp. 75-85. (Question 3).
4. Richhariya D, Sharma B. Textbook of Emergency Medicine including Intensive Care and Trauma, 2nd edition. New Delhi: Jaypee Brothers Medical Publishers (P) Ltd; 2022. pp. 669-73.
5. Richhariya D, Sharma B. Textbook of Emergency Medicine including Intensive Care and Trauma, 2nd edition. New Delhi: Jaypee Brothers Medical Publishers (P) Ltd; 2022. pp. 900-5. (Question 5).
6. Richhariya D, Sharma B. Textbook of Emergency Medicine including Intensive Care and Trauma, 2nd edition. New Delhi: Jaypee Brothers Medical Publishers (P) Ltd; 2022. pp. 1570-8. (Question 6).
7. Richhariya D, Sharma B. Textbook of Emergency Medicine including Intensive Care and Trauma, 2nd edition. New Delhi: Jaypee Brothers Medical Publishers (P) Ltd; 2022. pp. 785-90. (Question 7).
8. Richhariya D, Sharma B. Textbook of Emergency Medicine including Intensive Care and Trauma, 2nd edition. New Delhi: Jaypee Brothers Medical Publishers (P) Ltd; 2022. pp. 1602-10. (Question 8 and 9).
9. Richhariya D, Sharma B. Textbook of Emergency Medicine including Intensive Care and Trauma, 2nd edition. New Delhi: Jaypee Brothers Medical Publishers (P) Ltd; 2022. pp. 1078-100. (Question 10).

Emergency Medicine Paper 11

Devendra Richhariya

Question 1

A 30-year-old patient presents to the emergency department (ED) with fever and altered sensorium.

1. Enumerate differential diagnosis for fever and altered sensorium.

Acute-onset fever with altered mentation: This is a problem commonly encountered by the physician in the ED. "Acute febrile encephalopathy" is a term commonly used to identify this condition in which altered mental status either accompanies or follows a short febrile illness.

Fever and altered mental status/central nervous system (CNS) involvement: Cerebral malaria, arboviral encephalitis (e.g., Japanese encephalitis, West Nile virus), meningococcal meningitis, rabies, African trypanosomiasis, scrub typhus, angiostrongyliasis, and tickborne encephalitis.

2. Discuss the approach to the patient with fever and altered sensorium in the ED.

Fever and CNS symptoms: Specific neurological diagnoses in a traveler are rare. Fever and headache are common symptoms and are seen in systemic infections such as malaria, dengue, and chikungunya infection and rickettsial diseases. Malaria and meningitis are the most common treatable causes of fever and CNS symptoms and must always be excluded first. Cerebral malaria is caused by *Plasmodium falciparum* and can present with confusion, headache, seizures, or decreased consciousness. Any patient with neurological symptoms and a history of travel to a malaria-endemic region should be considered to have cerebral malaria and investigated. Other causes of fever and encephalopathy include bacterial infections (typhoid, Lyme disease, leptospirosis) and human immunodeficiency virus (HIV) seroconversion. Approach to the patient with fever and altered sensorium is shown in **Flowchart 1**.

Flowchart 1: Approach to the patient with fever and altered sensorium.

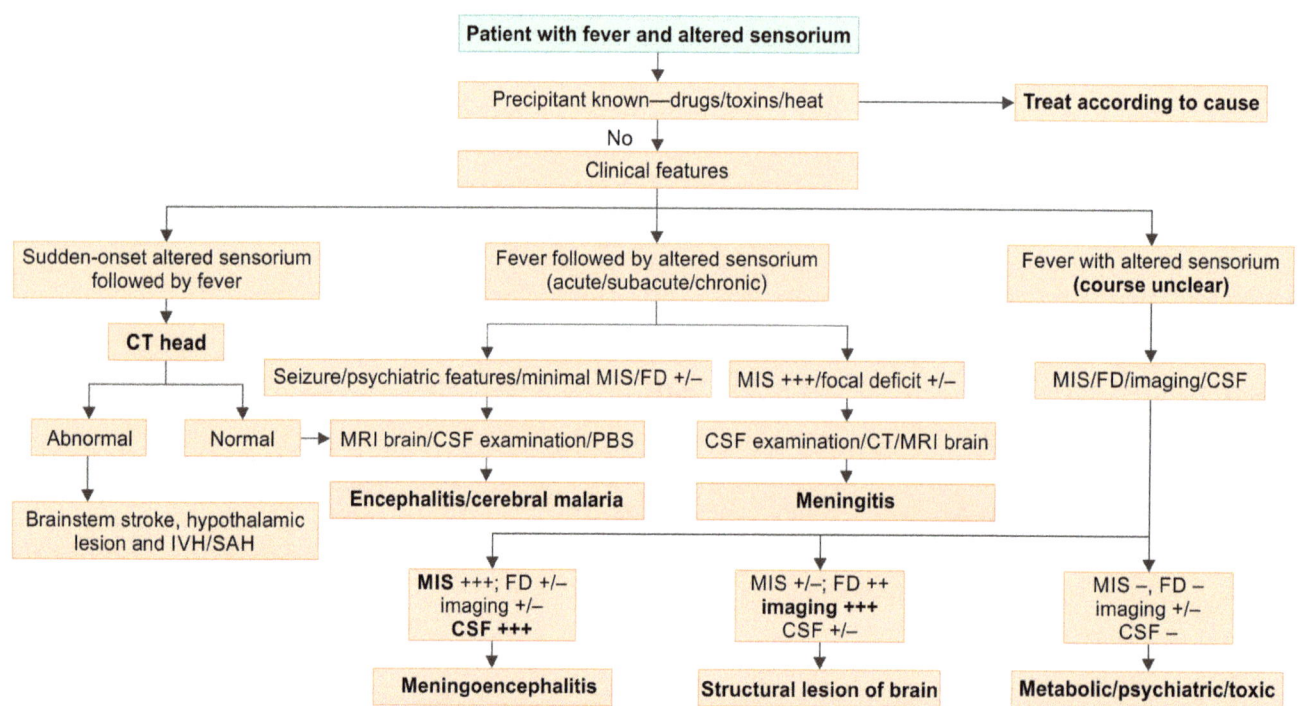

(CT: computed tomography; CSF: cerebrospinal fluid; FD: focal deficit; IVH: intraventricular hemorrhage; MIS: multisystem inflammatory system; MRI: magnetic resonance imaging; PBS: peripheral blood smear; SAH: subarachnoid hemorrhage)

Question 2

A 68-year-old male presents to ED with chest pain. His ECG shows ST-segment elevation in V2–V6.

1. Enumerate the causes of ST-segment elevation.

The causes of ST-segment elevation apart from acute myocardial infarction (MI) are myocarditis, pericarditis, stress cardiomyopathy (Takotsubo), benign early repolarization, acute vasospasm, spontaneous coronary artery dissection, left bundle branch block, various channelopathies, and electrolyte abnormalities. Causes of ST-segment elevation can be given by the mnemonic ELAVATION as follows:

E—Electrolyte abnormalities

L—Left-bundle branch block

A—Aneurysm of left ventricle

V—Ventricular hypertrophy

A—Arrhythmia (Brugada syndrome and ventricular tachycardia)

T—Treatment (iatrogenic pericarditis)

I—Injury (MI or cardiac contusion)

O—Osborne waves (hypothermia, hypocalcemia)

N—Nonatherosclerotic (vasospasm)

2. How will you manage this patient in the ED?

Patients with confirmed MI are admitted to hospital care immediately; antianginal, antiplatelet, and anticoagulant therapies are started. Nonenteric-coated, chewable aspirin (162–325 mg) is started immediately followed by maintenance dose (81–325 mg/day) indefinitely. Continuous ECG monitoring is conducted. Supplemental oxygen is started only if oxygen saturation is <90% or there are respiratory distress/other hypoxemia features. Lipid profile is obtained in the first 24 hours; high-intensity statins started, unless contraindicated. Beta-blockers (calcium channel blockers if beta-blockers contraindicated) can be started within the first 24 hours. Angiotensin-converting enzyme (ACE) inhibitors/angiotensin II receptor blocker (ARB) is recommended, especially for patients with impaired left ventricular ejection fraction (≤40%), early heart failure (HF), hypertension, and diabetes mellitus (DM). Patients remain on bed/chair rest with minimal ambulation.

3. Discuss HEART score and TIMI score in a patient with chest pain.

TIMI (thrombolysis in myocardial infarction) score **(Table 1)** and HEART (history, ECG, age, risk factors, and troponins) score **(Table 2)** are used for risk stratification in chest pain.

TABLE 1: Risk stratification: TIMI (thrombolysis in myocardial infarction) score—1 point for each positive score.

History	• Age >65 years • Three or more risk factors for CAD • Known CAD • Aspirin use in the past 7 days
Presentation	• Recent (<24 hours) severe angina • Positive cardiac biomarkers • ST deviation >0.5 mm

(CAD: coronary artery disease)

Note: Higher TIMI scores mandate admission. It predicts risk of an adverse cardiac outcome within 14 days of presentation with unstable angina or non-STEMI (ST-elevation myocardial infarction). *Vancouver chest pain rule*—used to determine very low-risk chest pain patients and help in early discharge.

TABLE 2: Risk stratification: HEART (history, ECG, age, risk factors, and troponins) risk score for chest pain patients in emergency department.

History	• Highly suspicious • Moderately suspicious • Slightly suspicious	2 1 0
ECG	• Significant ST-depression • Nonspecific repolarization changes • Normal	2 1 0
Age	• >65 years • 45–65 years • <45 years	2 1 0
Risk factors	• >3 risk • 1 or 2 • No risk	2 1 0
Troponins	• >3 × normal limit • 1–3 × normal limit • <Normal limit	2 1 0

HEART score	Risk of MACE	Recommendations
0–3	0.9%	ED discharge
4–6	12%	Observation
>6	65%	Cardiology admission

(ED: emergency department; MACE: major adverse cardiac event)

4. How will you decide between percutaneous coronary intervention and fibrinolytic therapy?

Reperfusion is indicated for all patients with ≤12-hour duration of symptoms and persistent ST-segment elevation. Fibrinolysis with tenecteplase, alteplase, or reteplase is recommended if revascularization is expected to be delayed beyond 2 hours. It is also important to distinguish between left ventricular MI (LVMI) and the right ventricular MI (RVMI) with the help of clinical features, ECG, and the hemodynamic features because mortality risk due to primary RV dysfunction is nearly as high as that due to LV dysfunction. Literature shows that primary percutaneous coronary intervention (PCI) is better in terms of reducing mortality, nonfatal MI, and stroke as compared with fibrinolysis if performed on time.

Primary PCI: Stenting is recommended over balloon angioplasty.

Question 3

A 30-year-old presents to the ED with an acute onset of breathlessness.

1. Enumerate the causes of acute onset of breathlessness.

Breathing difficulty (acute dyspnea) is the most common manifestation with which the patients come to the ED. It requires several steps for differentiation and the risk stratification of patients presenting with shortness of breath (SOB) **(Table 3)**.

TABLE 3: Differential diagnosis for acute dyspnea.

Head and neck	Cardiac	Miscellaneous
Angioedema	ACS	Hyperventilation
Anaphylaxis	Decompensated heart failure	Anxiety
Pharyngeal infection	Pulmonary edema (flash)	Pneumomediastinum
Deep neck infection	High output failure	Lung tumor
Foreign body	Cardiomyopathy	Massive pleural effusion
Neck trauma	Arrhythmia	Intra-abdominal process
Pulmonary	Valvular dysfunction	Ascites
COPD exacerbation	Cardiac tamponade	Pregnancy
BA exacerbation	Toxic/metabolic	Massive obesity
Pulmonary embolism	Organophosphate	Neurological
Pneumothorax	Salicylate	Stroke
Pneumonia	CO poisoning	Neuromuscular disease
ARDS	Toxic ingestion	Chest wall
Lung contusion or injury	DKA	Rib fracture
Hemorrhage	• Sepsis • Anemia	Flail chest

(ACS: acute coronary syndrome; ARDS: acute respiratory distress syndrome; BA: bronchial asthma; CO: carbon monoxide; COPD: chronic obstructive pulmonary disease; DKA: diabetic ketoacidosis)

2. In a patient with acute asthma, how do you classify his asthma attack based on the peak expiratory flow rate?

Symptoms and finding do not correlate well with the severity of symptoms so forced expiratory volume in 1 second and peak expiratory flow rate (PEFR) are important parameters in categorizing the severity of acute asthma. The other parameters to classify the severity of asthma are summarized in **Flowchart 2**.

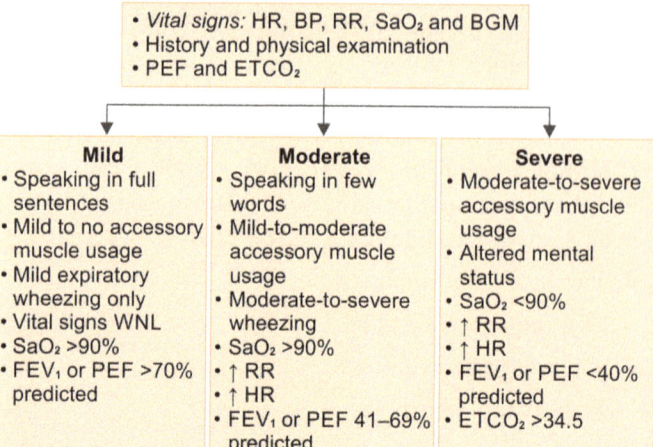

Flowchart 2: Categories of severity of asthma.

(BGM: blood glucose meter; BP: blood pressure; ETCO$_2$: end-tidal carbon dioxide; FEV$_1$: forced expiratory volume in 1 second; HR: heart rate; PEF: peak expiratory flow; RR: respiratory rate; SaO$_2$: oxygen saturation; WNL: within normal limit)

3. What are the indications for assisted ventilation in a patient with acute asthma?

Mechanical ventilation: Intubation can be considered in patients with the following:
a. *Noninvasive (NIV) failure:* Worsening of arterial blood gases (ABG) and/or pH in 1-2 hours; lack of improvement in ABG and/or pH after 4 hours
b. *Severe acidosis* (pH <7.25) and *hypercapnia* (PaCO$_2$ >60 mm Hg)
c. *Tachypnea* > 35 breaths/min
d. *Other complications:* Metabolic abnormalities, sepsis, pneumonia, pulmonary embolism, barotrauma, and massive pleural effusion.

4. What are the initial ventilator settings for invasive positive-pressure ventilation in acute asthma?

Mechanical ventilation in bronchial asthma: Severe bronchospasm causes longer time constant and severe inhomogeneity of time constant of lung units leading to air trapping; this is also called auto-positive end-expiratory pressure (PEEP). In other words, there is insufficient time for complete inspired air to flow out of the lungs before the next inspiration occurs. This can cause increased intrathoracic pressure and decreased venous return resulting in hemodynamic collapse. The target of ventilation in such patients should be to minimize air trapping and achieve hemodynamic stability. It can be achieved by providing long expiratory times which can be achieved by the following settings:

f = 8–10 breaths/min
VT = 4–8 mL/kg
T_I = ≤1 second
I:E ratio = 1:4–1:5
Gas flow = 80–100 L/min
PEEP = 0–5 cmH$_2$O (in case of severe asthma, it should be kept at zero)
Descending flow waveform pattern
P_{plat} <30 cmH$_2$O

Permissive hypercapnia refers to the strategy of accepting a higher PCO$_2$ while maintaining a pH >7.2. It aims to avoid air trapping. If P_{plat} >30 cmH$_2$O and PCO$_2$ >90 mm Hg, deeper sedation and/or paralysis should be considered.

Question 4

A 42-year-old male is brought to the ED with right arm and leg weakness with slurring of speech for the past 2 hours. His vitals are pulse rate (PR) 100 beats/min, blood pressure (BP) 200/130 mm Hg and oxygen saturation (SaO$_2$) 95%. He is fully conscious.

1. Describe stepwise assessment and management of this patient in ED.

Clinical signs of stroke depend upon the part of the brain involved. The American Heart Association/American Stroke Association (AHA/ASA) has popularized the FAST algorithm to diagnose stroke in the *prehospital setting*. FAST acronym stands for facial droop, arm weakness, slurred speech, and time of onset. Another easy way to remember the signs of stroke is the BEFAST method. This method also takes into account the symptoms of posterior circulation.

BEFAST: *B*alance (loss of balance/dizziness), *E*yes (disturbance of vision in one or both eyes), *F*ace (facial droop), *A*rm (weakness), and *S*peech (slurred) *T*est

All the symptoms need not be present to diagnose stroke. Any of the abovementioned symptoms can be present and is helpful in diagnosing ischemic as well as hemorrhagic stroke.

For complete assessment of a stroke patient, it is recommended to use the National Institutes of Health (NIH) stroke scale. According to the latest stroke metrics, a patient with acute stroke should be examined by a trained physician or a neurologist within 10 minutes of arrival at the emergency room. Urgent CT brain under stroke protocol with angiography of head and neck vessels is required. The most important early imaging test is noncontrast CT of the brain. This helps with one of the first branch points of therapy, which is distinguishing hemorrhagic stroke from ischemic stroke. Some hospitals use emergent MRI to evaluate patients with possible stroke, but this is much less common. Rapidly obtaining a noncontrast CT of the head should be a priority in working up the patient with suspected cerebrovascular accident (CVA). Head CT is the first and most important test when evaluating for thrombolysis and helps in differentiating hemorrhage, subdural hematoma, and tumor. On CT, most ischemic strokes eventually become visible as hypodensities of the brain parenchyma, but CT is largely normal for at least 6 hours. The earliest CT signs are loss of the cortical ribbon and gyral edema.

2. What are stroke mimics?

Common stroke mimics are shown in **Table 4**.

TABLE 4: Stroke mimics.

Toxic–metabolic	• Hypoglycemia or hyperglycemia • Hyponatremia or hypernatremia • Ingestion or overdose • Drug toxicity • Intoxication (alcohol, illicit drugs) • Hepatic encephalopathy
Intracranial hemorrhage	• Intracerebral hemorrhage • Subarachnoid hemorrhage • Subdural hematoma
Infectious	• Sepsis • Encephalitis • Meningitis
Structural lesions	• Brain mass or tumor • Spinal cord lesion
Others	• Demyelinating disease (i.e., multiple sclerosis) • Seizure or Todd paralysis • Migraine • Idiopathic intracranial hypertension • Reversible cerebral vasoconstrictive syndrome • Central nervous system vasculitis • Vestibular dysfunction • Hypertensive encephalopathy • Peripheral neuropathy • Dementia • Conversion disorder

3. What are the absolute and relative contraindications to fibrinolytic therapy?

Intravenous tissue plasminogen activator (tPA) infusion can only be given to eligible patients and there are strict inclusion and exclusion criteria **(Box 1)** as per stroke guidelines published in 2018.

> **BOX 1:** Inclusion and exclusion criteria for intravenous tPA infusion.
>
> *Inclusion criteria:*
> - Diagnosis of ischemic stroke causing measurable neurological deficit
> - Onset of symptoms <3 hours before beginning treatment
> - Aged ≥18 years
> - Exclusion criteria
> - Significant head trauma or prior stroke in previous 3 months
> - Symptoms suggest subarachnoid hemorrhage
> - Arterial puncture at noncompressible site in previous 7 days
> - History of previous intracranial hemorrhage
> - Intracranial neoplasm, arteriovenous malformation, or aneurysm
> - Recent intracranial or intraspinal surgery
> - Elevated blood pressure (systolic >185 mm Hg or diastolic >110 mm Hg)
> - Active internal bleeding
> - Acute bleeding diathesis
> - Platelet count <100,000/mm³
> - Heparin received within 48 hours, resulting in abnormally elevated aPTT greater than the upper limit of normal
> - Current use of anticoagulant with INR >1.7 or PT >15 seconds
> - Current use of direct thrombin inhibitors or direct factor Xa inhibitors with elevated sensitive laboratory tests (such as aPTT, INR, platelet count, and ECT; TT; or appropriate factor Xa activity assays)
> - Blood glucose concentration <50 mg/dL (2.7 mmol/L)
> - CT demonstrates multilobar infarction (hypodensity >1/3 cerebral hemisphere)
>
> *Relative exclusion criteria:*
> - Recent experience suggests that under some circumstances—with careful consideration and weighting of risk to benefit—patients may receive fibrinolytic therapy despite one or more relative contraindications. Consider risk to benefit of IV rtPA administration carefully if any of these relative contraindications are present:
>   – Only minor or rapidly improving stroke symptoms (clearing spontaneously)
>   – Pregnancy
>   – Seizure at onset with postictal residual neurological impairments
>   – Major surgery or serious trauma within previous 14 days
>   – Recent gastrointestinal or urinary tract hemorrhage (within previous 21 days)
>   – Recent acute myocardial infarction (within previous 3 months)
>
> (aPTT: activated partial thromboplastin time; ECT: ecarin clotting time; INR: international normalized ratio; PT: prothrombin time; rtPA: recombinant tissue plasminogen activator; TT: thrombin clotting time)

Question 5

1. What are the causes of acute onset of jaundice?

Viral infections are most common in acute hepatitis. Common viruses include hepatitis A, B, E, C, and D (super infection/coinfection with B) and uncommon viruses include cytomegalovirus, Epstein-Barr virus, herpes simplex virus (HSV), dengue fever, and transfusion transmitted virus (TTV).

Toxins and drugs: Drug-induced liver disease (DILI) includes paracetamol, carbon tetrachloride, isoniazid, phenytoin, amoxicillin-clavulanate, mushroom (*Amanita phyllodes*), ackee fruit, cycasin, aflatoxin (*Aspergillus flavus*), and sea anemone sting.

Acute liver failure (ALF): Its causes include abovementioned viruses and toxins, ischemic hepatopathy (cardiogenic shock, hypotension, heat stroke, and cocaine), vascular (Budd–Chiari syndrome, sinusoidal obstruction syndrome), Wilson's disease, HELLP (hemolysis, elevated liver enzymes, low platelet count) syndrome, acute fatty liver of pregnancy, primary graft nonfunction after liver transplantation, and malignant infiltration (breast cancer, small cell lung cancer). HSV hepatitis causes ALF in case of neonates, HIV coinfection, and pregnancy.

In India, 95% causes of ALF are viruses (hepatitis E ~40%, hepatitis B ~10–15%, hepatitis A ~1%) and DILI ~5%; while in America, viruses cause ~10% of ALF. Acetaminophen (paracetamol) overdose is a suicidal agent and a common cause of ALF (UK ~57%, USA ~45%, and France 22%). It appears that hepatitis C can cause ALF in the presence of hepatitis B coinfection.

2. List the complications of cirrhosis of liver.

When a significant amount of normal liver parenchyma is replaced by scar and fibrotic tissue, cirrhosis develops. Cirrhosis manifests as generalized weakness, abdominal pain, ascites, spontaneous bacterial peritonitis (SBP), electrolyte imbalance, and altered mental status due to development of hepatic encephalopathy. Cirrhosis is a progressive disease and is initially asymptomatic (compensated cirrhosis). With gradually declining liver functions, decompensation occurs, leading to different complications. A knowledge of these complications may help in prevention and successful treatment, thus improving quality of life of these patients.

3. Discuss briefly SBP.

Cirrhotic patients are more prone to infections. Common infections are SBP, urinary tract infections, pneumonia, cellulitis, and *Clostridium difficile* colitis. Use of proton-pump inhibitors, frequent use of urinary catheter, and antibiotics during admission make patients prone to these infections. SBP is diagnosed by presence of >250 polymorphonuclear leukocytes (PMN) in ascitic fluid and is monobacterial **(Table 5)**. It is usually caused by gram-negative organisms (*Escherichia coli*). Presence of polymicrobial infection or very high neutrophilic count in patients with localized abdominal symptoms suggests inflammation/perforation of an organ (secondary bacterial peritonitis). Usual presentation of SBP is with abdominal symptoms such as pain, diarrhea, vomiting, or ileus, or it may present with worsening of liver function, encephalopathy, gastrointestinal (GI) bleeding, or acute kidney injury (AKI).

TABLE 5: Diagnosis and treatment of spontaneous bacterial peritonitis.

Diagnosis	• Ascitic fluid cytology: 50 mL of ascitic fluid should be sent for cell count, Gram stain, and culture • Ascitic fluid WBC count >1,000/mm³ or polymorphonuclear cell >250/mL, or bacteria on Gram stain
Empiric treatment	• Oral fluroquinolone (in mild cases) • Intravenous fluroquinolones • Cefotaxime or ceftriaxone

(WBC: white blood cells)

4. Discuss briefly hepatorenal syndrome.

Acute kidney injury in cirrhosis is defined as rise in creatinine >50% over baseline or 0.3 mg more than baseline. It is present in around 20% patients with cirrhosis on admission. Common precipitating factors are infections, dehydration due to diuretics, lactulose overdose, non-steroidal anti-inflammatory drug (NSAID) and other nephrotoxic drugs, and large-volume paracentesis (LVP). Besides this, renal dysfunction may occur due to functional renal failure where no evidence of renal parenchymal abnormality is found and there is no response to initial fluid replacement and diuretic and nephrotoxic drug withdrawal. Functional renal failure is known as hepatorenal syndrome-AKI (HRS-AKI).

HRS-AKI is diagnosed by International Ascitic Club AKI Criteria (2015) as follows:
a. Patient of cirrhosis with ascites and AKI
b. No improvement in serum creatinine (S. Cr) on volume replacement (decrease to <1.5 mg/dL)
c. Absence of shock
d. No current or recent nephrotoxic drug use
e. Absence of parenchymal kidney disease as indicated by proteinuria (>500 mg/day), microhematuria [>50 red blood cells/high power field (RBC/HPF)], and/or abnormal renal findings on ultrasonography.

Treatment of AKI consists of stopping nephrotoxic drugs, NSAIDs and diuretics, optimizing dose of lactulose to avoid diarrhea, excluding intrinsic renal disease, treatment of infection, and correction of intravascular volume (1 g albumin/kg body weight – maximum 100 g/day). If no response to the above measures is seen, then vasoconstrictors should be added. Vasoconstrictors used are terlipressin, norepinephrine, and midodrine.

Question 6

1. Discuss the pathophysiology of AKI.

Acute kidney injury is defined as a sudden reduction in kidney function that is characterized by a diminished glomerular filtration rate (GFR) as manifested by an increased S. Cr or reduced urine output. AKI is further divided into three categories: (a) *Prerenal,* a kidney blood flow decrease; (b) *Intrarenal,* or kidney parenchymal injury; and (c) *Postrenal,* or urine flow obstruction. Intrarenal AKI is subdivided again on the basis of part of the kidney involved: glomeruli, vasculature, or interstitium. The patient seen in the emergency or acute setting is often diverse with complex medical histories and without effective primary care follow-up so an evidence-based approach for the management of AKI in the emergency setting is required. Most of the time, ED is the place where community-acquired AKI is identified for the first time. Thus, an emergency physician should identify and manage AKI appropriately in ED.

2. Discuss RIFLE criteria for acute kidney injury.

A variety of definitions for AKI are proposed in the literature. In 2012, the Kidney Disease: Improving Global Outcomes (KDIGO) group defined AKI based on the urine output and the S. Cr concentration. This definition is an increase in S. Cr of ≥0.3 mg/dL within 48 hours or an increase in S. Cr greater than 1.5 times baseline within 7 days or decreased urine output for 6 hours **(Table 6)**. Other classification systems of AKI, such as RIFLE (risk, injury, failure, loss, and end-stage) and Acute Kidney Injury Network (AKIN), can also be used but as per studies all three criteria are effective tools for predicting mortality without significant differences among them, but the advantage of KDIGO is that it covers parameters in AKIN and RIFLE.

TABLE 6: RIFLE (risk, injury, failure, loss, and end-stage) criteria.

AKI stage	Serum creatinine	Urine output
1	Increase in S. Cr ≥150% mg/dL	<0.5 mL/kg/h for 6–12 hours
2	Increase in S. Cr ≥200–300% mg/dL	<0.5 mL/kg/h for ≥12 hours
3	Increase in S. Cr 300% or creatinine >4 mg/mL with acute increase 0.5 mg/dL or initiation of renal replacement therapy	<0.3 mL/kg/h for ≥24 hours or anuria for ≥12 hours

3. Discuss the laboratory evaluation of acute kidney injury.

Acute kidney injury is diagnosed by evaluating laboratory values, urinalysis, urine sediment, and urine chemistries. Prerenal azotemia is considered when a high ratio of blood urea nitrogen (BUN) to creatinine is observed. In this setting, urine sodium concentration of <20 mEq/L as sodium is inappropriately retained and is also indicative of a prerenal cause.

Presence of renal disease can be identified by estimation of several novel biomarkers; clinical trials are currently underway to evaluate the efficacy of these markers. Several biomarkers are currently being evaluated in trials with the goal to identify a biomarker, or a panel of biomarkers, that would be helpful in the early diagnosis of AKI, and also able to differentiate between different types of renal injury, and could provide an accurate prognosis, all with a high degree of specificity and sensitivity. To that end, including serum measurements of cystatin C and neutrophil gelatinated-associated lipocalin (NGAL) and urine measurements of interleukin (IL)-18 and kidney injury molecule-1 (KIM-1) are a few examples of novel biomarkers though their use is not so widespread in clinical practice; however, they may represent the future for identification and assessment of the severity of renal disease. In spite of the well-known limitations described earlier, clinicians more frequently rely on BUN and S. Cr at the time of presentation and compare them with baseline values (when known) to help guide diagnosis and treatment.

4. What is radiocontrast-induced nephropathy?

A type of AKI that results within a few days of exposure to iodinated contrast for imaging studies is termed contrast-induced nephropathy. After hypoperfusion and nephrotoxic drugs, this is the third most common cause of new AKI in hospitalized patients. The contrast-induced nephropathy/AKI is self-limited but associated with increased mortality and even progression to chronic kidney disease. Patients with an estimated GFR <60 mL/min/1.73 m^2 are at higher risk for contrast-induced AKIs. In clinical practice, radiologists take detailed relevant history about comorbidities and other nephrotoxic medications before administering potentially harmful contrast. In a high-risk patient, use the lowest possible radiocontrast concentrations, administer IV hydration pre-exposure and postexposure, and minimize nephrotoxic agents, and renal replacement therapy (RRT) in critical cases should be considered. It is important to screen patients for reliable follow-up.

Question 7

A patient has come with suspected tetanus. Discuss the following.

1. Pathophysiology of tetanus.

Tetanus toxins act by a similar mechanism to botulinum toxin; tetanus toxin is taken up into nerve terminals of lower motor neurons, the nerve cells that activate voluntary muscles. Tetanus toxin is a zinc-dependent metalloproteinase that targets a protein [synaptobrevin/vesicle-associated membrane protein (VAMP)] that is necessary for the release of neurotransmitter from nerve endings through fusion of synaptic vesicles with the neuronal plasma membrane. Flaccid paralysis may be the initial symptom of local tetanus infection, caused by interference with vesicular release of acetylcholine at the neuromuscular junction, as occurs with botulinum toxin. Extensive retrograde transport of tetanus toxin occurs in the axons of lower motor neurons and tetanus toxin reaches the spinal cord or brainstem. Tetanus toxin crosses the synapses and is taken up by nerve endings of inhibitory GABAergic and/or glycinergic neurons that control the activity of the lower motor neurons. Once tetanus toxins reach inside the inhibitory nerve terminals, it cleaves VAMP, thereby inhibiting the release of GABA and glycine, resulting in functional denervation of the lower motor neurons, which leads to rigidity and spasms due to hyperactivity and increased muscle activity.

2. Control of muscle spasms.
3. Control of autonomic dysfunction.

Muscular rigidity and spasm often interfere with respiration and is a likely cause of death so treatment of these features is of vital importance. The patient also has severe pain due to rigidity and spasms, which stimulates muscle activity. Muscle relaxation is customarily achieved with benzodiazepines, which augment the effect of GABA on the GABAA (gamma-aminobutyric acid type A) receptors of lower motor neurons. *Baclofen* may also be effective, which acts on GABAB (gamma-aminobutyric acid type B) receptors; when given intrathecally, its sedative effect is avoided. In the setting of an intensive care unit, propofol, another GABAA receptor modulator, may be used, as may nondepolarizing muscle relaxants (pancuronium or pipecuronium), which act directly on the muscle motor end plates by competing for the acetylcholine binding site. *Magnesium*, a calcium antagonist, may be effective in relieving rigidity and spasms and acts both by reducing acetylcholine release and by reducing the muscle response to acetylcholine.

Magnesium also seems to reduce autonomic dysfunction, which is of importance, because antiadrenergic drugs, especially beta-blockers, may produce untoward effects, including cardiac arrest. *Dantrolene* reduces calcium mobilization and muscle contraction, by binding to the ryanodine receptor in muscle. To avoid the triggering of spasms by noise or other sensory stimulation, tetanus patients should be in a calm environment.

4. Immunotherapy and immunization.

Immunization: Tetanus toxoid 0.5 mL IM at presentation, then after 6 weeks, and then after 6 months.

Tetanus immunoglobulin 3,000–6,000 units IM (opposite arm of TT and some amount around the wound site), wound cleaning and antibiotic, is the mainstay of the acute treatment of tetanus which is based on eradication of *Clostridium tetani*, e.g., with *intravenous metronidazole*, 500 mg every 6 hourly, or penicillin, 100,000–200,000 IU/kg/day for 7–10 days. Tetanus immunoglobulin is given once intramuscularly to inactivate any free tetanus toxin; doses of 250 IU intramuscularly in an adult and 4 unit/kg in children are given as postexposure prophylaxis, while 3,000–6,000 IU intramuscularly is recommended for treatment clinical tetanus; though the tetanus immunoglobulin does not reduce the symptoms of tetanus, it may reduce the mortality. A part of tetanus immunoglobulin dose should also be infiltrated in and around the wound.

Question 8

1. Discuss the factors precipitating lithium toxicity.

Lithium is excreted almost completely by the kidneys and handled in the same manner as sodium, being freely filtered with 80% reabsorption at the proximal tubules.

Sodium intake and lithium clearance are directly related, and decreasing sodium intake may lead to decreased clearance of lithium. For this reason, lithium intoxication is more commonly encountered in low-salt diets, states of dehydration, or with a concurrent use of diuretics.

2. Discuss the toxic effects of chronic lithium poisoning.

Neurologic: Lithium is primarily a neurotoxin. The neurological symptoms form the predominant features of chronic lithium toxicity. Neurotoxicity does not correlate with serum concentrations; instead, it depends on the duration of exposure to an elevated concentration. Tremor, a common finding in patients undergoing chronic therapy, may increase with toxicity. Fasciculations, hyperreflexia, choreoathetoid movements, clonus, dysarthria, nystagmus, and ataxia are other findings. Altered mental status which could progress from confusion to stupor, coma, and seizures is also seen. The syndrome of irreversible lithium effectuated neurologic and neuropsychiatric toxicity (SILENT) defined as neurologic dysfunction caused by lithium in the absence of prior neurologic illness, persist for at least 2 month after cessation of the drug. In many instances, cerebellar dysfunction is a common feature along with hyperpyrexia. A feature which resembles neuroleptic malignant syndrome (NMS) or serotonin syndrome could be an indicator of severe lithium toxicity.

Renal: Polyurea and polydipsia (nephrogenic diabetes insipidus) are renal effects of chronic lithium poisoning. Chronic lithium therapy is also associated with chronic tubulointerstitial nephropathy, as manifested by the development of renal insufficiency with little or no proteinuria and biopsy findings of tubular cysts, renal tubular acidosis, and nephrotic syndrome.

Endocrine: Goiter along with hypothyroidism is the most common endocrine manifestation of chronic lithium therapy. Hyperthyroidism and frank thyrotoxicosis are also reported. The combination of hyperparathyroidism and hypercalcemia is frequently reported with chronic lithium therapy, especially in women.

Dermal: Dermatitis, localized edema, and ulcers

Respiratory system: Acute respiratory distress syndrome has been reported.

3. Discuss the management of chronic lithium poisoning.

a. The initial management should include stabilization of the patient with due care of airway, breathing, and circulation.
b. *Fluid and electrolyte balance*
   i. Restoration and maintenance of intravascular volume is the key in the management of acute poisoning.
   ii. Correction of blood volume with 0.9% normal saline (1.5–2 times the normal maintenance) will prevent lithium toxicity-induced renal dysfunction.
   iii. It also improves renal perfusion, GFR, and lithium elimination.
   iv. Correction of electrolyte abnormalities and monitoring of urine output is essential.
   v. Forced diuresis using loop diuretics, osmotic agents, carbonic anhydrase inhibitors, etc., should not be

tried as they may result in lithium retention rather than elimination.

vi. Sodium bicarbonate for urinary alkalinization should also be avoided.

c. *Extracorporeal drug removal (hemodialysis)*:
  i. Lithium is predominantly localized intracellularly and diffuses slowly across cell membranes. Clearance of lithium from the intravascular compartment by hemodialysis could be followed by a rebound phenomenon of redistribution from tissue stores and could lead to increased serum levels.
  ii. *Recommendations for hemodialysis*:
   • Absolute lithium concentration >4.0 mEq/L (mmol/L)
   • With any type of overdose or a concentration of >2.5 mEq/L with chronic toxicity
   • Patients who manifest severe signs and symptoms of neurotoxicity, such as alterations in mental status
   • Patients who have renal failure and show signs or symptoms of lithium toxicity.
   • Patients who show little or no sign of toxicity but who cannot tolerate sodium repletion therapy (congestive heart failure, liver failure, pancreatitis, or sepsis)
   • The dialysate bath should contain bicarbonate rather than acetate.
   • *Continuous arteriovenous hemodiafiltration* (CAVH): It has better efficacy than hemodialysis.

Question 9

1. Explain the process of regulation of body temperature.

Internal body temperature is regulated by the hypothalamus. The hypothalamus checks the current body temperature and compares it with the normal temperature of about 37°C. If our temperature is too low, the hypothalamus makes sure that the body generates and maintains heat. The body uses four mechanisms of heat exchange to maintain homeostasis: conduction, convection, radiation, and evaporation **(Fig. 1)**.

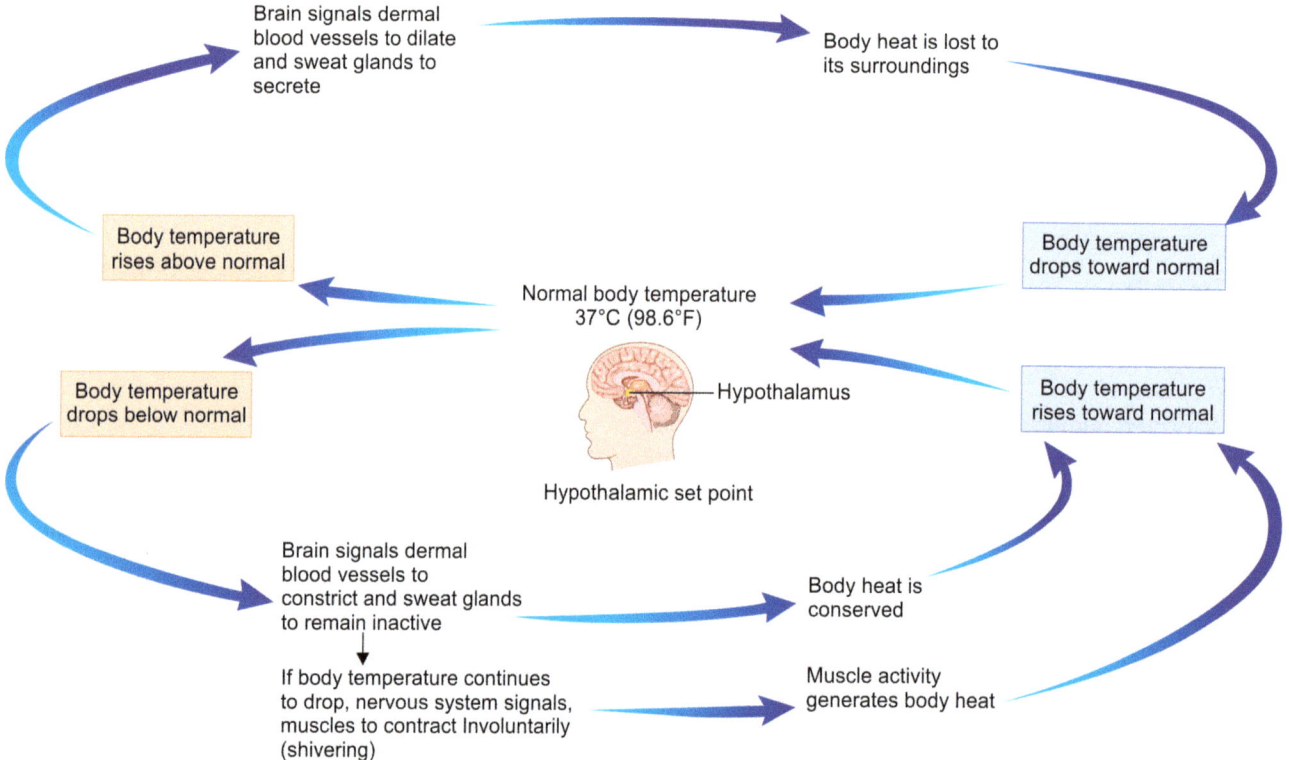

Fig. 1: Regulation of body temperature.

2. Explain the cooling techniques in heat stroke.

Treatment of heat stroke involves rapid mechanical cooling along with resuscitation measures. The body temperature must be lowered quickly. The patient should be moved to a cool area which is either indoor or in a shade and clothing may need to be removed to promote passive clothing. Active cooling methods include immersion in cold water, or a hyperthermia vest can be applied. Cold compresses to the torso, head, neck, and groin will help in bringing the body core temperature down. A fan or dehumidifying air-conditioning unit may be used to aid in evaporation of water.

3. What are the complications of heat stroke?

Heat stroke is usually seen in a young healthy individual who overexerts in the heat and humidity.
a. Respiratory alkalosis with lactic acid
b. Rhabdomyolysis
c. Renal failure
d. Disseminated intravascular coagulation (DIC)
e. Hyperuricemia which is frequently seen.

Question 10

1. What are the clinical features of myxedema crisis?

Severe hypothyroidism when left untreated for a prolonged duration may lead to a rare fatal disease, myxedema coma, in which the body's homeostasis goes haywire due to precipitating factors. These factors include infection, certain medications (amiodarone, anesthesia, barbiturates, β-blockers, diuretics, lithium, narcotics, phenothiazines, phenytoin, rifampin, and tranquilizers), and failure to reinstate thyroid replacement therapy during hospitalization, stroke, surgery, burns, hypoglycemia, hypothermia, GI hemorrhage, or trauma among others. Most (95%) of the myxedema coma cases occur due to primary hypothyroidism, while hypothalamic or pituitary causes account for the remaining (5%) cases.

Patients with myxedema coma generally present with altered sensorium, lethargy, confusion, and possibly obtundation rather than coma. Other characteristics include hypoglycemia, bradycardia, hypoventilation, hypotension, hypothermia (usually <95.9°F), hyponatremia, and increased levels of S. Cr and creatinine kinase.

2. List differential diagnosis of myxedema crisis.

The suspected diagnosis of myxedema coma includes clinical presentation of any patient with coma or compromised mental status with hypercapnia, hypothermia, and/or hyponatremia, and with decreased T3 and T4 concentrations. Measurement of serum cortisol is required to rule out coexisting adrenal insufficiency. However, there is a nonspecific presentation of clinical features in several instances such as altered mental status without coma, which makes it difficult to diagnose myxedema coma. Overall, altered mental status, hypothermia, and the presence of precipitating events are the three key features for the differential diagnosis of myxedema coma. Chiong and Mariash developed a tool as the diagnostic criterion for myxedema coma based on six common parameters of the disease, which is used by intensive care units of several hospitals.

3. Discuss the ED treatment of myxedema crisis.

Myxedema coma is a metabolic thyroid emergency condition, and the suspected patients should be administrated intensive care therapy for vital pulmonary, respiratory, and cardiovascular support. The mortality rate could be from 25 to 60% in myxedema coma patients despite the best treatment. Hence, the treatment for suspected myxedema coma should be initiated immediately rather than waiting for laboratory confirmation. Successful treatment depends upon the timely diagnosis, prompt treatment with thyroid hormones (intravenous levothyroxine is preferred over oral), supportive therapy (appropriate fluid management and correction of hypotension and dyselectrolytemia), and administration of steroid supplement (hydrocortisone) until coexisting adrenal insufficiency is ruled out, along with the aggressive treatment of precipitating factors.

■ SUGGESTED READING

1. Richhariya D, Sharma B. Textbook of Emergency Medicine including Intensive Care and Trauma, 2nd edition. New Delhi: Jaypee Brothers Medical Publishers (P) Ltd; 2022. p. 1299. (Question 1).
2. Richhariya D, Sharma B. Textbook of Emergency Medicine including Intensive Care and Trauma, 2nd edition. New Delhi: Jaypee Brothers Medical Publishers (P) Ltd; 2022. pp. 453-9. (Question 2).
3. Richhariya D, Sharma B. Textbook of Emergency Medicine including Intensive Care and Trauma, 2nd edition. New Delhi: Jaypee Brothers Medical Publishers (P) Ltd; 2022. pp. 266-577. (Question 3).
4. Richhariya D, Sharma B. Textbook of Emergency Medicine including Intensive Care and Trauma, 2nd edition. New Delhi: Jaypee Brothers Medical Publishers (P) Ltd; 2022. pp. 822-5. (Question 4).
5. Richhariya D, Sharma B. Textbook of Emergency Medicine including Intensive Care and Trauma, 2nd edition. New Delhi: Jaypee Brothers Medical Publishers (P) Ltd; 2022. pp. 674, 677-9. (Question 5).
6. Richhariya D, Sharma B. Textbook of Emergency Medicine including Intensive Care and Trauma, 2nd edition. New Delhi: Jaypee Brothers Medical Publishers (P) Ltd; 2022. pp. 744-7. (Question 6).
7. Richhariya D, Sharma B. Textbook of Emergency Medicine including Intensive Care and Trauma, 2nd edition. New Delhi: Jaypee Brothers Medical Publishers (P) Ltd; 2022. pp. 1314-6. (Question 7).
8. Richhariya D, Sharma B. Textbook of Emergency Medicine including Intensive Care and Trauma, 2nd edition. New Delhi: Jaypee Brothers Medical Publishers (P) Ltd; 2022. pp. 1525-34. (Question 8).
9. Richhariya D, Sharma B. Textbook of Emergency Medicine including Intensive Care and Trauma, 2nd edition. New Delhi: Jaypee Brothers Medical Publishers (P) Ltd; 2022. pp. 1692-6. (Question 9).
10. Richhariya D, Sharma B. Textbook of Emergency Medicine including Intensive Care and Trauma, 2nd edition. New Delhi: Jaypee Brothers Medical Publishers (P) Ltd; 2022. p. 883. (Question 10).

Emergency Medicine Paper 12

Devendra Richhariya

Question 1

1. Name two recent trials on control of blood pressure in patients with intracranial hemorrhage.

Intensive Blood Pressure Reduction in Acute Cerebral Hemorrhage-2 (INTERACT-2) and Antihypertensive Treatment of Acute Cerebral Hemorrhage-2 (ATACH-2) trials are focused on determining the clinical efficacy of early intensive systolic blood pressure (SBP) reduction in intracerebral hemorrhage (ICH) patients.

ATACH-2 trial: This trial was the latest phase 3 randomized controlled multicenter clinical trial aimed at studying the efficacy of early intensive reduction of SBP in ICH patients.

INTERACT-2 trial: This trial randomized 2,839 patients with ICH within 6 hours of symptom onset to intensive SBP reduction, with a target of <140 mm Hg within 1 hour, or guideline-recommended SBP reduction, with a target of <180 mm Hg using a variety of antihypertensive medications **(Table 1)**.

TABLE 1: Comparison between INTERACT-2 and ATACH-2 trials.

Variable	INTERACT-2	ATACH-2
Initial SBP criteria	SBP ≥150 mm Hg	SBP ≥180 mm Hg
Randomization	Within 6 hours from symptom onset	Within 4.5 hours from symptom onset
Treatment goal	*Intensive:* <140 mm Hg	*Intensive:* 110–139 mm Hg
	Standard: <180 mm Hg	*Standard:* 140–179 mm Hg
Antihypertensive treatment	Multiple	Single agent (intravenous nicardipine)
Mean SBP achieved	*Intensive:* 150 mm Hg	*Intensive:* 128.9 mm Hg
	Standard: 164 mm Hg	*Standard:* 141.1 mm Hg
Treatment failure rate in the intensive treatment group	67%	12.20%
Death or severe disability at 3 months	*Intensive:* 52.9%	*Intensive:* 38.7%
	Standard: 55.6% ($p = 0.06$)	*Standard:* 37.7% ($p = 0.72$)

(ATACH-2: Antihypertensive Treatment of Acute Cerebral Hemorrhage-2; INTERACT-2: Intensive Blood Pressure Reduction in Acute Cerebral Hemorrhage-2; SBP: systolic blood pressure)

2. Discuss any one of the abovementioned trials.

Two large clinical trials have evaluated the efficacy of the intensive lowering of blood pressure (BP) in patients with acute ICH. First, the INTERACT-2 trial evaluated 2,839 patients with SBPs between 150 and 220 mm Hg within 6 hours of ICH onset, who were randomized into groups with target SBPs of <140 or <180 mm Hg. The primary outcome was death or major disability, defined as a modified Rankin scale (mRS) score ≥3, which did not differ significantly between the two groups. This was evidenced by an odds ratio (OR) of 0.87 in the intensive treatment group, a 95% confidence interval (CI) of 0.75–1.01, and a $p = 0.06$. However, the intensive treatment group had better functional recovery and an improved physical and mental health-related quality of life compared to the standard treatment group. Additionally, the drastic reduction in BP did not cause serious adverse events. In concurrence with these results, the American Heart Association (AHA) and American Stroke Association (ASA) have provided evidence-based consensus guidelines which state that for patients with an SBP between 150 and 220 mm Hg and without contraindications, the acute lowering of SBP to 140 mm Hg is considered safe and may improve functional outcomes in patients with ICH.

3. Discuss briefly about drugs to control BP in patients with ICH.

The latest recommendation for the target point is SBP <140 mm Hg in ICH that should be achieved during the first hour using titratable agents to prevent the expansion of present hematoma. However, if elevated increase intracranial pressure (ICP) presents based on signs, symptoms, and radiologic findings, the physician should decrease BP to a point that cerebral perfusion pressure (CPP) remains in the range of 60–80 mm Hg. Intravenous labetalol and nicardipine are the first-line agents. Angiotensin-converting enzyme inhibitors (ACEIs) such as enalapril could be administered as the second-line option. It seems that nitroprusside and nitroglycerine may increase ICP, so they should be avoided.

In subarachnoid hemorrhage (SAH), the target point is SBP <160 mm Hg that could be achieved by various titratable agents such as nicardipine or labetalol to prevent stroke and rebleeding, and also by maintaining proper CPP. As mentioned in case of ICH, nitroprusside should also be avoided in SAH. Oral nimodipine improves neurological outcomes and should be administered to all patients with SAH.

Question 2

1. Discuss the triage of a victim of sexual assault.

Every hospital should have a standard operating procedure (SOP) for management of cases of sexual violence, and these must be printed and available to all staff of the hospital. The administrative guidelines regarding interdepartmental handling of such cases for examination and evidence collection should be clear to all the staff. Administration should simultaneously help clinical staff to inform police and complete medicolegal procedures. The hospital should have a uniform method of examination and evidence collection. A kit with required proforma along with the utilities such as nail cutters, syringes, swabs can be kept ready for immediate use. Health professionals need to maintain a clear and foolproof chain of custody of medical evidence collected and refer appropriate agencies for further assistance (e.g., legal support services and shelter services).

2. Discuss the assessment of a female victim of sexual assault.

Following are common injuries:
a. *Head:* Blow on head or head injury due to fall
b. *Neck:* Gripping of throat
c. Injuries on cheeks, lips, breast, and chest are common.
d. Generalized bruises, lacerations, contusions, bite marks, and nail marks
e. The marks of rope knots on the wrists and ankles

The examiner should strive to ascertain the following:
a. Whether these marks are of injuries or self-inflicted
b. Apparent development of the victim's body
c. Amount of resistance offered
d. Corroboration with statement of victim

Examination of nails: Scraping from the nail beds constitutes important evidence. Tags of epithelium, hairs, pieces of clothes, and bloodstains are important to collect.

Gait: The victim's gait must be made a note of. If consent is available, the victim's blood should be collected for grouping. This will help in ascertaining whether bloodstains are of the victim or assailant. A second examination after 48 hours may reveal deep bruises, which may not be evident at the first examination.

Examination of genitals: A gynecological examination should be conducted in lithotomy position and in good light. The history of the last menstrual period must be asked for to differentiate menstruation from bleeding due to injuries.

3. Discuss the treatment of a female victim of sexual assault.

Injuries: Hymen: Especially in a virgin victim, examination of hymen is important. Signs of recent rupture of hymen are ragged edematous edges of the hymen and hemorrhage.

Examination of vagina: Distensibility of vagina should be noted in relation to the number of fingers it admits. The character and extent of injury will vary in proportion to:
a. Disproportion of male and female organ
b. Whether the victim is a virgin or not
c. Extent of penetration
d. Amount of force.

Lacerations of posterior fourchette are very commonly associated with forceful intercourse, especially with a virgin. Finger penetration may lead to lateral vaginal wall tears. Bruising and lacerations in the vagina also must be recorded properly. Absence of injuries may be due to inability of the victim to offer resistance to the assailant because of intoxication or threats. Pictorial representation of these injuries can be very helpful for corroborative evidence.

Question 3

1. Discuss various steps to prepare a neonate for transport to other hospitals.

Every hospital must examine, treat, and stabilize anyone presenting to the emergency department (ED) for medical care. After the medical screening is completed, it may be determined that the patient requires care that exceeds the hospital's existing capabilities. At this time, they can make the decision to transfer the patient to a higher level of care. This decision to transfer cannot be based on the patient's ability to pay and must be within the hospital's own guidelines as well as the state and federal regulations. The referring hospital is responsible for contacting the receiving hospital to arrange the transfer. This initial contact should occur as early as possible in the case. The referring hospital needs to discuss with the family the reason for the transfer and should obtain verbal consent that they are in agreement with the transfer. All appropriate forms, records, labs, and imaging should also be transferred with the patient to comply with regulations. The best practice is for these referring hospitals to have established policies and agreements with the receiving hospitals. Any hospital cannot refuse to accept appropriately transferred patients when they have the capacity to treat and manage the patient. Most tertiary care pediatric hospitals have existing policies and procedures to expedite transfers from the referring hospitals. In addition, a majority of tertiary care pediatric hospitals have their own pediatric and neonatal transport teams in-house.

2. What are the special considerations in neonates when preparing for transport?

It is up to the referring facility to determine which pediatric or neonatal patient must be transferred to a higher level of care. Again, this is most common when the patient's needs have exceeded the medical care and resources for their facility. Below is a list of common situations that would require transfer:
a. Status postcardiopulmonary arrest
b. Respiratory distress or failure
c. Depressed or deteriorating neurologic examination or status
d. Patient in shock who is not responding adequately to treatment
e. Serious cardiac rhythm disturbances leading to inadequate perfusion
f. Children with severe electrolyte or metabolic disturbances [i.e., diabetic ketoacidosis (DKA)]
g. Children with life-threatening ingestion or exposure to toxic substances
h. Children who have sustained major traumatic injuries leading to circulatory, respiratory, or neurologic compromise.

The mode of transport for the patient should be determined in the communication between the referring and receiving facilities. It should take into account the condition of the patient and their risk for deterioration, distance between facilities, weather conditions, and cost. Air transport of a stable patient over a short distance is likely not necessary or cost effective. The main modes of transport are ground ambulance, rotor-wing aircraft (helicopter), or fixed-wing aircraft. Ground ambulance is the most often used mode of pediatric and neonatal transport. Together with determining the mode of transport, the type of team to transport the patient should be discussed between the referring and receiving facilities. These teams may be basic life support (BLS), advanced life support (ALS), or specialized pediatric and neonatal transport teams. All those involved in this discussion should have adequate knowledge of the capabilities of the particular teams in terms of pediatric equipment as well as procedural skills.

Question 4

A 7-year school-going boy came to ED with 1-day fever of 102.6°F and cold. Several cases of H1N1 influenza infection were reported during that period.

1. What standard precautions would you take in ED while examining a patient with suspected influenza infection?

Standard precautions are a group of infection prevention and control (IPC) practices applied to all patients, at every patient encounter, irrespective of their suspected or confirmed infection status. The basic principle is that all blood, body fluids, secretions, and excretions contain transmissible infectious agents. Hence, the implementation of standard precautions helps to maintain a physical, mechanical, or chemical barrier between microorganisms, the environment, and an individual, thus breaking the disease transmission cycle. These precautions include hand hygiene, use of personal protective equipment (PPE) (gloves, gown, mask, and protective eyewear), respiratory hygiene/cough etiquette by patients or healthcare workers (HCW), safe injection practices with proper disposal of sharp syringes, device sterilization, environmental cleaning, and disinfection. Wearing PPE is one such standard precaution, which creates a two-way protective barrier between the HCW and the patient by reducing the risk of transmitting microorganisms, which in turn, prevents hospital-acquired infections (HAI).

2. Define categories of patients with suspected H1N1 infection.

Category A: Patients with mild fever plus cough/sore throat with or without body ache, headache, diarrhea, and vomiting will be categorized as Category A. They do not require oseltamivir and should be treated for the symptoms mentioned above. The patients should be monitored for their progress and reassessed at 24–48 hours by the doctor. No testing of the patient for influenza is required. Patients should confine themselves at home and avoid mixing up with public and high-risk members in the family.

Category B: In addition to all the signs and symptoms mentioned under Category A,
a. If the patient has high-grade fever and severe sore throat, he may require home isolation and oseltamivir
b. Individuals having one or more of the following high-risk conditions shall be treated with oseltamivir:
   i. Children with mild illness but with predisposing risk factors
   ii. Pregnant women
   iii. Persons aged 65 years or older
   iv. Patients with lung diseases, heart disease, liver disease kidney disease, blood disorders, diabetes, neurological disorders, cancer, and HIV/AIDS
   v. Patients on long-term cortisone therapy.
   vi. No tests for influenza are required for Category B (a) and (b).

vii. All patients of Category B (a) and (b) should confine themselves at home and avoid mixing with public and high-risk members in the family.
viii. Broad-spectrum antibiotics as per the guideline for community-acquired pneumonia (CAP) may be prescribed.

Category C: In addition to the above signs and symptoms of Categories A and B, if the patient has one or more of the following, he can be grouped under Category C:
  i. Breathlessness, chest pain, drowsiness, fall in blood pressure, sputum mixed with blood, and bluish discoloration of nails.
  ii. Children with influenza-like illness who has a severe disease as manifested by the red flag signs (somnolence, high and persistent fever, inability to eat well, convulsions, shortness of breath, difficulty in breathing, etc.).
  iii. Worsening of underlying chronic conditions.

All these patients mentioned above in Category C require testing, immediate hospitalization, and treatment.

3. Discuss briefly the drugs used to treat a case of influenza infection.

Oseltamivir is the recommended drug for both prophylaxis and treatment for H1N1. In the current phase, if a person conforms to the case definition of suspect case, then he would be provided oseltamivir.

Dose for treatment is as follows: *By weight*:

For weight <15 kg, dose: 30 mg BD for 5 days
For weight 15–23 kg, dose: 45 mg BD for 5 days
For weight 24 to <40 kg, dose: 60 mg BD for 5 days
For weight >40 kg, dose: 75 mg BD for 5 days

For infants:

<3 months, dose: 12 mg BD for 5 days
3–5 months, dose: 20 mg BD for 5 days
6–11 months, dose: 25 mg BD for 5 days

Oseltamivir is also available as syrup (12 mg/mL).

If needed, dose and duration can be modified as per clinical condition.

4. How will you manage this child?

Supportive therapy comprises:
a. Intravenous fluids
b. Parenteral nutrition
c. Oxygen therapy/ventilatory support
d. Antibiotics for secondary infection
e. Vasopressors for shock
f. Paracetamol or ibuprofen is prescribed for fever, myalgia, and headache.
g. Patient is advised to drink plenty of fluids.
h. Smokers should avoid smoking.
i. For sore throat, a short course of topical decongestants, saline nasal drops, throat lozenges, and steam inhalation may be beneficial.
j. Salicylate/aspirin is strictly contraindicated in any influenza patient due to its potential to cause Reye's syndrome.
k. The suspected cases would be constantly monitored for clinical/radiological evidence of lower respiratory tract infection and for hypoxia (respiratory rate, oxygen saturation, and level of consciousness).

Question 5

1. Discuss the epidemiology, clinical features, complications, and recent observations about transmission of Zika virus infection.

Transmission: Zika virus is *transmitted primarily by Aedes mosquitoes*, which bite mostly during the day. Most people with Zika virus infection do not develop symptoms; those who do typically have symptoms including rash, fever, conjunctivitis, muscle and joint pain, malaise, and headache that last for 2–7 days.

Clinical presentation: In most cases, Zika virus infection causes a mild, self-limited illness. The incubation period is likely 3–12 days. Owing to the mild nature of the disease, more than 80% of Zika virus infection cases likely go unnoticed. The spectrum of Zika virus disease overlaps with other that of arboviral infections, but rash (maculopapular and likely immune-mediated) typically predominates. The rash in Zika virus infection is usually a fine maculopapular rash that is diffusely distributed. It can involve the face, trunk, and extremities, including palms and soles.

Management: There is no specific treatment available for Zika virus infection or disease. People with symptoms such as rash, fever, or joint pain should get plenty of rest, drink fluids, and treat symptoms with antipyretics and/or analgesics.

Question 6

Regarding ocular ultrasonography in the ED.

1. Discuss the uses of this technology in ED.

Point-of-care ultrasonography (POCUS) helps to detect a wide variety of ocular pathologies from trauma such as dislocated lens, globe disruption, vitreous hemorrhage, hyphemia, retinal detachment, orbital emphysema, and retrobulbar hemorrhage. Suspected globe rupture is a relative contraindication to ultrasonography (USG) examination due to risk of extruding globe contents with direct pressure on and around the eye.

Globe rupture: Distortion of normal shape of globe, decrease in size of globe, anterior chamber collapse, vitreous hemorrhage.

Lens dislocation: Highly reflective oval mass moving independent of the surrounding structure with eye movement.

Hyphemia: Echoic structure of variable echogenicity, depending on age of bleed.

Retrobulbar hemorrhage: Echolucent posterior to globe.

Ocular ultrasound plays an important role in differentiating orbital ultrasound from normal orbit **(Fig. 1A)**. It can also detect ocular injuries such as retrobulbar hemorrhage which is also known as guitar-pick sign **(Fig. 1B)**, retinal detachment **(Fig. 1C)**, and lens dislocation.

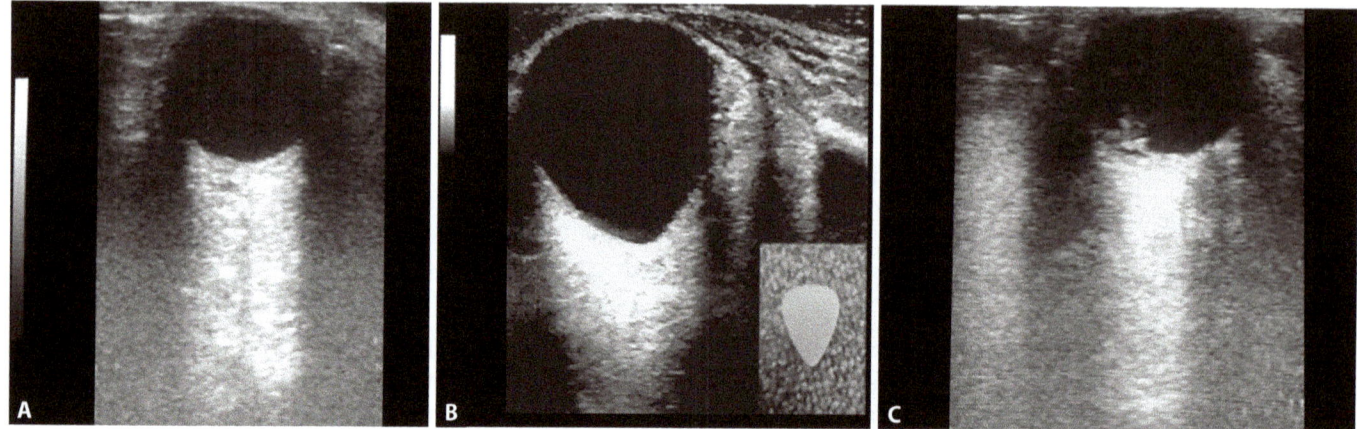

Figs. 1A to C: (A) Normal ocular ultrasonography; (B) Scan showing retrobulbar hematoma (guitar-pick sign); (C) Ocular scan showing retinal detachment.

2. Define normal values of optic nerve sheath diameter in adults.

Point-of-care optic nerve sheath ultrasound (ONSUS) is a bedside practice that can be used to evaluate for increased ICP. It has the advantages of being noninvasive, portable, and easily performed at bedside in minimum time. It can be repeated for reevaluation without risk of radiation. Systematic review and meta-analysis have shown that optic nerve sheath diameter (ONSD) of >5.00–5.70 mm has a concurrent ICP value >20 mm Hg. In healthy persons, the ONSD varies from 5.17 ± 1.34 to 3.55 ± 0.82 mm in different locations within the intraorbital space with no significant difference between sexes and age groups. The most stable results with lesser ONSD can be obtained if the diameter is measured 8–10 mm from the globe. The use of bedside ocular USG in measuring ONSD can be *a useful method for detecting raised ICP.*

3. List the pitfalls of this examination.

4. What are the precautions and contraindications of this test?

Ultrasound evaluation of ONSD has emerged in recent years as a useful noninvasive tool for estimating ICP or detecting intracranial hypertension. It is a safe technique that can be conducted at the bedside, in real time, and is reproducible, relatively low cost, and does not carry the risks of radiation. Several studies have described this technique, but none has validated its accuracy in comparison to the standard invasive measurement of ICP.

Recently, Aspide et al. studied the feasibility of using color Doppler to measure the ONSD as compared to 2D USG, having magnetic resonance imaging as the gold standard, and found that ONSD assessments using color Doppler yielded lower and less scattered measurements compared to 2D USG. The main contraindication to performing ophthalmic ultrasound is *if a patient has a globe rupture*. It is advised to refer any of these suspected patients immediately to an ophthalmologist.

Question 7

1. Discuss the diagnostic criteria and severity assessment for substance-use disorders based on the diagnostic and statistical manual of mental disorders.

These criteria fall under four basic categories: (1) Impaired control; (2) physical dependence; (3) social problems; and (4) risky use **(Box 1)**: The DSM-5-TR (Diagnostic and Statistical Manual of Mental Disorders, fifth edition, text revision) allows clinicians to specify how severe or how much of a problem the substance-use disorder is, depending on how many symptoms are identified **(Fig. 2)**. *Moderate*: Four or five symptoms indicate a moderate substance-use disorder. *Severe*: Six or more symptoms indicate a severe substance-use disorder.

> **BOX 1:** Four basic categories of severity assessment for substance-use disorders.
>
> *Impaired control:*
> - Substance is often taken in larger amounts or over a longer period than was intended
> - There is a persistent desire or unsuccessful efforts to cut down or control substance use
> - A great deal of time is spent in activities necessary to obtain the substance, use the substance, or recover from its effects
> - Craving, or a strong desire or urge to use the substance
>
> *Risky use of substance:*
> - Recurrent substance use in situations in which it is physically hazardous
> - Substance use is continued despite knowledge of having a persistent or recurrent physical or psychological problem that is likely to have been caused or exacerbated by the substance
>
> *Social impairment:*
> - Recurrent substance use resulting in a failure to fulfil major role obligations at work, school, or home
> - Continued substance use despite having persistent or recurrent social or interpersonal problems caused or exacerbated by the effects of the substance
> - Important social, occupational, or recreational activities are given up or reduced because of substance use
>
> *Pharmacological criteria:*
> - *Tolerance, as defined by either:* A need for markedly increased amounts of the substance to achieve intoxication or desired effect OR markedly diminished effect with continued use of the same amount of the substance
> - *Withdrawal, as manifested by either:* The characteristic withdrawal syndrome for the substance OR the substance (or a closely related substance) is taken to relieve or avoid withdrawal symptoms

DSM-5 outlines diagnostic criteria for AWS using two main components so that the AWS is diagnosed when the following two conditions are met:
1. A clear evidence of cessation or reduction in heavy and prolonged alcohol use
2. The symptoms of withdrawal are not accounted for by a medical or another mental or behavioral disorder.

Useful markers in an ED setting: According to various studies, a high-risk patient for severe AWS (delirium tremens) can be predicted on the basis of medical history, history of similar events, and if the patient is unconscious, laboratory markers are helpful in suspected cases. A summary of relevant markers in the emergency setting is given in **Table 2**. Severe AWS should be differentiated from hyponatremia, hepatic encephalopathy, infections (pneumonia, meningitis), thyrotoxicosis, head injury, psychosis, and drugs intoxication (tricyclic antidepressant, lithium, atropine). Neuroimaging is recommended to rule out any other neurologic condition, especially those associated with first-onset seizures or generalized tonic-clonic seizures.

Treatment of AWS is mainly based on control of agitation, autonomic hyperactive symptoms, and delirium tremens, later detoxification therapy, and motivation for prolong abstinence. Intravenous benzodiazepine is used as initial therapy. No specific benzodiazepine is superior to another **(Table 3)**.

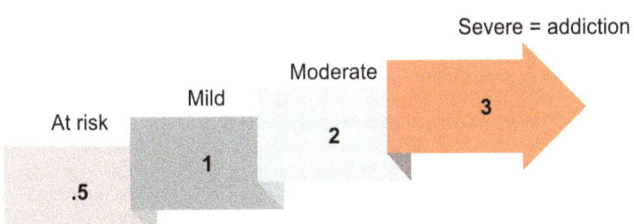

Fig. 2: Level of severity of substance-use disorder.

2. Enumerate different alcohol withdrawal syndromes (AWS).
3. Discuss the ED management of AWS.

Alcohol withdrawal syndrome occurs due to sudden stopping or reducing of chronic alcohol consumption which gives rise to a wide variety of clinical presentation ranging from nausea, vomiting, loss of appetite, diaphoresis, insomnia, tachycardia, anxiety, craving, hand tremors, fever, agitation, hyperexcitation, to more concerning features such as hallucination, seizures, and delirium tremens. Alcohol withdrawal starts after 6 hours of stopping the alcohol consumption and symptoms may last for 10–15 days.

TABLE 2: Relevant markers of alcohol-use disorder in an emergency department setting.

Markers	Significance
Ethanol	Estimated in breath, blood urine up to 6–24 hours, 90–95% specificity
Hypokalemia	Estimated in blood up to days to weeks 40% specificity serum levels <2.5 mEq/L indicate alcohol-use disorders
Thrombocytopenia	• Estimated in blood up to days to 10–12 days, 70–75% specificity • Rebound thrombocytosis after cessation of alcohol abuse
Mean corpuscular volume	• Estimated in blood up to days to months, specificity 80% • Dose-dependent increase
γ-glutamyl transferase	• Estimated in blood up to days to weeks, specificity 80% • Marker of liver injury due to alcohol-use disorder
Ratio AST/ALT >2	• Estimated in blood AST 18 hours, ALT 36 hours, specificity 80% • Marker of liver injury due to alcohol-use disorder

(ALT: alanine transaminase; AST: aspartate transaminase)

TABLE 3: Treatment for alcohol withdrawal syndrome.

Uncomplicated alcohol withdrawal symptoms	Complicated alcohol withdrawal symptoms	
	Alcohol withdrawal seizure	Alcohol withdrawal delirium tremens
• IV Diazepam 10–20 mg • IV Lorazepam 2–4 mg • IV Ondansetron 4 mg (if vomiting)	IV Lorazepam 2 mg	• IV Lorazepam 2–4 mg can be repeated with double dose till mild sedation • IV Diazepam 10–20 mg over 2 minutes can be repeated with double dose till mild sedation
• Lorazepam 2 mg orally • Diazepam 10–20 mg orally • Oxazepam 15–30 mg orally		• If symptoms are refractory to benzodiazepine • IV phenobarbital 65 mg every 30 minutes or propofol 5 µg/kg/min (requires intubation as respiratory depression is more than benzodiazepine)

(IV: intravenous)
Note: Alcohol-induced psychotic disorder is treated with antipsychotic drugs and abstinence from alcohol.

Question 8

A 2-year-old child was brought to ED with complaints of fever for 6 days associated with rash over the trunk and extremities. On examination, there was conjunctival congestion without any discharge and cervical lymphadenopathy.

1. **What is the most probable diagnosis?**
2. **What are the diagnostic criteria for this illness?**
3. **What are the complications?**
4. **How will you manage this child?**

A rash that develops along with fever can be caused by a variety of infectious diseases. Some illnesses involving both rash and fever include scarlet fever, measles, mononucleosis, and shingles. The most probable diagnosis is measles.

Differential diagnosis of measles includes rubella, roseola, Kawasaki syndrome, scarlet fever, and rickettsial, enteroviral, and adenoviral infections.

Complications of the disease include pneumonia and encephalitis, which can be fatal. Detection of measles immunoglobulin M (IgM) in a single serum sample is an indicator of acute measles infection. The gold standard for diagnostic serological assays is ≥ fourfold rise in titer for measles-specific immunoglobulin G (IgG) between acute and convalescent serum.

    There is no cure for measles. The virus must run its course, which usually takes about 10-14 days. The following measures should be taken:
a. Taking acetaminophen or ibuprofen for aches, pains, or fever
b. Getting plenty of rest
c. Drinking enough fluids
d. Gargling with salt water
e. Avoiding harsh light if your eyes hurt
f. Never give aspirin to children or teenagers unless your healthcare provider specifically tells you to because of the risk of Reye's syndrome.

Question 9

Discuss the following in a child with sickle cell disease (SCD): Vaso-occlusive crisis, fever, and neurologic complaints.

Sickle cell disease is an inherited blood disorder which is more commonly seen among people of African, Arabian, and Indian origin. SCD occurs in heterozygous form in about 8% of American blacks and in homozygous form in 1 in 400. The disease is largely not documented in India. The sickle hemoglobin was first described in India in the tribals of Nilgiri Hills in 1952. Emergency physicians need to be familiar with SCD and its complications as this can be one of the most common causes of ED visits.

1. Vaso-occlusive crisis

Acute pain in back and extremities is classical presentation due to vaso-occlusive crisis of SCD. Bone pain is quite common during sickle cell crisis usually involving the back and extremities. This pain diffuses without local signs of inflammation. Hence, if there are local signs, it suggests infection. The humeral or femoral heads are most commonly affected. Managing the pain on a priority basis is utmost important. Children may present with acute abdomen with acute splenic enlargement due to intrasplenic sickling and vascular obstruction. The child may be in shock. The emergency physician needs to be vigilant in differentiating uncomplicated crises from other more serious pathologic conditions. Investigations may be required to rule out other causes of acute abdomen, acute chest pains, or neurological complications.

2. Fever

Fever and infections: These patients are in a sort of immuno-compromised state as they are functionally asplenic after their early childhood. They are susceptible to infections from *Haemophilus influenzae, Streptococcus pneumoniae, Mycoplasma pneumonia, Salmonella typhimurium, Staphylococcus aureus,* and *Escherichia coli.*

3. Neurologic complaints

Both ischemic and hemorrhagic strokes are common in patients with SCD. Children with sickle cell anemia have >200 times greater risk of stroke than those without this disorder. It is unfortunate that these children are at 70–90% risk for recurrent stroke. Hence, chronic transfusion therapy is indicated in these children to prevent the recurrent strokes.

Question 10

1. Discuss briefly about mechanical cardiopulmonary resuscitation (CPR) devices.

Mechanical cardiopulmonary resuscitation device is a chest compression device composed of a constricting band and half backboard that is intended to be used as an adjunct to CPR during advanced cardiac life support by professional health care providers. The auto-pulse uses a distributing band to deliver the chest compressions **(Fig. 3)**. Theoretically, these mechanical devices should help eliminate the problems associated with fatigue, manpower, and CPR consistency, whether in the field or during transport. They also help free up the ambulance crew for other tasks related to resuscitation.

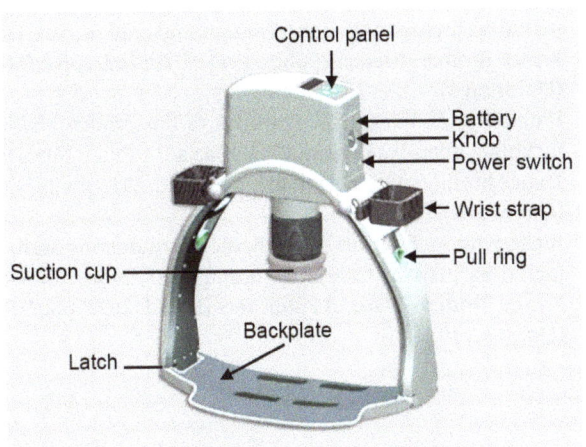

Fig. 3: Automated chest compression device.

2. What is an impedance threshold device (ITD) in CPR?

The impedance threshold device **(Figs. 4A and B)** is designed to enhance venous return and cardiac output during CPR by increasing the degree of negative intrathoracic pressure. Previous studies have suggested that the use of an ITD during CPR may improve survival rates after cardiac arrest. The noninvasive, single-use device prevents unnecessary air from entering the chest during CPR, creating a negative-pressure vacuum as the chest recoils.

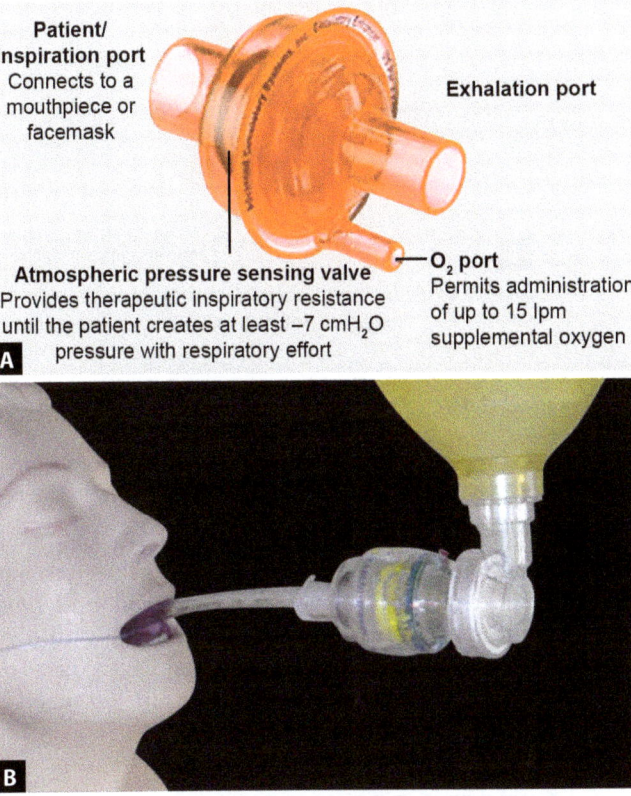

Figs. 4A and B: (A) Impedance threshold device; (B) One-way valve maintains negative pressure in the chest.

3. Discuss the techniques used in extracorporeal cardiopulmonary resuscitation (ECPR).

Extracorporeal cardiopulmonary resuscitation (ECPR) is a salvage procedure in which extracorporeal membrane oxygenation (ECMO) is initiated emergently on patients who have had cardiac arrest and on whom the conventional cardiopulmonary resuscitation (CCPR) has failed.

Extracorporeal cardiopulmonary resuscitation involves the application of percutaneous venoarterial ECMO (VA-ECMO) for management of cardiac arrest in the ED **(Figs. 5A and B)**. ECPR functions as a bridge therapy, enabling temporary systemic organ perfusion until the cause of cardiac failure can be definitively treated.

Extracorporeal cardiopulmonary resuscitation versus ECMO: The primary goals of ECMO are to stabilize hemodynamics, restore oxygen delivery, and carbon dioxide removal and to maintain normothermic physiologic processes to promote healing. The primary goal of ECPR is to address the reperfusion injury issue while preventing the patient's immediate death.

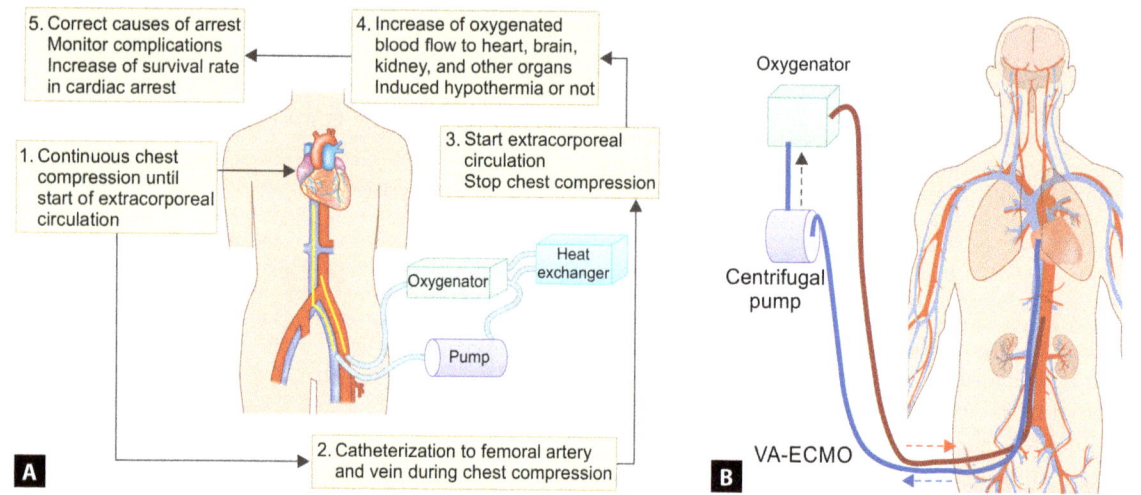

Figs. 5A and B: (A) Technique of extracorporeal cardiopulmonary resuscitation (ECPR); (B) Venoarterial extracorporeal membrane oxygenation (VA-ECMO) for management of cardiac arrest in the emergency department.

4. What do you understand by CPR feedback devices?

5. What are the recommendations for use of feedback devices during CPR?

Cardiopulmonary resuscitation feedback devices measure compression rate, depth, hand position, recoil, and chest compression fraction and provide real-time audio or visual feedback (or both) on these critical CPR skills. The recommended ratio of feedback devices is one per manikin (unless the device used is a manikin itself).

■ SUGGESTED READING

1. Richhariya D, Sharma B. Textbook of Emergency Medicine including Intensive Care and Trauma, 2nd edition. New Delhi: Jaypee Brothers Medical Publishers (P) Ltd; 2022. pp. 829-31. (Question 1).
2. Richhariya D, Sharma B. Textbook of Emergency Medicine including intensive Care and Trauma, 2nd edition. New Delhi: Jaypee Brothers Medical Publishers (P) Ltd; 2022. pp. 138-41. (Question 2).
3. Richhariya D, Sharma B. Textbook of Emergency Medicine including Intensive Care and Trauma, 2nd edition. New Delhi: Jaypee Brothers Medical Publishers (P) Ltd; 2022. pp. 1121-3. (Question 3).
4. Richhariya D, Sharma B. Textbook of Emergency Medicine including Intensive Care and Trauma, 2nd edition. New Delhi: Jaypee Brothers Medical Publishers (P) Ltd; 2022. pp. 68, 1158-68. (Question 4).
5. Centers for Disease Control and Prevention. (2002). Zika Virus. [online] Available from: https://www.cdc.gov/zika/index.html. [Last accessed May, 2023]. (Question 5).
6. Richhariya D, Sharma B. Textbook of Emergency Medicine including Intensive Care and Trauma, 2nd edition. New Delhi: Jaypee Brothers Medical Publishers (P) Ltd; 2022. p. 1555. (Question 6).
7. Richhariya D, Sharma B. Textbook of Emergency Medicine including Intensive Care and Trauma, 2nd edition. New Delhi: Jaypee Brothers Medical Publishers (P) Ltd; 2022. pp. 1443-54. (Question 7).
8. Richhariya D, Sharma B. Textbook of Emergency Medicine including Intensive Care and Trauma, 2nd edition. New Delhi: Jaypee Brothers Medical Publishers (P) Ltd; 2022. pp. 1158-60. (Question 8).
9. Richhariya D, Sharma B. Textbook of Emergency Medicine including Intensive Care and Trauma, 2nd edition. New Delhi: Jaypee Brothers Medical Publishers (P) Ltd; 2022. pp. 997-1000. (Question 9).
10. Richhariya D, Sharma B. Textbook of Emergency Medicine including Intensive Care and Trauma, 2nd edition. New Delhi: Jaypee Brothers Medical Publishers (P) Ltd; 2022. pp. 219-29. (Question 10).

Emergency Medicine Paper 13

Aysegul Bayir

Question 1

1. Draw neat labeled diagram of cerebral circulation.

Arterial blood circulation of the brain is provided by both internal carotid arteries (70%) and vertebral arteries (30%). The internal carotid arteries supply the cerebrum. Vertebral and basilar arteries and their branches supply the brainstem and cerebellum. The vertebral arteries originate from the subclavian arteries and two vertebral arteries join distally to form the basilar artery. The basilar arteries branch into the posterior cerebral arteries. The posterior cerebral arteries anastomose with the internal carotid arteries. This formation at the base of the brain is called the circle of Willis **(Fig. 1)**. The circle of Willis consists of three main arteries: (1) Anterior cerebral artery, (2) middle cerebral artery, and (3) posterior cerebral artery. These three main arteries branch into smaller arteries and arterioles and run through the brain tissue and provide blood supply to the relevant cerebral cortex. The anterior cerebral artery supplies the frontal cortex, parietal cortex, corpus callosum, medial cerebral hemispheric surface, and cingulate cortex. The middle cerebral artery is the largest branch of the internal carotid artery. The middle cerebral artery runs through the Sylvian fissure to the lateral surface of the brain. It is divided into four main surgical segments as M1, M2, M3, and M4. It supplies most of the brain, including the lateral frontal cerebral cortex, frontal and parietal lobes, capsula interna, and basal ganglia. The posterior cerebral artery supplies the occipital lobe, choroid plexus, lateral ventricle, inferomedial surface of the temporal lobe, and third ventricle.

2. How is cerebral autoregulation maintained?

Cerebral autoregulation is the ability of the cerebral vascular bed to keep stable of cerebral tissue blood flow despite changes in cerebral perfusion pressure (CPP). Cerebral blood flow (CBF) is regulated by the diameter changes in arterioles. Metabolic requirements, oxygen and glucose needs, and removal of cellular wastes are important for brain functions. The transport of glucose and oxygen to the brain tissue and the removal of cellular wastes are provided by adequate blood flow. The functions of the cerebral vascular bed are regulated by myogenic, neurogenic, endothelial, and vasogenic factors. CBF depends on CPP. CPP varies directly with mean arterial pressure (MAP) and inversely with intracranial pressure (ICP) and cerebral vasculary resistance (CVR). CPP is equal to the difference between MAP and ICP.

$$CBF = CPP/CVR = (MAP - ICP)/CVR$$

Smooth muscles in small arteries and arterioles respond to increased pressure by contraction. Astrocytes and microglia cells secrete vasoactive neurotransmitters. While acetylcholine and nitric oxide (NO) cause vasodilation, neuropeptide Y and serotonin play a role in autoregulation by vasoconstriction. Partial arterial carbon dioxide pressure ($PaCO_2$) is a metabolic regulatory factor in cerebral autoregulation. In hypoperfusion, anaerobic metabolism increases the $PaCO_2$ level and cerebral vasodilation occurs. In hyperperfusion, the $PaCO_2$ level decreases and vasoconstriction develops. In addition, mediators such as NO, thromboxane A2 and endothelin 1 secreted from endothelial cells also play a role in cerebral autoregulation by causing vasoconstriction or vasodilation.

3. Write about cerebral herniation syndromes.

Cerebral herniation is the pathological displacement of brain tissue. Its pathological displacement is a serious complication that results in dysfunction of the brainstem

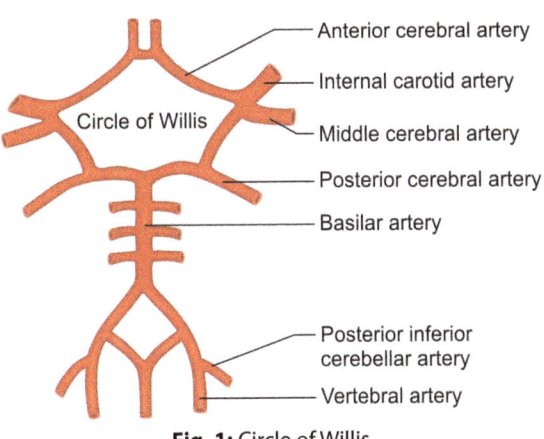

Fig. 1: Circle of Willis.

and cranial nerves. Herniation is usually caused by head trauma, Chiari malformation, hydrocephalus, brain abscess, ischemic cerebrovascular disease, intracerebral hemorrhage, and brain tumors. Because of the factors mentioned above secondary intracranial pressure increases, and give rise to brain herniation. High rate of mortality is associated with cerebral herniation thus emergency diagnosis and support are required.

Five types of herniation are as follows:
1. *Subfalcine herniation:* Frontal or as a result of parietal lesions, under falx cerebri herniation to the opposite side. Flow in the anterior cerebral artery may cause deterioration.
2. *Uncal herniation:* Supratentorial mass lesion of tentorial incisura of uncuspart of the uncus part of the temporal lobe herniation from its free edge. Mesencephalon and this due to compression of the pyramidal tract passing through the section. Paralysis of the nervus oculomotorius and motor in the contralateral body loss is typical. The degree of herniation, according to Duret, punctate hemorrhages in the brainstem is called bleeding. Posterior cerebral artery pressure can also develop. In advanced stages, corticospinal from the free edge of the contralateral tentorial incisura tract ipsilateral motor deficit occurs as a result of herniation. It is called *Kernohan sign.*
3. *Central herniation:* It describes the downward herniation of the diencephalon and mesencephalon through the tentorium opening. Cheyne–Stokes respiration can be observed in patients.
4. *Tonsillar herniation:* It occurs in posterior fossa lesions. It is the most common herniation we encounter. Your tonsils with herniation down the foramen magnum neck stiffness, torticollis, respiratory irregularity and sudden cardiac arrest can occur.
5. *Upward herniation:* Posterior fossa lesions or cerebellum after treatment of obstructive hydrocephalus from the tentorium opening of the vermis and central lobule upward correct herniation. Limitation of upward gaze in patients and unconsciousness may develop.

Question 2

1. Draw anatomy of shoulder joint.

Glenohumeral joint: It is the synovial joint between the humeral head and the glenoid fossa of the acromion **(Fig. 2)**. It is the joint with the widest range of motion in the shoulder complex. While this joint increases its range of motion, it makes it vulnerable to trauma. This joint is the most dislocated joint. Injuries are most commonly caused by falling on the abducted arm. Stabilization of the joint is provided by ligamentous structures and muscles.

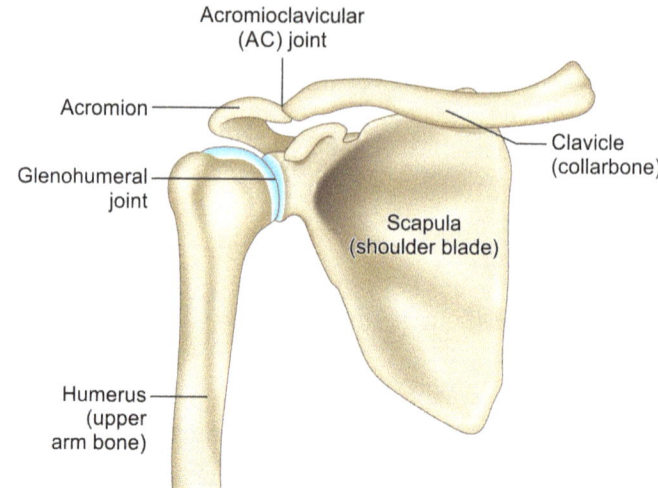

Fig. 2: Anatomy of shoulder joint.

2. Write pathophysiology of shoulder impingement syndrome.

It is an injury to subacromial structures as a result of narrowing of the subacromial space. Many mechanisms have been suggested in the formation of this pathology. These can be examined in two main groups as internal or intratendinous causes and external or extratendinous causes. Generally, pathology occurs with the combination of the intratendinous and extratendinous etiological factors. The main accepted intratendinous cause is in the rotator cuff decreased vascularity and blood supply especially older age. In older age group patients, repetitive tensile forces with decreased vascularity lead to rotator cuff pathologies. First, partial tears may turn into full-thickness tears over time. Repetitive contact of the hypovascular space with shoulder movements to the acromion and coracoacromial ligament is another proposed mechanism. The extratendinous mechanism is that protrusions and excesses in the anterior acromion cause compression of the rotator cuff. On the other hand, the coracoacromial ligament, which is hypertrophied or further calcified, also causes compression.

3. Discuss pathophysiology of rotator cuff tears.

Although the mechanism of formation of rotator cuff tears on the shoulder has not been fully revealed, generally accepted theories are—it is the formation of a tear after acute trauma or on the basis of chronic repetitive trauma. The tendon of the supraspinatus muscle is the most torn tendon. It has been suggested that the reason for this is the critical zone near the supraspinatus tendon attachment. The critical zone is less vascularized; it is the area about one centimeter away from the attachment site on the greater tubercle of the humerus. In a study conducted on cadavers, differences in shape and inclination of the acromion and osteophyte formations on the acromial part of the coracoacromial ligament and the lower surface of the anterior one-third of the acromion were described, and it was stated that these anatomical variations and degenerative changes were the source of the trauma to which the critical zone and the biceps tendon located just below it. During internal rotation, which is the most common position of the arm in daily life, the anatomical structures passing under the acromion come to the fore. With external rotation, the facet to which the supraspinatus tendon adheres falls to the lateral one-third anterior part of the acromion. Therefore, with the elevation of the shoulder in internal rotation or external rotation while in the anatomical position, the critical zone is damaged by remaining below the anterior one-third of the coracoacromial ligament or acromion.

Question 3

1. Write a short note on fundamentals of radiation physics.

Radiation can also be defined as rays and is a type of energy. It is defined as electromagnetic energy. Electromagnetic energy is in a broad spectrum. After the long wave, which has a very large wavelength, a very small frequency and a very small energy, the frequency of very small wavelengths such as radio, radiofrequency, microwave, infrared, visible light, ultraviolet (ultraviolet), X-ray, gamma ray; photon is very low. There are types of rays with large and very high energy characteristics. While there is no fear of nonionizing radiation, which basically does not remove electrons, very serious damage can occur from ionizing radiation, and the principles of radiation protection are very important; in the field of medicine, ionizing radiation such as ultraviolet, X-ray, gamma ray, photon; used in dermatology, nuclear medicine, medical imaging, and radiotherapy. While ionizing radiation moves through the material, it ionizes the environment by removing electrons from the orbits of the atoms, and as a result, undesirable damages occur in living matter. Radiofrequency and microwave are nonionizing and are used in physical therapy in the medical field. Other types of nonionizing radiations are used in technological fields such as radio, television, communication, heating. As the frequency increases, the energy increases and the ability to go deeper increases. As the wavelength increases, the energy decreases and the ability to go deep decreases. Electromagnetic energy makes wave motion, traveling at the speed of light. As the name suggests, it includes the concepts of electric and magnetic fields. As it moves through the medium and passes by the electron, it pulls or pushes the electron out of its orbit due to these electric and magnetic fields. Each electron in the atomic orbital has a binding energy to the nucleus. If the incoming EME is greater than this binding energy, it can eject electrons from the orbital.

Energy (E): Plank constant (h) × Frequency (f) or

Energy (E): $h \times 1/$wavelength (λ) or

Energy (E): Formulated as mass (m) × Speed of light $(c)^2$

2. Write about biologic effects of ionizing radiation.

Different types of radiation have different effects on living things. The impact on biological systems is very unpredictable. This effect is related to the total radiation dose, dose rate, radiation type, age of the system, many environmental and other factors. Depending on many complex parameters, the result that will occur when ionizing radiation transfers energy to the biological system is related to the absorbed dose. For complex organisms such as humans, there are two types of dose-effect relationships. In biological systems, ionizing radiation causes somatic and genetic effects. The somatic effect develops as a result of radiation absorption in the individual. Somatic influence can be deterministic (precise) or stochastic (uncertain). Early deterministic effects are erythema, pulmonary pneumonitis, and radiation sickness. Late effects usually occur >1 year after dosing. Late effects occur as keratosis, pulmonary fibrosis, cataracts, and obliterative endarteritis. The incidence of stochastic effects in the irradiated individual is not certain. Examples of these effects: Leukemia and cancer formations and have no threshold value. Genetic effects describe hereditary inherited genotypic changes that result in mutations in the chromosomes or genes of germ cells. They are considered in the stochastic effect group. The effect does not occur in the irradiated individual, but in subsequent generations of that individual. In order for the genetic effect to occur, the irradiated cell must survive and fertilize.

3. Discuss clinical features of acute radiation syndrome.

It has been stated that whole body or partial body exposure should be at least 1 Gy for the development of acute radiation syndrome. Acute radiation syndrome is not expected for exposures below 0.5 Gy. After exposure, 0–2 days are defined as the prodromal phase, 2–20 days as the latent phase, and 21–60 days as the disease phase. Early symptoms are nausea, vomiting, anorexia, apathy, diarrhea, fever, headache, and tachycardia. If these symptoms started within about 2 hours, it is considered that the patient was most likely exposed to high doses, and if they started within minutes, doses exceeding 10 Gy are considered. At such high-dose exposure, in patient develops cerebrovascular syndrome and possibly dying within a few days. If cerebrovascular syndrome does not develop and only gastrointestinal syndrome develops, then the patient may recover with appropriate medical intervention. Four different syndromes that may develop related to acute radiation syndrome have been defined as cerebrovascular, gastrointestinal, hematopoietic, and cutaneous syndromes. Cerebrovascular syndrome is usually seen in doses of 10 Gy and above. It is thought that this syndrome develops due to radiation-induced deterioration in cellular permeability and cerebrospinal fluid content, interstitial edema, and petechial hemorrhages. It has been reported that severe nausea and vomiting, confusion, disorientation, seizure, ataxia and papilledema can be seen in cerebrovascular syndrome.

Question 4

1. Discuss physiology of high-altitude acclimatization.

As the altitude increases, the partial pressure of oxygen in the atmosphere does not change (21%), but the oxygen pressure (the number of oxygen molecules in a unit volume of air) decreases in direct proportion to the atmospheric pressure. At 5,500 m, the oxygen pressure is about half that at sea level. At the summit of the Everest, this rate will drop to one-third. Due to the centrifugal effect caused by the earth's rotation, the atmosphere becomes thinner toward the poles. Low oxygen pressure at high altitude also means low oxygen pressure in the blood. The oxygen pressure in the blood at 5,500 m is about half that at sea level. Hemoglobin oxygen saturation decreases to approximately 70%. As you rise, the amount of oxygen in the atmosphere decreases, leading to an increase in the rate and depth of respiration. The most important stages that our body goes through while acclimatizing can be listed as—increase in pulmonary artery pressure, increase in cardiac output, increase in the number of red blood cells, increase in the oxygen carrying capacity of red blood cells and changes in body tissues in order to maintain their normal functions at low oxygen pressure.

2. List various high altitude illnesses.

In general, three diseases associated with climbing 2,500 m or higher are acute mountain disease, acute brain edema, and acute pulmonary edema, respectively. All three of these are collectively called acute high altitude disease.

Clinically, in acute mountain disease, at least one of the symptoms of fatigue, insomnia, vomiting or dizziness is observed in addition to headache after climbing to high altitude. The Lake Louise Acute Mountain Sickness Score has been defined for climbers and clinicians to recognize the disease, and the disease has been studied at three levels as mild, moderate, and severe. Acute brain edema is the name given to the more advanced and serious form of acute mountain disease. In other words, encephalopathy, altered consciousness or ataxia should be added in addition to acute mountain disease.

3. Discuss prevention of acute high altitude illnesses.

Gradually climbing is the most important approach to prevent acute mountain sickness and acute cerebral edema. In addition, the altitude at which the climber sleeps is considered more important than controlling the vertical distance traveled in a day (recommendation level 1B). If altitudes <3,000 m are to be climbed, the daily sleeping altitude should not be increased >500 m and a daily rest break should be given every 3–4 days. Acetazolamide is the most important medical prophylaxis in the prophylaxis of acute mountain sickness and acute brain edema. The daily dose is 2 × 125 mg in adults (level of recommendation 1A), although there are fewer studies in pediatric patients, the dose is 2 × 2.5 mg/kg PO (level of recommendation 1C). The recommended daily adult dose for dexamethasone use is 2 mg × 4 or 4 mg × 2. Higher doses are recommended in high-risk situations where climbing to 3,500 m or higher is required. However, it should not be used >10 days in order not to suppress the adrenal gland (recommendation level 1A). It is not recommended for use in the pediatric age group due to its potential side effects.

Question 5

1. Define vertigo.

Vertigo is the illusion of movement in which the patient feels the environment around him or himself spinning when the environment is stationary. It is divided into two as this unpleasant and uncomfortable sliding movement of the body (subjective vertigo) or feeling that the environment surrounding the person is spinning (objective vertigo). Vertigo is a symptom, not a disease. A diagnosis of the underlying disease is required for the proper management of vertigo. Vertigo may also be a component of the drowsiness or vertigo complaint expressed as dizziness. Dizziness is nonspecific and can result from a disorder in any organ system.

2. What is vestibulo-ocular reflex (VOR)?

The VOR includes reflexive eye movements that keep the visual field constant during head movement. For this purpose, there are four VOR arches—horizontal, vertical, indirect, and translational. In the horizontal vestibulo-ocular reflex (H-VOR) arc, the afferent fibers that have connections with the hair cells of the semicircular canal transmit the information they receive from here to the abducens and oculomotor nuclei that innervate the lateral and medial rectus muscles, thus ensuring the realization of H-VOR. The fibers forming the vertical VOR (V-VOR) reflex arc are mostly located lateral to the medial vestibular nucleus, vertical to the lateral vestibular nucleus, and in the center of the superior vestibular nucleus. Motor neurons that provide contralateral stimulation of the superior oblique and superior rectus muscles are important for the vertical VOR. Sensory information from the periphery is transmitted to the trochlear and oculomotor nuclei that innervate the superior oblique and superior rectus muscles, and to the ipsilateral abducens nucleus that innervates the lateral rectus muscle, thus ensuring the realization of V-VOR. The indirect VOR is responsible for corrective eye movements during rapid head movements between 0.1 and 8–10 Hz. Translational VOR (T-VOR) is responsible for the corrective movements of the head due to translational movements. T-VOR contributes to the formation of postural balance by transmitting the sensory inputs of the otolith organs to the vestibulospinal and vestibulocollic reflexes in order to stabilize the head and body.

3. How do you differentiate peripheral from central vertigo?

In peripheral vertigo, the pathology is mostly in the temporal bone, especially in the labyrinth. Central pathologies are the reflection of pathologies in the area extending from the vestibular system to the brain. The most important feature in distinguishing between central and peripheral vertigo is the features of nystagmus. Centrally derived nystagmuses are seen in brain and brainstem lesions. These may be in the horizontal plane, as in peripheral lesions, or in the form of vertical nystagmus. If a patient has a vertical nystagmus in the spontaneous gaze, that is, upward and downward, this always suggests a central lesion. In peripheral vertigo, auditory complaints, hearing loss, ringing, humming, and ear fullness may accompany the patient. Sometimes, as in vestibular neuritis, the patient may not have auditory findings. Auditory findings are not usually encountered in central vertigo. It is accompanied by remarkable findings such as vision loss, diplopia, coordination disorders, ataxia, and speech difficulties. Peripheral vertigo is usually described as spinning around, whereas in central vertigo, the feeling of instability and drunkenness is more prominent.

4. Discuss diagnostic approach to a patient with vertigo in emergency department (ED).

The most important point in diagnosis is history and physical examination. After a well-received history and physical examination, the diagnosis is largely approached. Bedside blood sugar should be checked while a history is taken from the patient and a physical examination is performed. Oral or intravenous (IV) glucose is given if the patient is hypoglycemic. ECG is taken to detect tachycardia, bradycardia, and dysrhythmia that may cause symptoms in the patient. Short PR, ischemia findings, prolonged QT interval, Wolf–Parkinson–White findings, QRS width are investigated on ECG. The patient's arterial blood pressure is measured and a pulse oximeter is inserted. The patient is monitored. The patient is examined with an otoscope. Bedside oculomotor examination provides important information for diagnosis. Oculomotor examination is done in two ways—dynamic and static. In static oculomotor examination, asymmetric eye movements and type of nystagmus are determined. In dynamic oculomotor examination, the oculomotor reflex is evaluated with the head impulse test and the head shaking test. Laboratory tests that should be requested for the patient are whole blood analysis, electrolytes, and β-hCG in women of childbearing age. If the physical examination findings support central pathologies or are suspicious, firstly, noncontrast brain tomography is taken. Diffusion-weighted MRI and MRI angiography are particularly important for detecting cerebrovascular disease of the brainstem and cerebellum.

Question 6

1. What is neurogenic shock?

Neurogenic shock is a type of distributive shock characterized by hypotension, bradycardia, and vasodilation with sympathetic denervation and increased vagal tone related to T6 and higher level medulla spinalis injuries.

2. Write pathophysiology of neurogenic shock.

Primary injury of the spinal cord is stretching, laceration and occurs with traumatic events that cause compression. Secondary damage develops within a few days or weeks after trauma due to hypotension, tissue edema, inflammation, electrolyte imbalances, shock, or tissue ischemia. The primary injury damages the intermediolateral nucleus, lateral gray matter, and anterior root axons and neural membranes. As a result, sympathetic tone is impaired.

With the effect of secondary damaging factors, progressive central hemorrhagic necrosis develops in the gray matter of the spinal cord region affected by trauma. In damaged cells develop excitotoxicity due to the accumulation of N-methyl-D-aspartate (NMDA), disturbances in electrolyte balance, mitochondrial damage, and reperfusion injury. Controlled and uncontrolled apoptosis increases. Capillary vasodilation, hypotension, bradycardia, disturbances of thermoregulation develop with loss of sympathetic tone and activation of the parasympathetic nervous system managed by the vagus nerve. Tissue perfusion is impaired as a result of decreased peripheral vascular resistance and vasodilation.

3. How will you differentiate neurogenic shock from spinal shock?

Spinal shock is a reversible clinical condition characterized by loss of spinal reflexes under the damaged cord. It refers to the physiological reflex response to trauma, not anatomical damage to the medulla spinalis. Under the damaged medulla spinalis, spinal cord functions are suppressed and sensorimotor functions are lost. In spinal shock seen flaccid paralysis under the damaged medulla spinalis region, loss of bulbocavernosus reflex, anal and urinary incontinence after trauma. Contrary to neurogenic shock, it can also be seen in spinal cord injuries below T6 level. It can take days or even months to return of spinal reflexes. Flask paralysis leaves its place to spasticity.

4. How do you manage neurogenic shock?

First, the patient's airway is opened, breathing and circulation are evaluated and supported, and a full neurological examination is performed [airway, breathing, circulation, disability, exposure (ABCDE)]. Measures should be taken against orthostatic hypotension (such as a stretcher that can provide inclination, elastic socks). Sufficient fluid resuscitation is done. At this time, a pulmonary artery catheter may be inserted to the patient to monitor hydration. Positive inotropic vasopressor agents such as dopamine, noradrenaline, and epinephrine are given intravenously. After resuscitation, the patient should be referred to a spine or trauma center. A general trauma assessment is made and differential diagnosis of other causes of hypotension (other types of shock) should be made. Treatment with rapid infusion of crystalloids in trauma patients is often also effective in the treatment of neurogenic shock. It will relatively correct hypovolemia. Since low blood pressure is not due to a true hypovolemia, care should be taken in fluid therapy in neurogenic shock. Uncontrolled fluid resuscitation can lead to heart failure and pulmonary edema. In addition, excessive fluid overload can cause cord edema and impaired tissue perfusion. If IV fluid therapy is not sufficient to maintain organ perfusion, positive inotropic vasopressor agents—dopamine (10–20 µg/kg/min), noradrenaline (2–20 µg/min) or epinephrine (1–10 µg/min)—are given intravenously. Atropine (0.5 mg every 4 hours), dopamine (2–10 µg/kg/min), epinephrine (1–10 µg/min), methylxanthine according to the patient's hemodynamics in the first few hours or days of spinal cord injury with predominant vagal tone to the heart (aminophylline, theophylline), propantheline is given. Pacing may be performed in some patients with symptomatic bradycardia with heart block. It is recommended to start methylprednisolone within the first 8 hours after the trauma in patients with spinal injuries with neurological deficits. First, methylprednisolone is given as an IV bolus of 30 mg/kg over 15 minutes. Then after 45 minutes start methyleprednisolone infusion 5.4 mg/kg over 24 hours starts. Consultation with neurosurgeons is made to relieve cord compression and plan surgical treatment.

Question 7

1. Write pathophysiology of pain.

All of the complex physiological events that end with the onset of active tissue damage and the perception of pain are called nociception. Nociception consists of four parts: (1) Transduction, (2) transmission, (3) modulation, and (4) perception. Transduction involves the conversion of noxious stimulus into electrical signals at sensory nerve endings and transmission to the spinal cord. Receptors that sense and transmit noxious stimuli are called nociceptors (pain receptors). These receptors convert specific modal energy into action potentials. Nociceptors are often referred to as "free nerve endings". These are unencapsulated nerve endings. They are activated by stimuli that threaten or cause tissue damage. All nociceptors are innervated by small diameter myelinated (Aδ) or unmyelinated nerve fibers (C6). Axons of primary afferents consist of myelinated and unmyelinated fibers. Peripheral nerves are classified according to their conduction velocity, diameter, degree of myelination or function. Pain occurs as a result of stimulation of free nerve endings due to a specific tissue damage or disease. Mediators such as bradykinin, substance P, prostaglandins, and histamine secreted from damaged tissues generate action potentials that are carried along the afferent nerves through the dorsal horn of the spinal cord. This action potential generates neuropeptides and neurotransmitters that transmit impulses to the thalamus and midbrain via the spinothalamic pathway causes release.

Nociceptive signals from the thalamus spread to the cortex, limbic system, frontal lobe, and parietal lobe. In these areas, the action potential is perceived as pain. Pain perception is subjective and emotional factors, stress, anxiety increase pain perception.

2. Discuss any three pain scales used in ED for adults.

Generally, "numeric rating scale (NRS)" and "visual analogue scale (VAS)" are used in adult ED patients who can communicate normally. These scales have been validated with similar specificity for pain severity assessment **(Fig. 3)**. Values of 7 and above on the numerical scale and 70 mm and above on the visual scale are in the category of severe pain. High doses of opioid analgesics may be required to relieve these patients. In addition, a 30% reduction in pain intensity is considered significant in sequential evaluations. It would be appropriate to use the PAINAD scale based on the opinion of the physician, especially in patients with dementia and patients with poor verbal communication. It is difficult to evaluate the severity of pain in sedated and unconscious patients. It is recommended to use the behavioral pain scale (BPS), which has been developed and validated for these patients.

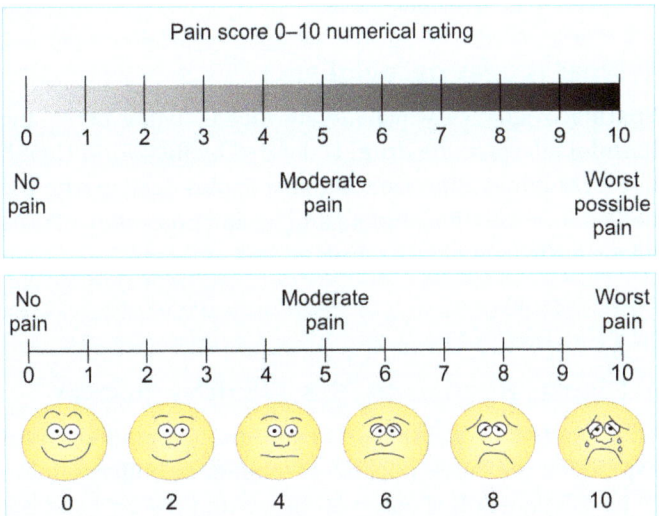

Fig. 3: Pain scales used in emergency department for adults.

3. Discuss complex regional pain syndrome (CRPS).

Complex regional pain syndrome is a painful clinical picture that may occur spontaneously or may develop after hemiplegia, heart attack and often trauma, and causes sympathetic, sensory, motor and trophic changes in the affected extremity. If there is no nerve injury in the clinical picture, it is called type 1, if there is, it is called CRPS type 2. It has also been classified as acute, dystrophic and atrophic, related to the present symptoms and the duration of the disease. Its annual incidence is in a wide range, ranging from 5.5 to 26.2 per 100,000 people. Different mechanisms have been implicated in its pathophysiology. Excessive inflammatory response to tissue injury, increase in cytokine level, oxidative stress markers and mast cell activity, neurogenic inflammation, excessive sympathetic response to painful stimuli are some of them. In its treatment, psychotherapy, physical therapy, spinal cord stimulator, sympathetic block, IV regional block, chemical and surgical sympathectomy and pharmacological treatment (antidepressants, anticonvulsants, opioid analgesics, calcitonin, bisphosphonates, membrane stabilizing agents, steroids, free radical scavengers) are used.

Question 8

1. Explain various gas laws relevant to hyperbaric oxygen therapy.

Hyperbaric oxygen therapy is used to treat disease in a closed system at higher than atmospheric pressure at sea level. It is a form of treatment applied by breathing 100% oxygen continuously or intermittently from a mask, headgear or environment at a high pressure. Atmospheric pressure at sea level is 1 ATA (1 ATA, atmosphere absolute = 760 mm Hg); 2 ATA at a depth of 10 m above sea level; and 3 ATA at 20 m depth. Hyperbaric oxygen therapy is based on the physiological and biochemical effects of hyperoxia and gas laws. According to Boyle–Mariotte's law, the volume and pressure of a gas are inversely proportional to each other at a constant temperature. In other words, the product of pressure and volume of a gas at a given temperature is always constant (pressure P_1, volume V_1 for the first equilibrium state of the gas; pressure P_2, volume V_2 for the second equilibrium state):

$$P_1 \times V_1 = P_2 \times V_2$$

Dalton's law states that each gas in a mixture creates a pressure in proportion to its amount in the mixture (P, gas pressure):

$$P_{total} = P_1 + P_2 + P_3 + \ldots + P_n$$

Henry's law, the amount of gas dissolved in a liquid or tissue at a constant temperature is directly proportional to the partial pressure of the gas with which the liquid or tissue is in contact (C is the concentration of the gas dissolved in the liquid; P is the partial pressure of the gas above the liquid; k is Henry's constant):

$$C = k \times P_{gas}$$

Physiologic effects of hyperbaric oxygen: Physiologic effects of hyperbaric oxygen are immune stimulation, bactericidal effect, reduction in tissue hypoxia, angiogenesis, fibroblast proliferation, increase of collagen synthesis, suppression of toxicity of harmful gases, and reduction in tissue edema.

2. Enumerate the indications of hyperbaric oxygen therapy.

a. Decompression sickness
b. Air or gas embolism
c. Carbon monoxide and cyanide poisoning, acute smoke inhalation
d. Gas gangrene
e. Necrotizing infections of soft tissue
f. Crush injuries, compartment syndrome, and other acute traumatic ischemia
g. Conditions where wound healing is delayed (diabetic and nondiabetic)
h. Chronic refractory osteomyelitis
i. Excessive blood loss
j. Radiation necroses
k. Suspicious skin flaps and grafts
l. Thermal burns
m. Brain abscess
n. Anoxic encephalopathy
o. Sudden hearing loss
p. Retinal artery occlusion
q. Skull bones, sternum and vertebrae acute osteomyelitis.

3. Write a note on one of the definitive indications of hyperbaric oxygen therapy.

Definitive indications for hyperbaric oxygen therapy: Carboxy hemoglobin (COHb) level above 25%, COHb level above 15% in pregnant females. In pregnant women, ischemic chest pain or ischemic change in EKG or troponin positivity in carbon monoxide (CO) toxicity, presence of neuropsychiatric examination findings or abnormal psychometric tests in CO toxicity patients, metabolic acidosis in CO toxicity.

Question 9

1. What is adverse drug reaction (ADR)?

Adverse drug reaction is defined as "harmful and unintended response to a drug" and can occur in various ways. Thus, according to the pharmacovigilance system, a drug is a serious ADR if it causes any of the following reactions—death, life-threatening, prolonged hospitalization or hospital stay, permanent or significant disability or incapacity, congenital anomaly or a congenital defect, and medically significant events.

2. Discuss the classification of ADRs.

Adverse drug reactions are divided into six classes according to time, duration and dose—type A, type B, type C, type D, type E, and type F.

Type A (augmented) ADRs: Frequent occurrence, exaggerated pharmacological exposure, predictable, dose dependent, and low mortality.

Type B (bizarre) ADRs: Rarity, unrelated to pharmacological action, unpredictable, dose independent, and high mortality.

Type C (chronic) ADRs: Rare, cumulative dose dependent, and time dependent.

Type D (delayed) ADRs: Rare, time dependent, usually dose dependent, and after using the drug manifestation.

Type E (end of use) ADRs: Rare and shortly manifest after discontinuation of the drug.

Type F (failure) ADRs: Common, dose dependent, and often caused by drug interactions.

3. Discuss pathophysiology of ADRs.

In pathophysiology of ADRs, allergy, hypersensitivity, immunological reactions, pharmacological side effects, intolerance or sensitivity, idiosyncrasy, toxicity, interactions, and pseudoallergies play roles.

4. What is pharmacovigilance?

Pharmacovigilance, which literally means "being alert to the harmful effects of the drug", is defined by the World Health Organization as "the science and activities dealing with the detection, evaluation, understanding and prevention of drug adverse effects, and other drug-related problems".

Question 10

1. Discuss Henderson–Hasselbalch equation.

The Henderson–Hasselbalch equation is a mathematical expression that allows the pH of a buffer or buffer solution to be calculated. It is based on the $pK\alpha$ of the acid and the ratio between the concentrations of conjugate base or salt and acid present in the buffer solution. The equation was first developed by Lawrence Joseph Henderson (1878-1942) in 1907. This chemist built the components of his equation based on carbonic acid as a buffer or buffer.

$$pH = pK\alpha + \log([A^-]/[HA])$$

In this equation, [HA] and [A$^-$] refer to the equilibrium concentrations of the conjugate acid-base pair used to create the buffer solution. When [HA] = [A$^-$], the solution pH is equal to the $pK\alpha$ of the acid.

2. Describe Kassirer–Bleich equation.

The Kassirer–Bleich equation is obtained by inserting known constants into the Henderson–Hasselbalch equation, then taking the antilog of each side. This equation is very useful for understanding clinical acid–base interactions.

Kassirer–Bleich equation: $H^+ = 24 \times PCO_2/HCO_3^-$

3. Discuss pathophysiology of respiratory acidosis.

Metabolic acidosis occurs by three main mechanisms: (1) increased acid production, (2) loss of bicarbonate, or (3) decreased renal acid excretion. In addition to these three pathological mechanisms, it is possible to collect metabolic acidosis under two subheadings according to the gap in serum anions: Metabolic acidosis with high anion gap and normal anion gap.

Metabolic acidosis due to increased acid production:
a. *Lactic acidosis:* Plasma lactate level above 4 mmol/L; it is one of the most common causes of metabolic acidosis. In type A lactic acidosis, tissue oxygenation is impaired and lactate production is increased as a result of anaerobic respiration. It can be seen in conditions such as hypovolemia, heart failure, and sepsis. Type B lactic acidosis is a nonsystemic acidosis observed as a result of regional tissue ischemia, cancer patients, alcoholism, toxic alcohol intoxication, and drug-induced mitochondrial dysfunction. D-lactic acidosis is a type of lactic acidosis observed in some malabsorption syndromes and some diabetic ketoacidosis patients. It occurs after the absorption of lactic acid, which is released as a result of glucose fermentation by bacteria in the intestine.
Ketoacidosis: It occurs in patients with uncontrolled diabetes, after excessive alcohol consumption or as a result of malnutrition. Increased acidity due to oral or IV intakes: Methanol, ethylene glycol intoxications, salicylic acid intoxication, chronic acetaminophen use and toluene exposure seen in the dye industry and those who breathe honey can be given as examples.
b. *Metabolic acidosis with loss of bicarbonate:* Patients with severe diarrhea may have other electrolyte deficits as well as acidosis due to loss of bicarbonate. It can be observed especially in elderly patients, patients with impaired oral intake, and those with prolonged diarrhea, in patients with a spare bladder created from the sigmoid colon, and in patients with proximal renal tubular acidosis (type 2) with impaired renal bicarbonate absorption.
c. *Metabolic acidosis with decreased renal acid excretion:* Acidosis due to decrease in glomerular filtration rate (mechanism observed in acute and chronic renal failure); type 1 and type 4 renal tubular acidosis.

4. Explain the adaptation of chronic respiratory acidosis.

Lungs remove 15,000 mmol of CO_2 daily from the body. If there is a problem in the removal of carbon dioxide by the lungs, carbon dioxide accumulates in the body and the plasma pH tends to decrease. As a result, any situation that reduces/inhibits the excretion of carbon dioxide from the lungs can cause respiratory acidosis (alveolar hypoventilation).

Respiratory center depression: Brain tumor, chronic narcotic-tranquilizer use.

Neuromuscular disorders: Poliomyelitis, multiple sclerosis, acid maltase deficiency, myxedema, muscular dystrophy, malnutrition, hypothyroidism, corticosteroid use.

Airway obstruction: Chronic bronchitis, emphysema, asthma, cystic fibrosis.

Reactive patients: Interstitial fibrosis, diaphragmatic paralysis, kyphoscoliosis, hydrothorax, prolonged pneumonias. Pickwickian syndrome causes chronic respiratory acidosis. It is the balance between the functioning of the lungs and kidneys that determines the plasma pH. In order to maintain the acid-base balance, if the kidneys deteriorate the lungs, and if the lungs deteriorate, the kidneys step in and try to maintain this ratio and keep the plasma pH constant. An average 4 mmol/L increase in (HCO_3^-) occurs for every 10 mm Hg increase in PCO_2 from the reference value of 40 mm Hg. For example, if arterial PCO_2 has risen from 40 mm Hg to 60 mm Hg (due to decreased alveolar ventilation) and remained elevated for several days, then this chronic rise of "2 tens" (i.e., 60 − 40 = 20 mm Hg rise = 2 rises of 10 mm Hg) results in a rise of plasma bicarbonate by 8 from its reference value of 24 mmol/L up to 32 mmol/L. Consequently, if this chronic respiratory acidosis was the only base disorder present, then plasma bicarbonate would be 32 mmol/L. The renal response within by 6–12 hours with a maximal effect reached by 3–4 days. This maximal effect is not sufficient to return plasma pH to normal, but because of the additional renal contribution, the pH is returned toward normal much more than occurs in an acute respiratory acidosis.

■ SUGGESTED READING

1. Richhariya D, Sharma B. Textbook of Emergency Medicine including Intensive Care and Trauma, 2nd edition. New Delhi: Jaypee Brothers Medical Publishers (P) Ltd; 2022. pp. 1557-60. (Question 1).

2. Richhariya D, Sharma B. Textbook of Emergency Medicine including Intensive Care and Trauma, 2nd edition. New Delhi: Jaypee Brothers Medical Publishers (P) Ltd; 2022. p. 1604. (Question 2).
3. Richhariya D, Sharma B. Textbook of Emergency Medicine including Intensive Care and Trauma, 2nd edition. New Delhi: Jaypee Brothers Medical Publishers (P) Ltd; 2022. p. 191. (Question 3).
4. Richhariya D, Sharma B. Textbook of Emergency Medicine including Intensive Care and Trauma, 2nd edition. New Delhi: Jaypee Brothers Medical Publishers (P) Ltd; 2022. pp. 1708-11. (Question 4).
5. Richhariya D, Sharma B. Textbook of Emergency Medicine including Intensive Care and Trauma, 2nd edition. New Delhi: Jaypee Brothers Medical Publishers (P) Ltd; 2022. pp. 801-3. (Question 5).
6. Richhariya D, Sharma B. Textbook of Emergency Medicine including Intensive Care and Trauma, 2nd edition. New Delhi: Jaypee Brothers Medical Publishers (P) Ltd; 2022. p. 1576. (Question 6).
7. Richhariya D, Sharma B. Textbook of Emergency Medicine including Intensive Care and Trauma, 2nd edition. New Delhi: Jaypee Brothers Medical Publishers (P) Ltd; 2022. pp. 355-62. (Question 7).
8. Richhariya D, Sharma B. Textbook of Emergency Medicine including Intensive Care and Trauma, 2nd edition. New Delhi: Jaypee Brothers Medical Publishers (P) Ltd; 2022. pp. 249-52. (Question 8).
9. Richhariya D, Sharma B. Textbook of Emergency Medicine including Intensive Care and Trauma, 2nd edition. New Delhi: Jaypee Brothers Medical Publishers (P) Ltd; 2022. pp. 1025-31. (Question 9).
10. Richhariya D, Sharma B. Textbook of Emergency Medicine including Intensive Care and Trauma, 2nd edition. New Delhi: Jaypee Brothers Medical Publishers (P) Ltd; 2022. pp. 303-10. (Question 10).

Emergency Medicine Paper 14

Aysegul Bayir

Question 1

1. Classify fractures.

Types and classification of fracture:
a. *According to bone tissue strength:*
   i. Traumatic fracture in normal bone
   ii. Pathological fracture in diseased
   iii. Bone stress fracture
b. *Accordingly whether the fracture line is in contact with the external environment through the skin or mucous membrane surrounding the bone or not:*
   i. Closed fractures
   ii. Open fractures
c. *According to the force that creates the fracture:*
   i. Fractures with direct mechanism
   ii. Fractures with indirect mechanism
   iii. Fractures with a combination of direct and indirect mechanisms
d. *According to the number of fractures:*
   i. Single broken line
   ii. Multiple fracture line
e. *According to the degree of fracture and fracture line:*
   Separated (displaced) fractures:
   i. Transverse fracture
   ii. Oblique fracture
   iii. Spiral broken
   iv. Shear fracture
   v. Fragmented fracture
   Nondisplaced fractures:
   i. Crack (fissure, linear fracture)
   ii. Green stick fracture
   iii. Torus fracture
   iv. Compression fractures
   v. Dented (impacted) fractures
   vi. Undifferentiated fractures of the epiphysis
f. *According to the anatomical localization of the fracture in the bone:*
   i. Proximal region fractures (proximal epiphyseal and metaphyseal region; trochanteric, femoral neck, tibia condyle, etc.)
   ii. Body (shaft) fractures (diaphyse region; expressed as 1/3 upper, 1/3 middle, 1/3 lower region)
   iii. Distal region fractures (distal epiphyseal and metaphyseal region; supracondylar, malleolar, pilon, Colles' fractures, etc.)
   iv. Fractures of the pineal region (in children, epiphysis and metaphyseal fractures affecting the physis line are understood in the period before the physis is closed)
   v. Fracture—dislocations (dislocation of the joint where the broken bone joins with the fracture)
g. *According to the histological structure of the broken bone:*
   i. Spongios region
   ii. Fractures of cortical
   iii. Region fractures

2. How do fractures heal?

Fracture healing starts from the moment of fracture and consists of following three stages:
  I. Inflammatory period
 II. Reparation period
III. Remodeling period

These three periods continue before one ends and the other begins, and the longest period is the remodeling period. During the inflammatory phase (24–72 hours), vasoactive mediators, growth factors, and other cytokines are released from injured tissues and platelets. Cytokines affect cell migration, proliferation, differentiation, and matrix synthesis. Growth factors recruit fibroblasts, mesenchymal cells, and osteoprogenitor cells to the fracture site. Macrophages, polymorphous nucleosides, and mast cells reach the fracture site to initiate the removal of tissue debris. Vasoactive substances (nitric oxide and the factor that stimulates endothelial angiogenesis) cause neovascularization and local vasodilation during the recovery phase, which lasts from 2 days–2 weeks. Undifferentiated mesenchymal cells migrate to the fracture site and may develop into cells that will lead to cartilage, bone, and fibrous tissue replacement. Fracture hematoma organizes and fibroblasts and chondroblasts appear between the bone ends and cartilage is formed (type II collagen). Remodeling occurs within 1–7 years after the repair period, excess bone tissue around the fracture is resorbed, medullary channels are opened and normal bone structure is gained. Remodeling happens according to Wolff's laws. If there is a convexity and concavity outside of the normal, stretching and bone resorption on the convex side, compression and new bone formation on the concave side occur. It has been determined that resorption and bone formation occur according to the electrical activity that occurs here.

3. How will you describe radiographic appearance of a long bone fracture?

Bidirectional radiographs should be taken, especially in extremity injuries. With this approach, the probability of detecting existing pathologies increases and it is possible to better understand some pathologies. Diagnosis should not be attempted with nonstandard radiographs. It is common in emergency departments to pull two adjacent joints, which are likely to be injured, without proper positioning. However, it is important to visualize the joints proximal and distal to the bone with suspected fracture. In order to define pathology on a radiograph, it is necessary to have a good grasp of anatomy. Segmented and displaced fractures are easily seen. Long bone fractures are recognized as a radiolucent image that also distorts the cortical structure on direct graphy. Mostly, feeding arteries in long bones may appear broken, but the radiolucent line formed by the artery is mostly oblique and is observed in a single cortex.

4. Write the principles of splinting of long bone fractures.

Circular casts or splints are used to stabilize the extremity in connective tissue trauma or bone long fractures until the fractured bones heal and the soft tissue inflammation, edema, and damage heal. They are medical materials that keep the broken bone ends fixed in order to ensure that the healing takes place as desired in long bone fractures and to prevent the broken bone ends from damaging the surrounding vein and nerve tissue. Splints and plasters are applied to cover an upper and a lower joint in the area of the fracture. The splint should be made to prevent the movement of the extremity and stabilize the broken bone ends, but should not impede circulation. Splints that prevent circulation can cause compartment syndrome. Therefore, circulation should be checked frequently after splint application.

Question 2

1. Enumerate various fractures of radius bone.

Galeazzi fracture, Colles' fracture, Smith's fracture, radius body fracture, radius head fracture.

2. Discuss the clinical and radiological features of Smith's fracture.

A Smith's fracture is a distal radius fracture in which the distal fragment is displaced to the volar side and the proximal fragment is displaced to the dorsal side. Fracture occurs when the elbow is in extension, the wrist is in flexion, or the forearm is in supination, and the wrist is in dorsal flexion, as a result of a fall or direct trauma. In physical examination, this image in which the distal part is displaced to the volar side and the proximal part to the dorsal side is called "gardener's knife deformity".

3. Explain the complications of Smith's fracture.

Complications of Smith's fractures **(Fig. 1)** are malunion, leading to a garden spade deformity or carpal tunnel syndrome, as well as complex regional pain syndrome or extensor pollicis longus rupture.

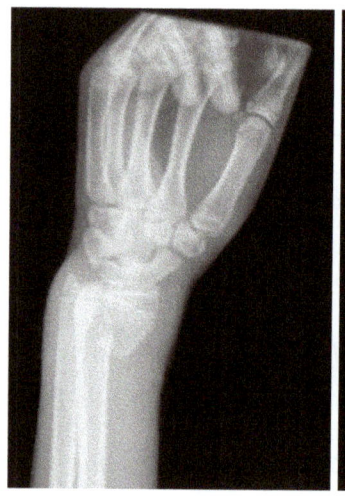
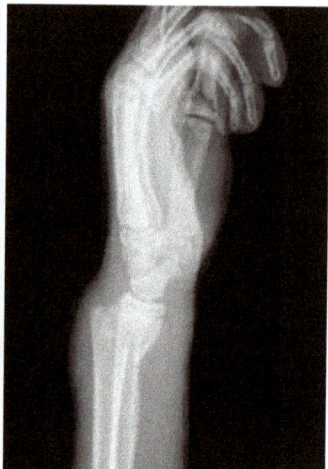

Fig. 1: X-ray of Smith's fracture.

4. How do you manage this fracture in emergency department?

Smith's fracture is treated with 3 weeks of closed reduction with a splint or circular cast, and physical therapy.

Question 3

1. Classify supracondylar fractures of humerus.

Gartland classification:
a. *Type I:* Undifferentiated fractures (Type I-a if there is no medial impact here, crush in the coronal plane, slight hyperextension in the sagittal plane classified as Type I-b if any).
b. *Type II:* Dissociated fractures; but posterior, cortex it is solid.

c. *Type III:* Dissociated fractures in which both the anterior and posterior cortex are not intact.
d. *Type IV:* Both anterior and posterior cortex. They are dissociated fractures that are not intact and completely unstable.

2. Explain the clinical presentation of supracondylar fractures.

Patient in humerus supracondylar fractures presents to the emergency department with the symptoms of swelling, pain, inability to move, and crepitation in the elbow. Vascular and nerve examination must be done in detail and recorded. The color and temperature of the fingers and the presence of peripheral circulation should be carefully evaluated.

3. What are the early and late complications of supracondylar fractures?

Its early complications are brachial artery, median and ulnar nerve injury, and compartment syndrome. Late complications are malunion, infection, myositis ossificans, cubitus varus, and joint stiffness.

4. Discuss the diagnosis and management of compartment syndrome.

The most important diagnostic tool in compartment syndrome is physical examination and clinical findings. The earliest and most common finding is pain disproportionate to the severity of the injury. Patients generally describe the pain as a deep, burning pain, and the intensity of pain increases with passive stretching. Later, paresthesia, sensory deficits, and focal motor deficits may develop. After necrosis develops, the pain may regress in the later period. One of the early findings in the examination is that the muscle in the affected compartment is painful with passive stretching. The affected compartment is tense, hard, and edema may be observed. There may also be a decreased pulse or capillary filling. Decreased sensation, muscle weakness, and paralysis are late findings. Compartment pressure measurement is an important diagnostic procedure in the diagnosis of compartment syndrome. This may not be possible in hospitals where there is not enough equipment. However, fasciotomy can be planned based on the patient's history and physical examination without measuring pressure. Although acute compartment syndrome is a diagnosis made by clinical findings and measurement of compartment pressure, conditions such as creatine kinase (CK) increase and myoglobinuria may develop since it is a process with muscle destruction. However, surgical consultation should not be delayed in the suspected patient to wait for laboratory results. If creatine phosphokinase is >1,000 U/mL, Compartment syndrome may develop. Things that may cause external pressure such as splints, plasters, and bandages should be removed. The affected extremity should be kept at the level of the heart to prevent the decrease of arterial flow. Analgesia should be well provided. Hypotension should be avoided as it will cause a decrease in perfusion, and if necessary, a bolus of fluid should be given. Definitive treatment is fasciotomy. A single pressure measurement can cause an unnecessary fasciotomy with a 35% false positive 20; a delay in fasciotomy can cause amputation and increase morbidity. Continuous pressure monitoring for at least 2 hours and frequent evaluation are recommended for the patient who cannot be examined and a reliable anamnesis cannot be obtained.

Question 4

A 35-year-old man sustained blunt trauma to hip by lateral collision. His blood pressure (BP) at arrival is 70 mm Hg. He has no other obvious injury. You are strongly suspected pelvic fracture.

1. How will you examine this patient with regard to suspected pelvic fracture?

On physical examination and inspection of pelvic area hematoma, dermabrasion, limb inequality, abnormal pelvic internal or external; the presence of rotation deformity is investigated. The presence of blood at the outlets of the urethral meatus, vagina, or rectum points to the possibility of concomitant injuries in these areas. Tenderness with palpation and crepitation is sought; rotational instability with gentle internal and external rotation movements by grasping the iliac wings; vertical instability is investigated with careful push-pull maneuvers by holding the leg. All these challenging maneuvers should be performed once and carefully to avoid disrupting the pelvic hematoma and causing new bleeding. A rectal and vaginal digital examination should be performed with every female patient to avoid missing any latent open fractures or accompanying injuries. In men, high prostate on rectal examination and blood in the urinary meatus suggest urethral injury, while vaginal or rectal tears due to incision of bone fragments can lead to open fractures with very high mortality. It is characterized by the separation of the skin-subcutaneous tissue from the underlying fascia by shearing forces on examination; Morel—Lavallée lesions, which are encountered with high infection rates, should not be missed.

2. How do you classify of pelvic fractures?

According to the Tile classification, pelvis fractures are classified as **Type A, Type B, and Type C**. Type A fractures are also divided into two subgroups. A1 fractures are those that do not involve the pelvic ring, such as spinals or ischial tuberosity fractures. A2 fractures are minimal displacement fractures caused by low-energy trauma.

Type B1 fractures result from anterior-posterior (AP) compression and opening of the anterior pelvis with symphysis diastasis or ramus fracture. The posterior sacroiliac and interosseous ligaments are intact. In type B1.1, diastasis is <2.5 cm and the sacrospinous ligament is intact. In B1.2 type, diastasis is >2.5 cm and the sacrospinous ligament and anterior sacroiliac ligament are torn. Type B2.1 fractures are ipsilateral anterior and posterior pelvic ring fractures with lateral compression. Type B2.2 fractures are "bucket handle type" fractures with contralateral anterior and posterior lesions. B3 fractures are fractures formed by bilateral and AP compression.

Type C fractures are unstable in all planes. These are vertical shear fractures and AP compression type fractures in which all ligaments are severed. Type C1 fractures are unilateral, C2 group is vertically unstable on one side and rotationally unstable bilaterally on the other side, C3 fractures are bilateral vertically unstable fractures.

3. How will you investigate this patient for pelvic fracture?

In the evaluation of pelvic fractures, "inlet and outlet" radiographs described by Pennal et al. should be taken in addition to AP radiographs. While rotational deformities, openings in the sacroiliac joint and symphysis, and displacement in the AP plane are better observed in the "inlet" graphy, in which the X-ray tube is directed 40° caudally; on the other hand, sacrum pathologies, vertical displacement, and anterior pelvis pathologies can be seen in the "outlet" radiograph taken at 40° cephalad. Computed tomography is especially valuable in investigating posterior injuries that cannot be recognized by direct radiography, evaluating the spinal canal and foramen, recognizing low-grade AP, and rotational displacements, and examining whether fractures extend into the acetabulum.

4. After taking care of ABCD, how will you manage this patient in the emergency department if he is found to have a pelvic fracture?

In the emergency treatment of hemodynamically unstable patients, application of pelvic bandage helps to control bleeding by narrowing the pelvic volume and providing temporary stability, especially in AP compression type fractures. It has problems such as causing pressure sores in long-term use and making it difficult to approach the patient. In some countries, especially during the transportation of patients, the pneumatic antishock trousers have disadvantages such as preventing the approach to the abdomen and lower extremities, disrupting the circulation of the leg in some cases and causing compartment syndrome after a while. External fixators, which are accepted as the gold standard in acute management, provide fracture stabilization and clot formation. They can control most low-pressure hemorrhages, as they facilitate and also narrow the pelvic volume. With this approach, the patient, it has been reported that, while early mobilization is provided, many complications, especially pulmonary and thromboembolic are reduced. In the emergency approach to the bleeding patient, when the external fixation or posterior stabilization Ganz clamp and C clamp are insufficient, or in the treatment of major arterial hemorrhages, angiography and selective embolization are life-saving when the necessary conditions are quickly met.

Question 5

1. Enumerate the emergencies in the first 20 weeks of pregnancy.

Complete abortion, incomplete abortion, missed abortion, vaginal bleeding, ectopic pregnancy, urinary infection, gestational trophoblastic disease, emesis, and hyperemesis gravidarum.

2. Discuss pathophysiology of ectopic pregnancy.

Normally, fertilization takes place in the fallopian tubes. The fertilized egg travels through the fallopian tube to the uterus and is embedded in the uterus to develop. If there is a problem that prevents the fertilized egg from passing through the fallopian tubes (occlusion), it is buried in the fallopian tube (95–99%), peritoneal cavity or cervix instead of the uterus. These regions are not regions where the embryo can complete its development. Embryo located in the fallopian tube begins to grow. The wall of the fallopian tubes cannot withstand the destruction and pressure and ruptures. The most important causes of obstruction in the tubes and inability of implantation in uterus are severe pelvic inflammatory disease, previous tubal surgeries and interventions, endometriosis, intrauterine devices, and tubal ligation. An ectopic pregnancy rupture can cause life-threatening bleeding.

3. Explain the diagnosis of ectopic pregnancy.

Especially with the use of beta-human chorionic gonadotropin (β-hCG) and transvaginal ultrasonography, the diagnosis of ectopic pregnancy can be made easily and without delay. Abdominal tenderness, inguinal pain, adnexal mass, uterine enlargement, rupture and peritoneal irritation findings depending on the extent of bleeding, tachycardia, tachypnea and orthostatic changes may occur. β-hCG is absolutely positive in cases of ectopic pregnancy. In a normal pregnancy, β-hCG is measured every 36–48 hours, and this regular increase is not observed in an ectopic pregnancy. Apart from this, values such as serum progesterone, CK, relaxin, prorenin can also be checked. The gold standard in the diagnosis of ectopic pregnancy is the detection of an ectopic pregnancy focus in laparoscopy.

4. Write the management of a patient with ectopic pregnancy.

The aim of the treatment of ectopic pregnancy is to correct the existing pathology, and to ensure that the fertility of the patient is not damaged if there is a demand for fertilization. The treatment is planned surgically or medically according to the rupture of the ectopic pregnancy focus, the condition of the intact tuba, and the patient's desire for fertilization. Methotrexate is used in medical treatment. Generally, medical treatment can be applied in cases of ectopic pregnancy that has not ruptured, the gestational sac is <4 cm, and there is no fetal heart movement. The treatment dose is 50 mg/m^2 or 1 mg/kg for methotrexate. Laparoscopy and laparotomy can be applied in surgical treatment. Linear salpingostomy, partial salpingectomy, tubal milking can be performed with laparoscopy. Laparotomy in ectopic pregnancy is preferred because of severe bleeding, insufficient visualization of the adnexa during laparoscopy, or ectopic pregnancy in abdominal, interstitial, or cornual ovarian localization.

Question 6

1. Enumerate various cold injuries.

Systemic and local cold injuries are systemic hypothermia, frostbite, frostnip, trench (immersion) foot, chilblain (perniones).

2. Enumerate the risk factors precipitating frostbite.

Frostbite is common in soldiers and mountaineers. Precipitating factors are homelessness, psychiatric illnesses, alcohol and drug use, multisystem trauma, and fatigue.

3. How do you classify frostbite injuries?

Frostbite are classified into four categories:
1. In first-degree frostbite, centrally located white plaque with loss of sensation and erythema are seen around it.
2. Second-degree erythema and edema as well as bullae are seen. These bullae fill with a serous or milky fluid within the first 24 hours.
3. Third-degree hemorrhagic bullae are seen, which, after a 2-week period, lead to the development of a hard black eschar tissue.
4. It is associated with fourth degree total necrosis and tissue loss.

4. How do you manage victims of frostbite in emergency department?

First of all, treat hypothermia. The tissue is rapidly heated in circulating water at 40°–42°C until it softens/starts to stretch or becomes erythematous. Clear bullae are debrided (controversial), hemorrhagic bullae are aspirated (to prevent extra edema increase). Renew tetanus immunoprophylaxis. Pain management—initially parenteral opiates followed by oral non-steroidal anti-inflammatory drugs (NSAIDs), (the purpose of NSAIDs is not only analgesia, but also arachidonic acid and stops the prostaglandin production cascade). Wound care, dressing, limb splint and elevation; apply topical aloe vera every 6 hours. After superficial frostbite, the patient can be discharged with a close doctor. In deep injuries, the patient is hospitalized. Use of oral antibiotic, topical antibiotic ointment, and silver sulfadiazine is controversial.

Question 7

1. What are the causes of otalgia?

Pain caused by the disease of the ear itself is called otodynia, pain originating from another organ in the head and neck is called referred otalgia—reflected ear pain. External ear tract infections (otitis externa) and otitis media are the most common local causes of ear pain. Any inflammatory, traumatic or tumoral disease in the regions innervated by trigeminal nerve, facial nerve, nervus facialis, glossopharyngeal nerve, vagus nerve, and C2 or C3 nerves may cause referred otalgia in the same ear.

2. Discuss pathophysiology and microbiology of otitis media.

Otitis media are an infection and inflammation of the air spaces of the middle ear and temporal bone, and of the mucosa lining the Eustachian. Otitis media begins following viral infection of the nasopharynx, nasal mucosa, Eustachian tube, and upper airway. Inflammation, increased edema, and secretions cause obstruction in the narrowest part of the esophagus and prevent aeration. Bacterial colonization and suppuration then take place in this region. Although mostly viral agents play a role in its emergence (especially through viral upper respiratory tract infections), otitis media are generally bacterial diseases. Bacteria accompanying the event may be present in the upper respiratory tract flora or may have come from outside this region. There is a different bacteriological profile specific to each clinical picture. Knowing these will guide us in empirical antibiotic therapy. *Streptococcus pneumoniae*, *Haemophilus influenza*, and *Moraxella catarrhalis* constitute the majority of microorganisms in the etiology of acute otitis media. In a significant part of the middle ear aspirates, no growth can be detected.

3. Explain the complications of otitis media.

In general, otitis media may present with some complications depending on the virulence of the pathogen, host resistance, stage of the disease and whether there are additional diseases.

Intratemporal: Tympanic membrane perforation, acute coalescent mastoiditis, facial nerve palsy, acute labyrinthitis, petrositis, acute necrotic otitis, chronic otitis media.

Intracranial: Meningitis, encephalitis, brain abscess, otitis hydrocephalus, subarachnoid abscess, subdural abscess, sigmoid sinus thrombosis.

Systemic: Bacteremia, septic arthritis, bacterial endocarditis.

4. Discuss emergency department treatments of otitis media.

Antibiotic treatment and treatment for otalgia are applied. Nonsteroidal anti-inflammatories and paracetamol are preferred as analgesics. The use of antibiotics in early otitis media is controversial. Antibiotic treatment is definitely given in suppurative otitis media. High-dose amoxicillin or second-generation cephalosporins are the first choices. For patients who do not benefit from high-dose amoxicillin therapy, treatment is changed to amoxicillin-clavulanic acid (90 mg/kg amoxicillin, 6.4 mg/kg clavulanic acid in two doses). In patients with tympanic membrane rupture, topical antibiotics used in the middle ear containing ofloxacin are preferred rather than systemic antibiotics. Treatment should be continued for 10–15 days. If there is a history of penicillin allergy, azithromycin (10 mg/kg single dose) or clarithromycin (15 mg/kg divided two doses) can be used.

Question 8

1. Enumerate the causes of acute pain in the right lower quadrant of abdomen.

Appendicitis, intestinal obstruction, diverticulitis, cholecystitis, perforated ulcer, rectus hematoma, ectopic pregnancy, ovarian cyst or torsion, salpingitis, mittelschmerz, endometriosis, ureteral stone, renal colic, seminal vesiculitis, psoas abscess, inguinal hernia.

2. Discuss the clinical features of acute appendicitis.

Typical symptoms of acute appendicitis are anorexia and epigastric or periumbilical pain followed by right lower quadrant pain, nausea, and vomiting. It may also be accompanied by symptoms such as fever, constipation or diarrhea, dysuria, pyuria, and hematuria.

3. Discuss Alvarado score for acute appendicitis.

Following are the signs/symptoms in Alvarado score (**Table 1**):

TABLE 1: Alvarado score.

Sign/Symptom	Score
Migration of pain	1
Anorexia	1
Nausea	1
Tenderness of right lower quadrant	2
Rebound pain	1
High body temperature	1
Leukocytosis	2
Shift of white blood cell count to left	1
Total	10

Score <4: Acute appendicitis unlikely
Score 5–6: Possible acute appendicitis
Score 7–8: Likely acute appendicitis
Score 9–10: Highly likely acute appendicitis

4. Write briefly about the role of ultrasound in diagnosis of acute appendicitis.

Ultrasonography (USG) in the diagnosis of acute appendicitis is a preferred imaging method especially for young adult women because it does not have the risk of ionizing radiation, can be applied at the bedside, and is reproducible. If it is done by an experienced practitioner in thin people with thin adipose tissue, an easy diagnosis is made with USG. The main findings are that the outer diameter of the appendix is >6 mm, the lumen cannot be compressed with the probe, the target mark, fecalitis in the appendix lumen, periappendicular fluid, and the appendix wall is >3 mm.

Question 9

A 20-year-old adult man was hit by a cricket ball and sustained blunt trauma to right eye while playing. He presented to an emergency department with severe pain in the eye.

1. What are the possible ocular injuries sustained?

Periorbital bone fractures, traumatic lens injury, corneal abrasion, globe perforation, retrobulbar hemorrhage, retinal detachment, carotid cavernous fistula, optic nerve injury, choroidal rupture, preretinal hemorrhage, vitreous hemorrhage, commotio retina.

2. How will you evaluate this case?

First of all, the patient's periorbital region is reviewed for gross pathology. Injury of the eyelid, periorbital ecchymosis and hematomas, tenderness and crepitation in the periorbital bone tissue are evaluated. Corneal abrasions, foreign body in the cornea are evaluated. If necessary, wash with sterile saline. Vision should be measured and recorded. If there is pain, local anesthetic "Alcain" should be dripped. Visual field should be evaluated with the confrontation method. Comparative size and responses of the pupil (direct-indirect and "Marcus–Gunn response") should be evaluated. Eye movements should be evaluated. In addition, consultation from an ophthalmologist should be requested and detailed ophthalmologic examination should be provided. It should be evaluated by the ophthalmologist with anterior segment (biomicroscopy) and posterior segment (fundoscopy) and intraocular pressure (IOP) should be measured.

3. Evaluate ruptured eye globe.

First of all, the patient's airway should be opened; his breathing and circulation should be controlled and stabilized. A complete physical examination should be performed for other accompanying systemic injuries. Patients will often have decreased visual acuity, and this can be assessed using a Snellen chart or near card. In patients with severe visual impairment, acuity evaluation is by the patient's ability to count fingers, see a moving hand, or flashes of light. Inspection of the eye using a slit lamp enhances the ability to detect penetrating foreign bodies, scleral or corneal lacerations, uveal prolapse, or iris abnormalities such as peaked or "tear-drop" pupil. A Seidel sign may also be present when performing fluorescein staining of the cornea and sclera as a stream of clear aqueous fluid originating from the globe wound site, although the globe can be open even if this sign is negative. Seidel testing is contraindicated in cases of obvious globe rupture. A maxillofacial computed tomography scan can aid in the management of globe rupture, although it should never replace an ophthalmic evaluation. Magnetic resonance imaging of the globe is contraindicated because of the possibility of foreign body.

4. Discuss management of ruptured eye globe.

The treatment of other injuries that threaten the patient's life is a priority. In the meantime, emergency ophthalmology consultation is requested for the patient with suspected glob. Oral intake of the patient is discontinued. Tetanus prophylaxis, if necessary, antiemetic and analgesic treatment is applied. All applications that increase intraocular pressure should be avoided. Foreign bodies in the eye should not be tried to be removed until they go to the operating room. The patient's eyeball should be closed and protected using a sterile Fox shield, cup, or another protective device. The head is elevated 30° to reduce intraocular pressure.

Question 10

A 55-year-old diabetic patient presents with redness and swelling in right leg for two days.

1. Enumerate the possible causes.

Cellulitis, deep vein thrombose, lymphangitis, soft tissue abscess, thrombophlebitis, Baker's cyst and rupture, intra-knee pathologies, muscle ruptures, trauma.

2. What is role of ultrasound in this patient?

Doppler USG is an important imaging method in investigating vascular and nonvascular causes of lower extremity swelling. It is the most preferred radiological diagnosis method because it is inexpensive, can be applied at the bedside, is noninvasive, does not require contrast material, and does not carry the risk of ionizing radiation. Deep vein thrombosis (DVT) can be diagnosed with venous Doppler USG with high sensitivity (95%) and specificity (100%). In patients with DVT, the presence of thrombus in the venous lumen on USG, the inability to compress the lumen when pressed with a probe, and the absence of colored flow of venous filling make the diagnosis. Diffuse soft tissue edema can be detected in patients with acute cellulitis. In addition, traumatic lesions, septic arthritis, Baker's cyst rupture, muscle contusion, and hematomas, abscesses can also be detected by USG.

3. Explain the clinical features of any two causes.

In DVT, the patient has complaints of swelling, redness, and pain in the leg. Physical examination findings are not always clear in DVT. The most common physical examination findings are leg redness, swelling, Homans sign (pain when the foot is dorsiflexed) and a positive Pratt test (pain with calf squeezing and patting). These findings are detected after a completely obstructing DVT. It is difficult to diagnose clinically, especially since the majority of DVT that occurs after arthroplasty is not completely obstructed. Only 1% of all DVT cases are clinically manifested.

Cellulitis progresses with increased temperature in the related soft tissue, edema, redness, tenderness, pain, irritation, itching, sometimes blister formation on the lesion and systemic fever.

4. Discuss management of such patients in emergency department.

First of all, the differential diagnosis of diseases such as DVT and cellulitis with life-threatening complications such as pulmonary embolism or sepsis that may cause swelling and redness in the leg should be made. For this, whole blood examination, D-dimer, infection markers, biochemical tests, venous Doppler USG should be requested. Anticoagulant prophylaxis should be initiated to prevent pulmonary embolism in patients with suspected acute DVT. For this, low molecular weight heparin, heparin or oral anticoagulants are used. Thus, the growth of the thrombus is also prevented. Thrombolytic therapy can be given for recanalization of the thrombosed vessel. Vena cava filters are another method for the prevention of pulmonary embolism. In the treatment of cellulite, elevation of the extremity should be performed. Predisposing factors should be controlled. The most common agents for cellulitis are *Staphylococcus aureus* and *Group A beta hemolytic streptococci*. Antibiotic treatment should be planned for these factors.

SUGGESTED READING

1. Richhariya D, Sharma B. Textbook of Emergency Medicine including Intensive Care and Trauma, 2nd edition. New Delhi: Jaypee Brothers Medical Publishers (P) Ltd; 2022. pp. 1616-35. (Question 1).
2. Richhariya D, Sharma B. Textbook of Emergency Medicine including Intensive Care and Trauma, 2nd edition. New Delhi: Jaypee Brothers Medical Publishers (P) Ltd; 2022. pp. 1615-20. (Question 2).
3. Richhariya D, Sharma B. Textbook of Emergency Medicine including Intensive Care and Trauma, 2nd edition. New Delhi: Jaypee Brothers Medical Publishers (P) Ltd; 2022. p. 1673. (Question 3).
4. Richhariya D, Sharma B. Textbook of Emergency Medicine including Intensive Care and Trauma, 2nd edition. New Delhi: Jaypee Brothers Medical Publishers (P) Ltd; 2022. p. 1635. (Question 4).
5. Richhariya D, Sharma B. Textbook of Emergency Medicine including Intensive Care and Trauma, 2nd edition. New Delhi: Jaypee Brothers Medical Publishers (P) Ltd; 2022. pp. 1072-7. (Question 5).
6. Richhariya D, Sharma B. Textbook of Emergency Medicine including Intensive Care and Trauma, 2nd edition. New Delhi: Jaypee Brothers Medical Publishers (P) Ltd; 2022. pp. 1686-91. (Question 6).
7. Richhariya D, Sharma B. Textbook of Emergency Medicine including Intensive Care and Trauma, 2nd edition. New Delhi: Jaypee Brothers Medical Publishers (P) Ltd; 2022. pp. 908-14. (Question 7).
8. Richhariya D, Sharma B. Textbook of Emergency Medicine including Intensive Care and Trauma, 2nd edition. New Delhi: Jaypee Brothers Medical Publishers (P) Ltd; 2022. pp. 699-704. (Question 8).
9. Richhariya D, Sharma B. Textbook of Emergency Medicine including Intensive Care and Trauma, 2nd edition. New Delhi: Jaypee Brothers Medical Publishers (P) Ltd; 2022. pp. 899-902. (Question 9).
10. Richhariya D, Sharma B. Textbook of Emergency Medicine including Intensive Care and Trauma, 2nd edition. New Delhi: Jaypee Brothers Medical Publishers (P) Ltd; 2022. p. 537. (Question 10).

Emergency Medicine Paper 15

Shweta Ashok

Question 1

A 22-year-old male presented with fever and jaundice of 5 days duration. Clinical examination shows moderate jaundice and splenic enlargement.

1. Enumerate differential diagnosis of fever with jaundice.

Following is the list of differential diagnosis for fever with jaundice (**Table 1**):

TABLE 1: Differential diagnosis for fever with jaundice.

Hepatic and biliary causes	• Acute cholangitis, acute cholecystitis • Acute pancreatitis • Primary sclerosing jaundice
Infections	• Malaria (*Plasmodium falciparum*), viral Hepatitis—B, C, D • Leptospirosis, dengue, yellow fever, brucellosis, rickettsia, cytomegalovirus, tuberculosis, Epstein–Barr virus, amebic liver disease
Neoplasms	Hodgkin's lymphoma, chronic myeloid leukemia myelofibrosis
Inflammation	Septic thrombophlebitis
Hemolytic	Sickle cell crisis, hemolytic uremic syndrome

2. What are the various forms of complicated malaria?

Malaria is described as severe or complicated when it includes one or more of the following features along with the presence of asexual forms of *Plasmodium falciparum* in peripheral smear (**Table 2**).

TABLE 2: Criteria for severe and complicated malaria.

Complication	Definition
Cerebral malaria	Impaired consciousness, unarousable coma
Repeated generalized convulsions	Two convulsions within 24 hours
Severe anemia	Hb <5 g/dL
Renal failure	Serum creatinine >3 g/dL, oliguria

Contd...

Contd...

Complication	Definition
Respiratory distress	• Acidotic breathing, pulmonary edema • Acute respiratory distress syndrome
Hypoglycemia	Blood glucose <40 mg/dL
Circulatory collapse or shock	Systolic blood pressure <90 mm Hg, rapid thready pulse
Disseminated intravascular coagulopathy (DIC)	Bleeding from different sites of body
Acidosis	Blood pH <7.25
Black water fever	Macroscopic hemoglobinuria (cola-colored urine)
Jaundice	Bilirubin >3 mg/dL
Hyperparasitemia	>5% of erythrocytes infested by parasites

3. How will you confirm your diagnosis of malaria?

Diagnosis is based on:
a. History of potential exposure in a malarious area.
b. Clinical symptoms
c. Microscopic examination—thick and thin blood films.
d. Immunodiagnosis
e. Additional laboratory studies.

Microscopic Examinations

Thin blood film:
a. A standard hematologic blood smear (fixed with methanol and stained with Giemsa) allows a single sheet of intact red cells to be scrutinized for the percentage of red cells parasitized, from which the number of parasites per microliter can be calculated.
b. A thin film identifies the morphology of both parasites (especially species of *Plasmodium*) as well as the red blood cells, since the red cells are not destroyed.
c. Thin films are useful for counting very heavy infections.

Thick blood film **(Figs. 1A to D):**
a. Place a small drop of blood (5 µL) on a microscope slide, spread it evenly to a diameter of approximately 1 cm, allow it to dry and then stain without initial fixation, with Field's or Giemsa stain.
b. Record the result as the number of parasites seen per oil-immersion field or per 200 white cell nuclei counted.
c. A thick blood film contains several layers of red cells, lysed by staining procedure, allowing parasitism's down to 40/µL to be detected under microscope.

Quantitative buffy coat (QBC) test: A QBC is a quick and direct test to make the identification of malaria **(Fig. 2)**.
a. Highly sensitive test for malarial parasite.
b. It is based on acridine-orange staining of blood samples from peripheral circulation centrifuged in micro-hematocrit tubes (QBC) and the examination under ultraviolet lighting source (fluorescence microscope).
c. It can easily detect low levels of parasitemia (two parasites/mL).

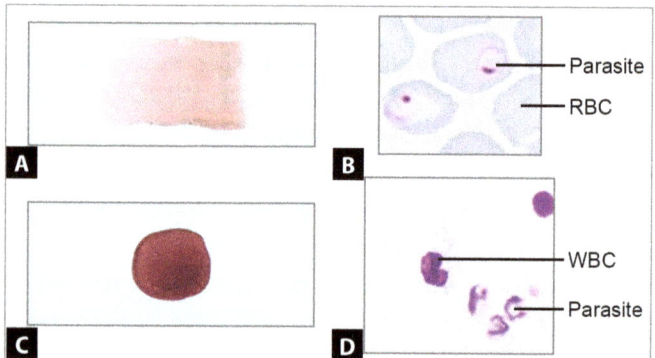

Figs. 1A to D: (A) Thin blood film; (C) thick blood film; (B) and (D) blood smear showing *Plasmodium falciparum* parasites infecting some of the patient's red blood cells (RBC). (WBC: white blood cells)

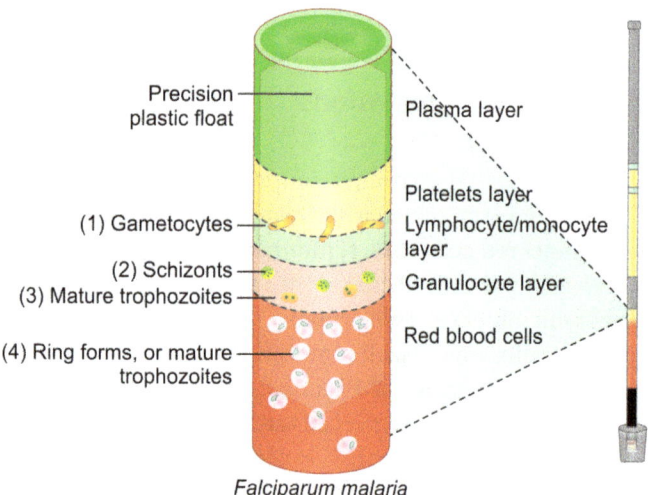

Falciparum malaria
Fig. 2: Falciparum malaria in quantitative buffy coat.

Rapid diagnostic test (RDT): A RDT is an alternate way of quickly establishing the diagnosis of malaria infection by detecting specific malaria antigens in a person's blood.

Immunodiagnosis: Malarial antibodies can be detected by serological techniques such as immunofluorescent assay (IFA) or enzyme-linked immunosorbent assay (ELISA).

The IFA procedure can be used to determine if a patient has been infected with *Plasmodium*.
- Because of the time required for development of antibody and also the persistence of antibodies, serologic testing is not practical for outline diagnosis of acute malaria.

ELISA also has been used as a tool to screen blood donors, but have a limited sensitivity due to use of only *Plasmodium falciparum* antigen instead of antigens of all four human species.

Additional laboratory test:
a. Polymerase chain reaction (PCR) testing for parasite messenger ribonucleic acid (RNA) or deoxyribonucleic acid (DNA).
b. Normochromic normocytic anemia, thrombocytopenia and raised erythrocyte sedimentation rate (ESR).
c. Total leukocyte count is low to normal, but neutrophil leukocytosis may be seen in several infections.
d. Plasma viscosity and C-reactive protein levels are high.
e. Prothrombin time (PT) and partial thromboplastin time may be prolonged in severe infections. Antithrombin III levels are reduced.
f. In complicated malaria, there may be metabolic acidosis and low plasma concentrations of glucose, sodium, bicarbonate, calcium, magnesium, and albumin. Lactate, blood urea nitrogen (BUN), creatinine, muscle and liver enzymes, bilirubin and gamma globulin levels may be elevated.
g. Neuroimaging in patients with cerebral malaria may demonstrate brain swelling, cortical infarcts, and hyperintense areas in white matter.

4. Discuss the emergency department management of the present case if he was found to have malaria.

Patients should be admitted to an appropriate level of intensive care. Both supportive and specific antimalarial therapies are crucial for the patient's survival.

Supportive management:
a. Initial resuscitation may require oxygen for hypoxia.
b. Fluid replacement
c. Intravenous (IV) glucose for hypoglycemia.
d. Blood or platelet transfusion for severe anemia or for disseminated intravascular coagulation

e. Intubation for severe respiratory distress or suspected raised intracranial pressure with altered mental status.
f. Monitor to identify and treat seizures, hyperpyrexia, acute respiratory distress syndrome (ARDS), or acute renal failure.
g. Culture blood samples for bacterial infections, and give immediate parenteral antibiotics.

Specific antimalarial chemotherapy:
a. Initiate parenteral therapy with an efficacious antimalarial drug without delay.
b. Artesunate is considered the drug of choice for severe malaria by the World Health Organization. Dose—2.4 mg/kg IV at 0, 8, and 24 hours, then daily. Artesunate can be given intramuscular (IM) if necessary.
c. Quinidine gluconate —6.25 mg base (= 10 mg salt)/kg IV load over 2 hours, follow with 0.0125 mg base (= 0.02 milligram salt)/kg/min continuous infusion.
d. Quinidine is given along with doxycycline or clindamycin.
e. Doxycycline—2.2 mg/kg IV (up to adult dose of 100 mg) every 12 hours for 7 days.
f. In children under age 8 years, clindamycin 10 mg base/kg loading dose IV followed by 5 mg base/kg IV every 8 hours for 7 days.
g. Quinine dihydrochloride is an alternative to quinidine gluconate. Dose—20 mg (salt)/kg infused IV over 2-4 hours, then 10 mg/kg every 8 hours, can be given IM if necessary, as 50 mg/mL solution.
h. An unstable patient with a clinical or travel history suggesting malaria should be started on artesunate or quinidine gluconate until diagnosis of malaria can be ruled out.

Special considerations
Pregnancy: Artemisinin drugs are safe during the second and third trimester of pregnancy.
a. Quinidine and quinine can be used in pregnancy but carry a greater risk of causing hypoglycemia through stimulation of insulin secretion from hypertrophied pancreatic beta cells.

Question 2

1. Define hypoglycemia.

Hypoglycemia is more often a complication of diabetic mellitus management (either in oral form or insulin therapy). It is clinically defined as:
a. Symptoms consistent with the diagnosis.
b. Symptoms associated with a low glucose level (generally, plasma glucose concentration of ≤70 mg/dL or 3.9 mmol/L)
c. Symptoms resolve with glucose administration.

2. Enumerate the causes for hypoglycemia.

Hypoglycemia is very common among patients using insulin therapy and some long-acting sulfonylureas such as chlorpropamide, glyburide (glibenclamide), and glipizide. It is rarely encountered in patients using metformin. Some risk factors for severe hypoglycemia in type 2 diabetes mellitus (T2DM) patients include—age, past history of vascular disease, renal failure, decreased food intake, alcohol consumption, and drug interactions. In nondiabetics, consider critical illness like sepsis or liver failure, adverse effects of drugs and alcohol, factitious hypoglycemia, tumors such as insulinoma or nonislet cell, and hormone deficiencies like adrenal insufficiency or hypopituitarism **(Table 3)**.

TABLE 3: Causes of hypoglycemia.

Hypoglycemia in diabetic patients	Hypoglycemia in nondiabetic patients
• Elderly age group	• Critical illness like sepsis or liver failure
• Past history of vascular disease	• Adverse effects of drugs and alcohol
• Renal failure	• Factitious hypoglycemia
• Decreased food intake	• Tumors such as insulinoma or non-islet cell
• Alcohol consumption	• Hormone deficiencies such as adrenal insufficiency or hypopituitarism
• Drug interactions	

3. Discuss the clinical features of hypoglycemia.

The clinical features of hypoglycemia are divided into two broad categories—neuroglycopenic and autonomic **(Table 4)**.

TABLE 4: Common clinical features of hypoglycemia.

Neuroglycopenic manifestations	Autonomic manifestations	
	(i) *Adrenergic symptoms:*	(ii) *Cholinergic symptoms:*
• Alteration in consciousness	• Anxiety	• Sweating
• Lethargy	• Nervousness and Irritability	• Hunger
• Confusion		• Paresthesia
• Combativeness	• Nausea/vomiting	
• Agitation	• Palpitations	
• Seizures	• Tremors	
• Focal neurologic deficits		

4. How do you manage sulfonylurea-induced hypoglycemia?

Management of hypoglycemia in emergency department or a prehospital setup, includes prompt diagnosis and per oral (PO) or IV administration of rapidly metabolized carbohydrates (glucose or dextrose).
a. In patients with altered mental status, 50% dextrose in water is administered IV as a bolus dose of 50 mL, which provides 25 g of glucose.
b. After 15 minutes, if hypoglycemia persists, repeat the dose.

c. If the patient regains consciousness, and blood sugar is >70 mg/dL, continue carbohydrates (PO administration of long-acting carbohydrates) to prevent recurrence.
d. If the blood sugars have normalized but the patient is still unconscious or drowsy, continue IV infusion of dextrose (5% dextrose in water), to maintain capillary blood glucose (CBG) >100 mg/dL.
e. Check CBG every 30 minutes for the first 2 hours, looking for rebound hypoglycemia.
f. Infusion can be reduced or eventually withdrawn, if hypoglycemia is maintained by slow administration of dextrose.

For sulfonylurea-induced hypoglycemia, *octreotide is the treatment of choice.*

Octreotide:
a. Octreotide, a somatostatin analog and is able to suppress insulin secretion immediately and negates the effects of the sulfonylurea.
b. *Dose:* 50–100 µg, subcutaneous for a single episode. If recurrent episodes—50–100 µg subcutaneous once every 6–8 hours or constant infusion of 125 µg/h.
c. Octreotide is given after the initial glucose therapy is inadequate. It is primarily given to reduce the risk of recurrent hypoglycemia.

Diazoxide:
a. Also used in treatment of refractory sulfonylurea-induced hypoglycemia.
b. *Mechanism of action (MOA):* Acts directly by inhibiting insulin secretion from pancreatic β cells.
c. *Dose:* 300 mg over 30 minutes every 4 hours as a slow IV infusion.
d. May cause hypotension.

Question 3

1. Enumerate various diving-related emergencies.

Injuries related to diving are classified into **(Table 5)**:

TABLE 5: Diving-related injuries.	
Barotrauma of descent	• Otic barotrauma or ear squeeze (barotitis) • Inner and external ear barotrauma (external squeeze) • Sinus barotrauma or sinus squeeze • Facial barotrauma or mask squeeze
Barotrauma of ascent	• Alternobaric vertigo • Pulmonary barotrauma or pulmonary over inflation syndromes • Arterial gas embolism • Decompression sickness
Injuries related to prolonged exposure to depths	Nitrogen narcosis or rapture of the deep

a. Injuries associated with descent
b. Injuries associated with ascent
c. Injuries related to prolonged exposure to significant depths.

2. Discuss the pathophysiology of decompression sickness.

Decompression sickness may occur in divers breathing compressed air, caisson workers, high altitude pilots or astronauts. The pathophysiology is related to obstructive and inflammatory effects of inert gas bubbles in tissues and the vascular system. As the diver descends, there is an ambient pressure rise and nitrogen gas dissolves in the body's tissues. During a rapid onset, falling ambient pressures lead to formation of nitrogen bubbles as the gas expands and comes out of solution. Bubbles obstruct blood flow leading to direct ischemia. Air blood and air endothelial interfaces initiate a variety of inflammatory and thrombotic processes which activate the endothelium leading to neutrophil adhesions and activation, changing the permeability of the endothelium causing third spacing of fluid.

3. Explain the classification of decompression sickness.

Decompression sickness (DCS) is commonly classified into three types:
1. Type I or pain—only DCS
2. Type II or serious type DCS
3. Type III or combination of DCS and arterial embolism.

Type I DCS, also called **"Pain-only"** sickness, involves the joints, extremities and skin (**"cutis marmorata"**). Lymphatic obstruction can occur, causing lymphedema, which usually takes days to resolve despite recompression therapy.

Type II DCS involves the central nervous system (CNS), mainly the spinal cord in compressed air divers and the brain in high-altitude decompressions, vestibular symptoms (**"staggers"**), and the cardiopulmonary symptoms (**"chokes"**).

Type III DCS, also known as **decompression illness**, occurs when an arterial gas embolism causes inert gas to come out of solution after a dive profile.

4. Discuss the clinical features of DCS.

The onset of DCS may usually occur within minutes to several hours after surfacing. Rarely, symptoms may take up to days after diving **(Table 6)**.

TABLE 6: Clinical features of decompression sickness (DCS).

Classification	DCS Type I (Pain—only)	DCS Type II (Serious DCS)	DCS Type III (Decompression illness)
Clinical features	• Deep pain in joints and extremities, usually single joint, commonly knees and shoulders • Lymphedema • Skin changes—mottling, pruritus, color changes	• *Central nervous system:* Sensation of truncal constriction, ascending paralysis • *Vestibular symptoms (staggers):* Vertigo, tinnitus, disequilibrium • *Cardiopulmonary (chokes):* Cough, hemoptysis, dyspnea, substernal chest pain, cardiovascular collapse	• Combination of type II DCS along with arterial gas embolism • Symptoms of DCS type II + variety of stroke syndromes—loss of consciousness, seizures, blindness, disorientation, hemiplegia

Question 4

1. Enumerate the causes for ARDS.

Acute respiratory distress syndrome can result from indirect, extrapulmonary or direct pulmonary lung injury. The most common risk factors are sepsis, pneumonia, aspiration pneumonitis, trauma, acute lung injury (TRALI), inhalational injuries or burns **(Fig. 3)**.

2. What are Berlin diagnostic criteria for ARDS?

Acute respiratory distress syndrome is an acute form of diffuse lung injury occurring in patients with predisposing risk factors. ARDS can be diagnosed once cardiogenic pulmonary edema and alternative causes of acute hypoxemic respiratory failure and bilateral infiltrates have been excluded. Berlin's diagnostic criteria define the patient to have ARDS, if he meets all of the following criteria—onset within 1 week of a known clinical insult or new/worsening respiratory symptoms.

Presence of bilateral opacities on chest radiograph or CT scan. These opacities are not fully explained by pleural effusion, lobar collapse, lung collapse, or pulmonary nodules.

Patient's respiratory failure is not explained by cardiac failure or fluid overload.

Presence of hypoxemia: A moderate-to-severe impairment of oxygenation must be present, as defined by the ratio of arterial oxygen tension to fraction of inspired oxygen (PaO_2/FiO_2). The severity of the hypoxemia defines the severity of the ARDS:

a. *Mild ARDS:* The PaO_2/FiO_2 is >200 mm Hg, but ≤300 mm Hg, on ventilator settings that include positive end-expiratory pressure (PEEP) or continuous positive airway pressure (CPAP) ≥5 cmH_2O.
b. *Moderate ARDS:* The PaO_2/FiO_2 is >100 mm Hg, but ≤200 mm Hg, on ventilator settings that include PEEP ≥5 cmH_2O.
c. *Severe ARDS:* The PaO_2/FiO_2 is ≤100 mm Hg on ventilator settings that include PEEP ≥5 cmH_2O.

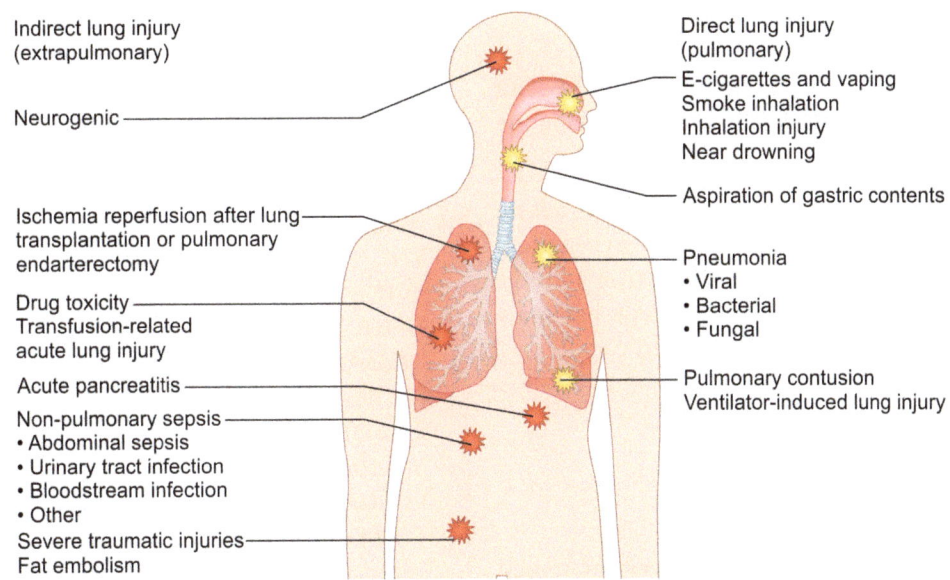

Fig. 3: Causes of acute respiratory distress syndrome.

3. Discuss ventilator management of ARDS.

Acute respiratory distress syndrome is a serious respiratory condition that can lead to respiratory failure if not managed properly. Ventilator management plays a critical role in the treatment of ARDS. The goal of ventilator management is to support the patient's respiratory function while allowing the lungs to heal.

Mechanical ventilatory support after endotracheal intubation is initially started with volume cycled mechanical ventilators with **low tidal volumes**. Here are some key aspects of ventilator management in ARDS:

FiO_2 titration: The initial ventilator setting could be FiO_2 as 1.0 (or a lower value can achieve a PaO_2 >60 mm Hg and oxygen saturation >90%).

Low tidal volume: In ARDS, lungs are often stiff and prone to damage. Using low tidal volume ventilation (6–8 mL/kg of ideal body weight) can help prevent further lung injury by minimizing the amount of pressure delivered to the lungs during each breath.

Positive end-expiratory pressure: PEEP less than or equal to 5 cm of water and inspiratory flow 760 L/min. High PEEP may be applied to increase lung volume and keep the alveoli open. PEEP is applied in small increments of 3–5 cmH_2O up to a maximum of 15 cmH_2O to achieve maximum oxygen saturation of >90% with low nontoxic FiO_2 levels.

Rate: Ventilatory rate of 20–25 breaths/min is needed to keep $PaCO_2$ and pH normal.

Other ventilatory strategies: In some patients, high frequency ventilation or partial liquid ventilation and lung replacement therapy with extracorporeal membrane oxygenation has shown promising results.

Prone position: In situations where maximum PEEP with FiO_2 of 1.0 does not supply sufficient oxygen, placing the patient in a prone position has been found to be useful.

Monitoring and adjusting: Ventilator management in ARDS requires close monitoring of patient's oxygenation, ventilation, and lung compliance. Ventilator settings may need to be adjusted frequently to maintain adequate oxygenation and prevent further lung injury.

Question 5

1. Explain the clinical features of tricyclic antidepressant (TCA) overdose.

Clinical features of TCA overdose or toxicity vary from mild antimuscarinic symptoms to severe cardiotoxicity secondary to sodium channel blockage. Symptoms can occur within a few minutes to hours of ingestion **(Table 7)**.

A Glasgow Coma Scale score of <8 in emergency department is a strong predictor of serious complications such as seizures and cardiac dysrhythmias.

TABLE 7: Clinical features of tricyclic antidepressant overdose.	
Mild-to-moderate toxicity	Drowsiness, confusion, slurred speech, ataxia dry mucous membranes and axillae, sinus tachycardia, mild hypotension urinary retention, decreased bowel sounds and ileus myoclonus, hyperreflexia
Serious toxicity	Coma, cardiac conduction delays, supraventricular tachycardia, hypotension, respiratory depression, ventricular tachycardia, seizures
Secondary complications from serious toxicity	• Aspiration pneumonia • Pulmonary edema • Anoxic encephalopathy • Hyperthermia • Rhabdomyolysis

2. What are the electrocardiogram (ECG) changes in a patient with TCA overdose?

Tricyclic antidepressant overdose can cause a number of changes on an ECG, reflecting the drug's effects on the heart. ECG changes usually develop within 6 hours of ingestion and typically resolve over 36–48 hours in moderate to severe levels of toxicity. TCA overdose can occur any time after ingestion, and may not be present initially. Therefore, serial ECG monitoring is recommended in patients with suspected TCA overdose.

The most common ECG findings in TCA overdose include **(Fig. 4)**:

a. *Widening of the QRS complex:* This is the most specific ECG finding in TCA overdose. QRS widening occurs due to blockade of sodium channels in the myocardium, leading to slowed conduction through the heart.
b. *Prolongation of the QT interval:* TCA overdose can cause prolongation of the QT interval, which is associated with an increased risk of ventricular arrhythmias and sudden cardiac death.
c. *T-wave inversion:* T-wave inversion is a common finding in TCA overdose and can be seen in leads II, III, aVF, and V4–V6.
d. *ST-segment changes:* ST-segment depression or elevation can be seen in TCA overdose, although this is less specific than QRS widening.
e. *Sinus tachycardia:* TCA overdose can cause an increase in heart rate, leading to sinus tachycardia.
f. *Ventricular arrhythmias:* TCA overdose can cause ventricular arrhythmias, such as ventricular tachycardia or ventricular fibrillation, which can be life-threatening.

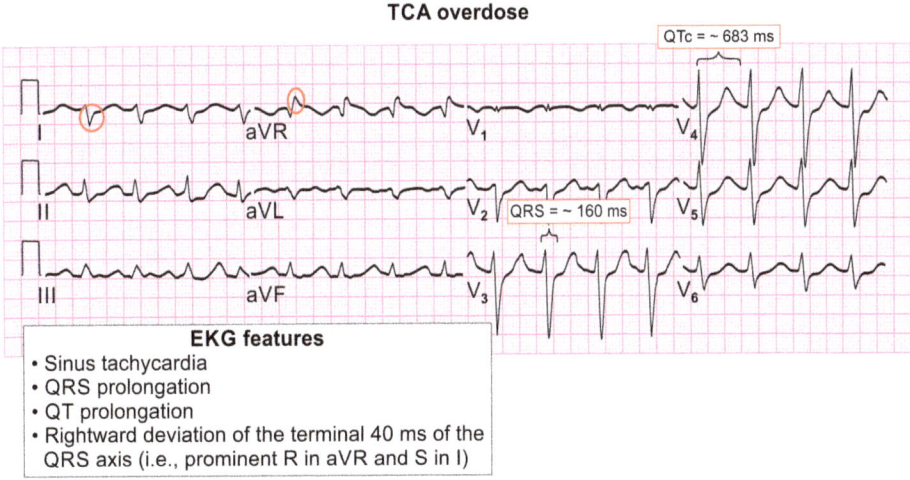

Fig. 4: Electrocardiogram changes in tricyclic antidepressant (TCA) toxicity.

3. How do you manage a patient with TCA overdose?

a. The treatment of TCA overdose in ED should be managed aggressively.
b. Establish an IV line, initiate continuous cardiac monitoring.
c. Evaluate for alterations of consciousness, hemodynamic instability, and respiratory impairment.
d. Gastrointestinal (GI) decontamination is warranted in all patients presenting early to emergency department (presents within 1 hour of ingestion), and is awake with patent airways, due to decreased GI tract motility.
e. Gastric lavage is followed by ingestion of activated charcoal. Give a single PO dose of activated charcoal @1 g/kg (50–100 g).
f. Ingestion of TCA with serious cardiac toxicity requires treatment with alkalinization with sodium bicarbonate 1–2 mEq/kg IV bolus given over a few minutes. Repeat bolus or add 150 mEq to 1 L 5% dextrose in water given @2–3 mL/kg/h.
g. In mechanically ventilated patients, hyperventilation can be used to raise the pH. Goal is to maintain blood pH between 7.35 and 7.45.
h. If serum potassium <3.5 mEq/L, replace potassium as needed, either PO or IV form.
i. Seizures or agitation can be treated with benzodiazepines (IV diazepam @ 0.1 mg/kg). Phenobarbital (10–15 mg/kg) can be given for seizures refractory to benzodiazepines.
j. Hypotension to be treated with normal saline given as bolus of 10–30 mL/kg. If hypotension is refractory to normal saline, start inotropes such as noradrenaline or adrenaline.
k. In case of torsades de pointes or refractory dysrhythmias, treat with IV magnesium sulfate 2 g over a few minutes, 3% saline 1–3 mL/kg IV over 10 minutes; transcutaneous or transvenous pacing in case of any cardiac atrioventricular (AV) blocks.

Question 6

1. Discuss the clinical features of neuroleptic malignant syndrome (NMS).

a. Neuroleptic malignant syndrome is a rare but potentially fatal complication of a therapeutic range of short drug therapy with antipsychotic drugs.
b. NMS patients are commonly seen among young adult males (20–25 years age).
c. Typically develops over a period of 1–3 days after ingestion.
d. Characterized by a **tetrad** of **altered mental status, muscular rigidity, fever and sympathetic nervous system lability.**
e. Along with the tetrad, other features are recent dopamine antagonist exposure or dopamine agonist withdrawal and negative evaluation of other causes.
f. **Autonomic nervous system instability:** Tachypnea, tachycardia, diaphoresis, flushing skin, pallor, and bowel and bladder incontinence.
g. Muscle rigidity is typically described as **lead pipe** and **cogwheel rigidity**.
h. Along with muscle rigidity, tremor, chorea, akinesia, opisthotonos, trismus, blepharospasm can be expected.
i. Other symptoms such as dysphagia, dyspnea, abnormal reflexes, mutism, as well as seizures can be present.

Laboratory abnormalities: Elevated creatinine kinase levels, leukocytosis, elevated levels of hepatic transaminases, hypo or hypernatremia, metabolic acidosis, myoglobinuria, elevated BUN, and creatinine levels, and decreased serum iron level.

2. Describe any one diagnostic criteria for NMS.

Following are the diagnostic criteria for NMS (**Table 8**):

TABLE 8: Diagnostic criteria for neuroleptic malignant syndrome.

Major features	• Fever >38°C (100.4°F), measured orally on at least two occasions
	• Psychomotor slowing and altered mental status
	• Lead pipe rigidity
	• Sympathetic nervous system lability (two or more features)
	  – Elevated blood pressure
	  – Blood pressure fluctuation
	  – Diaphoresis
	  – Urinary incontinence
	• Recent dopamine antagonist exposure or dopamine agonist withdrawal

Minor features	• Increased creatine kinase level (>4 × upper limit) or myoglobinuria • Tachycardia • Tachypnea • Hypersalivation (more prominent with clozapine or amisulpride) • Tremor • Muscle cramps
Exclusion criteria	No other infectious, toxic, metabolic or neurologic cause identified

3. How do you differentiate between NMS and serotonin syndrome?

The differentiation between serotonin syndrome and NMS is given in **Table 9**.

TABLE 9: Differentiation between serotonin syndrome and neuroleptic malignant syndrome.

Serotonin syndrome	Neuroleptic malignant syndrome
No increased leukocytes	Leukocytosis
No increased creatine phosphokinase (CPK)	Increased CPK
Gastrointestinal (GI) symptoms such as nausea, vomiting, diarrhea will be present	GI symptoms not present
Motor features such as ataxia, myoclonus, hyperreflexia, other than muscle rigidity	Primarily lead pipe or cogwheel muscle rigidity

4. Explain the treatment of a case with NMS.

Treatment of NMS in emergency department:
a. Withdraw any antipsychotic and potentiating drugs, such as anticholinergics, antihistamines, or lithium.
b. Intravenous hydration to restore circulating volume and maintain urine output.
c. Reduce the patient's temperature with external cooling methods like ice packs, cooling blankets, etc.
d. Sedation with a benzodiazepine, such as lorazepam, 1-2 mg IV every 2-4 hours as needed.
e. *Airway protection:* Consider early intubation and mechanical ventilation, especially if hypersalivation is present.
f. Use nondepolarizing neuromuscular blocking agents such as rocuronium, over depolarizing agents.
g. Prompt reduction in muscle rigidity can be expected to minimize the occurrence of complications such as rhabdomyolysis, renal failure, respiratory failure, disseminated intravascular coagulation, and cardiovascular collapse.
h. Agents to reduce severe muscle rigidity are given here:

Dantrolene: A direct-acting skeletal muscle relaxant that is primarily used in severe NMS cases where the rigidity is very prominent.

Dose: 1.0-2.5 mg/kg IV load, followed by 1 mg/kg IV every 6 hours up to a maximum dose of 10 mg/kg/day.

Should not be used along with calcium, as it increases the risk of cardiovascular collapse.

Dantrolene is discontinued once symptoms resolve.

Bromocriptine: A centrally acting dopamine agonist that can reduce fever and muscle rigidity in NMS and shorten the duration.

Dose: Starting with 2.5 mg PO 3-4 times a day and increase dose by 2.5 mg every 24 hours up to maximum dose of 45 mg/day.

Adverse effect: Hypotension, vomiting, and worsening of psychosis.

Bromocriptine is maintained for at least 10 days for NMS related to oral neuroleptics and for about 2-3 weeks for depot neuroleptics.

Amantadine: Similar to bromocriptine, only available in enteral form and less likely to cause hypotension.

Dose: 100 mg PO 3 times a day.

Patients are given continuous monitoring and care in the intensive care unit. Most patients recover in 2-14 days.

Question 7

1. Enumerate various generalized skin disorders.

Some generalized skin disorders are:
a. Erythema multiforme
b. Toxic epidermal necrolysis (TEN)
c. Exfoliative erythroderma
d. Staphylococcal and Streptococcal toxic shock syndrome

e. Staphylococcal scalded skin syndrome
f. Pemphigus vulgaris
g. Rocky Mountain spotted fever
h. Disseminated viral/gonococcal infection
i. Purpura fulminans.

2. Explain the clinical features of erythema multiforme.

The common characteristic features of erythema multiforme are:
a. Erythematous macules, papules
b. Target lesions
c. Urticaria or vesiculobullous lesions.

Erythema multiforme minor presents with localized papular eruptions of the skin with acral distribution and involving target lesions and/or raised edematous papules.

Erythema multiforme major is a severe form of this disease presenting along with:
a. Multisystem involvement
b. Vesiculobullous lesions
c. Erosions of mucous membranes (especially involving one or more mucous membrane areas and epidermal detachment of <10% total body surface area) **(Fig. 5)**.

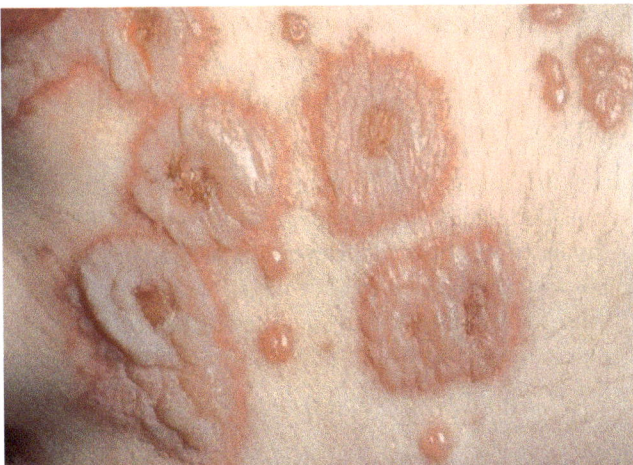

Fig. 5: Erythema multiforme major target lesion (central vesicle with the edematous ring).

Stevens-Johnson syndrome is considered as a severe form of erythema multiforme major, with high incidence among young adults (20-40 years). Patients present with the following symptoms:
a. Fever, malaise, myalgia
b. Arthralgia
c. Diffuse pruritus or generalized burning sensation over skin prior to eruption of the lesion.
d. Maculopapular and target or iris lesions are most characteristic.
e. Erythematous papules appear symmetrically on the dorsum of hands and feet and on the extensor surfaces of the extremities.
f. Maculopapule evolves into target lesion within the next 24-48 hours.
g. As maculopapular lesions enlarge, the central area becomes cyanotic, occasionally accompanied by central purpura or a vesicle.
h. Urticarial plaques may occur.
i. Vesiculobullous lesions, which are pruritic and painful, develop within preexisting maculopapule or plaques, usually on the extensor surface of the arms and legs. Also found on the mucosal surfaces including eyes, mouth, vagina urethra, and anus.
j. Lesions develop over a period of 2-4 weeks and heal over 5-7 days.

3. Discuss the clinical features of TEN.

Toxic epidermal necrolysis is an explosive dermatosis, characterized by:
a. Tender erythema
b. Bullae formation
c. Mucous membrane lesions
d. Exfoliation

Symptoms include 1-2 week prodrome:
a. Malaise
b. Anorexia
c. Arthralgias
d. Fever or symptoms of upper respiratory tract infection
e. Skin tenderness, pruritus, tingling, or burning sensation.

Characteristic skin signs of TEN are:
a. Warm, tender erythroderma
b. Vesicles and bullae
c. Exfoliation
d. Involvement of mucous membranes—initially involving eyes, nose, mouth, and genitalia, later becomes generalized.
e. The erythematous areas become tender and confluent within hours.
f. Flaccid, ill-defined bullae appear within the areas of erythema.
g. *Nikolsky sign* is a slippage of the epidermis from the dermis when slight rubbing pressure is applied to the skin.
h. The bullae form along the cleavage plane between the epidermis and the dermis. The epidermis is then shed into large sheets, which leave raw, denuded areas of exposed dermis.
i. The average time taken for the onset of the lesions postexposure from the precipitating factors or agents is 2 weeks. Cutaneous extension follows between 24 hours and 15 days, with some severe cases developing within 24 hours.

Other clinical features include:
a. Perilabial blistering and erosive lesions are disfiguring and impair adequate oral intake leading to hypovolemia.
b. Ocular complications such as purulent conjunctivitis, painful erosions and potential blindness.
c. Anogenital lesions are common.
d. Mucous membranes of the GI, urinary and respiratory tracts can also be involved.
e. Infections and hypovolemia with electrolyte disorders are the leading cause of deaths among the patients with TEN.

4. Enumerate the management of a patient with TEN.

Toxic epidermal necrolysis requires hospitalization in an intensive care or burn unit.
a. Stabilize the airways, prefer advanced airways at the earliest, as sloughing of airways and respiratory epithelium may occur.
b. Hypovolemia and electrolyte abnormalities to be corrected with IV fluids @10–30 mL/kg bolus followed by maintenance fluids. In case of hypotension, start inotropes such as norepinephrine or epinephrine infusion.
c. Prompt, aggressive, and early administration of antibiotics in suspected infection or sepsis.
d. Remove any triggering agent, if identified.
e. Pain management as appropriate.

Question 8

A 22-year-old medical student presented with an attempted suicide. He had attempted suicide twice before but was unsuccessful. He says, "He feels depressed".

1. How will you assess suicide risk in this patient?

The most important part of the evaluation of depression is the assessment of suicide risk.
a. Use straight forward, nonjudgmental questions regarding the patient's suicide or homicidal thoughts or intent, and seek corroborative information from the family members, friends, first responders, etc.
b. Evaluate the patient based on the decision support tool given by the suicide prevention resource center.

A "yes" response to any question below indicates the need for emergency psychiatric consultation:

a. *Thoughts of carrying out a plan:* Have you been thinking about how you might kill yourself?
b. *Suicide intent:* Do you have intention of killing yourself?
c. *Past suicide attempt:* Have you ever tried suicide in the past?
d. *Significant mental health conditions:* Have you had treatment for mental health problems?
e. *Substance use disorder:* Do you have a history of alcohol or substance abuse? Have you used drugs or medication for nonmedical reasons in the past months?
f. *Irritability/Agitation/Aggression:* Have you been feeling anxious or agitated? Having conflicts or getting into fights? Is there direct evidence of irritability, agitation, or aggression?

Check the score: A "yes" response is equal to 1.

Score 0: If every item (a–f) is "no" discharge may be appropriate following one or more emergency department-based brief suicide prevention interventions.

Score >1: If the responses to the transition question and any item 1–6 are "yes", consider consulting a mental health specialist during the emergency department visit for further evaluation, including a comprehensive suicide risk assessment. Consider the immediate safety needs of the patient and design a treatment plan accordingly.

2. How will you plan emergency department disposition?

Once a risk assessment is done, next step is to educate the patients and family and provide reassurance **(Fig. 6)**.
a. Involve the patient in the decision-making process.
b. Disposition is based on the assessment of harm to self or others, the ability to care for one's self, level of supportive environment at home and complicating medical or substance abuse problems.
c. Antidepressants are usually prescribed by the primary care physicians or psychiatrist for depression, neurogenic pain, or smoking cessation.
d. Follow appointment scheduled for a date within 1 week of discharge.
e. Barriers and solutions to be discussed.
f. Crisis center or emergency contact number to be provided.
g. Written instructions and education materials provided, including what to do if the patient's condition worsens and when to return to the ED.
h. Patient confirms his or her understanding of the patient care plan and senses the provider's care and concern.

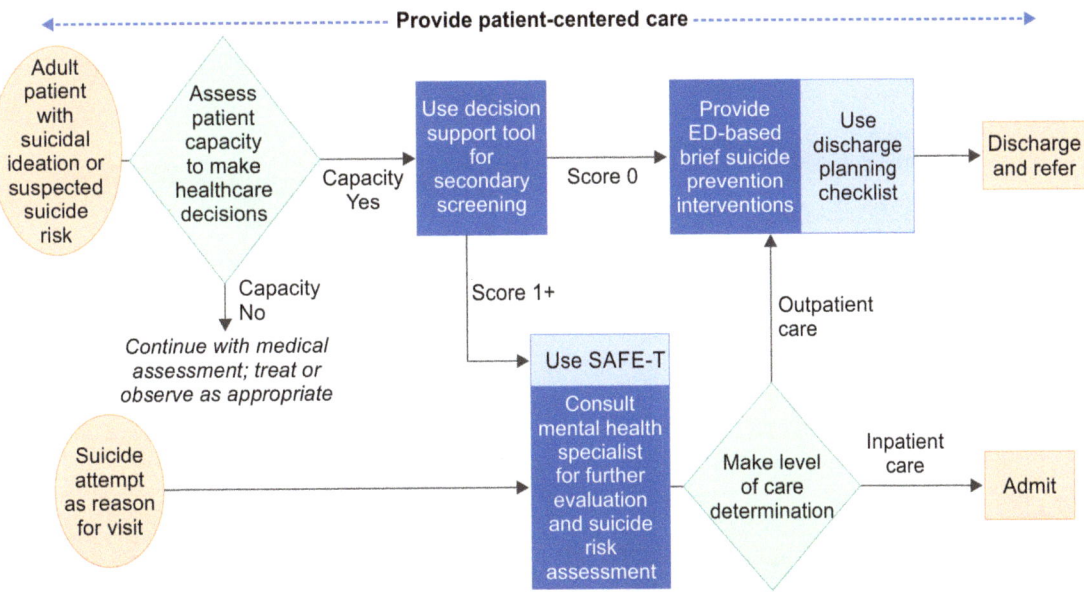

Fig. 6: Process for care and discharge of patients with suicide risk from emergency department (ED).

Question 9

1. Enumerate inherited and acquired clotting disorders (thrombophilia).

Following is the list of hypercoagulable states (**Table 10**):

TABLE 10: Hypercoagulable states.	
Inherited	**Acquired**
Activated protein C resistance due to factor V Leiden mutation	*Medications:* Oral contraceptives/hormone replacement therapy, tamoxifen, lenalidomide
Prothrombin gene mutation 20210A	Pregnancy
Protein C deficiency	Malignancy
Protein S deficiency	Heparin-induced thrombocytopenia
Antithrombin deficiency	Antiphospholipid syndrome
Severe hyper-homocysteinemia	Hyperviscosity syndromes
ABO blood type (non-0)	Human immunodeficiency virus (HIV)

2. Discuss the pathophysiology of hemophilia A.

Hemophilia is the most common hereditary disorder of hemostasis. They manifest with prolonged and excessive bleeding either spontaneously or after insignificant trauma (**Figs. 7A and B**).

a. It is an X-linked, recessive hemorrhagic trait that manifests as a congenital absence or decrease in plasma clotting Factor VIII, a pro-coagulation cofactor, and initiator of thrombin (clotting cascade), for generation of fibrin to form a platelet-fibrin plug at sites of endothelial disruption.

b. Female hemophilia gene carriers do not manifest the symptoms of hemophilia A.

Pathophysiology:

a. When the vascular endothelium sustains an injury, the hemostatic process initiates the coagulation cascade to restore vascular integrity and prevent further bleeding.

b. Platelet activation occurs at the site of vascular rupture initiating promulgation of clotting factors and fibrin formation resulting in a platelet-fibrin plug to inhibit further bleeding.

c. Factor VIII, the deficit of which causes hemophilia A, provides essential enhancement of thrombin generation and promulgation of fibrin formation to inhibit further bleeding.

d. Factor VIII adheres to the Von Willebrand factor to protect it from proteolytic degradation.

e. Bleeding in hemophilia results from defective fibrin stabilization secondary to inadequate fibrin generation, which results in a failure of secondary hemostasis.

f. Insufficient thrombin in the coagulation cascade results in a deficiency of fibrin.

3. Explain the clinical features of hemophilia A.

Bleeding is the primary effect of hemophilia A. Bleeding can occur without any injury or after any mild or severe injury. The condition causes internal and external bleeding. Internal bleeding can cause bruises, lumps in the body, joint swelling, joint damage and potentially, organ damage.

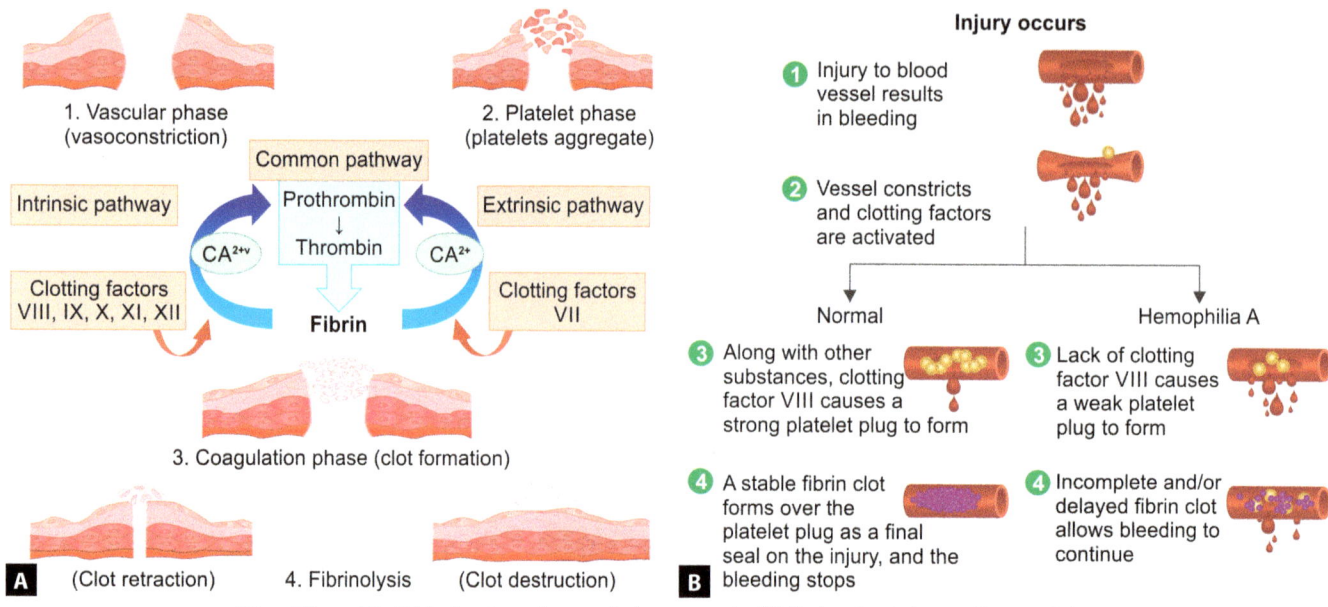

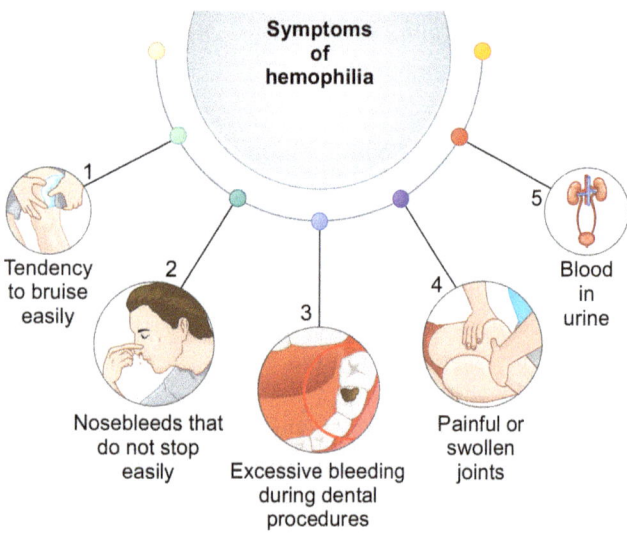

Figs. 7A and B: (A) Activation of coagulation cascade; (B) Pathophysiology of hemophilia.

Fig. 8: Symptoms of hemophilia.

Common symptoms include **(Fig. 8):**
a. Nosebleeds
b. Bleeding of the gums or in the mouth
c. Swollen joints and joint stiffness
d. Bruises
e. Heavy menstrual bleeding
f. Gastrointestinal bleeding with blood in stool.
g. Blood in urine
h. Coughing blood or vomiting blood.

4. Discuss the management of a patient with hemophilia presenting with hemarthrosis.

Treatment for hemarthrosis depends on the cause and may include simple home remedies, medication for the relief of pain and swelling, removal of the blood, and/or medication to prevent bleeding.

a. Treatment with rest, ice, compression, and elevation (RICE) is often used for the management of pain and swelling.
b. Avoid blood thinners. Do not take any pills for pain relief unless recommended or prescribed by your healthcare provider.
c. For large bleeds, joint aspiration may be done within 2 days of the bleed to prevent damage that the blood can cause in the joint.
d. Surgeries such as synovectomy (removal of the joint lining), meniscectomy, and osteotomy have been used for the treatment of hemarthrosis.
e. Tailored physical therapy, designed to use your joints while avoiding overuse or damaging motions, can help recover and prevent deformities.
f. Electrical therapy with transcutaneous electrical nerve stimulation (TENS) has been used for pain control.
g. As a preventive measure, blood-clotting medication (prophylactic blood-clotting factors) may be suggested if the hemarthrosis is due to hemophilia.

Question 10

1. Enumerate the causes of rhabdomyolysis.

Other causes of rhabdomyolysis are **(Table 11) (Fig. 9):**

Anesthesia related:
a. Malignant hyperthermia
b. Muscular dystrophies
c. Muscle channelopathies
d. Propofol infusion syndrome

TABLE 11: Causes of rhabdomyolysis.	
Acquired	**Genetic**
Drugs/toxins	*Metabolic muscle disorder:* Disorders of fatty acid metabolism, glutaric aciduria, disorders of glycogen metabolism-glycogen storage disorder
• Ethanol • Infectious/sepsis	*Mitochondrial disorders:* Complex I, complex II, cytochrome b, tRNA mutations, deoxyguanosine kinase gene
• Extreme physical exertion • Crush injury/compartment syndrome	*Muscular dystrophies:* Duchenne muscular dystrophy, Becker muscular dystrophy
• Ischemia/metabolic disorders • Primary neurological disorder—status epilepticus	Disorders of intramuscular calcium release and excitation-contraction coupling
Idiopathic	Miscellaneous—tRNA splicing endonuclease 54 gene

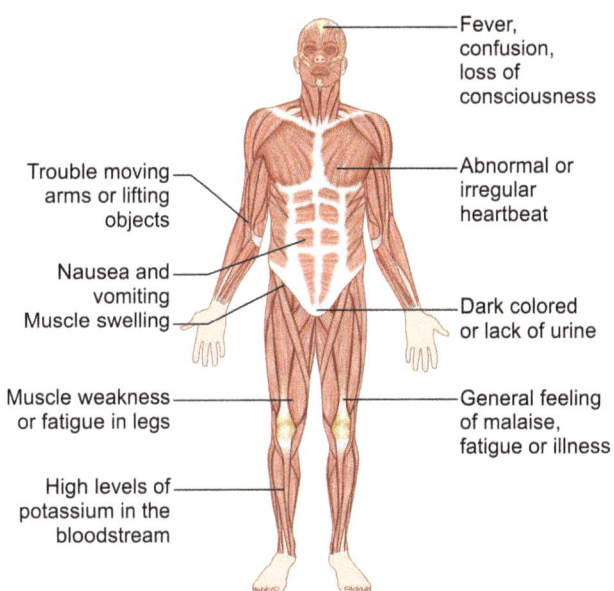

Fig. 10: Symptoms of rhabdomyolysis.

BOX 1: Other symptoms of rhabdomyolysis.

Patients may have other symptoms like:
a. Muscular pain and tenderness
b. Decreased muscle strength
c. Fever, dyspnea, pedal edema
d. Soft tissue swelling
e. Skin changes consistent with pressure necrosis
f. Nausea/vomiting
g. Oliguria/anuria
h. Confusion, agitation, delirium
i. Arrhythmias
j. Electrolyte abnormalities are prominent features of rhabdomyolysis
k. Hyperphosphatemia
l. Hyperkalemia
m. Hypercalcemia
n. Hyperuricemia
o. Hypoalbuminemia

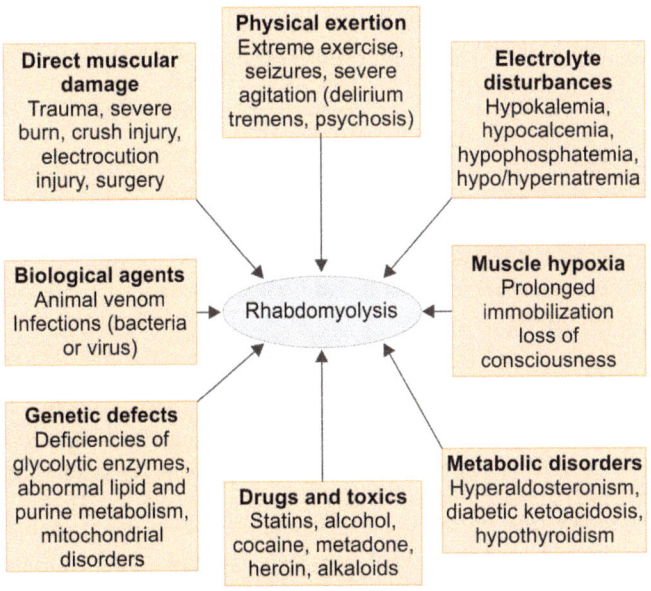

Fig. 9: Principal causes of rhabdomyolysis.

2. Explain the clinical features of rhabdomyolysis.

The classic characteristics of rhabdomyolysis comprises of:

a. Myalgia
b. Generalized weakness
c. Darkened/brown urine
d. Elevated serum muscle enzymes, like creatine kinase.

Following are some symptoms of rhabdomyolysis **(Fig. 10)** **(Box 1)**:

3. Discuss the diagnosis of rhabdomyolysis.

The diagnostic evaluation should be performed in patients with myalgias and pigmenturia.

History and examination: The history should focus on the factors that may cause or predispose to rhabdomyolysis, including traumatic, nontraumatic exertional and non-traumatic nonexertional etiologies. Examination should focus on signs that suggest muscle injury, including muscle weakness and tenderness, limb edema, and evidence of trauma or compartment syndrome.

Laboratory studies: Obtain the following key diagnostic laboratory studies:

a. Serum creatine kinase, the standard biomarker for rhabdomyolysis.

b. Urinalysis for reddish-brown urine as evidence of myoglobinuria.
c. Complete blood count, differential, and platelet count, for the evidence of infection or hemolysis.
d. Blood urea nitrogen, and creatinine, for renal function and evidence of acute kidney injury.
e. Routine electrolytes plus calcium and phosphate, for hyperkalemia, hypocalcemia, and hypophosphatemia.
f. Elevated levels of aspartate aminotransferase (AST) and alanine aminotransferase (ALT) may suggest release from muscle due to rhabdomyolysis.
g. PT, activated partial thromboplastin time (aPTT), D-dimer, and fibrinogen for evidence of disseminated intravascular coagulation.
h. Arterial blood gas for metabolic acidosis.
i. Serum albumin, for hypoalbuminemia, which can be seen with systemic capillary leak syndrome.
j. Electrocardiography, for cardiac dysrhythmias secondary to hyperkalemia and hypocalcemia.
k. Blood cultures and infection work-up if febrile or suspecting infection.
l. Alcohol level and toxicology screen, if suspicion for alcohol or drugs as primary or contributing cause of rhabdomyolysis.
m. Additional testing such as electromyography (EMG), magnetic resonance imaging (MRI), molecular genetic studies, or muscle biopsy is done on those suspected to have underlying myopathy.

4. Explain the treatment of rhabdomyolysis in emergency department.

Once the patient is in emergency department:
a. *Recognize and manage fluid and electrolyte abnormalities*:
   Aggressive IV rehydration for the next 24–72 hours.
   i. Rapid correction of the fluid deficit with IV crystalloids followed by infusion of 4 mL/kg/h.
   ii. Maintaining a minimum urine output of 3–4 mL/kg/h.
   iii. Ringer lactate is the preferred fluid for resuscitation in nontraumatic rhabdomyolysis.
   iv. Place a urinary catheter in patients in critical condition and those with acute kidney injury to monitor their urine output.
   v. Cardiac monitoring to recognize any dysrhythmias.
   vi. For patients with heart disease, preexisting renal diseases, elderly or with comorbid conditions, hemodynamic monitoring to avoid fluid overload.
   vii. Hypocalcemia observed in early rhabdomyolysis requires no treatment.
   viii. If hypercalcemia is symptomatic, continue saline diuresis.
   ix. Hyperkalemia which is severe in the initial 12–36 hours, can be treated with calcium. Use of ion-exchange resins (e.g., sodium polystyrene sulfonate) may be effective.
   x. Treat hyperphosphatemia with oral phosphate binders when serum levels are >7 mg/dL.
   xi. Dialysis (hemodialysis or peritoneal) may be needed.
b. *Identification of the specific causes* and the use of appropriate countermeasures directed at the triggering events, including discontinuation of drugs or other toxins.
c. *Prompt recognition, evaluation, and treatment of compartment syndrome* in patients in whom it is present.

SUGGESTED READING

1. Richhariya D, Sharma B. Textbook of Emergency Medicine including Intensive Care and Trauma, 2nd edition. New Delhi: Jaypee Brothers Medical Publishers (P) Ltd; 2022. pp. 1328-35. (Question 1).
2. Richhariya D, Sharma B. Textbook of Emergency Medicine including Intensive Care and Trauma, 2nd edition. New Delhi: Jaypee Brothers Medical Publishers (P) Ltd; 2022. pp. 867-70. (Question 2).
3. Richhariya D, Sharma B. Textbook of Emergency Medicine including Intensive Care and Trauma, 2nd edition. New Delhi: Jaypee Brothers Medical Publishers (P) Ltd; 2022. pp. 1697-700. (Question 3).
4. Richhariya D, Sharma B. Textbook of Emergency Medicine including Intensive Care and Trauma, 2nd edition. New Delhi: Jaypee Brothers Medical Publishers (P) Ltd; 2022. pp. 570-3. (Question 4).
5. Richhariya D, Sharma B. Textbook of Emergency Medicine including Intensive Care and Trauma, 2nd edition. New Delhi: Jaypee Brothers Medical Publishers (P) Ltd; 2022. pp. 1425-30. (Question 5).
6. Richhariya D, Sharma B. Textbook of Emergency Medicine including Intensive Care and Trauma, 2nd edition. New Delhi: Jaypee Brothers Medical Publishers (P) Ltd; 2022. pp. 1425-30. (Question 6).
7. Richhariya D, Sharma B. Textbook of Emergency Medicine including Intensive Care and Trauma, 2nd edition. New Delhi: Jaypee Brothers Medical Publishers (P) Ltd; 2022. pp. 1013-38. (Question 7).
8. Richhariya D, Sharma B. Textbook of Emergency Medicine including Intensive Care and Trauma, 2nd edition. New Delhi: Jaypee Brothers Medical Publishers (P) Ltd; 2022. pp. 1047-55. (Question 8).
9. Richhariya D, Sharma B. Textbook of Emergency Medicine including Intensive Care and Trauma, 2nd edition. New Delhi: Jaypee Brothers Medical Publishers (P) Ltd; 2022. pp. 1002-10. (Question 9).
10. Richhariya D, Sharma B. Textbook of Emergency Medicine including Intensive Care and Trauma, 2nd edition. New Delhi: Jaypee Brothers Medical Publishers (P) Ltd; 2022. p. 750. (Question 10).

Emergency Medicine Paper 16

Shweta Ashok

Question 1

1. What is HAZMAT?

HAZMAT or "Hazardous materials" are substances in quantities or forms that may pose a reasonable risk to health, property, or the environment.
a. HAZMATs include such substances as toxic chemicals, fuels, nuclear waste products, and biological, chemical, and radiological agents.
b. HAZMATs may be released as liquids, solids, gases, or combination or form of all three, including dust, fumes, gas, vapor, mist, and smoke.

2. How will you recognize a HAZMAT event?

A HAZMAT (hazardous materials) event can occur in various ways, such as a spill, leak, explosion, or release of dangerous substances into the environment. Here are some common signs that may indicate a HAZMAT event:
a. *Unusual odors:* Hazardous materials often emit strong, unpleasant odors that can be easily detected in the surrounding area. These smells can range from a sweet or chemical-like scent to a foul, rotten odor.
b. *Visible haze, fog, or smoke:* A HAZMAT event can also produce a visible plume of smoke, haze, or fog in the air. This can be caused by a chemical reaction, a spill, or a release of gas or vapor.
c. *Unusual noise:* Some HAZMAT events, such as explosions or chemical reactions, can produce loud noises that are easily audible from a distance.
d. *Emergency vehicles:* In the event of an HAZMAT event, you may notice a significant presence of emergency vehicles, such as fire trucks, ambulances, and police cars. These vehicles may be responding to the incident or helping to evacuate the area.
e. *Evacuation orders:* If you receive an evacuation order from local authorities or emergency services, it is a clear indication that a HAZMAT event is occurring, and you should follow the evacuation procedures immediately.

If you suspect that there is a HAZMAT event occurring in your vicinity, take immediate action to protect yourself and those around you. You should follow any emergency instructions given by local authorities, avoid the affected area if possible, and seek medical attention if you experience any symptoms of exposure to hazardous materials.

3. What are the various control zones for decontamination in the field?

In the HAZMAT field, there are various control zones for decontamination. These zones are established to ensure the safety of personnel and the public during hazardous materials incidents. The following are the different control zones for decontamination:

Hot zone: This is the area where the hazardous materials are located, and it is the most dangerous zone. Only trained and equipped personnel should be allowed to enter this zone.

Warm zone: This is the area surrounding the hot zone where decontamination takes place. Personnel who have been in the hot zone must go through decontamination before entering the warm zone. This zone may also be used for equipment staging and other support activities.

Cold zone: This is the area furthest from the hot zone and is considered a safe zone. This area is where command and control functions take place and where decontaminated personnel and equipment are located.

Support zone: The support zone is typically located a safe distance away from the incident site, and is used as a staging area for personnel, equipment, and supplies. It may also serve as a decontamination area for those who have been exposed to the hazardous materials, and may include facilities for medical treatment or other support services.

The purpose of the support zone is to ensure the safety and well-being of emergency responders and other personnel, as well as to facilitate an effective response to the hazardous materials incident. Responders must be trained on the proper use and management of the support zone, in order to minimize the risk of injury or exposure to hazardous materials.

The boundaries of these zones can change depending on the specific incident and the type of hazardous material involved. The use of these zones helps to ensure that personnel and the public are protected during hazardous materials incidents.

Question 2

A 7-month-old male child presented to the emergency department with episodes of crying spells and red colored stools. His mother noticed a mass in the right lower quadrant of abdomen.

1. What are the possible diagnoses?

Based on the given information, there are several possible diagnoses that could explain the symptoms of the 7-month-old male child. Here are a few:

Intussusception: This is a medical emergency that occurs when a portion of the intestine telescopes into an adjacent part, causing obstruction, inflammation, and potentially leading to tissue damage. The classic triad of intussusception includes abdominal pain, vomiting, and bloody stool. Intussusception is most common in children between 6 months and 3 years of age.

Meckel's diverticulum: This is a congenital abnormality that results from incomplete closure of the omphalomesenteric duct during fetal development. Meckel's diverticulum can cause gastrointestinal bleeding, abdominal pain, and a palpable mass in the lower right quadrant of the abdomen. Meckel's diverticulum is most common in children <2 years of age.

Infectious gastroenteritis: This is a common condition in young children that is caused by a viral or bacterial infection of the digestive system. Symptoms may include abdominal pain, vomiting, diarrhea, and fever. In some cases, infectious gastroenteritis can cause blood in the stool.

Cow's milk protein intolerance: This is a condition in which the child's immune system reacts to the proteins in cow's milk, leading to gastrointestinal symptoms such as abdominal pain, diarrhea, and bloody stool.

Allergic colitis: This is a condition in which the child's immune system reacts to certain foods, leading to inflammation, and damage to the lining of the colon. Symptoms may include abdominal pain, diarrhea, and bloody stool.

These are just a few possible diagnoses based on the given information. However, a proper diagnosis can only be made by a qualified healthcare professional after a thorough physical examination and appropriate diagnostic tests.

2. How do you investigate this child?

When a 7-month-old male child presents to the emergency department with episodes of crying spells, red-colored stools, and a mass in the right lower quadrant of the abdomen, the following investigations may be considered:

Physical examination: The child should be thoroughly examined, including the abdomen, to assess for the presence of a mass, tenderness, or distension. A digital rectal examination may also be performed to assess for the presence of blood.

Laboratory tests: Blood tests may be done to evaluate the child's complete blood count (CBC) to assess for signs of infection or anemia, electrolytes, and kidney function.

Imaging tests: Imaging tests may be used to visualize the mass in the abdomen and diagnose the underlying condition. These may include abdominal X-rays, ultrasound, computed tomography (CT) scan, or magnetic resonance imaging (MRI).

Stool tests: Stool tests may be done to evaluate for the presence of blood, bacteria, viruses, or parasites.

Diagnostic procedures: A diagnostic procedure, such as an endoscopy or colonoscopy, may be performed to directly visualize the gastrointestinal tract and assess for abnormalities.

The investigations will depend on the suspected diagnosis and the findings of the initial physical examination. It is important to note that any diagnostic procedure or imaging test should be done with caution in a young child and only after weighing the risks and benefits. A pediatrician or pediatric gastroenterologist should be consulted for further management and treatment.

3. How do you manage the child in emergency department?

The management of a 7-month-old male child who presents to the emergency department with episodes of crying spells, red-colored stools, and a mass in the right lower quadrant of the abdomen will depend on the underlying cause of the symptoms. Here are some general approaches to managing the common conditions that may be responsible for these symptoms:

Intussusception: A child suspected of having intussusception should be promptly treated with intravenous (IV) fluids and antibiotics through an IV line, and imaging tests will be done to confirm the diagnosis. Treatment may involve a procedure called an air or barium enema to correct the intussusception. In some cases, surgery may be necessary.

Meckel's diverticulum: The management of Meckel's diverticulum may involve surgery to remove the abnormality, especially if it is causing symptoms such as gastrointestinal bleeding or obstruction.

Infectious gastroenteritis: Treatment of infectious gastroenteritis may involve supportive care, such as fluid and electrolyte replacement and symptomatic relief of diarrhea and vomiting. Antibiotics may be prescribed if there is a bacterial infection.

Cow's milk protein intolerance and allergic colitis: Management of these conditions may involve dietary changes, such as switching to a hypoallergenic formula or eliminating specific foods from the child's diet. In some cases, medications may be prescribed to manage symptoms such as inflammation and pain.

In all cases, it is important to closely monitor the child's symptoms and follow-up with a pediatrician or pediatric gastroenterologist for appropriate management and treatment. It is also important to provide adequate nutrition and hydration, and to prevent complications such as dehydration and electrolyte imbalances.

Question 3

1. What are the key changes in recent 2018 Advanced Trauma Life Support (ATLS) guidelines compared to the previous ATLS guidelines?

Here are some of the key changes in the 2018 ATLS guidelines compared to the previous ATLS guidelines:

Emphasis on the need for teamwork and communication: The 2018 ATLS guidelines place a greater emphasis on the importance of communication and teamwork in trauma care. This includes the need for clear and concise communication between team members, as well as the importance of effective leadership and coordination of care.

Updated approach to airway management: The 2018 ATLS guidelines recommend a more aggressive approach to airway management in patients with trauma. This includes a focus on early recognition and intervention for airway obstruction and the use of advanced airway techniques such as video laryngoscopy and intubation.

Focus on early identification of hemorrhage: The 2018 ATLS guidelines emphasize the importance of early identification and control of hemorrhage in trauma patients. This includes the use of point-of-care ultrasound and other diagnostic tools to identify sources of bleeding, as well as the use of early resuscitation strategies such as tranexamic acid and early blood product administration.

Greater emphasis on damage control surgery: The 2018 ATLS guidelines recommend a greater emphasis on damage control surgery in the management of severely injured patients. This includes a focus on rapid control of hemorrhage and contamination, as well as the use of staged surgical interventions to minimize the risk of complications.

Updated approach to spinal immobilization: The 2018 ATLS guidelines recommends a more selective approach to spinal immobilization in trauma patients. This includes a focus on identifying patients who are at high risk for spinal injury and avoiding unnecessary immobilization in low-risk patients, as well as the use of alternative immobilization techniques such as cervical collars and vacuum mattresses.

2. Classify hemorrhagic shock as per 2018 ATLS guidelines.

The physiologic effects of hemorrhage are divided into four classes based on clinical signs, useful for estimating the acute blood loss. The following classification system is useful in emphasizing the early signs and pathophysiology of the shock state **(Table 1)**:

a. *Class I hemorrhage:* <15% blood volume loss (usually occurs in those donated 1 unit of blood).
b. *Class II hemorrhage:* 15–30% blood volume loss (uncomplicated mild hemorrhage for which crystalloid fluid resuscitation is required).
c. *Class III hemorrhage:* 31–40% blood volume loss (complicated moderate hemorrhagic state in which at least crystalloid infusion is required and also blood replacement).
d. *Class IV hemorrhage:* >40% blood volume loss (severe hemorrhage form in which patient will need aggressive resuscitative measures. Blood transfusion is required).

TABLE 1: Signs and symptoms of hemorrhage by class based on ATLS 2018 guidelines.

Parameter	Class 1	Class II (Mild)	Class III (Moderate)	Class IV (Severe)
Approximate blood loss	<15%	15–30%	31–40%	>40%
Heart rate	↔	↔/↑	↑	↑/↓↓
Blood pressure	↔	↔	↔/↓	↓
Pulse pressure	↔	↓	↓	↓
Respiratory rate	↔	↔	↔/↑	↑
Urine output	↔	↔	↓	↓↓
Glasgow Coma Scale score	↔	↔	↓	↓
Base deficit	0 to –2 mEq/L	–2 to –6 mEq/L	–6 to –10 mEq/L	–10 mEq/L or less
Need for blood products	Monitor	Possible	Yes	Massive transfusion protocol

Question 4

1. What is BLUE protocol for ultrasound (USG) in emergency department?

Bedside lung ultrasound in emergency (BLUE) is a basic point-of-care ultrasound (POCUS) examination performed for identifying undifferentiated respiratory failure at the bedside, immediately after the physical examination, and before any radiography.
a. The protocol is simple and takes only a few minutes to perform.
b. It analyzes three standardized points on each hemithorax in patients with acute respiratory failure, by establishing the presence or absence of:
   i. Lung sliding
   ii. Anterior lung rockets
   iii. Posterior and/or lateral alveolar and/or pleural syndrome (PLAPS)
   iv. A noncompressible deep vein.
c. Lung ultrasonography is becoming a standard tool in critical care, due to its very high sensitivity and specificity to diagnose common chest pathologies.

2. Describe different profiles in lung USG.

Ultrasound profile (Fig. 1)
a. *Left panel:* The A profile is defined as predominant A lines plus lung sliding at the anterior surface in supine or half-sitting patients (stage 1/1).
   i. This profile suggests chronic obstructive pulmonary disease (COPD), embolism, and some posterior pneumonia. Pulmonary edema is nearly ruled out.
b. *Middle:* The B profile is defined as predominant B lines in stage 1.
   i. This profile suggests cardiogenic pulmonary edema, and nearly rules out COPD, pulmonary embolism, and pneumothorax.
c. *Right panel:* An AB profile, massive B lines at the left lung, A lines at the right lung.
   i. This profile is usually associated with pneumonia.

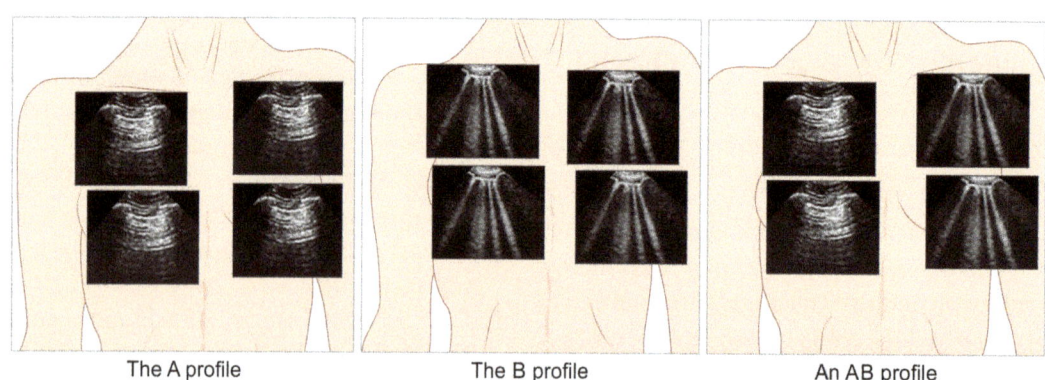

Fig. 1: Ultrasound profiles.

3. Explain the role of USG in diagnosis of lung parenchymal diseases.

Lung parenchymal diseases refer to conditions that affect the tissue and structures within the lungs themselves. While USG is not typically the first choice of imaging modality for evaluating lung parenchymal diseases, instead, other imaging modalities like chest X-ray, CT, and MRI are preferred. However, in certain situations, such as when a patient is critically ill and cannot be moved, or when a patient cannot tolerate a CT scan due to radiation exposure, an ultrasound may be used as an alternative imaging modality.

Parenchymal disease can be detected by ultrasonography as long as there is no air between the probe and the lesion and the beam reaches the pleura. Some lung parenchymal diseases that may be detected on ultrasound include:

a. *Pleural effusion:* This occurs when fluid accumulates in the pleural space, the area between the lung and the chest wall. On ultrasound, pleural effusion appears as a black area between the lung and the chest wall.
b. *Pneumothorax:* This occurs when air enters the pleural space, causing the lung to collapse. On ultrasound a pneumothorax can be used to diagnose a collapsed lung (pneumothorax) by detecting the absence of lung sliding or the presence of lung point on the ultrasound image.
c. *Interstitial lung diseases:* Ultrasound may be used to evaluate for interstitial lung diseases, which are a group of conditions that affect the lung tissue, including pulmonary fibrosis. On ultrasound, interstitial lung diseases may appear as areas of increased or decreased lung density.
d. *Lung consolidation:* This is a condition where the lung tissue becomes filled with fluid, pus, or other substances,

making it denser and less elastic. Ultrasound can help detect areas of consolidation in the lungs, which may be indicative of pneumonia or other lung infections.

e. *Lung abscess:* This refers to a collection of pus within the lung tissue. On USG, a lung abscess may appear as a hypoechoic (dark) area within the lung.
f. *Lung cancer:* While USG is not typically used to diagnose lung cancer, it may be used to guide the placement of a needle during a biopsy to obtain a tissue sample for diagnosis.

Question 5

1. What is sudden infant death syndrome (SIDS)?

Sudden infant death syndrome is the sudden and unexplained death of an apparently healthy infant <1 year of age, usually during sleep. SIDS is sometimes called "crib death" because the infants often die in their cribs.

The cause of SIDS is not known, but it is believed to be related to abnormalities in the part of an infant's brain that controls breathing and arousal from sleep.

There are several risk factors associated with SIDS, including placing an infant to sleep on their stomach or side, soft bedding in the crib, overheating, exposure to secondhand smoke, premature birth or low birth weight, and maternal smoking during pregnancy.

2. Enumerate various causes for SIDS.

The cause of SIDS is not known, but it is believed to be related to abnormalities in the part of an infant's brain that controls breathing and arousal from sleep.

A combination of genetic, environmental, and lifestyle factors which can increase the risk of sudden and unexplained death in apparently healthy infants. Some of the potential causes of SIDS include:

Abnormalities in the brainstem: The brainstem controls vital functions such as breathing, heart rate, and blood pressure, and some research suggest that abnormalities in this area may contribute to SIDS.

Respiratory issues: Some infants who die from SIDS may have problems with their breathing, including episodes of apnea (a pause in breathing) or hypopnea (shallow breathing).

Cardiac abnormalities: Certain heart conditions may increase the risk of SIDS, such as long QT syndrome, a condition that affects the heart's electrical activity.

Environmental factors: Exposures to environmental toxins, such as cigarette smoke, may increase the risk of SIDS.

Sleeping position: Placing infants on their stomachs or sides to sleep has been associated with an increased risk of SIDS.

Overheating: Infants who become overheated during sleep may be at higher risk for SIDS.

Maternal factors: Some maternal factors, such as young maternal age, smoking, substance use, and inadequate prenatal care, may increase the risk of SIDS.

It is important to note that while these factors may increase the risk of SIDS, the exact cause of SIDS remains unknown in most cases.

3. What are the risk factors for SIDS?

There are several risk factors associated with SIDS, including placing infants to sleep on their stomach or side, soft bedding in the crib, overheating, exposure to secondhand smoke, premature birth or low birth weight, and maternal smoking during pregnancy. Following are some risk factors that may increase the likelihood of SIDS occurring:

Age: SIDS most commonly occurs in infants between 1 and 4 months of age.

Sleeping position: Infants who are placed on their stomachs or sides to sleep have a higher risk of SIDS than those who are placed on their backs.

Soft bedding: The use of soft bedding, such as blankets, pillows, or stuffed animals, in the infant's sleep area has been linked to an increased risk of SIDS.

Prematurity and low-birth weight: Infants who are born prematurely or have a low-birth weight have a higher risk of SIDS.

Maternal factors: Maternal smoking during pregnancy, as well as exposure to secondhand smoke after birth has been linked to an increased risk of SIDS. Other maternal factors, such as young maternal age, poor prenatal care, and substance abuse, may also increase the risk.

Family history: Infants with siblings or other family members who have had SIDS have a higher risk of SIDS.

Overheating: Infants who become too warm during sleep may be at higher risk for SIDS.

Male sex: Male infants have a slightly higher risk of SIDS than female infants.

It is important to note that most infants who have one or more of these risk factors do not develop SIDS, and infants who do not have any of these risk factors can still develop SIDS. However, taking steps to reduce these risk factors can help to lower the risk of SIDS.

4. How will you prevent SIDS?

While the exact cause of SIDS is not fully understood, there are several steps that parents and caregivers can take to help reduce the risk of SIDS. These include:
a. Always placing infants on their backs to sleep, both for naps and at night. Infants who sleep on their stomachs or sides are at a higher risk of SIDS.
b. Using a firm and flat sleep surface, such as a crib or bassinet, with a tight-fitting sheet. Soft surfaces, such as couches or adult beds, are not safe for infants to sleep on.
c. Keeping soft objects, loose bedding, and other hazards out of the sleep area. This includes pillows, blankets, stuffed animals, and crib bumpers.
d. Avoiding overheating by dressing infants in lightweight clothing and keeping the room at a comfortable temperature. Infants who become too warm during sleep are at a higher risk of SIDS.
e. Offering a pacifier at naptime and bedtime. This has been shown to reduce the risk of SIDS, although it is not clear why.
f. Avoiding exposure to smoke, both during pregnancy and after birth. Infants who are exposed to cigarette smoke are at a higher risk of SIDS.
g. Providing a safe sleep environment for infants when they are away from home. This includes using a safe sleep surface, such as a portable crib or play yard.
h. *Breastfeeding infants:* Breastfeeding has been associated with a lower risk of SIDS.

It is important to note that while these steps can help to reduce the risk of SIDS, there is no way to completely prevent SIDS.

Question 6

1. What are the revised diagnostic criteria for sepsis and septic shock?

The new definitions emphasize the importance of organ dysfunction as the primary indicator of sepsis and septic shock, rather than relying solely on systemic inflammatory response syndrome (SIRS) criteria.

Here are the diagnostic criteria for sepsis and septic shock according to Sepsis-3:

Sepsis: Suspected or confirmed infection.

An acute change in sequential (sepsis-related) Organ Failure Assessment (SOFA) score of 2 or more points, which is a measure of organ dysfunction.

The SOFA score ranges from 0 to 24 and includes assessments of six organ systems–respiratory, cardiovascular, renal, hepatic, coagulation, and neurological.

Septic shock: Sepsis as defined above.

Vasopressor therapy required to maintain a mean arterial pressure (MAP) of 65 mm Hg or greater serum lactate level >2 mmol/L (18 mg/dL) despite adequate fluid resuscitation.

The revised diagnostic criteria focus on early recognition and management of sepsis and septic shock by identifying patients with organ dysfunction, rather than relying solely on inflammatory markers. This shift in emphasis allows for earlier intervention and potentially better outcomes for patients with sepsis and septic shock.

2. Explain Quick Sequential Organ Failure Assessment (qSOFA) scoring of sepsis.

Quick Sequential Organ Failure Assessment (qSOFA) is a simplified version of the SOFA score that can be used at the bedside to quickly identify patients with suspected infection who are at higher risk for poor outcomes. It consists of three criteria, with one point assigned for each of the following:
1. Respiratory rate of 22 breaths per minute or higher
2. Altered mentation (e.g., confusion or decreased level of consciousness)
3. Systolic blood pressure of 100 mm Hg or lower

Patients with a qSOFA score of 2 or higher are considered at increased risk of poor outcomes and should prompt clinicians to investigate for the presence of organ dysfunction, initiate appropriate therapy, and consider referral to critical care if necessary.

Quick Sequential Organ Failure Assessment is not a substitute for clinical judgment, and it should be used in conjunction with other clinical information to guide decision-making. It is also important to recognize that qSOFA is not a diagnostic tool for sepsis, but rather a screening tool to identify patients at increased risk of poor outcomes who may require further evaluation and management.

3. What are the recent surviving sepsis bundles guidelines?

The most recent version of the Surviving Sepsis Campaign (SSC) guidelines is the 2021 update. The 2021 SSC guidelines continue to emphasize the importance of early recognition and management of sepsis, with a focus on the use of protocols and bundles to improve outcomes. Some key recommendations from the guidelines include:
a. *Use of the quick qSOFA* score to identify patients at high risk of poor outcomes from sepsis.
b. *Administration of broad-spectrum antibiotics within 1 hour* of sepsis recognition.
c. *Aggressive fluid resuscitation* in patients with sepsis-induced hypotension or elevated serum lactate levels.

d. *Use of vasopressors* in patients with persistent hypotension despite adequate fluid resuscitation.
e. *Early initiation of source control measures,* such as drainage of abscesses or removal of infected tissue.
f. Use of *lung-protective ventilation strategies* in patients with sepsis-induced respiratory failure.
g. Use of *renal replacement therapy* in patients with sepsis-induced acute kidney injury.

Question 7

1. What are the causes of abdomen pain in neonates and young infants?

Young infants typically tend to eat every second hourly. So incessant cries and fatigue with poor feeding are the signs of serious illness. Intermittent, colicky pain is often associated with intussusception, colic, and gastroenteritis. Necrotizing enterocolitis and volvulus are more typically associated with continuous pain. Pain after feeds may be caused by gastroesophageal reflux. Pyloric stenosis causes progressive painless projectile vomiting followed by renewed interest in feeding.

There are many possible causes of abdominal pain in neonates and young infants.

Some of the most common causes include:

Colic: This is a common condition that causes excessive crying and fussiness in babies. It is not clear what causes colic, but it usually resolves on its own within a few months.

Gastroesophageal reflux (GERD): GERD occurs when stomach acid flows back into the esophagus. The symptoms include spitting up, vomiting, and irritability.

Constipation: Infants may experience abdominal pain and discomfort if they are constipated. The signs of constipation include infrequent bowel movements, hard stools, and straining during bowel movements.

Intussusception: This is a condition in which a portion of the intestine folds into itself, causing a blockage. The symptoms include abdominal pain, vomiting, and bloody stools.

Gastrointestinal infections: Infants may experience abdominal pain and diarrhea as a result of a viral or bacterial infection.

Milk protein intolerance: Some babies are intolerant to cow's milk protein, which can cause abdominal pain, vomiting, and diarrhea.

Hernia: A hernia occurs when an organ or tissue protrudes through a weak spot in the surrounding muscle or connective tissue. In infants, a hernia may be visible as a bulge in the abdomen.

Meconium ileus: This is a blockage in the intestine caused by thick, sticky meconium. It is more common in babies with cystic fibrosis.

Urinary tract infection: Infants with a urinary tract infection may experience abdominal pain, fever, and frequent urination.

2. What are the major life-threatening causes of abdominal pain in neonates and young infants?

Abdominal pain in neonates and young infants can be a sign of a serious medical condition. Some of the major life-threatening causes of abdominal pain in this population include:

Intestinal obstruction: This is a blockage that prevents food or fluids from passing through the small or large intestine. It can be caused by a variety of factors such as meconium ileus, volvulus, and intussusception.

Necrotizing enterocolitis: This is a serious condition that occurs when the lining of the intestinal wall becomes inflamed and dies. It is most common in premature infants and can lead to perforation of the bowel.

Malrotation with midgut volvulus: This is a condition in which the intestine twists around its mesentery, leading to obstruction and ischemia.

Gastrointestinal perforation: This is a hole in the stomach or intestine that can be caused by a variety of factors such as trauma, infection, or inflammation. It can lead to peritonitis and sepsis.

Acute appendicitis: This is an inflammation of the appendix that can lead to perforation and peritonitis.

Hernias: These are protrusions of abdominal contents through a weakness in the abdominal wall. In infants, inguinal hernias are the most common.

Mesenteric adenitis: This is an inflammation of the lymph nodes in the mesentery that can mimic the symptoms of appendicitis.

Urinary tract infections: These can cause abdominal pain in infants, particularly if there is associated fever.

Question 8

A 2-year-old child presented with fever, drooling of saliva, and stridor.

1. Enumerate the causes of stridor in infants and children.

Stridor in infants and children can have several different causes, including:

Croup: This is a viral infection that causes inflammation of the upper airway, which can result in a barking cough, hoarseness, and stridor.

Epiglottitis: This is a bacterial infection that causes inflammation and swelling of the epiglottis, which can lead to difficulty breathing and stridor.

Foreign body aspiration: This occurs when a child inhales a foreign object, such as a toy or food, which can cause obstruction of the airway and stridor.

Anaphylaxis: This is a severe allergic reaction that can cause swelling of the throat and airway, leading to difficulty breathing and stridor.

Trauma to the neck or airway: This can occur as a result of a fall, car accident, or other injury, and can lead to obstruction of the airway and stridor.

Vocal cord dysfunction: This occurs when the vocal cords do not function properly, causing difficulty breathing and stridor.

Tonsillitis: Inflammation of the tonsils can cause difficulty breathing and stridor.

Congenital abnormalities: Infants may be born with structural abnormalities in the airway that can cause stridor, such as laryngomalacia or tracheomalacia.

2. What is croup?

Croup (*viral laryngotracheobronchitis*) is the most common cause of stridor outside the neonatal period, commonly affecting children 6 months–3 years old. It is caused by a viral infection that inflames the upper airways, including the larynx, trachea, and bronchi. The most common causes are: Parainfluenza virus rhinovirus.

Other causes are: Influenza respiratory syncytial virus (RSV) metapneumovirus enterovirus coronavirus.

3. Discuss the clinical presentation of croup.

The clinical features of croup may vary in severity from mild to severe, and typically develop over a period of several days. The common signs and symptoms of croup include:
a. A barking cough that may sound like a seal or dog barking.
b. Hoarse voice or changes in voice quality.
c. Difficulty breathing, which may cause a high-pitched or wheezing sound when inhaling.
d. Rapid, shallow breathing.
e. Stridor, a harsh, high-pitched sound that occurs when breathing in.
f. Mild-to-moderate fever.
g. Runny or stuffy nose.
h. Irritability or restlessness.

In some cases, croup may also cause other symptoms such as:
a. Bluish or grayish skin around the nose, mouth, or fingernails due to a lack of oxygen.
b. Dehydration, especially if the child is having difficulty drinking fluids.
c. Fatigue or lethargy.

Most cases of croup are mild and can be treated at home conservatively with rest and fluids. Though the symptoms usually last for about 3–7 days, the cough can linger for up to 2 weeks. Most children recover fully without any lasting complications.

4. What is the diagnosis of croup?

Diagnosis is clinical based on the history as given by parents and the signs on examination.

X-ray radiograph of neck demonstrates subglottic narrowing, referred to as "steeple sign" **(Fig. 2)**.

Severity: Croup is classified as mild, moderate, and severe depending on the degree of airway obstruction.

Modified Westley croup score is one of the commonly used scoring guidelines in clinical practice. It is the sum of points assigned for five factors—level of consciousness, cyanosis, stridor, air entry, and retractions. The points given for each factor is listed in **Table 2**, and the final score ranges from 0–17.

A total score of <4 points indicates mild croup: The characteristic barking cough and hoarseness may be present, but no stridor at rest. *A score of 3–5 points indicates moderate croup.* It presents with easily heard stridor, and few other signs. *A total score of 6–11 points indicates severe croup.* It presents with obvious stridor along with marked chest wall indrawing. *A score of >12 points indicates impending respiratory failure.* The barking cough and stridor may not be prominent at this stage. Severe croup is rare and seen among <1% of children presenting to the emergency department.

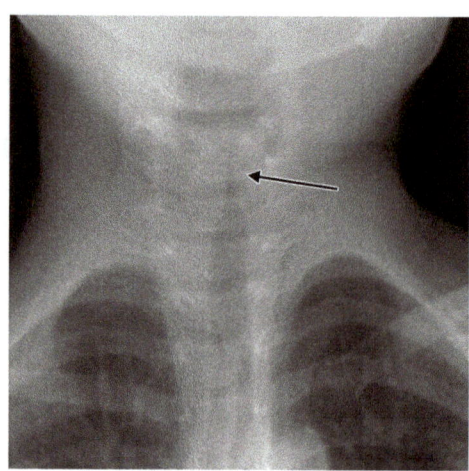

Fig. 2: The steeple sign as seen on an anteroposterior (AP) neck X-ray of a child with croup.

TABLE 2: Modified Westley croup score.

Clinical features	Assigned score
Inspiratory stridor	• None = 0 point • With agitation only = 1 point • At rest = 2 points
Intercostal retractions	• Mild = 1 point • Moderate = 2 points • Severe = 3 points
Air entry	• Normal = 0 point • Slightly decreased = 1 point • Severely decreased = 2 points
Cyanosis	• None = 0 point • With agitation only = 4 points • At rest = 5 points
Level of consciousness	• Normal = 0 point • Altered = 5 points

5. Discuss the treatment of croup.

The treatment of croup depends on the severity of the symptoms. In most cases, croup is a self-limited illness that improves on its own within a few days. The following treatments may be recommended to help alleviate symptoms and improve the child's comfort:

Humidifier: Using a cool-mist humidifier in the child's bedroom can help to relieve cough and ease breathing. Alternatively, taking the child into a steamy bathroom for a few minutes can also be effective.

Rest: Encouraging the child to rest and limiting physical activity can help to reduce the strain on the respiratory system and promote healing.

Fluids: Making sure the child drinks plenty of fluids can help to prevent dehydration, thin out mucus secretions, and make coughing more productive.

Medications: Over-the-counter pain relievers, such as acetaminophen or ibuprofen, can be given to help reduce fever and relieve pain. Oral steroids may be prescribed to help reduce inflammation in the airways and improve breathing, hence, reducing the duration of the disease. Recommended is dexamethasone single dose of 0.6 mg/kg per oral.

Emergency care: In rare cases of severe croup, where the child is struggling to breathe, hospitalization may be necessary. In the hospital, the child may receive supplemental oxygen, nebulized medications, and other treatments to help alleviate symptoms and improve breathing.

For severe croup with persistent respiratory failure despite medical therapy, endotracheal intubation may be necessary. There is insufficient evidence to determine whether nebulized beta agonists are beneficial with croup, as it causes vasodilation, which may worsen upper airway edema. Hence, beta-agonists are not recommended in croup.

Question 9

A 12-year-old child presented to your emergency department with fever and severe headache. The attending physician suspected him to be suffering from Nipah virus infection. Discuss the following with regard to Nipah virus infection:

1. History and epidemiology.

Nipah virus is classified as a zoonotic virus, meaning that it is transmitted from animals to humans. The primary reservoir of the virus is fruit bats of the *Pteropodidae* family, and transmission to humans can occur through direct contact with infected animals or consumption of contaminated food or water.

Nipah virus was first discovered in 1999 following an outbreak of disease in pigs and people in Malaysia and Singapore. The first Nipah virus outbreak occurred in India in the year 2001 at Siliguri. The second outbreak happened at Nadia in 2007. Nipah virus exhibits neurological and pneumonic tropism with the predominant clinical presentation being encephalitis in humans. The epidemiology of Nipah virus outbreaks is complex, as it involves multiple factors, including the ecology of the virus, the behavior of the reservoir host (fruit bats), and the interactions between humans, animals, and the environment. Outbreaks of Nipah virus are often linked to agricultural practices that bring humans and domestic animals into close contact with bats, as well as the consumption of contaminated food or water.

2. Transmission of infection.

Nipah virus is primarily transmitted to humans from animals, specifically fruit bats of the *Pteropodidae* family. The virus can be transmitted to humans through direct contact with infected bats, their urine or saliva, or through consumption of food or water contaminated with bat excretions.

Transmission of Nipah virus can also occur through contact with infected animals, such as pigs, which can act as intermediate hosts for the virus. Humans can contract the virus through direct contact with infected pigs, or by consuming contaminated pork products.

Human-to-human transmission of Nipah virus has also been reported, particularly in healthcare settings where there is close contact between infected individuals and healthcare workers. The virus can be transmitted through respiratory secretions, such as droplets, or through contact with contaminated surfaces. Preventing transmission of

Nipah virus requires strict biosecurity measures, particularly in regions where the virus is known to be present. This includes avoiding direct contact with infected animals, wearing protective clothing and equipment, implementing proper hand hygiene, and implementing proper food safety practices. In summary, Nipah virus is primarily transmitted to humans through contact with infected animals, particularly fruit bats and pigs. Human-to-human transmission can also occur through close contact with infected individuals. Preventing transmission requires strict biosecurity measures and proper hygiene practices.

3. Clinical features of Nipah virus.

The clinical features of Nipah virus infection can vary widely, ranging from asymptomatic or mild respiratory illness to severe encephalitis with a high case fatality rate.

The incubation period of Nipah virus infection is typically between 5 and 14 days. The initial symptoms of the infection are often nonspecific and can include fever, headache, myalgia (muscle pain), vomiting, and sore throat. In some cases, patients may also experience cough, abdominal pain, and diarrhea.

As the infection progresses, patients may develop neurological symptoms, including seizures, disorientation, and altered consciousness. In severe cases, patients may develop encephalitis, which can lead to coma and death.

The case fatality rate of Nipah virus infection varies between outbreaks, with reported rates ranging from 40–90%. Factors that may affect the severity of the disease include the virulence of the virus strain, the age and immune status of the patient, and the time to initiation of appropriate medical treatment.

4. Management of Nipah virus.

Currently, there is no specific treatment or vaccine for Nipah virus infection, and supportive care is the primary form of management. The management of Nipah virus infection involves a multidisciplinary approach, including clinical management, infection control, and public health measures.

Clinical management of Nipah virus infection involves supportive care, such as respiratory support, fluid and electrolyte management, and treatment of complications such as seizures. Patients with severe neurological symptoms may require intensive care and mechanical ventilation.

Infection control measures are critical for preventing the spread of Nipah virus. Strict isolation precautions, including contact and droplet precautions should be implemented for suspected or confirmed cases of Nipah virus infection. Healthcare workers should wear personal protective equipment, including gloves, gowns, masks, and eye protection, when caring for patients with suspected or confirmed Nipah virus infection. Public health measures, including active surveillance, contact tracing, and outbreak investigation, are critical for controlling Nipah virus outbreaks. Public health authorities should implement strict biosecurity measures in areas where the virus is known to be present, and should provide public education about the risks of Nipah virus infection and how to prevent transmission.

Question 10

1. Discuss the odds ratio giving an example.

The odds ratio is a statistical measure used to quantify the association between two binary variables. It is the ratio of the odds of an event occurring in one group to the odds of the same event occurring in another group. In other words, it tells us how much more or less likely it is for an outcome to occur in one group compared to another group. Here is an example to illustrate how odds ratio works:

Suppose a study is conducted to investigate the association between smoking and lung cancer. The researchers divide the participants into two groups—smokers and nonsmokers. They find that out of 100 smokers, 30 develop lung cancer, while out of 100 nonsmokers, only 5 develop lung cancer.

The odds of developing lung cancer in the smoker group are calculated as the ratio of the number of smokers who developed lung cancer (30) to the number of smokers who did not develop lung cancer (70). This gives an odd of 0.43 (30/70).

Similarly, the odds of developing lung cancer in the nonsmoker group are calculated as the ratio of the number of non-smokers who developed lung cancer (5) to the number of non-smokers who did not develop lung cancer (95). This gives an odd of 0.05 (5/95).

The odds ratio is then calculated as the ratio of the odds of developing lung cancer in the smoker group to the odds of developing lung cancer in the nonsmoker group. This gives an odds ratio of 8.6 (0.43/0.05).

This means that smokers are 8.6 times more likely to develop lung cancer compared to nonsmokers. In other words, the odds of developing lung cancer are 8.6 times higher in smokers than non-smokers.

The odds ratio is a useful measure because it allows us to compare the strength of association between two groups even if the baseline risk of the outcome is different in the two groups. In the above example, the baseline risk of developing lung cancer is much higher in the smoker group than in the non-smoker group. However, the odds ratio takes this into account and provides a meaningful comparison of the strength of association between smoking and lung cancer in the two groups.

2. Discuss the likelihood ratio giving an example.

In statistics, the likelihood ratio is a measure of the strength of evidence provided by the data in favor of one statistical hypothesis over another. It is defined as the ratio of the likelihoods of two different hypotheses, given the same observed data. The likelihood ratio is often used in hypothesis testing, model selection, and parameter estimation. Here is an example to illustrate the concept of likelihood ratio: Suppose we have a medical test for a rare disease, which affects only 1% of the population. The test has a sensitivity of 90% (i.e., it correctly identifies 90% of the people who have the disease) and a specificity of 95% (i.e., it correctly identifies 95% of the people who do not have the disease). We want to know how strong the evidence is in favor of a positive test result indicating the presence of the disease, compared to a negative test result indicating the absence of the disease.

Let H0 be the null hypothesis that the person does not have the disease, and let H1 be the alternative hypothesis that the person does have the disease. The likelihood of observing a positive test result, given H0, is 0.010.05 + 0.990.05 = 0.0595. The likelihood of observing a positive test result, given H1, is 0.010.9 + 0.990.1 = 0.108. The likelihood ratio in favor of H1 over H0 is therefore:

Likelihood ratio = Likelihood (H1)/Likelihood (H0)
= 0.108/0.0595 = 1.82.

This means that observing a positive test result is 1.82 times more likely if the person has the disease (H1) than if the person does not have the disease (H0). We can use this likelihood ratio to calculate the odds ratio, which is a commonly used measure of the strength of association between a risk factor and a disease:

Odds ratio = Likelihood ratio/(1 – prior odds)

where the prior odds are the odds of having the disease before the test result is known. For example, if the prior odds are 1:100 (i.e., the person has a 1% chance of having the disease before the test), then the odds ratio is:

Odds ratio = 1.82/(1/100) = 182

■ SUGGESTED READING

1. Richhariya D, Sharma B. Textbook of Emergency Medicine including Intensive Care and Trauma, 2nd edition. New Delhi: Jaypee Brothers Medical Publishers (P) Ltd; 2022. pp. 55-62. (Question 1).
2. Richhariya D, Sharma B. Textbook of Emergency Medicine including Intensive Care and Trauma, 2nd edition. New Delhi: Jaypee Brothers Medical Publishers (P) Ltd; 2022. pp. 1235-42. (Question 2).
3. Richhariya D, Sharma B. Textbook of Emergency Medicine including Intensive Care and Trauma, 2nd edition. New Delhi: Jaypee Brothers Medical Publishers (P) Ltd; 2022. pp. 1518-32. (Question 3).
4. Richhariya D, Sharma B. Textbook of Emergency Medicine including Intensive Care and Trauma, 2nd edition. New Delhi: Jaypee Brothers Medical Publishers (P) Ltd; 2022. pp. 364-73. (Question 4).
5. Mayo Clinic. 2022. [online] Available from: https://www.mayoclinic.org/diseases-conditions/sudden-infant-death-syndrome/symptoms-causes/syc-20352800 [Last accessed April, 2023]. (Question 5).
6. Richhariya D, Sharma B. Textbook of Emergency Medicine including Intensive Care and Trauma, 2nd edition. New Delhi: Jaypee Brothers Medical Publishers (P) Ltd; 2022. pp. 319-27. (Question 6).
7. Richhariya D, Sharma B. Textbook of Emergency Medicine including Intensive Care and Trauma, 2nd edition. New Delhi: Jaypee Brothers Medical Publishers (P) Ltd; 2022. pp. 1169-75. (Question 7).
8. Richhariya D, Sharma B. Textbook of Emergency Medicine including Intensive Care and Trauma, 2nd edition. New Delhi: Jaypee Brothers Medical Publishers (P) Ltd; 2022. pp. 1185-89. (Question 8).
9. National Centre for Disease Control. (2023). [online] Available from: https://ncdc.mohfw.gov.in/index1.php?lang=1&level=1&sublinkid=238&lid=242 [Last accessed April, 2023]. (Question 9)
10. Richhariya D, Sharma B. Textbook of Emergency Medicine including Intensive Care and Trauma, 2nd edition. New Delhi: Jaypee Brothers Medical Publishers (P) Ltd; 2022. pp. 81-90. (Question 10).

Emergency Medicine Paper 17

Devendra Richhariya

Question 1

1. Discuss jugular venous pulsations, waves, and its clinical significance.

At the bedside, the jugular venous pulse (JVP) is often observed at the right side of the patient's neck **(Fig. 1)**; more specifically, it can be seen passing diagonally over the top of the sternocleidomastoid muscle. The jugular venous pressure is usually assessed by observing the right side of the patient's neck. The normal mean jugular venous pressure, determined as the vertical distance above the midpoint of the right atrium, is 6–8 cmH$_2$O. Clinical significance of JVP is given in **Table 1**.

2. Discuss basic hemodynamic monitoring in a patient admitted in the ICU.

The methods for assessing the volume status are broadly categorized into static (traditional) and dynamic measurements **(Table 2)**.

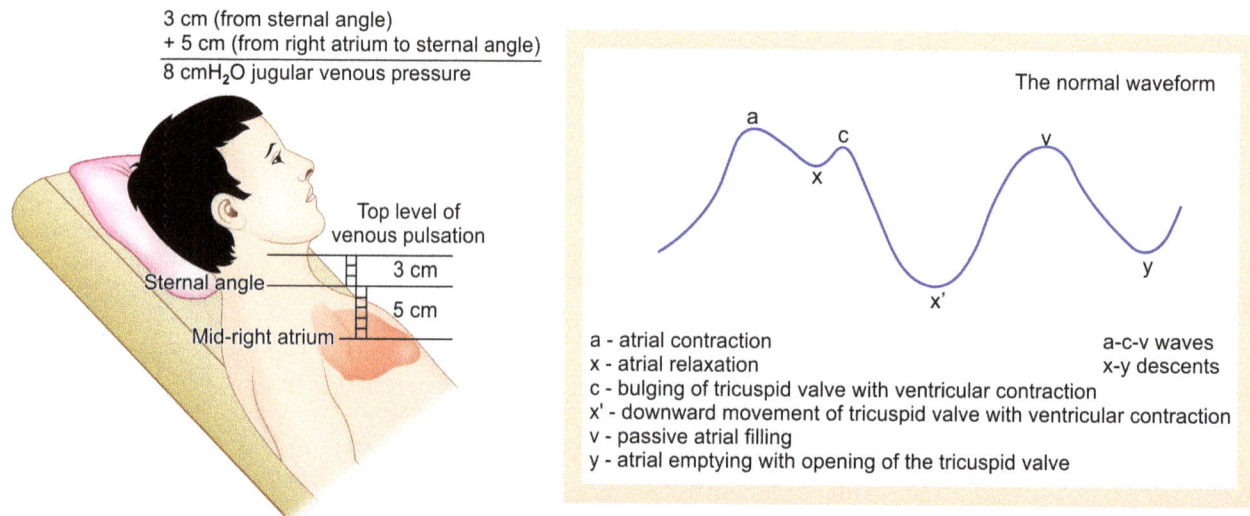

Fig. 1: Jugular venous pulse.

TABLE 1: Jugular venous pulse (JVP): Clinical significance.	
A wave	• Prominent in • RV hypertrophy • Pulmonary stenosis • Pulmonary hypertension • Tricuspid stenosis • Absence in atrial fibrillation and tricuspid regurgitation • Canon wave-complete AV block atrial flutter, ventricular asystole
C wave	• Prominent in tricuspid regurgitation • Absent in constrictive pericarditis
V wave	Prominent in constrictive pericarditis

(AV: atrioventricular; RV: right ventricular)

TABLE 2: Assessing the volume status (static and dynamic measurement).

Static measurement	Dynamic measurement
Mean arterial pressure	PPV or SVV
Central venous pressure	IVC DI
Pulmonary artery occlusion pressure	End-expiratory occlusion test
Mixed venous oxygen saturation	PLR
Mixed venous PCO$_2$	• *Limitations of dynamic indices:* To predict accurate volume responsiveness by IVC DI, PPV, or SVV methods, the patient must be mechanically ventilated with a tidal volume of at least 8 mL/kg of ideal body weight, no spontaneous breaths of the patient, no cardiac arrhythmias
Arterial pH base excess and HCO$_3$	
Echocardiographic parameters: IVC size, LVEDP	• *PLR:* Is the only dynamic index to date that has the ability to predict the response to fluids in a spontaneously breathing patient (no need to mechanically ventilate the patient)
Hemodynamic monitors	
Invasive monitors	PAC
Minimally (less) invasive monitors	• LiDCO PiCCO (calibrated transpulmonary thermodilution) • Flotrac, LiDCO rapid (noncalibrated)
Noninvasive monitors	• USCOM (ultrasonic cardiac output monitors) • NICOM (noninvasive cardiac output monitors) • Bioreactance • Bioimpedance

(IVC DI: inferior vena cava distensibility index; LiDCO: lithium dilution cardiac output; LVEDP: left ventricular end diastolic pressure; PAC: pulmonary artery catheters; PCO$_2$: carbon dioxide tension; PiCCO: pulse contour cardiac output; PLR: passive leg raise; PPV: pulse pressure variation; SVV: stroke volume variation)

Question 2

1. Enumerate the causes of hyponatremia.

The causes of hyponatremia are as follows:

a. Diarrhea and vomiting
b. Diuretics (most common thiazides)
c. Chronic heart failure and cirrhosis
d. Nephrotic syndrome
e. Acute or chronic kidney disease
f. Syndrome of inappropriate antidiuretic hormone (SIADH)
g. Hypothyroidism
h. Glucocorticoid deficiency
i. Mineralocorticoid deficiency
j. Salt-losing nephropathies
k. Cerebral salt wasting

2. Write the approach to diagnose such cases.

a. *Mild hyponatremia:* Serum sodium level is 130–134 mEq/L.
b. *Moderate hyponatremia:* Serum sodium level is 129–125 mEq/L.
c. *Severe hyponatremia:* Serum sodium level is <125 mEq/L. Hyponatremia is also classified as hypovolemic, euvolemic, and hypervolemic hyponatremia according to its volume reserve. Once again, it is divided into hypotonic, isotonic, and hypertonic hyponatremia according to osmolality **(Flowchart 1)**. According to the duration of hyponatremia occurrence, it is called acute if it occurs in <48 hours, and chronic hyponatremia if it appears in >48 hours.

3. Write about the management of life-threatening hyponatremia in ICU.

Patients with acute severe central nervous system findings due to life-threatening hyponatremia should immediately be treated with 100 mL of 3% NaCl. If the clinical findings do not change, infuse two more doses of 100 mL 3% NaCl IV. A total of three doses can be applied. Since the risk of herniation is low in moderate or mild symptomatic patients, 3% NaCl is infused at a rate of 0.5–2 mL/kg/h. Patients with chronic hyponatremia are at a risk of osmotic demyelination syndrome (ODS), which can sometimes be irreversible. Patients who are in the high-risk group, especially for ODS, are patients accompanied by alcoholism, chronic hepatic disease, cirrhosis, hypokalemia, and malnutrition.

In a patient with low risk of ODS, a maximum of 10–12 mEq/L increase should be achieved in 24 hours. In patients with a high risk of ODS, a maximum of 4–6 mEq/L improvement should be achieved in 24 hours.

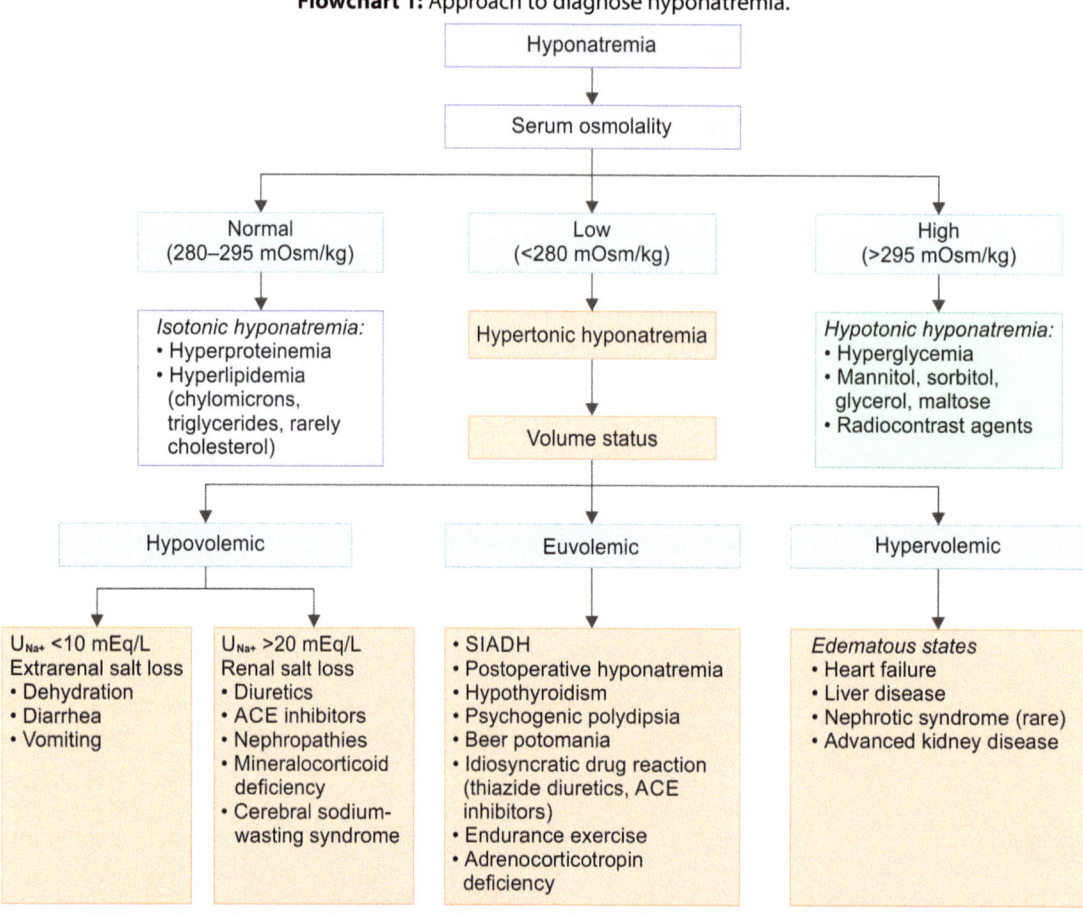

Flowchart 1: Approach to diagnose hyponatremia.

(ACE: angiotensin converting enzyme; SIADH: syndrome of inappropriate antidiuretic hormone)

If chronic hyponatremia is severe, i.e., serum sodium is <125 mEq/L or symptomatic (lethargy, confusion, seizure), 3% NaCl is recommended for treatment as in acute hyponatremia. Initially, 3% NaCl is given to these patients to raise the basal sodium level to 4-6 mEq. If the urine/serum electrolyte ratio is <0.5, water is restricted or vasopressin antagonists are given. If this ratio is >1, salt tablets are added to the diet and loop diuretics are also given.

The serum sodium level should be closely monitored during treatment. To find the amount of fluid required to close the sodium deficit, and how much the liquid given in the treatment raises serum sodium, Na deficit = (total body water) TBW × (desired Na − actual Na) can be used.

Each 1 mL/kg of 3% NaCl administered increases serum sodium by approximately 1 mEq/L. It is this calculation rather than others that is recommended to be followed by international guides.

Specific precautions in hyponatremia treatment:
a. If patients present with acute hyponatremia, severe central nervous system findings, and herniation risk, their serum sodium level should be improved rapidly by giving 3% 100 mL NaCl IV three times.
b. In moderate or mild symptomatic patients, serum sodium is corrected by infusing 3% NaCl at 0.5-2 mL/kg/h.
c. The underlying cause should be treated in patients with chronic hyponatremia. Serum sodium should be corrected slowly due to the risk of ODS.
d. In patients with hypotonic hyponatremia, sodium should be corrected up to 10 mEq in 24 hours and 18 mEq in 48 hours.

Question 3

1. Discuss the physiology of temperature regulation in human.

Thermoregulation is the process by which an organism maintains its internal body temperature within a certain range, despite changes in external conditions. For the human body, it ranges between 36.5 and 37.5°C. The main purpose of thermoregulation is to keep the enzyme systems of the body working properly **(Flowchart 2)**.

Flowchart 2: Physiology of temperature regulation.

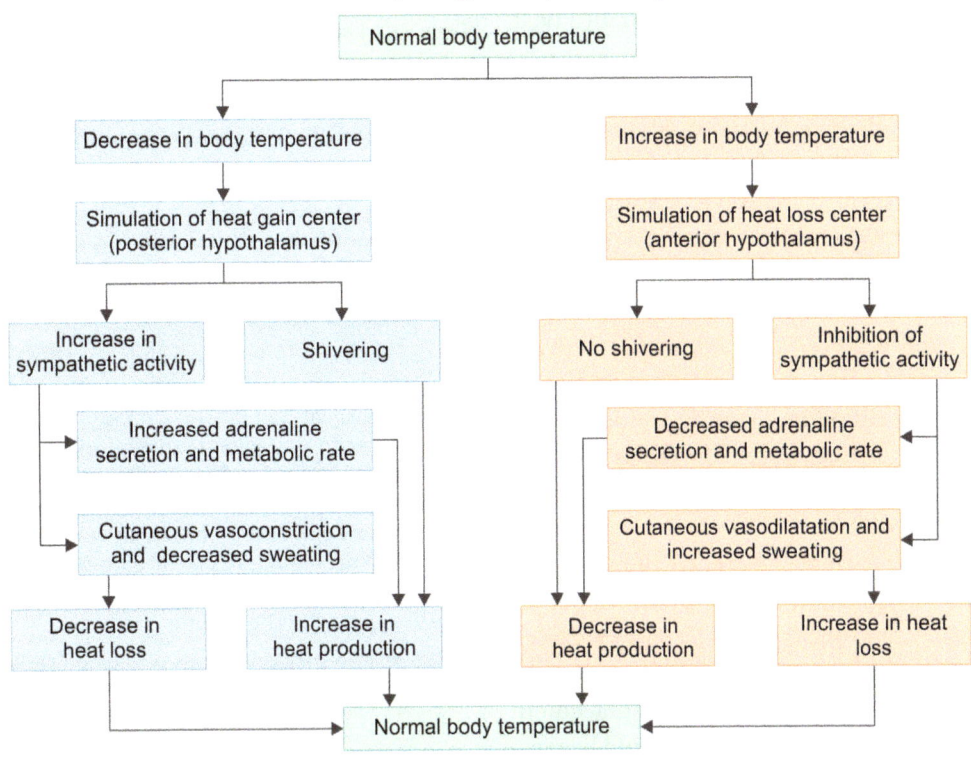

2. Enumerate heat emergencies.
3. Write about their clinical presentation.

Heat emergencies/illness is a spectrum of disorders due to environmental exposure to heat. It ranges from minor conditions such as heat cramps, heat syncope, and heat exhaustion to a more severe condition known as heat stroke. A number of heat illnesses exist across a broad spectrum of presentations **(Table 3)**.

TABLE 3: Classification of heat illness.	
Type	**Characteristic feature**
Heat cramps	Muscular pain which happens after exercise in hot conditions
Heat edema	Cutaneous condition characterized by dependent edema from vasodilatory pooling
Heat rash	Irritation of the skin that results from excessive sweating during hot and humid weather
Heat tetany	A result of short periods of stress in intense heat. Symptoms may include hyperventilation, respiratory problems, numbness or tingling, or muscle spasms
Heat syncope	Dizziness as a result of excess heat
Heat exhaustion	A precursor of a heatstroke, which includes heavy sweating, rapid breathing, and a fast, weak pulse
Heat stroke	A core body temperature of >40°C (104°F) due to environmental heat exposure with either a lack or dysfunction of the central and peripheral thermoregulation center. Symptoms include dry skin, rapid, strong pulse, and dizziness

4. Write about the management of such cases in the emergency department (ED).

Investigations: Important recommended investigations are complete blood count (CBC), liver function tests (LFTs), urea and electrolytes (U&E), and glucose levels.

Urate maybe a predictor of acute kidney injury. Creatine kinase may be a predictor of rhabdomyolysis. Coagulation studies may indicate arterial blood gases. Urinalysis may show myoglobinuria and impending acute kidney injury. Electrocardiogram (ECG) and chest X-ray (CXR) are done to check for aspiration/pulmonary edema.

Treatment:
a. Maintain airway, breathing, and circulation and cardiac monitoring. Monitor core body temperature regularly.
b. Treatment of heat stroke involves rapid mechanical cooling along with resuscitation measures. The body temperature must be lowered quickly.
c. The patient should be moved to a cool area which is either indoor or in a shade and clothing may need to be removed to promote passive clothing.
d. Active cooling methods include immersion in cold water, or a hyperthermia vest can be applied. Cold compresses to the torso, head, neck, and groin will help in bringing the core body temperature down. A fan or dehumidifying air-conditioning unit may be used to aid in evaporation of the water.

e. Immersion should be avoided for an unconscious person, but if there is no alternative, the patient's head must be held above water.
f. Dantrolene, a direct-acting paralytic which abolishes shuddering and is effective in many other forms of hyperthermia, has no individual or additive effects on cooling in the context of heat stroke, showing a lack of endogenous thermogenic response to cold water immersion. Aggressive ice water immersion is the gold standard for life-threatening heat stroke.
g. Adequate hydration is an essential adjunct to cool the temperature. In mild cases of dehydration, hydration can be achieved by drinking water or isotonic sport drinks. In exercise- or heat-induced dehydration, an imbalance of electrolytes can occur and is exacerbated by overconsumption of water.
h. Hyponatremia can be corrected by intake of hypertonic fluids. Absorption is rapid and complete in most people but in the event of confusion, impaired conscious level, or if the patient is unable to tolerate oral fluid, then an intravenous rehydration and electrolyte replacement may be required. The person's condition should be reassessed at regular intervals including the vital signs to ensure stability.

Question 4

1. Write about medical oxygen therapy in the ED.

Supplemental oxygen: A reasonable goal is to achieve arterial oxygen tension (PaO_2) of 65–70 mm Hg with oxygen saturation of >90%. Various devices are used to deliver oxygen. They are divided into low- or high-flow systems, or open or closed systems. This depends upon their capacity to deliver oxygen at sufficient flow rates so as to meet the patient's flow demands. In a low-flow system, the lower the oxygen flow, and the higher the patient's flow requirements, the higher the probability of entraining room air leading to lower fraction of inspired oxygen (FiO_2). Examples of low-flow systems are nasal cannula or facemask. Examples of high-flow devices are venturi masks, facemasks with reservoir bag, and resuscitation bag–mask–valve unit. Venturi mask is a fixed performance device ensuring delivery of precise oxygen concentrations from 24% to 60%. These are extremely useful in chronic obstructive pulmonary disease (COPD) patients where oxygen saturation has to be carefully titrated so as not to blunt the hypoxic drive of the patients.

2. Enumerate causes of type 1 respiratory failure.

Type I (hypoxemic) respiratory failure: It is characterized by PaO_2 <60 mm Hg (8.00 kPa) with normal or low arterial CO_2 tension ($PaCO_2$). This is the most common form of respiratory failure. Causes of type 1 (hypoxemic) respiratory failure are shown in **Box 1**.

> **BOX 1:** Causes of type 1 respiratory failure.
>
> - *Low FiO_2:* High altitude
> - *Airways:* COPD, asthma, postintubation laryngeal edema, mucus plug, bronchiectasis, vocal cord paralysis
> - *Lung parenchyma:* Pulmonary edema, ARDS, pulmonary hemorrhage, lung contusion, pneumonia, alveolar proteinosis, hypersensitivity pneumonitis, transfusion-related lung injury, lung resection, aspiration, radiation injury
> - *Interstitial:* Pulmonary fibrosis, viral or atypical pneumonia
> - *Pulmonary vasculature:* Pulmonary veno-occlusive disease, pulmonary embolism, intracardiac or intrapulmonary shunt
> - *Pleural:* Pneumothorax, pleural effusion
> - *Chest wall:* Kyphoscoliosis, thoracoplasty, massive obesity, chest wall trauma, flail chest, burns
>
> (ARDS: acute respiratory distress syndrome; COPD: chronic obstructive pulmonary disease)

3. Enumerate causes of type 2 respiratory failure.

Type 2 (hypercapnic) respiratory failure results when there is an imbalance between ventilatory demand and ventilatory capacity. Excessive increase in load or a drastic fall in capacity may precipitate it. It may also occur when there is coexistent increased load and reduced capacity, though each may be of moderate severity. Pure hypoventilation as a sole cause can be identified by the presence of normal alveolar–arterial oxygen gradient ($AaDO_2$). Hypercapnia can also occur as a part of hypoxic failure if the gas exchange derangements are quite severe. Causes of type 2 (hypercapnic) respiratory failure are shown in **Box 2**.

> **BOX 2:** Causes of type 2 respiratory failure.
>
> - *Respiratory drive (reduced):* Ondine's curse, drug overdose, obesity hypoventilation syndrome, traumatic brain injuries, carotid body resection, metabolic alkalosis
> - *Neural transmission* (reduced)
> - *Spinal cord:* Cervical spine injury, tumor
> - *Anterior horn cells:* Poliomyelitis, amyotrophic lateral sclerosis
> - *Peripheral nerves:* Phrenic nerve injury, Guillain–Barré syndrome, critical illness polyneuropathy, Lyme disease, beriberi, diphtheria
> - *Neuromuscular junction:* Neuromuscular blocking agents, tick paralysis, organophosphorus poisoning, botulism, tetanus, myasthenia gravis, Eaton–Lambert syndrome
> - *Respiratory muscles:* Muscular dystrophy, polymyositis, malnutrition, dyselectrolytemia, hypothyroidism
> - *Chest wall:* Kyphoscoliosis, thoracoplasty, fibrothorax, flail chest, ankylosing spondylitis, asphyxiating thoracic dystrophy

4. Enumerate the prerequisites for putting patients on noninvasive ventilatory treatment.

Noninvasive ventilation (NIV): It is defined as a process of delivering positive-pressure ventilation through a noninvasive interface (nasal mask, face mask). It can be delivered through either the modern ventilators or portable NIV devices. It has been found to be useful in acute exacerbation of COPD, immunocompromised patient with respiratory failure, acute cardiogenic pulmonary edema, postextubation support, and postoperative respiratory failure. Both NIV and continuous positive airway pressure (CPAP) have proven clinical benefit in the above situations. They, however, have been found to have no impact on outcome in patients with acute respiratory distress syndrome (ARDS) or pneumonia. In fact, a therapeutic trial with either of them in these two conditions may actually cause unnecessary delay in intubation. NIV has been found to obviate the need for intubation in >50% of properly selected patients.

Question 5

1. Describe cardiac biomarkers of importance in the ED.

Biomarkers are fundamental in establishing the diagnosis and managing cardiovascular diseases (CVD), the leading cause of morbidity and mortality in the world. The delicate nature and time sensitivity of CVD, in which minutes can hugely impact the outcome, have made biomarkers an area of continuous research and development. Cardiac troponin and B type cardiac natriuretic peptides are the two best markers utilized in clinical settings due to their major role in diagnosis and risk stratification in acute coronary syndromes (ACS) and heart failure.

Ideal cardiac biomarker: Biomarkers can have several roles, and it is an ideal situation if a single biomarker provides multiple information which is pivotal to the management in the ED. An ideal cardiac biomarker is thus expected to have most of the attributes such as early detection in blood, highly specific for cardiac injury, low cost, and availability of a sensitive assay to detect it. Clearly, no such ideal cardiac biomarker exists and usually a multimarker strategy is practiced depending on the clinical scenario, for optimal outcomes.

2. How will you set up "point-of-care" laboratory in the ED? Write the rationale behind that.

Point-of-care testing (POCT) is now a proven approach that can provide faster turnaround time (TAT) of laboratory test results. POCT is currently routine in all hospitals and has become the standard for patient care in a variety of other health care settings. Therefore, a quality assurance program is vital to managing errors and the reliability of POCT results **(Flowchart 3)**.

Rationales for setting up a point-of-care laboratory in ED:
a. Capital savings
b. Faster results
c. Faster therapeutic action
d. Increasing nursing efficiency
e. Limit opportunities for error
f. Improved patient adherence
g. Improved patient outcome

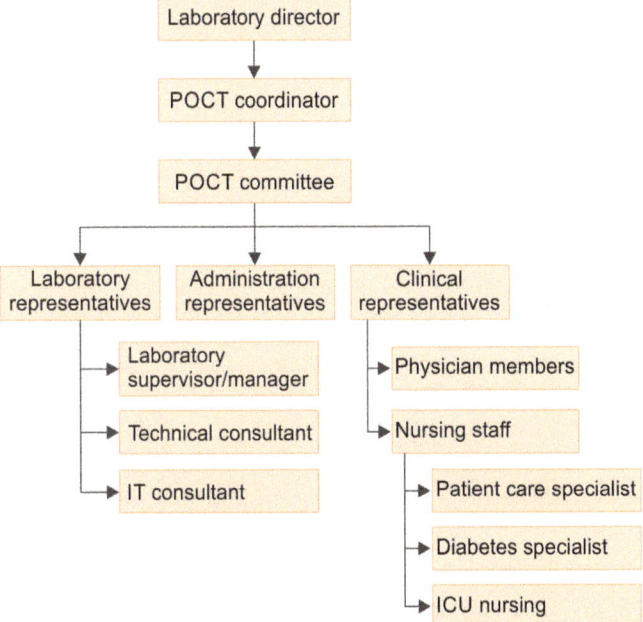

Flowchart 3: Administrative requirements for setting up a POCT laboratory.

(ICU: intensive care unit; IT: information technology; POCT: point-of-care testing)

Question 6

1. Discuss the basic principles of splinting and traction.

Acute trauma to bone leads to fracture. Acute pain and deformity prompt the patient to visit the ED. Pain management, reduction of fracture, and immobilization are the key elements in the management of factures **(Table 4)**. Many patients who sustain blunt trauma also incur injuries to the musculoskeletal system. These injuries often appear to be dramatic but only infrequently cause immediate threat to life or limb. However, musculoskeletal injuries have the potential to distract team members from more urgent resuscitation priorities. Major musculoskeletal injuries indicate that the body sustained significant forces.

TABLE 4: Common orthopedic injury and splinting procedure in the emergency department.

Injury	Orthopedic procedure/spilt
Distal phalanx fracture of the hand	Finger protector splint
Boxer's fracture	Ulnar gutter splint
Metacarpal fracture	Radial or ulnar gutter splint
Scaphoid fracture	Thumb spica splint
Carpal fracture	Dorsal splint of the forearm
Radius and ulna fracture	Sugar-tong splint
Elbow dislocation	Posterior long arm (elbow) splint
Supracondylar fracture of the humerus	Posterior long arm (elbow) splint
Proximal humerus fracture	Coaptation splint, sling, and swathe
Shoulder dislocation	Shoulder immobilizer or sling and swathe
Metatarsal fracture	Posterior short leg (posterior ankle) splint
Ankle sprain	Posterior short leg (posterior ankle) splint
Ankle dislocation	Trilaminar ankle splint
Distal tibia/fibula fracture	Trilaminar ankle splint
Knee dislocation	Knee immobilizer or knee splint
Patellar dislocation	Knee immobilizer or knee splint

Skin traction: It is used for elderly neck femur fractures and distal femur fractures as a temporary method of immobilization till a definitive method such as fixation is done.

Skeletal traction is used for effective traction for a longer period of time, through Steinmann pin or Denham (threaded) pin.

2. What are the devices used in the ED and prehospital care for splinting?

Crammer wire/malleable splints: Crammer wire is made up of malleable aluminum wires attached to a strong but flexible aluminum rod. Splint can bend easily at any angle. The main purposes are to keep the upper or lower limb in a desired position and preoperative management of patient for immobilization.

Thomas splint: It was devised by Hugh Owen Thomas. Initially used for tuberculosis of knee, it is now commonly used for immobilization of hip and thigh injuries.

Inflatable splints: These serve as good first aid and temporary measure for immobilization of fractures which surround the extremity including the digits. Few disadvantages are involved such as risk of occlusion of blood vessels become greater in the extremity in which blood supply is already compromised and unwanted high pressure may lead to necrosis of the digits. It is a plastic piece of first-aid equipment that is premade in the shape of a limb.

Coaptation splint: It is an over-the-shoulder splint to immobilize the shoulder and humerus. This splint is most commonly used for midshaft humerus fractures, which have a tendency to fall into varus angulation. By incorporating a valgus bump at the level of medial elbow, angulation can be avoided.

3. Write about types of immobilization dressings.

Upper extremities immobilization:

a. *Long arm splint and long arm cast:* These are used to immobilize distal humerus and elbow and upper forearm.
b. *Sugar-tong splint:* It is a long forearm splint to immobilize elbow and wrist. The slab is cut for thenar eminence and stops at mid-palmar crease. It is used for immobilizing Colles fracture. The reduction of a wrist is held by a long, curved mold applied to the splint, maintaining radial height and restoring volar tilt.
c. *Ulnar gutter splint:* It is a forearm splint used to immobilize wrist and 4th/5th digits.
d. *Short arm cast:* It is a way of durable immobilization of forearm and wrist.
e. *Thumb spica cast:* It immobilizes first metacarpophalangeal (MCP) and wrist joints.

Lower extremity immobilization:

a. *Long leg splinting:* It is a long, well-padded splint for immobilization of both knee and ankle.
b. *Robert Jones bulky dressing:* It implies relative knee immobilization using soft roll. It can be used for any joint though. Wrap knee with soft roll beginning over the proximal tibia and extending to the distal femur.

Question 7

1. Write about the anatomical differences in adult and child airway related to endotracheal intubation.

The relatively larger tongue and smaller oral cavity mean that, in the child, the tongue is more likely to obstruct the airway than in the adult. This makes it essential that there is correct positioning of the head and jaw to open the airway **(Table 5)**.

TABLE 5: Anatomical differences in adult and child airway.

Anatomy	Pediatric	Adult
Tongue	Large	Normal
Epiglottis shape	Floppy, omega-shaped	Firm, flatter
Epiglottis level	Level of C3–C4	Level of C5–C6
Trachea	Smaller, shorter	Wider, longer
Larynx shape	Funnel-shaped	Column
Larynx position	Angle posteriorly away from glottis	Straight up and down
Narrowest point	Subglottic region	At the level of vocal cord
Lung volume	250 mL at birth	600 mL as adult

2. Enumerate its immediate complications.

Two dangerous emergent issues in the immediate post-RSI (rapid-sequence intubation) phase are hypoxia and hypotension which should be addressed as quick as possible. Look for DOPE in all cases of post-RSI hypoxia or hypotension:

D—displacement (tube)/drugs
O—obstruction
P—pneumothorax
E—equipment failure

3. List the long-term complications of endotracheal intubation.

Complications following endotracheal intubation are given in **Table 6**.

TABLE 6: Complications of endotracheal intubation.

Traumatic	• Dental damage, perforation, or laceration of pharynx, larynx, trachea, esophagus, or vocal cord injuries • Dislocation of arytenoid cartilage
Hemodynamic and others	• Mainstem bronchus intubation • Aspiration • Hypotension • Arrythmias • Hypoxia • Hypercarbia • Laryngeal spasm • Bronchospasm
Late	• Vocal cord palsy/paresis/ulceration • Arytenoid cartilage trauma • Dysphagia • Anterior glottic web • Aspiration/aspiration pneumonia

Question 8

1. Define disaster.

As per Disaster Management Act, 2005, disaster is defined as "A catastrophe, mishap, calamity or grave occurrence in any area, arising from natural or man-made causes, or by accident or negligence which results in substantial loss of life or human suffering or damage to, and destruction of property, or damage to, or degradation of environment and is of such a nature or magnitude as to be beyond the coping capacity of the community of the affected area."

2. Write about factors that may hinder ED response to disaster.

Disaster disrupts the large number of people of a normal functioning society. It causes damage of property and loss of human life. Disaster management requires external help to manage the disaster. The following steps are important to minimize the losses:

a. *Reliability of system which detects the disaster early:* Reliable and early detection of an emergency and careful planning
b. *Coordination within the team:* Coordination and along with efficient, trained personnel
c. *Manpower:* Resources for handling emergencies
d. *Promptness:* Appropriate emergency response actions
e. *Communication:* Effective notification and communication facilities
f. *Training:* Proper training of concerned personnel.
g. *Drill:* Regular mock drill/rehearsal
h. *Corrective action:* Regular review and updating plan

3. Write about the components of hospital emergency operation plan.

Establishing the emergency operation center (EOC): It serves as central command post during a disaster, generally established outside the ED. It should be large enough for key people and support staff. It should be located in a safe area.

How to activate and when to activate incident command center (ICS) **(Table 7):**

a. Determine who will activate the ICS
b. Notifying the hospital personnel
c. Briefing all core members regarding assignments and clear immediate direction
d. Activation of ICS should be announced using standardized codes, such as "Disaster Code"

TABLE 7: Overall responsibilities of the head of incident command center.

Logistic (provide support)	Planning (prepare action plan)	Finance (cost accounting and procurement)	Operations (direct tactical action)
Responsible for acquisition and maintenance of facilities, services, personnel, equipment, and materials	• Collect, analyze, display information • Prepare incident action plan • Maintain situation and resource status • Maintain incident documentation • Prepare demobilization • Promote continuity of operations	• Monitor incident costs • Maintain financial records • Administer procurement contracts	Carry out the medical objective to the best of their ability

Other important command staff

Public information officer	Safety officer	Liaison officer
Provides information to the news media, serves as the central point for information dissemination	Monitors the facility and anticipates, detects, and corrects unsafe situations	Function as an incident contact person for representatives from other assisting and cooperating agencies

4. Describe ED disaster response including triage.

Disaster response is the immediate intervention or provision during the disaster or just after the disaster to preserve the human life and provide basic necessities to affected people. In view of complexity of the disaster, response would vary and depends on the sudden/slow onset of disaster, place of disaster (rural, urban, mountain, coastal, or marine), and magnitude of disaster (managed with local authority or need central government assistance). Components are assignment of task, strategies to handle the situation, coordination, and communication policy **(Table 8)**. Triaging [START (simple triage and rapid treatment) or SALT (sort, assess, lifesaving interventions, treatment/transport) for adult and jumpSTART for pediatric)] of mass casualty and their treatment should be followed.

TABLE 8: Sequence of activities in the ED during mass casualty management.

Assignments	Strategies	Coordination
• Assembly of team • Roles and responsibilities • Personal protection • Equipment distribution	• Patient identifications • Triage tagging • Documentation	• With command center • Use of mobile

Mass casualty: Triaging and treatment
- Victim identification
- Rapid vitals assessment and physical examination
- Tagging according to triage categories
- Care priorities
- Documentation
- Disposition
- Regular communication with emergency command center (EOC)

Debriefing
- Evaluation of triaging decisions and evaluation of strategies
- Assessment of medical and diagnostic performance
- Discussion about communication and management skills

Question 9

1. Discuss the basic principles of decontamination in cases of poisoning.

Decontamination: Personal protective equipment (gown, gloves, goggles) should be used by healthcare providers while undressing the patients who are exposed to toxic substances. Plenty of water is used to clean the patient. Clothing of the patient should be collected, sealed, and disposed of properly. If eyes are exposed to the toxins, they should be washed with plenty of crystalloid solution and the patient may require local anesthetics and ophthalmologist consultation.

Gastric decontamination: Emesis, orogastric lavage, single-dose activated charcoal, and whole bowel irrigation are the methods used for gastric decontamination. None of the methods of gastric decontamination showed positive effects on clinical outcome in the management of the poisoned patient. There is no role of induction of emesis by ipecac syrup for emptying the stomach of the poisoned patient.

Urinary alkalinization: It is useful for weak acids and moderate to severe salicylate toxicity when criteria for initiation of hemodialysis are not fulfilled. Correct the hypokalemia before starting the urinary alkalinization. Forced diuresis has no role in treatment of any poisoning, toxicity, or overdose.

Extracorporeal removal of poison: Hemodialysis, hemoperfusion, and continuous renal replacement therapy can be used as per availability but have limited indications.

2. What is ocular decontamination?

When something toxic gets into the eye, flushing with large amounts of room-temperature liquids can reduce injury to the cornea and help with systemic absorption, if that is an issue. Normal saline is preferred for use in the eyes. However, with the duration that most eyes must be flushed, tepid tap water is good to use but not the best solution. For most liquids, 10 minutes of flushing is ideal. However, for caustic substances, 15–20 minutes of flushing is absolutely essential.

3. What is gastric decontamination?

Gastric lavage: Gastric lavage, once very popular for removal of the ingested poison, is now rarely indicated. There is no evidence that gastric lavage changes the outcome in poisoned patients. Gastric lavage should be considered for life-threatening poison if presentation is within a few minutes (<1 hour) of ingestion. Similarly, single-dose activated charcoal or multidose activated charcoal are also not beneficial in specific or undifferentiated poison. They can be used within <1 hour of ingestion of poison. 50 g of activated charcoal is sufficient. Whole bowel irrigation is rarely used now and is unpleasant for both the patient and the staff.

The role of gastric lavage is highly controversial. While the western literature is bluntly stating this as a harmful procedure, one needs to consider the regional variation in the poisoning scenario. While India is still suffering from poisonings such as organophosphorus compounds (OPC), weedicides, and many plant poisons which are lethal with prolonged toxicity, Western countries have almost switched to tablet overdoses which are quickly absorbed into the circulation and the availability of antidotes and easy access to extracorporeal removal made their researchers conclude that gastric lavage is either harmful or contraindicated in a patient who was brought to the emergency room after an hour of drug overdose or poison. But even Western literature suggests gastric lavage in sustained-release tablets or preparations. The most common agricultural poison, OPC, remains in enterohepatic circulation for longer duration and its prolonged toxicity cannot be ruled out. Considering the variation in the poisoning scenario, unavailability of antidotes, and nature of poisons, I still feel that agricultural poisons deserve a good gastric lavage and late presentation tablet overdoses do not require lavage. As we practice in a country with a mixed culture, we should justify the role of lavage appropriately on an individual basis.

Question 10

You are the ED in-charge. One of your doctors/staff had a needle-stick injury while he was doing invasive lifesaving procedures on an HIV- and HBsAg-positive victim in the ED. How will you guide him?

1. What are the immediate actions to be taken?

Do not panic. Do not put cut/prick finger.

Post-HIV exposure management/prophylaxis: It is necessary to determine the status of the exposure and the HIV status of the exposure source before starting postexposure prophylaxis (PEP).

Immediate measures: Wash with soap and water. There is no added advantage with antiseptic/bleach.

Next step: Prompt reporting. Postexposure treatment should begin as soon as possible, preferably within 2 hours. It is not recommended after 72 hours.

2. What are the initial baseline investigations to be done?

Initial baseline investigations of exposed human immunodeficiency virus (HIV) I and II, hepatitis B surface antigen (HBsAg), hepatitis C virus (HCV), and hepatitis B surface antibody (anti-HBs).

The health care provider should be tested for HIV as per the following schedule:
a. *Baseline HIV test:* At the time of exposure
b. *Repeat HIV test:* At 6 weeks following exposure
c. *Second repeat HIV test:* At 12 weeks following exposure

On all three occasions, health care workers (HCW) must be provided with a pre-test and post-test counseling. HIV testing should be carried out on three test kits or antigen preparations, namely ERS [enzyme-linked immunosorbent assay (ELISA)/rapid/simple)]. The HCW should be advised to refrain from donating blood, semen, or organs/tissues and abstain from sexual intercourse. In case sexual intercourse is undertaken, a latex condom should be used consistently. In addition, women HCW should not breastfeed their infants during the follow-up period.

3. Which medicines/injections you would like to give him immediately?

The decision to start PEP is made on the basis of degree of exposure to HIV and the HIV status of the source from whom the exposure/infection has occurred.

Basic regimen: Zidovudine (AZT)—600 mg in divided doses (300 mg/twice a day or 200 mg/thrice a day) for 4 weeks + Lamivudine (3TC)—150 mg twice a day for 4 weeks.

Expanded regimen: (4 weeks therapy) Basic regimen + Indinavir—800 mg/thrice a day, or any other protease inhibitor.

4. Describe how to follow him up.

Postexposure prophylaxis should be started, as early as possible, after an exposure. It has been seen that PEP started after 72 hours of exposure is of no use and hence is not recommended. The optimal course of PEP is not unknown, but 4 weeks of drug therapy appear to provide protection against HIV. If the HIV test is found to be positive at any time within 12 weeks, the HCW should be referred to a physician for treatment.

SUGGESTED READING

1. Richhariya D, Sharma B. Textbook of Emergency Medicine including Intensive Care and Trauma, 2nd edition. New Delhi: Jaypee Brothers Medical Publishers (P) Ltd; 2022. pp. 296-300. (Question 1).
2. Richhariya D, Sharma B. Textbook of Emergency Medicine including Intensive Care and Trauma, 2nd edition. New Delhi: Jaypee Brothers Medical Publishers (P) Ltd; 2022. pp. 312-3. (Question 2).
3. Richhariya D, Sharma B. Textbook of Emergency Medicine including Intensive Care and Trauma, 2nd edition. New Delhi: Jaypee Brothers Medical Publishers (P) Ltd; 2022. pp. 1692-6. (Question 3).
4. Richhariya D, Sharma B. Textbook of Emergency Medicine including Intensive Care and Trauma, 2nd edition. New Delhi: Jaypee Brothers Medical Publishers (P) Ltd; 2022. pp. 570-4. (Question 4).
5. Richhariya D, Sharma B. Textbook of Emergency Medicine including Intensive Care and Trauma, 2nd edition. New Delhi: Jaypee Brothers Medical Publishers (P) Ltd; 2022. pp. 434-7. (Question 5).
6. Richhariya D, Sharma B. Textbook of Emergency Medicine including Intensive Care and Trauma, 2nd edition. New Delhi: Jaypee Brothers Medical Publishers (P) Ltd; 2022. pp. 1621-35. (Question 6).
7. Richhariya D, Sharma B. Textbook of Emergency Medicine including Intensive Care and Trauma, 2nd edition. New Delhi: Jaypee Brothers Medical Publishers (P) Ltd; 2022. pp. 214-6. (Question 7).
8. Richhariya D, Sharma B. Textbook of Emergency Medicine including Intensive Care and Trauma, 2nd edition. New Delhi: Jaypee Brothers Medical Publishers (P) Ltd; 2022. pp. 172-9. (Question 8).
9. Richhariya D, Sharma B. Textbook of Emergency Medicine including Intensive Care and Trauma, 2nd edition. New Delhi: Jaypee Brothers Medical Publishers (P) Ltd; 2022. pp. 1394-5. (Question 9).
10. Richhariya D, Sharma B. Textbook of Emergency Medicine including Intensive Care and Trauma, 2nd edition. New Delhi: Jaypee Brothers Medical Publishers (P) Ltd; 2022. p. 1373. (Question 10).

Emergency Medicine Paper 18

Devendra Richhariya

Question 1

1. Enumerate causes of acute pancreatitis.

Gallstone disease and alcohol are the most common causes of acute pancreatitis across the world **(Table 1)**. Differential diagnosis includes perforation, myocardial infarction, acute cholecystitis, choledocholithiasis, intestinal obstruction, bowel ischemia, etc.

2. Describe the methods to assess the severity of acute pancreatitis in the ED.

The most important aspect of managing an acute pancreatitis patient is assessment of severity. It is always a challenge to talk to the relatives about severity of an attack and the likely outcome, i.e., the prognosis. There are various scales available to assess the severity such as Ranson's, Imrie's, and APACHE II (acute physiology and chronic health evaluation), etc., but BISAP (bedside index for severity in acute pancreatitis) score is the easiest to use at bedside **(Table 2)**. The entire exercise of assessment is to know which patients have organ failure because the outcome depends on the number of organs involved **(Table 3)**.

TABLE 1: Causes of acute pancreatitis.

Common causes	• Gallstones • Alcohol • Hypertriglyceridemia • ERCP • Drugs [azathioprine, 6-mercaptopurine, sulfonamides, estrogen, tetracycline, valproic acid, anti-HIV medications, 5-ASA] • Trauma (especially blunt abdominal trauma) • Postoperative (abdominal and nonabdominal operations)
Uncommon causes	• Vascular causes and vasculitis (ischemic-hypoperfusion states after cardiac surgery) • Connective tissue disorders and TTP • Cancer of the pancreas • Hypercalcemia (hyperparathyroidism) • Periampullary diverticulum • Pancreas divisum • Hereditary pancreatitis • Viral and parasitic (mumps, coxsackievirus, cytomegalovirus, echovirus, *Ascaris*) • Autoimmune
Recurrent acute pancreatitis without an obvious cause	• Microlithiasis, biliary sludge • Drugs • Alcohol abuse (hidden) • Hypertriglyceridemia, hypercalcemia • Pancreas divisum with minor papilla stenosis • Pancreatic cancer • Intraductal papillary mucinous neoplasm IPMN • Cystic fibrosis • Idiopathic

(5-ASA: 5-aminosalicylic acid; ERCP: endoscopic retrograde cholangiopancreatography; HIV: human immunodeficiency virus; IPMN: intraductal papillary mucinous neoplasm; TTP: thrombotic thrombocytopenic purpura)
Note: In about 20% of patents, causes still remain idiopathic after all investigations.

TABLE 2: BISAP (bedside index in severity of acute pancreatitis) score.

BUN	BUN >25 mg/dL (8.9 mmol/L)	1 point
Impaired mental status	Abnormal mental status with a Glasgow coma score <15	1 point
SIRS	Evidence of SIRS	1 point
Age	Age >60 years old	1 point
Pleural effusion	Imaging study reveals pleural effusion	1 point

(BUN: blood urea nitrogen; SIRS: systemic inflammatory response syndrome)
Note: Score: 0–2 points: Lower mortality (<2%); 3–5 points: Higher mortality (>15%).

TABLE 3: Markers of severe acute pancreatitis.

Risk factors for severity	• Age >60 years • Obesity, BMI >30 kg/m^2 • Comorbid disease (Charlson comorbidity index)
Markers of severity at admission or within 24 hours	• *SIRS:* Defined by presence of two or more criteria: • Core temperature <36°C or >38°C • Heart rate >90 beats/min • Respirations >20 breaths/min or PCO$_2$ <32 mm Hg • White blood cell count >12,000/μL, <4,000/μL, or 10% bands • APACHE II • Hemoconcentration (hematocrit >44%), admission, BUN (>22 mg/dL) • BISAP score ≥3
Markers of severity during hospitalization	• Persistent organ failure • Pancreatic necrosis

(APACHE: acute physiology and chronic health evaluation; BISAP: bedside index for severity of acute pancreatitis; BMI: body mass index; BUN: blood urea nitrogen; PCO$_2$: partial pressure of carbon dioxide)

3. Write about only diagnostic studies in patients with suspected acute pancreatitis.

a. Diagnosis should be considered in any patient who comes with severe abdominal pain in upper abdomen/back/chest, is apparently in distress, and has vomiting, tachycardia, epigastric tenderness, and pain that is not easily controlled with analgesics. He may be an alcoholic or there may be a past history of pancreatitis/biliary colic.
b. Investigations in the emergency department (ED) that would help to differentiate all these are electrocardiogram (ECG), complete blood count (CBC), liver function test (LFT), amylase, creatinine, abdominal X-ray (both erect and supine), and ultrasonography (USG). No laboratory test is gold standard of acute pancreatitis. Amylase or lipase values should be at least three times the upper limit of the normal values according to the current recommendations.
c. *Lipase* is more specific for pancreatic injury, remains elevated for longer period of time, and is less associated with nonpancreatic disease. *Urine trypsinogen-2 dipstick test* is a noninvasive rapid test with high sensitivity and specificity, which is less in use because of limited availability.
d. In case of diagnostic dilemma, it is best to do contrast-enhanced computed tomography (CECT) scan of the abdomen within few hours in the ED itself. But if the diagnosis of acute pancreatitis is clear based on blood test and imaging, then it is wise to delay CT scan for 3–4 days as necrosis is not picked up early and you will anyway have to repeat a CT scan on day 4 or day 5.

Question 2

1. Describe the pathophysiology of otitis media.

The outer one third of the external auditory canal has an incomplete cartilage whereas the inner two third is composed of bone with a tight overlying skin attachment that easily injures due to a minute trauma.

The blood supply is from the superior temporal vessels in the anterior part and the posterior auricular vessels in its posterior part. The connection of the posterior auricular vein to the sigmoid sinus is a source of the intracranial spread of infections.

2. Write about the microbiology of otitis media.

The most common bacterial pathogens recovered in adults with *acute otitis media (OM)* are *Streptococcus pneumoniae, Haemophilus influenzae*, methicillin-sensitive *Staphylococcus aureus*, and *Pseudomonas aeruginosa*. Young adults remain protected from all *Haemophilus* strains as they have received the *H. influenzae* type b vaccine. The predominant organisms involved in *chronic OM* are *S. aureus, P. aeruginosa, Aspergillus*, and anerobic bacteria (less common). *Viral OM* caused predominantly by respiratory syncytial virus and rhinovirus occurs in those under the age of 10 years.

3. Write about the acute and long-term complications of OM.

Complications of OM are tympanic membrane perforation, hearing loss, acute serous labyrinthitis, facial nerve paralysis, acute mastoiditis, lateral sinus thrombosis, cholesteatoma, and intracranial complications (meningitis and brain abscess).

Question 3

1. Enumerate various causes of acute scrotal pain.

The presentation of an acute scrotum can be broken down into four subcategories: (1) painful swollen testicle, (2) painless swollen testicle, (3) erythematous testicle, and (4) traumatic testicle. Within each of these groups, there is a diagnosis that cannot be missed. However, not all scrotal emergencies present with pain in the genital area. It is important to rule out scrotal emergencies in patients presenting with lower abdominal pain **(Table 4)**.

TABLE 4: Differential diagnoses for acute scrotal pain.	
Ischemic	Testicular torsion, torsion of the testicular appendage
Infectious	Epididymitis, epididymoorchitis, orchitis, scrotal cellulitis, scrotal abscess, Fournier's gangrene, Hansen's disease, filariasis
Traumatic	*Blunt:* Testicular contusion, testicular rupture, penetrating testicular rupture, hematocele, scrotal degloving
Inflammatory	Henoch-Schönlein purpura
Idiopathic	Idiopathic scrotal swelling
Oncologic	Testicular tumors
Other	Strangulated/incarcerated inguinal hernia, referred pain from abdominal pathology, e.g., ruptured abdominal aortic aneurysm or nephrolithiasis

2. Write how to differentiate clinically important causes of acute scrotal pain.

The differential diagnosis of painful scrotal swelling is given in **Table 5**.

3. Discuss the treatment option for testicular torsion in ED.

a. Testicular torsion is a time-sensitive emergency. Manual detorsion can be attempted before surgical intervention but should not delay surgical intervention. *Trials of manual detorsion* have been found to decrease ischemia time. Even if the testicle is manually detorsed, surgery is still required. Surgical exploration is the definitive management for testicular torsion. Before performing manual detorsion, it must be explained that the procedure is painful but, if successful, it will alleviate the pain. Analgesic medication, local analgesia injection (i.e., local lidocaine), or procedural sedation should be administered.

b. Stand at the foot of the bed or to the right of the patient. Holding the testicle between the thumb and index finger, rotate it in an outward direction (like opening a book) from medial to lateral. The initial attempt should be with one and a half full rotations (540°). Relief from pain is a positive end point. You can also reassess with bedside USG. If the pain worsened with detorsion in the medial to lateral rotation, detorse in the lateral to medial direction, because one third of testicular torsions occur with medial to lateral rotation.

c. After manual detorsion, the patient still requires emergent surgical intervention. The urologist will expose the scrotum in the operating room and examine the testicle for viability after detorsion of the spermatic cord. If viable, the testicle is sutured into the inner scrotal lining (also known as an orchiopexy). The noninvolved testicle is also sutured into the lining to prevent torsion. If the testicle is found to be nonviable, the patient will undergo unilateral orchiectomy.

TABLE 5: Comparing testicular torsion, epididymitis, and appendage torsion.			
History	**Testicular torsion**	**Epididymitis**	**Appendage torsion**
Age	Neonates and adolescents	Adolescents and young adults	Prepubertal
Pain onset	Acute	Gradual progressive	Acute to subacute
Associated symptoms	Nausea and vomiting	Dysuria	
Physical examination		Fever	
Cremasteric reflex	Absent	Present/absent	Present/absent
Testicles	Testicular swelling, progressive to diffuse hemiscrotal involvement, high riding, transverse alignment	Epididymal swelling progressing to diffuse hemiscrotal involvement, normal position	Head of the affected testicle or epididymis, normal position

Question 4

1. Write about the anatomy of importance related to epistaxis.

Nasal mucosa has a very rich blood supply from internal carotid artery (ICA) and external carotid artery (ECA). Kiesselbach's plexus (Little's area) is situated anteriorly and formed by anterior and posterior ethmoidal arteries (branches of ICA), sphenopalatine artery, and branches of internal maxillary artery (branches of ECA). Posteriorly, nasal mucosa gets blood supply from the posterior branches of the sphenopalatine artery **(Fig. 1)**. Pathology behind epistaxis is erosion of mucosa and rupture of superficial arteries or veins. Nearly 90% of the patients present with anterior epistaxis from Little's area. Rest 10% of the patients present with posterior epistaxis that is more serious than anterior epistaxis and more commonly seen in old age patients with comorbidities.

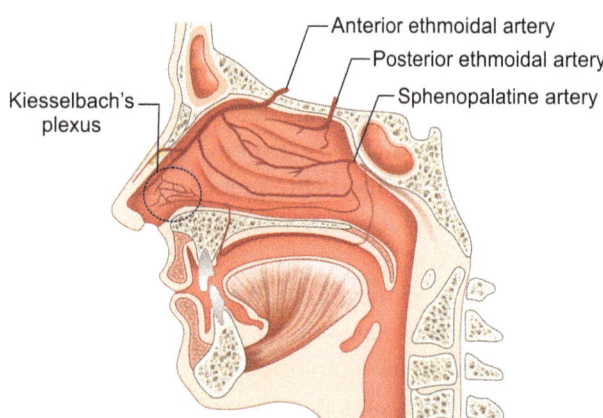

Fig. 1: Nasal anatomy.

2. Write about the ED management of such cases.

a. *History:* For stable patients, nasal and systemic history are important. Specific questions regarding duration, severity, frequency, location, laterality, precipitating factors of epistaxis and methods used to stop epistaxis need to be asked. Past medical history, use of medication [especially aspirin, warfarin, nonsteroidal anti-inflammatory drugs (NSAIDs), heparin, ticlopidine, dipyridamole], and family history should be documented.
b. *Physical examination:* Check vitals of the patient. Make the patient stable if any abnormality is observed. Nasal examination requires nasal examination instruments including nasal speculum, adequate illumination, and proper suction, topical medicines, cauterization, and packing material ready.
c. *Topical vasoconstrictor* (0.05% oxymetazoline) is beneficial in hemorrhage control and localizing bleeding point. Clots should be suctioned out for better examination. The nasal floor should be parallel to the room floor. Tilted head would restrict visualization to the anterior and upper part of the nasal cavity only. Nasal speculum is used for internal examination.
d. *Posterior epistaxis:* It should be suspected in patients with constant posterior pharyngeal trickling even after placing anterior packing; epistaxis from both nares and location of bleed cannot be visualized from anterior examination. Fiberoptic endoscopy by an experienced consultant is an advanced option for better visualization of nasal cavity and nasopharynx. Throat examination would complete examination in patients with epistaxis. Trickling of blood on the posterior pharyngeal wall would indicate posterior epistaxis and ongoing bleeding.
e. *Blood investigations:* These are not routinely indicated in single infrequent cases. For recurrent bleeding or for a patient with other comorbidities, few routing blood tests can be done, i.e., complete blood count (CBC), PT-INR (prothrombin time-international normalized ratio), activated partial thromboplastin time (aPTT), liver function tests (LFTs), etc. CT scan or MRI is indicated to evaluate surgical anatomy or local pathology. Angiography is rarely required.
f. *Treatment:* First stage of treatment is to maintain hemodynamic instability. Hypotension or hypertension should be managed accordingly. Local treatment of epistaxis is divided into *surgical and nonsurgical management*. The aim of management is to identify and control the source of bleeding. There are various methods to control bleeding:
   i. Manual hemostasis
   ii. Cauterization
   iii. Nasal packing: Anterior and posterior nasal packing
   iv. Surgical treatment.

Question 5

A 46-year-old patient was brought to the ED after 1 hour of accident. On presentation, he is talking incomprehensible words. His vitals are respiratory rate (RR) 32 breaths/min, oxygen saturation (SpO$_2$) 92% on room air, pulse rate (PR) 118 beats/min, and blood pressure (BP) 88/60 mm Hg. He is opening his eyes to painful stimuli. He withdraws right upper and lower limb on painful stimuli with no movement of the left side. The right pupil is fixed and dilated.

1. What is his Glasgow Coma Scale (GCS)?

Talking incomprehensible words—score 3
Opening his eyes to painful stimuli—score 2
Withdraws right upper and lower limb on painful stimuli—score 4

Total score—score 9

Category: Moderate-to-severe traumatic brain injury (TBI)

2. Describe a stepwise approach to the patient in ED.

Moderate and severe TBI: A patient with moderate TBI has a GCS score of 9–13. The patient can present with a variety of clinical features such as worsening headache, nausea, confusion, seizure, and loss of consciousness. The patient may present with isolated facial trauma or polytrauma associated with focal neurologic deficits.

a. The emergency physician should be more cautious while managing this type of patient. Initially, patients are able to talk but gradually their GCS score deteriorates significantly and consistently with severe TBI. Most of the patients have extra-axial hematoma: epidural or subdural. These patients have better clinical outcomes if the TBI is detected early and treated rapidly.
b. Successful management depends upon frequent assessment of GCS score, close observation for minor mental status changes, focal neurologic findings, frequent use of CT scanning, and early neurosurgical intervention.
c. In the (ED) if the patient presents with moderate TBI with herniation, immediate intervention like hyperventilation and osmotic therapy should be initiated and consideration should be given for surgical evacuation of hematoma before transferring to a definitive care unit. All moderate TBI patients should undergo CT scan and admitted to the observation unit for frequent neurological examination and monitoring and repeat CT scan should be done if required.

Severe TBI is when the patient presents acutely with a GCS score of 8 or less. Any intracranial contusion, hematoma, or brain laceration is considered as a severe TBI. Patients with severe TBI and with increase in intracranial pressure (ICP) present with symptoms of progressive hypertension, bradycardia, and shallow or irregular respiration (Cushing's reflex/phenomenon). These features represent the life-threatening raised ICP and require urgent ICP management such as hyperventilation, osmotic therapy, and surgical decompression.

ED Care

Assessment of all head injuries of the patients should be done within 15 minutes of arrival:
a. Airway, breathing, and circulation (ABC) assessment and management
b. Assessment of risk factors
c. CT scan of head and cervical spine imaging and other body areas
d. Consciousness of patient should be assessed immediately
e. An anesthetist or critical care physician should provide appropriate airway management and assist with resuscitation in a patient with GCS of 8 or less.
f. A standard head injury proforma should be used for documentation.

3. How will you prevent further brain injuries?

Airway, breathing, and circulation: Head trauma management starts with assessment and stabilization of the airway, breathing, and circulation, like for any other critically ill patient.

a. Rapid-sequence endotracheal intubation with in-line stabilization of the cervical spine should be considered for airway protection for patients with a GCS < 8.
b. Maintain partial pressure of arterial oxygen (PaO_2) >60 mm Hg and SpO_2 >90%. Hypoxia and hypotension are associated with the increase in mortality.
c. Maintain normocarbia [partial pressure of arterial carbon dioxide ($PaCO_2$) around 35 mm Hg] and avoid hyperventilation in patients with TBI; hyperventilation produces vasoconstriction and further ischemia which decreases cerebral perfusion.
d. Similarly, hypercarbia produces vasodilation, raised intracranial tension, and clinical deterioration.
e. Use of hyperventilation should be restricted only to acutely herniating and deteriorating patients while arranging for emergency craniotomy.

Fluid resuscitation: Choosing the right fluid is an important aspect for head trauma management. Maintain normovolemia by intravenous fluid, blood, and blood products.

a. Ringer's lactate and normal saline are ideal solutions for resuscitation of TBI. Hypotonic and glucose-containing fluids should not be used.
b. Normal serum sodium level should be maintained.
c. Hyponatremia causes brain edema. Vasopressor can be used in neurogenic shock due to spinal cord injury.

Measures to maintain ICP: It is important to maintain equal volume of each compartment [brain, blood, and cerebrospinal fluid (CSF)] of the skull. ICP monitoring is preferred in severe traumatic injury by placing external ventricular drain which is helpful in measuring the global ICP and controlling it by CSF drainage.

a. Mannitol is helpful in reducing the raised ICP. It should not be used in hypotensive patients. It is highly recommended as bolus (1 g/kg) in an acutely deteriorating and herniating patient provided the patient is normovolemic and normotensive.

b. Hypertonic saline is also helpful in reducing the raised ICP. 3% concentration is frequently used and hypertonic saline can be used in a hypotensive patient.
c. Barbiturates are also helpful in reducing the raised ICP, but should not be used in a hypotensive and hypovolemic patient. So these are not helpful in the acute resuscitative phase.
d. Hypothermia is also helpful in reducing the raised ICP.
e. Prophylactic hypothermia is neuroprotective and its beneficial effects are seen in severe TBI.

Anticonvulsant: Possibility of seizure in head trauma increases with increase of severity of head injury. Patients with severe TBI are more prone to seizures. Seizures can be controlled by anticonvulsants such as phenytoin, fosphenytoin, diazepam, and lorazepam.

Scalp wound: This should be inspected carefully and cleaned adequately. Stop hemorrhage by applying direct pressure or bleeding vessels ligation. Sutures or staples can be applied. CT scan of the head should be performed to exclude or confirm the skull fracture.

A *neurosurgeon's advice* should be taken for all cases of open/depressed skull fracture.

Question 6

1. Describe incomplete spinal cord syndrome.

Incomplete spinal cord syndrome (ISCS) occurs when lesions involve specific structural and/or functional anatomic regions of the cord, with some preservation of sensory and/or motor function below the lesion **(Fig. 2)**.

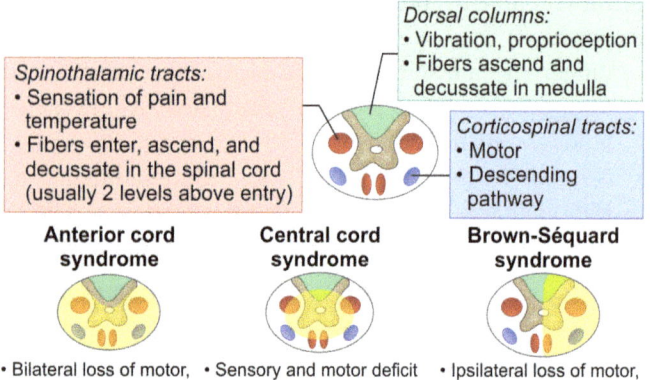

Fig. 2: Types of incomplete spinal cord syndrome.

The clinical presentation of the ISCS is largely determined by the involvement of the three tracts: (1) Corticospinal tract, (2) spinothalamic tract, and (3) posterior column of the spinal cord. There are eight types of ISCS based on the clinical presentations: (a) Central cord syndrome, (b) Brown-Séquard syndrome (unilateral cord syndrome), (c) anterior cord syndrome, (d) posterior syndrome, (e) caudal equine syndrome, (f) conus medullaris syndrome, (g) subacute combined degeneration myelopathy, and (h) cruciate paralysis.

Central cord syndrome occurs due to syringomyelia. Anterior cord syndrome occurs due to anterior spinal artery occlusion. Posterior cord syndrome occurs due to posterior spinal artery occlusion.

2. Discuss the management of neurogenic shock.

Neurogenic shock and spinal shock: In spinal cord injury (SCI), there are two conditions, namely *neurogenic shock* and *spinal shock*. Neurogenic shock is a cardiovascular event. It occurs when there is a SCI above the T6 level. The sympathetic nerve gets affected and due to peripheral vasodilatation, there is hypotension. Patients cannot develop tachycardia as the sympathetic nerves to the heart are affected. This is treated with fluids followed by vasopressors if necessary. *Spinal shock* is the state of complete paralysis due to SCI. There is flaccid paralysis with loss of reflexes including anal wink and bulbocavernosus reflex. This will recover as the neurological condition improves. SCI is often overlooked in (a) head injury, (b) intoxication, and (c) polytrauma. Maintaining mean arterial pressure (MAP) at 85–90 mm Hg for 7 days has been found to improve outcomes. The presence of bradycardia with hypotension can be due to neurogenic shock, while head injury produces hypertension and bradycardia.

Use of steroids: The 2016 Cochrane review recommended against the use of steroids. But the AO Spine 2017 guidelines recommend the use of steroids, i.e., methylprednisolone intravenously within 8 hours of cervical spine injury and continued for 24 hours. The dose of steroid should be 30 mg/kg bolus followed by 5.4 mg/kg/h for 23 hours. An increased risk of sepsis (pneumonia or septicemia) was noted with 48-hour steroid administration.

Question 7

A 56-year-old male whose weight is 70 kg has been brought to the ED with second-degree burns involving both upper limbs. He had an unsuccessful attempt trying to save his wife from fire within a closed compartment having cool garments. He is highly agitated and coughing black sputum.

1. What are the initial concerns in managing this case?

Treatment protocol: Remove all clothing immediately. Areas exposed to source of burns should be washed with water at 20–25°C temperature to avoid hypothermia.

a. *Circulation, airway, and breathing:* A burn patient is treated as any trauma patient; treatment guidelines should be followed as per advanced trauma life support (ATLS) protocol. Primarily, endotracheal intubation should be done where it is suspected or needed. In worst case scenario, tracheostomy must be done to secure airway at the earliest and ensure oxygen supply.
b. *Establish an intravenous access:* In cases of larger surface area burns, it is imperative to secure a "central" catheterization. It is better to access the subclavian vein than the femoral vein.
c. If central catheterization is difficult, a 16–18-gauge needle (spinal needle is compatible) is approached from distal femoral or proximal tibial bone marrow under local anesthesia. Intravenous fluid administration can be initiated at 100 mL/h. During this, other sites for peripheral access can be established by other medical ED personnel.
d. *Avoid systemic hypothermia:* In order to prevent systemic hypothermia, intravenous fluids need to be administered at temperature closer to the body temperature.
e. *Polytrauma:* In higher percentage of burns, the victim is likely to endure other injuries, in some cases due to subsequent fall or trauma associated with the event. Serial examinations of upper and lower limbs and TBI must be carried out. If any concomitant injury is present, the designated department should be involved. A burns surgeon needs to be followed up with for management of burns.
f. *Ocular injury:* Both eyes are irrigated well to remove all irritants, dust, and debris. An ophthalmologist is consulted for further treatment.

Maintaining analgesia for the burns patient:
a. Exposed areas are kept under running water for both pain relief and to prevent further heat from being dissipated to the underlying tissues.
b. In order to prevent hypothermia, the patient needs to be covered well even in unburnt areas. Avoid using ice coolants for local application.
c. Pain relief is administered immediately to relieve anxiety and stress. Intravenous administration is preferred due to vasoconstriction as compared to intramuscular or subcutaneous routes.
d. Steady increments of morphine on an hourly basis are preferred to establish the most preferred method of pain relief. In a patient associated with respiratory injury, opioids can only be used with close monitoring of ventilation.
e. Careful and precise titration of drugs on infusion should be done. One must look out for respiratory and hemodynamic changes.
f. In order to perform escharotomy/fasciotomy, it is done ideally in the burns center. Analgesics such as tramadol and ketamine are most used in these surgical approaches.
g. General anesthesia is preferred for children or stressed adults for surgical interventions.

2. How will you manage various inhalational injuries produced by smoke?

Inhalation injuries cause formation of casts, reduction of available surfactant, increased airway resistance, and decreased pulmonary compliance. These patients require aggressive measures to keep airway free of mucus and other secretions such as chest physiotherapy, airway suctioning, therapeutic serial bronchoscopies, and early aggressive ambulation. Bronchodilators that are useful in the treatment of inhalation injury include albuterol or levalbuterol for wheezing/bronchospasm, and racemic epinephrine for stridor or retractions, typically administered every 4 hours **(Table 6)**.

TABLE 6: Smoke inhalation injury.

Injury subtype	Mechanism	Clinical consequences	Treatment
Upper airway injury	Thermal burn from heat transfer	Airway edema and obstruction	• Titrate humidified oxygen to maintain saturation >90% • If airway obstruction, definitive airway management • Bronchodilators • Fiberoptic bronchoscopy to evaluate lower respiratory tract inhalation injury • Respiratory physiotherapy and mucolytics • Weaning ventilation • Extubation planning
Lower airway parenchyma	Chemical and particulate irritants	• Fibrin cast obstructs the airways • Inflammation • Ventilation–perfusion mismatch • Atelectasis • Bronchospasm	
Systemic cellular dysfunction due to carbon monoxide and cyanide exposure	Asphyxia and hypoxia	• Lactic acidosis • CNS insult • CVS insult	

(CNS: central nervous system; CVS: cardiovascular system)

3. Discuss Parkland formula for fluid resuscitation in such cases.

The following formulas are recommended by guidelines for estimating the fluid requirement in a burn patient; however, fluid therapy can be modified according to the condition of the patient and prognosis of the injuries.

Adult: Fluid requirement is calculated for the initial 24 hours from the onset of burns by Parkland formula given below and total fluid is given over 24 hours as shown in **Flowchart 1**:

Parkland formula: Lactated Ringer's solution, 4 mL/kg of body weight × %TBSA (total body surface area)

Modified Brooke's formula: 2 mL/kg of body weight/%TBSA

Flowchart 1: Distribution of adequate fluid resuscitation over 24 hours.

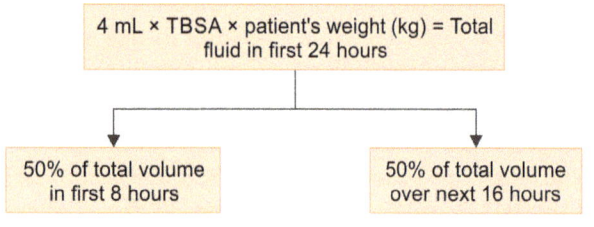

Question 8

A 30-year-old patient is brought to the ED with acute loss of vision.

1. Enumerate causes if the patient has painful vision loss.

2. Enumerate causes if he has painless loss of vision.

Painful diminution of vision, e.g., acute angle closure glaucoma, acute iridocyclitis, and acute keratitis/corneal ulcer. Retinal vein occlusion is one of the most common causes of sudden unilateral painless loss of vision **(Table 7)**.

TABLE 7: Causes of painful and painless vison loss.		
	Unilateral	Bilateral
Painful vision loss	• Corneal abrasion • Acute angle closure glaucoma • Inflammation • Cavernous sinus thrombosis • Toxic/caustic exposure • Trauma	• Keratitis • Toxic/caustic exposure • Trauma
Painless vision loss	• Retinal detachment • Vitreous detachment/hemorrhage • Retinal artery/vein occlusion • Lens dislocation • Ischemic optic neuropathy	• Stroke • Medication • Metabolic derangement • Psychogenic

Question 9

1. Enumerate emergencies in the first 20 weeks of pregnancy.

Obstetric emergencies can arise at any point in time, and it is important to diagnose the condition and institute prompt treatment as needed. The early half of the pregnancy can have complications related to miscarriages or infections arising as a result of unsafe abortions. In the second half of the pregnancy, antepartum hemorrhage complicates 3–5% of pregnancies. Of these, there are two types: placenta previa, where the placenta is implanted partially or completely in the lower uterine segment, and abruptio placenta **(Table 8)**.

TABLE 8: Emergencies during pregnancy	
First 20 weeks of pregnancy	Nausea, vomiting, hyperemesis gravidarum, spontaneous abortion, and septic abortion

After 20 weeks of pregnancy	• *Chronic and gestational hypertension:*
	  – Preeclampsia
	  – HELLP
	  – Eclampsia
	• Placenta previa
	• Vasa previa
	• Premature rupture of membrane
	• Preterm labor

(HELLP: hemolysis, elevated liver enzymes, low platelet count)

2. Write in detail about the management of a patient presenting with ectopic pregnancy.

Rapid fluid resuscitation: Ectopic pregnancy is a time-specific emergency. Immediate ABC assessment should be done and volume status should be supported by intravenous fluid, blood, and blood products. Further management decisions should be taken on the basis of USG and beta human chorionic gonadotropin (β-hCG).

Surgical treatment: Generally laparoscopy/sometimes laparotomy—this decision will depend upon the patient's condition, doctor's expertise, availability of team, sonography findings, etc. Sometimes, intraoperative bleeding or frozen pelvis during laparoscopy leads to laparotomy.

Medical management with methotrexate: If minimal symptoms, patient is stable, normal baseline LFT and renal function test (RFT), tubal mass <3.5 cm in diameter, no fetal heart, no evidence of rupture, and future fertility is desirable *Do not forget to administer anti-D (50 μg) if Rh-negative* (alloimmunization can occur even with 0.1 mL fetal blood admixing) If β-hCG to start with is very low (<1,000) and shows a falling trend, then just serial assays without any active treatment can be done till the levels drop to zero. Treatment plan is summarized in **Flowchart 2**.

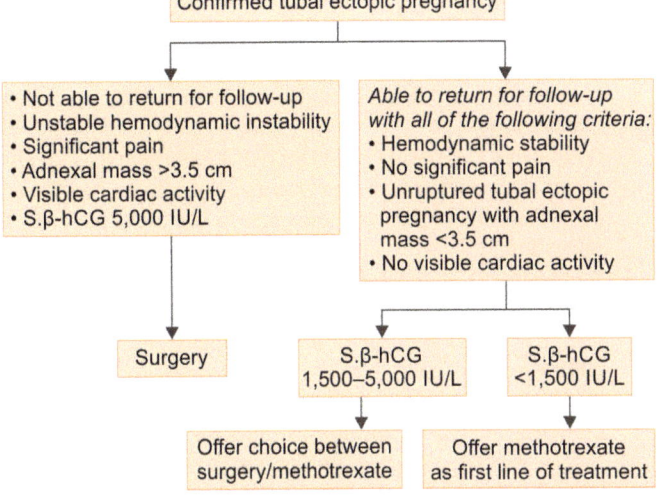

Flowchart 2: Treatment plan for ectopic pregnancy.

- Tight bandage
- Postsurgery

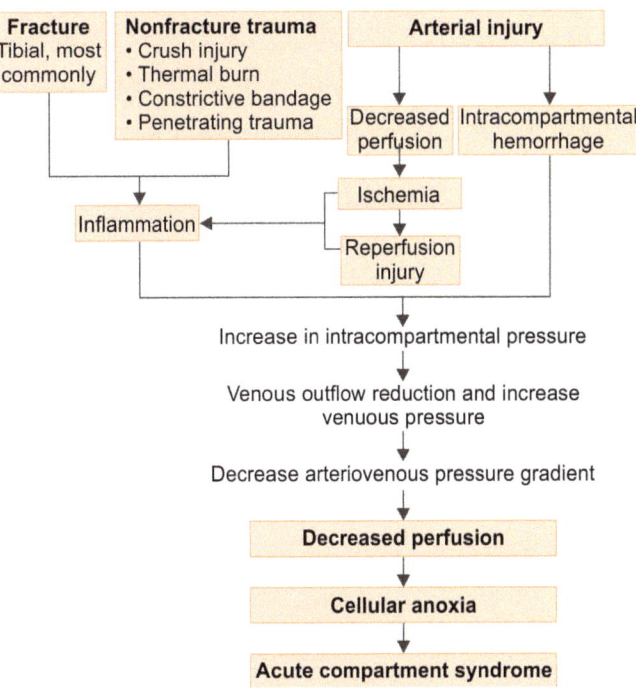

Flowchart 3: Compartment syndrome.

Question 10

1. Define compartment syndrome.

Compartment syndrome is a painful condition that occurs when pressure within the muscles builds up to dangerous levels. This pressure can decrease blood flow, which prevents nourishment and oxygen from reaching nerve and muscle cells. Compartment syndrome results when injured muscle cells increase in size with intracellular fluid uptake while total space remains constant. This swelling results in increases in intracompartmental pressures. As pressure increases, blood flow to the damaged tissue decreases resulting in tissue ischemia and eventually necrosis. It is classically taught that increased pressures, resulting in tissue ischemia for more than 6–8 hours, result in permanent damage **(Flowchart 3)**.

2. List the settings in which it occurs.

- Trauma
- Crush injury
- Fracture (open/closed) fracture tibia and high energy fracture shaft femur and forearm
- Bleeding
- Prolonged vascular occlusion
- Burns
- Venomous bite
- Intraosseous fluid replacement
- IV fluid extravasation

3. List its clinical presentation.

Compartment syndrome: Clinical diagnosis
- Pain out of proportion
- Palpable tense compartment
- Pain with passive stretch
- Paresthesia/hypoesthesia
- Paralysis
- Pulselessness or pallor

4. Discuss the management of a case of suspected compartment syndrome in case of fracture shaft tibia on the right side.

The treatment for compartment syndrome is fasciotomy **(Flowchart 4)**. This procedure allows the swelling muscle to expand outside of its compartment, thereby preserving afferent blood flow. Fasciotomy continues to be a controversial subject in the realm of crush syndrome management. Some authors argue that this is a lifesaving intervention that also decreases the risk for complications related to crush syndrome. Other studies have not shown such profound benefits with fasciotomy. The benefits of fasciotomy must be compared with the outcomes related to localized wound infection, sepsis, subsequent amputations, and increased mortality.

Flowchart 4: Approach to management of compartment syndrome.

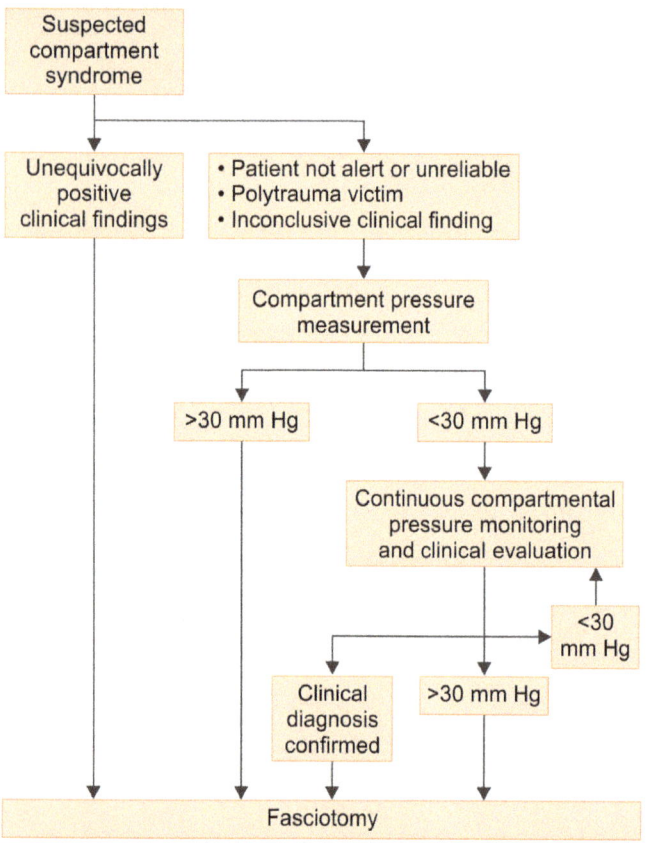

SUGGESTED READING

1. Richhariya D, Sharma B. Textbook of Emergency Medicine including Intensive Care and Trauma, 2nd edition. New Delhi: Jaypee Brothers Medical Publishers (P) Ltd; 2022. pp. 669-73. (Question 1).
2. Richhariya D, Sharma B. Textbook of Emergency Medicine including Intensive Care and Trauma, 2nd edition. New Delhi: Jaypee Brothers Medical Publishers (P) Ltd; 2022. pp. 910-1. (Question 2).
3. Richhariya D, Sharma B. Textbook of Emergency Medicine including Intensive Care and Trauma, 2nd edition. New Delhi: Jaypee Brothers Medical Publishers (P) Ltd; 2022. pp. 784-90. (Question 3).
4. Richhariya D, Sharma B. Textbook of Emergency Medicine including Intensive Care and Trauma, 2nd edition. New Delhi: Jaypee Brothers Medical Publishers (P) Ltd; 2022. pp. 915-9. (Question 4).
5. Richhariya D, Sharma B. Textbook of Emergency Medicine including Intensive Care and Trauma, 2nd edition. New Delhi: Jaypee Brothers Medical Publishers (P) Ltd; 2022. pp. 1560-4. (Question 5).
6. Richhariya D, Sharma B. Textbook of Emergency Medicine including Intensive Care and Trauma, 2nd edition. New Delhi: Jaypee Brothers Medical Publishers (P) Ltd; 2022. pp. 1570-2. (Question 6).
7. Richhariya D, Sharma B. Textbook of Emergency Medicine including Intensive Care and Trauma, 2nd edition. New Delhi: Jaypee Brothers Medical Publishers (P) Ltd; 2022. p. 1678. (Question 7).
8. Richhariya D, Sharma B. Textbook of Emergency Medicine including Intensive Care and Trauma, 2nd edition. New Delhi: Jaypee Brothers Medical Publishers (P) Ltd; 2022. p. 905. (Question 8).
9. Richhariya D, Sharma B. Textbook of Emergency Medicine including Intensive Care and Trauma, 2nd edition. New Delhi: Jaypee Brothers Medical Publishers (P) Ltd; 2022. pp. 1075, 1079. (Question 9).
10. Richhariya D, Sharma B. Textbook of Emergency Medicine including Intensive Care and Trauma, 2nd edition. New Delhi: Jaypee Brothers Medical Publishers (P) Ltd; 2022. p. 1673. (Question 10).

Emergency Medicine Paper 19

Rahul Solanki

Question 1

1. Enumerate cerebral stroke mimics.

Cerebral stroke mimics are listed in **Table 1**.

TABLE 1: Stroke mimics.	
Toxic-metabolic	• Hypoglycemia or hyperglycemia • Hyponatremia or hypernatremia • Ingestion or overdose • Drug toxicity • Intoxication (alcohol, illicit drugs) • Hepatic encephalopathy
Intracranial hemorrhage	Intracerebral hemorrhage, subarachnoid hemorrhage, subdural hematoma
Infectious	• Sepsis • Encephalitis • Meningitis
Structural lesions	• Brain mass or tumor • Spinal cord lesion
Others	• Demyelinating disease (i.e., multiple sclerosis), seizure or Todd's paralysis • Migraine • Idiopathic intracranial hypertension • Reversible cerebral vasoconstrictive syndrome • Central nervous system vasculitis • Vestibular dysfunction • Hypertensive encephalopathy • Peripheral neuropathy • Dementia • Conversion disorder

2. Write cerebral stroke thrombolysis-inclusion criteria.

3. Enumerate exclusion criteria.

Inclusion and exclusion criteria for ischemic stroke thrombolysis are given in **Box 1**.

4. Which investigations are must before doing stroke thrombolysis?

As per the stroke guidelines of finger stick glucose is an essential test before thrombolysis is started. Following basic tests can be considered in special patient groups but the start of thrombolytic therapy if indicated should not be delayed unless the patient has a history of bleeding disorder, is taking anticoagulants or has history of thrombocytopenia. After completion of acute management of stroke other lab tests such as liver function, kidney function, etc., can be done.

- Electrocardiogram (this should not delay the noncontract brain CT)
- Complete blood count including platelets
- Troponin
- Prothrombin time and international normalized ratio (INR)
- Activated partial thromboplastin time
- Ecarin clotting time, thrombin time, or appropriate direct factor Xa activity assay (if the patient is taking new oral anticoagulants).

5. Enumerate the medicines and their dose used in thrombolysis.

Dose of tissue plasminogen activator (tPA): As per the guidelines infuse 0.9 mg/kg (maximum dose 90 mg) over 60 minutes, with 10% of the dose given as a bolus over 1 minute.

For treatment within 3 hours of stroke onset, alteplase led to a good outcome for 33%, versus 23% for control [odds ratio (OR) 1.75, 95% CI 1.35–2.27]. The number needed to treat (NNT) for one additional patient to achieve a good outcome was 10.

For treatment from 3 to 4.5 hours, the proportion with a good outcome in the alteplase and control groups was 35 and 30% (OR 1.26, 95% CI 1.05–1.51, NNT 20).

The benefit of intravenous (IV) defibrinogenating agents and of IV fibrinolytic agents other than alteplase and tenecteplase is unproven; therefore, their administration is not recommended outside a clinical trial. Tenecteplase administered as a 0.4-mg/kg single IV bolus has not been proven to be superior or noninferior to alteplase but might be considered as an alternative to alteplase in patients with minor neurological impairment and no major intracranial occlusion.

BOX 1: Inclusion and exclusion criteria for intravenous (IV) tPA infusion.

- Inclusion criteria
- Diagnosis of ischemic stroke causing measurable neurological deficit
- Onset of symptoms <3 hours before beginning treatment
- Aged ≥18 years
- Exclusion criteria
- Significant head trauma or prior stroke in previous 3 months
- Symptoms suggest subarachnoid hemorrhage
- Arterial puncture at noncompressible site in previous 7 days
- History of previous intracranial hemorrhage
- Intracranial neoplasm, arteriovenous malformation, or aneurysm
- Recent intracranial or intraspinal surgery
- Elevated blood pressure (systolic >185 mm Hg or diastolic >110 mm Hg)
- Active internal bleeding
- Acute bleeding diathesis
- Platelet count <100,000/mm^3
- Heparin received within 48 hours, resulting in abnormally elevated aPTT greater than the upper limit of normal
- Current use of anticoagulant with INR >1.7 or PT >15 seconds
- Current use of direct thrombin inhibitors or direct factor Xa inhibitors with elevated sensitive laboratory tests (such as aPTT, INR, platelet count, and ECT, TT, or appropriate factor Xa activity assays)
- Blood glucose concentration <50 mg/dL (2.7 mmol/L)
- CT demonstrates multilobar infarction (hypodensity >1/3 cerebral hemisphere)
- Relative exclusion criteria

Recent experience suggests that under some circumstances—with careful consideration and weighting of risk to benefit—patients may receive fibrinolytic therapy despite one or more relative contraindications. Consider risk to benefit of IV rtPA administration carefully if any of these relative contraindications are present:

- Only minor or rapidly improving stroke symptoms (clearing spontaneously)
- Pregnancy
- Seizure at onset with postictal residual neurological impairments
- Major surgery or serious trauma within previous 14 days
- Recent gastrointestinal or urinary tract hemorrhage (within previous 21 days)
- Recent acute myocardial infarction (within previous 3 months)

[aPTT: activated partial thromboplastin time; CT: computed tomography; ECT: ecarin clotting time (ECT used to monitor patient on Hirudin anticoagulation therapy); INR: international normalized ratio; rtPA: recombinant tissue plasminogen activator; tPA: tissue plasminogen activator; TT: thrombin time]

Question 2

1. How does a patient of chronic obstructive pulmonary disease (COPD) with acute exacerbation present in emergency department (ED)?

Clinical manifestations: The three cardinal symptoms of COPD are: (1) Chronic cough, (2) sputum production, and (3) dyspnea. Symptoms which are less common include wheezing and chest tightness. History of decreasing level of activity or reduction in the speed of walking should be enquired. Other symptoms include weight loss or weight gain, anxiety, and depression.

Triggers: Respiratory infections are estimated to trigger approximately 70% of COPD exacerbations. Viral and bacterial infections cause most exacerbations, whereas atypical bacteria are a relatively uncommon cause. The remaining 30% are due to environmental pollution, pulmonary embolism, or have an unknown etiology. Some COPD exacerbations of unknown etiology may be related to other medical conditions, such as myocardial ischemia, heart failure, aspiration, or pulmonary embolism.

2. How to classify them according to severity?

Severity of exacerbation:

- *Mild:* Mild tachypnea (RR 20–30/min), no accessory muscle of respiration, no altered sensorium, hypoxia easily correctable with low flow oxygen, no hypercarbia.
- *Moderate:* Tachypnea (RR >35/min), accessory muscle of respiration active, no altered sensorium, hypoxia easily correctable with low flow oxygen (venturi 28–40%), rise in PCO_2 above usual PCO_2 or between 50 and 60 mm Hg.
- *Severe:* Tachypnea (RR >35/min), accessory muscle of respiration active, altered sensorium present, hypoxia not easily correctable with low flow oxygen (requiring >40% venturi), rise in PCO_2 above 60 mm Hg or respiratory acidosis (pH <7.25).

3. Discuss ED management of such cases.

Management of COPD exacerbation goals: Reversing airflow limitation with inhaled short-acting bronchodilators and systemic glucocorticoids, treating infection, ensuring adequate oxygenation, and averting intubation and mechanical ventilation. Other goals of care are to prevent complications of immobility, such as thromboembolic and deconditioning, improve nutritional status, and aid patients who smoke with smoking cessation.

Oxygen therapy: Supplemental oxygen is a critical component of acute therapy. Because of the risk of worsening hypercapnia use controlled oxygen to maintain a pulse oxygen saturation (SpO_2) of 88–92% or an arterial oxygen tension (PaO_2) of approximately 60.

High flow nasal cannula (HFNC): It provides supplemental oxygen (adjustable FiO_2) at a high flow rate (up to 60 L/min), resulting in a low level of continuous positive airway pressure. The specific indications for HFNC remain unclear, and robust comparisons of HFNC with noninvasive ventilation (NIV) in patients with COPD exacerbations are lacking.

Beta (β) adrenergic agonist: These medications may be administered via a nebulizer or a metered dose inhaler (MDI) with a spacer device and may be combined with a short acting antimuscarinic agent (e.g., albuterol, levalbuterol). Typical doses of albuterol for this indication are 2.5 mg (diluted to a total of 3 mL) by nebulizer every 1–4 hours as needed, or four to eight puffs (90 µg/puff) by MDI with a spacer every 1–4 hours as needed. Increasing the dose has not been shown to confer an advantage in COPD and can cause side effects.

Anticholinergic agents: These agents are typically used with SABA (Short-Acting B2 Agonist) for patients who require hospital-based treatment of a COPD exacerbation. Typical doses of ipratropium in this situation are 500 µg by nebulizer every 4 hours as needed. Alternatively, two to four puffs (18 µg/puff) can be administered by MDI with a spacer every 4 hours as needed.

Systemic glucocorticoids: Addition of glucocorticoids to above therapies improves symptoms, lung function, and decreases the length of hospital stay. The optimal dose of systemic glucocorticoids for treating a COPD exacerbation is unknown. The Global Initiative for Chronic Obstructive Lung Disease (GOLD) guidelines advises using the equivalent of prednisone 40 mg once daily for the majority of COPD exacerbation.

Antibiotics: Most clinical practice guidelines including GOLD guidelines recommend antibiotics for patients having a moderate to severe COPD exacerbation that requires hospitalization. It has shown to shorten time to recover, reduce risk of early relapse, treatment failure, and hospitalization.

Therapy without documented evidence: Mucoactive agents, methylxanthines, and mechanical techniques to augment sputum clearance have not been shown to confer benefit for patients with a COPD exacerbation.

Chest physiotherapy: Mechanical techniques to augment sputum clearance, such as directed coughing, chest physiotherapy with percussion and vibration, intermittent positive pressure breathing, and postural drainage, have not been shown to be beneficial in COPD and may provoke bronchoconstriction.

Supportive care: Supportive care for patients hospitalized with an exacerbation of COPD may include one or more of the following therapies—cigarette smoking cessation, thromboprophylaxis, nutritional support.

Question 3

1. Explain the clinical presentation of a case of diabetic ketoacidosis (DKA).

Clinical features of DKA:
- Polyuria and nocturia
- Thirst
- Weight loss
- Weakness
- Blurred vision
- Acidotic (Kussmaul) respiration
- Abdominal pain, especially in children
- Leg cramps
- Nausea and vomiting
- Confusion and drowsiness
- Coma

2. Discuss laboratory investigations of importance in such case (DKA).

Laboratory investigations in DKA:

Venous blood: Glucose Na^+, K^+, Cl^-, HCO_3^- urea (BUN), creatinine ketone bodies, calcium anion gap, lactate, if significant lactic academia suspected visual inspection of plasma (hypertriglyceridemia).

Arterial or capillary blood: pH, standard HCO_3^-, base excess PCO_2, PO_2.

Others: Electrocardiogram (ECG), cardiac enzymes full blood count, chest radiograph, blood, urine culture for sputum.

3. Explain the management of such cases in ED (DKA).

Successful treatment of DKA aims for correction of dehydration, hyperglycemia, and electrolyte imbalances and identification of comorbid precipitating events, and above all, frequent patient monitoring (**Flowchart 1**).

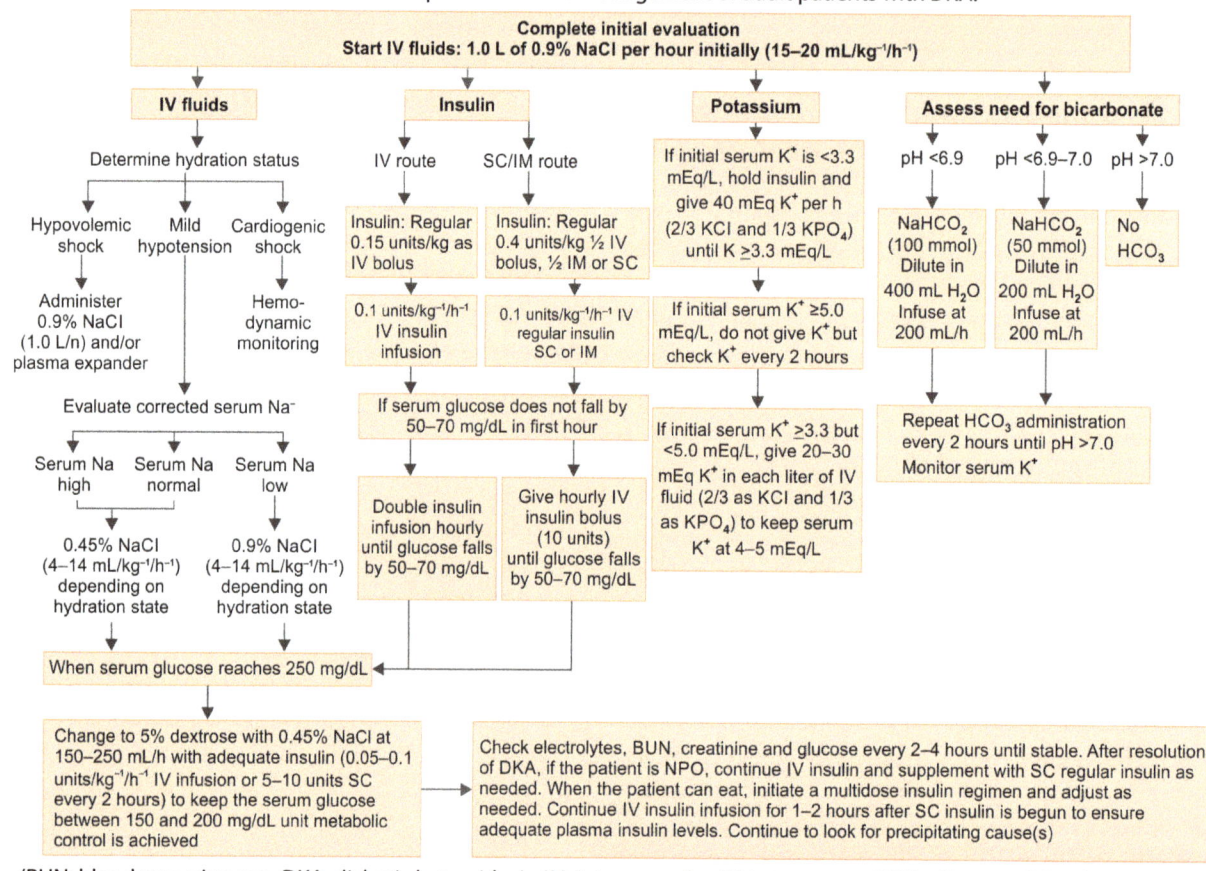

Flowchart 1: The protocol for the management of adult patients with DKA.

(BUN: blood urea nitrogen; DKA: diabetic ketoacidosis; IM: intramuscular; IV: intravenous; NPO: nil per os; SC: subcutaneous)

Question 4

1. Write about emergency psychiatric assessment steps.

It is a focused *mini mental state exam (MMSE)* to review the patient's attention, memory, and executive function. The ease of incorporation and relatively short amount of time needed to complete assessment makes the MMSE one of the more relevant tools to integrate into ED examinations for altered mental status. An impaired cognitive ability may signify dysfunction secondary to dementia or delirium. The unpredictable and changeable pattern of delirium may be better identified using the *confusion assessment method (CAM)*. The CAM diagnostic algorithm looks at four features: (1) Acute onset and fluctuating course, (2) Inattention, (3) Disorganized thinking, and (4) Altered level of consciousness. The diagnosis of delirium is then made when both features 1 and 2 are present along with either one of 3 or 4.

2. Write about medical evaluation of psychiatric patient.

Assessment at triage: The psychiatric patient may present to the ED in a variety of ways. These patients are often either referred by existing psychiatric and primary care providers, or they are brought in by police or emergency medical services due to acutely agitated, self-harming, disruptive or intoxicated states. Occasionally, patients with psychiatric complaints will refer themselves to the ED, and there are even instances where psychiatric disease is newly uncovered by the emergency physician while evaluating the patient for a separate medical condition.

Evaluation: The initial ED assessment for a psychiatric patient frequently aims to identify the presence of a medical condition that may be causing or worsening the patient's mental health before addressing the psychiatric issue. The American College of Emergency Physicians (ACEP) recommends a focused medical assessment in the ED whereby any organic causes of disease can be identified through relevant diagnostic evaluation as needed based on the patient's presenting signs and symptoms. Routine laboratory testing and diagnostics are not recommended to exclude medical causes for the patient's condition. Investigations may be useful, however, in those patients over 45 years of age with new onset of psychiatric symptoms, those with cognitive impairment, delirium, substance abuse or withdrawal, decreased levels of consciousness, abnormal vital signs or advanced age (≥65 years).

3. How to assess potential harm to self and others in acute psychiatric emergency?

Self-harm is described as an intentional injury or poisoning of oneself, which may or may not include suicidal ideation or attempt. It is usually a manifestation of a maladjusted emotional response to distressing stimuli or triggers. Patients of self-harm are often particularly vulnerable and distraught, with the extreme nature of the phenomenon making them more likely to present to EDs. Current standards of assessment for self-harm in the ED are highly variable and risk assessment tools for suicide are underdeveloped and often not properly utilized, increasing the likelihood that many patients with substantial risks are missed or undetected. Protect the patient first by placing him/her in a private room without any dangerous objects, de-escalate any acute agitation as needed and perform a focused medical assessment to search for any underlying organic condition. Patients should undergo risk assessment for suicide and safety for discharge. Communication plays a vital role in exploring the frequency and intensity of suicidal ideation, and the physician should attempt to ascertain the presence of a prepared plan, history of previous attempts and patient's beliefs on self-harm to thoroughly comprehend the risk of suicide. Most patients with considerable risk of suicide will typically be admitted to the hospital. However, any patients discharged after being deemed to be low risk should cautiously and comprehensively document their decision-making, risk assessment, findings, rationale, and any consultations as appropriate.

Question 5

Write short notes on:
1. Toxic epidermal necrolysis (TEN).
2. Stevens–Johnson syndrome (SJS).

Stevens–Johnson syndrome and TEN synonyms:
Lyell syndrome: SJS and TEN are blistering diseases of the skin. In 1922 Stevens and Johnson described a condition which was characterized by disseminated cutaneous eruption with central necrosis, febrile erosive stomatitis, and severe purulent conjunctivitis. Adverse reactions of drugs are the common cause of these complex conditions (SJS and TEN). Adverse drug reaction is the cause in about >80% of the TEN and 50% cases in SJS. Condition is associated with widespread erythema, necrosis, and bullous detachment of extensive areas of epidermis. SJS is considered as erythema multiform major. Epidermal detachment in SJS is <10% while epidermal detachment in TEN is >30%. A total of 10–30% cases overlap between SJS and TEN. Diagnosis is mostly clinical.

Clinical presentation: The patient with SJS/TEN presents with fever, malaise, muscle and joint pain with purpuric lesions which occur on the face, upper torso, and proximal limbs. Lesions gradually involve other body parts eventually turning into fluid filled blisters. Hemorrhagic crust on lips is characteristic. Ocular manifestations include conjunctivitis, clouding, symblepharon, corneal erosions, and photophobia. Erosion can spread to GI tract and respiratory tract giving rise to symptoms such as dysphagia, diarrhea, pulmonary edema, and bronchopneumonia. Glomerulonephritis represents renal involvement.

Management: Indian Association of Dermatologist, Venerologist, and Leprologist (IADVL) consensus treatment guidelines for SJS/TEN.

Immediate management:
- Stop all drugs
- Fluid replacement
- Nutritional support
- Sterile vaseline or paraffin gauze dressing
- Temperature regulation
- Antacids and analgesics
- Initiation of disease specific therapy—corticosteroids, cyclosporine, IV immunoglobulin, plasmapheresis
- Other drugs—cyclophosphamide, thalidomide, N-acetyl cysteine, pentoxifylline.

Continued management:
- Ophthalmic and oral care
- Pulmonary care
- Antibiotics.

Question 6

1. Discuss thyroid function test of importance in ED.

Thyroid hormone changes are a common feature in emergency patients with no known thyroid dysfunction. A decrease in triiodothyronine (T3) is frequently observed with normal levels of free thyroxine (fT4) and thyroid-stimulating hormone (TSH), a condition known as euthyroid sick syndrome (ESS), nonthyroidal illness syndrome (NTIS), or low T3 syndrome. Interpretation of thyroid function test is given in **Table 2**.

TABLE 2: Interpretation of thyroid function test.

TSH	Free T4	Free T3	Interpretation
Normal	Normal	Normal	None
Low	High	High	Hyperthyroidism
Low	Normal	normal	Subclinical hyperthyroidism
Low	Normal	High	T3 toxicosis
Low	High	Normal	Thyroiditis T4 ingestion hyperthyroidism in older adults or in comorbid conditions
Low	Low	Low	Euthyroid sick syndrome central hypothyroidism
High	Normal	Normal	Subclinical hypothyroidism recovery from euthyroid sick syndrome

(T3: triiodothyronine; T4: thyroxine; TSH: thyroid stimulating hormone)

In myxedema coma: The suspected diagnosis of myxedema coma includes clinical presentation of any patient with coma or compromised mental status with hypercapnia, hypothermia, and/or hyponatremia, and with decreased T3 and T4 concentrations **(Table 3)**. Measurement of serum cortisol is required to rule out co-existing adrenal insufficiency.

In thyrotoxicosis and thyroid storm: Serum TSH is usually the test of choice and when suppressed to unmeasurable levels (<0.05 µIU/mL) is a sensitive marker for the suspicion of thyrotoxicosis. Thorough history and clinical examination often provide valuable clues for the diagnosis of thyrotoxicosis which can be further confirmed by FT3 and FT4 levels. Diagnosis can be confirmed by the presence of TSH receptor antibodies, measured by ELISA, which has a high sensitivity and specificity of 98% and 99% respectively as compared to anti-thyroid peroxidase (anti-TPO) antibodies, which are present in only 75% cases of Graves' disease. If antibody levels are inconclusive, radioactive iodine uptake (RAIU) can be helpful in differentiating various causes of thyrotoxicosis. Thyroid storm is unrecognized, undertreated, life-threatening form of severe thyrotoxicosis. Thyroid storm is rare and mostly acute reaction to thyroid and nonthyroid surgery, trauma infections contrast media, amiodarone, after delivery in preexisting hyperthyroidism. Other risk factors are acute coronary syndrome, pulmonary embolism, and DKA. Prompt recognitions and treatment are warranted as mortality is almost 100%.

2. Explain the clinical presentation of a case of myxedema coma.

Patients with myxedema coma generally present with altered sensorium, lethargy, confusion, and possibly obtundation rather than coma. Other characteristics include hypoglycemia, bradycardia, hypoventilation, hypotension, hypothermia, (usually <95.9°F), hyponatremia, increased levels of serum creatinine and creatinine kinase. The clinical presentation of myxedema coma is shown in **Table 4**.

TABLE 3: Importance of thyroid function test in diagnosing myxedema coma.

Parameter	Glasgow Coma Scale Score				TSH (mU/L)		Free T4 levels <0.6 ng/dL	Body temperature <95°F	Heart rate <60	Precipitating event*
	0–10	11–13	14	15	>30	15–30				
Point	4	3	2	0	2	1	1	1	1	1
Scoring	Myxedema coma ≥7 points, likely 5–7 points, and unlikely <5 points									

*Burns, carbon monoxide retention, gastrointestinal hemorrhage, infection, sepsis, medications, stroke, surgery, trauma, etc.
(T4: thyroxine; TSH: thyroid-stimulating hormone)

TABLE 4: Clinical presentation of myxedema coma.

System	Clinical presentation
Central nervous system (CNS)	• Decreased mental status—may be due to decreased cerebral blood flow and cerebral glucose metabolism • Confusion, apathy, lethargy, obtundation, and coma • Cognitive impairment and psychiatric disorders can also be seen • Hyponatremia • Hypoglycemia (~25% patients)
Respiratory system	• Respiratory depression • Fluid accumulation—pleural effusion • Obstructive sleep apnea—obesity and weight gain • Myxedematous infiltration of the pharynx and tongue requiring mechanical ventilation
Cardiovascular system (CVS)	• Bradycardia, low cardiac output, and decreased blood volume • Increased systemic peripheral resistance and pericardial effusion
Renal system	• Severe renal impairment—reduced blood flow and low glomerular filtration rate (GFR) • Elevated creatinine • Decreased sodium reabsorption leading to hyponatremia

Contd...

Contd...

System	Clinical presentation
Gastrointestinal tract (GIT)	Decreased intestinal mobility—constipation, anorexia, nausea, abdominal pain and distension
Skin and hair	• Myxedematous facies—generalized puffiness, ptosis, macroglossia, coarse and sparse hair, and periorbital edema • Dry, pale, and thickened skin with nonpitting edema (myxedema) • Dry and brittle hair • Hoarseness in voice
Metabolic	Hypothermia (up to 75°F)
Laboratory and others	• Reduced T4 and T3 • Elevated TSH—primary hypothyroidism; normal/low TSH—central/secondary hypothyroidism • Respiratory acidosis • ECG—bradycardia, decreased voltage, prolonged QT interval, nonspecific ST-T changes and Osborn waves in cases of hypothermia • Chest radiograph—pleural effusions and cardiomegaly

(ECG: electrocardiogram; T3: tri-iodothyronine; T4: thyroxine; TSH: thyroid-stimulating hormone)

3. Discuss ED management of the patient of myxedema coma.

Successful treatment depends upon the timely diagnosis, prompt treatment with thyroid hormones (IV levothyroxine is preferred over oral), supportive therapy (appropriate fluid management and correction of hypotension and dyselectrolytemia), administration of steroid supplement (hydrocortisone) until coexisting adrenal insufficiency is ruled out, along with the aggressive treatment of precipitating factors. The treatment of myxedema coma is detailed in **Flowchart 2**.

Flowchart 2: Approach to treatment of myxedema coma.

Treatment of myxedema coma				
Thyroid replacement therapy		**Supportive therapy**		**Precipitating event**
Large initial IV dose: T4 (200–400 µg); maintenance dose: 1.6 µg/kg/d IV/PO	Alternative: Initial IV T4 (200–300 µg) in combination with T3 (10–25 µg)	Hypocortisolemia	IV hydrocortisone (100 mg q8h) until the possibility of coexisting adrenal insufficiency is excluded	Identification and elimination by specific treatment, use of empirical antibiotics
			Follow-up steroid therapy: Discontinue if cortisol level >25 µg/dL or corticotropin-stimulating testing if <25 µg/dL	
T3 loading dose: 5–20 µg IV/NG once Maintenance dose: 2.5–10 q8h IV/PO		Hypoventilation	Intubation and mechanical ventilation	Selected cases
		Hypothermia	Passive rewarming with a blanket	Respiratory acidosis: Assisted mechanical ventilation
		Hyponatremia	Free-water restriction and normal saline	
		Hypotension	Fluids and vasopressor drugs	Pulmonary edema: IV furosemide
		Hypoglycemia	IV dextrose or glucose	

(IV: intravenous; T3: tri-iodothyronine; T4: thyroxine)

Question 7

1. Discuss clinical features, laboratory investigations, and management of acute lithium toxicity cases.

Lithium is a monovalent cation such as sodium and potassium. At the cellular level, lithium competes with these cations and displaces them, leading to intracellular metabolic changes. Lithium salts are mainly used for the treatment of manic-depressive psychosis (bipolar disorder) and depressive disorders. Amelioration of neutropenia induced by chemotherapy, prevention of cluster headaches, and alcohol abuse are the other therapeutic uses.

Clinical features: Since the therapeutic to toxic index of lithium is very narrow, there is always been an overlap between the clinical features of adverse effect of the drug on therapeutic doses to toxic effects due to over doses.

Adverse effects:
- Thirst, polyuria, tremor, acne, hypothyroidism, dysarthria, ataxia, alopecia, and exacerbation of psoriasis
- Nephrogenic diabetes insipidus (10% of the patients)
- Gastrointestinal (GI) adverse effects—mild and reversible (10–20% of the patients)
  - Diarrhea, vomiting, abdominal pain, nausea, and anorexia
- Exophthalmos, restlessness, and anxiety
- Parkinsonian syndrome characterized by tremor, fasciculations and cogwheel rigidity
- Hypercalcemia with cardiac rhythm disturbances
- Leukocytosis with neutrophilia is a common occurrence
- *Toxicities in new-born babies of mothers who are on lithium:* Hypotonicity, lethargy, and cyanosis (floppy baby syndrome).

Lithium toxicity due to overdosage: Having a prolonged redistributive phases and tissue burdens, lithium exposure can be divided into three main categories of toxicity—(1) acute, (2) acute-on-chronic, and (3) chronic.

Acute toxicity:
- Acute ingestions of lithium containing preparations produce clinical findings similar to that of ingestions of other metal salts, with predominant early GI symptoms—nausea, vomiting, and diarrhea
- Lightheadedness and dizziness due to orthostatic hypotension
- Neurologic manifestations are a late finding in acute toxicity as the lithium redistributes slowly into the central nervous system
- Frequent ECG abnormalities which include T wave inversions, prolonged QT, sinoatrial dysfunction and bradycardia. But serious cardiac events are a rarity.

Diagnosis: Leukocytosis, serum lithium levels, electrolytes like Na_2, K^+

A therapeutic lithium level is somewhere between 0.6 and 1.2 milliequivalents per liter (mEq/L). Lithium levels 1.5 mEq/L or more, symptoms of toxicity begin to show up.

The levels of toxicity are classified as: Mild: 1.5–2.5 mEq/L, Moderate: 2.5–3.5 mEq/L, Severe: above 3.5 mEq/L and potentially fatal.

Treatment: The initial management should include stabilization of the patient with due care of airway, breathing, and circulation.

Gastrointestinal decontamination: Gastric lavage and activated charcoal are not much of use. Whole bowel irrigation with polyethylene glycol electrolyte lavage solution (2L/h for 5 hours) has shown a good efficacy in eliminating lithium in early stages.

Sodium polystyrene sulfonate (SPS) is a cationic exchange resin often used for the treatment of severe hyperkalemia has found to be useful in the decontamination by reduction of absorption of lithium:
- *Dose:* Adults—60 mL suspension (15 g) orally four times a day
- 120–200 mL of suspension (30–50 g) given rectally as retention enema following a cleansing enema
- *Dose:* Children—1 g/kg/every 6 hours orally or every 2–6 hours rectally.

Fluid and electrolyte balance: Correction of blood volume with 0.9% normal saline (1.5–2 times the normal maintenance) will prevent lithium toxicity induced renal dysfunction.

It also improves renal perfusion, glomerular filtration rate, and lithium elimination. Correction of electrolyte abnormalities and monitoring of urine output are essential.

Extra corporeal drug removal:
Hemodialysis: Recommendations for hemodialysis
- Absolute lithium concentration above 4.0 mEq/L (mmol/L)
- With any type of overdose or a concentration of >2.5 mEq/L with chronic toxicity
- Patients who are manifesting severe signs and symptoms of neurotoxicity, such as alterations in mental status
- Patients who have renal failure and show signs or symptoms of lithium toxicity
- Patients who show little or no sign of toxicity but who cannot tolerate sodium repletion therapy (congestive heart failure, liver failure, pancreatitis or sepsis)

Continuous arteriovenous hemodiafiltration (CAVH): It has better efficacy than hemodialysis.

Question 8

1. Define status epilepticus.

Status epilepticus was earlier defined as a continuous seizure lasting >30 minutes, or two or more seizures without full recovery of consciousness between any of them. Later the definition was modified as: Status epilepticus is defined as a seizure with 5 minutes or more of continuous clinical and/or electrographic seizure activity or recurrent seizure activity without recovery between seizures.

2. Define refractory status.

Refractory/malignant status epilepticus: Refractory status epilepticus and the continuous or repetitive seizures are unresponsive to first- and/or second-line antiepileptic drug therapy with a benzodiazepine and other anticonvulsant in adequate loading dose.

3. Discuss stepwise approach to the management of a case of status epilepticus in ED.

Stabilization phase (0-5 minutes seizure activity) airway and breathing: Consider nasopharyngeal airway, suction and supplemental oxygen.

Circulation: Secure IV access. Check blood glucose levels. If sugar levels <60 mg/dL, start IV dextrose (D50W) 50 mL.

Initial therapy phase (5-20 minutes):
Benzodiazepines are the first therapy of choice:
a. 10 mg for >40 kg, 5 mg for 13-40 kg of intramuscular (IM) midazolam single dose OR
b. 0.1 mg/kg/dose, maximum: 4 mg/dose of IV lorazepam, may repeat dose once OR
c. 0.15-0.2 mg/kg/dose, maximum: 10 mg/dose IV diazepam, may repeat dose once.

If none of the above benzodiazepines are available any one of the following may be administered:
a. 15 mg/kg/dose of IV phenobarbital single dose OR
b. Intranasal midazolam, buccal midazolam OR
c. 0.2-0.5 mg/kg, maximum: 20 mg/dose of rectal diazepam single dose.

Second therapy phase (20-40 minutes): At this point, a response to the therapy administered in the previous phase should be evident. If there is a lack of response, the following can be administered as a single dose:
a. *20 mg PE/kg, maximum:* 1,500 mg PE/dose of IV fosphenytoin single dose OR
b. *IV levetiracetam 60 mg/kg, maximum:* 4,500 mg/dose, single dose OR
c. *40 mg/kg, maximum:* 3,000 mg/dose of IV valproic acid, single dose.

If none of the options are available, IV phenobarbital 15 mg/kg, single dose can be administered. Consider definitive airway protection by endotracheal intubation and mechanical ventilation.

Third therapy phase (40-60 minutes): If the seizure persists, any drug of the second line therapy may be repeated or administered anesthetic doses of:
a. Thiopental 100-250 mg bolus with repeat bolus of 50 mg ever 2-3 minutes till seizures are controlled followed by infusion of 3-5 mg/kg/h OR
b. Propofol 2 mg/kg IV bolus followed by 5-10 mg/kg/h infusion OR
c. Midazolam 0.1-0.3 mg/kg bolus followed by infusion at 0.05-0.4 mg/kg/h.

If patient needs third line therapy then the airway must be protected by endotracheal intubation and mechanical ventilation. The patient should undergo continuous electroencephalogram (EEG) monitoring.

Question 9

1. Discuss clinical presentation of a patient with acute nontraumatic intracranial bleed.

Subarachnoid hemorrhage (SAH) is usually present with severe thunderclap headache but may also present with syncope, decreased level of consciousness, neck pain, nuchal rigidity, seizure, and other nonspecific symptoms. The range of symptoms of spontaneous intracerebral hemorrhage (ICH) is even wider, and depending on the site of bleeding and the volume, may vary from a mild headache to a deep coma with/without focal neurologic deficits. An important point is that over first hours, the symptoms may worsen or rarely improve. Taking everything into account, there is no definite finding in terms of diagnosis of hemorrhagic stroke patients, and diagnostic certainty always needs brain imaging.

2. Explain the ED management of such cases of acute nontraumatic intracranial bleed.

Subarachnoid hemorrhage and ICH have some same and also specific management in terms of both surgical and nonsurgical interventions. All patients with SAH need neurological surgeon's consultation. Patients with ICH are generally managed medically by neurologists, though there are few indications for surgical intervention.
- Airway management
- Blood pressure control
- Blood sugar control
- Reversal of anticoagulation
- Antifibrinolytic
- Seizure management
- Intracranial pressure (ICP) control
- Surgical interventions
- Other managements.

3. How to manage raised ICP in ED?

The hematoma itself or the surrounding edema can result in elevated increased ICP, which can precipitate secondary brain injury and neurologic deterioration. Elevation of the head of the bed and providing the patient with adequate analgesia and sedation are the mainstay of preventing ICP elevation in ICH. The patients should be treated with normal saline and hypotonic fluids should be avoided.

In case of elevated ICP, osmotic agents such as mannitol and hypertonic saline are the first line agents. Though the care should be taken while achieving a mild serum hyperosmolality (300–310 mOsm/kg), maintain normovolemia and prevent marked hyperosmolality and hypernatremia. Using the barbiturate anesthesia is the next step in managing raised ICP. Nevertheless, the physician should be aware of its adverse effects including hypotension. Hyperventilation ($PaCO_2$: 25-30 mm Hg) decreases ICP markedly. However, its effect is temporary and in the cost of decreasing cerebral perfusion pressure. Therefore, it should be avoided generally and only be used when the aforementioned steps failed to decrease ICP.

Neuromuscular blockade can reduce ICP. However, due to its potential adverse effects including pneumonia, it is generally avoided. Glucocorticoids are ineffective in reducing or preventing increased ICP in ICH.

Question 10

1. Enumerate poisonous snakebites in India.

Most common venomous snake species in India "known as big four (refers to the four)" are: (1) spectacled cobra (*Naja naja*), (2) saw-scaled viper (*Echis carinatus*), (3) Russell's viper (*Daboia russelii*), and (4) common krait (*Bungarus caeruleus*).

2. Discuss clinical presentation of a case of poisonous snakebite.

Signs of local toxicity at the bite site would suggest envenomation. Signs of systemic toxicity of Viperid and Elapid species are as listed in **Tables 5 and 6**.

3. Explain the management of such cases of snakebites.

The management of snakebite includes firstly ascertaining whether it was a snakebite at all, if yes as whether venomous or not as also looking for signs and symptoms suggestive of both local and systemic envenomation. Evidence of venomous snakebite per se does not establish envenomation as a good number of bites especially with cobra species could be dry (bite without injection of venom).

Take brief history and perform physical examination, first aid, triaging, whole blood clotting test.

Differentiating hematotoxic (Viperid) and neurotoxic (Elapid) bites: Hemostatic abnormalities are prima facie evidences of Viperid bite, give a history of snakebite. All Viperid bites can potentially cause renal failure. Syndromic approach of snakebite is described in **Figure 1**.

Antisnake venom (ASV): The only treatment available for venomous snakebite is ASV.

TABLE 5: Signs and symptoms suggestive of Viperid bite (hematotoxic).

Clinical signs	Symptoms Biochemical parameters suggesting envenomation
Presence of fang marks with significant local signs at the bite site such as swelling, pain, erythema, cyanosis, etc.	Nausea, recurrent vomiting, abdominal pain
Tender lymphadenopathy of the nodes draining the bite site	
Hemoptysis, epistaxis, hematuria, hematemesis and melena, chemosis, macular bleed, excessive menstrual bleed, bleeding from the bite site or cannula, bleeding into the muscles, gingival sulci bleed, bleeding into the skin and mucous membranes showing as purpura or petechia	• Deranged hemostatic profile evidenced by either of or all of an abnormal • WBCT (whole blood clotting test) • PT (prothrombin time) >1.5 times control • APTT (activated plasma thromboplastin time), 1.5 times above normal
Abdominal tenderness	Low back ache or loin tenderness
Hypotension resulting from hypovolemia or direct vasodilatory effect of venom	Muscle pain indicating rhabdomyolysis
Lateralizing signs suggestive of an intracerebral bleed	Low platelet count <100,000/cmm Crenated red blood cells in peripheral smear
Bilateral parotid enlargement (viper head appearance)	Rise in serum urea/creatinine, 30% over that of baseline
Conjunctival edema and subconjunctival hemorrhage	Proteinuria
Confusional state	Raised D Dimer
Jaundice	Raised liver enzymes—AST (aspartate aminotransferase), ALT (alanine transaminase)
Ptosis (Russell's viper bite)	Decreased fibrinogen
	Dysgeusia with a metallic taste in the mouth
	Passage of reddish or dark-colored urine or a reduction in the amount of urine

TABLE 6: Signs and symptoms suggestive of elapid bite—cobra and krait (neurotoxic).

Clinical signs	Symptoms Biochemical parameters suggesting envenomation
Fang marks, swelling, necrosis, blistering and local reaction at the bite site, lymphangitis	Pain, swelling, and inflammation of the bitten part
Descending paralysis, initially of muscles innervated by cranial nerves, commencing as a ptosis, diplopia or an ophthalmoplegia (the eyelid feels heavy with a difficulty in focusing)	Diplopia, dysphagia, dysgeusia (tingling sensation in the tongue with a loss of taste), dysphonia, dyspnea (5Ds)
"Broken neck" sign due to paralysis of neck muscles	Descending paralysis
Diaphoresis, circumoral pallor and paresthesia	Abdominal pain and vomiting
Miosis (pupillary constriction)	Profound thirst
Painful lymphadenopathy	Palpitation, breathlessness and chest pain
Paralysis of jaw and tongue may lead to upper airway obstruction and aspiration of pooled secretions as the victim is unable to swallow	Confusional state usually due to cerebral hypoxia
Bulbar paralysis and respiratory failure can cause cyanosis, altered sensorium and coma	Fall in tidal volume/respiratory volumes
Krait bite often presents in the early morning with paralysis that can often be mistaken for a stroke	

Syndrome-1	• Local swelling with bleeding and clotting abnormalities—all species of **Viperidae** • Local swelling with bleeding, clotting abnormalities with shock or acute kidney injury, dark brown urine, facial paralysis, ptosis ophthalmoplegia—**Russel viper (India and Sri Lanka)** • With conjunctival edema (chemosis) and acute pituitary insufficiency—**Russel viper (Myanmar)**
Syndrome-2	• Local swelling with paralysis—**cobra/king cobra** • Minimum or no local swelling with paralysis, bitten on ground while sleeping—**krait**
Syndrome-3	• Bitten on land—**Russel viper** • Bitten on land while sleeping indoor—**krait** • Bitten in water—**sea snake**

Fig. 1: Syndromic approach to snakebite.

Types of ASV available are—polyvalent-liquid/dry lyophilized. Dose in victim is same in all age group, child, pregnant, elderly.

Indications of ASV: Rapid developing swelling in more than half of the affected limb, enlarged and tender lymph node.

Coagulation abnormalities—epistaxis hemoptysis hematuria gum bleeding.

Neurotoxic features—ptosis, ophthalmoplegia, regurgitation, nasal voice bulbar palsy.

Cardiotoxic feature—hypotension, shock, and arrhythmia.

Acute kidney injury (renal failure)—features of rhabdomyolysis hyperkalemia dark brown urine oliguria or anuria, raised urea creatinine.

Doses of ASV: Start with 10 vials of ASV diluted in 100 mL of normal saline. Start ASV at 10–15 drops/min for the first 15 minutes, watch for allergic reactions. If there is no evidence of reaction to the ASV, continue with the ASV at a constant speed such as to finish in 1 hour. Continue to monitor the vital signs at 5-minute intervals for the first 30 minutes and then at 15-minute intervals for 2 hours.

Further requirement of doses: Repeat doses of ASV are given as 10 vials, 6 hours after the first dose in case of Viperid bites as the liver takes up to 6 hours to replenish the coagulation factors. Very rarely does one require doses of >20 vials in Elapid bites. *Mechanical ventilation would be required in patients with respiratory failure.*

Neostigmine and cobra envenomation: Cobra venom is α-bungarotoxin, which reversibly blocks postsynaptic acetylcholine receptors. Neostigmine is an anticholinesterase that prolongs the half-life of acetylcholine and can therefore reverse respiratory paralysis and neurotoxic symptoms. It is particularly effective for postsynaptic neurotoxins such as that of Naja naja venom. Despite the fact that the neostigmine test (neostigmine 0.5 mg IM with atropine 0.6 mg IV) was actually an Indian discovery, it is still poorly used in India. There is doubt over its efficacy against presynaptic neurotoxins such as those of the Bungarus caeruleus and the Daboia russelii.

In case of neuroparalysis, *neostigmine:* 0.5–2.5 mg in adults and 0.025 mg/kg in children IV infused over 5 minutes. Give concurrent administration of atropine 0.6–1.2 mg IV in adults and 0.01 mg/kg of atropine IM or subcutaneous in children, if the neostigmine test is positive, same is repeated at half hourly intervals to a total of five doses. This is followed up by repeat injections at increasing intervals of 2–12 hours. If there is no improvement in symptoms after 1 hour, neostigmine should be stopped.

Supportive care: In victims presenting with hematemesis, a Ryle's tube is passed into the stomach and in patients with a likelihood of progression to renal failure it is prudent to have an indwelling Foley's catheter. Both this be done early in the course of hospitalization as the likelihood of traumatic bleed is considerable in case of Viperid bites.

Pain management: Nonsteroidal anti-inflammatory drugs (NSAIDs) are avoided in venomous snakebite especially Viperid. Paracetamol could be given orally; in case of severe pain, one could use tramadol hydrochloride.

Antibiotics: A wide range of antibiotics have been used as prophylaxis against secondary infection especially in cases of significant necrosis at the bite site. Combination of amoxicillin with clavulanic acid can be used for the same.

SUGGESTED READING

1. Richhariya D, Sharma B. Textbook of Emergency Medicine including Intensive Care and Trauma, 2nd edition. New Delhi: Jaypee Brothers Medical Publishers (P) Ltd; 2022. pp. 820-7. (Question 1).
2. Richhariya D, Sharma B. Textbook of Emergency Medicine including Intensive Care and Trauma, 2nd edition. New Delhi: Jaypee Brothers Medical Publishers (P) Ltd; 2022. pp. 583-91. (Question 2).
3. Richhariya D, Sharma B. Textbook of Emergency Medicine including Intensive Care and Trauma, 2nd edition. New Delhi: Jaypee Brothers Medical Publishers (P) Ltd; 2022. pp. 871-6. (Question 3).
4. Richhariya D, Sharma B. Textbook of Emergency Medicine including Intensive Care and Trauma, 2nd edition. New Delhi: Jaypee Brothers Medical Publishers (P) Ltd; 2022. pp. 1047-55. (Question 4).
5. Richhariya D, Sharma B. Textbook of Emergency Medicine including Intensive Care and Trauma, 2nd edition. New Delhi: Jaypee Brothers Medical Publishers (P) Ltd; 2022. pp. 1025-32. (Question 5).
6. Richhariya D, Sharma B. Textbook of Emergency Medicine including Intensive Care and Trauma, 2nd edition. New Delhi: Jaypee Brothers Medical Publishers (P) Ltd; 2022. pp. 882-92. (Question 6).
7. Richhariya D, Sharma B. Textbook of Emergency Medicine including Intensive Care and Trauma, 2nd edition. New Delhi: Jaypee Brothers Medical Publishers (P) Ltd; 2022. pp. 1525-34. (Question 7).
8. Richhariya D, Sharma B. Textbook of Emergency Medicine including Intensive Care and Trauma, 2nd edition. New Delhi: Jaypee Brothers Medical Publishers (P) Ltd; 2022. pp. 833-7. (Question 8).
9. Richhariya D, Sharma B. Textbook of Emergency Medicine including Intensive Care and Trauma, 2nd edition. New Delhi: Jaypee Brothers Medical Publishers (P) Ltd; 2022. pp. 828-31. (Question 9).
10. Richhariya D, Sharma B. Textbook of Emergency Medicine including Intensive Care and Trauma, 2nd edition. New Delhi: Jaypee Brothers Medical Publishers (P) Ltd; 2022. pp. 1720-8. (Question 10).

Emergency Medicine Paper 20

Rahul Solanki

Question 1

1. Discuss recent advances in management of a difficult airway.

A difficult airway is considered in whom anatomical irregularities/deviation predict difficulty in securing the airway. A failed airway is considered in which the chosen technique has failed, and rescue technique is implemented. Obviously, there is much overlap, but it is important to keep the two notions distinct. *Difficult airway can be divided into two categories—an anatomically difficult airway and a physiologically difficult airway.* The anatomical difficult airway requires anatomical or logistical manipulation for successful intubation, whereas the physiologic difficult airway requires optimization of overall patient management (correction of low oxygen saturation, blood pressure, or metabolic derangement, such as severe metabolic acidosis). Difficult airway can be a difficulty in bag mask ventilation, intubation, insertion supraglottic airway or front of neck access to airway. This can be an anticipated or unexpected airway difficulty. The perception of a difficult airway is relative, and many emergency intubations could be considered difficult. Systematic approach can be adopted for identifying the potentially difficult airway by LEMON, MOANS, RODS, and SMART assessments.

- Extraglottic devices such as the laryngeal mask airway-pro-seal (LMA)
- New extraglottic devices Laryngeal Tube, the Cobra perilaryngeal airway (PLA)
- Rigid fiber-optic devices—video-laryngoscope, angulated video-intubation laryngoscope.

Clinical impact of new airway technologies: With the development of these effective new intubation and ventilation devices, together with an improved understanding of the predictors of difficulty in all aspects (bag-mask, extraglottic device, intubation, and cricothyrotomy) of airway manage.

2. Enumerate the methods of percutaneous tracheostomy.

Percutaneous cricothyroidotomy (Seldinger technique): This is performed by using "cricothyroidotomy kit" **(Fig. 1)** available commercially and by using a Seldinger technique. A finder needle attached to a syringe is substituted for the intravenous (IV) cannula catheter and steps of needle cricothyroidotomy are followed. Syringe is removed from the needle and the guide wire is advanced through the needle. The needle is removed once the guide wire is in place. A small stab incision is made using the scalpel in the skin close to the guide wire. Airway catheter along with dilator is inserted over the wire. The dilator and the guide wire both are removed once the airway tube is placed in the trachea. Placement is confirmed through observation of chest rise, auscultation, and assessment of end-tidal CO_2. The tube is secured in place with appropriate tape. The cannula is then connected to high flow oxygen at 15 L/min (50–60 psi) with a Y-connector. Intermittent insufflation, 1 second on for inspiration and 4 seconds off for exhalation, should be done by placing the thumb over it. In this fashion, patient may be adequately ventilated for 30–45 minutes using this technique. Because of the inadequate exhalation, CO_2 slowly accumulates and thus limits the use of this technique for longer time, especially in head injury patients. Significant barotrauma can occur and may convert simple pneumothorax into tension pneumothorax. Therefore, careful and frequent monitoring must be done till definitive airway achieved either by intubation or tracheostomy.

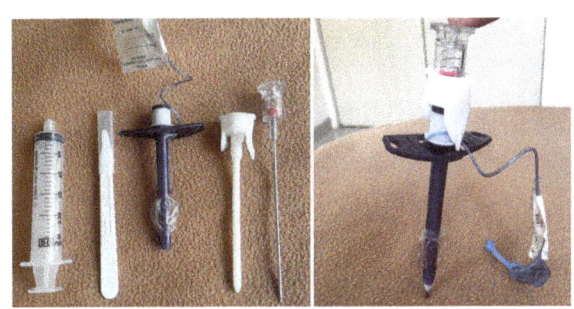

Fig. 1: Percutaneous cricothyroidotomy by "cricothyroidotomy kit".
Courtesy: Dr Amit D Nabar.

Question 2

Write about RUSH protocol in ICU: (a) Indications, (b) Methods, (c) Techniques, and (d) Pitfalls.

Indications: RUSH protocol (rapid ultrasound for shock and hypotension) is a rapid evaluation of cardiac function, key vascular structures, and likely sources of hypotension. Stroke volume is an established important value to assess in the setting of shock, allowing the provider to predict the patient's response to treatment.

Methods: The RUSH exam involves a 3-part bedside physiologic assessment simplified as "the pump," "the tank," and "the pipes." The components of the RUSH exam are: Heart, inferior vena cava (IVC), Morrison's/FAST abdominal views, aorta, and pneumothorax (HI-MAP). The *RUSH exam* can be remembered by the HI-MAP mnemonic (goal is to increase the patient's MAP): Heart, IVC, Morrison's pouch (and complete the FAST), aorta, and pneumothorax. The examination should be undertaken in the *HI-MAP order* and should be done in a timely manner at bedside in the emergency department (ED).

Techniques: The RUSH exam sequencing is shown in **Figure 2** and done in stepwise approach **(Table 1)**. Identification of various shock and findings by RUSH protocols are summarized in **Table 2**.

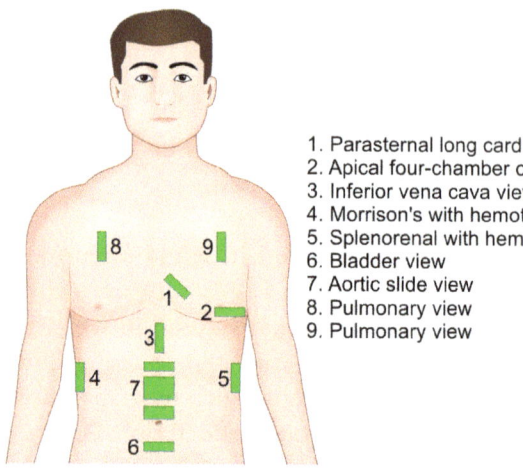

1. Parasternal long cardiac view
2. Apical four-chamber cardiac view
3. Inferior vena cava view
4. Morrison's with hemothorax view
5. Splenorenal with hemothorax view
6. Bladder view
7. Aortic slide view
8. Pulmonary view
9. Pulmonary view

Fig. 2: RUSH exam sequencing.

TABLE 1: Stepwise approach in RUSH protocol.

	Step 1	Step 2	Step 3
Pump	Pericardial effusion: (a) Effusion present? (b) Signs of tamponade? Diastolic collapse of R vent +/− R atrium?	Left ventricular contractility: (a) Hyperdynamic? (b) Normal? (c) Decreased?	Right ventricular strain: (a) Increased size of RV? (b) Septal displacement from right to left?

Tank	Tank volume:
	(1) Inferior vena cava:
	  (a) Large size/small Insp collapse?
	   —CVP high—
	  (b) Small size/large Insp collapse?
	   —CVP Low—
	(2) Internal jugular veins: (a) Small or large?
		Tank leakiness:
		(1) E-FAST exam:
		  (a) Free fluid Abd/Pelvis?
		  (b) Free fluid thoracic cavity?
		(2) *Pulm edema:* Lung rockets?
			Tank compromise: Tension pneumothorax?
			(a) Absent lung sliding?
			(b) Absent comet tails?

Pipes	Abdominal aorta aneurysm: Abd aorta >3 cm?	Thoracic aorta aneurysm/dissection:
		(a) Aortic root >3.8 cm?
		(b) Intimal flap?
		(c) Thor aorta >5 cm?
			(1) Femoral vein DVT?
			   Noncompressible vessel?
			(2) Popliteal vein DVT?
			   Noncompressible vessel?

(Abd: abdomen; CVP: central venous pressure; DVT: deep vein thrombosis; Insp: inspiratory; Pulm: pulmonary)

TABLE 2: Identification and findings of various shock by RUSH protocol.

RUSH exam	Hypovolemic shock	Distributive shock	Obstructive shock	Cardiogenic shock
Pump	Hyperdynamic heart	Hyperdynamic heart (early sepsis) Poor contractility (late sepsis)	Pericardial tamponade RV strain Poor contractility	Poor contractility
Tank	• Small, collapsing IVC • Peritoneal or pleural fluid	• Normal/small IVC • Pleural or peritoneal fluid	• Large, non-collapsing IVC • Absent lung sliding	• Large, non-collapsing IVC • Lung rockets, pleural effusion
Pipes	AAA or dissection	Normal	DVT	Normal

(AAA: abdominal aortic aneurysm; DVT: deep vein thrombosis; IVC: Inferior vena cava; RV: right ventricular)

Pitfalls: In limited field and point-of-care ultrasound, common errors are usually due to limited access, misdiagnosis as a result of wrong timing, unsuitable patient conditions, limited transducer options, satisfaction of search, and unfamiliarity with pediatric sonography. Misdiagnoses due to inexperience may lead to errors in the treatment that may worsen patients' outcomes or even be fatal.

Question 3

1. Discuss recent/last updates in basic life support (BLS) and advanced cardiac life support (ACLS) guidelines.

The American Heart Association (AHA) guidelines for adult, pediatric, neonatal, and resuscitation are revised in year 2020. These guidelines are helpful for the resuscitation providers and instructors during cardiac arrest resuscitation and also result in changes in resuscitation training and practice. The changes in the 2020 AHA guidelines for cardiopulmonary resuscitation (CPR) are summarized below.

- Easy to remember resuscitation scenarios, algorithms, and visual aids guidance for BLS and ACLS are developed.
- Re-emphasis is given on the importance of early initiation of CPR by lay rescuers
- Early epinephrine administration has been reaffirmed, with emphasis such as previous guidelines.
- Use of real-time audio-visual feedback is suggested as a means to maintain CPR quality.
- To improve CPR quality, continuous measure of arterial blood pressure and end tidal carbon dioxide ($ETCO_2$) during ACLS resuscitation is emphasized.
- Routine use of double sequential defibrillation is not recommended as per recent evidences.
- For medication administration during ACLS resuscitation, IV access is the preferred route but intraosseous (IO) access is acceptable if IV access is not available.
- After return of spontaneous circulation (ROSC), patient care requires close attention to oxygenation, blood pressure control, evaluation for percutaneous coronary intervention, targeted temperature management, and multimodal neuroprognostication.
- Postcardiac arrest recovery is long and continuous process after the initial hospitalization, patients should have formal assessment and support for their physical, cognitive, and psychosocial needs.
- Debriefing after resuscitation for lay rescuers, Emergency Medical Services providers, and hospital-based healthcare workers is beneficial to support their mental health and well-being.
- Management of cardiac arrest in pregnancy focuses on maternal resuscitation improves the chances of successful resuscitation of the mother with preparation for early perimortem cesarean delivery if necessary to save the infant.

The changes in algorithms and other performance aids are:

- A sixth link, *Recovery,* is added to the resuscitation—chains of survival **(Fig. 3)**.
- The emphasis is given on the role of early epinephrine administration for patients with non-shockable rhythms in the universal adult cardiac arrest algorithm (modified now).
- Two new algorithms for opioid-associated emergency have been added for lay rescuers and trained rescuers.
- The postcardiac arrest care algorithm was updated to emphasize the need to prevent hyperoxia, hypoxemia, and hypotension.
- In postcardiac arrest care section new diagram is added to guide and inform neuroprognostication.
- A new algorithm has been added to address cardiac arrest in pregnancy.

2. Explain the recent updates in advanced trauma life support (ATLS) guidelines.

The ATLS program recently released its 10th edition, which contains several key changes based upon recent literature updates. The main changes are highlighted in this article on a chapter-by-chapter basis **(Table 3)**.

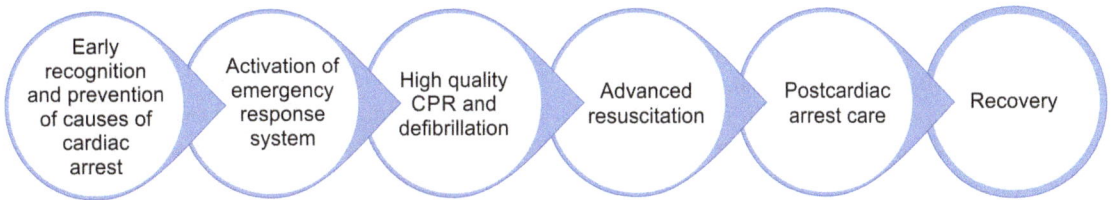

Fig. 3: Resuscitation—updated chain of survival. (CPR: cardiopulmonary resuscitation)

TABLE 3: Recent updates in advanced trauma life support.

Chapter	New recommendations
Initial assessment	Restriction to only 1 L of crystalloid fluid during initial assessment
Airway and ventilation	• Drug-assisted intubation has now replaced rapid sequence intubation (RSI) • Video laryngoscopy highlighted as useful
Shock	• Early use of blood products advocated. • Tranexamic acid is now recommended within 3 hours
Thoracic trauma	• Flail chest replaced by tracheobronchial tree injury as a life-threatening injury • New location for needle thoracocentesis in adults • Modified FAST recommended for identification of pneumothorax • Traumatic circulatory arrest algorithm introduced
Abdominal and pelvic trauma	• Prostate examination no longer recommended as part of the evaluation • Preperitoneal pelvic packing included in hemorrhage protocol
Head trauma	• Anticoagulation reversal table is now included in the guidance • Revised version of the GCS introduced
Spine and spinal cord trauma	• CCR and NEXUS guidelines are now recommended • "Spinal immobilization" has been replaced with "spinal motion restriction." Prolonged backboard usage (>2 hours) should be avoided
Thermal injuries	New fluid resuscitation formula (2 mL/kg/%TBSA)
Musculoskeletal trauma	• The use of a tourniquet to control severe extremity bleeding is now recommended • Antibiotics dosing regimens for open fractures introduced
Pediatric trauma	The PECARN traumatic brain injury algorithm now recommended
Geriatric trauma	• Lower threshold for imaging in the elderly population is now recommended • High-risk preexisting conditions highlighted
Trauma in pregnancy	Vaginal fluid pH >4.5 is an indicator of amniotic fluid leakage
Transfer to definitive care	• CT scans should now be avoided in the primary hospital • SBAR communication tool now recommended

(CCR: Canadian C-spine rules; CT: computed tomography; GCS: Glasgow Coma Scale; NEXUS: National Emergency X-Radiography Utilization Study; PECARN: Pediatric Emergency Care Applied Research Network; SBAR: situation, background, assessment and recommendation; TBSA: total body surface area)

Question 4

1. Discuss etiology of meningitis in children.

Risk factors and etiology: Common pathogens for community-acquired disease are *Streptococcus pneumoniae*, *Haemophilus (H.) influenzae* meningitis, and *Neisseria meningitides*. However, *H. influenza* meningitis is seen less in vaccinated child.

- Age—elderly and younger child
  - *Neonates (<1 week):* Escherichia (E.) coli, Listeria (L.) monocytogenes, Group B Streptococcus
  - *Neonates (>1 week):* L. monocytogenes
  - *Infants and children:* N. meningitidis, S. pneumoniae
  - *Young adults:* Meningitides, S. pneumoniae
  - *Elderly:* N. meningitidis, S. pneumoniae, L. monocytogenes
- Malnutrition, overcrowding, and low social economic status, exposure to epidemic.
- Head and neck infections—otitis media, mastoiditis
- Major medical illness—liver disease, renal disease, DM
- Immuno-compromised—patients on steroids, chemotherapy, cancer patients, complement deficiency, splenectomy patients.
  - *S. pneumoniae, H. influenzae, and Listeria monocytogenes.*
- *Patients with cochlear implant or basilar skull fracture:*
  - *S. pneumoniae, H. influenzae, Group A beta hemolytic streptococci*
- *Patient with neurosurgery or basilar skull fracture:*
  - *Staphylococcus aureus*, coagulase negative *Staphylococci, Pseudomonas*
- *Viral causes:*
  - Common viruses which can cause meningitis are arboviruses, herpes simplex virus (HSV), coxsackieviruses, echoviruses, human enteroviruses, human immunodeficiency virus (HIV), varicella zoster, Epstein–Barr virus.
- Subacute causes of meningitis—tuberculosis, fungal, autoimmune disorders such as SLE, malignancy, drugs—are uncommon.

2. Explain the clinical features, physical examination, laboratory evaluation, and ED treatment of bacterial meningitis in this age group.

Clinical presentation: Clinical features may vary depending on duration and severity of illness, causative organism and host characteristics. Initial symptoms may be nonspecific and comprise of a prodrome such as fever, malaise, and headache. Hence emergency physician must have low threshold to suspect meningitis. Patients lying in extremes of age group, immunocompromised patient and partially treated may not have classical symptoms. Presentation of subacute meningitis such as fungal and tuberculous meningitis is also obscure. The classic triad of *fever, altered mental status, and neck stiffness* is seen in <50% of patients with meningitis. At least two of four symptoms of fever, altered mental status, neck stiffness, and headache will be present in 95% patient. Associated symptoms—genitourinary complaints, rash, cough.

Enquire about—immunization history, associated comorbidities.

Travel history—e.g., Japanese B infection is common in south-East Asia.

Social history—e.g., residence in closed dormitories is risk factor for meningococcal meningitis.

History of tuberculosis

Physical examination: Kernig's signs—with the patient lying supine and hip flexed to right angle, attempt to straighten the leg to full extension—inability to do so is a positive Kernig's sign.

Brudzinski's signs—with the patient in supine position attempt to passively flex the neck cause flexion at hip joint.

Head jolt test: The patient is asked to move his/her head back and forth in the horizontal plane at a rate of 2–3 turns/second. If the patient's headache worsens, it is considered positive.

Signs of brain parenchymal irritation: Altered mental status, seizures, personality changes, and focal neuro deficit. In advanced stages of meningitis cerebral edema develops which causes symptoms such as vomiting, headache, and cranial nerve abnormalities.

Investigations: Complete blood count—total leucocyte count may be increased in bacterial meningitis. However, a normal total leukocyte count does not rule out meningitis. Measure blood sugar levels frequently. Coagulation profile will be required before performing lumbar puncture.

Chest X-ray: A total of 50% of patient with pneumococcal meningitis have evidence of chests infection in initial X-ray. Blood cultures are to be collected as soon as possible in a patient suspected with meningitis. Blood cultures are positive in 50–80% cases of bacterial meningitis.

Other ancillary tests: Liver function tests, renal function test. Blood biomarkers of inflammation such as procalcitonin, CRP can be used to guide treatment.

Neuroimaging: It is not mandatory to perform neuroimaging before initiating treatment in clinically suspected meningitis. Urgent CT brain should be performed in patients with signs of increased intracranial tension before performing lumbar puncture.

Cerebrospinal fluid (CSF) analysis: At least three sterile tubes containing 1–1.5 mL of CSF each should be collected. Parameters to be assed in CSF-opening pressure, turbidity, xanthochromia, glucose, protein, CSF lactate, CSF to serum glucose ratio, cell counts, gram staining, acid fast staining, CSF culture. CSF findings in different types of meningitis are summarized in **Table 4**.

Emergency department treatment of bacterial meningitis in this age group: Choice of empirical antibiotics will depend on the infection suspected based on patient's age and premorbid condition **(Table 5)**. Dexamethasone may attenuate the inflammatory response and its consequences like vasculitis, cerebral edema, etc., and shown to reduce overall mortality and neurological sequelae. First dose of dexamethasone should be administered at least 10–20 minutes before administration of antibiotics. Dose is 0.15 mg/kg. It is continued every 6 hours for next 4 days. Other corticosteroids have poor central nervous system (CNS) penetrations, hence not to be used. All patients with meningitis have to be hospitalized and started on IV antibiotic therapy.

TABLE 4: Cerebrospinal fluid (CSF) findings in different types of meningitis.

	Normal	Bacterial	Viral	Fungal	Tubercular
Opening pressure (cm CSF)	<170 mm	>300	200	300	Raised
Appearance	Clear	Turbid/purulent	Clear	Clear	Clear
CSF WBC (cells/μL)	<5	1,000–5,000	5–1,000	5–100	5–100
Predominant cells	None	Neutrophil	Lymphocytes	Lymphocytes	Lymphocytes
CSF protein	28–32 mg/dL	Raised	Normal-mildly raised	Markedly raised	Raised
CSF glucose (mg/dL)	45	Very low	Normal/slightly low	Very low	Low
CSF plasma glucose ratio	0.66	Very low	Normal/slightly low	Very low	Low
CSF lactates	normal	>35 mg/dL	Normal	>25 mg/dL	
% of PMNs	0	>80%	1–50%	1–50%	<30%

(PMNs: polymorphonuclear leukocytes; WBC: white blood cells)

TABLE 5: Empirical antibiotic therapy for meningitis.

Age group	Empirical antibiotic therapy
Neonates	Ampicillin (150 mg/kg/day) + 3rd generation cephalosporin, e.g., cefotaxime (100–150 mg/kg/day)
Infant and children	Cefotaxime or ceftriaxone (80–100 mg/kg/day) + vancomycin (60 mg/kg/day)
Adults	Ceftriaxone (80–100 mg/kg/day) + vancomycin (30–60 mg/kg/day)
Immunocompromised patient	Cefotaxime (8–12 g/day) or ceftriaxone (4 g/day) + ampicillin (12 g/day) vancomycin (30–60 mg/kg/day)
Suspected nosocomial infection	Vancomycin (30–60 mg/kg/day) + ceftazidime (6 g/day) or cefepime (6 g/day) or meropenem (6 g/day)

Question 5

1. Define sepsis.

The definition as sepsis-3 in 2016, defines sepsis as a *"life-threatening organ dysfunction caused by dysregulated host response to infection."* Whereas septic shock is recognized as, *"A subset of sepsis in which underlying circulatory and cellular metabolism abnormalities are profound enough to substantially increase mortality."*

2. Discuss qSOFA score in ED.

Sepsis-3 definition suggests clinical criteria to operationalize and rapidly categorize patients according to new definition. A qSOFA score of ≥2 points **(Table 6)** or a worsening sequential organ failure assessment (SOFA) score of ≥2 point is taken as marker of organ dysfunction and in event of suspected infection qualifies for sepsis.

3. Describe recent surviving sepsis guidelines including 1-hour and 6-hour bundles.

The 1-hour bundle is composed of the following five elements—measuring the lactate level, obtaining blood culture prior to administration of antibiotics, administering broad-spectrum antibiotics, beginning rapid administration of 30 mL/kg crystalloid fluid for hypotension or lactate ≥4 mmol/L **(Table 7)**.

TABLE 6: qSOFA score.

H	**H**ypotension: SBP less than or equal to 100 mm Hg
A	**A**ltered mental status (any GCS <15)
T	**T**achypnea: Respiratory rate greater than or equal to 22/min

(GCS: Glasgow Coma Scale; SBP: systolic blood pressure; SOFA: sequential organ failure assessment)

TABLE 7: Surviving sepsis guidelines.

HOUR-1 bundle of surviving sepsis campaign	
Bundle elements to be completed within 1st hour	• Measure lactate level. Remeasure if initial lactate is >2 mmol/L • Obtain blood cultures prior to administration of antibiotics. Best practice statement • Administer broad-spectrum antibiotics, strong recommendation • rapidly administer 30 mL/kg crystalloid for hypotension or lactate ≥4 mmol/L • Apply vasopressors if patient is hypotensive during or after fluid resuscitation to maintain MAP ≥65 mm Hg
"Time zero" or "time of presentation"	Time of triage at the first point of contact or, if patient is referred from another care location, represents the time when sepsis is first identified through chart review
HOUR-6 bundle	
• Repeat lactic acid if initial lactic acid >2 • Vasopressors if hypotensive • Repeat physical examination	

(MAP: mean arterial pressure)

Question 6

1. Enumerate the causes of vomiting by age.

Differential diagnosis of vomiting in the pediatric age **(Table 8)** group may be a result of a range of causes, including gastrointestinal (GI) (i.e., obstructive and inflammatory) etiologies, CNS disease, pulmonary problems, renal disease, endocrine/metabolic disorders, drugs (either as side effects or in overdose), psychiatric disorders.

2. Discuss clinical guidelines for assessing dehydration in children.

Child with dehydration (diarrhea vomiting) should be assessed for: (1) Dehydration, (2) Blood in diarrhea, (3) Coexisting malnutrition, and (4) Serious non-intestinal infections.

TABLE 8: Causes of acute vomiting in infants and children.

Infants	Children
Viral gastroenteritis	Viral gastroenteritis
Gastroesophageal reflux	Sepsis
Pyloric stenosis	Meningitis/encephalitis
Intussusception	Appendicitis/pyelonephritis
Sepsis	Hepatitis
Malrotation	Raised Intracranial tension
Food intolerance	Toxic ingestion
Metabolic disorders	Adverse drug reactions
	Cyclic vomiting syndrome

History should focus on—duration of diarrhea and number of watery stools per day; volume of water in stool; presence of blood in the stool; frequency of urination; presence of vomiting, fever, cough or seizures; pre-illness feeding practices; fluids, food and drugs taken during illness and immunization history. Examination should include—general condition of child; signs of dehydration; nutritional status (weight/weight for height/MAC) and severity of malnutrition if any; presence of blood in stool besides general physical and systemic examination. Classification of dehydration **(Table 9)** is of utmost importance in the management.

3. How will you treat a case of mild-to-moderate dehydration in children?

Plan of treatment for acute diarrhea has been shown in **Table 10**. Management of acute vomiting consists of assessment and correction of dehydration and correction of specific etiology besides symptomatic management. Since acute vomiting is mostly seen as a part of acute gastroenteritis, our discussion here will be focused on that.

Objectives: (1) Prevent and treat dehydration, (2) Drugs (antibiotics, Zinc), (3) Nutritional management, and (4) Education.

Indications for hospital admission are: (1) Shock, (2) Severe dehydration, (3) Neurological abnormalities (lethargy, seizures), (4) Intractable or bilious vomiting, (5) Failure of oral rehydration, (6) Suspected surgical condition, and (7) Conditions for a safe follow-up and home management are not met.

TABLE 9: Classification of dehydration.

Severe (Two of the following are present)	Some (Two of the following are present)	No dehydration
Lethargy/unconscious	Restless, irritable	Not enough signs to classify some or severe dehydration
Sunken eyes	Sunken eyes	
Not able to drink/drinking poorly	Drinks eagerly, thirsty	
Skin pinch goes back very slowly	Skin pinch goes back slowly	

TABLE 10: Plan of treatment for dehydration.

Severe dehydration	Some dehydration	No dehydration
Plan C	Plan B	Plan A
Urgent care in hospital	Treat dehydration with ORS/IV fluid	Home care

(IV: intravenous; ORS: oral rehydration solution)

Question 7

1. Describe pediatric seizure disorder.

A seizure is a single event characterized by the abnormal excessive synchronized firing of cortical neurons which causes involuntary muscle contractions with or without alteration in mental status. Focal seizure starts from unilateral area of brain while generalized seizures arise from both cerebral hemispheres at once. The manifestations of focal seizures depend on the area of the brain involved. Neonatal seizures are typically subtler than seizures in older children and adults, in view of the immature nervous system of the neonate. Benign febrile seizures (convulsions) are an inherited predisposition to developing a tonic-clonic seizure with a high fever. The description is limited to convulsions associated with high fever in children under the age of 5 (usually between 6 and 36 months of age), with no cause for the seizure other than the fever. Benign febrile seizures are common, occurring in 3–5% of children under the age of 5. Most patients have only one or two seizures. Recent genetic analysis of families with febrile convulsions has defined specific associated gene defects.

2. Write about their presentation.

Clinical presentation: Depending upon the area in the brain where the seizure initiates and how it propagates symptoms could vary widely.

- Generalized seizures cause loss of consciousness along with purposeless full-body tonic (sustained)-clonic (interrupted) movements, atonia, and/or myoclonic jerking.
- Focal seizures can manifest as disturbances in motor/sensory/autonomic function, emotional state, cognition, behavior, or memory with or without alteration in consciousness.
- At the cessation of seizure activity, the patient will enter the postictal period, characterized by confusion, fatigue, lethargy, and/or irritability.
- Neonatal seizures may present with subtle findings, such as ocular movement or lip smacking or abnormal vitals.
- Nonconvulsive status epilepticus can present as altered mental status, mild confusion, and subtle physical movements, inexplicable sudden changes in mental status or delayed recovery after a seizure.
- *Clinical features of concern (red flags) are:* Seizure in clinically unwell child such as symptoms of infection, meningeal signs, dehydration, complex febrile, seizure, altered level of consciousness, additional risks for serious bacterial infection—(age <6 months or >60 months with first febrile seizure, age <12 months with incomplete or unknown immunization history, febrile status epilepticus).

3. Write its ED management.

Immediate measures for a seizing child in ED, should be taken and they are secure airway, give high flow oxygen, assess breathing and circulation, assess vital signs, check blood glucose, secure IV access in a large vein, place patient on full monitor, followed by medications depending on seizure type and underlying cause.

Treatment of febrile seizure: Antipyretic therapy is to be given to relive symptoms of associated febrile illness but they do not reduce seizure activity. Supportive therapy is usually sufficient for seizures lasting <15 minutes as most of the seizures are brief and self-limiting. Rectal diazepam can be used. Seizures lasting ≥15 minutes are treated in the line of status epilepticus. Maintenance drug therapy is usually not indicated.

Treatment of neonatal seizure: Maintain airway, breathing, circulation, and temperature. Collect blood for biochemistry. Check blood glucose immediately, correct glucose and calcium, administer IV phenobarbitone 20 mg/kg. Repeat in 5 mg/kg boluses every 15 minutes if seizure continues up to a maximum dose of 40 mg/kg. IV phenytoin 15–20 mg/kg diluted in same amount of normal saline at a maximum rate of 1 mg/kg/min over 35–40 minutes. IV lorazepam (0.05–0.1 mg/kg) or diazepam (0.25 mg/kg bolus or 0.5 mg/kg rectal) or IV midazolam as a continuous infusion (an initial IV bolus of 0.15 mg/kg, followed by continuous infusion (1 µg/kg/min) increasing by 0.5 to 1 µg/kg/min every 2 minutes until a favorable response or a maximum of 18 µg/kg/min 100 mg pyridoxine IV or oral (if IV not available) should be given.

Treatment of status epilepticus: In *the community-prolonged* (lasting 5 minutes or more) or repeated (3 or more in an hour), generalized, convulsive (tonic-clonic, tonic or clonic) seizures in the community should receive immediate emergency care. If history of previous episode of prolonged or serial convulsive seizures is present buccal midazolam or rectal diazepam can be given. Care must be taken to secure airway and assess respiratory and cardiac function. *Patient in ED-convulsive status* epilepticus can lead to permanent neuronal injury. Majority of the seizures are brief and self-limiting. If a seizure activity lasts for >5 minutes the chances are more that the seizure is likely to be prolonged. Keeping that in mind all the status treatment protocols have used a 5-minute definition. Early treatment minimizes risk of seizures reaching 30 minutes and subsequent neuronal damage. Moreover, the adverse outcomes associated with needlessly intervening on brief, self-limited seizures are eliminated by avoiding aggressive therapy before 5 minutes.

Question 8

1. Discuss transmission, clinical presentation, and management of Nipah virus (NiV).

- *Transmission:* Nipah virus is a zoonotic virus, meaning that it can spread between animals and people. Fruit bats, also called flying foxes, are the animal reservoir for NiV in nature. NiV is also known to cause illness in pigs and people. Infection with NiV is associated with encephalitis (swelling of the brain) and can cause mild-to-severe illness and even death. Outbreaks occur almost annually in parts of Asia, primarily Bangladesh and India. NiV infection can be prevented by avoiding exposure to sick pigs and bats in areas where the virus is present, and not drinking raw date palm sap which can be contaminated by an infected bat. During an outbreak, standard infection control practices can help prevent person-to-person spread in hospital settings. NiV is transmitted to humans either from animals (contact with urine, saliva or contaminated materials) or from other humans.
- *Clinical presentation* ranges from asymptomatic infection to fatal encephalitis. Some people can also experience atypical pneumonia and acute respiratory distress. Early diagnosis of NiV infection can be challenging due to the nonspecific early symptoms of the illness. Later in the course of illness and after recovery, testing for antibodies is conducted using an enzyme-linked immunosorbent assay (ELISA).
- *Management:* Currently there are no licensed treatments available for NiV infection. Treatment is limited to supportive care, including rest, hydration, and treatment of symptoms as they occur. There are, however, immunotherapeutic treatments (monoclonal antibody therapies) that are currently under development and evaluation for treatment of NiV infections.

2. Explain the transmission, clinical presentation, and management of Zika virus (ZIKV).

Transmission: Zika virus is *transmitted primarily by Aedes mosquitoes*, which bite mostly during the day. Most people with ZIKV infection do not develop symptoms; those who do typically have symptoms including rash, fever, conjunctivitis, muscle and joint pain, malaise and headache that last for 2–7 days.

Clinical presentation: In most cases, ZIKV infection causes a mild, self-limited illness. The incubation period is likely 3–12 days. Owing to the mild nature of the disease, >80% of ZIKV infection cases likely go unnoticed. The spectrum of

ZIKV disease overlaps with other that of arboviral infections, but rash (maculopapular and likely immune-mediated) typically predominates. The rash in ZIKV infection is usually a fine maculopapular rash that is diffusely distributed. It can involve the face, trunk, and extremities, including palms and soles.

Management: There is no specific treatment available for ZIKV infection or disease. People with symptoms such as rash, fever or joint pain should get plenty of rest, drink fluids, and treat symptoms with antipyretics and/or analgesics.

Question 9

A 2-year-old child presented with fever, drooling of saliva, and stridor.

1. Enumerate the causes of stridor in infants and children.

Causes of stridor: In newborn and infants, the most common cause is laryngomalacia, a condition in which tissues located in the throat above the vocal cords are too soft and flop into the airway. This causes inspiratory stridor, meaning the symptoms of noisy breathing occur when a child inhale **(Table 11)**.

TABLE 11: Most common causes of stridor in infants and children.

	Nasopharyngeal	Laryngeal	Tracheal
Neonates	• Rhinitis • Choanal atresia or stenosis • Craniofacial abnormalities • Micrognathia	• Laryngomalacia • Intubation trauma • Reflux laryngitis • Laryngotracheal stenosis • Vocal cord palsy	• Tracheal bronchomalacia • Tracheal stenosis • Vascular compression
Children	• Allergic rhinitis • Adenoiditis • Adenotonsillar hypertrophy • Foreign bodies	• Croup • Hemangioma • Papillomatosis • Intubation trauma • Vocal cord palsy	• Foreign bodies • Tracheal stenosis

2. Write short notes on the following:
   a. **Croup**
   b. **Clinical presentation of croup**
   c. **Diagnosis of croup**
   d. **Treatment of croup**

Croup: Croup or viral laryngotracheobronchitis (LTB) is one of the frequent causes of stridor. Stridor is a high pitched, harsh sound which occurs during inspiration. Wheeze is a musical sound that occurs during expiration, due to lower airway obstruction. Croup is a syndrome that includes spasmodic croup (recurrent croup), laryngotracheitis (viral croup), LTB, and laryngotracheobronchopneumonitis. However, recurrent and viral croup account for most cases.

Viral infections: Parainfluenza types 1 and 3 accounts for >70% of viral LTB cases; other viruses—influenza A, influenza B, adenovirus, respiratory syncytial virus, and metapneumovirus.

Clinical presentation: Viral croup symptoms usually start like an upper respiratory tract infection, with low-grade fever and coryza followed by a barking cough and various degrees of respiratory distress (e.g., nasal flaring, respiratory retractions, and stridor). The symptoms subside quickly with resolution of the cough usually within 2 days, although the cough may persist for up to 1 week. Symptoms can increase and decrease in the same child, becoming worse at night and when the child is agitated. Symptoms also vary from child to child based on host factors, such as immunity and the anatomy of the subglottic space. Many children with croup may come to the ED because symptoms begin abruptly, causing parental concern.

Diagnosis: The diagnosis of croup is based on clinical assessment. Diagnosis also involves closely assessing the severity of croup by evaluating respiratory status and rate, retractions, stridor, heart rate, use of accessory muscles, and mental status. The most reliable findings to assess severity are the presence of stridor and the severity of retractions (*Westley croup scoring*). Pulse oximetry can also be used to assess the severity of disease. Laboratory and imaging evaluation are not essential, but may be used to rule out other illnesses in selected patients with an atypical or severe presentation. A complete blood count (neutrophilic leukocytosis) and high C-reactive protein (CRP) may help distinguish croup from bacterial etiologies of stridor (e.g., bacterial tracheitis, epiglottitis, peritonsillar abscess, and retropharyngeal abscess), but it is nonspecific. Lateral neck radiography may be considered if the diagnosis is in doubt because it could help detect epiglottitis (thickened epiglottis), retropharyngeal abscess (widening of the retropharyngeal soft tissues), and bacterial tracheitis (thickened trachea). Endoscopy may also be needed in patients with recurrent croup.

Management:
- *General care:* Keeping a symptomatic child calm by avoiding distressing procedures is important because agitation may worsen airway obstruction.
- *Humidification therapy* has long been used as a treatment for croup. However, it has not been shown to reduce croup severity, hospitalization, additional medical care, or epinephrine and corticosteroid use in patients with mild to moderate illness in the ED.

- *Corticosteroid therapy* benefits patients with croup presumably by decreasing edema in the laryngeal mucosa, and is usually effective within 6 hours of treatment. Corticosteroid therapy decreases the need for additional medical care, hospital stays, and intubation rates and duration. Administer dexamethasone single dose 0.6 mg/kg.
- *Epinephrine:* A number of small randomized controlled trials have shown that nebulized epinephrine is an effective treatment for moderate to severe croup, with benefits such as reduction in croup severity, various objective pathophysiologic measures, and need for intubation. The recommended dose 0.5 mL/kg (maximal dose: 5 mL) of L-epinephrine 1:1,000 via nebulizer, which may be available in clinical settings along with other resuscitation supplies. Using a nebulizer is equally as effective as using intermittent positive pressure ventilation.

Question 10

1. Enumerate the medicines used in rapid sequence intubation (RSI) (also known as drug-assisted intubation).

Rapid sequence intubation is the most widely used technique for emergency intubation of patients without identifiable difficult airway attributes, with recent large registry data showing that it is used in 85% of all ED intubations. This approach provides optimal condition for intubation with minimal risk of aspiration of gastric content. This procedure (RSI) is performed with the help of induction agents (potent sedative) and neuromuscular blocking agents (NMBA) (succinylcholine or rocuronium). RSI is based on the concept that with the help of neuromuscular paralytic agent, conscious spontaneously breathing patient is taken to a state of unconsciousness with complete neuromuscular paralysis. Thus positive-pressure ventilation is avoided until the endotracheal tube (ETT) is placed correctly in the trachea, with the cuff inflated **(Table 12)**.

2. Write about pharmacology of importance of medicines used in RSI as per recent updates.

Common sedative agents used during RSI include *etomidate, ketamine, and propofol*. Commonly used NMBA are succinylcholine and rocuronium. Certain induction agents and paralytic drugs may be more beneficial than others in certain clinical situations **(Table 13)**.

TABLE 12: Drugs for rapid sequence intubations.

Drugs: Pretreatment, induction and paralysis (PIP)		
Pretreatment—LOAD	Induction	Paralysis
L—Lignocaine	Etomidate	Suxamethonium
O—Opioids–Fenatnyl	Propofol	Rocuronium
A—Atropine	Ketamine	Vecuronium
D—Defasciculating agents	Midazolam	Atracurium

TABLE 13: Pharmacology of importance of medicines used in rapid sequence intubation.

Agent	Standard dose (mg/kg)	Dose if hemodynamic compromise	Comments
Etomidate	0.2–0.3	0.1–0.2	Rapid onset, short duration. Few hemodynamic effects. Preferred for hypotensive patients with head injury or coronary artery disease
Ketamine	1.0–2.0	No difference	Longer duration. Sympathetic stimulation, bronchodilation, dreams, salivation. Preferred for patients with asthma
Propofol	2.0–2.5 mg/kg given 40 mg every 10 seconds	No difference	Slow infection preferred over rapid bolus administration. Rapid bolus may result in cardiorespiratory depression. Titrate dose to response. Maintenance doses by infusion are preferred 0.3–3 mg/kg/h for prolonged sedation. Avoid in patients with hypovolemia
Fentanyl and midazolam	Fentanyl 1.0–4.0 µg/kg for *pain:* Midazolam 5.0–10.0 mg for sedation	Reduce by 50% if hemodynamically compromised	Can cause respiratory depression during initial administration. Excellent for prolonged sedation and pain control, but monitor vital signs often
Succinylcholine	0.6–1.5	No difference	Short-acting. Many contraindications and adverse effects. Clinical duration 4–6 minutes
Rocuronium	0.6–1.5	No difference	Onset time equal to succinylcholine. Clinical duration 30–60 minutes
Vecuronium	0.08–0.10	No difference	Onset time 2–3 minutes. Clinical duration 25–40 minutes

SUGGESTED READING

1. Centers for Disease Control and Prevention. (2022). Areas with Risk of ZIKA. [online] Available from: https://www.cdc.gov/zika/index.html [Last accessed May, 2023]. (Question 8).
2. Centers for Disease Control and Prevention. (2022). Nipah virus (NiV). [online] Available from: https://www.cdc.gov/vhf/nipah/index.html [Last accessed May, 2023]. (Question 8).
3. Richhariya D, Sharma B. Textbook of Emergency Medicine including Intensive Care and Trauma, 2nd edition. New Delhi: Jaypee Brothers Medical Publishers (P) Ltd; 2022. p. 205. (Question 1).
4. Richhariya D, Sharma B. Textbook of Emergency Medicine including Intensive Care and Trauma, 2nd edition. New Delhi: Jaypee Brothers Medical Publishers (P) Ltd; 2022. p. 395. (Question 1).
5. Richhariya D, Sharma B. Textbook of Emergency Medicine including Intensive Care and Trauma, 2nd edition. New Delhi: Jaypee Brothers Medical Publishers (P) Ltd; 2022. p. 364. (Question 2).
6. Richhariya D, Sharma B. Textbook of Emergency Medicine including Intensive Care and Trauma, 2nd edition. New Delhi: Jaypee Brothers Medical Publishers (P) Ltd; 2022. p. 227. (Question 3).
7. Richhariya D, Sharma B. Textbook of Emergency Medicine including Intensive Care and Trauma, 2nd edition. New Delhi: Jaypee Brothers Medical Publishers (P) Ltd; 2022. pp. 844-8. (Question 4).
8. Richhariya D, Sharma B. Textbook of Emergency Medicine including Intensive Care and Trauma, 2nd edition. New Delhi: Jaypee Brothers Medical Publishers (P) Ltd; 2022. p. 321. (Question 5).
9. Richhariya D, Sharma B. Textbook of Emergency Medicine including Intensive Care and Trauma, 2nd edition. New Delhi: Jaypee Brothers Medical Publishers (P) Ltd; 2022. pp. 1177-80. (Question 6).
10. Richhariya D, Sharma B. Textbook of Emergency Medicine including Intensive Care and Trauma, 2nd edition. New Delhi: Jaypee Brothers Medical Publishers (P) Ltd; 2022. pp. 1208-13. (Question 7).
11. Richhariya D, Sharma B. Textbook of Emergency Medicine including Intensive Care and Trauma, 2nd edition. New Delhi: Jaypee Brothers Medical Publishers (P) Ltd; 2022. pp. 1275-89. (Question 8).
12. Richhariya D, Sharma B. Textbook of Emergency Medicine including Intensive Care and Trauma, 2nd edition. New Delhi: Jaypee Brothers Medical Publishers (P) Ltd; 2022. p. 1186. (Question 9).
13. Richhariya D, Sharma B. Textbook of Emergency Medicine including Intensive Care and Trauma, 2nd edition. New Delhi: Jaypee Brothers Medical Publishers (P) Ltd; 2022. pp. 209-18. (Question 10).

Emergency Medicine Paper 21

Pradeep Kumar Botsa

Question 1

1. Discuss pathophysiology of bomb blast injuries.

There are four main types of blast effects **(Fig. 1)**. A primary injury is caused by a direct effect of blast wave overpressure on tissue. Primary blast injury mostly affects air-filled structures such as the lungs, ears, and gastrointestinal (GI) tract, by the following mechanisms—spalling, shearing, and implosion. Spalling is displacement and fragmentation of a dense medium into a less dense medium. Shearing is a stress caused by the blast wave traveling through different tissue densities at different velocities. Implosion is where the less dense material is displaced into denser material. A secondary blast injury is due to collateral damage from flying objects and sharps. Tertiary blast injury results from the victim being propelled through the air and striking stationary objects. A quaternary blast injury is a result of burns, smoke inhalation, or chemical agent release.

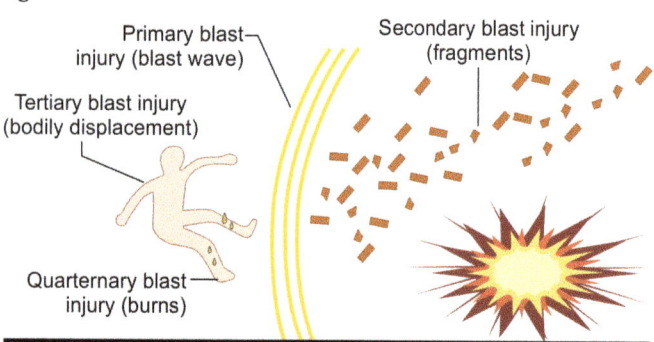

Fig. 1: Pathophysiology of bomb blast.

2. Enumerate the factors affecting bomb blast injuries.

Distance of victim from explosion: Proximity of the victim to the explosion is an important factor in a primary blast injury.

Enclosed versus open space: The effects of an explosion in a closed space such as a room, bus, or train are much greater than in an open space. Injuries are more severe, and mortality is greater.

Surrounding environment: Blast waves are reflected by solid surfaces; thus, a person standing next to a wall may suffer increased primary blast injury.

Quantity of explosive: A greater quantity of explosive produces greater potential for damage at any distance.

Type of explosive: Explosives are commonly classified as either low-order or high-order. Low-order explosives burn rapidly and produce a blast wave of <1,000 m/s. Black powder is an example of a low-order explosive. High-order explosives detonate causing an almost instant transformation of the original explosive material into gases occupying the same volume of space under extremely high pressure. These high-pressure gases expand rapidly, compress the surrounding medium, and produce a supersonic, overpressure blast wave, moving at >4,500 m/s, followed closely by a negative pressure wave.

Embedded sharps: Many terrorists purposefully embed multiple pieces of metal and plastic in the explosive, maximizing the number and severity of secondary injuries.

3. Explain field triage in bomb blast injuries.

Field triage is used to identify priority for treatment of mass casualties. **Figure 2** shows how they are sorted to ensure that those who need immediate life-saving intervention receive this promptly, whilst identifying those less severely injured who can wait. Traumatic arrest in the context of the battlefield is unlikely to be survivable. Diverting resources when under fire, or in the context of mass casualties to the arrested patient is likely to result in further deaths. If resources permit during tactical evacuation, it may be that more specialist interventions, such as resuscitative thoracotomy, could be considered.

4. What is emergency department (ED) triage in bomb blast injuries?

Triaging of bomb blast injuries in ED can be done as given in **Flowchart 1**.

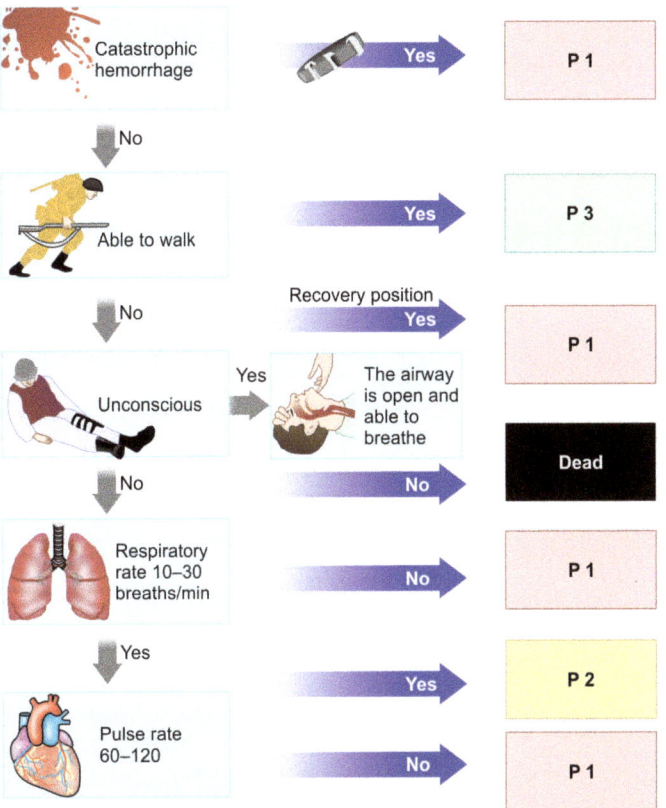

Fig. 2: Field triage of mass casualties. P1 (Priority 1) = Immediate life-saving interventions required; P2 (Priority 2) = Interventions can be delayed but urgent care required within 2 hours; P3 (Priority 3) = It requires medical intervention that can be delayed without risk to patient.

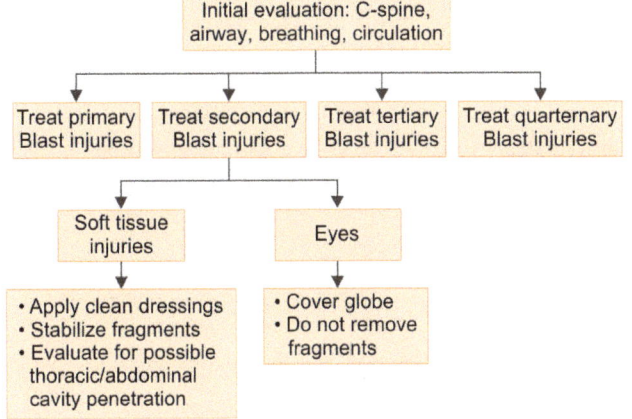

Flowchart 1: Triaging of bomb blast injuries in emergency department.

Question 2

1. Discuss control zones of a chemical release event at a scene.

Control zones of a chemical release event at a scene **(Fig. 3)**:

- *Hot zone (the contaminated area or site of release):* The immediate area where the suspected chemicals and victims of exposure are located is designated the hot zone. Only trained personnel in fully encapsulated protective gear should be allowed to enter. Their primary role is rescue of victims by removing them from further exposure.
- *Warm zone:* A surrounding corridor through which each victim is washed off and decontaminated is created outside the hot zone and is designated the warm zone. This is located uphill and upwind of the hot zone.
- *Cold zone:* A clean area where the victims who are free of external liquid contamination are received. Here, a lower level of protective equipment is necessary and a very low risk of secondary contamination exists.

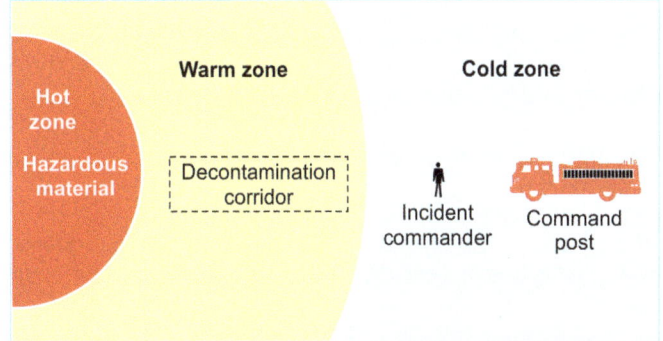

Fig. 3: Control zones of a chemical release event at a scene.

2. How do you suspect chemical terrorism?

- Rapid onset of symptoms, within minutes to days.
- Multiple simultaneous victims are affected with similar symptoms without signs of trauma.
- Most common symptom often noted is respiratory distress.
- There is no typical history of fever or rash or bleeding.
- There are complaints of neuromuscular effects and vesicles based on the chemical agents used.
- The patients do not respond to specific antibiotic drugs.
- There might be many unexplained deaths of humans, animals, fish, or plants.

3. Classify the chemical agents as per their actions.

Chemicals are usually introduced into the body by inhalation, absorption, ingestion, or inoculation, rapidly acting or with delayed effects. The principles of management after exposure to chemical agents centers around the removal of the patient from further exposure to the toxin, attention to ABCs, prior to evacuation, and during decontamination. Rapid identification of the offending agent based on history and/or examination can allow for the initiation of specific antidotes for reversal of symptoms as outlined above. Therapeutic measures are otherwise largely supportive, depending on the organ system affected, and include antibiotic coverage to prevent secondary bacterial infection where appropriate **(Table 1)**.

TABLE 1: Classification and characteristics of chemical agents.

Agent class	Examples of agents	Mechanism of action	Route of exposure	Clinical characteristics
Nerve agents	• *G-agents:* Sarin, cycloserine, tabun, and soman • *V-agents:* VE, VG, VM, VR, and VX	Inhibition of acetylcholinesterase leads to accumulation of acetylcholine in body	Inhalation or skin	• *Symptoms:* Miosis, hypersalivation, runny nose, diaphoresis, bronchospasm, muscle excitation, arrhythmias, seizures, respiratory paralysis • *Management:* Supportive +/− Seizure control. Atropine + Pralidoxime
Vesicants (blister agents)	• *Mustards:* Mustard gas, nitrogen mustard • *Arsenicals:* Lewisite • Phosgene oxime	• *Mustards:* DNA alkylation leads to cell death • *Arsenicals:* Enzyme inhibition causes NADPH and glutathione oxidation, resulting in disruption of metabolism and cell death • *Phosgene oxime:* Unknown	Inhalation or skin	• *Onset:* Hallmark of mustards is post-exposure latency (symptom-free period) for several hours. Arsenical exposure—immediate pain • *Symptoms:* Corneal irritation/erosion, skin erythema/blistering, rhinorrhea, hoarseness of voice, cough. Phosgene oxime causes wheals followed by eschars (no blisters) • *Management:* Mainly supportive. No antidote for mustards or phosgene • *Antidote for arsenicals (Lewisite):* Dimercaprol/British anti-Lewisite (BAL)
Blood agents (cyanogenic agents)	Hydrogen cyanide, cyanogen chloride	Inhibition of cytochrome oxidase in cells, preventing oxygen utilization	Skin, inhalation, or ingestion	• *Symptoms:* Confusion, nausea, weakness, cyanosis, CNS excitation followed rapidly by depression, convulsions, coma, and cardiorespiratory arrest. • *Antidotes for cyanide toxicity:* Hydroxocobalamin, sodium nitrite followed by sodium thiosulfate
Choking agents (pulmonary agents)	Phosgene, diphosgene, chloropicrin, chlorine	• *Chlorine:* Acidification of gas causes irritation/necrosis of respiratory tract mucosa/lung tissue → pulmonary edema/ARDS • *Phosgene/diphosgene:* Disruption of alveolar surface tension → pulmonary edema	Inhalation	• *Symptoms:* Nose and throat irritation, dyspnea, wheezing, cough with increased secretions, hypoxia on room air is a sign of ARDS-like lung injury • *Management:* Mainly supportive with high-flow oxygen/mechanical ventilation as needed. Possible role of corticosteroids, bronchodilators and/or inhaled sodium bicarbonate
Incapacitating agents (tear gases)	Chloroacetophenone (CN), O-chloroben-zylidene malononitrile (CS), oleoresin of capsicum (OC), and dibenz 1: 4-oxazepine (CR)	Direct toxicity, possibly through NADH-dependent receptors of skin and mucosa	Inhalation or skin	• *Symptoms:* Lachrymators—conjunctivitis, tearing of eye, blepharospasm • Sternutators—sneezing, upper respiratory tract irritation • Vomiting agents—nausea/vomiting • *Management:* Immediate decontamination + supportive treatment

(ARDS: acute respiratory distress syndrome; CNS: central nervous system; DNA: deoxyribonucleic acid; NADH: nicotinamide adenine dinucleotide hydrogenase; NADPH: nicotinamide adenine dinucleotide phosphate hydrogen)

4. Discuss personal protective equipment (PPE).

The use of PPE to protect airway, skin, and eyes is an indispensable component of emergency response. Limitations to the use of PPE are the restriction of physical activity, dehydration, heat-related illness, and psychological effect. These limitations can be avoided by training emergency personnel to use PPE appropriately **(Fig. 4)**.

Level A PPE should be used when the highest level of respiratory, skin, eye, and mucous membranes protection is needed. A typical Level A conveys a chemical resistant fully encapsulated suit, over-gloves, and boots integrated into the suit. Respiratory protection is a self-contained breathing apparatus. Level A protection is required for entry into an unknown hazardous environment.

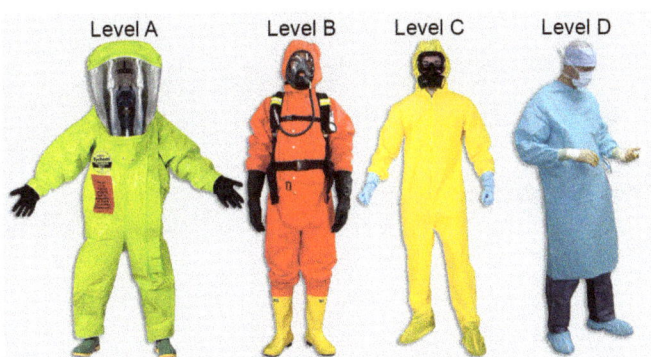

Fig. 4: Personal protective equipment level.

Level B PPE is used when the highest level of respiratory protection is needed, but lesser protection to skin and eyes needed. It represents a chemical resistant hooded suit, double gloves, over-boots, and a self-contained breathing apparatus, and may be used for decontamination procedures for an unknown substance and for entry into hot zones where the agent is not caustic.

Level C PPE is utilized when the type of airborne substance is known and identified, similar to Level B, but uses an air-purifying respirator instead of a self-contained breathing apparatus. Level C PPE can be used only after the hazardous substance has been identified, and upon verification of adequate oxygen in the environment.

Level D PPE is used for droplet precautions, consists of a gown, head cover, mask, gloves, and shoe covers. A more enhanced mask with higher filtration rate can be utilized in case of known airborne substance.

Question 3

1. Discuss pathophysiology of coagulopathy observed in trauma victims.

The pathophysiology of trauma-induced coagulopathy consists of coagulation activation, hyperfibrino(geno)lysis, and consumption coagulopathy **(Flowchart 2)**. These pathophysiological mechanisms are the characteristics to disseminated intravascular coagulation (DIC) with the fibrinolytic phenotype.

2. Explain the role of thromboelastography (TEG) in coagulopathy.

Thromboelastography is a noninvasive test that quantitatively measures the ability of whole blood to form a clot. TEG is used to assess viscoelastic changes in clotting whole blood under low shear conditions after adding a specific coagulation activator **(Fig. 5)**.

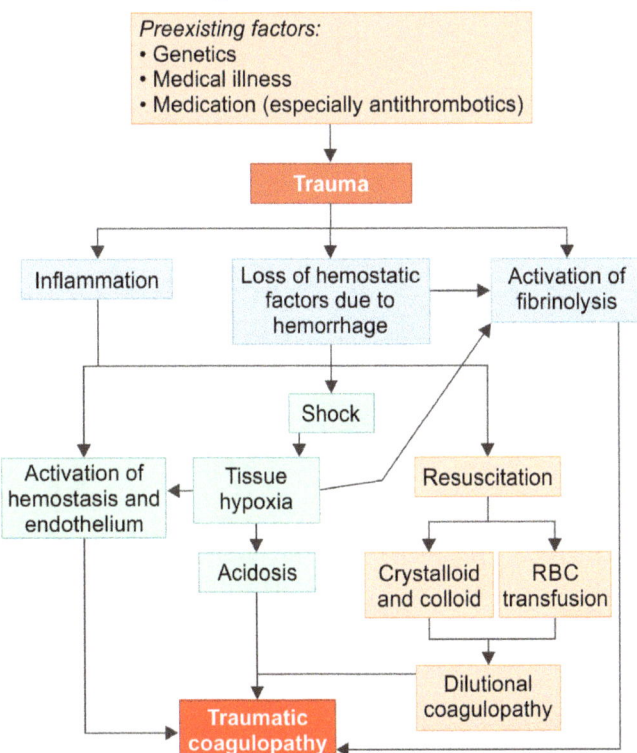

Flowchart 2: Pathogenesis of trauma-induced coagulopathy.

- A technique used for the characterization and quantification of the status of a patient's coagulation state.
- It can be used to measure hemostasis by studying the strength and elasticity of the clot and how quickly the clot breaks up.
- TEG can be viewed in real-time and management decisions about blood products and can be tailored based on the patient's clinical state.

3. Discuss damage control resuscitation.

Damage control resuscitation (DCR) is a strategy that emphasizes to maintain or restore homeostasis in trauma patients. The name "damage control" was coined from naval tactics aimed to keep a damaged ship as combat-capable as possible until definite repair can be done. The concept goes hand in hand with damage control surgery. The major threats in damage control resuscitation are acidosis, coagulopathy, and hypothermia which makes a forward feedback loop that leads to progressive worsening of a patient's hemodynamic status and eventually death. Damage control resuscitation is also known as hypotensive resuscitation and hemostatic resuscitation. Appropriate fluid administration might help to maintain homeostasis.

Aim: To limit blood loss and prevent coagulopathy by combining hypotensive resuscitation, early airway control and early and balanced use of blood products and other hemostatic agents.

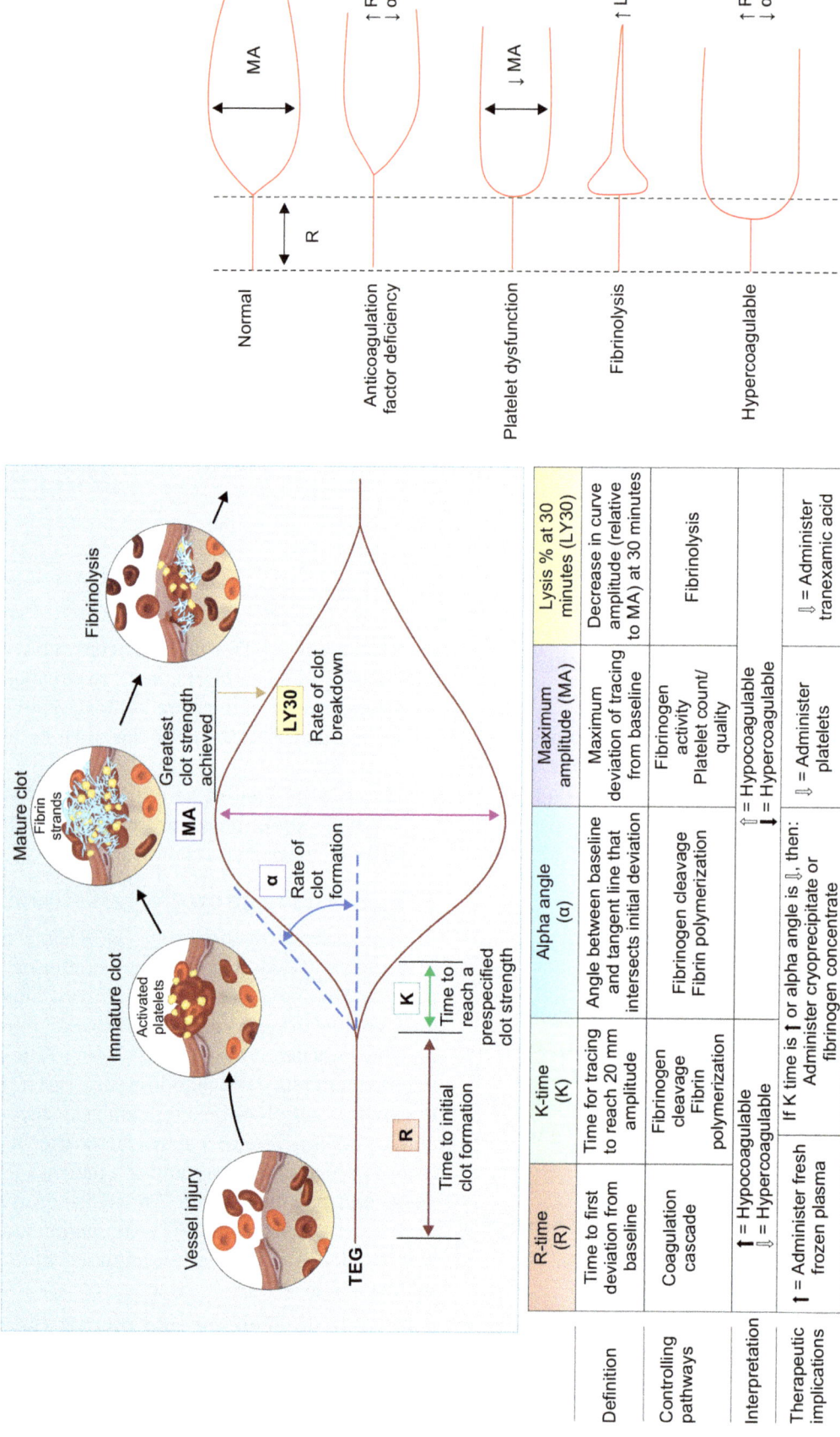

Fig. 5: Thromboelastography (TEG).

Phases (**Fig. 6**):
- Control of life-threatening hemorrhage and contamination
- Complete resuscitation
- Correction of physiologic derangements

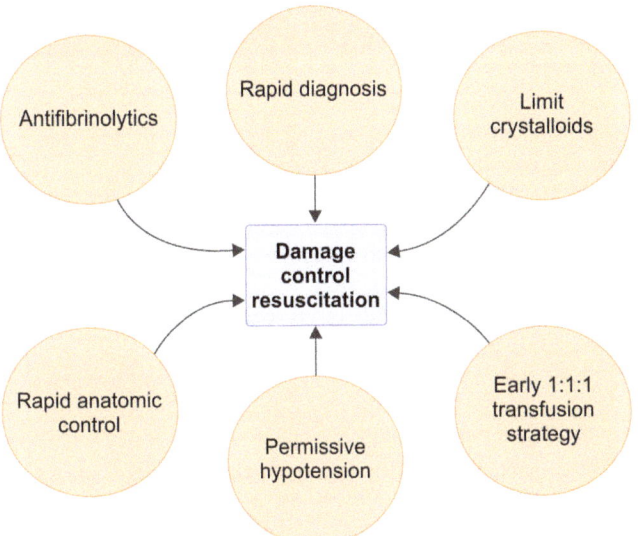

Fig. 6: Damage control resuscitation.

Question 4

1. What are the clinical criteria for anaphylaxis?

Acute onset of an illness (minutes to several hours) with the involvement of skin and mucosal tissues and either of these: (a) Respiratory compromise (dyspnea, wheeze, bronchospasm, strider, reduced peak expiratory flow, hypoxemia); (b) Reduced blood pressure or signs and symptoms of end organ dysfunction (hypotonia, collapse, syncope, incontinence).

Two or more of the following that occur rapidly after exposure to an antigen:
- Skin or mucosal tissue involvement
- Respiratory compromise
- Reduced blood pressure or associated signs and symptoms
- Persistent GI signs and symptoms (crampy abdominal pain, vomiting)

Systolic blood pressure <90 mm Hg >30% decrease in the patient's baseline in adults.

Age-specific low systolic blood pressure in children <70 mm Hg from 1 month-old infants up to 1 year <70 mm Hg + (2[age]) from 1 to 10 years; children <90 mm Hg in 11–17 year-old children.

2. Enumerate pathophysiology of anaphylaxis.

Anaphylaxis is a severe systemic hypersensitivity reaction that is rapid in onset; characterized by life-threatening airway, breathing, and/or circulatory problems; and usually associated with skin and mucosal changes. Because it can be triggered in some persons by minute amounts of antigen (e.g., certain foods or single insect stings), anaphylaxis can be considered the most aberrant example of an imbalance between the cost and benefit of an immune response. Current understanding of the immunopathogenesis and pathophysiology of anaphylaxis (**Flowcharts 3A and B**), focusing on the roles of IgE and IgG antibodies, immune effector cells, and mediators thought to contribute to examples of the disorder. Anaphylaxis causes the immune system to release a flood of chemicals (**Table 2**) that can cause you to go into shock—blood pressure drops suddenly and the airways narrow, blocking breathing. Signs and symptoms include a rapid, weak pulse; a skin rash; and nausea and vomiting.

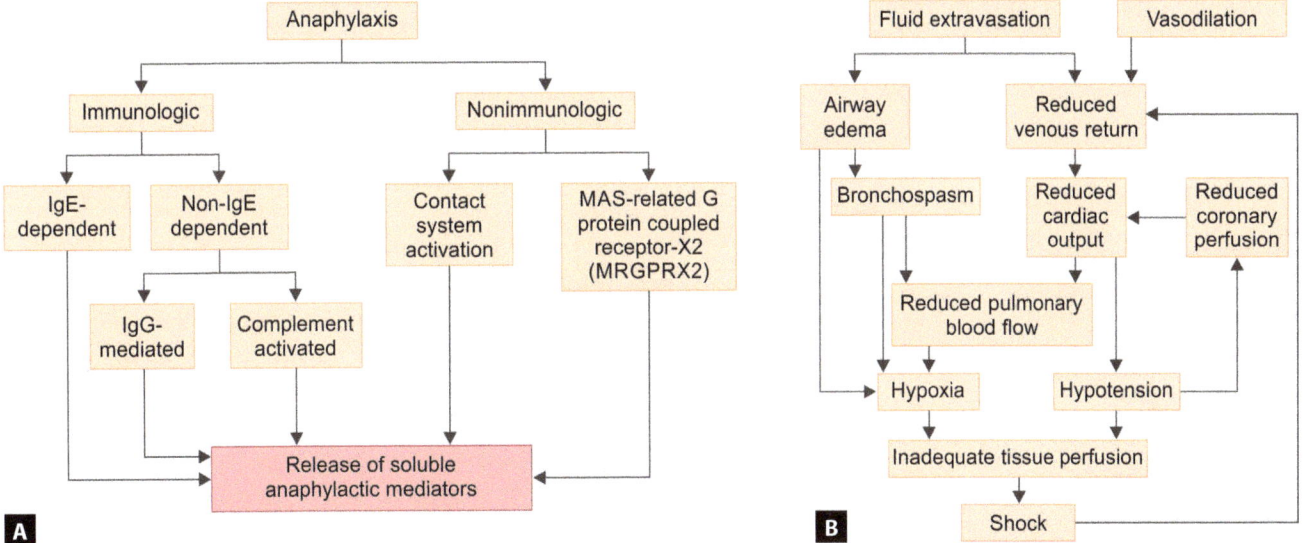

Flowcharts 3A and B: (A) Immunopathogenesis; (B) Pathophysiologic mechanism of anaphylactic shock.

(MRGPRX2: MAS-related G protein coupled receptor-X2)

TABLE 2: Release of chemical mediators by activation of immune system.

	Chemical mediator	Action
Arachidonic acid metabolites	• Cysteinyl leukotrienes • Prostaglandins • Platelet activating factor	Bronchoconstriction, coronary vasoconstriction increased vascular permeability, mucus hypersecretion, eosinophil activation and recruitment
Chemokines	• IL-8 • MIP-1α • Eosinophil chemotactic factors	Neutrophil and eosinophil chemotaxis, inflammatory cell recruitment, activation of NADPH oxidase
Cytokines	• GM-CSF • IL-3, -4, -5, -6, -10, and -13 • TNF-α	Eosinophil chemotaxis and activation; inflammatory cell activation and recruitment, induction of Ig E-receptor expression, induction of apoptosis
Proteases	• Chymase • Tryptase • Carboxypeptidase A	Cleavage of complement proteins and neuropeptides, inflammatory-cell chemoattractant, conversion of angiotensin I to angiotensin II, activation of protease-activated receptor-2
Proteoglycans	• Chondroitin sulfate • Heparin	Anticoagulation, complement inhibition, eosinophil chemoattractant, kinin activation
Others	• Histamine • Nitric oxide	• Vasodilation, bronchial and gastrointestinal smooth muscle contraction, mucus hypersecretion • Vasodilation, increased vascular permeability

(GM-CSF: granulocute-macrophage colony stimulating factor; IL: interleukin; MIP: macrophage inflammatory protein; NADPH: nicotinamide adenine dinucleotide phosphate hydrogen; TNF: tumor necrotic factor)

3. Discuss current treatment of anaphylaxis.

Oxygenation: It is done through face mask or endotracheal intubation, if needed. Mechanical ventilation is indicated for severe bronchospasm, apnea or cardiac arrest.

Epinephrine: The universally recommended drug; intramuscular dose 0.3–1 mL and intravenous dose 3–5 mL of 1:10,000 dilutions.

Mechanism of action: It increases intracellular cyclic adenosine monophosphate (cAMP) levels in leukocytes and mast cells which inhibits the histamine release. It has beneficial effects on myocardial contractility and peripheral vascular tone and bronchial smooth muscle also.

Intravenous (IV) fluids and inotropes: The treatment of choice—norepinephrine infusion, methoxamine, phenylephrine, vasopressin, and methylene blue-tried in refractory cases.

Nebulization: With salbutamol in cases where bronchospasm is seen. Aminophylline 5–6 mg/kg IV is given over 30 minutes. Ketamine, magnesium sulfate also can be used in severe cases of asthma.

Question 5

1. Discuss physiologic changes in pregnancy affecting resuscitation.

Resuscitation in pregnancy has few unique aspects and consideration when compared to normal adult resuscitation as it involves resuscitation of two patients—pregnant woman and fetus. It is important to be familiar with the physiological changes in pregnancy which impact the resuscitation. The resuscitation modifications begin as early as in first trimester which peaks at the second trimester and stays the same until labor. These are based on the anatomical and physiological and anatomical changes during the course of pregnancy. The changes during pregnancy and their implications are tabulated in **Table 3**.

Cardiovascular:
- Cardiac output increases 30–50%
- Peripheral resistance—decreases 20%
- Blood pressure—decreases 10–15 mm Hg systolic in first half of pregnancy; then back to baseline
- Blood volume—100 cc/kg or 6–7 L
- Central venous pressure—may be increased up to 10 mm Hg
- Central venous oxygen saturation—increases as high as 80%
- Plasma volume—increases 30–50%

Hematologic: Fibrinogen, factors V, VII, VIII, X, von Willebrand factor-increase, with heightened risk for venous thromboembolism in second half of pregnancy

Respiratory and pulmonary:
- Upper airway edema, hyperemia, and friability due to estrogen and volume effects; can result in difficult airway
- Diaphragm elevation
- Higher thoracostomy tube insertion site during pregnancy;
- Hemoglobin F has greater affinity for oxygen than maternal hemoglobin, so, fetal oxygen maintained at expense of maternal oxygenation; maintain maternal oxygen saturation >95%
- Respiratory rate—no change, tidal volume, minute ventilation-increase

TABLE 3: Anatomical, physiological changes in pregnancy and their associated implications.

Systems	Changes during pregnancy	Implications
Airway	• Edema/friability of upper airway • Edema to pharynx, larynx	• Difficult to perform bag mask ventilation • Difficulty in laryngoscopy • Small diameter ET tube may be needed
Breathing	• Diaphragm elevation by 4 cm • Reducing FRC • Oxygen consumption is increased by 20% to meet the oxygen demands of maternal and fetal organs • Increased tidal volume and minute ventilation	• High thoracostomies • Hypoxia can develop quickly • Hypoxia develops soon • Hence maintain saturation >94% • Partial pressure of carbon dioxide is reduced leading to respiratory alkalosis. Normal $PaCO_2$ can mean impending respiratory failure
Circulation	• Cardiac output increased by 30–40% • Increased heart rate • Plasma volume increased by 30% • Uterine blood flow increased by 10–20% • Blood pressure reduces in the second trimester • Aortocaval compression starting from 20 weeks • Diaphragmatic elevation, apex of heart moved to left	• Masking the effecting of sepsis • Hypotension on supine position • Avoid access in lower extremities • Decreases the effectiveness of CPR • Changes in ECG—left axis deviation • Q waves in lead III • ST depressions in inferolateral leads • T wave changes—flattened or inverted
Other changes	• Relaxation of lower esophageal sphincter • Changes in bile composition (lithogenic) • Plasma volume increase by 50% and 30% increase in red cell mass • Increase in clotting factors, vWF • Dilatation of ureteropelvic system—physiological hydroureteronephrosis and increased vesicoureteric reflex • Vaginal pH decreases	• Risk of aspiration • Prone for cholelithiasis • Physiological anemia leading reduced oxygen carrying capacity to tissue, more impact during CPR • Hypercoagulable state—increased risk of venous thromboembolism • Increased pyelonephritis • Increased chance of chorioamnionitis

(CPR: cardiopulmonary resuscitation; ECG: electrocardiogram; ET: endotracheal; FRC: functional residual capacity; vWF: von Willebrand factor)

Renal and urinary:
- Progesterone dilates renal collecting system
- Ureteral peristalsis decreases
- Renal US may show mild hydronephrosis
- Increased risk for ascending infection.

Gastrointestinal:
- Alkaline phosphatase rises from placental production
- Bile is more lithogenic
- Increased risk of cholecystitis/cholelithiasis
- Decreased lower esophageal tone
- Decreased gastric emptying
- Increased likelihood of aspiration of gastric contents.

Uteroplacental unit:
- 25% of blood flow directed to uteroplacental unit; no autoregulation of blood flow
- Enlarging uterus can compress vena cava and vessels below the diaphragm
- Supine hypotension syndrome can occur after 30 minutes of supine position
- Place patient in left lateral tilt position during third trimester; replace volume adequately to account for increased blood and plasma volume in pregnancy; avoid femoral and lower extremity site for blood and volume.

2. How will you resuscitate a 26-week pregnant woman who is in cardiac arrest?

- One person should provide manual left lateral displacement of the uterus in the supine position while another is performing cardiopulmonary resuscitation (CPR).
- Chest compression should be performed slightly above the center of the sternum.
- Airway management in pregnant patients is more difficult. Bag mask ventilation with high flow oxygen before intubation is important. Early intubation with cricoid pressure will decrease the risk of Mendelson's syndrome.
- Drugs are given the same as per the normal advanced cardiac life support protocol. Defibrillation is also normally performed as per the protocol, where adhesive defibrillation pads are preferred over the paddles because of breast enlargement. Fetal or uterine monitors should be removed before defibrillation.
- Emergency cesarean section is performed at 5 minutes after maternal cardiac arrest if there is no return of spontaneous circulation in the mother as the fetus is of viable gestational age (>24 weeks).

- A midline vertical incision from umbilicus to symphysis pubis is required
- Continue maternal CPR during the perimortem cesarean delivery.
- Do not delay cord clamping if the baby requires immediate resuscitation. Once the baby is delivered, the resuscitation of the mother and baby should be continued.
- The chance of a neurologically intact neonate is increased with a more rapid delivery. Maternal pulses can return after delivery, once aortocaval compression is relieved.

Question 6

1. Discuss the various methods to confirm correct position of endotracheal tube.

Visualize: Watch for the passage of the tip of the endotracheal tube through the vocal cords at intubation, whenever possible.

Observe: For the continuous rise and fall of the chest symmetrically on ventilation.

Auscultate: Confirm air entry using a stethoscope by means of five-point auscultation.

Auscultation of sounds over the stomach, if not heard, confirms tracheal intubation.

Auscultation over both sides, i.e., the axilla and lung bases shall confirm the tracheal intubation, if heard equally. If heard unilaterally, it may indicate endobronchial intubation.

Capnography: CO_2 in the exhaled air is a reliable indicator of correct tube placement.

Oximetry: Saturation probe always helps to confirm correct tube placement and thereby adequate oxygenation. Visualization and capnography are the most reliable for correct tube placement.

2. Draw and label the normal capnogram.

A healthy patient with normal lungs when ventilated via a patent tracheal tube or tracheostomy, the continuous waveform produces a typical **"square wave"** capnography trace and provides visual breath-by-breath assessment of a patient's airway and ventilation. Morphology of capnography traces are shown in **Figure 7**.

Phase I (Inspiratory phase) represents inspiratory phase, so no CO_2 is detected

Phase II (expiratory upstroke) represents expiration of both dead space gas and alveolar gas from the respiratory bronchioles and alveoli.

Phase III (alveolar plateau) represents phase of expiration of alveolar gases.

Phase IV (expiratory downstroke) represents the beginning of the next breath, with the CO_2 content returning rapidly to zero. Healthy patients with normal respiratory function will produce a capnography trace with this form.

3. Write on the role of capnography variations in assessment of ventilator abnormalities.

Ventilatory abnormalities and capnography variations are shown in **Figure 8**.

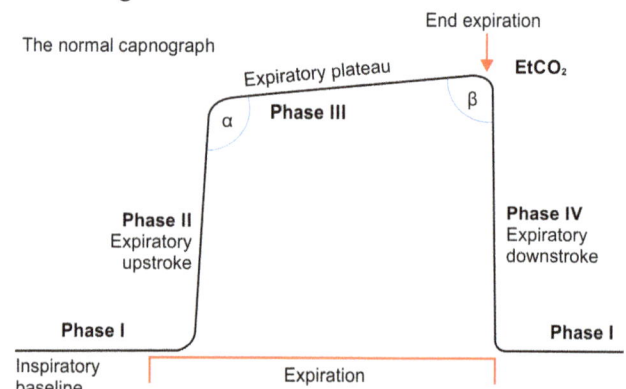

Fig. 7: Morphology of normal capnography wave.

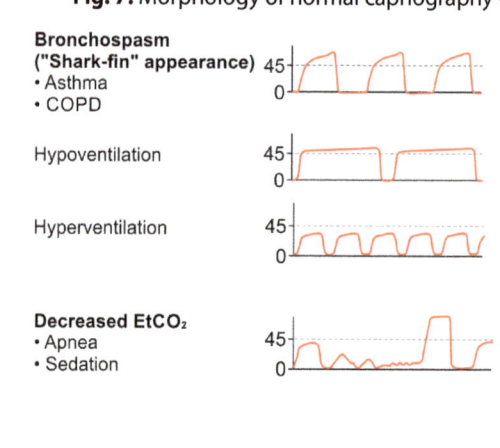

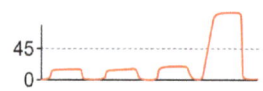

Fig. 8: Ventilatory abnormalities and capnography variations. (COPD: chronic obstructive pulmonary disease; CPR: cardiopulmonary resuscitation; ET: endotracheal)

Question 7

1. Discuss pathophysiology of tumor lysis syndrome (TLS).

Metabolic derangement caused by rapid breakdown of cancer cells as a consequence of therapy. This causes the release of intracellular contents, thus causing hyperuricemia, hyperphosphatemia, hyperkalemia, and hypocalcemia. This also causes the release of nucleic acids and intracellular proteins **(Flowchart 4)**.

2. Explain the clinical features of TLS.

Tumor lysis syndrome refers to metabolic consequences resulting from sudden release of intracellular metabolites, nucleic acids and proteins from tumor cells undergoing death spontaneously or posttreatment. It is divided into two groups, i.e., laboratory and clinical based on *Cairo–Bishop definitions*.

Laboratory TLS is defined as presence of ≥2 of following laboratory abnormalities, i.e., uric acid ≥8 mg/dL, potassium ≥6 mEq/L, phosphorus >4.5 mg/dL in adults (≥6.5 mg/dL in children) and calcium ≤7 mg/dL or 25% change in these laboratory values from baseline, present within 3 days before or 7 days after initiation of therapy.

Clinical TLS is defined as laboratory TLS accompanied with ≥1 of the following—serum creatinine ≥1.5 times the upper limit of normal, seizure, cardiac dysrhythmia or death.

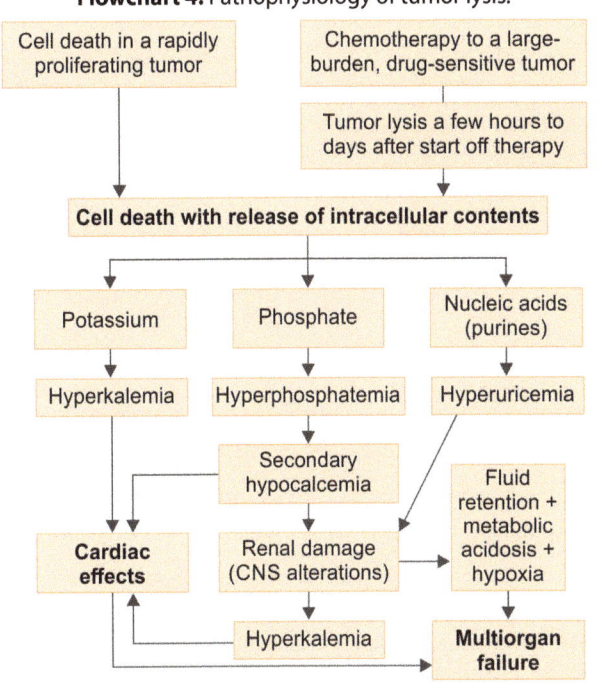

Flowchart 4: Pathophysiology of tumor lysis.

(CNS: central nervous system)

The clinical manifestations noted are acute kidney injury, seizures, and cardiac dysrhythmias or cardiac arrest. Renal failure occurs due to the precipitation of uric acid within renal tubules. Phosphorus released from cells may combine with calcium and get precipitated in renal tubules and parenchyma also. Hyperkalemia causes cardiac dysrhythmias or cardiac arrest. Hypocalcemia may cause tetany and seizures and can lead to dysrhythmias. Hypovolemia can further precipitate renal failure.

3. Discuss the management of TLS.

Treatment:

- *Aggressive intravenous hydration:* Prophylactic allopurinol and maintaining good hydration can reduce the risk of TLS developing.
- Aggressive IV fluid administration to increase urinary excretion of the released intracellular solutes.
- *Correction of electrolyte disturbances:* Hypocalcemia to be treated only if symptomatic. Calcium administration is done only when there are cardiovascular abnormalities or severe tetany.
- *Treatment of hyperkalemia:* β-adrenergic agonists, sodium bicarbonate, and dextrose-insulin therapy.
- Hyperphosphatemia is managed with phosphate binders (limited effect) or by the administration of dextrose and insulin, hemodialysis or continuous renal replacement therapy is also preferred due to the increased phosphate load.
- *Hemodialysis:* If there is persistent hyperkalemia, intractable hyperphosphatemia and hypocalcemia (calcium phosphate product ≥70 mg^2/dL^2), intractable fluid overload and oliguria or anuria (in absence of hypovolemia).
- *Rasburicase:* 0.2 mg/kg/day. Allopurinol to be used only in case of rasburicase hypersensitivity or glucose-6-phosphate dehydrogenase (G6PD) deficiency.

Question 8

1. Draw a labeled diagram of cardiac conduction system.

Cardiac conduction system is made up of five elements **(Fig. 9)**:

1. The sinoatrial (SA) node
2. The atrioventricular (AV) node
3. The bundle of His
4. The left and right bundle branches
5. The Purkinje fibers.

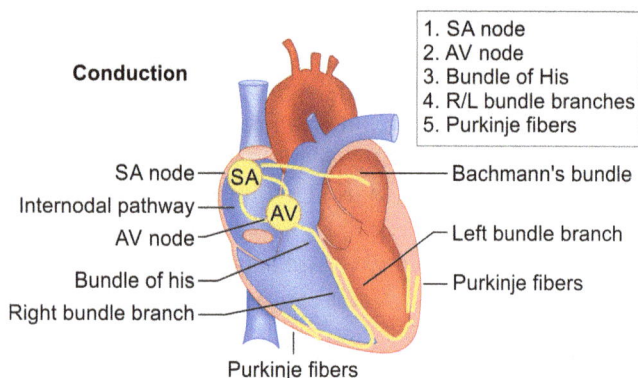

Fig. 9: Cardiac conducting system.

2. Classify cardiac arrhythmias.

Dysrhythmias are classified according to their electrophysiologic origin, appearance on the electrocardiogram, and underlying ventricular rate.
- Bradycardias
- Extrasystoles
- Narrow-complex (QRS <0.12 second) tachycardias (regular and irregular)
- Wide-complex (QRS ≥ 0.12 second) tachycardias (regular and irregular).

Another classification is based on:
- Rate (bradycardia or tachycardia)
- Rhythm (regular or irregular)
- Origin of impulse (supraventricular, ventricular, or artificial pacemaker)
- Intraventricular conduction (narrow or wide-complex QRS).

3. Classify antiarrhythmic agents.

Vaughan–Williams classification:

Class I: Sodium (fast) channel blockers—slow depolarization with varying effects on repolarization. These drugs have membrane-stabilizing effects.
- *IA:* Moderate slowing of depolarization and conduction; prolong repolarization and action potential duration; procainamide, quinidine, and disopyramide
- *IB:* Minimally slow depolarization and conduction; shorten repolarization and action potential duration; lidocaine, phenytoin, tocainide, and mexiletine
- *IC:* Markedly slow depolarization and conduction; prolong repolarization and action potential duration; flecainide, propafenone (shares properties with class IA agents), vernakalant (atrial-specific, investigational).

Class II: β-adrenergic blockers; propranolol, esmolol, metoprolol, and atenolol.

Class III: Prolong action potential duration and refractory period duration; bretylium, amiodarone, dofetilide, ibutilide, sotalol, dronedarone.

Class IV: Calcium (slow) channel blockers; verapamil diltiazem miscellaneous—digoxin, magnesium sulfate, adenosine.

4. Discuss various mechanisms of cardiac arrhythmias.

These are: (1) Induced automaticity, (2) leading center, (3) triggered activity by the mechanism of early afterdepolarization, and (4) triggered automaticity by the mechanism of delayed afterdepolarization **(Fig. 10)**.

- Enhanced automaticity—spontaneous depolarization in non-pacemaker cells or depolarization at an abnormally low threshold in pacemaker cells.
  Example: The idioventricular rhythms of severe hyperkalemia or myocardial ischemia and the atrial or junctional tachycardias (JTs) associated with digoxin toxicity.
- *Triggered activity* refers to abnormal impulse(s) resulting from afterdepolarizations. Afterdepolarizations are fluctuations in membrane potential that occurs as the resting potential is restored. These fluctuations may precipitate another depolarization just before the full resting potential is reached (early afterdepolarizations) or after full resting potential is reached (delayed afterdepolarizations). Example for early afterdepolarization is acquired torsades de pointes.

For delayed afterdepolarization, noted with rapid heart rates and intracellular Ca^{2+} overload, is seen with digoxin toxicity or reperfusion therapy for acute myocardial infarction.

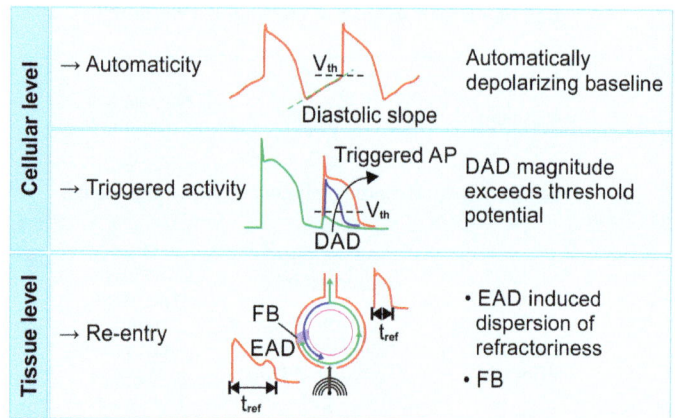

Fig. 10: Mechanisms of cardiac arrhythmias. (AP: action potential; DAD: Delayed after depolarization; EAD: early after depolarization; FB: functional block)

Question 9

1. Discuss anatomy of knee joint.

The knee joint is a synovial joint that connects three bones—the femur, tibia, and patella. It is a complex hinge joint composed of two articulations—the tibiofemoral joint and patellofemoral joint. The tibiofemoral joint is an articulation between the tibia and the femur, while the patellofemoral joint is an articulation between the patella and the femur **(Fig. 11)**.

Articular surfaces: Tibiofemoral joint—lateral and medial condyles of femur, tibial plateaus.

Patellofemoral joint: Patellar surface of femur, posterior surface of patella.

Ligaments and menisci:
- *Extracapsular ligaments:* Patellar ligament, medial and lateral patellar retinacula, tibial (medial) collateral ligament, fibular (lateral) collateral ligament, oblique popliteal ligament, arcuate popliteal ligament, anterolateral ligament (ALL)
- *Intracapsular ligaments:* Anterior cruciate ligament (ACL), posterior cruciate ligament (PCL), medial meniscus, lateral meniscus.

Innervation: Femoral nerve (nerve to vastus medialis, saphenous nerve) tibial and common fibular (peroneal) nerves, posterior division of the obturator nerve.

Blood supply: Genicular branches of lateral circumflex femoral artery, femoral artery, posterior tibial artery, anterior tibial artery, and popliteal artery.

Movements: Extension, flexion, medial rotation, lateral rotation.

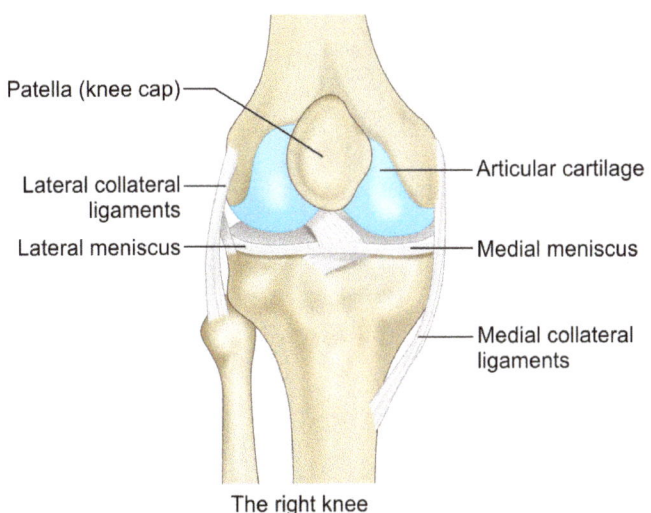

Fig. 11: Anatomy of knee joint.

2. What are the clinical tests for diagnosing cruciate ligament injuries of the knee joint?

The anterior drawer test: It identifies the tears of the ACL. The test is performed with the patient in a supine position, hip flexed at 45°, and knee flexed at 90°.

While stabilizing the patient's foot, the examiner places his or her thumbs over the joint line while pulling the tibia forward. The thumbs are used to palpate for any translation of the tibia relative to the femur. A positive test result is defined as greater anterior translation of the tibia relative to the femur as compared with the other knee.

The Lachman test—specific for ACL injury: It is done with the knee flexed 20°–30° while the examiner uses one hand to grasp and stabilize the femur. The tibia is then pulled anteriorly, and the examiner notes tibial excursion. The examiner records "firmness" or a "soft end point." The end point can be graded as 1+ (0–5 mm more displacement than on the normal side), 2+ (5–10 mm), or 3+ (>10 mm).

Posterior drawer test: It assesses for PCL injury. The posterior drawer test can be accomplished with the patient's knee flexed at 90° and the foot stabilized by the examiner. A smooth backward force is applied to the tibia. Posterior displacement of the tibia >5 mm, or a soft end point, indicates injury to the PCL.

The posterior sag sign test: It also indicates PCL integrity. The patient is placed in a supine position, and a pillow is placed under the distal thigh for support resting the heel on the stretcher. The knee is flexed to 45° or 90°. If the tibia sags backward, the test result is positive, indicating PCL insufficiency.

Question 10

1. Discuss blood supply of spinal cord.

The main blood supply to the spinal cord is via the single anterior spinal artery and the two posterior spinal arteries (PSA) **(Fig. 12)**. The anterior spinal artery is formed by the vertebral arteries which originate from the first part of the subclavian artery and travels caudally down the spinal cord through the anterior sulcus. The anterior spinal artery provides blood to the anterior two-thirds of the spinal cord, and the PSA deliver blood to the posterior one-third of the spinal cord. The anterior spinal artery and PSA are fed additional arteries throughout their course down the spinal cord at each spinal level through the intervertebral foramen, which are called segmental spinal arteries. The largest segmental medullary artery is the artery of Adamkiewicz and supplies a large area of the thoracolumbar region and thus considered a watershed area.

2. Show a labeled diagram of transverse section of spinal cord at T6 vertebral level.

Importance: T-6 through T-12 nerves affects *abdominal and back muscles*. These nerves and muscles are important for balance and posture, and they help you cough or expel foreign matter from your airway **(Fig. 13)**.

3. Explain the various rules for imaging cervical spine in a trauma patient.

Nexus criteria and Canadian C-spine rule are followed in a trauma patient.

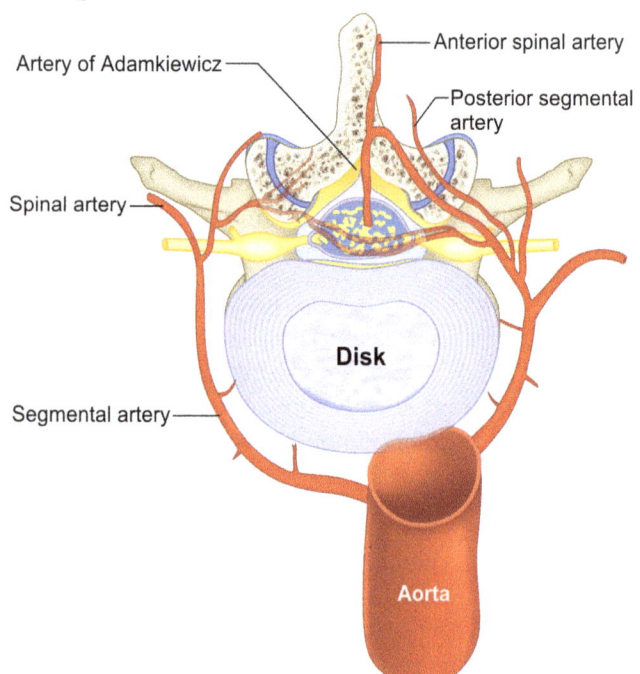

Fig. 12: Blood supply of spinal cord.

Nexus criteria (National emergency X-radiography utilization study):
a. Absence of midline cervical tenderness.
b. Normal level of alertness and conscious level.
c. No evidence of intoxication.
d. Absence of focal neurologic deficit.
e. Absence of painful distracting injury.

Cervical spine imaging is not needed in patients who lack any one of above five clinical criteria.

Canadian cervical spine rule for radiography: Cervical imaging is not required who meet these three criteria. Canadian rule consists of three assessments, which are asked in sequential order. To proceed to the next assessment, the answer to the previous assessment must be "Yes." If the answer to any assessments is "No," then imaging is immediately performed.

Assessment 1: There are no high-risk factors that mandate radiography.

Assessment 2: There are low risk factors that allow a safe assessment of range of motion.

Assessment 3: The patient is able to rotate his/her neck 45° to the left and to the right, regardless of the pain.

High risk factors include—age 65 years or older, dangerous mechanism of injury, and presence of paresthesia in the extremities.

Low risk factors include—simple rear end motor vehicle crashes, patient able to sit up in the ED, patient ambulatory at any time, delayed onset of pain, and absence of midline cervical spine tenderness.

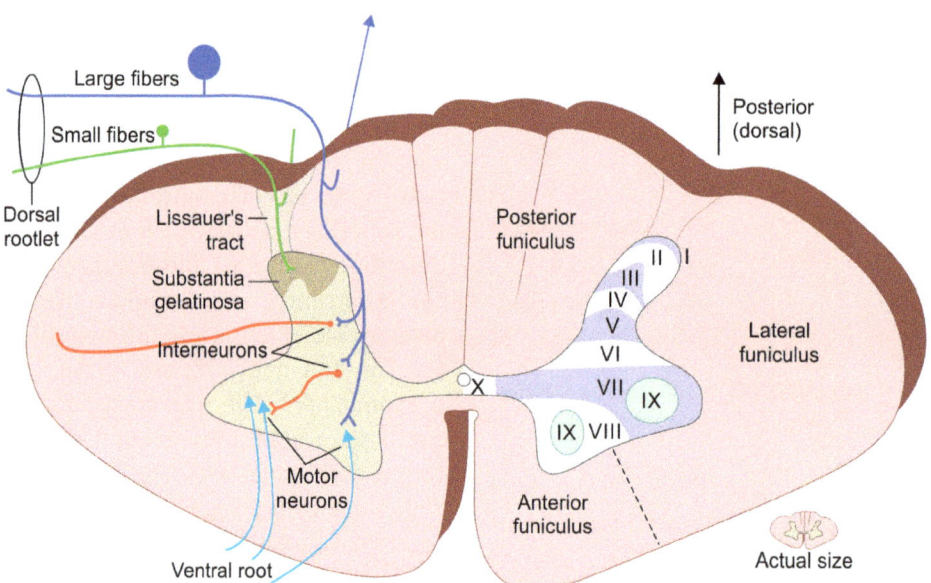

Fig. 13: Transverse section of spinal cord at T6 level.

SUGGESTED READING

1. Richhariya D, Sharma B. Textbook of Emergency Medicine including Intensive Care and Trauma, 2nd edition. New Delhi: Jaypee Brothers Medical Publishers (P) Ltd; 2022. pp. 185-94. (Question 1).
2. Richhariya D, Sharma B. Textbook of Emergency Medicine including Intensive Care and Trauma, 2nd edition. New Delhi: Jaypee Brothers Medical Publishers (P) Ltd; 2022. pp. 187-8. (Question 2).
3. Richhariya D, Sharma B. Textbook of Emergency Medicine including Intensive Care and Trauma, 2nd edition. New Delhi: Jaypee Brothers Medical Publishers (P) Ltd; 2022. p. 1537. (Question 3).
4. Whyte AF, Soar J, Dodd A, Hughes A, Sargant N, Turner PJ. Emergency treatment of anaphylaxis: concise clinical guidance. Clin Med. 2022;22(4):332-9. (Question 4).
5. ASCIA. (2023). ASCIA guidelines- acute management of anaphylaxis. [online] Available from: https://www.allergy.org.au/hp/papers/acute-management-of-anaphylaxis-guidelines. [Last accessed May, 2023]. (Question 4).
6. Richhariya D, Sharma B. Textbook of Emergency Medicine including Intensive Care and Trauma, 2nd edition. New Delhi: Jaypee Brothers Medical Publishers (P) Ltd; 2022. p. 1115. (Question 5).
7. Richhariya D, Sharma B. Textbook of Emergency Medicine including Intensive Care and Trauma, 2nd edition. New Delhi: Jaypee Brothers Medical Publishers (P) Ltd; 2022. p. 217. (Question 6).
8. Richhariya D, Sharma B. Textbook of Emergency Medicine including Intensive Care and Trauma, 2nd edition. New Delhi: Jaypee Brothers Medical Publishers (P) Ltd; 2022. p. 971. (Question 7).
9. Richhariya D, Sharma B. Textbook of Emergency Medicine including Intensive Care and Trauma, 2nd edition. New Delhi: Jaypee Brothers Medical Publishers (P) Ltd; 2022. pp. 473-80. (Question 8).
10. Richhariya D, Sharma B. Textbook of Emergency Medicine including Intensive Care and Trauma, 2nd edition. New Delhi: Jaypee Brothers Medical Publishers (P) Ltd; 2022. pp. 1634-5. (Question 9).
11. Richhariya D, Sharma B. Textbook of Emergency Medicine including Intensive Care and Trauma, 2nd edition. New Delhi: Jaypee Brothers Medical Publishers (P) Ltd; 2022. pp. 1570-1. (Question 10).

Emergency Medicine Paper 22

Ajay Singh Thapa

Question 1

A 27-year-old man was found to be involved in a car accident. After taking care of ABCD, he was stabilized. Now on secondary survey, you are strongly suspecting genitourinary trauma.

1. How will you differentiate between extraperitoneal bladder rupture and intraperitoneal bladder rupture?

Bladder injury is broadly divided into extraperitoneal and intraperitoneal injuries. Extraperitoneal bladder injuries generally occur with pelvic fractures, while intraperitoneal bladder injuries occur with high-energy impact to an overdistended bladder. Intraperitoneal rupture requires surgical repair while extraperitoneal injuries may be treated conservatively with a urinary catheter. The presence of other renal tract injuries involving the ureters or urethra may require separate intervention **(Table 1)**.

2. How do you treat extraperitoneal bladder rupture?

Most extraperitoneal bladder leaks can be effectively managed with maximal bladder drainage per urethral or suprapubic catheter. Depending on the presumed size of the bladder defect, the bladder should be drained for 10–14 days and then assessed for healing via cystogram. Immediate surgical repair of an extraperitoneal bladder injury is appropriate in the setting of intravesical bone spicules, rectal or vaginal laceration, and bladder neck injuries in order to minimize the risks of fistula formation, abscess, urine leak, and incontinence **(Flowchart 1)**.

3. What are the indications for operative treatment for extraperitoneal bladder rupture?

Absolute indications: Blunt or penetrating external trauma with gross hematuria and a known pelvic fracture.

Relative indications: Penetrating injury to buttocks, pelvis or lower abdomen with any degree of microscopic hematuria. Widening of pubic symphysis >1 cm and/or widening of obturator ring >1 cm.

TABLE 1: Differentiation between extraperitoneal bladder rupture and intraperitoneal bladder rupture.

Extraperitoneal bladder rupture	Intraperitoneal bladder rupture
Most common form of bladder injury	Less common than extraperitoneal bladder rupture
Causes separation of fascial planes between bladder and pelvis	Secondary to injury of bladder dome, communication between bladder and peritoneal cavity
• *Simple:* Extravasated contrast solution is limited to perivesical space • *Complex:* Extravasated contrast solution extends to high scrotum perineum	Extravasated contrast solution often appears less concentrated relative to contrast solution in the bladder
Treatment: Most often urinary drainage via Foley's catheter more severe injury may require injury	*Treatment:* Most often surgical intervention

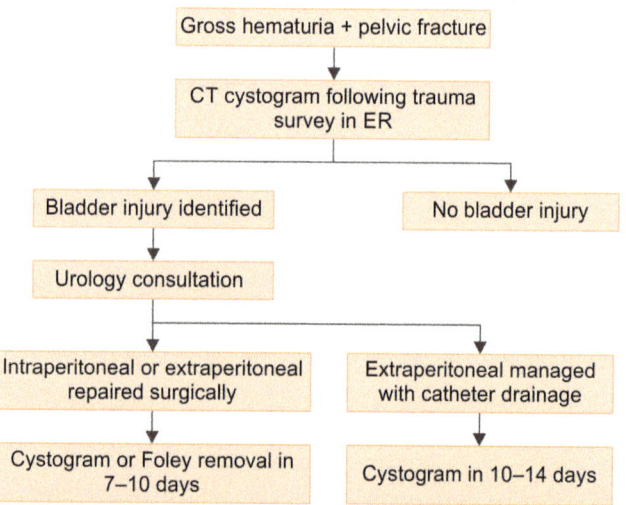

Flowchart 1: Approach to treatment bladder rupture.

(CT: computed tomography; ER: emergency room)

4. Discuss clinical features of urethral injuries.

Blood at the urethral meatus is the most important sign of a urethral injury. The most common symptoms of urethral injuries include blood at the tip of the penis in men or the urethral opening in women, blood in the urine, an inability to urinate, and pain during urination. Bruising may be visible between the legs or in the genitals. Other symptoms may arise when complications develop. Symptoms of urethral injuries include pain with voiding or inability to void. Additional signs include perineal, scrotal, penile, and labial ecchymosis, edema, or both.

5. Explain the diagnosis of urethral injuries.

Retrograde urethrogram remains the preferred initial diagnostic modality to evaluate a suspected urethral injury. Retrograde urethrography (RUG) or ascending urethrography is used to image male anterior urethra in cases of blunt perineal trauma to assess for urethral disruption, suspected urethral stricture and fistulas. The patient is positioned in a 45° oblique position and water-soluble iodinated contrast media are gently instilled into a stretched penis through a 12–16 gauge Foley catheter positioned with its balloon in the fossa navicularis and spot films are taken.

Question 2

1. Enumerate the causes of acute pain in right upper quadrant of abdomen.

Biliary: Cholecystitis, cholangitis, cholelithiasis

Colic: Colitis, diverticulitis, ileitis, retrocecal appendicitis, perforated duodenal ulcer

Hepatic: Abscess, hepatitis, masses, hepatic congestion

Pulmonary: Pneumonia, pulmonary embolism

Renal: Nephrolithiasis, pyelonephritis.

2. Discuss clinical features of acute cholecystitis.

Presentation of acute cholecystitis is like an extended biliary colic where pain starts in epigastrium, is usually severe, may radiate to right shoulder or back, may be associated with vomiting often associated with low-grade fever and ileus. Patient may give a history of similar pain in past but used to subside in 30–40 minutes and his/her interpretation is usually a "gas block" in past. On examination about 50% patient will have right upper quadrant (RHQ) tenderness and a sudden holding of breath during deep inspiration (Murphy's sign). Ultrasonography is usually diagnostic showing stone, thickening of gallbladder (GB) wall, and pericholecystic collection of fluid.

3. Explain the diagnosis of acute cholecystitis.

Acute cholecystitis means inflammation of GB which most commonly occurs due to gall stones. It occurs when a stone gets lodged in neck of GB or cystic duct leading to mechanical distension, ischemia of wall and bacterial infection. Usual organisms are gram-negative bacteria such as *Escherichia coli* or *Klebsiella* **(Table 2)**.

TABLE 2: Criteria for diagnosis of acute cholecystitis.

Local examination	Right upper quadrant mass pain or tenderness, Murphy's signs
Systemic features	Fever, raised C reactive protein, elevated WBC count
Imaging	• USG—sonographic Murphy's signs, GB thickening, distension, pericholecystic fluid • CT—GB wall thickening, distension, hyperdense GB wall pericholecystic fluid, and fat stranding
Diagnosis	• One local + one systemic = suspected • One local + one systemic + imaging finding = definitive diagnosis

(CT: computed tomography; GB: gallbladder; WBC: white blood cells)

4. Discuss emergency department (ED) management of acute cholecystitis.

Treatment of acute cholecystitis is urgent laparoscopic cholecystectomy unless patient is unfit for surgery in which case you can plan for an early cholecystectomy within 4–6 weeks. In sick patients USG-guided PTGBD (percutaneous transhepatic gallbladder drainage) is a good procedure to tide over the crisis. Lap cholecystectomy in presence of acute cholecystitis carries a complication rate of 1–3% but one must understand that perforation/empyema GB with sepsis has a mortality of 15–30%. So in an acute case if you decide to go for conservative treatment, patient can progress to one of these complications. Hence urgent laparoscopic cholecystectomy is preferred. Complications after lapchole are common bile duct (CBD) injury, bile leak, local hematoma, atherosclerosis, biliary stricture, etc., all of which require treatment in specialized centers. There are no long-term complications of removing GB except mild diarrhea in about 10% of patients due to bile acid malabsorption.

Question 3

1. What are the anatomic boundaries and structures of the anterior neck zones (horizontal zones)?

Neck is divided into three zones: Zone 1, Zone 2, and Zone 3 **(Table 3)**. In penetrating trauma, zone designations have anatomic, diagnostic, and management implications. Since the zone system is helpful in guiding management decisions, it is preferable to employ the zone system when describing traumatic injuries. Understanding of the anatomy of the neck, especially the location of important structures, is essential to providing optimal care **(Fig. 1)**.

TABLE 3: Anatomical zones of the neck and their structures.

	Zone I	Zone II	Zone III
Anatomic landmarks	Clavicle/sternum to cricoid cartilage	Cricoid cartilage to the mandible	Superior angle of the mandible
Anatomic structures in zone	• Proximal common carotid artery • Subclavian artery • Vertebral artery • Lung apices • Trachea • Thyroid • Esophagus • Thoracic duct • Spinal cord	• Carotid artery • Vertebral artery • Jugular vein • Pharynx • Trachea • Esophagus • Larynx • Vagus nerve • Recurrent laryngeal nerve • Spinal cord	• Vertebral artery • Distal carotid artery • Distal jugular vein • Salivary and parotid glands • Cranial nerves IX–XII • Spinal cord

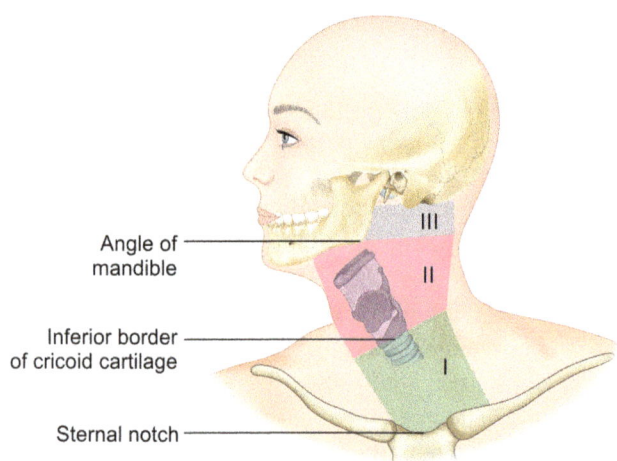

Fig. 1: Anatomical zones of the neck.

2. Discuss features of airway compromise in neck injuries.

- Respiratory distress
- Stridor hoarseness
- Hemoptysis
- Subcutaneous emphysema
- Sucking wound.

3. Explain the treatment options for airway management in a patient with neck trauma.

Airway: As always, the priority is airway stabilization, particularly in patients with neck trauma, while maintaining cervical spine immobilization. Remember that in-line stabilization should always be maintained when there is a concern for a cervical spine injury. Up to 10% of patients with penetrating neck injuries may present with airway compromise. Be aware that despite a stable initial appearance, airway compromise can ensue rapidly.

Beware that swelling, distorted anatomy, and hematoma formation may contribute to impending airway obstruction in facial or neck trauma. Therefore, early airway control should be considered as the conditions may rapidly worsen.

The goal of prehospital adult airway management is to obtain an open airway to oxygenate and ventilate the patient. This can generally be achieved with noninvasive methods of jaw thrust, nasopharyngeal airway (NPA), oropharyngeal airway (OPA), supplemental oxygen, and bag-valve-mask (BVM) ventilation. Tracheostomy, fiberoptic bronchoscopy (FOB) guided intubation and direct laryngoscopy are the standard methods used to secure the airway in these patients, but sometimes they may aggravate the underlying injury. Technique of choice depends upon patient's condition, urgency, and experience of anesthesiologist and surgeon.

4. What is "no-zone" targeted diagnostic work-up in penetrating neck injuries?

The current "no zone" algorithm for penetrating neck trauma focuses on identifying **hard signs** of injury and assessing patient stability rather than looking to the zone of injury for management (**Table 4**).

TABLE 4: Clinical features of concern in neck trauma.

Hard signs	• Airway compromise • Expanding and pulsatile hematoma • Active, brisk bleeding • Hemorrhagic shock • Hematemesis • Neurologic deficit • Massive subcutaneous emphysema • Air bubbling through wound
Soft signs	• Hemoptysis • Oropharyngeal blood • Dyspnea • Dysphagia • Dysphonia • Nonexpanding hematoma • Chest tube air leak • Subcutaneous or mediastinal air • Vascular bruit or thrill • Crepitus

Question 4

1. Enumerate the causes of vaginal bleed in a woman at 32 weeks of pregnancy.

Obstetrics causes: Placenta previa, abruptio placentae, vasa previa, disseminated intravascular coagulation, uterine rupture.

Nonobstetrics causes: Cervical cancer, cervicitis, cervical polyp, vaginitis, vaginal laceration.

2. What is HELLP (hemolysis, elevated liver enzymes, and low platelets) syndrome?

This (HELLP syndrome) is an acronym for hemolysis, elevated liver enzymes, and low platelet counts and occurs in about 7.5% of all pregnancies, more commonly in those complicated by severe preeclampsia and eclampsia. It may develop during the antepartum period more so in the third trimester and also in the postpartum period. Majority (80%) of women with HELLP have hypertension and proteinuria. In symptomatic women there may be hypertension and proteinuria with epigastric or right upper quadrant pain, nausea, vomiting, headache, edema, weight gain, and rarely jaundice. Maternal complications such as eclampsia, acute renal failure, disseminated intravascular coagulopathy, placental abruption, cerebral hemorrhage, pulmonary edema, hepatic infarction or parenchymal hemorrhage and subcapsular hematoma may occur. Mortality can occur in 1–3% cases. Neonatal morbidity and mortality are also increased. There is a higher incidence of growth restriction, prematurity, perinatal asphyxia, and stillbirths. Neonatal thrombocytopenia also occurs in a few cases. Mortality is higher in preterm deliveries.

Management of HELLP is largely supportive. Careful observation of parameters and correction of anemia and coagulopathy is required. Antihypertensives to control blood pressure in women with preeclampsia are needed to prevent worsening. Delivery is the definitive therapy for HELLP. In mild cases, pregnancy may be continued with meticulous monitoring till reasonable fetal maturity is achieved. Corticosteroids for fetal lung maturation should be used in pregnancy <34 weeks gestation. Those presenting early on with HELLP (<26 weeks gestation) are advised termination. Prolonged conservative management may have poor fetal and maternal outcomes. Large hepatic hematomas or those presenting with rupture and hemodynamic instability may need surgery or hepatic artery embolization for management. Liver transplant is a last resort in those who do not respond to standard management.

3. Discuss criteria to diagnose preeclampsia.

The diagnosis of preeclampsia is made by the presence of new onset hypertension >140/90 mm Hg after 20 weeks gestation either with proteinuria and/or evidence of maternal acute kidney injury, liver dysfunction, neurological features, hemolysis or thrombocytopenia, fetal growth restriction. Some cases may be diagnosed for the first time in intrapartum or early postpartum period **(Table 5)**.

4. Explain the management of eclampsia.

Eclampsia: Preeclampsia complicated by generalized tonic-clonic seizures is eclampsia and has poor implications for maternal and perinatal outcome. Usually preceded by severe preeclampsia, convulsions can occur in the antenatal or postnatal period. In the antenatal period, eclampsia occurs usually in the last 3 months of pregnancy closer to term. In postnatal period, seizures occur usually within 48 hours of birth though cases have been reported even 7 days after delivery. All pregnant women presenting with seizures should be considered to be eclampsia until proven otherwise. In women presenting with focal neurological deficits, atypical eclamptic seizures and prolonged comatose state, alternate diagnosis should be sought.

TABLE 5: Criteria of diagnosing the preeclampsia.

Criteria	Diagnosis of preeclampsia	Comments
Blood pressure	• >140/90 mm Hg after 20 weeks • Confirm by repeat blood pressure measurement in a few hours	Previously normotensive woman
Proteinuria	• ≥300 mg/24 hours • Urine protein: creatinine ratio ≥0.3 • Dipstick 1+ persistent	Automated dipstick recommended, if not available visual dipstick used
Hematological complications	Thrombocytopenia—platelet count below 150,000/mm^3, DIC, hemolysis	
Renal disease	Creatinine level >1.1 mg/dL or doubling of baseline	No history of previous renal disease
Liver involvement	Serum transaminases double of normal	With or without right upper quadrant or epigastric pain
Pulmonary edema		
Cerebral or visual symptoms	*Headache or visual disturbances:* Eclampsia, altered mental status, blindness, stroke, clonus, severe headaches, persistent visual scotomata	
Uteroplacental dysfunction	Fetal growth restriction, abnormal umbilical artery Doppler waveform analysis, or stillbirth	

(DIC: disseminated intravascular coagulation)

TABLE 6: MgSO$_4$ regimen for eclampsia treatment.

	Intramuscular regimen (Pritchard regimen)	Intravenous regimen (Zuspan regimen)
Loading dose	• 4 g MgSO$_4$ as 20% v/w solution intravenously at rate not exceeding 1 g/min • Follow promptly with 10 g MgSO$_4$ 50% v/w solution, 5 g as deep intramuscular in upper outer quadrant of each buttock by 3 inch 20 gauge needle	4–6 g MgSO$_4$ in 100 mL normal saline over 15–20 minutes
Repeat convulsions after 15 minutes	Give additional 2 g MgSO$_4$ as 20% v/w solution intravenously at rate not exceeding 1 g/min	
Maintenance dose	Every 4 hours, 5 g MgSO$_4$ 50% v/w solution as deep intramuscular in alternate buttock	1–2 g/h maintenance in 100 mL intravenous fluid/infusion
Prerequisites for maintenance doses	• Patellar reflex is present • Respiration is not depressed • Urine output over last 4 hours is >100 mL	• Deep tendon reflexes present • Serum magnesium levels done 4–6 hourly to maintain between 4 and 7 mEq/L • Serum magnesium levels if creatinine >1 mg/dL
Maternal observations	• Respiratory rate and blood pressure every 30 minutes, maternal pulse hourly • Urine output hourly, deep tendon reflexes 2 hourly, fetal heart rate continuous monitoring	
Pain relief	1 mL of 2% lidocaine can be added to the intramuscular preparation	
Discontinue	24 hours after delivery or last fit whichever is later	24 hours after delivery or last fit whichever is later

Treatment: Delivery of the fetus is the definitive treatment of preeclampsia and eclampsia. However, when the woman has convulsed, it is important to stabilize her condition before termination of pregnancy which is done irrespective of ability of the fetus to be salvaged.

The mainstay of eclampsia treatment is use of magnesium sulfate to prevent further convulsions or even forestall convulsions in severe preeclampsia. It is administered either by intramuscular route as intermittent injections or intravenous route as continuous infusion; the doses used are same for eclampsia and preeclampsia. The treatment has to be continued till 24 hours after delivery or last seizure, whichever is later **(Table 6)**.

Question 5

1. Discuss causes of acute lower abdominal pain in a nonpregnant female and etiopathogenesis of pelvic inflammatory disease (PID).

The female pelvis comprises organs of the reproductive system—vagina, uterus, fallopian tubes, and ovaries; urinary system—ureters and urinary bladder; gastrointestinal (GI) system—sigmoid colon and rectum; as well as components of the musculoskeletal system. Acute pelvic pain can originate from the reproductive organs or from any structures that lie next to or pass through the pelvis. The pelvic organ nerve innervation is from T9–L1 and S2–S4 spinal nerves. Pain may be initiated by inflammation, distention, or ischemia of an organ, or by spillage of blood, pus, or other material into the pelvis. The dull aching or the visceral pain is a result of the overlap of afferent innervation supplying the pelvic organs and the appendix, ureters, and colon, making their precise localization difficult. On the other hand, sharp stabbing like results pain when the afferent nerves in the parietal peritoneum adjacent to an affected organ are stimulated. Further characteristics of pelvic pain along with features and differential diagnoses are illustrated in **Table 7**.

2. Discuss clinical features of PID.

Many episodes of PID go unrecognized. While some cases are asymptomatic, others get misdiagnosed due to mild or nonspecific symptoms or signs such as abnormal bleeding, dyspareunia, and vaginal discharge.

3. Explain the ED management of PID.

Pelvic inflammatory disease encompasses a spectrum of inflammatory disorders of the upper female genital tract, including any combination of endometritis, salpingitis, tubo-ovarian abscess, and pelvic peritonitis. The common organisms causing PID are *Neisseria gonorrhoeae*, *Chlamydia trachomatis*, microorganisms that comprise the vaginal flora such as anaerobes, *Gardnerella vaginalis*, *Haemophilus influenzae*, enteric gram-negative rods, and *Streptococcus agalactiae*; cytomegalovirus (CMV), *Mycoplasma hominis*, *Ureaplasma urealyticum*, and *Mycoplasma genitalium*. Furthermore, women younger than 25 years, multiple sexual partners, not using condom, recent treatment for sexually transmitted infection, or HIV-positive status are the risk factors for PID. Many episodes of PID go unrecognized **(Table 8)**.

TABLE 7: Characteristics of acute pelvic pain with corresponding features and differential diagnoses.

Pain characteristics	Features	Differential diagnoses
Site of pain	Right lower quadrant of the abdomen	Acute appendicitis, pyelonephritis, ectopic pregnancy, ovarian cyst or torsion, ureteric colic, inguinal hernia, mittelschmerz, musculoskeletal pain
	Left lower quadrant of the abdomen	Diverticulitis, ectopic pregnancy, ovarian cyst or torsion, pyelonephritis, ureteric colic, perirectal abscess, inguinal hernia, mittelschmerz, musculoskeletal pain
	Lower abdomen	Cystitis, bowel obstruction, inflammatory bowel disease dysmenorrhea, ectopic pregnancy, uterine perforation or myomas, abortion, pelvic inflammatory disease (PID), endometritis, ovarian hyperstimulation syndrome, placental abruption, ovarian vein thrombosis, incarcerated/strangulated hernia, displaced intrauterine device, somatization disorder, musculoskeletal pain
Onset of pain	Acute	Vascular, obstructive, viscus perforation causes
	Subacute	Inflammatory causes
	Chronic	Malignancy, inflammatory causes
Character of pain	Tearing like	Dissection of aorta or its branches
	Stabbing like	Irritation of parietal peritoneum
	Colicky	Obstruction of tubular organ, smooth muscle spasms, e.g., ureteric colic
	Dull	Visceral pain
Radiation of pain	Loin to groin	Nephrolithiasis
	Migration of pain from umbilicus to right lower abdomen	Acute appendicitis
	Radiation to back	Aortic dissection, PID, cystitis
Associating factors of pain	Hypotension or signs of shock	Ruptured ectopic pregnancy, leaking aortic aneurysm, aortic dissection
	Fever	Acute appendicitis, PID, pyelonephritis
	Diarrhea, nausea, vomiting, anorexia	Gastrointestinal pathology
	Vaginal bleeding or discharge, dyspareunia, cervical motion tenderness	Sexually transmitted infection (STI), PID, tubo-ovarian abscess (TOA)
	Vaginal bleeding	Placental abruption, miscarriage, mittelschmerz
	Urinary frequency or hesitancy, hematuria	Nephrolithiasis, urinary tract infection (UTI)
	Pressure like feeling in perineum	Uterine prolapse
Time course or pattern of the pain	Mid-cycle vaginal bleeding	Mittelschmerz
	During and post coital pain	PID, gynecological malignancy
	Infertility treatment	Ovarian hyperstimulation syndrome (OHSS), ovarian torsion
	Urogenital procedure or surgery	Wound infection or sepsis, venous thrombosis, venous thrombophlebitis, thermal injury
	Trauma	Sexual assault, intimate partner violence, female genital mutilation
Aggravating factors	Change in posture	Musculoskeletal pain
	Menstruation	Endometriosis, adenomyosis
	Dyspareunia	PID, TOA
	Bouncy movements such as jumping or travelling over bumpy road	Peritonitis
Relieving factors	Laying still	Peritonitis, musculoskeletal pain
	Passage of urine	Acute urinary retention
Severity	Mild discomfort	PID, UTI, mesenteric ischemia, hernia
	Moderate pain	Peritonitis, aortic aneurysmal leak or dissection, appendicitis, ovarian or adnexal cyst, miscarriage, placental abruption, strangulated or incarcerated hernia, musculoskeletal pain
	Uncontrollable	Ovarian or adnexal torsion, ureteric colic, labor pain

TABLE 8: Management of pelvic inflammatory disease (PID)—diagnosis, treatment, and disposition.

PID	Diagnosis	Treatment	Disposition
Mild-to-moderate PID	PID without any mass or tubo-ovarian abscess (TAO)	Ceftriaxone 250 mg intramuscularly once PLUS Doxycycline 100 mg twice a day orally for 14 days With or Without Metronidazole 500 mg twice a day for 14 days	Outpatient follow-up with instructions to abstain from sexual intercourse until treatment is complete and until their partner or partners have been treated
Severe PID	PID with mass or (TAO)	Cefotetan 2 g intravenously twice a day OR Cefoxitin 2 g intravenously 4 times a day PLUS Doxycycline 100 mg twice a day orally or intravenously *For tubo-ovarian abscess (TAO), to the above therapy, add the following:* Clindamycin 900 mg intravenously thrice a day PLUS Gentamycin loading dose (2 mg/kg), followed by a maintenance dose (1.5 mg/kg) intravenously thrice a day or substituted with a single daily dosing (3–5 mg/kg) OR Ampicillin/Sulbactam 3 g intravenously 4 times a day PLUS Doxycycline 100 mg orally or intravenously twice a day	Inpatient treatment to ensure clinical stability and improvement in cases of hemodynamic instability, peritonitis, severe systemic symptoms, concern for treatment failure of oral antibiotics (no clinical improvement after 72 hours of initiation of oral therapy), pregnancy and inability to tolerate oral antibiotics

Question 6

1. Explain differentiating temporary teeth from permanent teeth.

Primary teeth are smaller and look whiter than permanent teeth because they have thinner enamel. Their roots are also shorter and thinner **(Table 9)**.

TABLE 9: Differentiating temporary teeth from permanent teeth.

Temporary teeth (primary)	Permanent teeth
Develops 6 month–6 years lighter in color smaller in dimension	6 years onward, grayish in color, larger in dimensions
Develops directly from dental lamina	Develops from extension of dental lamina
Mesiodistal dimension of crown is more than cervico-incisal length	Cervico-incisal length is more than mesiodistal diameter of crown

2. Discuss Ludwig's angina.

Ludwig's angina is a potentially life-threatening condition with rapid progression within hours, the cellulitis starts from the submandibular space and spreads to the connective tissues of floor of mouth and neck. Odontogenic polymicrobial cellulitis mostly caused by *viridans group streptococci (VGS), Staphylococcus aureus,* and anaerobes. *Dental pathologies:* Dental caries, recent dental procedures, poor oral hygiene. *Trauma:* Mandibular fractures, facial fractures, piercings of tongue. *Other causes:* Submandibular sialadenitis, oral malignancy, systemic illness with immunocompromised status [acquired immunodeficiency syndrome (AIDS), diabetes mellitus, post-transplant patients]. Patients mostly present with neck pain and swelling, along with dysphagia. Other symptoms include dysphonia "hot potato" muffled voice, drooling of saliva, pain over floor of mouth, tongue swelling, restricted neck movement, and fever. Red flags (serious clinical features) are **T**oxic general appearance, **A**ltered mental status, **A**irway obstruction, **P**oor hydration status, **P**oor oral acceptance.

Investigations: Clinical presentation forms the base of diagnosis, though no specific laboratory tests are indicated, CT scan of neck with IV contrast enhancement is the study of choice, as it gives a details of airway compromise, soft tissue swelling, and involvement of mediastinum.

Treatment: Comforting the patient's posture, maintaining airway patency and oxygenation should be the priority, wide bore IV access should be immediately secured and crystalloid fluid should be administered. Advanced airway should be placed without any delay in case of compromised airway.

Antibiotic therapy: Broad-spectrum empirical antibiotics should be administered with priority. Both aerobic and anaerobic coverage should be given. Patients with less severe symptoms and patent airway may be treated with oral antibiotics. Oral penicillin VK and amoxycillin are first line choice while levofloxacin, cefuroxime, and amoxicillin-clavulanate are the second line choice. While patients with suspicion of deep neck infections should be treated with IV piperacillin/tazobactam, imipenem-cilastatin, and ertapenem. Surgical drainage should be done if computed tomography suggests abscess.

3. Explain dental avulsion.

Dental avulsion is described as a complete displacement of a tooth from its socket in the alveolar bone, and it is one of the most traumatic dental injuries which originate exposure of the cells of the periodontal ligament to the external environment as well as disruption of the blood supply to the pulp **(Table 10)**.

TABLE 10: Dental avulsion.

Traumatic injuries to teeth are very common and usually associated with road traffic accidents, contact sports like boxing, taekwondo, karate, etc., or fights. This is very common with children than adults while playing or falling.	
Pathophysiology	Pain due to trauma can be because of exposure of pulp, avulsion, or luxation
Clinical presentation	Pain is severe like pulpitis but associated with bleeding
Red flags	Fractured crown of tooth
History	It is very important for clinician to know cause of injury, angle of impact, and object of impact to know the extent of injury
Physical examination	Mobility of tooth is very common, sometimes fracture can occur at the root which is very painful but show no sign clinically. Radiographs are helpful in such cases
Investigations	Radiographs OPG or IOPA are most commonly done
Treatment	• If the fracture is at crown of the tooth exposing the pulp of tooth then root canal treatment is done followed by restoration of the tooth • If there is luxation, splinting is done • In case of avulsion, teeth can be replanted under half an hour of injury if the tooth is preserved in saliva or milk and periodontal ligament fibers are intact

(IOPA: intraoral periapical; OPG: orthopantomogram)

Question 7

1. Enumerate the causes of lower GI bleed.

- Diverticular disease
- Malignancy (colon and rectum)
- Inflammatory bowel disease
- Colitis (infective, radiation, ischemia)
- Vascular malformation
- Hemorrhoids
- Anal fissure
- Rectal varices.

2. How will you differentiate upper GI bleed from lower GI bleed?

The GI bleed is defined as bleeding in the GI tract from mouth to anus. It is further divided into upper GI bleed (bleed that occurs from source in esophagus to ligament of Treitz in duodenum) and lower GI bleed (bleed that occurs from source distal to ligament of Treitz).

Upper GI bleed: It typically presents with hematemesis and or/melena and can present with hematochezia if the bleeding is brisk. Strong supporting features are positive gastric lavage blood urea nitrogen (BUN)/Cr ration >30 (SI units) risk factors, cirrhosis, alcohol, non-steroidal anti-inflammatory drug (NSAID), *Helicobacter pylori,* hiatal hernia.

Lower GI bleed: It typically presents with hematochezia can present with melena if source is small intestine or ascending colon. Strong supporting feature is—blood clots mixed with stool; refuting feature—hemodynamic instability.

3. Discuss ED evaluation of a patient with lower GI bleed and management of a patient with lower GI bleed.

Initial evaluation history: Every patient with history of black stool should be evaluated as soon as possible to assess the severity of bleeding, to ascertain source of the bleeding. Information collected from the initial evaluation is helpful in resuscitation, diagnostic, and treatment. Mostly melena occurs if GI bleeding proximal to ligaments of Treitz. Past medical history about hematemesis abdominal pain dyspepsia dysphagia should be obtained. History of smoking, alcohol, and liver disease should be documented. History of use of NSAID antiplatelets and anticoagulants or iron tablets are important.

Physical examination: In cases of upper GI bleed (hematemesis, melena) physical examination is the key to check hemodynamic status. Signs of hypovolemia such as low pulse pressure, tachycardia cold clammy extremities postural hypotension should be addressed on priority basis. Palmer erythema, jaundice, spider angioma, and gynecomastia give clue for existing liver disease. Abdominal examination is performed for any tenderness organomegaly mass and ascites. Rectal examination may also give some clue for diagnosis.

Investigations: Initial laboratory work-up starts with complete hemogram, knowing the status of baseline hemoglobin, and obtaining the blood grouping and typing; other test helpful are—lactate level, coagulation profile, liver function test, kidney function test. Patient with upper GI bleed usually have raised BUN—creatinine or urea—creatinine ratio. Electrocardiograph cardiac enzyme should be obtained in the high-risk group patient like elderly.

Management triage: Hemodynamic stabilization is the key for initial management. Aggressive resuscitation in patient with hemorrhagic shock, two large bore cannulas should be inserted immediately, typed and crossmatched blood transfusion as soon as possible. Airway management should be considered in patient with respiratory difficulties and altered mental status. Elective intubation further decreases the risk of aspiration.

Fluid resuscitation and blood transfusion: Patient with active bleeding and or with the unstable hemodynamic parameters should receive IV fluid (normal saline or ringer lactate 500 mL in 30 minutes) till the blood is arranged. Initially base line hemoglobin level should be obtained later hemoglobin level is diluted by movement of extravascular fluid to vascular space and also by IV fluid during resuscitation. Most of the guidelines suggested to keep the hemoglobin level >7 g in active bleeding patient and >9 g in patient with unstable coronary artery disease. Avoid transfusing the blood in variceal bleed patient as it can worsen the bleeding from the varices. Platelet and fresh frozen plasma transfusion should be considered in patient with low platelet count and deranged coagulation profile (INR >1.5). Platelet transfusion should also be considered in patient on antiplatelet therapy.

Nasogastric lavage: Nasogastric lavage is not beneficial in all patient of upper GI bleed. Nasogastric lavage is helpful in removing the particulate matter, blood clot, fresh blood from the stomach which facilitate the endoscopy.

Endoscopy: For upper GI bleed endoscopy is diagnostic modality of choice. Endoscopy is helpful in identifying in bleeding lesion and after that hemostasis can also be achieved in bleeding lesion by therapeutic endoscopy. Early endoscopy is recommended in patient with upper GI bleed.

Question 8

1. How do you classify fractures of proximal femur?

They are classified on the basis of anatomical location of fracture into—neck of femur fracture, intertrochanteric fracture and subtrochanteric fracture **(Fig. 2A)**. Each of these fracture types requires special methods of treatment and has its own set of complications and controversies regarding the optimal method of management **(Fig. 2B)**.

2. What are the clinical features of proximal femur fractures?

- Radiating pain to the knee.
- Inability to bear weight.
- Shortening or sideways rotation of the affected leg.
- Increased pain in the hip during rotation of the leg.
- Swelling on the side of the hip.

3. Discuss ED management of proximal femur fracture.

Initial management of any orthopedic emergency is aimed at control of pain and reduction of swelling.

In prehospital setting or with minor injuries rest, ice, compression, and elevation (RICE) method has been proven to provide relief:

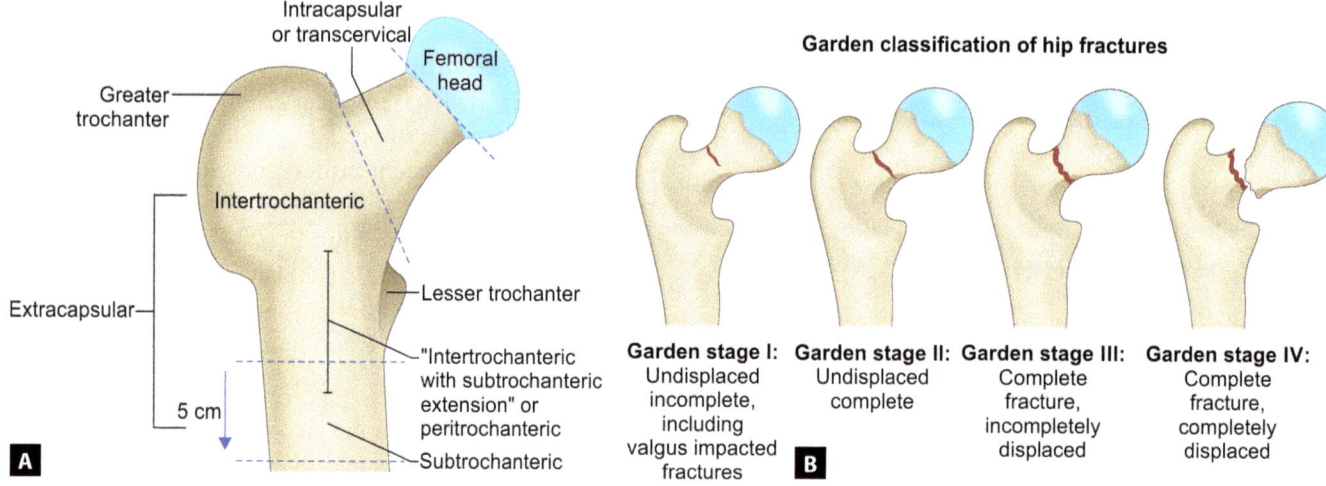

Figs. 2A and B: Anatomical classification fractures of proximal femur.

- **R**est: Reduction of movement reduces pain and prevents further bleeding
- **I**ce: Cold compress causes local vasoconstriction and thus reduces swelling
- **C**ompression: Wrapping the part in elastic compression bandages helps reduce swelling
- **E**levation: Raising the affected part at or above the heart level improves venous return and reduces swelling.

Pain control: Analgesics—NSAIDs or narcotic analgesia should be used early for pain control. It can be given intravenously or intramuscularly.

Peripheral nerve blocks: Digital nerve blocks, wrist or ankle blocks are used for hand and feet injuries. Femoral or axillary nerve blocks can be used for proximal injuries.

Procedural sedation: Use of sedatives such as propofol, midazolam or ketamine is needed for painless manipulation of fracture in ED.

Fracture hematoma blocks: This is used for reduction of fractures of distal radius or ulna. A total of 10–20 mL of 2% xylocaine is infiltrated into the hematoma which allows easy and painless reduction.

Surgery: Proximal femur fractures are *treated with surgery*. Proximal femur fractures are treated by using IM nail or an extramedullary sliding hip screw (SHS) or hip arthroplasty methods depending on the condition of the patient or the choice of the surgeon.

4. Explain the complications of proximal femur fracture.

- Deep vein thrombosis and pulmonary embolism
- Malunion
- Delayed union
- Nonunion
- Avascular necrosis
- Fixation failure
- Prosthesis dislocation.

Question 9

1. What are the causes of red eye?

Conjunctivitis is the most common cause of red eye. Other common causes include blepharitis, corneal abrasion, foreign body, subconjunctival hemorrhage, keratitis, iritis, glaucoma, chemical burn, and scleritis. Six serious causes of red eye which may cause visual loss are acute angle closure glaucoma, keratitis scleritis iritis, penetrating eye injury and embedded foreign bodies, acid or alkali eye burn.

2. How will you evaluate a patient with red eye?

History and physical examination: Location, quality, severity, timing, context-associated symptoms modifying factors. Inspection of whole patient visual acuity each eye and pin hole, periauricular lymphadenopathy, conjunctiva corneal globe tenderness, pupil shape reaction to light accommodation, eye movement fundoscopy.

3. Discuss management of a patient with red eye.

Treatment is supportive; avoid the allergen where possible, avoid rubbing the eyes, and apply a cool or warm compress to relieve symptoms. Treatment of red eye from a corneal or conjunctival foreign body consists of removal of the foreign body. Ophthalmologist advice is sought if there is any serious cause of red eye.

Question 10

1. How do you examine radial, median, and ulnar nerve injuries at elbow and at wrist?

Ulnar nerve entrapment at the elbow (cubital tunnel syndrome) and wrist (Guyon's canal syndrome) occurs due to repetitive compression, from leaning on the elbows or wrists (cyclist's palsy) and prolonged elbow flexion. It can also occur from trauma, swelling, fractures, and vascular and bony pathologies/abnormalities.

Ulnar nerve injury at wrist: Tap finger over the ulnar nerve at the wrist to determine whether this causes a tingling sensation (Tinel sign), which is a sign of nerve compression, because the ulnar nerve also travels through a narrow tunnel at the elbow.

The median nerve is usually damaged at either the elbow, due to a fracture of the humerus bone of the upper arm, or the wrist, due to either carpal tunnel syndrome or a wrist laceration or gashing. If the median nerve is damaged at the elbow region, it is known as a proximal injury to the median nerve. *If radial nerve damaged at the axilla*, there will be a loss of extension of the forearm, hand, and fingers. Thus, this usually presents with a wrist drop on physical examination. There will be a sensory loss in the lateral arm.

2. What is nursemaid injury? Describe the methods to manage nursemaid injury.

Nursemaid's elbow (radial head subluxation) **(Fig. 3A)** is a common injury among toddlers' early childhood. It happens when a ligament slips out of place and gets caught between two bones in the elbow joint. Nursemaid's elbow (also called a pulled elbow) causes arm pain, avoid moving arm, support arm from other hand, unable to rotate palm.

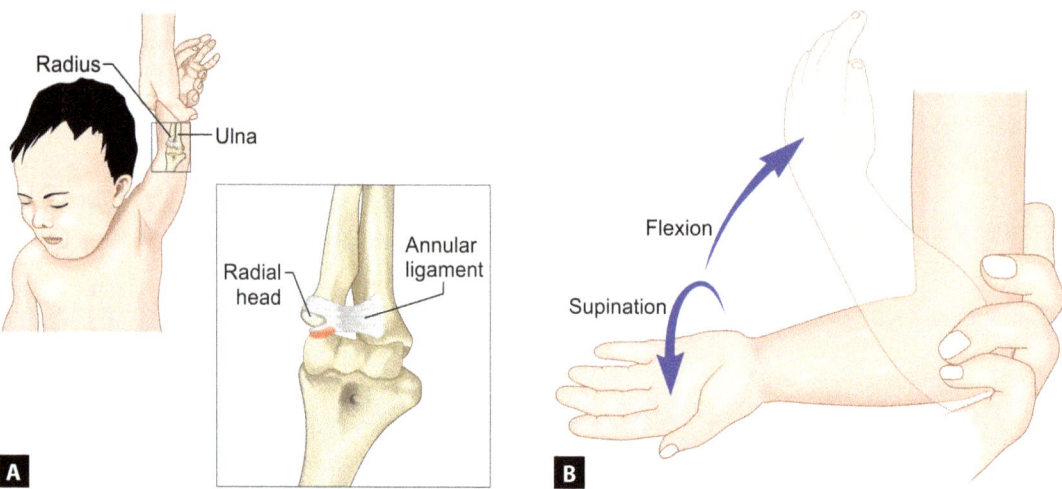

Figs. 3A and B: (A) Nursemaid injury; (B) Management (reduction procedure).

Management by reduction (Fig. 3B):
- Apply pressure at radial head
- Grasp wrist and apply slight traction
- Supinate wrist while to flexing elbow 90°.

SUGGESTED READING

1. Richhariya D, Sharma B. Textbook of Emergency Medicine including Intensive Care and Trauma, 2nd edition. New Delhi: Jaypee Brothers Medical Publishers (P) Ltd; 2022. pp. 1597-1600. (Question 1).
2. Richhariya D, Sharma B. Textbook of Emergency Medicine including Intensive Care and Trauma, 2nd edition. New Delhi: Jaypee Brothers Medical Publishers (P) Ltd; 2022. pp. 670-1. (Question 2).
3. Richhariya D, Sharma B. Textbook of Emergency Medicine including Intensive Care and Trauma, 2nd edition. New Delhi: Jaypee Brothers Medical Publishers (P) Ltd; 2022. p. 1565. (Question 3).
4. Richhariya D, Sharma B. Textbook of Emergency Medicine including Intensive Care and Trauma, 2nd edition. New Delhi: Jaypee Brothers Medical Publishers (P) Ltd; 2022. pp. 1089-96. (Question 4).
5. Richhariya D, Sharma B. Textbook of Emergency Medicine including Intensive Care and Trauma, 2nd edition. New Delhi: Jaypee Brothers Medical Publishers (P) Ltd; 2022. p. 1062. (Question 5).
6. Richhariya D, Sharma B. Textbook of Emergency Medicine including Intensive Care and Trauma, 2nd edition. New Delhi: Jaypee Brothers Medical Publishers (P) Ltd; 2022. pp. 931, 941, 1215. (Question 6).
7. Richhariya D, Sharma B. Textbook of Emergency Medicine including Intensive Care and Trauma, 2nd edition. New Delhi: Jaypee Brothers Medical Publishers (P) Ltd; 2022. pp. 657-60. (Question 7).
8. Richhariya D, Sharma B. Textbook of Emergency Medicine including Intensive Care and Trauma, 2nd edition. New Delhi: Jaypee Brothers Medical Publishers (P) Ltd; 2022. pp. 1615-19. (Question 8).
9. Richhariya D, Sharma B. Textbook of Emergency Medicine including Intensive Care and Trauma, 2nd edition. New Delhi: Jaypee Brothers Medical Publishers (P) Ltd; 2022. pp. 900-5. (Question 9).
10. Richhariya D, Sharma B. Textbook of Emergency Medicine including Intensive Care and Trauma, 2nd edition. New Delhi: Jaypee Brothers Medical Publishers (P) Ltd; 2022. p. 1615. (Question 10).

Emergency Medicine Paper 23

Ajay Singh Thapa

Question 1

1. How will you differentiate pyelonephritis from cystitis?

Pyelonephritis: Pyelonephritis is upper urinary tract infection which involves kidney and ureter. In contrast to cystitis, patient with pyelonephritis presents with more systemic symptoms than local such as fever, vomiting, nausea, abdominal pain, flank pain. For diagnosis of pyelonephritis, ultrasonography (USG) kidney ureter bladder (KUB) or noncontrast computed tomography (NCCT KUB) should be done. Urine culture and blood culture should be sent from emergency before administration of antibiotic is ideal approach.

Cystitis: Cystitis is superficial infection of urinary bladder. Patient who has cystitis presents with localized symptoms such as dysuria, urinary frequency, hesitancy, hematuria or suprapubic pain. It is more common in woman than man. Usually patient with cystitis has no fever with only abovementioned localized symptoms. It is necessary to evaluate regarding sexually transmitted disease (STD) by proper history such as urethral discharge, vaginal discharge, vaginal bleeding, new sexual partner, sexual partner with STD, etc. All these symptoms are more suggestive of STD than cystitis. Man with >50 years of age, prostatic abnormality, and history of previous instrumentation can present with cystitis.

2. What is the difference between uncomplicated urinary tract infection and complicated urinary tract infection?

Acute uncomplicated pyelonephritis: As pyelonephritis is infection on renal parenchyma, antibiotics which penetrate in tissue can be considered as initial treatment. Fluoroquinolones are initial choice of antibiotic. But being emergency physician you must consider to start outpatient or inpatient treatment. Indications for admission are inability to maintain oral hydration, unable to take oral medicines, severe sepsis, acute renal failure, immunocompromised, pregnancy, etc., if patient allergic to fluoroquinolones, oral or intravenous (IV) amoxicillin can be started if low local resistance to organism. If the patient can be treated as outpatient treatment oral fluoroquinolone is initial treatment of choice.

Acute complicated pyelonephritis: As mentioned above patients with pyelonephritis associated with structural and functional abnormality of genitourinary tract, immunocompromised status, and signs of sepsis are considered as complicated pyelonephritis. These patients require as early as possible broad-spectrum IV antibiotics. Take culture before administration of antibiotics. Recently, ceftozolone/tazobactam and ceftazidime/avibactam newer antibiotics are on trial for complicated UTI.

3. Discuss urine analysis in urinary tract infection.

After urine dip stick test, urine routine and microscopic examination is most commonly used test to diagnose UTI in emergency department. Urine microscopic examination provides information regarding presence of bacteria, white blood cells (WBC), red blood cells (RBC), and epithelial cells in urine. The WBC count >5 per high power field in symptomatic patient indicates abnormal result. If counts are less but history and clinical examination findings are suggestive of UTI, first rule out false negative causes. Presence of WBC and RBC indicates other causes such as vaginal bleeding or bleeding from genitourinary tract and do further diagnosis accordingly. Presence of epithelial cells indicates contaminated specimen.

4. Comment on antimicrobial regime for adult female having complicated cystitis.

These patients required as early as possible broad-spectrum IV antibiotics. Take culture before administration of antibiotics. Recently, ceftozolone/tazobactam and ceftazidime/avibactam newer antibiotics are on trial for complicated UTI.

Doses:
- IV cefepime 1 g twice a day
- IV piperacillin/tazobactam 4.5 g three times a day
- IV imipenem 500 mg four times a day
- IV ciprofloxacin 400 mg twice a day
- IV vancomycin 15 mg/kg twice a day.

Question 2

1. What are the sources of carbon monoxide (CO) poisoning?

Fire-related smoke inhalation is the major cause for CO poisoning. Other potential sources of CO are poorly functioning heating systems, improperly vented fuel-burning equipment (kerosene heaters, charcoal grills, camping stoves, and gasoline-powered generators) and motor vehicles working in poorly ventilated areas (e.g., ice rinks, warehouses, parking garages), methylene chloride (dichloromethane), an industrial solvent, and a component of paint remover.

2. Discuss the pathophysiology of CO poisoning.

Carbon monoxide is a colorless, tasteless, odorless, and nonirritating gas formed by hydrocarbon combustion. The concentration in atmospheric for CO is generally <0.001%, but it may be more in urban areas or enclosed environments. CO binds to hemoglobin with very high affinity than oxygen, forming carboxyhemoglobin (COHb) and resulting in impaired oxygen transport and utilization. CO can also produce an inflammatory cascade that may lead to central nervous system (CNS) lipid peroxidation and delayed neurologic sequelae.

Inhaled or ingested methylene chloride is converted to CO by the liver, can also cause CO toxicity in the absence of ambient CO. CO diffuses very rapidly across the pulmonary capillary membrane and binds to the iron moiety of heme with around 240 times more affinity of oxygen. Once CO binds to the heme, an allosteric change occurs that greatly reduces the ability of the other three oxygen binding sites to release oxygen to peripheral tissues. This leads to a leftward shift of the oxyhemoglobin dissociation curve and impairment in tissue oxygen delivery. CO also reduces the peripheral oxygen utilization. Around 10–15% of CO is extravascular and bound to molecules such as myoglobin, cytochromes, and nicotinamide adenine dinucleotide phosphate (NADPH) reductase, leads to an impairment of oxidative phosphorylation at the mitochondrial level.

3. Explain the diagnosis of CO poisoning.

Acute CO poisoning is usually suspected on the basis of history and physical examination because the diagnosis of chronic CO intoxication is very much difficult without strong clinical suspicion. Routine pulse oximetry (SpO_2) cannot screen for CO intoxication, as it cannot differentiate carboxyhemoglobin from oxyhemoglobin.

Mild-to-moderate CO-toxicity patients present with headache (the most common presenting symptom), nausea, and dizziness, malaise. Patients may also present with symptoms ranging from mild confusion to coma. Some may have a "cherry red" appearance of the lips.

Severe CO toxicity can present with neurologic symptoms such as seizures, syncope, or coma, and also cardiovascular manifestations such as myocardial ischemia, ventricular arrhythmias, and lung problems such as breathlessness, pulmonary edema, and metabolic disorder such as profound lactic acidosis.

Delayed neuropsychiatric syndrome: Nearly 40% of patients with severe CO toxicity, a syndrome of delayed neurologic sequelae (DNS) can arise after apparent recovery within a year. The development of DNS poorly correlates with COHb levels, although majority of cases are associated with loss of consciousness during acute intoxication.

The diagnosis of CO poisoning is based upon high COHb level measured by cooximetry of an arterial blood gas (ABG) sample. In hemodynamically stable patients, venous samples are also accurate and commonly used to avoid arterial prick and it may be very useful when handling large number of patients in major disasters. Nonsmokers can have up to 3% of baseline COHb; in smokers, this is about 10–15%, levels more than these values are diagnostic of CO poisoning. A carboxyhemoglobin measurement is essential for diagnosis, but levels may not correlate with the degree of poisoning and are not predictive of DNS.

4. Discuss the role of hyperbaric oxygen (HBO) in CO poisoning.

Indications for HBO
- CO level >25%
- CO level >20% in pregnant patient
- Loss of consciousness or low Glasgow coma scale (GCS)
- Severe metabolic acidosis (pH <7.1)
- Evidence of end-organ damage (e.g., ECG changes, chest pain, or altered mental status).

Hyperbaric oxygen treatment involves exposing patients to 100% O_2 under supra-atmospheric conditions. This leads to a reduction in the half-life of COHb, from about 90 minutes on 100% normobaric oxygen to about 30 minutes during HBO. The amount of oxygen dissolved in the blood also rises from 0.3–6.0 mL/dL, which substantially increases the release of non-hemoglobin-bound O_2 to the tissues. HBO treatment may be beneficial in preventing the late neurocognitive deficits associated with severe CO toxicity.

Question 3

1. How to classify severity of asthma exacerbation in adults?

Severity of asthma: The *assessment of severity can be done based on GINA guidelines*. On physical examination, cyanosis, nasal flaring, use of accessory muscles of respiration leading to intercostal or supraclavicular indrawing, tachycardia, tachypnea, hypotension, and altered level of consciousness are at higher risk of fatal asthma and need special attention. On auscultation bilateral Ronchi can be presented silent chest without wheezing indicated severe airflow obstruction. Symptoms and finding do not correlate well with severity of symptoms so forced expiratory volume in 1 second and peak expiratory flow rate (PEFR) are important parameters in categorizing the severity of acute asthma. The other parameters to classify severity of asthma are summarized in **Flowchart 1**.

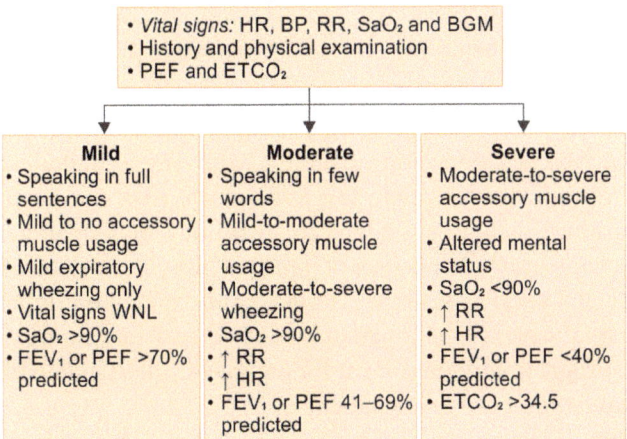

Flowchart 1: Categories of severity of asthma.

(BGM: blood glucose meter; BP: blood pressure; $ETCO_2$: end-tidal carbon dioxide; FEV_1: forced expiratory volume in 1 second; HR: heart rate; PEF: peak expiratory flow; RR: respiratory rate; SaO_2: oxygen saturation; WNL: within normal limit)

2. Explain the ED treatment of acute asthma.

Status asthmaticus *or acute severe asthma (FEV_1 OR PEFR <25 % of predicted)* is clinically characterized by hypoxemia, tachypnea, tachycardia, accessory muscle use wheezing impending respiratory arrest, and usual dose of bronchodilators and steroid does not improve the clinical conditions. Rapid and aggressive treatment is required to prevent the cardiopulmonary arrest. Adjuncts treatment is also required apart from the bronchodilators and early corticosteroid.

Magnesium—1–2 g IV over 30 minutes; nebulized magnesium is also added along with aggressive bronchodilators and inhaled corticosteroid therapy and effective in improving the pulmonary functions. Doses for nebulization magnesium sulfate 95 mg are in four divided doses 20 minutes apart.

Admission to intensive care unit (ICU): If the patient's condition further deteriorates (persistent respiratory distress, inability to maintain oxygen level above 90%, persistent hypercapnia, abnormal ABG–PaO_2 <60 mm Hg and/or $PaCO_2$ >60 mm Hg, alteration of mental status, acute confusion and drowsiness) even after above said measures then the patient can be shifted to ICU and noninvasive positive pressure (NIV) should be tried.

Noninvasive ventilation (NIV)—for patients with respiratory failure assisted mode of ventilation must be given first trial through noninvasive mode and if patients do not tolerate it or noncooperative then invasive mode of ventilation is applied after endotracheal intubation.

3. Describe the indications for mechanical ventilation in acute asthma.

Mechanical ventilation: Intubation can be considered in patients with the following:
- *NIV failure:* Worsening of ABG and or pH in 1–2 hours; lack of improvement in ABG and or pH after 4 hours.
- *Severe acidosis* (pH <7.25) and hypercapnia [$PaCO_2$ >60 mm Hg].
- *Tachypnea* >35 breaths/min.

Other complications: Metabolic abnormalities, sepsis, pneumonia, pulmonary embolism, barotrauma, massive pleural effusion.

4. How will you manage a patient of acute asthma who is on a ventilator?

There are three ventilator strategies that can be used to reduce hyperinflation and auto-PEEP in the intubated asthmatic patient: (1) Reduction of the respiratory rate, (2) reduction of tidal volume, and (3) shortening of inspiration by increasing inspiratory flow to allow greater time for exhalation with each respiratory cycle.

As a starting point for ventilating patients with severe asthma, recommendations are that the ventilator initially be used in pressure control mode, setting the pressure to achieve a tidal volume of 6–8 mL/kg, respiratory rate of 11–14 breaths/min and PEEP at 0–5 cmH_2O. We use these settings with a goal of obtaining a pH, in general, above 7.2 and a P_{plat} under 30 cmH_2O.

Question 4

1. What is syncope?

Syncope is defined as transient loss of consciousness (TLOC) due to transient global cerebral hypoperfusion; it has three important features rapid onset, short duration, and complete recovery.

2. Discuss the causes of syncope.

Very important to identify the life-threatening etiology such as acute coronary syndrome (ACS), aortic dissection, leaking aortic aneurysm (AAA), SAH, ruptured ectopic pregnancy and gastrointestinal (GI) bleed which may present as syncope in about 15% of cases: Missed diagnosis in these conditions can lead to medicolegal action inpatients presenting as syncope. The physician evaluating a patient with TLOC should be alert for the possibility of this disease in addition to cardiovascular diagnosis of ominous significance.

- *Cardiac syncope:* Cardiac causes which are associated with syncope include arrhythmia, ischemia, structural/valvular abnormalities (e.g., aortic stenosis), cardiac tamponade, and pacemaker malfunction. Bradycardia and tachycardia are second commonest reasons of syncope after reflex syncope.
- *Hemorrhage:* Large blood loss because of acute severe bleed can manifest as syncope. Important potential causes include—trauma, GI bleed, leaking aortic aneurysm, ruptured ovarian cyst, ectopic pregnancy rupture, and ruptured spleen.
- *Massive pulmonary embolism:* Hemodynamically significant pulmonary embolism is an uncommon but well documented cause of syncope.
- *Subarachnoid hemorrhage:* Patients presenting with syncope following a headache require evaluation for a possible subarachnoid hemorrhage.

3. Explain the ED evaluation of a patient with syncope.

There are two main objectives for evaluation of a patient with syncope in emergency department:
1. To identify the syncope so that an effective specific treatment strategy can be given.
2. To assess the prognosis in view of death, severe adverse events, and syncope recurrence.

During ED evaluation the differential diagnosis of syncope is extensive, main focus remains on the treatment of underlying cause when this is obvious. However, the cause of syncope often remains unclear. First challenge during evaluation of syncope is to differentiate it from seizure. Epilepsy, stroke, and head trauma may present with TLOC and syncope such as situations. Taking careful history alone can narrow down the diagnosis. History of previous seizure, head injury, tongue bite, the presence of a tonic-clonic activity, abnormal posturing, incontinence of bowel or bladder, missed antiepileptic medication, and postictal confusion gives clue about seizure; while syncope associated with sweating or nausea and rapid return of orientation upon awakening. Supine and upright blood pressure measurement, 12 lead ECG monitoring followed by additional testing including carotid sinus massage, echocardiography, tilt-table test, coronary angiography, CT angiography, EP study can be done in selected subgroup of patient.

4. How will you differentiate syncope from seizure?

Syncope is a common, disabling, and often challenging symptom. It can cause fall and injury, and can be the warning sign before sudden cardiac death. Differentiation of syncope from other causes of transient loss of consciousness (TLOC) such as seizure **(Table 1)** and "syncope mimics" (pseudoseizure, nonsyncopal TLOC, and psychological disorder) is very important for emergency physician while evaluating such type of patient.

TABLE 1: Differentiation of syncope caused by neurally mediated hypotension, arrhythmias, seizures, and psychogenic causes.

	Neurally mediated hypotension	Arrhythmia	Seizures	Psychogenic
Demographics and clinical settings	• Female > Male • Younger age (<55 years) • >2 episodes • Standing • Warm room • Emotional upset	• Male > Female • Older age groups • Fewer episodes (<3), during exertion or supine position • Family history of sudden death	Younger age <45 years Any setting	• Female > Male • Younger age • Occurs in the presence of gathering, often many episodes in a day, no identifiable trigger
Premonitory symptoms	Longer duration >5 sec with palpitation, blurred vision, nausea, warmth, diaphoresis, light-headedness	• Shorter duration (<6 sec) • Palpitation less common	Sudden onset or brief aura	Usually, absent
Observation during events	Pallor, diaphoresis, dilated pupil, slow pulse, low BP, Incontinence may occur, brief clonic movement may occur	Blue not pale, incontinence can occur, brief clonic movement can occur	Blue face, no pallor frothing from mouth prolonged syncope, tongue bite, eye deviation, incontinence more likely, increase in heart rate and blood pressure	• Normal color • No diaphoresis • Eye closed • Normal heart rate and blood pressure • No incontinence, prolonged duration
Residual symptoms	• Residual symptoms common • Prolonged fatigue common, oriented	Residual symptoms uncommon unless prolonged unconsciousness, oriented	Residual symptoms common, aching muscle, disoriented, Fatigue headache, slow recovery	• Residual symptoms uncommon, oriented

Question 5

1. Define acute hepatic encephalopathy.

Presence of abnormal neuropsychiatric manifestations in cirrhosis is called hepatic encephalopathy (HE). About 50–75% patients with cirrhosis develop HE.

2. Explain the clinical features of acute hepatic encephalopathy.

It can vary from trivial changes in cognitive abilities on psychometric testing (minimal HE) to overt encephalopathy (lethargy and coma). Encephalopathy can be episodic, recurrent, or persistent. *Grading of HE* is done according to *"West Heaven criteria"*. Encephalopathy occurs due to increase in ammonia and various other toxins and systemic inflammation. However, blood ammonia levels do not correlate with grade of encephalopathy. There are several factors which precipitate HE. Constipation, large protein meal, uremia, infections, sedatives, electrolyte imbalance and GI bleed are the usual precipitating factors.

3. Discuss ED treatment of acute hepatic encephalopathy.

- Supportive care of unconscious or confused patient
- Identification and treatment of concomitant disease
- Careful search for and correction of precipitating factors
- Reduction of ammonia production and absorption
    - Lactulose, lactitol, lactose orally or in enema form
    - Restriction of dietary protein
    - Disaccharide inhibitors
    - Probiotics
- Promotion of nitrogen excretion
    - L-ornithine—aspartate IV and PO
    - Sodium benzoate IV and PO
- Correction of neurotransmitter abnormalities in the brain
    - Flumazenil
    - Branched—chain amino acid—enriched formulations
    - Zinc replication (many possible modes of action)
- Portosystemic shunt suppression
- Liver support systems: Liver transplantation

4. Define acute-on-chronic liver failure (ACLF).

Acute-on-chronic liver failure is a syndrome characterized by acute decompensation of chronic liver disease associated with organ failures and high short-term mortality. Alcohol and chronic viral hepatitis are the most common underlying liver diseases.

Question 6

1. Enumerate the risk factors for venous thromboembolism.

The role of the emergency physician is to identify potentially life-threatened patients, who would benefit from early intervention and treatment, and to stabilize and treat accordingly **(Table 2)**.

2. Discuss the diagnostic testing for venous thromboembolism.

Most routine investigations including basic blood work, chest radiograph, ECG, cardiac troponins, brain natriuretic peptide (BNP), and arterial blood gas (ABG), are of limited value; CT pulmonary angiography and V/Q scan, compression ultrasonography (CUS), pulmonary angiography.

3. What are the scores for pulmonary embolism?

Scoring systems, such as the *pulmonary embolism severity index (PESI), the simplified pulmonary embolism severity index (sPESI)*, the Hestia score, and the Geneva score, incorporate medical history, and clinical criteria into a score that establishes patients at either low or very low risk for adverse outcomes. Both the PESI and sPESI have demonstrated sufficient sensitivity to indicate outpatient or observation management in patients with low scores. Likewise, a Hestia score of zero indicates low risk.

TABLE 2: The classic risk factors for PE can be memorized by a mnemonic "THROMBOSIS".

T	Trauma/Travel
H	Hypercoagulable states/Hormonal replacement therapy
R	Recreational drug use
O	Older
M	Malignancy
B	Birth control
O	Obesity/Obstetrical (risk highest from second week of pregnancy to first 6 weeks postpartum)
S	Surgery
I	Immobilization
S	Sickness

Inherited risk factors: Factor V Leiden mutation, Antiphospholipid antibody syndrome, Antithrombin III deficiency, Protein C deficiency, Protein S deficiency, Prothrombin gene mutation, Increased factor VIII activity, Activated protein C (APC) resistance, Dysfibrinogenemia, Hyperhomocysteinemia.

Question 7

1. Define acute kidney injury (AKI).

A variety of definitions for AKI proposed in literature. In 2012, the Kidney Disease: Improving Global Outcomes (KDIGO) group defined AKI based on the urine output and the serum creatinine (SCr) concentration. *This definition is an increase in SCr of greater than or equal to 0.3 mg/dL within 48 hours or an increase in SCr >1.5 times baseline within 7 days or decreased urine output for 6 hours.*

AKI is defined as a sudden reduction in kidney function that is characterized by a diminished GFR as manifested by an increased SCr or reduced urine output. AKI is further divided into three categories: (1) *Prerenal,* a kidney blood flow decrease; (2) *Intrarenal,* or kidney parenchymal injury; and (3) *Postrenal,* or urine flow obstruction.

2. Explain the stages of AKI.

Classification systems of AKI, such as RIFLE (risk, injury, failure, loss, end-stage) and acute kidney injury network (AKIN), can also be used, but as per studies all three criteria are effective tools for predicting mortality without significant differences among them but advantage of KDIGO is that it covers parameters in AKIN and RIFLE **(Table 3)**.

TABLE 3: KDIGO guidelines for acute kidney injuries kidney disease: Improving global outcomes (KDIGO) guidelines.

AKI stage	Serum creatinine	Urine output
1	1.5–1.9 × baseline OR ≥0.3 mg/dL increase	<0.5 mL/kg/h for 6–12 h
2	2.0–2.9 × baseline	<0.5 mL/kg/h for >12 h
3	3.0 × baseline OR initiation of renal replacement therapy	<0.3 mL/kg/h for ≥24 h OR anuria for ≥12 h
Risk, injury, failure, loss, end-stage (RIFLE) criteria		
1	Increase in SCr ≥150% mg/dL	<0.5 mL/kg/h for 6–12 h
2	Increase in SCr ≥200–300% mg/dL	<0.5 mL/kg/h for ≥12 h
3	Increase in Cr 300% OR creatinine >4 mg/mL with acute increase 0.5 mg/dL or initiation of renal-replacement therapy	<0.3 mL/kg/h for ≥24 h OR anuria for ≥12 h

Source: Adapted from Moore PK, Hsu RK, Liu KD. Management of acute kidney injury: core curriculum. Am J Kidney Dis. 2018;72(1):136-48.

3. Explain the investigations in a patient with AKI.

For assessment of patients with AKI, creatinine clearance is better tool for assessing AKI as it measures effectiveness of the glomeruli to filter creatinine from the plasma and is a close approximation of the GFR. Dilution, volume overload states, and reductions of creatinine production during the acute phases of an illness are confounding factors during estimation of SCr values. In critical and acute care settings patient's body muscle mass also fluctuates which alters the relative SCr levels. For these reasons, and to apply steady-state kinetics more accurately, other biomarkers are being studied as potential surrogates for acute kidney function such as serum cystatin C, neutrophil gelatinase-associated lipocalin, kidney injury molecule-1. However, in the acute setting, SCr remains the most validated estimation of GFR to determine kidney function.

4. What is contrast-induced nephropathy?

Contrast-induced AKI: A type of AKI that results within a few days of exposure to iodinated contrast for imaging studies is termed as contrast-induced nephropathy. After hypoperfusion and nephrotoxic drugs this is the third most common cause of new AKI in hospitalized patients. The contrast-induced nephropathy/AKI is self-limited but associated with increased mortality and even progression to chronic kidney disease. Patients with an estimated GFR <60 mL/min/1.73 m^2 are higher risk for contrast-induced AKIs. In clinical practice, radiologists take detail relevant history about comorbidities, other nephrotoxic medications before administering potentially harmful contrast. In high-risk patient, use the lowest possible radiocontrast concentrations, administer IV hydration preexposure and postexposure, minimize nephrotoxic agents and renal replacement therapy (RRT) in critical cases should be considered. It is important to screen patients for reliable follow-up.

Question 8

1. Discuss the pathogenesis of tetanus.

Tetanus toxins act by similar mechanism such as botulinum toxin, tetanus toxin is taken up into nerve terminals of lower motor neurons, the nerve cells that activate voluntary muscles. Tetanus toxin is a zinc-dependent metalloproteinase that targets a protein (synaptobrevin/vesicle-associated membrane protein—VAMP) that is necessary for the release of neurotransmitter from nerve endings through fusion of synaptic vesicles with the neuronal plasma membrane. Flaccid paralysis may be the initial symptom of local tetanus infection, caused by interference with vesicular release of acetylcholine at the neuromuscular junction, as occurs with botulinum toxin. Extensive retrograde transport of tetanus toxin occurs in the axons of lower motor neurons and tetanus toxin reaches the spinal cord or brainstem. Tetanus toxin crosses the synapses and taken up by nerve endings of inhibitory GABAergic and/or glycinergic neurons that control the activity of the lower motor neurons. Once tetanus toxins inside the inhibitory nerve terminals, it cleaves VAMP, thereby inhibiting the release of gamma-aminobutyric acid (GABA) and glycine, resulting functional denervation of the lower motor neurons, which leads to rigidity and spasms due to hyperactivity and to increased muscle activity.

2. Explain the clinical features of tetanus.

Tetanus toxin causes rigidity and spasms due to hyperactivity of voluntary muscles. Rigidity is the tonic, involuntary contraction of muscles, while spasms are short lasting muscle contractions that can be elicited by sensory stimulation or by stretching of the muscles; they are termed reflex spasms. A highly reduced ability to open the mouth as rigidity of the temporal and masseter muscles leads to trismus (lockjaw). Tetanus typically manifests as trismus/lockjaw, risus sardonicus, dysphagia, neck stiffness, abdominal rigidity, and opisthotonos, i.e., hyperactivity of muscles of the head, neck, and trunk. The limbs tend to be less severely affected, but with full opisthotonos, decorticate posture occurs (flexion of the arms and extension of the legs). In both local/cephalic and generalized tetanus, trismus is frequently the initial symptom but the tetanus may present in any form described above. In addition, general muscle ache, focal flaccid paralysis, and an array of unusual symptoms reflecting unusual patterns of neuronal inactivation, including diplopia, nystagmus, and vertigo, may occur. The tetanus toxin affects not only motor system but autonomic system also. Episodes of tachycardia, hypertension, and sweating, sometimes rapidly alternating with bradycardia and hypotension are common autonomic dysfunction, especially in generalized tetanus. Autonomic symptoms usually occur a week after the occurrence of motor symptoms. Tetanus-mediated respiratory insufficiency is a treatable condition with the availability of modern intensive care, autonomic dysfunction has become a major cause of death in tetanus victims. Sensory nerves may also become invaded by tetanus toxin, causing altered sensation, such as pain and allodynia.

3. Describe the treatment of tetanus.

Treatment of tetanus is supportive and is consist of identification of wound and debridement, removal of spores and further toxin production can be prevented. As disease itself does not provide the immunity so tetanus immunization should be provided. Patient with respiratory compromise should be admitted in intensive care unit for immediate neuromuscular blockade and intubation support. Treatment is summarized in **Table 4**.

TABLE 4: Summary of tetanus treatment.

Steps	Interventions
Wound	Identify wound and wound debridement
Antibiotic therapy	Metronidazole 500 mg IV 6 hourly, theoretically penicillin can enhance the effect of tetanospasm
Immunization	• Tetanus toxoid 0.5 mL IM at presentation then after 6 weeks and then after 6 months • Tetanus immunoglobulin 3,000–6,000 units IM (opposite arm of TT and some amount around the wound site)
Muscle relaxation	Diazepam
Respiratory distress management	Sedation neuromuscular blockade (succinylcholine/vecuronium for intubation) mechanical ventilation
Autonomic dysfunction management	• Magnesium sulfate loading dose 40 mg/kg IV then continuous infusion 2 g/h or • Labetalol 0.25–1 mg/min IV infusion • Morphine sulfate 0.5–1 mg/kg/h • Clonidine 300 µg every 8 hourly

TABLE 5: Tetanus prophylaxis in routine wound management (>18 years).

Tetanus immunization	Clean minor wound		All other wound	
	Td	TIG	Td	TIG
<3 dose or uncertain	Yes	No	Yes	Yes
>3 dose				
Last dose within 5 years	No	No	No	No
Last dose within 5–10 years	No	No	Yes	No
Last dose >10 years	Yes	No	Yes	No

(All other wounds: contaminated wounds (feces, dirt, saliva, soil), puncture wounds, avulsions, burns, crush injuries, and frostbite; Td: tetanus-diphtheria toxoid; TIG: tetanus immune globulin)

4. Discuss tetanus immunization.

Tetanus immunization must be done especially for patients who have either never been vaccinated (250 U of intramuscular human tetanus immune globulin) or did not have tetanus shots in the last 10 years [intramuscular or subcutaneous tetanus toxoid (0.5 mL)] **(Table 5)**.

Question 9

1. What are the precipitating factors for thyroid storm?

Thyroid storm is unrecognized, undertreated, life-threatening form of severe thyrotoxicosis. Thyroid storm is rare and mostly acute reaction to thyroid and nonthyroid surgery, trauma infections contrast media, amiodarone, after delivery in preexisting hyperthyroidism. Other risk factors are acute coronary syndrome, pulmonary embolism, and diabetic ketoacidosis.

2. Explain the clinical features of thyroid storm.

Clinical features of thyroid storm are typical and include hyperpyrexia, out of proportion tachycardia, altered mental status (agitation, delirium coma) along with clinical picture of hyperthyroidism. Classic features of thyroid storm include fever, marked tachycardia, heart failure, tremor, nausea and vomiting, diarrhea, dehydration, restlessness, extreme agitation, delirium, or coma. Fever is typical and may be >105.8°F (41°C). Prompt recognitions and treatment are warranted as mortality is almost 100%. The causes of mortality in patient of thyroid storm: Sepsis multiorgan failure, congestive heart failure arrhythmias, and disseminated intravascular coagulation.

3. Discuss the management of thyroid storm.

Management of thyroid storm is summarized in **Table 6**.

TABLE 6: Management of thyroid storm.	
B-adrenergic blockers	• Propranolol 60–80 mg orally every 4 h (IV 0.5–1.0 mg as test dose then repeat 1–2 mg every 15 minutes till desired effect then 1–2 mg every 3 h) or • Metoprolol 25–50 mg orally every 6 h or • Esmolol 50–100 µg/kg/min infusion
Inhibition of thyroid hormone synthesis	Propylthiouracil 500–1,000 mg loading then 250 mg every 4 h or methimazole 60–80 mg/day
Inhibition of thyroid hormone release	• Saturated potassium iodide solution (50 mg/drops) 1–2 drops orally or per rectally or • Lugol's solution (8 mg iodide/drop) 5–7 drops
Corticosteroid	Hydrocortisone 300 mg IV then 100 mg every 8 h
Treatment of underlying precipitant	Empirical antibiotics
Supportive measures	Volume resuscitation cooling blankets, fan ice packs/lavage
Others	Lorazepam, diazepam

Question 10

1. Draw intrinsic and extrinsic coagulation pathways and fibrinolysis pathway.

Physiology of hemostasis: The normal hemostatic system consists of a complex process that limits blood loss through the formation of a platelet (primary hemostasis) and the production of cross-linked fibrin (secondary hemostasis), which strengthens the platelet plug. These reactions are counterregulated by the fibrinolytic system **(Fig. 1)**. Hemostasis is a process of balance between the coagulation and the fibrinolytic system. The coagulation system consists of two main components primary and secondary hemostasis.

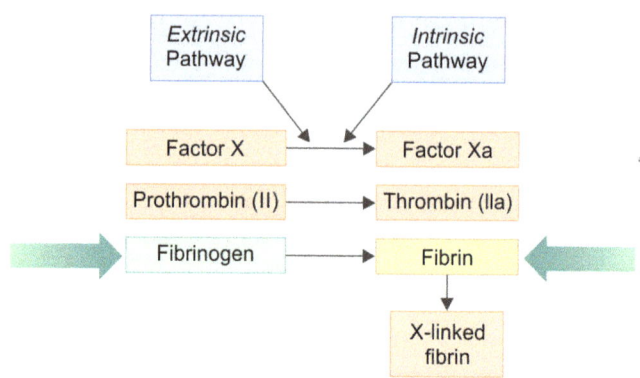

Fig. 1: Physiology of hemostasis extrinsic and intrinsic pathways.

Primary hemostasis: In a normal adult, when the vascular subendothelial surface is exposed due to injury to a vessel, platelets interact with the exposed collagen forming a platelet plug at the site of injury to arrest the initial site of ooze, with the help of von Willebrand factor which connects the platelet to the vascular subendothelium and fibrinogen that helps in binding of platelets together. This process occurs within 20 seconds of injury and needs to be stabilized by secondary hemostasis.

Secondary hemostasis (coagulation cascade): The secondary hemostasis consists of two different pathways named intrinsic and extrinsic pathway.

The intrinsic pathway begins by the activation of factor XII by the damaged vascular surface that further results in activation of factors XI, IX, and finally factor X. The extrinsic pathway is activated by the conversion of factor VII to its activated form, which directly helps in activation of factor X. These pathways finally merge at the point of factor X activation. Following the activation of the factor X, a common pathway is followed that results in formation of cross-linked fibrin clot which on deposition stabilizes the primary homeostasis.

2. Explain the complications of heparin.

Thrombocytopenia, bleeding events, and osteopenia are the three most common drug-related problems associated with heparin and low molecular weight heparin (LMWH) therapy. These side effects often complicate treatment and increase the overall cost of care. Hyperkalemia and hypersensitivity reactions are also noticeable adverse effects.

3. Discuss the management of warfarin-induced bleeding.

The reversal of warfarin needs immediate and sustained therapy. Immediate reversal is achieved by the therapy of prothrombin complex concentrates (PCC) and fresh frozen plasma (FFP), and sustained reversal is achieved through vitamin K administration **(Table 7)**.

TABLE 7: Management of vitamin K antagonists-induced high INRs and bleeding.

Condition	Interventions
Raised INR but <5; absent significant bleeding	Lower/omit dose. Increase frequency of monitoring. Resume therapy at a lower dose if INR more than minimally supratherapeutic
INR ≥5.0 but ≤10.0; absent significant bleeding	Omit 1–2 doses. Increase frequency of monitoring. Resume therapy when INR therapeutic Or Omit dose. Give 1.0–2.5 mg oral vitamin K. If the patient is at increased risk of bleeding, If requires more rapid reversal for a surgical procedure, give 2–4 mg oral vitamin K; the INR should decrease within 24 hours If the INR remains elevated, additional vitamin K (1–2 mg orally) may be given
INR >10; absent significant bleeding	Hold warfarin therapy. Give 5–10 mg oral vitamin K; the INR should decrease within 24–48 hours. Increase frequency of monitoring. Administer additional vitamin K if necessary. Resume therapy when INR within therapeutic range
Serious or life-threatening bleeding	Hold warfarin therapy. Give 10 mg vitamin K by slow IV infusion, in addition to 4-factor PCC or FFP. Vitamin K may be given every 12 hours.

(FFP: fresh frozen plasma; INR: international normalized ratio; PCC: prothrombin complex concentrate)

SUGGESTED READING

1. Richhariya D, Sharma B. Textbook of Emergency Medicine including Intensive Care and Trauma, 2nd edition. New Delhi: Jaypee Brothers Medical Publishers (P) Ltd; 2022. pp. 766-71. (Question 1).
2. Richhariya D, Sharma B. Textbook of Emergency Medicine including Intensive Care and Trauma, 2nd edition. New Delhi: Jaypee Brothers Medical Publishers (P) Ltd; 2022. pp. 1496-7. (Question 2).
3. Richhariya D, Sharma B. Textbook of Emergency Medicine including Intensive Care and Trauma, 2nd edition. New Delhi: Jaypee Brothers Medical Publishers (P) Ltd; 2022. pp. 575-82. (Question 3).
4. Richhariya D, Sharma B. Textbook of Emergency Medicine including Intensive Care and Trauma, 2nd edition. New Delhi: Jaypee Brothers Medical Publishers (P) Ltd; 2022. pp. 415-22. (Question 4).
5. Richhariya D, Sharma B. Textbook of Emergency Medicine including Intensive Care and Trauma, 2nd edition. New Delhi: Jaypee Brothers Medical Publishers (P) Ltd; 2022. pp. 477-81. (Question 5).
6. Richhariya D, Sharma B. Textbook of Emergency Medicine including Intensive Care and Trauma, 2nd edition. New Delhi: Jaypee Brothers Medical Publishers (P) Ltd; 2022. pp. 521-8. (Question 6).
7. Richhariya D, Sharma B. Textbook of Emergency Medicine including Intensive Care and Trauma, 2nd edition. New Delhi: Jaypee Brothers Medical Publishers (P) Ltd; 2022. pp. 743-50. (Question 7).
8. Richhariya D, Sharma B. Textbook of Emergency Medicine including Intensive Care and Trauma, 2nd edition. New Delhi: Jaypee Brothers Medical Publishers (P) Ltd; 2022. pp. 1314-6, 1657. (Question 8).
9. Richhariya D, Sharma B. Textbook of Emergency Medicine including Intensive Care and Trauma, 2nd edition. New Delhi: Jaypee Brothers Medical Publishers (P) Ltd; 2022. p. 891. (Question 9).
10. Richhariya D, Sharma B. Textbook of Emergency Medicine including Intensive Care and Trauma, 2nd edition. New Delhi: Jaypee Brothers Medical Publishers (P) Ltd; 2022. pp. 537, 543. (Question 10).

Emergency Medicine Paper 24

Devendra Richhariya

Question 1

1. Discuss the use of resuscitative endovascular balloon occlusion of the aorta (REBOA) in emergency department.

Resuscitative endovascular balloon occlusion of the aorta has recently come up as a minimally invasive alternative to open aortic cross-clamping in the management of nonresponsive category of polytrauma patients. It will help in controlling noncompressible hemorrhage arising below the diaphragm. It is being used in both blunt and penetrating abdominal trauma. The use of REBOA provides for temporary hemorrhage control and improved hemodynamics until definitive surgical/endovascular control of hemorrhage achieved (**Fig. 1**). REBOA is being used in Zone I and III of the aorta. Zone I of the aorta extends from the left subclavian artery to the celiac artery. Zone II continues from the celiac artery to the renal artery. Zone III extends from the origin of the lowest renal artery to the aortic bifurcation (infrarenal aorta). Zone I occlusion is utilized in patients in cardiac arrest or those in hemorrhagic shock with evidence of noncompressible hemorrhage arising below the diaphragm. Zone II is considered to be a no-occlusion zone. Zone III occlusion is reserved for patients without evidence of intra-abdominal hemorrhage but with evidence of a pelvic fracture.

2. Explain the use of extracorporeal membrane oxygenation (ECMO) in emergency department.

Extracorporeal membrane oxygenation is a modified cardiopulmonary bypass form providing artificial respiration and/or mechanical circulatory support in critically ill patients in intensive care units (ICUs) (**Fig. 2**). It is a mechanical cardiopulmonary form that can provide prolonged life support in patients unresponsive to conventional management. Conventional cardiopulmonary bypass devices provide support for patients undergoing surgery for minutes to hours, while ECMO provides support for days to weeks for patients with respiratory, cardiac or combined cardiopulmonary failure. Indications for ECMO have been extended for longer use in ICUs and for both heart and lung transplants and lung resections in unstable patients. Venovenous ECMO (VV-ECMO) typically provides support for patients with isolated respiratory failure, while venoarterial ECMO (VA-ECMO) is used in both cardiac and cardiopulmonary failure.

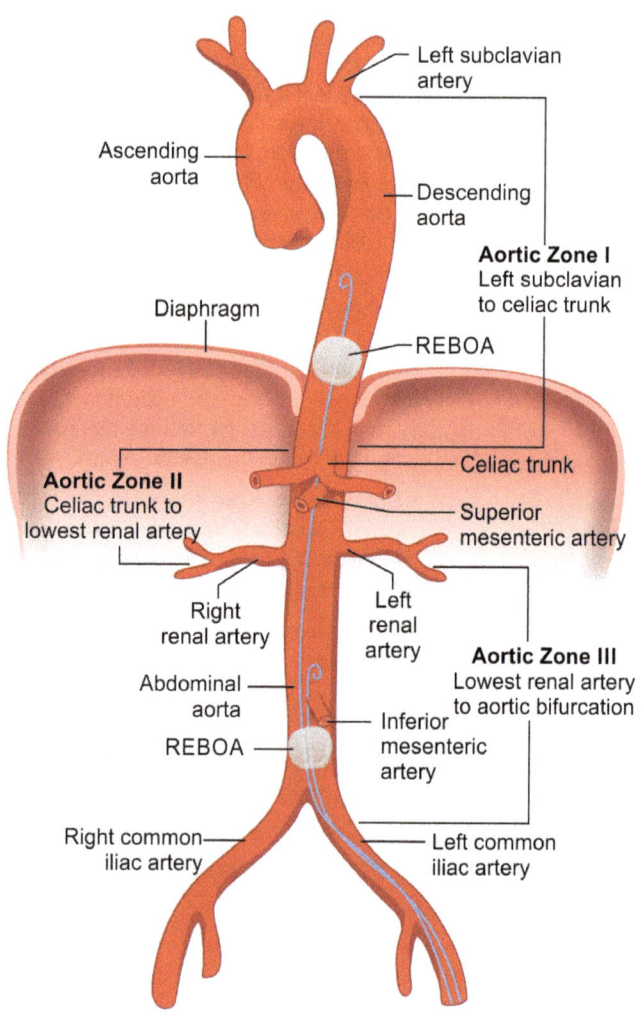

Fig. 1: Resuscitative endovascular balloon occlusion of the aorta (REBOA).

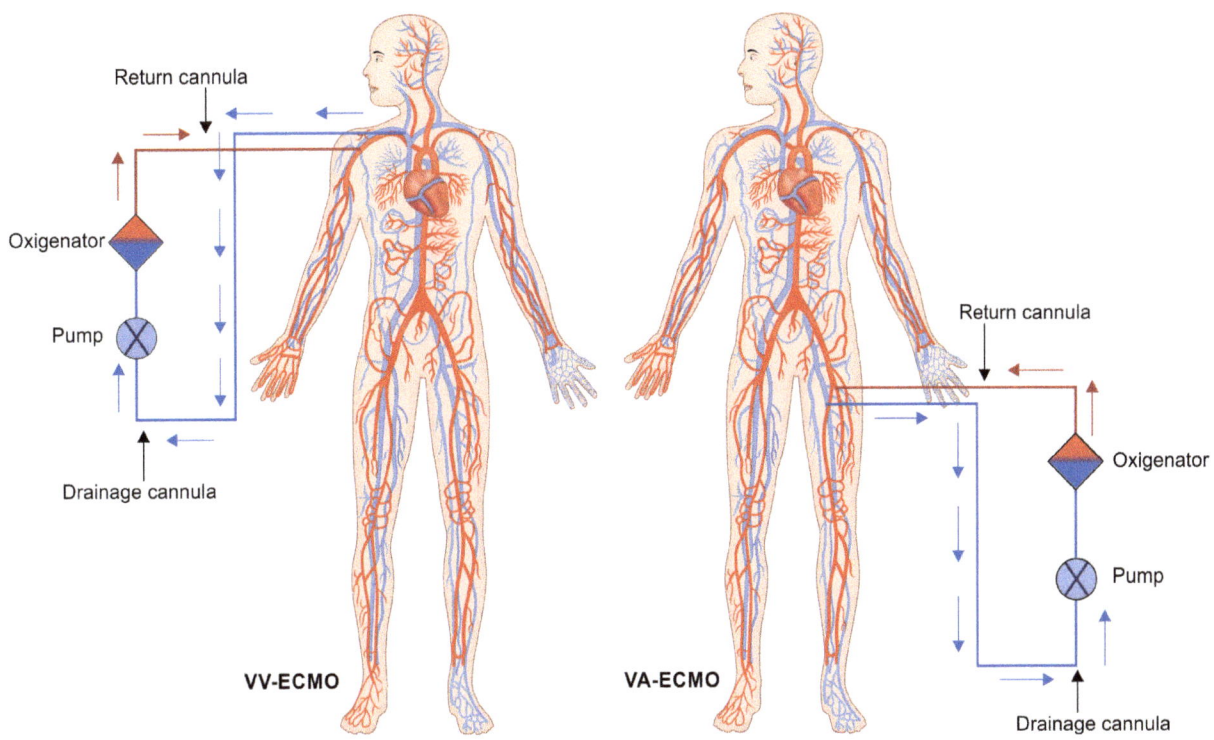

Fig. 2: Typical schematic illustration of VV-ECMO and VA-ECMO supports. (VA-ECMO: venoarterial extracorporeal membrane oxygenation; VV-ECMO: Venovenous extracorporeal membrane oxygenation)

Question 2

1. What is routine newborn care?

Whenever the parent's perception that something is wrong with the newborn infants, they may present to the emergency department for various reasons. The role of the emergency physician is important to recognize abnormality and, if no abnormality detected, address the concerns of the parent. It is very important to differentiate conditions that are self-limited or are variants without physiologic consequence from potential to worsen. Illness in the newborn is often subtle and early detection can be lifesaving. Therefore, the emergency physician should be familiar and comfortable with performing a newborn examination **(Table 1)**. Because of the time constraints in the emergency department, it may not possible to complete physical examination; a systematic approach can allow a thorough examination in a matter of minutes.

TABLE 1: Head-to-toe approach for normal newborn examination.

Head	• Shape • Fontanelle • Lesions/swelling
Eyes	• Red reflex • Extraocular movement • Pupillary shape/size

Contd...

Ears	• Positioning • Tags
Nose	Nasal patency
Mouth	• Palate • Dentition • Oral lesions
Neck	Swelling/cysts
Chest	• Asymmetric chest rise with respirations retractions • Accessory respiratory muscle use
Lungs	• Symmetric air entry • Breath sounds
Heart	Murmur
Abdomen	• Hepatosplenomegaly • Cord vessels at birth
Genital	• Inguinal masses • Testicular/scrotal asymmetry • Genital hypertrophy/lesions • Rectal patency
Extremities	• Tenderness • Extremity use/range of motion • Additional digits/tags Hip click
Neurology	• Tone • Suckling • Palmar/plantar • Moro

2. Discuss the steps of neonatal resuscitation.

a. Newborn or neonatal mortality contributes to an estimated total of 2.5 million deaths annually, with most of these deaths occurring in low-resource countries. Newborn babies are far more likely to need resuscitation due to respiratory cause.
b. Therefore, all healthcare providers present during the delivery of infants have to be well-versed in strategies to recognize and manage situations requiring resuscitation of the neonate.
c. Prepare for delivery by anticipating perinatal risk and organizing the environment. Effective communication with immediate access to essential supplies and at least one person dedicated to the care of the newborn should be present in the delivery room.
d. Care of the term infant upon delivery with good tone and normal breathing and or crying proceeds by drying the baby and placing them skin-to-skin with the mother.
e. Observe breathing, activity, and color. Delayed cord clamping beyond 30 seconds is reasonable in these infants. Delayed cord clamping is associated with less need for transfusion, less necrotizing enterocolitis, and intraventricular hemorrhage (IVH) of any grade.
f. If, however, the infant is not of a term gestation or does not have an appropriate tone or breathing on delivery, they are placed in a radiant warmer.
g. Stabilize initially and prevent hypothermia by warming (wet babies lose heat rapidly), rub the baby dry to stimulate spontaneous breaths or crying, position to open airway (neutral position, place a folded towel under the shoulders.
h. Preterm babies may require a plastic wrap, cap, radiant warmer, adjusted room temperature, thermal mattress, and warm humidified gases to prevent hypothermia.
i. Clear secretions (blood, meconium or other fluid) from mouth and nose by gentle suctioning as appropriate.
j. If, despite the above, there is abnormal breathing or a heart rate <100 beats per minute begins rescue breathing within 1 minute of an initial assessment. Use positive pressure ventilation (soft face mask and t-piece or self-inflating bag-valve) and oxygenate using room air or supplemental oxygen with SpO_2 monitoring (titrate to achieve a preductal oxygen saturation approximating the interquartile range), possibly including positive end-expiratory pressure (PEEP) of 5 cmH_2O.
k. Seek expert help if not already requested. Persistent deterioration should prompt administration of intravenous (IV) or intraosseous infusion (IO) epinephrine at 0.01–0.03 mg/kg (or 0.05–0.1 mg/kg through the endotracheal tube), volume replacement (10 mL/kg of fluid or blood), investigation, and management of other possible causes of arrest, such as pneumothorax.

3. Explain vascular access in the newborn.

Since the 1940s the umbilical vein regular use in neonates, but because of high rate of complications compels central and peripheral routes being used for infusion of fluid, nutrients, and drugs. Nowadays peripheral venous access is preferred except for high volume fluid resuscitation, reliable infusion of irritant drugs, and long-term parenteral nutrition. Intraosseous infusion provides a reliable alternative to peripheral veins for rapid infusion of fluid. Long, thin silastic catheters can be inserted through a peripheral venous cannula for parenteral nutrition or other central venous infusions as an alternative to direct central venous cannulation using the Seldinger or other techniques. When central venous cannulation is needed for >6 weeks, Broviac or Hickman catheters, is inserted through a subcutaneous tunnel are considered. The most common serious complication of vascular access is infection. Infection associated with central venous catheters is reduced by prophylactic vancomycin or teicoplanin. Other complications of central venous infusion are associated with cannula mispositioning, bleeding, and thrombosis. Distal hypoperfusion may follow arterial cannulation. Modern emergency and intensive care pediatrics is impossible without adequate venous and arterial vascular access.

Question 3

1. How will you clinically evaluate dehydration in children?

Child with diarrhea **should be assessed** for (1) Dehydration, (2) Blood in diarrhea, (3) coexisting malnutrition, and (4) Serious nonintestinal infections.

History should focus on—duration of diarrhea and number of watery stools per day; volume of water in stool; presence of blood in the stool; frequency of urination; presence of vomiting, fever, cough or seizures; pre-illness feeding practices; fluids, food and drugs taken during illness and immunization history. **Examination** should include—general condition of child; signs of dehydration; nutritional status [weight/weight for height/mid-arm circumference (MAC)] and severity of malnutrition if any; presence of blood in stool besides general physical and systemic examination. The classification of dehydration **(Table 2)** is of utmost importance in the management.

TABLE 2: Classification of dehydration.

Severe (Two of the following are present)	Some (Two of the following are present)	No dehydration
Lethargy/unconscious	Restless, irritable	Not enough signs to classify some or severe dehydration
Sunken eyes	Sunken eyes	
Not able to drink/drinking poorly	Drinks eagerly, thirsty	
Skin pinch goes back very slowly	Skin pinch goes back slowly	

2. Discuss the treatment of dehydration according to severity.

Assessment and correction of dehydration and correction of specific etiology are besides symptomatic management **(Table 3)**. Since acute vomiting is mostly seen as a part of acute gastroenteritis, its *objectives are:* (1) Prevent and treat dehydration, (2) Drugs (antibiotics, Zinc), (3) Nutritional management, (4) Education.

Indications for hospital admission are: (1) Shock, (2) Severe dehydration, (3) Neurological abnormalities (lethargy, seizures), (4) Intractable or bilious vomiting, (5) Failure of oral rehydration, (6) Suspected surgical condition, (7) Conditions for a safe follow-up and home management are not met.

TABLE 3: Plan of treatment for dehydration.

Severe dehydration	Some dehydration	No dehydration
Plan C	Plan B	Plan A
Urgent care in hospital	Treat dehydration with ORS/IV fluid	Home care

(IV: intravenous; ORS: oral rehydration solutions)

3. What are the compositions of reduced World Health Organization (WHO) oral rehydration solutions (ORS)?

The compositions of oral rehydration solution are given in **Table 4** below:

TABLE 4: Compositions of standard and low osmolarity oral rehydration solutions (ORS).

	Standard ORS solution (mEq)	Low osmolarity ORS (mmol/L)
Glucose	111	75
Sodium	90	75
Chloride	80	65
Potassium	20	20
Citrate	10	10
Osmolarity	311	245

4. Discuss the maintenance phase for successfully rehydrated children.

Maintenance fluid requirements **(Table 5)** are determined by many mechanisms for children, when calculating maintenance fluids, emergency physician must aware about factors that may affect fluid balance. Maintenance fluid requirements are increased in hospitalized children due to their illness and associated problems such as fever, burn injuries, hypermetabolic states, pain, asthma, and increased intestinal losses. Holliday–Segar method is most commonly used technique to calculate maintenance fluids for children. The Holliday–Segar method is usually preferred due to its ease of calculation.

TABLE 5: Holliday–Segar method for calculating maintenance fluid requirements in children.

	Holliday–Segar method	Holliday–Segar estimate
First 10 kg	100 mL/kg/day	4 mL/kg/h
Second 10 kg	50 mL/kg/day	2 mL/kg/h
Every kilogram thereafter	20 mL/kg/day	1 mL/kg/h

Question 4

1. Discuss types of neglect in children.

a. *Physical neglect:* A child's basic needs, such as food, clothing or shelter, are not met or they are not properly supervised or kept safe.
b. *Educational neglect:* A parent does not ensure their child is given an education.
c. *Emotional neglect.*
d. *Medical neglect.*

2. Explain the risk factors for child maltreatment.

Children <4 years of age: Children with special needs that may increase caregiver burden (e.g., disabilities, mental health issues, and chronic physical illnesses) **(Table 6)**.

TABLE 6: Risk factors for child maltreatment.

Individual risk factors	Family risk factors	Community risk factors
Caregivers with the following issues: • Drug or alcohol issues • Mental health issues, including depression • Who do not understand children's needs or development • Caregivers who are young or single parents or parents with many children • Low education or income high levels of parenting stress or economic stress	• Families that have household members in jail or prison • Families that are isolated from and not connected to other people (extended family, friends, neighbors) • Families experiencing other types of violence, including relationship violence • Families with high conflict and negative communication styles	Communities with high rates of: • Violence and crime • Poverty and limited educational and economic opportunities • High unemployment rates • Easy access to drugs and alcohol • Low community involvement among residents

3. Discuss the diagnosis of physical abuse in child.

Factors that may be considered in determining child abuse include: **Physical examination, including evaluating injuries or signs and symptoms of suspected abuse or neglect, lab tests, X-rays or other tests, information about the child's medical and developmental history.** The differential diagnosis of child abuse varies depending upon the clinical manifestations. Familiarity with the medical conditions or cultural practices that mimic child abuse can facilitate arrival at the correct diagnosis, initiation of appropriate therapy, and avoidance of the consequences of an unnecessary evaluation for and/or report of suspected child abuse. One helpful distinguishing feature is that many abused children present with multiple types of injuries (e.g., bruising and fractures).

Varieties of physical maltreatment: Blunt trauma thermal injury, Shaking trauma syndrome, Munchausen syndrome by proxy.

Question 5

1. Explain the causes of jaundice in neonates and infants.

Neonatal Jaundice (Table 7)
a. Physiologic
b. Pathological
c. Conjugated hyperbilirubinemia
d. Unconjugated hyperbilirubinemia

2. Discuss the pathogenesis of various causes of jaundice in children.

Jaundice either due to increased bilirubin production owing to decreased bilirubin clearance **(Table 8)**.

TABLE 7: Causes of jaundice.

<24 hours	24 hours–2 weeks	>2 weeks—unconjugated	>2 weeks—conjugated
Rhesus hemolytic disease	Physiological	Physiological	Sepsis
ABO incompatibility	Breast milk jaundice	Breast milk jaundice	TPN
G6PD deficiency	Infection	Infection	Neonatal hepatitis
Spherocytosis	Hemolytic disorders	Hypothyroidism	Cystic fibrosis
Congenital infection	Bruising	Hemolytic disorders	Bile duct obstruction

(ABO: blood grouping system; G6PD: glucose-6-phosphate dehydrogenase; TPN: total parenteral nutrition)

TABLE 8: Various causes of jaundice in children.

Increased bilirubin production:	Decreased bilirubin clearance:

• *Hemolytic disease:*
  – Immune mediated (Ph alloimmunization, ABO incompatibility)
  – Heritable (spherocytosis, G6PD deficiency, pyruvate kinas deficiency)
• Polycythemia
• Extravasation of blood (cephalohematoma, intraventricular hemorrhage)
  – Sepsis with disseminated intravascular coagulation (DIC)
	• Prematurity
	• *Increased enterohepatic circulation:*
	  – Breast milk jaundice
	  – Pyloric stenosis
	  – Small or large bowel obstruction
	• Inborn errors of metabolism (Gilbert syndrome, Crigler–Najjar syndrome)
	• Metabolic disorder (hypothyroidism, hypopituitarism)

3. Explain the approach to a child with jaundice.

Approach to child with jaundice is summarized here (**Flowcharts 1A and 1B**).

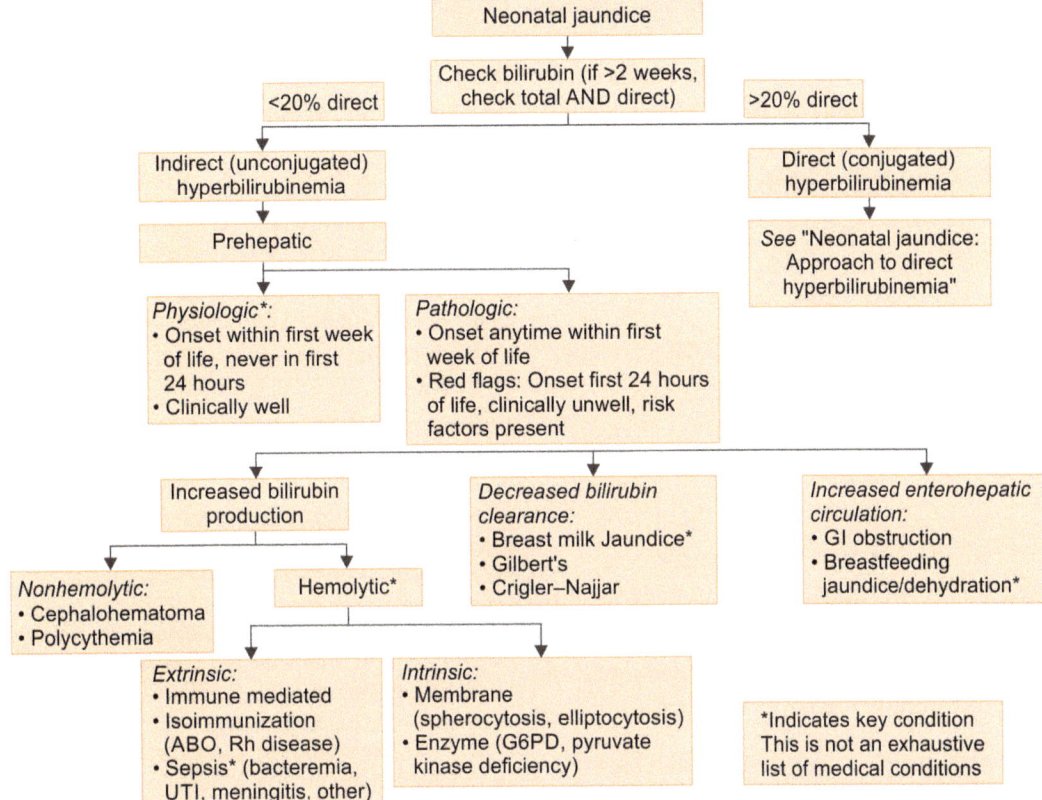

Flowchart 1A: Approach to a child with jaundice (indirect hyperbilirubinemia).

(ABO: blood grouping system; G6PD: glucose-6-phosphate dehydrogenase; GI: gastrointestinal; UTI: urinary tract infection)

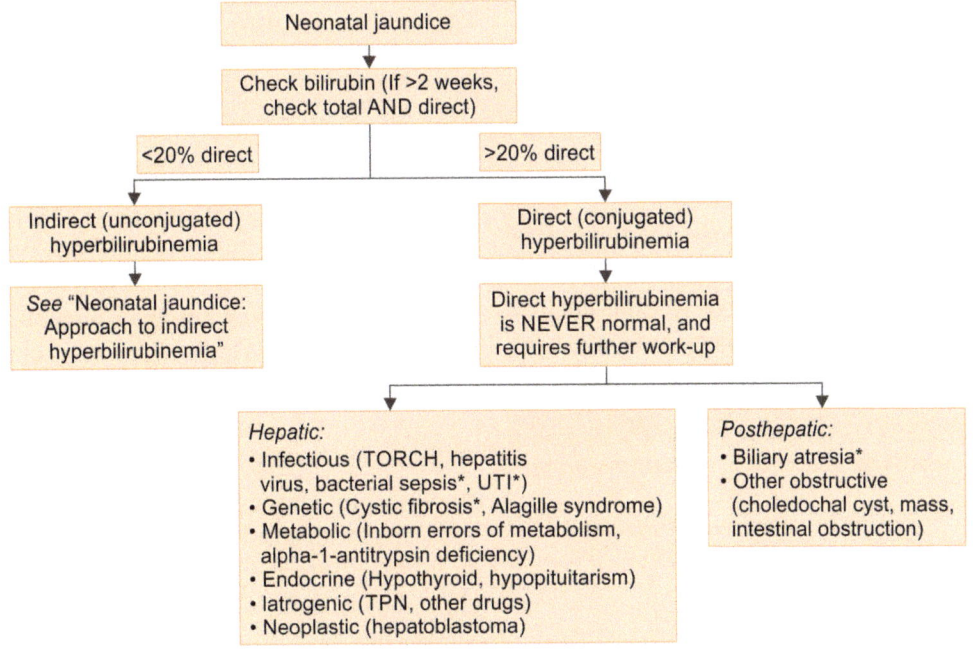

Flowchart 1B: Approach to a child with jaundice (indirect hyperbilirubinemia).

Question 6

1. Discuss confidence interval.

A confidence interval is the mean of estimate plus and minus the variation in that estimate. This is the range of values we expect our estimate to fall between if we redo our test, within a certain level of confidence. Confidence, in statistics, is another way to describe probability. In frequentist statistics, a confidence interval is a range of estimates for an unknown parameter. A confidence interval is computed at a designated confidence level; the 95% confidence level is most common, but other levels, such as 90% or 99%, are sometimes used.

$$CI = \bar{x} \pm z \frac{s}{\sqrt{n}}$$

CI = confidence interval
x = sample mean
z = confidence level value
s = sample standard deviation
n = sample size

2. Positive and negative predictive values.

Positive predictive value is the probability that subjects with a positive screening test truly have the disease. *Negative predictive value* is the probability, which subjects with a negative screening test truly do not have the disease.

3. What are triple-blinded, randomized studies?

To avoid any bias in the study, the blinding is resorted to which means "concealing or masking of the subjects-assignment to a study group (control or treatment) from those participating in the study".

The blinding could be single blinded, double blinded, or triple blinded.

Single blinded: The study subjects will not know whether he/she would receive the treatment (test intervention) or control (placebo).

Double blinded: Neither the study subjects or experimenter will know which of the subjects are in the treatment (test intervention) or control (placebo) group.

Triple blinded: Neither of the study subjects, experimenter, and observer will know which of the subjects are in the treatment (test intervention) or control (placebo) group **(Table 9)**.

TABLE 9: Type of blinding studies.

Type of blinding	Concealment about allocation of subjects to a group (√ – Yes; X – No)		
	Subjects	Experimenter	Observer
Single	√	X	X
Double	√	√	X
Triple	√	√	√

Question 7

1. What are LVADs (left ventricular assist devices)?

Mechanical circulatory support (MCS) devices are mechanical pumps designed to assist or replace the function of either the left (LVAD) or the right ventricle, or both ventricles, of the heart. *European Society of Cardiology 2016 Recommendations for implantation of mechanical circulatory support in patients with refractory heart failure are as* Bridge to transplant, and as Destination Therapy. The presence of portal hypertension with liver cirrhosis is a contraindication to initiating MCS support. High fixed pulmonary vascular resistance (PVR) (thresholds vary from 3–6 Wood units) is a contraindication to heart transplantation and consequently to use of LVAD.

2. What are the indications of LVADs?

Indications of left ventricular assist devices are summarized in **Box 1**.

BOX 1: Eligibility criteria for implantation of left ventricular assist device (LVAD).

Patients with >2 months of severe symptoms despite optimal medical and device therapy and more than one of the following:
- LVEF <25% and, if measured, peak VO_2 <12 mL/kg/min
- ≥3 HF hospitalizations in previous 12 months without an obvious precipitating cause
- Dependence on intravenous inotropic therapy
- Progressive end organ dysfunction (worsening renal and/or hepatic function) due to reduced perfusion and not to inadequate ventricular filling pressure (PCWP ≥20 mm Hg and SBP ≤80–90 mm Hg or CI ≤2 L/min/m²).
- Absence of severe right ventricular dysfunction together with severe tricuspid regurgitation.

(CI: cardiac index; HF: heart failure; LVEF: left ventricular ejection fraction; PCWP: pulmonary capillary wedge pressure; SBP: systolic blood pressure; VO_2: oxygen consumption)

3. How do LVADs function?

Left ventricular assist device (LVAD) is implanted in the chest. It helps pump blood from the lower left heart chamber (left ventricle) to the rest of the body. A control unit and battery pack are worn outside the body and are connected to the LVAD through a small opening (port) in the skin **(Fig. 3)**.

4. Explain the medical complications of LVADs.

As with any surgical procedure, LVAD implantation is associated with an adverse event profile. Such complications of LVAD therapy include bleeding, infection, pump thrombosis, right heart failure, device malfunction, and stroke **(Box 2)**.

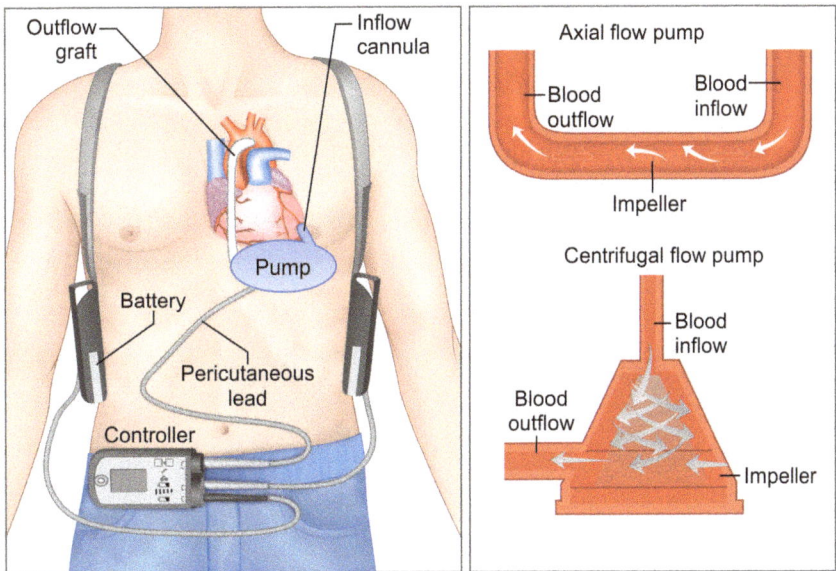

Fig. 3: Configuration of current era durable left ventricular assist devices (LVADs). Durable LVADs are implanted with the inflow cannula of the pump positioned at the left ventricular apex connected to either an axial flow or centrifugal flow device. The outflow graft is positioned in the aorta to provide flow via a continuous flow mechanism.

BOX 2: Complications of left ventricular assist device (LVAD).

Intrinsic to the pump and its constituents:
- Pump malfunction, controller faults, driveline faults, short-shield malfunction
- Related to the patient's native heart condition
- Arrhythmias, valve insufficiency, RV failure
- Pump-patient interface
- GI bleeding (acquired Von Willebrand disease, infection, pump thrombosis), Anemia (from bleeding or hemolysis due to erythrocyte destruction from pump), Thromboembolism (stroke, pulmonary embolism, mesenteric ischemia especially in suboptimal anticoagulation).
- Treatment of infection is on lines of sepsis management with volume resuscitation and antibiotics. In general, LVAD-related bloodstream infections are difficult to eliminate and frequently require pump exchange or transplantation.

(GI: gastrointestinal; RV: right ventricular)

Question 8

1. What are the two different classes of novel oral anticoagulants (NOAC)? Enumerate commonly used drugs of each class.

Direct thrombin inhibitors were developed to overcome the limitations of vitamin K antagonist. Used in high-risk patient including stroke and with atrial fibrillation. Currently five direct acting oral anticoagulants are available.

a. *Dabigatran: Oral direct thrombin inhibitor,* which is used to reduce the risk of stroke and systemic embolism with nonvalvular atrial fibrillation; it has more predictable pharmacology activity than warfarin and broad therapeutic window. It is safer than warfarin, with notable exception of higher risk of major gastrointestinal (GI) bleeding. For practical purposes, a normal *thrombin clotting time* excludes a significant coagulopathy due to dabigatran.

b. *Apixaban, Rivaroxaban Betrixaban, and Edoxaban:* These oral *direct factor Xa inhibitors* have predictable pharmacological properties that do not require routine laboratory monitoring. Currently used for prevention of thromboembolism in patients undergoing hip or knee replacement surgery and reduction of systemic embolism in non-valvular atrial fibrillation. Currently available *anti-factor Xa activity assay* can be used specifically for their activity.

2. Discuss the role of NOAC in patients with atrial fibrillation.

Patients with atrial fibrillation (AF) benefit from anticoagulation to reduce stroke risk. The Food and Drug Administration (FDA) approved four novel oral anticoagulants (NOACs) for AF treatment—(1) dabigatran, (2) rivaroxaban, (3) apixaban, and (4) edoxaban. These agents offer several advantages over warfarin, including straightforward dosing regimens, no requirement for monitoring, and lower risk of intracranial hemorrhage.

a. Edoxaban, dabigatran—require additional lead in therapy with UH/LMWH for 5 days.
b. Apixaban, rivaroxaban—do not require bridging/lead in therapy with parenteral anticoagulation.
c. Preferred over warfarin in patients with nonvalvular AF
d. Patients who cannot be relied upon to get their international normalized ratio (INR) levels checked or
e. Patients who cannot adhere to diet restrictions required when taking warfarin.

3. Explain CHA_2DS_2-VASc score and HAS-BLED score.

The CHA_2DS_2-VASc score for atrial fibrillation stroke risk calculates stroke risk for patients with atrial fibrillation. CHA_2DS_2-VASc score ≥2: recommends oral anticoagulation. A HAS-BLED score of ≥3 indicates that caution is warranted when prescribing oral anticoagulation and regular review is recommended **(Table 10)**.

TABLE 10: Risk stratification for anticoagulation therapy in atrial fibrillation patient.

CHA_2DS_2-VASc scoring system		HAS-BLED score	
Components	**Score**	**Components**	**Score**
Congestive heart failure	1	Hypertension	1
		Abnormal liver and kidney	1
Diabetes	1	Stroke	1
Hypertension	1	Bleeding predisposition	1
Stroke/TIA/Thromboembolism	2	Labile INR	1
Age >75 years	2	Elderly >65	1
Age 65–174	1	Drugs (use of antiplatelet and alcohol)	1
Sex—Female	1		

Total Maximum Score 9: AHA recommends oral anticoagulation for a score of 2 or greater.
Aspirin is recommended in known CAD patients even with a score of zero.
A score of 3 or greater indicates a high risk of bleeding.
(AHA: American Heart Association; CAD: coronary artery disease; TIA: transient ischemic attack)

Question 9

1. What is ocular ultrasound?

Ocular ultrasound plays important role differentiating orbital ultrasound from normal orbit **(Fig. 4A)**. It can also detect ocular injuries like retrobulbar hemorrhage which is also known as Guitar pick sign **(Fig. 4B)**, retinal detachment **(Fig. 4C)**, and lens dislocation.

2. What is fluid administration limited by lung sonography (FALLS) protocol? Discuss.

The FALLS-protocol is a tool proposed for the management of unexplained shock, mainly using lung ultrasound. However, giving only an indirect idea of the mechanism of shock, they are not fully designed to provide a diagnosis **(Flowchart 2)**.

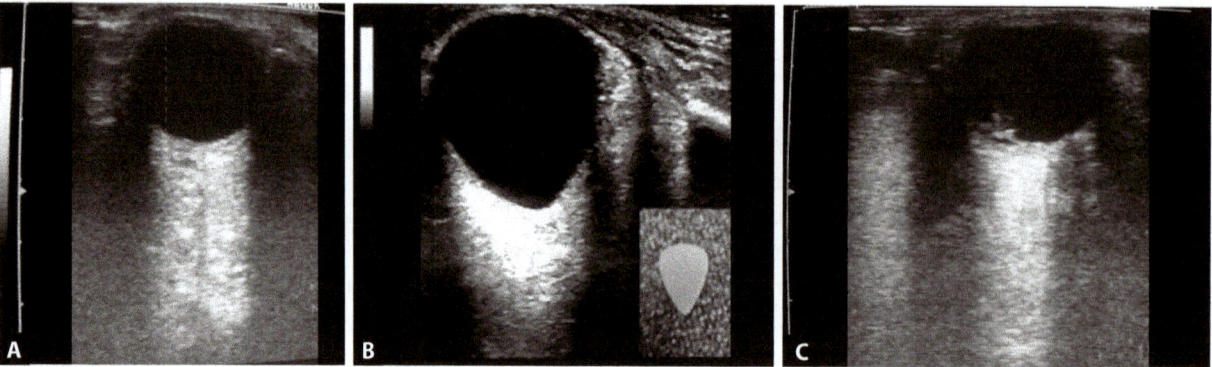

Figs. 4A to C: (A) Normal occular ultrasonography; (B) Scan showing retrobulbar hematoma (Guitar pick sign); (C) Ocular scan showing retinal detachment.

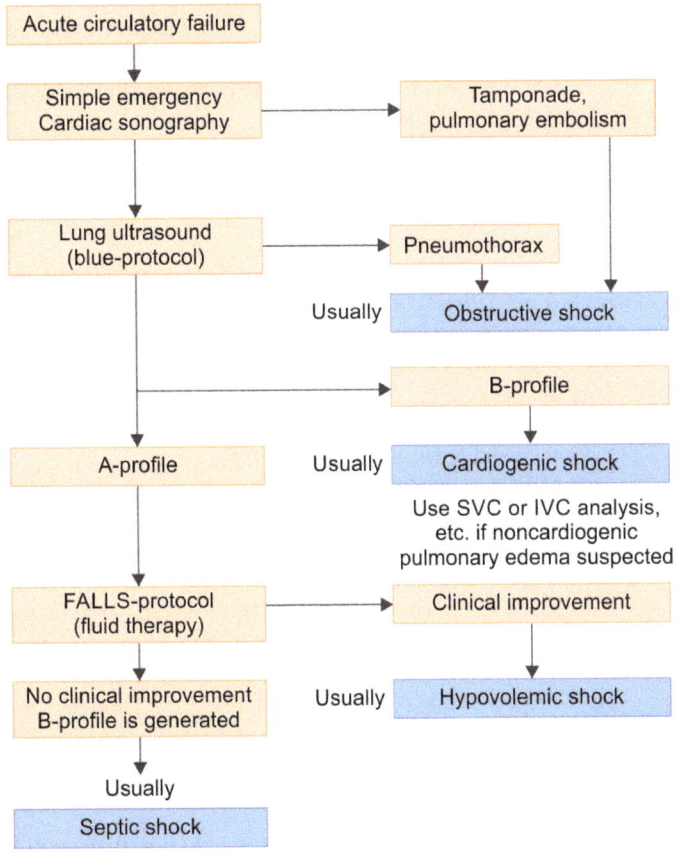

Flowchart 2: FALLS protocol (Schematic decision tree).

from the pleural line, reach the edge of the screen and erase A lines. These artifacts are defined as B lines and when more than three are present per longitudinal scan area constitute an interstitial syndrome. B lines correlate with extravascular lung water and may be suggestive of interstitial or alveolar fluid. They may be seen in a variety of disease states such as pulmonary edema, acute respiratory distress syndrome (ARDS), pneumonia, pulmonary fibrosis.

C lines: Pleural tissue thickening and tissue image touching the surface, with a size on the centimeter scale or less, roughly pyramidal or cupola shaped (hence the C for cupola), may be suggestive of pneumonia in the right context. Additionally, lung tissue takes the appearance of liver tissue in alveolar consolidation, an ultrasound finding known as **hepatization**.

Question 10

1. Discuss high sensitivity troponin.

High-sensitivity cardiac troponin (hs-cTn T and I), has substituted the old cardiac troponin (cTn) tests. It can detect troponin at concentrations 10 to 100 folds lower than the old assays, with higher sensitivity, precision and NPV at an earlier point of time. Cardiac troponins are detected in the serum by the use of highly specific monoclonal antibodies. The European Society of Cardiology and American College of Cardiology consensus document recommends using laboratory cut-offs at the 99th centile of normal with 10% coefficient of variation. This will make serum cTnI values from 0.1–2 µg/L indicative of myocyte necrosis. American College of Emergency Physicians (ACEP) and American Heart Association (AHA) guidelines recommend the use of troponin as level A class 1 in diagnosis of acute coronary syndrome (ACS). Cardiac troponin also has a prognostic value in mortality and adverse cardiac events.

2. Explain HEART pathway.

The HEART score identifies patients at low, intermediate, and high risk for short-term adverse outcome resulting from ACS **(Table 11)**.

3. Discuss ADvISED trial in aortic dissection.

The ADvISED trial was an international multicenter prospective observational study of a novel diagnostic strategy that integrated the Aortic Dissection Detection Risk Score (ADD-RS) and D-Dimer in an ED population to rule out Acute Aortic Syndrome (AAS). Acute aortic syndromes include aortic dissection, intramural aortic hematoma,

3. Explain ultrasound finding in pneumonia.

The Ultrasound Appearance of Pneumonia

Where fluid-filled alveoli are surrounded by air-filled lung; B lines, a form of short path reverberation artefact, result. In the appropriate clinical setting a localized patch of numerous B lines, often with tiny areas of sub pleural consolidation, suggests early pneumonia.

A lines: Acoustic impedance between the pleura and the surrounding lung parenchyma creates typical horizontal artifacts known as A lines. The most usual artifact, A lines are roughly horizontal, hyperechoic (bright), and parallel to the pleural line and arise below it, at an interval that is exactly the interval between the skin and pleural line. These may be present in normal lungs. However, they may be accentuated in disease states such as asthma and chronic obstructive pulmonary disease (COPD). Simply, A lines indicate air, whether physiologic or pathologic.

B lines: When there is a variation in normal tissue and pleura interface, such as may occur in with fluid presence in the lung, vertical artifacts moving with lung sliding arise

TABLE 11: Risk stratification-HEART risk score for chest pain patients in emergency department.

History	Highly suspicious	2
	Moderately suspicious	1
	Slightly suspicious	0
ECG	Significant ST depression	2
	Nonspecific repolarization changes	1
	Normal	0
Age	>65 years	2
	45–65 years	1
	<45 years	0
Risk factors	>3 risk	2
	1 or 2	1
	No risk	0
Troponins	>3 × normal limit	2
	1–3 × normal limit	1
	<normal limit	0

Heart Score	Risk of MACE	Recommendations
0–3	0.9%	ED discharge
4–6	12%	Observation
>6	65%	Cardiology admission

(ECG: electrocardiogram; MACE: major adverse cardiovascular events)

penetrating aortic ulcer and aortic rupture. AAS are rare but life-threatening cardiovascular emergencies with nonspecific clinical presentations, which results in over testing and misdiagnosis. The ADvISED trial introduces a new clinical strategy that combines a pre-test probability assessment with a D-dimer to help physicians reduce over-testing and misdiagnosis of AAS.

SUGGESTED READING

1. Richhariya D, Sharma B. Textbook of Emergency Medicine including Intensive Care and Trauma, 2nd edition. New Delhi: Jaypee Brothers Medical Publishers (P) Ltd; 2022. pp. 345-9, 1594. (Question 1).
2. Richhariya D, Sharma B. Textbook of Emergency Medicine including Intensive Care and Trauma, 2nd edition. New Delhi: Jaypee Brothers Medical Publishers (P) Ltd; 2022. pp. 1124-34. (Question 2).
3. Richhariya D, Sharma B. Textbook of Emergency Medicine including Intensive Care and Trauma, 2nd edition. New Delhi: Jaypee Brothers Medical Publishers (P) Ltd; 2022. pp. 1175-80. (Question 3).
4. BMJ Best Practice. (2023). Child abuse. [online] Available from: https://bestpractice.bmj.com/topics/en-us/846 [Last accessed April, 2023]. (Question 4).
5. Cleveland Clinic. (2023). Jaundice in Newborns. [online] Available from: https://my.clevelandclinic.org/health/diseases/22263-jaundice-in-newborns [Last accessed April, 2023]. (Question 5).
6. Richhariya D, Sharma B. Textbook of Emergency Medicine including Intensive Care and Trauma, 2nd edition. New Delhi: Jaypee Brothers Medical Publishers (P) Ltd; 2022. pp. 80-90. (Question 6).
7. Richhariya D, Sharma B. Textbook of Emergency Medicine including Intensive Care and Trauma, 2nd edition. New Delhi: Jaypee Brothers Medical Publishers (P) Ltd; 2022. pp. 483-5. (Question 7).
8. Richhariya D, Sharma B. Textbook of Emergency Medicine including Intensive Care and Trauma, 2nd edition. New Delhi: Jaypee Brothers Medical Publishers (P) Ltd; 2022. pp. 22 & 537. (Question 8).
9. Richhariya D, Sharma B. Textbook of Emergency Medicine including Intensive Care and Trauma, 2nd edition. New Delhi: Jaypee Brothers Medical Publishers (P) Ltd; 2022. pp. 364-73. (Question 9).
10. Richhariya D, Sharma B. Textbook of Emergency Medicine including Intensive Care and Trauma, 2nd edition. New Delhi: Jaypee Brothers Medical Publishers (P) Ltd; 2022. pp. 20, 435, 530. (Question 10).

Emergency Medicine Paper 25

Devendra Richhariya

Question 1

1. Discuss the pathophysiology of hemorrhagic shock in trauma.

Pathophysiology of hemorrhagic shock is described in **Figure 1**.

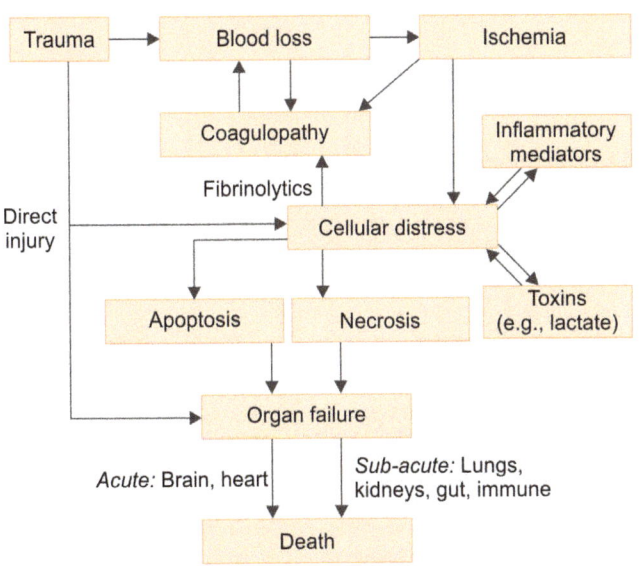

Fig. 1: Pathophysiology of hemorrhagic shock.

2. Discuss permissive hypotension and its indications and contraindications.

Permissive hypotension implies accepting an adequate, not normal, blood pressure. It is employed in an actively bleeding patient until hemostasis is obtained, after which point definitive resuscitation begins. During resuscitation of a patient with hemorrhagic shock, volume infusion in the face of continued blood loss results in dilutional coagulopathy and hypothermia, while the transient elevation in blood pressure contributes to further bleeding from wounds and vessels. This approach may be associated with organ dysfunction, abdominal compartment syndrome, and death in major trauma patients. Permissive hypotension, therefore, can facilitate an environment that optimizes coagulation, albeit at the potential expense of optimal tissue perfusion pressure, until repair restores the integrity of the system.

Permissive hypotension is the act of maintaining a blood pressure lower than physiologic levels in a patient who has suffered from hemorrhagic blood loss. The practice is employed in order to maintain adequate vasoconstriction and organ perfusion, and to prevent undesired coagulopathy during initial fluid resuscitation. Permissive hypotension is contraindicated in patients with traumatic brain injury because reduced perfusion pressure and oxygenation can lead to secondary brain injury. In such situations, a mean arterial pressure (MAP) of >80 mm Hg (a cerebral perfusion pressure of approximately 60 mm Hg) is required in order to maintain cerebral perfusion pressure.

3. Discuss the classifications of hemorrhagic shock in trauma.

The classification of hemorrhagic shock in trauma is given in **Table 1**.

TABLE 1: Classification of hemorrhagic shock in trauma.				
	Class I	Class II	Class III	Class IV
Absolute blood loss	<750 mL	750–1,500 mL	1,500–2,000 mL	>2,000 mL
Relative blood loss	<15%	15–30%	30–40%	>40%
Pulse rate	<100	100–120	120–140	>140
Blood pressure	Normal	Normal	Decreased	Decreased
Pulse pressure	Normal/increased	Decreased	Decreased	Decreased
Capillary refill	Normal	Decreased	Decreased	Decreased
Respiratory rate	14–20	20–30	30–40	>35
Urine output (mL/hr)	>30	20–30	5–15	Negligible
CNS mental status	Slightly anxious	Anxious	Confused	Confused lethargic
Fluid replacement	Crystalloid	Crystalloid	Crystalloid + blood	Crystalloid + blood

(CNS: central nervous system)

4. Describe the ABC score for massive blood transfusion protocol.

The assessment of blood consumption (ABC) score in trauma was developed to assist clinicians in discerning when massive transfusion would be required to resuscitate trauma patients. Hemorrhage is the most common cause of early death in trauma patients. Massive transfusion protocols (MTPs) have been designed to accelerate the release of blood products but can result in waste if activated inappropriately. The ABC score **(Table 2)** has become a widely accepted score for MTP activation.

TABLE 2: Trigger for MTP: ABC score ≥2 (accuracy of prediction of MTP 75%).

Components	Points
Penetrating injury	1
FAST positive	1
Heart rate >100/min	1
Systolic BP <90 mm Hg	1

(ABC: assessment of blood consumption; BP: blood pressure; FAST: focused assessment with sonography in trauma; MTP: massive transfusion protocol)

Question 2

1. Discuss the pathophysiology of sepsis and septic shock.

Pathogenesis of sepsis is characterized by an inflammatory cascade. The cascade has humoral, cellular, complement, and cytokine components. This is a complex host and pathogen interaction model that if remains unchecked and dysregulated ultimately leads to final common pathway of cell injury and death. The endothelial cell is the focal point of interactions between the inflammatory events and disordered hemostasis. Vascular bed-specific factors and endothelial cell injury can shift the balance between antithrombotic and prothrombotic states. The mediators ultimately lead to microvascular plugging and vasoconstriction. The resultant hypoperfusion/ischemia leads to acute organ dysfunction. Uninterrupted, a vicious cycle ensues that can end in death. Disease course is the result of several innate, immunological, and external factors. Disease progression in sepsis is highly heterogeneous and unpredictable. Sepsis is a dynamic disease which may progress to septic shock and organ failure which is associated with high mortality.

2. What are the various scoring systems for early identification of sepsis in emergency?

Scoring systems for early identification of sepsis in the emergency department (ED) are given in **Tables 3 and 4**.

TABLE 3: Screening tool to rule in/out sepsis in the emergency department.

This is a simplified tool that can be used to screen patients for sepsis in the ED or in critical care unit

1. Obtain proper history for any potential source of infection	Lung infections, kidney infections such as urinary tract infection, infection lingering in the abdomen, meningitis, and endocarditis, skin and soft-tissue infection, wound infection, catheter-related infections, or bloodstream infections	Yes/no
2. Search for signs and symptoms that would indicate	Fever >38.3°C or temperature <36°C, altered mental status with a GCS <15, heart rate >90 bpm (tachycardia), respiratory rate >20 bpm (tachypnea), leukocytosis or leukopenia (WBC count >12,000 μ/L or <4,000 μ/L, respectively)	Yes/no

If both of the above are answered YES, suspicion of infection is present.
Laboratory investigations that should be ordered are complete blood count with differential, blood lactate and cultures, and basic metabolic panel. Ultrasound of the abdomen, CT scan, chest X-ray, amylase, lipase, ABG, and procalcitonin should be obtained according to the signs and symptoms and according to physician discretion.

3. Whether the organ dysfunction criteria are present?	If suspicion of infection and organ dysfunction is present, the patient's condition is labeled as septic shock and should be entered into the protocol.	Yes/no

(ABG: arterial blood gas; GCS: Glasgow Coma Scale; WBC: white blood cells)

TABLE 4: qSOFA (quick sequential organ failure assessment) score.

H	Hypotension: SBP ≤100 mm Hg
A	Altered mental status (any GCS <15)
T	Tachypnea: Respiratory rate ≥22/min

(GCS: Glasgow Coma Scale; SBP: systolic blood pressure)

3. Discuss the pathway of lactate production and its significance for an emergency physician.

Sepsis and septic shock are associated with a stress response that includes increased release of epinephrine (adrenalin). This hormone stimulates the membrane-bound enzyme Na^+/K^+-ATPase, which utilizes adenosine triphosphate (ATP) generated by aerobic glycolysis to provide the energy necessary to "pump" ions into and out of the cells. Na$^+$/K$^+$-ATPase stimulation increases aerobic glycolysis and thereby lactate production. The traditional use of lactate measurement as a marker of inadequate tissue perfusion and tissue hypoxia in critical care is somewhat limited because of the increasing realization over the past decade that trauma victims and others suffering potential critical illnesses may have raised lactate production despite adequate tissue perfusion. The pathway of lactate production is summarized in **Figure 2**.

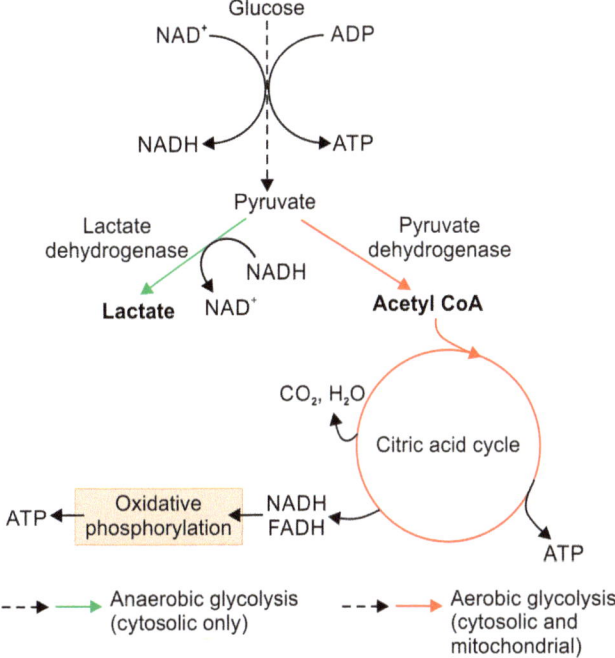

Fig. 2: Pathway of lactate production. [ADP: adenosine diphosphate; ATP: adenosine triphosphate; CoA: coenzyme A; FADH: flavin adenine dinucleotide; NAD$^+$: nicotinamide adenine dinucleotide; NADH: nicotinamide adenine dinucleotide (NAD) plus hydrogen]

Question 3

1. Discuss the mechanism of blood flow during cardiopulmonary resuscitation (CPR).

The "cardiac compression" theory of forward blood flow during chest compressions for cardiac arrest presumes that blood is squeezed from the heart into the arterial and pulmonary circulations, with closure of the mitral and tricuspid valves, preventing retrograde blood flow, and opening of the aortic and pulmonary valves in response to forward blood flow. Air is thought to move freely in and out of the lungs, so that the intrathoracic pressure does not significantly rise and the pulmonary circulation is not adversely affected by chest compressions. With the relaxation of chest compression, the heart fills with blood and air passively returns to the lungs.

2. What is resuscitative thoracotomy?

Resuscitative thoracotomy is nearly always performed in the emergency department (ED) and involves gaining rapid access to the heart and major thoracic vessels through an anterolateral chest incision to control exsanguinating hemorrhage or other life-threatening chest injuries. A resuscitative thoracotomy is a thoracotomy performed to resuscitate a major trauma patient who has sustained severe thoracic or abdominal trauma followed by cardiac arrest **(Table 5)**.

TABLE 5: Indications for resuscitative thoractomy Eastern Association for the Surgery of Trauma (EAST) recommendations

Recommendation	Mechanism	Location	Signs of life (SOL)
Strong	Penetrating	Thoracic	With SOL
Conditional	Penetrating	Thoracic	Without SOL
	Penetrating	Extrathoracic (noncranial)	With SOL
	Penetrating	Extrathoracic (noncranial)	Without SOL
	Blunt	–	With SOL
Conditional (against)	Blunt	–	Without SOL

3. What is therapeutic hypothermia?

Studies suggest that after achieving return of spontaneous circulation (ROSC) (period of global cerebral hypoxia–ischemia), mild induced hypothermia is used as neuroprotective and outcome improving measures. Mild induced hypothermia suppresses the many pathological processes leading to delayed cell death, including apoptosis (programmed cell death). Hypothermia reduces the release of excitatory amino acids and free radicals and decreases the cerebral metabolic rate for oxygen (CMRO$_2$) by about 6% for each 1°C reduction in the core temperature. Hypothermia reduces the inflammatory response associated with the postcardiac arrest syndrome. *The previous term therapeutic hypothermia is replaced by the new term "targeted temperature management" (TTM).* Temperature is maintained between 32 and 36°C with a temperature control monitoring system. The minimum duration of TTM should be at least 24 hours.

Methods of inducing and/or maintaining TTM include the following:
a. The first inexpensive method is by simply applying ice packs and/or wet towels; for nursing staff, this method

is time consuming; also temperature fluctuations will be more, and controlled rewarming is not possible.
b. Cooling blankets or pads
c. Water- or air-circulating blankets
d. Water-circulating gel-coated pads
e. Transnasal evaporative cooling—large multicenter randomized controlled trials are needed
f. Intravascular heat exchanger, placed usually in the femoral or subclavian veins
g. Extracorporeal circulation [e.g., cardiopulmonary bypass, extracorporeal membrane oxygenation (ECMO)].

Question 4

1. Draw a well-labeled diagram of circle of Willis.

The structure of the circle of Willis includes left and right internal carotid arteries, left and right anterior cerebral arteries, and left and right posterior cerebral arteries **(Fig. 3)**.

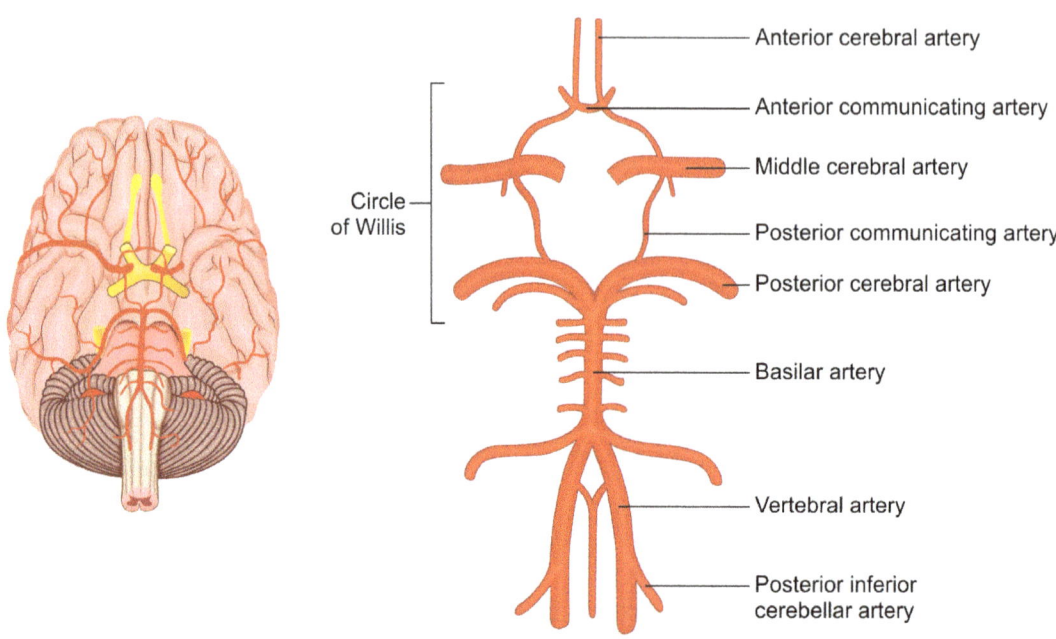

Fig. 3: Circle of Willis.

2. Describe Monro–Kellie doctrine and autoregulation.

Understanding cerebral blood flow mechanics is crucial to realizing the importance of optimal blood pressure targets following traumatic brain injury (TBI) **(Fig. 4)**. In 1783, Alexander Monro applied the principles of physics to the intracranial contents creating what came to be known as the Monro–Kellie hypothesis. This principle had substantial implications for cerebral blood flow during periods of intracranial pressure changes. In a healthy state, cerebral perfusion pressure **(Fig. 5)** remains constant due to changes in flow related to intact cerebrovascular autoregulation (CAR).

Monro–Kellie doctrine:
a. The brain is enclosed in a nonexpandable case of bone.
b. The substance of the brain is nearly incompressible.
c. The volume of the brain in the cranial cavity is therefore constant or nearly constant.
d. A continuous outflow of venous blood from the cranial cavity is required to make space for the continuous incoming arterial blood.

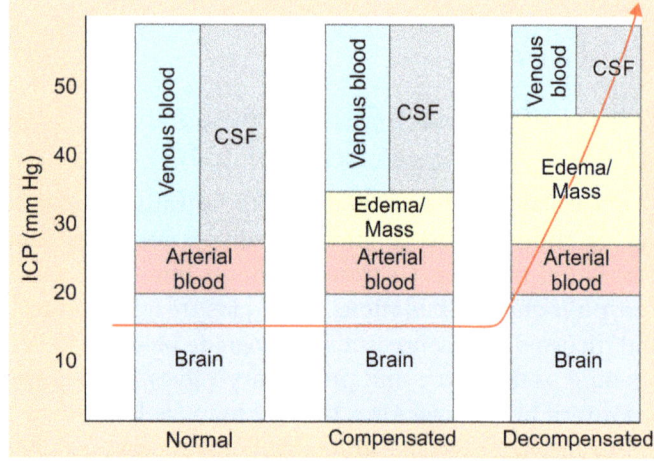

Fig. 4: Cerebral blood flow and intracranial pressure.
(CSF: cerebrospinal fluid; ICP: intracranial pressure)

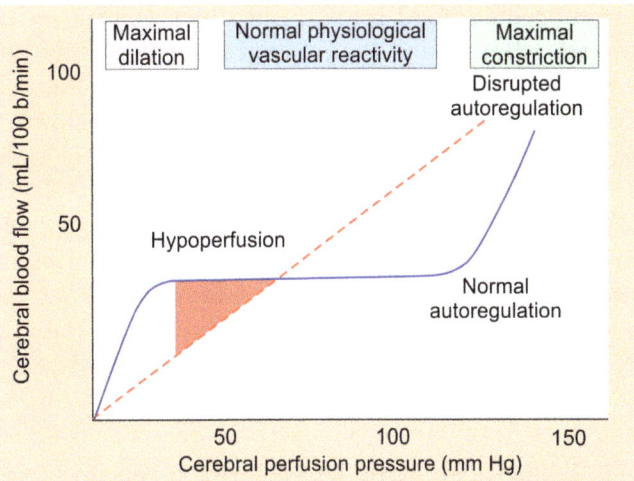

Fig. 5: Cerebral blood flow and cerebral perfusion pressure.

3. Enumerate anatomical and physiological risk factors for acute ischemic stroke.

Risk factors for acute ischemic stroke are given in **Table 6**.

TABLE 6: Anatomical and physiological risk factors for acute ischemic stroke.

Nonmodifiable	Modifiable	Risk factors for embolic stroke
• Age • Race • Sex • Ethnicity • History of migraine headaches • Fibromuscular dysplasia • *Heredity:* Family history of stroke or transient ischemic attacks (TIAs)	• Hypertension • Diabetes mellitus • Cardiac disease • High cholesterol • Previous stroke • Carotid stenosis • Hyperhomocysteinemia • *Lifestyle issues:* Excessive alcohol intake, tobacco use, illicit drug use, physical inactivity • Obesity • Oral contraceptive use/postmenopausal hormone use	• Arrhythmias • Valvular heart diseases • Thrombus and structural lesions • Structural heart diseases

Question 5

1. Draw a well-labeled diagram of the anatomy of the ankle joint and describe the assessment of Lisfranc injury.

Anatomy of the ankle joint is shown in **Figure 6**.

Assessment of Lisfranc injury:
a. A Lisfranc injury is a tarsometatarsal fracture dislocation characterized by traumatic disruption between the articulation of the medial cuneiform and the base of the second metatarsal.
b. Diagnosis is confirmed by radiographs which may show widening of the interval between the first and the second rays.
c. Treatment is generally operative with either open reduction and internal fixation (ORIF) or arthrodesis.

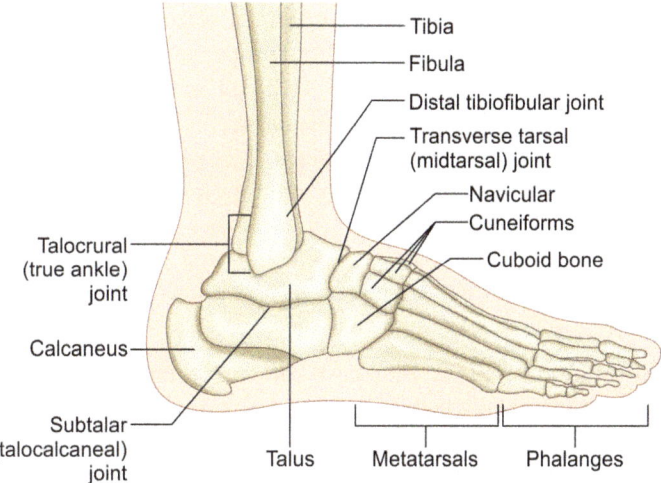

Fig. 6: Anatomy of ankle joint.

2. Draw a well-labeled diagram of the anatomy of shoulder joint and describe various types of shoulder dislocations.

Anatomy of shoulder joint is shown in **Figure 7**.

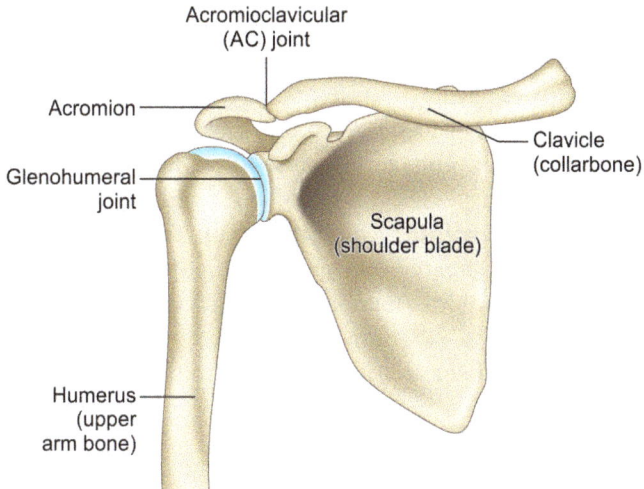

Fig. 7: Anatomy of shoulder joint.

Types of shoulder dislocation:
Anterior dislocation: It is the most common form of shoulder dislocation. It is possible to reduce the dislocation with analgesics and intra-articular block or sedation. Lay patient supine with affected arm adducted to the side with elbow extended. Stand on the affected side and grip hand, pilling axial traction and making small, short vertical oscillations,

as though shaking their hand. Gradually, move the abducted arm with continued oscillations at 90° of abduction, externally rotate the shoulder, and continue abduction and oscillations. Reduction should occur by 120° of abduction.

Posterior dislocation: This type of dislocation is much less common; classic mechanisms include seizure and electric shock. It is difficult to treat without proper sedation. Forward and flex the affected arm to 90°. Abduct across midline and internally rotate. The assistant standing on the contralateral side of the body can pull axial traction while the humeral head is milked anteriorly. External rotation can sometimes help with final reduction.

3. Describe the assessment of scaphoid lunate dislocation.

Scapholunate dissociation, also known as rotary subluxation of the scaphoid, refers to an abnormal orientation of the scaphoid relative to the lunate and implies severe injury to the scapholunate interosseous ligament and other stabilizing ligaments.

Carpal dissociation implies carpal instability, which has important clinical implications; thus, it is essential to identify this finding on imaging. Note that the absence of dissociation does not exclude ligamentous injury, as lower-grade injuries that result in dynamic instability may present with normal radiographic carpal alignment.

The typical pattern of scapholunate dissociation consists of:
a. Relative flexion (volar rotation) of the scaphoid
b. Relative extension (dorsal rotation) of the lunate.

Acute nondisplaced and chronic asymptomatic injuries may be treated conservatively with nonsteroidal anti-inflammatory drugs (NSAIDs) and immobilization.

Surgical repair or reconstruction of the scapholunate interosseous ligament is normally required to prevent long-term complications, namely proximal migration of the capitate between the scaphoid and lunate with a resultant degenerative disease known as scapholunate advanced collapse.

Question 6

1. Describe the pathophysiology of fever in pediatrics and elderly population.

Body temperature is regulated by thermosensitive neurons which are located in the anterior hypothalamus, which responds to any change in temperature of blood and also through the warm and cold receptors located on the skin and muscles. To maintain the temperature, either the blood flow is redirected to or from the cutaneous vascular bed, regulating the extracellular fluid volume and also by increasing or decreasing the sweating. There are *three main mechanisms* for producing fever: (a) In response to the pyrogens, production of heat is in excess to the loss and defective mechanism of heat loss. Endogenous pyrogens are mainly cytokines such as interleukins (IL)-1 and 6, tumor necrosis factor-α (TNF-α), and interferons β and γ. Other endogenous pyrogens include leukemia inhibitory factor-M (LIF), ciliary neurotrophic factor (CNTF), and oncostatin-M. Many exotoxins such as drugs, malignancies, and inflammatory diseases can also produce fever by production of endogenous pyrogens. (b) Another mechanism in which the heat production is in excess to the release is in case of salicylate poisoning and malignant hyperthermia. (c) The third mechanism, where the loss of heat is defective, is seen in cases of ectodermal dysplasia and victims of severe heat exposure.

2. Discuss about antipyretics and analgesics used in the ED.

Antipyretic agents act upon the arachidonic acid pathway. Their main action is to competitively bind on COX enzymes' catalytic site competing with arachidonic acid, hence inhibiting the production on prostaglandin 2.

Paracetamol: It is recommended in doses of 10–15 mg/kg at 4–6 hourly intervals (maximum 60 mg/kg/day). Antipyretic effect takes 30–60 minutes to initiate. Paracetamol helps in reduction of body temperature by 1–2°F within 2 hours of administration. The greater the initial temperature, the greater the fall of temperature after the drug intake.

Ibuprofen: This drug can be used at a dose of 10 mg/kg, as a first-line antipyretic. No great differences have been shown in safety and efficacy as compared to paracetamol. Although a combination of these two can be more effective, it is not recommended routinely in children because of associated improper drug dosages.

Mefenamic acid: This is an effective antipyretic, mainly in controlling the high-grade fever at the dose of 6–7 mg/kg/dose (20 mg/kg/day is maximum). A common practice is to give one dose of mefenamic acid for high temperature and then subsequently followed by paracetamol.

3. Elaborate the pathophysiology of hypothermia and enumerate the causes of hypothermia in adults.

Resting metabolism and neurological functions are decreased as a result of cooling. Even when the core temperature is normal, skin cooling induces shivering which directly increases the metabolism by increased muscle activity and indirectly by increased ventilation and cardiac output. As the core temperature decreases, shivering increases and reaches the maximum level when the core temperature is about 32°C and stops by about 30°C. With decreasing temperature metabolism generally decreases below 32°C.

Causes of hypothermia in adults:
a. *Disturbance of thermoregulating mechanisms:*
   i. Trauma
   ii. Hypovolemic shock
   iii. Substantia nigra pars compacta (SNC) lesions
   iv. Extreme age points
   v. General or neuroaxial anesthetic
   vi. Related illnesses (diabetes, cardiac failure)
   vii. Alcohol or antidepressant use
b. *Extreme heat loss:*
   i. Prolonged exposure to the environment
   ii. Blood perfusions and intravenous drips
   iii. Burns
   iv. General or neuroaxial anesthetic.

Question 7

1. Describe the pathophysiology of acute respiratory distress syndrome (ARDS) in dengue and malaria.

a. Plasma leak from capillaries into the extravascular compartment: Rise in hematocrit count that may progress to shock
b. Signs of respiratory distress secondary to fluid overload
c. Fluid overload in pulmonary or gastrointestinal system: Pleural effusion/ascites
d. Signs of bleeding due to thrombocytopenia
e. Decreased adequate perfusion leading to severe organ impairment.

2. Enumerate the steps of drug-assisted intubation of a trauma victim.

The steps of drug-assisted intubation are given in **Table 7**.

3. Discuss high-flow oxygen therapy and its indications, contraindications, and proven benefits.

High-flow oxygen therapy is a breathing support. Continuous, warmed (to 37°C), and humidified oxygen is given through a tube placed in the nostrils. It is only offered if traditional oxygen therapy is not helping. High-flow oxygen therapy helps reduce the effort your body needs to put into breathing. Indication, contraindication, and proven benefits are given in **Box 1**.

TABLE 7: Steps of drug-assisted intubation.

Step	Time interval (min)	Pharmacologic agents
Preoxygenation	0–3	Oxygen, including addition of nasal cannula
Premedication	3	Induction agent ± fentanyl, lidocaine, atropine, defasciculating agents (vecuronium, rocuronium; usually one-tenth the induction dose)
Paralysis	3.5–5.5	Midazolam, ketamine, etomidate, propofol, or other induction agents followed by succinylcholine or rocuronium
Placement	6–6.5	Oxygen
Performance	7–7.5	Oxygen
Postintubation management	7.5+	Oxygen, sedatives, analgesics, etc.

BOX 1: Indications for high-flow oxygen therapy.

- ARDS and acute hypoxemic respiratory failure
- Hypoxemia induced by severe heart failure
- Postextubation respiratory compromise
- Airway instrumentation (as an adjunct during manipulation of the airway, e.g., bronchoscopy, and during intubation in patients with both low and high risk, i.e., hypoxemia, morbid obesity)
- Immune compromise
- End-of-life care

Contraindications:
- Critically ill infants and children requiring a higher level of respiratory support
- Upper airway obstruction
- Central apnea
- Asthma
- Trauma, facial trauma
- Pneumothorax
- Decreased level of consciousness

Proven benefits: HFNC has been gaining attention as an alternative respiratory support for critically ill patients after few large randomized clinical trials. Initial data of published trials are mostly available for neonates. In seriously ill adults, however, evidence for use of HFNOT is not even because the studies included conditions of varying etiology, such as hypoxemic respiratory failure, exacerbation of COPD, postextubation, pre-intubation oxygenation, sleep apnea, acute heart failure, and conditions entailing do-not-intubate orders.

(ARDS: acute respiratory distress syndrome; COPD: chronic obstructive pulmonary disease; HFNC: high-flow nasal cannula; HFNOT: high-flow nasal oxygen therapy)

Question 8

1. Describe various clinical decision-making rules for management and disposition of low-risk chest pain.

Clinical decision rules (CDRs), also known as decision "aids," are evidence-based tools or the protocols to assist the emergency physician/clinicians in decision-making for common complaints in the ED. These CDRs are often helpful in the ED setting, to identify patients who might be at higher risk for serious conditions, such as pulmonary embolism (PE) or subarachnoid hemorrhage (SAH), or to prevent overuse of unnecessary testing **(Table 8)**.

TABLE 8: Risk stratification: HEART risk score for chest pain patients in ED.

History	Highly suspicious	2
	Moderately suspicious	1
	Slightly suspicious	0
ECG	Significant ST-depression	2
	Nonspecific repolarization changes	1
	Normal	0
Age	>65 years	2
	45–65 years	1
	<45 years	0
Risk factors	>3 risk	2
	1 or 2	1
	No risk	0
Troponins	>3× normal limit	2
	1–3× normal limit	1
	< Normal limit	0
Heart score	**Risk of MACE**	**Recommendations**
0–3	0.9%	ED discharge
4–6	12%	Observation
>6	65%	Cardiology admission

(ECG: electrocardiograph; ED: emergency department; MACE: major adverse cardiac event)

2. Describe the anatomy of coronary circulation.

The two main coronary arteries are the left main and right coronary arteries **(Fig. 8)**.

Left main coronary artery (LMCA): It supplies blood to the left side of the heart muscle (the left ventricle and left atrium). LMCA divides into the following branches:
a. The left anterior descending artery branches off the left coronary artery and supplies blood to the front of the left side of the heart.

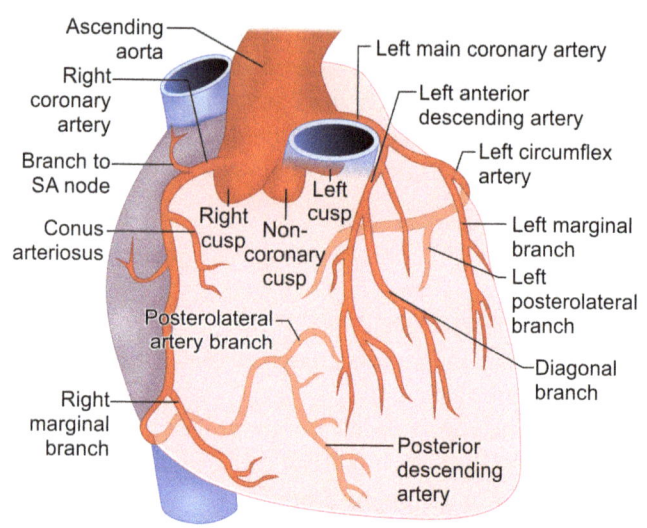

Fig. 8: Anatomy of coronary circulation. (SA: sinoatrial)

b. The circumflex artery branches off the left coronary artery and encircles the heart muscle. This artery supplies blood to the outer side and back of the heart.

Right coronary artery (RCA): It supplies blood to the right ventricle, the right atrium, and the sinoatrial (SA) and atrioventricular (AV) nodes, which regulate the heart rhythm. The right coronary artery divides into smaller branches, including the right posterior descending artery and the acute marginal artery. Together with the left anterior descending artery, the right coronary artery helps supply blood to the middle or septum of the heart.

3. Draw Einthoven's triangle.

Einthoven's triangle is an imaginary formation of three limb leads in a triangle used in electrocardiography, formed by the two shoulders and the pubis. The shape forms an inverted equilateral triangle with the heart at the center. It is named after Willem Einthoven, who theorized its existence **(Fig. 9)**.

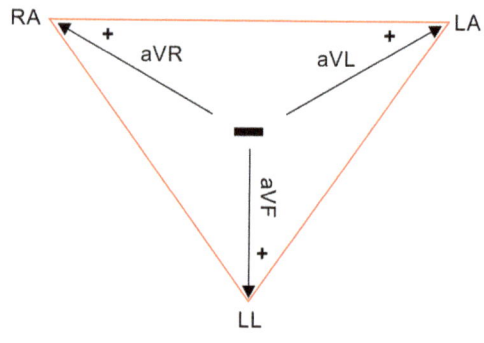

Fig. 9: Einthoven's triangle. (LA: left arm; LL: left leg; RA: right arm)

Question 9

1. Enumerate the causes and diagnostic algorithm of hypernatremia.

Hypernatremia occurs when the serum sodium level is measured over 145 mmol/L and a clinical picture is related to this. Tonicity shows the activity of solutes that cannot easily penetrate the cell membrane and provides the transcellular distribution of water. It is the most effective anion that provides osmolality of extracellular fluid. Hypernatremia is accompanied by hypertonicity, decreased cell volume, and usually dehydration. If hypernatremia develops within 48 hours, it is called acute hypernatremia and if it develops over 48 hours, it is called chronic hypernatremia (Flowchart 1).

2. Describe the approach to diagnosis of mixed acid–base disorder from arterial blood gas (ABG) analysis.

Mixed acid–base disorder: It means simultaneous presence of more than one acid–base disorder. Mixed acid–base disorders can be suspected from the patient's history, from a lesser- or greater-than-expected compensatory respiratory or renal response, and from analysis of the serum electrolytes and anion gap. Always correlate with the patient's history (Flowchart 2).

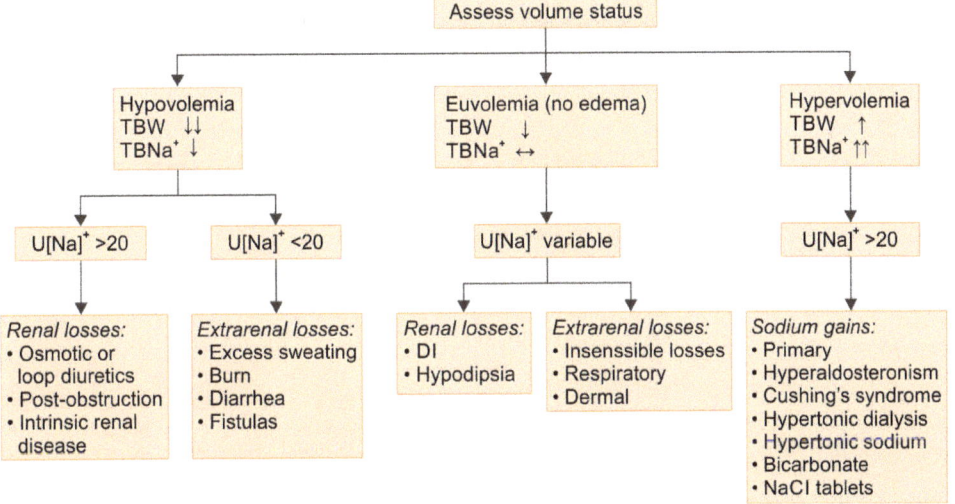

Flowchart 1: Algorithm to evaluate hypernatremia.

(DI: diabetes insipidus; TBW: total body water)

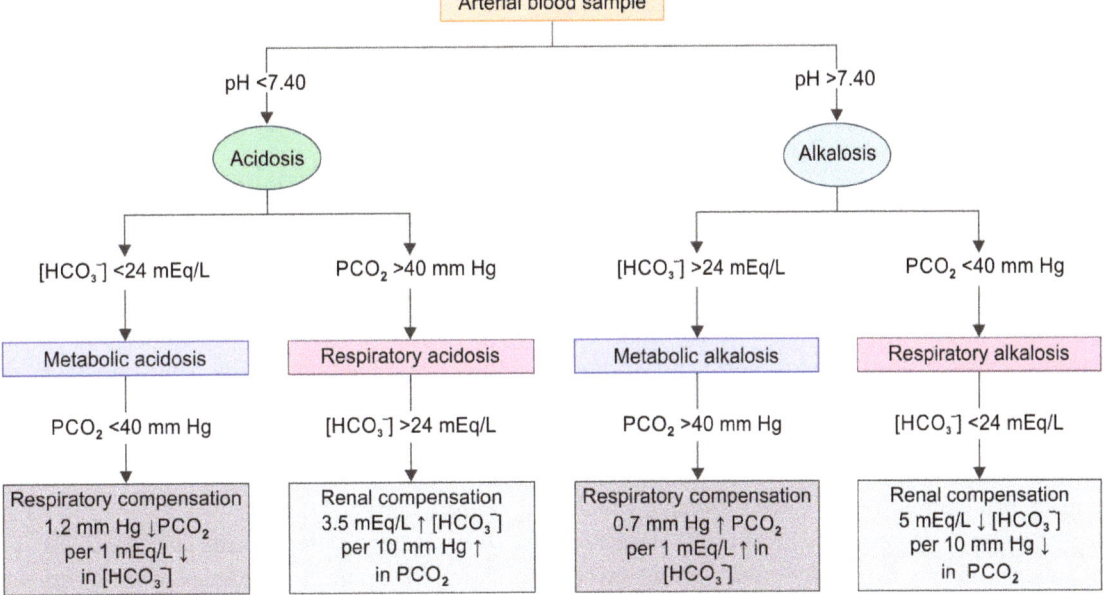

Flowchart 2: Mixed acid–base disorder evaluation.

(PCO_2: partial pressure of carbon dioxide)

3. Describe the physiology and pathophysiology of potassium homeostasis.

Potassium homeostasis denotes the maintenance of the total body potassium content and plasma potassium level within narrow limits in the face of potentially wide variations in dietary potassium intake. It involves two concurrent processes: external and internal **(Table 9)**.

TABLE 9: Pathophysiology of potassium homeostasis.

	Increased intake	*Reduced loss*	*Redistribution to extracellular fluid*
K⁺ ↑	Supplements intake	Severe or end-stage renal failure	Acidosis
	Potassium infusion	ACE inhibitors	Beta-blockers
		Angiotensin receptor blockers	Cellular necrosis
		Mineralocorticoid receptor antagonists	Trauma
		Heparins	Hypermagnesemia
		NSAIDs	
	Reduced intake	*Increased loss*	*Redistribution to intracellular fluid*
K⁺ ↓	Malnutrition	Vomiting	Alkalosis
		Sweating	Beta-agonists
		Acute tubular necrosis	Alpha-antagonists
		Loop diuretics	Insulin
		Thiazides	Hypomagnesemia
		Corticosteroids	Hypothermia

(ACE: angiotensin-converting enzyme ; NSAIDs: non-steroidal anti-inflammatory drugs)

Question 10

1. Describe the pulse-echo principle.

Two basic principles need to be understood regarding how ultrasound is generated and an image is formed. The first is the *piezoelectric effect*, which explains how ultrasound is generated from ceramic crystals in the transducer. An electric current passes through a cable to the transducer and is applied to the crystals, causing them to deform and vibrate. This vibration produces the ultrasound beam. The frequency of the ultrasound waves produced is predetermined by the crystals in the transducer.

The second key principle is the *pulse-echo principle*, which explains how the image is generated. Ultrasound waves are produced in pulses, not continuously, because the same crystals are used to generate and receive sound waves, and they cannot do both at the same time. In the time between the pulses, the ultrasound beam enters the patient and is bounced or reflected back to the transducer. These reflected sound waves, or echoes, cause the crystals in the transducer to deform again and produce an electrical signal that is then converted into an image displayed on the monitor. The transducer generally emits ultrasound only 1% of the time; the rest of the time is spent receiving the returning echoes.

2. Describe the ALARA principle.

ALARA stands for "as low as reasonably achievable". It means *avoiding exposure to radiation that does not have a direct benefit to you, even if the dose is small.* To do this, you can use three basic protective measures in radiation safety: time, distance, and shielding. ALARA is not only a sound-safety principle, but also a regulatory requirement for all radiation safety programs. Radiation safety programs attempt to lower the doses received by radiation workers by utilizing practical, cost-effective measures **(Fig. 10)**.

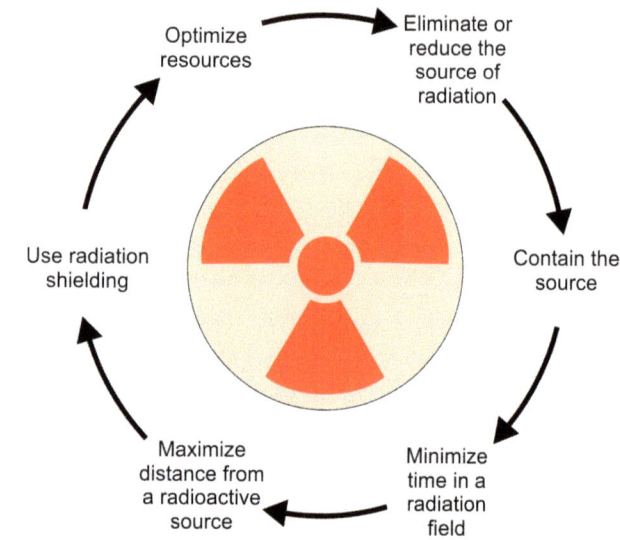

Fig. 10: Six fundamental principles of ALARA.

3. Discuss the role of lung ultrasound in diagnosis of critical clinical conditions. Enumerate the artifacts observed.

A sonographic, physiologic assessment for shock, often described as the RUSH (rapid ultrasound in shock) examination, has gained popularity. This framework organizes the potential etiologies of shock into three broad, sonographically assessable systems that drive hemodynamics, which can be simplified as:

a. *Pump:* Cardiac function
b. *Tank:* Intravascular volume status
c. *Pipes:* Vascular emergencies in the venous and arterial systems.

Careful evaluation of these components can enable clinicians to quickly identify the underlying etiology of shock in patients with undifferentiated hypotension and subsequently allow early initiation of the most appropriate treatment.
a. Pericardial effusion
b. Global left ventricular (LV) contractility
c. Right ventricular (RV) strain
d. Intravascular volume status to assess the inferior vena cava (IVC)
e. A FAST examination is performed to evaluate for fluid in the peritoneal and thoracic cavities
f. To assess for a tension pneumothorax
g. Aortic aneurysms and dissection.

4. Describe the utility of low-frequency probes during resuscitation.

The utility of various low-frequency probes during resuscitation is given in **Table 10**.

TABLE 10: Indications of various low-frequency probes are required for imaging at greater depths.

Linear	Curvilinear	Phased array
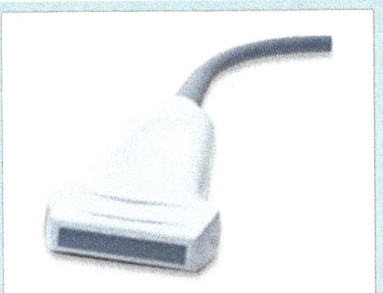	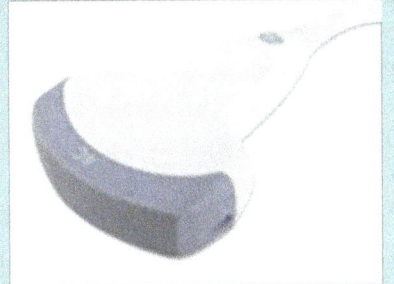	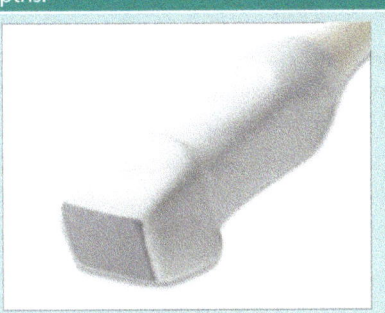
a. "Vascular probe" b. High frequency (5–10 MHz) c. Lower penetration d. Great image quality e. Big footprint f. Bad for movement g. *Uses:* Vascular, pleural, optic nerve, venous access	a. "Abdominal probe" b. Low frequency (2.5–5 MHz) c. Higher penetration d. Lose image quality e. Big footprint f. Bad for movement g. *Uses:* Abdominal, FAST, E-FAST, lung, pleural, gyn	a. "Cardiac probe" b. Low frequency (2–8 MHz) c. Higher penetration d. Lose image quality e. Small footprint f. Great for movement g. *Uses:* Cardiac, lung, pleural, FAST, EFAST, TCD

(FAST: focused assessment with sonography in trauma; E-FAST: extended focused assessment with sonography in trauma; TCD: transcranial Doppler)

■ SUGGESTED READING

1. Richhariya D, Sharma B. Textbook of Emergency Medicine including Intensive Care and Trauma, 2nd edition. New Delhi: Jaypee Brothers Medical Publishers (P) Ltd; 2022. pp. 1557-64. (Question 1).
2. Richhariya D, Sharma B. Textbook of Emergency Medicine including Intensive Care and Trauma, 2nd edition. New Delhi: Jaypee Brothers Medical Publishers (P) Ltd; 2022. pp. 319-27. (Question 2).
3. Richhariya D, Sharma B. Textbook of Emergency Medicine including Intensive Care and Trauma, 2nd edition. New Delhi: Jaypee Brothers Medical Publishers (P) Ltd; 2022. p. 237. (Question 3).
4. Richhariya D, Sharma B. Textbook of Emergency Medicine including Intensive Care and Trauma, 2nd edition. New Delhi: Jaypee Brothers Medical Publishers (P) Ltd; 2022. pp. 1557-60. (Question 4).
5. Richhariya D, Sharma B. Textbook of Emergency Medicine including Intensive Care and Trauma, 2nd edition. New Delhi: Jaypee Brothers Medical Publishers (P) Ltd; 2022. pp. 1602-9. (Question 5).
6. Richhariya D, Sharma B. Textbook of Emergency Medicine including Intensive Care and Trauma, 2nd edition. New Delhi: Jaypee Brothers Medical Publishers (P) Ltd; 2022. pp. 1159, 1687. (Question 6).
7. Richhariya D, Sharma B. Textbook of Emergency Medicine including Intensive Care and Trauma, 2nd edition. New Delhi: Jaypee Brothers Medical Publishers (P) Ltd; 2022. p. 245. (Question 7).
8. Richhariya D, Sharma B. Textbook of Emergency Medicine including Intensive Care and Trauma, 2nd edition. New Delhi: Jaypee Brothers Medical Publishers (P) Ltd; 2022. pp. 18-20. (Question 8).
9. Richhariya D. Sharma B. Textbook of Emergency Medicine including Intensive Care and Trauma, 2nd edition. New Delhi: Jaypee Brothers Medical Publishers (P) Ltd; 2022. pp. 311-5. (Question 9).
10. Richhariya D, Sharma B. Textbook of Emergency Medicine including Intensive Care and Trauma, 2nd edition. New Delhi: Jaypee Brothers Medical Publishers (P) Ltd; 2022. pp. 364-73. (Question 10).

Emergency Medicine Paper 26

Devisha Varma Jhunjhunwala

Question 1

A 35-year-old male bike rider presents to the emergency department (ED) with a history of head-on collision with a motor vehicle. He is drowsy and sonorous, responding with "aaah-uggh" on painful stimuli and extensor response in lower limbs. Pulse is 120 beats/min, blood pressure (BP) 80/60 mm Hg, and oxygen saturation 70%. On examination, his mouth is full of blood and breath sounds are not heard over the left lung.

1. How will you approach and manage this case?

The patient is a case of trauma. Hence, as per advanced trauma life support (ATLS), we will approach the patient with ABCDE (airway, breathing, circulation, disability, exposure).

Airway: We will give supplemental oxygen to the patient and look for any foreign body or secretions to be suctioned out, and put a cervical collar to prevent cervical injury.

Breathing: Look for any asymmetrical chest rise to rule out pneumothorax, flail chest, etc. Call for chest X-ray imaging. History and findings suggestive of left lung pneumothorax or hydropneumothorax.

Circulation: 1 liter warm isotonic IV fluid should be started and blood transfusion if required.

Disability: Assess the level of consciousness and pupillary reflexes along with plantar reflexes. Act accordingly.

Exposure: Preserve hypothermia.

2. Describe Le Fort classification and management algorithm of maxillofacial injuries.

LeFort classification and management of maxillofacial injury is summarized in **Figure 1**.

Le Fort I: Body of maxilla separated from the pterygoid plate and nasal septum. Teeth and hard palate move.

Le Fort II: Pyramidal fracture across the central maxilla and hard palate.

Le Fort III: Entire face is separated from the skull by fractures of zygomatic suture line, across orbits, and base of nose and ethmoids.

Le Fort IV: Includes Le Fort III and frontal bone.

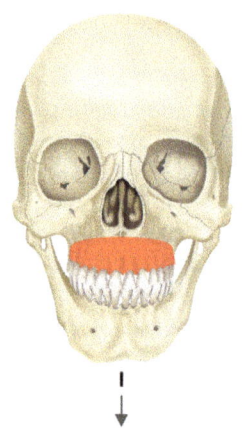
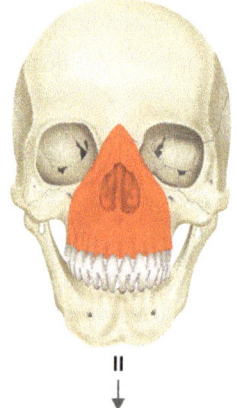
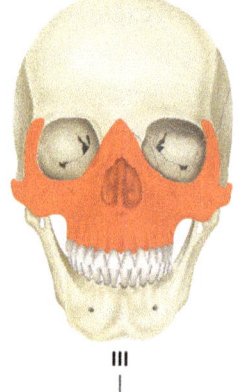

Le Fort I
- Horizontal fracture of maxilla at the level of nasal fossa
- Maxilla moves while the nasal bridge is stable
- No hypesthesia
- Facial edema and malocclusion of teeth are present

Le Fort II
- Pyramidal fracture involving maxilla, nasal bones, and medial aspect of the orbits
- Movement of upper jaw with nose
- Marked facial edema is present with nasal flattening, traumatic telecanthus, epistaxis, or CSF rhinorrhea

Le Fort III
- Craniofacial dissociation involving maxilla, zygoma, nasal bones, ethmoid bones, and bones of base of skull
- Movement of the entire face with distraction
- High risk of airway obstruction
  – Dish-face deformity
  – Facial flattening and elongation
  – Swollen eyes
  – Protrusion of mandible

Fig. 1: Types of Le Fort fracture. (CSF: cerebrospinal fluid)

Management: To protect airway from hemorrhage and mechanical obstruction **(Flowchart 1)**, remove avulsed teeth or foreign bodies. Emergency Physician should be ready to manage difficult airway, bag mask ventilation should be effective and alternate airway device should be ready. Keep cricothyrotomy as a backup if other airway securing methods fail.

Hemorrhage: Control posterior nasal epistaxis early with nasal tampon, dual-balloon device, or Foley's catheter placement. After intubation, oral packing might be needed for severe facial bleeding.

3. Discuss the role of point-of-care ultrasound (POCUS) in this case.

Point-of-care ultrasound is a noninvasive way to speed up diagnosis and treat patient. By using POCUS in this case, we can find lung sliding, B-lines, or comet tail artifacts. A-lines and lung point sign can be seen to detect pneumothorax over the left lung. Ocular ultrasound plays an important role in differentiating orbital ultrasound from normal orbit.

eFAST: Evaluation of the thorax is also added later on in the traditional FAST (focused assessment with sonography in trauma) examination to detect pneumothorax. The protocol for evaluation of shock, respiratory distress, and cardiac arrest is also added, e.g., *Protocol for evaluation of dyspnea*: BLUE [bedside lung ultrasonography (USG) in emergency] and RADIUS (rapid assessment of dyspnea with USG). The BLUE protocol includes only lung USG for detection of pneumothoraxes, as well as pulmonary edema, consolidation, and effusion. RADIUS protocol is similar to BLUE but also includes cardiac and inferior vena cava (IVC) evaluation.

The *RUSH* (rapid USG for shock and hypotension) protocol is simplified and described as an examination of the (a) pump, (b) tank, and (c) pipes for better understanding. The "pump" evaluation includes parasternal long and short axes of the heart, plus subxiphoid and apical views. The "tank" evaluation involves interrogation of the IVC, FAST examination of the abdomen including pleural views, and ultrasound of the lung. The "pipes" portion of RUSH involves visualization of the suprasternal, parasternal, epigastric, and supraumbilical aorta, with additional scans of the femoral and popliteal veins for deep venous thrombosis. The RUSH examination is not specifically for trauma patients; thus, the "pipes" portion of the protocol is usually not necessary in the setting of acute trauma. The number of different protocols for evaluation of the critically injured patients is a source of confusion. Most practical and time-efficient of these protocols is the eFAST examination, which includes evaluation for pneumothorax, and portions of the RUSH examination, which includes a brief subcostal view of the heart and evaluation of the IVC.

Flowchart 1: Management of maxillofacial injuries.

```
• Primary survey
• Airway
• Breathing
• Circulation
        ↓
Other life-/limb-threatening injuries
        ↓
Secondary survey
```

Sinuses	Nose Ear	Major bones	Eyes/Orbit	Lacerations
• Associated intracranial injuries • Disruption or crepitance near orbit • Depressed skull fracture • Inspect for foreign body	• Asymmetry • Widening of nasal bridge • Tenderness, crepitus • Bimanual palpation test • Nasal septal hematoma, auricular hematoma • Battle sign • Hemotympanum • CSF rhinorrhea, otorrhea	• Complete inspection • Palpate the major facial bones for crepitus • Look for associated intracranial or spinal injuries • Tongue blade test for mandible fracture • TMJ dislocation	• Check visual acuity, light perception • Hyperesthesia • Exophthalmos or enophthalmos • Raccoon eyes • Check facial stability • Neo fractures • Ocular ultrasound	• Look for entrapment injuries, avulsion, intraoral lacerations • Seek surgical consultation for eyelid, lip, ear, penetrating and contaminated wounds

(CSF: cerebrospinal fluid; TMJ: temporomandibular)

Question 2

1. Describe Full Outline of Unresponsiveness (FOUR) scale in comparison to Glasgow Coma Scale (GCS) score.

Full outline of unresponsiveness is a new validated coma scale as an alternative to GCS in evaluation of the level of consciousness. The FOUR scale remains testable in critically ill patients who are intubated **(Table 1)**.

TABLE 1: Grading of Full outline of unresponsiveness (FOUR) coma scale in comparison to Glasgow Coma Scale (GCS) score.

GCS	FOUR score
Eye opening response: • Spontaneously, 4 • To speech, 3 • To pain, 1	*Eye response:* • Open and tracking or blinking to command, 4 • Open but not tracking, 3 • Closed but open to loud voice, 2 • Closed but open to pain, 1 • Closed with pain, 0
Best verbal response: • Oriented, 5 • Disoriented, 4 • Inappropriate words, 3 • Incomprehensible sounds, 2 • No response, 1	*Motor response:* • Thumbs up, fist, or peace sign, 4 • Localizes pain, 3 • Flexion response to pain, 2 • Extension response to pain, 1 • No response to pain or myoclonic status, 0
Best motor response: • Obeys commands, 6 • Localizes pain, 5 • Withdrawal from pain, 4 • Decorticate flexion, 3 • Decerebrate extension, 2 • No movement, 1	*Brainstem reflexes:* • Pupil and corneal reflexes present, 4 • One pupil wide and fixed, 3 • Pupil or corneal reflexes absent, 2 • Pupil and corneal reflexes absent, 1 • Absent pupil, corneal, and cough reflex, 0 *Respiration:* • Not intubated, regular pattern, 4 • Not intubated, Cheyne–Stokes pattern, 3 • Not intubated, irregular breathing, 2 • Breathes above the ventilator rate, 1 • Breathes at the ventilator rate or apnea, 0

2. Describe pediatric emergency care applied research network (PECARN) rule.

Pediatric emergency care applied research network prediction rule is used to identify children with minor head injury who are at a very low risk of clinically significant intracranial injury.

Low-risk criteria for infants and children with minor head injury:

a. *Age <2 years clinical criteria:* Normal mental status, no scalp hematoma except frontal, loss of consciousness for <5 seconds, no severe mechanism, no palpable skull fracture, normal behavior as per parents.

b. *Age >2 years clinical criteria:* Normal mental status, no loss of consciousness, no vomiting, no severe mechanism, no sign of basilar skull fracture, and no severe headache.

3. Describe optic nerve sheath diameter (ONSD) and its clinical significance.

Intracranial pressure (ICP) evaluation is measuring ONSD 3 mm behind the eye. Less than 5 mm is normal. Ultrasound is used for assessment of papilledema in cases of increased ICP. Bedside ocular USG for measuring ONSD can be used as an early test for diagnosing raised ICP as it is a noninvasive, cost-effective bedside test, which can be repeated for re-evaluation.

4. What is Cushing's reflex?

Elevations in ICP are life-threatening and known as Cushing's reflex.

It includes hypertension, bradycardia, and respiratory irregularity.

Question 3

1. Enumerate the causes of acute-onset abdominal pain in the epigastric region. Discuss the investigations to be sent from the ED to reach the most probable diagnosis.

Causes of epigastric abdominal pain are esophagitis, peptic ulcer disease, perforated ulcer, pancreatitis, and biliary tract disease. Blood tests include amylase and lipase for pancreatitis, electrolytes for dehydration, liver function tests (LFTs) for cholecystitis or hepatitis, and electrocardiogram (ECG) for ischemia or infarction.

2. Describe the clinical features and management of acute appendicitis.

Diagnosis should be considered in any patient who comes with severe abdominal pain in the upper abdomen/back/chest, who is apparently in distress, or who has vomiting, tachycardia, epigastric tenderness and pain that is not easily controlled with analgesics. He may be an alcoholic or there may be a past history of pancreatitis/biliary colic.

Right lower quadrant pain, flank pain, nausea, vomiting, worsening of pain on deep inspiration due to peritoneal irritation, and rebound tenderness and guarding suggest peritonitis.

Rovsing's sign: Pain over McBurney's point while palpating the descending colon in the left lower quadrant.

Psoas sign: Elicited if abdominal pain is produced with extension of right leg at the hip while the patient lies on the left side. Obturator test elicits pain with internal and external rotation of flexed right thigh at the hip.

Investigations in ED that would help to differentiate all these are ECG, complete blood count (CBC), LFT, amylase, creatinine, abdominal X-ray (both erect and supine), and USG. No laboratory test is gold standard of acute pancreatitis. Amylase or lipase values should be at least three times the upper limit of the normal values according to the current recommendations. Treatment of acute appendicitis is summarized in **Table 2**.

TABLE 2: Treatment of acute appendicitis.

Airway, breathing, circulation	Supplemental oxygen, vital signs, and pulse oximetry monitoring (every 2 hourly)
Pain control	Parenteral analgesics and narcotics
Crystalloid therapy	Ringer's lactate 250–500 mL/hr or 5–10 mL/kg/hr (2.5–4 L), monitor hematocrit, creatinine, heart rate MAP 65–85 mm Hg, urine output 0.5–1 mL/kg/hr
Electrolyte therapy	Correction of low ionized calcium and low magnesium, and control hyperglycemia
Antiemetics and antibiotics	• Control of nausea and vomiting, NPO status with early resumption of oral feeding, placing of nasogastric tube, and suctioning not indicated • Antibiotics not indicated prophylactically or in mild pancreatitis; antibiotics only indicated in strongly suspected infection
Gastroenterologist consultation	In diagnosed biliary obstruction and cholangitis, ERCP is indicated in the first 24 hours

(ERCP: endoscopic retrograde cholangiopancreatography; MAP: mean arterial pressure; NPO: nil per os)

Question 4

1. Enumerate the causes of vaginal bleeding in a 16-year-old female.

a. Ectopic pregnancy
b. Menstrual cycle irregularity due to polycystic ovarian disease
c. Threatened abortion
d. Molar pregnancy
e. Endometriosis
f. Sexual assault/trauma
g. Urinary tract infection
h. Ovarian torsion

2. Describe abruptio placenta, its pathophysiology, clinical presentation, and ED management.

Abruption of placenta means premature separation of placenta.

Symptoms: Abdominal pain, bleeding, severe shock.

Signs: Shock spasm of uterus, fetal part hard to feel, often no fetal heart sound. All emergency protocols should be considered while shifting the patient to the obstetric emergency unit.

a. *Pathophysiology:* Abruptio placenta is premature separation of normal implanted placenta from the uterine lining. Spontaneous abruptio placenta occurs between 24 and 28 weeks.
b. *Clinical presentation:* Mild abruption has mild uterine tenderness, no or mild vaginal bleeding, normal maternal vital signs, no coagulopathy, and fetal distress.

   Severe abruption has no or severe vaginal bleeding, fetal distress, coagulopathy, severe uterine pain or tenderness, continuous uterine contractions, maternal hypotension or shock, nausea, or vomiting.
c. *ED management includes:*
   i. Maternal stabilization
   ii. Electronic fetal monitoring (cardiotocodynamometry) to identify fetal distress
   iii. Emergency obstetrician consultation
   iv. Place two large-bore IV lines
   v. Obtain CBC, coagulation panel, fibrin degradation product, and crossmatch maternal blood
   vi. Administer anti-D Ig intramuscularly if the mother is Rh negative.
   vii. Transvaginal scan for retroplacental clot
   viii. Immediate delivery indicated.

3. Enumerate the salient features of perimortem cesarean section. What are the additional features of maternal cardiopulmonary resuscitation (CPR)?

Perimortem C-section: Shift focus from a typical cardiac arrest scenario to one that focuses on both maternal CPR and rapid delivery of the baby **(Table 3)**.

Features of maternal CPR:

a. During the procedure, continue CPR. Step away if defibrillating the patient during resuscitation.
b. Left lateral tilt position **(Figs. 2A and B)** if compressions can be performed. Else supine.
c. *Maternal preparation:* Splash abdomen with povidone iodine to avoid delay.
d. Drain bladder for better visualization and also decrease bladder injury.

e. Make a vertical incision with scalpel below umbilicus to symphysis pubic.
f. Linea nigra is guide for midline.
g. Use fingers to bluntly separate rectus muscles laterally.
h. *Enter peritoneum:* Expose uterus; while the assistant retracts above the bladder, make a vertical incision on the midline of uterus. When the anterior placenta is encountered, proceed to deliver the baby.
i. Rupture amniotic sac and have wall suction ready to evacuate fluid.
j. *Fetal delivery:* Steady pressure to the fundus to assist baby delivery in vertex position.
k. If breech presentation, deliver buttocks first followed by both legs and body.
l. *Placental delivery and uterine care:* Manually remove placenta. If an obstetrician is available, then complete closure with their help; if not available, then exteriorize the uterus and clean the uterine cavity with sponges until cleared. Close the uterus with one or two running stitches of number 0 or 1 vicryl.

TABLE 3: Steps in perimortem cesarean section.

Recommended equipment	Steps of resuscitative hysterotomy
• Sterile gloves • Fixed blade scalpel • Sterile scissors • Umbilical cord clamps • Antiseptic	a. With continuing maternal resuscitation and manual left uterine displacement, if antiseptic solution is available, pour over the abdomen b. Make an incision over the abdomen—vertical incision (preferred over Pfannenstiel) from xiphisternum to pubic symphysis as it allows more space for visualization c. Incision from skin to peritoneum d. Make vertical incision over the uterus from fundus to lower segment of uterus e. Stretch the uterine incision through fingers to allow easy access to the delivery f. Deliver the baby after cutting the cord between the two umbilical clamps. Hand over the baby to a neonatologist g. Deliver the placenta h. Uterus to be closed in layers followed by closure of abdomen as done in a regular manner i. Oxytocin and antibiotics can be considered j. Foley's catheter can be placed

Incisions

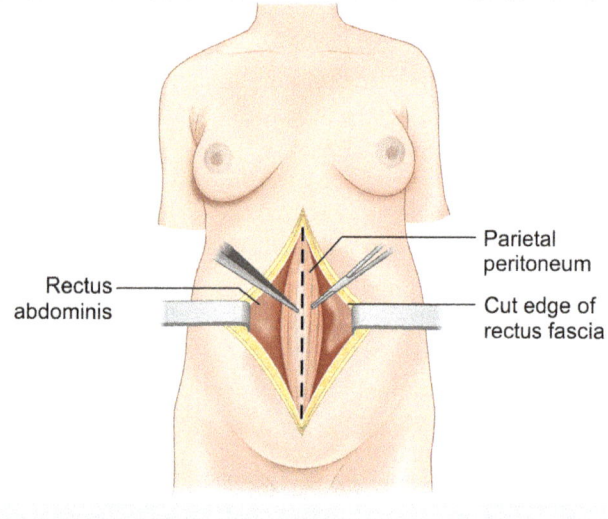

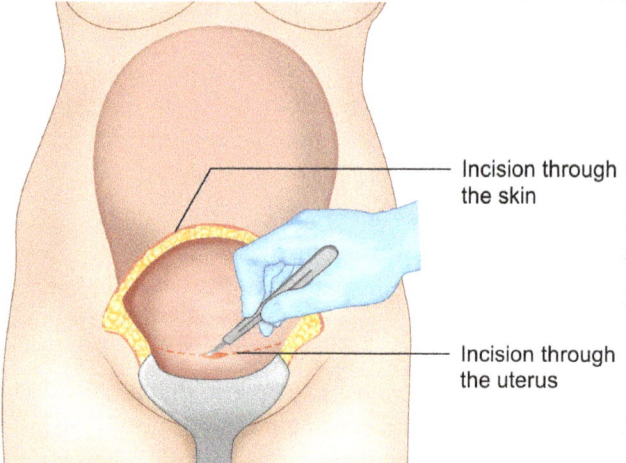

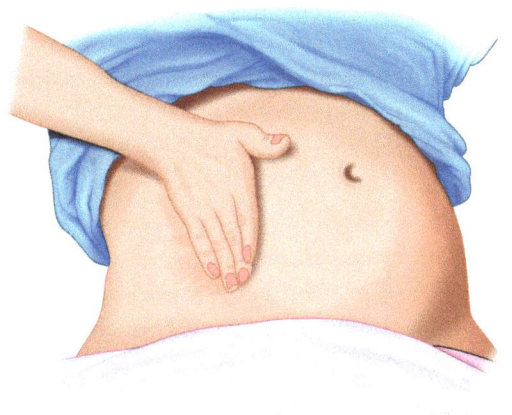
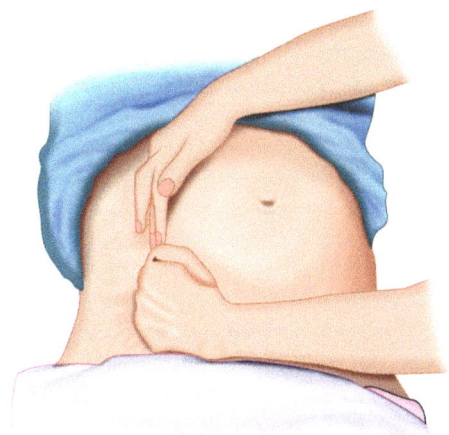

Figs. 2A and B: *Left lateral tilt position:* (A) One-handed technique; (B) Two-handed technique.

Question 5

1. Discuss the evaluation and management of penetrating eye injury in a young boy.

Evaluation: Examine early before swelling of eyelids or use retractors, document visual acuity, systematically examine eye from front to back, check pupil for tear drop sign pointing globe rupture and hyphema, and conduct swinging flashlight test for afferent papillary effect.

Fat through wound indicates orbital septal perforation. Check intraocular pressure for evidence of orbital compartment syndrome in absence of globe injury. Binocular double vision suggests entrapment of extraocular muscles, whereas monocular double vision suggests lens dislocation.

Management: Airway management is done during primary survey of eye trauma which is likely seen in facial trauma. Do not administer paralytics unless the patient can be bagged effectively or alternate airway devices are in place. Apply direct pressure to external wounds to control hemorrhage.

2. Enumerate the causes of keratoconjunctivitis and its management in the ED.

The causes of keratoconjunctivitis are as follows:
a. *Viral:* Pharyngoconjunctival fever presents with fever, conjunctivitis, pharyngitis, and preauricular adenopathy. *Epidemic keratoconjunctivitis* presents with eye pain, photophobia, subepithelial defects, and pseudomembranes over conjunctiva. Topical antibiotics should NOT be prescribed because there is no evidence of protection against secondary infections.
b. *Bacterial: Haemophilus* species, *Streptococcus pneumoniae, Moraxella catarrhalis,* and *Staphylococcus aureus.*

Management: Topical antibiotic such as fluoroquinolones (ciprofloxacin and ofloxacin) and bacitracin-polymyxin.

Allergic conjunctivitis: Management includes allergen avoidance, topical antihistamines, and mast cell stabilizers.

3. What is Seidel sign?

Fluorescein is instilled in eye. It binds to damaged corneal epithelium and looks green under Wood's lamp. A positive Seidel test shows aqueous humor leaking through a full-thickness corneal wound. Aqueous wound will turn fluorescein lime green under a cobalt blue light as it oozes through the wound while being observed through a slit lamp. The Seidel test can be negative with a small or spontaneously sealing corneal laceration.

4. Discuss the approach to orbital cellulitis in a 65-year-old diabetic female.

Orbital cellulitis is extension of sinus infection into orbit or traumatic inoculation.
a. Bacteria: *S. pneumoniae, H. influenzae, M. catarrhalis, S. aureus, Streptococcus pyogenes,* and bacteroides
b. Seen as erythema and swelling around eye
c. Suspect if eyelid or periorbital inflammation is accompanied by any of the following: Ptosis, impaired extra ocular movements, pain with eye movement, chemosis, or afferent papillary defect
d. Inpatient management, possible surgical drainage
e. Oral antibiotics to complete 3 weeks' course
f. Cefuroxime (50 mg/kg IV every 8 hours)
g. Ampicillin–sulbactam (50 mg/kg IV every 6 hours)
h. If anaerobic infection, suspect clindamycin (10 mg/kg every 6 hours).

Question 6

1. Compare and contrast the two major classifications of pelvic fractures.

2. Discuss the clinical presentation and patient profile for pelvic fractures.

3. Discuss the management of unstable pelvic fractures in the ED.

Different pattern of pelvic fracture based on mechanism of injury and direction of causative force are given in **Table 4**.

Clinical presentation of a pelvic fracture patient is given in **Table 5**.

Management principles include:
a. Unstable patient, stabilize with bedsheet or pelvic binding device to reduce pelvic volume and stabilize fracture ends.
b. Resuscitate with crystalloid, blood, and blood products.
c. Retroperitoneal bleeding may complicate pelvic fractures.
d. Up to 4 L blood can be accommodated in pelvis, until vascular pressure is overcome and tamponade occurs.
e. If FAST reveals free intraperitoneal fluid, then computed tomography (CT) scan is needed to determine the next step.
f. If a pelvic fracture patient is unstable and other sources of bleeding have been excluded through CT or laparotomy, angiography with embolization is done.

TABLE 4: Classifications of pelvic fractures.

Category	Characteristics	Severe hemorrhage	Bladder rupture	Urethral injury
Lateral compression fracture	Transverse fracture of pubic rami, ipsilateral or contralateral to posterior injury	60	20	20
Anterior posterior fracture (open book)	• Symphyseal diastasis and/or longitudinal rami fractures • Secondary injured structures vary based on the severity of AP pelvic fracture • Minimal widening of SI joint with intact posterior ligaments • Complete SI joint widening with disruption of posterior ligaments	1 53	8 14	12 36
Vertical shear fracture	Separation of symphysis and/or SI joint with vertical displacement anteriorly or posteriorly, occasionally through iliac wing and/or sacrum	75	15	25
Mixed patterns	Combination of other injury patterns, lateral compression or vertical shear being common	58	6	21

(AP: anteroposterior; SI: sacroiliac)

TABLE 5: Clinical presentation and patient profile for pelvic fractures.

Fracture	Clinical findings
Iliac wing (Duverney)	Swelling tenderness over iliac wing, abdominal pain, ileus, acetabular fractures
Single ramus of pubis or ischium	Local pain and tenderness, may have inability to ambulate
Ischium body	Local pain, tenderness, pain with hamstring movement
Sacral fracture	Pain on rectal examination, sacral root injury with upper transverse fracture, vertical fracture may transect pelvic ring
Coccyx fracture	Pain, tenderness over sacral region, pain on compression during rectal examination
Anterior superior iliac spine	Pain with hip flexion and abduction
Anterior inferior iliac spine	Pain in groin, pain with hip flexion
Ischial tuberosity	Pain with sitting or flexing the thigh

Question 7

1. Describe the clinical features and management of acute necrotizing ulcerative gingivitis.

a. Acute necrotizing ulcerative gingivitis is a progressive infection of gingiva and presents with pain, edema, ulceration, fever, halitosis, decreased appetite, and generalized malaise.
b. Poor hygiene, smoking, immunosuppression, viral infections, stress, and sleep deprivation.
c. It is mixed infection which includes spirochetes (*Prevotella intermedia*).
d. Ludwig's angina is when this gingivitis spreads beyond gingiva to involve deeper tissues/mouth floor.
e. *Treatment:* Analgesia, better oral hygiene, antimicrobial oral rinses, extensive disease require local debridement, and parenteral antibiotic therapy.

2. Discuss the clinical features and management of peritonsillar abscess.

Peritonsillar abscess is a deep oropharyngeal infection. It occurs in adolescents and young adults. Pus is formed between tonsillar capsule and superior constrictor muscle.

Bacteria: Beta hemolytic streptococci, *S. aureus*, *H. influenzae*

Clinical features: Sore throat, fever, chills, trismus, voice change (hot potato voice), ipsilateral ear pain, may be torticollis

Treatment: Trial of oral antibiotics (ampicillin, sulbactam, clindamycin), prompt aspiration or incision and drainage using local anesthetics at ED.

3. Discuss the management of temporomandibular joint dislocation in ED.

Management of temporomandibular joint dislocation (Fig. 3): The head should be firmly placed against the wall. Few layers of gauze should be placed over gloved thumbs for protection. Emergency Physician should be facing the patient. Insert gloved thumb in patient's mouth over mandibular molar as deep as possible. Curve fingers beneath the angle and body of mandible. Apply pressure downward and backward toward the patient. Alternatively reduction can be done by examiner standing behind and above the reclined patient, thumbs are inserted on molors and downward and backward is applied.

4. Discuss the nerve blocks of face.

a. Provide analgesia with little or no distortion to face.
b. Topical anesthetic applied to mucosa should be used before the intraoral approach for infraorbital and mental nerve blocks.
c. *Supraorbital and supratrochlear nerve blocks:* The purpose of these blocks is to provide anesthesia to the entire forehead up to the vertex of scalp and down the ridge of nose.
d. *Infraorbital nerve block:* The purpose of this block is to provide anesthesia to lower lid, medial cheek, ipsilateral side of nose and ipsilateral upper lip.
e. *Mental nerve block:* The purpose of this block is to provide anesthesia to labial mucosa, gingiva, and lower lip adjacent to incisors and canines.
f. *Auricular block:* The purpose of this block is to provide anesthesia to the entire ear.

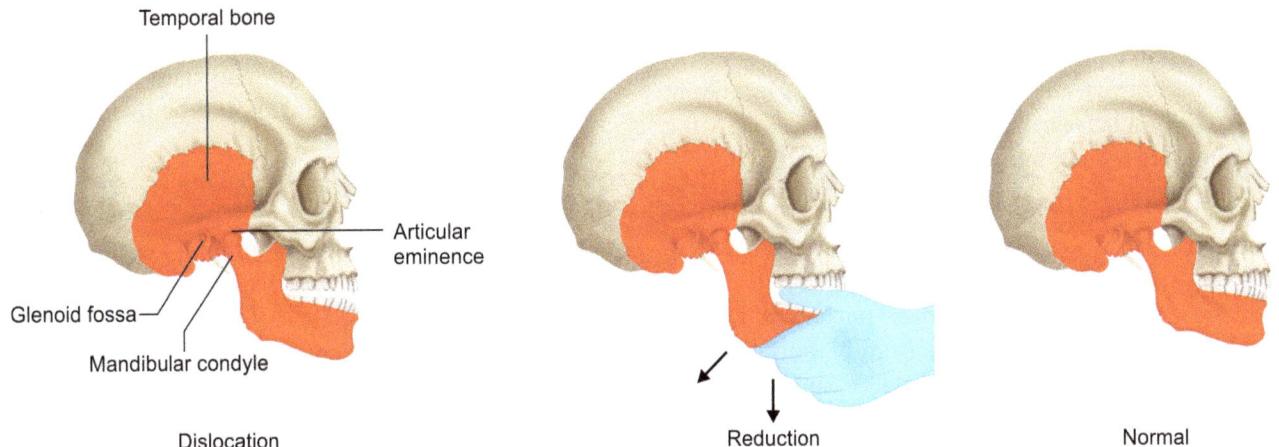

Fig. 3: Technique of managing temporomandibular joint dislocation.

Question 8

1. Discuss the assessment and management of lip laceration.

Assessment: The cosmetically important junction of skin and red portion of lips is the vermillion border. Orbicularis oris muscle surrounding the mouth is responsible for retaining saliva inside the mouth and producing bilabial sounds of speech and facial expressions.

a. Identify missing, impacted or fractured teeth, and exposed bone of maxilla or mandible.
b. If teeth are missing, after adequate anesthesia, explore the wound to find out any broken pieces embedded in laceration.
c. If laceration crosses vermillion skin and/or vermillion mucosal border.

Management: Intraoral mucosa lacerations may not need sutures if they are isolated and wound edegs spontaneously approximate (<1 cm in length).

a. Larger gaping needs to be sutured with 5-0 rapidly absorbable suture carefully to evert edges including only mucosa with entrance 2-3 mm from wound edges. Irrigate.

b. Next, approximate orbicularis oris muscle with 4-0 or 5-0 absorbable sutures with simple interrupted or horizontal mattress. Irrigate again.
c. Later, suture skin with 6-0 nonabsorbable monofilament suture in a simple interrupted fashion.
d. Skin adhesive can also be used as an alternative.
e. Wounds which cross the vermillion border should be repaired by placing the first stitch with 6-0 nonabsorbable monofilament suture to precisely align the edges of the vermillion border. After this, repair vermillion with 6-0 material and mucosa with 5-0 absorbable suture.
f. Prescribe antibiotics and analgesics and follow-up for wound healing.

2. Discuss the evaluation and management of necrotizing fasciitis of leg.

In necrotizing fasciitis of leg, there is direct invasion of subcutaneous tissue from external trauma (IV, surgical incision, abscess, insect bite, or ulcer) or direct spread from perforated viscus (colon, rectum, or anus).

Infection can spread as fast as 1 in/hr. Type 1 occurs in extremities, caused by polymicrobial infections, gram-positive cocci, gram-negative rods, anaerobes, and *Clostridium*.

Symptoms: Severe pain out of proportion, anxiety, diaphoresis, and tenderness beyond erythema.

Crepitus brawny edema due to bacterial gas may be present. Low-grade fever, bullae, hypotension, gas on X-ray, and crepitus are seen in some patients but not all.

Management: Immediate surgical intervention is recommended for successful management followed by broad-spectrum antibiotics. Aggressive fluid resuscitation should be followed. Transfusion of packed red blood cells is required if there is anemia from hemolysis. Avoid vasoconstrictors because they will decrease perfusion to already ischemic tissue.

Surgery: Fasciotomy, amputation, and debridement are decided by the surgeon.

Mortality is higher if debridement is delayed by >24 hours.

3. Discuss the evaluation and management of bleeding scalp wounds.

a. Look for intracranial injury before definitive wound care.
b. Control scalp hemorrhage by applying direct pressure or clamping involved vessel at wound edges until complete assessment.
c. Gently palpate with gloved finger to assess depth, galeal laceration, or depressed skull fracture.
d. If depression is found, then a CT scan should be done.
e. *Management:* Shaving increases the risk of wound infection. For better vision, brush hair or matt it down with ointment (bacitracin zinc or petroleum). Sometimes, trim adjacent scalp hair with scissors.
f. Suture accessible lacerations to galea to prevent subgaleal hematoma.
g. Close scalp with surgical staples or simple interrupted percutaneous sutures using nonabsorbable monofilament or rapidly absorbable material.
h. Leave suture tails long for easy removal later.
i. Hair braiding is a technique for combing hair apposition and tissue adhesive.
j. Pressure dressing over scalp wounds for 24 hours to prevent wound hematoma.

4. Describe the clinical features and management of local anesthesia-induced systemic toxicity.

Local anesthesia-induced systemic toxicity is dose-related clinical progression of sodium channel blockade in non-target tissues, primary in brain and heart.

a. Toxicity can be characterized by subtle neurologic symptoms to refractory seizures or cardiovascular collapse.
b. Risk can be reduced by reducing dose limitation and applying techniques to minimize systemic absorption.
c. Seizures are treated by benzodiazepines.
d. Vasopressin and tachyarrhythmias agents (beta blockers, calcium channel agonists) should be avoided in such toxicity.
e. IV 20% lipid emulsion 1.5 mL/kg infused over 1 minute with continuous infusion or repeat dose (maximum 10 mL/kg over the initial 30 minutes) is effective treatment for local anesthesia toxicity as bupivacaine has high lipid solubility.
f. Prilocaine and benzocaine cause oxidation of ferrous form, creating methemoglobin that becomes visible as cyanosis if methemoglobin concentration exceeds 1.5 g/dL.

Question 9

1. Discuss the differential diagnosis and management of acute onset of scrotal pain.

a. *Testicular torsion:* Sudden-onset pain and happens in neonates and adolescents.
Undescended testicle and rapid increase in testicular size are risk factors.
High riding transverse alignment of testicle is seen.
Testicular detorsion is done by standing at the foot of or on the right side of the patient's bed. Torsed testis is detorsed similar to opening a book, right testis is rotated counterclockwise, and left is rotated clockwise.

b. *Epididymitis:* Gradual onset of pain and happens in adolescents and young adults.
Risk factors are sexual activity, genitourinary anomalies and genitourinary instrumentation.
Normal position/vertical alignment of testicles is seen.
Oral antibiotics are as follows:
Age <35 years: Treat for gonorrhea and chlamydia with Ceftriaxone 250 mg IV/IM + Doxycyvcline 100 mg PO twice a day for 10 days
Age >35 years: Treat gram-negative bacilli, ofloxacin 300 mg PO twice a day for 10 days, levofloxacin 500 mg PO every day for 10 days.
c. *Appendage torsion:* Variable pain and happens in prepubertal.
Risk factor is presence of appendages.
Normal position/vertical alignment is seen.
Blot dot sign: Pain is localized to the upper pole of testis or epididymis; blue spot is observed through the scrotal skin. Analgesics, bed rest, and supportive underwear are recommended.

2. Describe the clinical features and management of zipper entrapment injury.

Zipper entrapment injury occurs when circumferential objects surrounding penis occlude veins and arterial supply.

Dismantling zipper with wire clutters or trauma shears or surgical interventions such as circumcision are recommended.

Clean the affected area with povidone–iodine, 1–2% lidocaine, and the zipper area with mineral oil or nontoxic lubricant. If not, then cut the zipper away from clothing to make the zipper easier to handle.

Question 10

1. Describe the clinical features and management of intussusception in a child.

Intussusception in a child occurs when one segment of the intestine intertwines into the other, e.g., ileum into colon. Constriction of mesentery leads to engorgement of intussuscepted mass and bowel ischemia. Intussusception is the most common cause of intestinal obstruction in children < 2 years of age.

Clinical features: Intermittent abdominal pain and lethargy (insensitive signs).

Intermittent intussusception: It occurs in 5–12-month-old infants. Pain causes legs drawn to the chest and then pain free in between untill the next episode of pain. Bilious vomiting occurs after 6–12 hours.

Management: High suspicion cases need intermediate air-contrast enema (both diagnostic and therapeutic), bolus of normal saline due to decreased intake, vomiting and intestinal edema, and antiemetics with antibiotics with increased white blood cells (WBC).

Surgeon should be notified. Free air on X-ray is suggestive of peritonitis. Crescent sign on X-ray of the abdomen means that the curved edge of one segment of bowel visibly protrudes into another or an obstructive pattern.

Immediate surgical intervention is required for children who are in shock.

2. Describe the clinical features and management of supracondylar fracture.

Supracondylar fracture is the most common fracture in children <8 years of age.

Pointing finger sign: Injury to anterior interosseous nerve. Classification is based on the extent of the fracture fragment displaced:
a. *Type 1:* Anterior or posterior pad sign on X-ray finding. No displacement or angulation
b. *Type 2:* Angulation at varying degrees, humerus posterior cortex intact
c. *Type 3:* Completely displaced, no cortical contact
    i. *3a:* Distal fragment posteromedially rotated, impinging against the radial nerve
    ii. *3b:* Posterolaterally rotated. There is a risk of injury to the brachial artery and median nerve. Compartment syndrome can develop.

Management:
a. Level of displacement and prereduction manages supracondylar fractures.
b. Analgesics
c. Immobilization
d. Double sugar-tong splint
e. Long arm posterior splint with elbow 90° and forearm pronated or neutral rotation for 3 weeks
f. Operative pinning for types 2 and 3.

3. What is Salter–Harris classification?

Salter–Harris classification of fracture line to the physis and prognosis for growth disturbance **(Fig. 4)**:

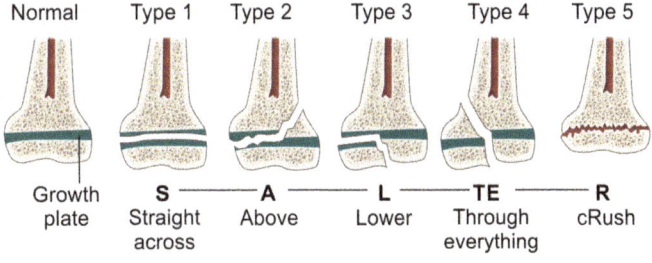

Fig. 4: Salter–Harris classification of fracture.

a. *Type 1:* Epiphysis is separated from metaphysis. There are no associated fragments of bone as thick periosteal attachments surrounding physis remain intact. There is a low incidence of growth disturbance.
b. *Type 2:* Fracture line extends along the hypertrophic cell zone of physis and then out through a piece of metaphyseal bone. Periosteum over the metaphyseal fragment remains intact while the opposite fracture is torn away and adhered to epiphysis but away from diaphysis. On X-ray, a triangular-shaped fragment of metaphysis is seen. Closed reduction of displacement and immobilization, splint, ice, elevation, and analgesia are recommended.
c. *Type 3:* Fracture lines extend intra-articularly from epiphysis, through the hypertrophic zone of physis with cleavage plane along physis to periphery. The X-ray appearance of epiphyseal fragment is not associated with an apparent metaphyseal fracture. Conduct a CT or MRI scan to see the extent of fracture/articular movement. Open reduction to ensure alignment.
d. *Type 4:* Fracture line starts at the articular surface and extends into epiphysis, entire thickness and through metaphysis. The X-ray identifies epiphyseal and metaphyseal fragments. Open surgical reduction is required to treat.
e. *Type 5:* It involves knee or ankle. There is crushing of chondrocytes due to compressive force into physis. Displacement of epiphysis is minimal but significant damage is done to the physis. X-ray mostly looks normal or focal narrowing of physeal plate is seen. There is typical joint effusion. Cast is recommended, and watch for bone growth arrest.

SUGGESTED READING

1. Richhariya D, Sharma B. Textbook of Emergency Medicine including Intensive Care and Trauma 2nd edition. New Delhi: Jaypee Brothers Medical Publishers (P) Ltd; 2022. pp. 1551-5. (Question 1).
2. Richhariya D, Sharma B. Textbook of Emergency Medicine including Intensive Care and Trauma, 2nd edition. New Delhi: Jaypee Brothers Medical Publishers (P) Ltd; 2022. pp. 1551-5. (Question 2).
3. Richhariya D, Sharma B. Textbook of Emergency Medicine including Intensive Care and Trauma, 2nd edition. New Delhi: Jaypee Brothers Medical Publishers (P) Ltd; 2022. pp. 699-70. (Question 3).
4. Richhariya D, Sharma B. Textbook of Emergency Medicine including Intensive Care and Trauma, 2nd edition. New Delhi: Jaypee Brothers Medical Publishers (P) Ltd; 2022. pp. 1114-20. (Question 4).
5. Richhariya D, Sharma B. Textbook of Emergency Medicine including Intensive Care and Trauma, 2nd edition. New Delhi: Jaypee Brothers Medical Publishers (P) Ltd; 2022. pp. 899-905. (Question 5).
6. Richhariya D, Sharma B. Textbook of Emergency Medicine including Intensive Care and Trauma, 2nd edition. New Delhi: Jaypee Brothers Medical Publishers (P) Ltd; 2022. p. 1635. (Question 6).
7. Richhariya D, Sharma B. Textbook of Emergency Medicine including Intensive Care and Trauma, 2nd edition. New Delhi: Jaypee Brothers Medical Publishers (P) Ltd; 2022. pp. 928-42. (Question 7).
8. Richhariya D, Sharma B. Textbook of Emergency Medicine including Intensive Care and Trauma 2nd edition. New Delhi: Jaypee Brothers Medical Publishers (P) Ltd; 2022. p. 1667. (Question 8).
9. Richhariya D, Sharma B. Textbook of Emergency Medicine including Intensive Care and Trauma, 2nd edition. New Delhi: Jaypee Brothers Medical Publishers (P) Ltd; 2022. pp. 773-90. (Question 9).
10. Richhariya D, Sharma B. Textbook of Emergency Medicine including Intensive Care and Trauma, 2nd edition. New Delhi: Jaypee Brothers Medical Publishers (P) Ltd; 2022. pp. 1237, 1615. (Question 10).

Emergency Medicine Paper 27

Susmeet Mishra

Question 1

1. Discuss various scoring systems to predict outcome in acute onset chest pain.

There are various scoring systems to predict outcome in acute onset chest pain but the important ones are mentioned here for comparison. Chest pain is one of the most common causes of presentation to the emergency room. The diagnosis of non-ST-elevation acute coronary syndrome (NSTE-ACS) typically causes uncertainty.

- Classical considerations for risk stratification are history, electrocardiogram (ECG), age, risk factors and troponin (HEART). Each can be scored with zero, one or two points, depending on the extent of the abnormality. The HEART score facilitates accurate diagnostic and therapeutic choices **(Table 1)**. The HEART score is an easy, quick, and reliable predictor of outcome in chest pain patients.
- Another score for reliably predicting outcome is GRACE score. The GRACE score is a prospectively studied scoring system which risk stratifies patients with diagnosed acute coronary syndrome (ACS) to estimate their in-hospital and 6-month to 3-year mortality.
- The thrombolysis in myocardial infarction (TIMI) risk score is a tool used to predict the chances of having or dying from a heart event for people with—unstable angina, a heart condition that causes chest pain, non-ST-segment elevation myocardial infarction (NSTEMI), and a type of heart attack **(Table 2)**.

TABLE 1: Risk stratification—HEART risk score for chest pain patients in ED.

History	• Highly suspicious • Moderately suspicious • Slightly suspicious	2 1 0
ECG	• Significant ST depression • Nonspecific repolarization changes • Normal	2 1 0
Age	• >65 years • 45–65 years • <45 years	2 1 0
Risk factors	• >3 risk • 1 or 2 • No risk	2 1 0
Troponins	• >3 × normal limit • 1–3 × normal limit • < normal limit	2 1 0

Heart Score	Risk of MACE	Recommendations
0–3	0.9%	ED discharge
4–6	12%	Observation
>6	65%	Cardiology admission

(ECG: electrocardiogram; MACE: major adverse cardiac event)

TABLE 2: Risk scores for risk stratification of acute coronary syndrome.

TIMI risk score for STEMI	TIMI risk score for NSTE-ACS	GRACE risk score for entire spectrum of ACS
Score: 0–14 (scores ≥3: high risk)	Score: 0–7 (scores ≥3: high risk)	Range: 1–372 Low risk: <109 Intermediate risk: 109–140 High risk: >141
Based on below variables at admission: 1. ≥65 years 2. Risk factors: Diabetes mellitus, angina, hypertension 3. SBP <100 4. Heart rate >100 5. Weight <67 kg 6. Anterior STE or LBBB 7. Treatment start >4 hours	Based on one point each for seven variables at admission: 1. ≥65 years of age 2. ≥3 risk factors for CAD 3. Prior ≥50% coronary stenosis 4. ST deviation on ECG 5. ≥2 anginal events in prior 24 hours 6. Aspirin use in prior 7 days 7. Elevated cardiac biomarkers	Based on eight variables at admission: 1. Age 2. Heart rate 3. SBP 4. Serum creatinine 5. Killip class 6. Cardiac arrest 7. ST-segment deviation on ECG 8. Elevated cardiac enzymes/markers

(ACS: acute coronary syndrome; ECG: electrocardiogram; LBBB: left bundle branch block; NSTE-ACS: non-ST elevation ACS; SBP: systolic blood pressure; STE: ST-segment elevation; STEMI: ST-elevation myocardial infarction)

2. Explain ECG findings requiring immediate coronary intervention. Enumerate other causes of ST elevation.

Coronary interventions in a center with catheterization laboratory facilities are decided upon by various factors in ECG changes are considered as one of the topmost priorities.
a. ST elevation if elevated >1 mm in 2 limb leads or >2 mm in two chest leads
b. Reciprocal ST depression
c. T wave inversion typically deeply inverted, symmetrical and pointed
d. Pathological Q waves
e. Conduction problems

Other causes of ST elevation: Coronary vasospasm, pericarditis benign early repolarization, left bundle branch block, left ventricular hypertrophy, ventricular aneurysm, Brugada syndrome, ventricular paced rhythm, raised intracranial pressure, takotsubo cardiomyopathy.

3. Describe the utility of cardiac biomarkers in emergency department (ED).

Cardiac biomarkers are used for the diagnosis and risk stratification of patients with chest pain and suspected ACS and for management and prognosis in patients with acute heart failure, pulmonary embolism, and other disease states. Cardiac markers can be classified into those that signify myocardial necrosis [creatine kinase-myoglobin binding (CK-MB) fraction, myoglobin, and cardiac troponins], those that indicate myocardial ischemia (ischemia modified albumin), those that suggest myocardial stress (natriuretic peptides), and those markers of inflammation and prognosis [C-reactive protein (CRP), soluble CD40 ligand (sCD40L), and homocysteine].

The cardiac troponins, in particular, have become the cardiac markers of choice for patients with ACS, eclipsing CK-MB, and myoglobin in terms of clinical value. Indeed, cardiac troponin is central to the definition of acute myocardial infarction (MI) in the consensus guidelines from the European Society of Cardiology (ESC) and the American College of Cardiology (ACC): These guidelines recommend that cardiac biomarkers should be measured at presentation in patients with suspected MI, and that the only biomarker that is recommended to be used for the diagnosis of acute MI at this time is cardiac troponin due to its superior sensitivity and accuracy **(Table 3)**.

4. Discuss classification of acute myocardial infarction.

Acute myocardial infarction is classified as ACS differs with the type of clinical setting **(Table 4)** and the ACS sub-category of (STEMI/NSTE-ACS).

TABLE 3: Cardiac markers trends relative to time.

Cardiac biomarker	Time to appear	Time to peak	Time to return normal
cTn	6–12 hours	24 hours	Up to 14 days
cTn I/T	3–4 hours	24 hours	4–10 days
CK-MB	4–6 hours	24 hours	48–72 hours
Myoglobin	2–4 hours	6–12 hours	24–36 hours

(CK-MB: creatine kinase-myoglobin binding)

TABLE 4: Types of ACS presentation.

Type	Clinical setting	Etiology/findings
Type 1	Spontaneous MI	• Rupture, ulceration, fissuring, erosion or dissection of atherosclerotic plaque OR • Distal platelet emboli with resultant myocyte necrosis.
Type 2	MI secondary to ischemic imbalance	Non-CAD related condition such as arrhythmia, coronary embolus, coronary endothelial dysfunction, coronary artery spasm, anemia, tachycardia, respiratory failure, pulmonary embolism, severe aortic stenosis, hypotension, hypertension, sepsis, use of cardiotoxic drugs, stress, cocaine and tobacco use.
Type 3	MI resulting in death when biomarker values are unavailable	• Death due to cardiac arrest before blood samples could be obtained or before cardiac biomarkers could rise • ECG shows new ischemic changes or new LBBB
Type 4a	MI related to PCI (recurrent MI)	cTn elevation to >5 times the 99th percentile of URL or >20% in patients with normal pre-PCI values AND one of the following: • Angina • ECG—new ischemic changes • Angiography—either reduced blood flow or blockage • Imaging studies—new regional wall motion abnormality
Type 4b	MI related to stent thrombosis (recurrent MI)	• Stent thrombosis on angiography or autopsy AND • Rise and/or fall in cardiac biomarker levels
Type 5	MI related to CABG (recurrent MI)	Cardiac biomarkers values >10 times with 99th percentile of URL in patients with normal pre-CABG values AND one of the following: • ECG—new pathological Q waves or LBBB • Angiography—occlusion of a new graft or native coronary artery • Imaging—new regional wall motion abnormality

(CABG: coronary artery bypass surgery; CAD: coronary artery disease; cTn: cardiac troponin; ECG: electrocardiogram; LBBB: left bundle branch block; MI: myocardial infarction; PCI: percutaneous coronary intervention; URL: upper reference level)

Question 2

1. Describe etiopathogenesis clinical features and management of acute kidney injury (AKI).

Acute kidney injury is defined as a sudden reduction in kidney function that is characterized by a diminished glomerular filtration rate (GFR) as manifested by an increased serum creatinine (SCr) or reduced urine output. AKI is further divided into three categories: **(1) Prerenal**, a kidney blood flow decrease; **(2) Intrarenal**, or kidney parenchymal injury; and **(3) Postrenal**, or urine flow obstruction. Intrarenal AKI is subdivided again on the basis of part of the kidney is involved: Glomeruli, vasculature, or interstitium.

A sudden decrease in kidney function that is characterized by a diminished GFR as manifested by an increased SCr or reduced urine output.

Etiopathogenesis: Four important steps in the renal function are: (1) Glomerulus receives blood flow delivered through circulation. (2) An ultrafiltrate is formed in the glomeruli and then delivered to the renal tubules. (3) Renal tubules reabsorb the solutes and/or water. (4) Tubular fluid (now urine) exits the tubules, draining to the renal pelvis, the ureters and then to the bladder and urine is then expelled via urethra. Any process that interferes with any of the above four structures or steps involved in this process causes renal disease. Rapid decline in the process leads to AKI.

Signs and symptoms of AKI include:
- Decreased urine output (although occasionally, urine output remains normal)
- Chest pain or pressure
- Jugular vein distention
- Fluid retention, causing edematous legs, ankles, or feet
- Shortness of breath
- Confusion
- Nausea
- Seizures or coma in severe cases.

Investigations: For decades, the standard tests for assessing renal function have been blood urea nitrogen (BUN), SCr, GFR, and urine output measurement.

Although BUN has long been considered a marker of kidney injury, it can be affected by many factors, including drug therapy, nutritional status, gastrointestinal (GI) bleeding, trauma, and infection.

New diagnostic biomarkers: More accurate, real-time diagnostic biomarkers to allow early detection of AKI; the emphasis is shifting from biomarkers indicating kidney failure to those that signal a change in kidney function. Research shows that even small changes in kidney function significantly affect outcomes in patients with AKI. Promising biomarkers include the following:

- Neutrophil gelatinase-associated lipocalin (NGAL).
- *Cystatin C:* Elevated serum levels have been found to be early AKI predictors.
- Tissue inhibitor metalloproteinase-2 (TIMP-2). In one study, urinary TIMP-2 testing showed certain patients had seven times the risk of developing AKI.
- *GFR:* This biomarker is reflected directly in urine output. It is one of the best real-time indicators of current kidney function.

Treatment: The timely identification of the at risk patients, timely diagnosis, and early treatment of all the AKI cases are essential part of the general management of individual patients who might be suffering from AKI. The initial principle of AKI management is specifically to treat its causative factor or trigger, such as treating infection in sepsis-associated AKI. The second principle of management and specific treatments according to the underlying cause of AKI syndromes such as hepatorenal syndrome, cardiorenal syndrome, glomerulonephritis, interstitial nephritis, vasculitis, and multiple myeloma, etc. Currently, there are no effective pharmacotherapies for treating acute tubular necrosis (ATN). The third principle is based on ensuring that there is avoidance of any additional insults of AKI. There is a need to optimize hemodynamic that are systemic based, so that even in the absence of some other triggers, additional damage is not experienced and correct perfusion pressure and renal perfusion are adequately maintained. The fourth principle is to apply provide supportive care to prevent and treat complications. Renal replacement therapy (RRT) is a spectrum of dialysis modalities employed in management of renal dysfunction.

2. Discuss sodium bicarbonate therapy.

Administration of sodium bicarbonate in patients with AKI has been controversial. Acidemia and serum pH improved after administration of sodium bicarbonate without reversing the cause of acid production. Patients with severe metabolic acidosis may require sodium bicarbonate therapy as a temporizing measure while the clinician attempts to reverse the underlying cause. Bicarbonate therapy may be helpful in stabilizing the hemodynamic and improve vasopressor sensitivity in patients with a pH <7.1. The recently published BICAR-ICU trial (Sodium Bicarbonate Therapy for Patients with Severe Metabolic Acidosis in the Intensive Care Unit) found no difference between 28-day mortality or organ failure at 7 days between treatment and control groups. However, patients with severe AKI did show a trend toward decreased need for renal replacement therapy who received bicarbonate therapy. Clinicians should be aware of some clinically significant side effects of sodium bicarbonate therapy. A transient increase in arterial PCO_2 can occur as sodium bicarbonate ultimately gets metabolized to CO_2, which may be detrimental for patients with an already extreme minute ventilation.

Indications: Cardiac conduction delays QRS prolongation (e.g., tricyclic antidepressant poisoning) metabolic acidosis related to: Severe renal disease, uncontrolled diabetes, severe primary lactic acidosis, circulatory insufficiency due to shock, severe dehydration, extracorporeal circulation of blood, cardiac arrest, drug toxicities, barbiturates salicylate toxic alcohols urine alkalization, severe diarrhea with HCO_3 loss. Nebulized sodium bicarbonate is an excellent option to treat chemical injuries resulting from chlorine gas, especially within the pulmonary mucosa.

Side effects of sodium bicarbonate therapy: Hypokalemia ionized hypocalcemia prolongation of QTc interval, hypercapnia hemodynamic instability during hemodialysis, and increase in urinary sodium excretion.

3. Discuss urine analysis in ED.

Urine analysis is a very common and the oldest performed procedure in ED which can diagnose a lot more things. It is done in ED to look for:
- Renal disease such as glomerulonephritis, nephritic syndrome, pyelonephritis and renal failure
- Diagnosis of urinary tract infection
- Metabolic disorders such as diabetes mellitus
- Differential diagnosis of jaundice
- Diagnosis of plasma cell dyscrasias
- *Diagnosis of pregnancy:* It is a must for all women in the reproductive age group with amenorrhea and pain abdomen.

4. What are the indications for RRT in ED?
- Diuretic-resistant pulmonary edema
- Hyperkalemia (refractory to medical therapy)
- Metabolic acidosis (refractory to medical therapy)
- Uremic complications (pericarditis, encephalopathy, bleeding)
- Dialyzable intoxications (e.g., lithium, toxic alcohols, and salicylates).

Question 3

1. Discuss clinical features and management of pediatric meningitis.

Clinical features: Fever irritability, headache, projectile vomiting, shrill cry, bulging fontanelle, seizures, altered sensorium, photophobia, neck rigidity, generalized hypertonia, diplopia, ptosis, squint, poor feeding, and refusal to suck.

Kernig's sign: Extension of knee is restricted to <135° when the hip is 90° flexed position.

Brudzinski's sign: On flexing the neck there is flexion of hips and knees.

Management Investigations: Complete blood count—total leukocyte count may be increased in bacterial meningitis. However, a normal total leukocyte count does not rule out meningitis. Measure blood sugar levels frequently. Coagulation profile will be required before performing lumbar puncture.

Chest X-ray: A total of 50% of patient with pneumococcal meningitis have evidence of chests infection in initial X-ray. Blood cultures are to be collected as soon as possible in a patient suspected with meningitis. Blood cultures are positive in 50–80% cases of bacterial meningitis.

Other ancillary tests: Liver function tests, renal function test. Blood biomarkers of inflammation like procalcitonin, CRP can be used to guide treatment.

Neuroimaging: It is not mandatory to perform neuroimaging before initiating treatment in clinically suspected meningitis. Urgent CT brain should be performed in patients with signs of increased intracranial tension before performing lumbar puncture.

Treatment: Priority of treatment is prompt administration of antibiotics.

Bacterial meningitis: After stabilization of airway, breathing and circulation appropriate empirical antibiotics must be administered. If the clinical suspicion is high, empirical antibiotics should be started before performing lumbar puncture. Choice of empirical antibiotics will depend on the infection suspected based on patient's age and premorbid condition **(Table 5)**. Dexamethasone may attenuate the inflammatory response and its consequences such as vasculitis, cerebral edema, etc., and shown to reduce overall mortality and neurological sequelae. First dose of dexamethasone should be administered at-least 10–20 minutes before administration of antibiotics. Dose is 0.15 mg/kg. It is continued every 6 hours for next 4 days. Other corticosteroids have poor central nervous system (CNS) penetrations, hence not to be used. All patients with meningitis have to be hospitalized and started on intravenous antibiotic therapy.

Viral meningitis: There is no specific treatment for viral meningitis and the treatment is largely supportive. Acyclovir 10 mg/kg 8 hourly can be given in herpes simplex virus (HSV) meningitis/encephalitis. Other aspects which may need emergent management in meningitis are septic shock, metabolic complications such as hypoglycemia, acidosis, hypokalemia, raised intracranial tension, seizure, coagulopathy.

TABLE 5: Empirical antibiotic therapy for meningitis.

Age group	Empirical antibiotic therapy
Neonates	Ampicillin (150 mg/kg/day) + 3rd generation cephalosporin, e.g., cefotaxime (100–150 mg/kg/day)
Infant and children	Cefotaxime or ceftriaxone (80–100 mg/kg/day) + vancomycin (60 mg/kg/day)
Adults	Ceftriaxone (80–100 mg/kg/day) + vancomycin (30–60 mg/kg/day)
Immunocompromised patient	Cefotaxime (8–12 g/day) or ceftriaxone (4 g/day) + ampicillin (12 g/day) + vancomycin (30–60 mg/kg/day)
Suspected nosocomial infection	Vancomycin (30–60 mg/kg/day) + ceftazidime (6 g/day) or cefepime (6 g/day) or meropenem (6 g/day)

2. Explain the approach and management of coma in a young adult.

The overall goal of the examination in a comatose patient is to identify key clinical findings that will help narrow our differential diagnosis **(Table 6)** of the patient's comatose state. In addition, it is useful to accurately document the patient's current condition so that subsequent examinations can accurately describe any dynamic changes in clinical status.

Investigations: Complete blood count (CBC), Coagulation panels liver enzymes, renal function test, arterial blood gases (ABG), thyroid stimulating hormone (TSH), urinalysis, cerebrospinal fluid (CSF) studies, toxic screen ECG, CXR, CT brain (noncontract)—the mainstay of ED imaging for/coma, CT angiography/venography—if available can help to diagnose vertebral or basilar artery occlusion, intracerebral aneurysm, venous sinus thrombosis, or AV malformation.

TABLE 6: Causes of coma-differential diagnosis.

Structural CNS diseases	Nonstructural cause		Coma mimics
	Metabolic	Toxic	
• Intracranial hemorrhage • Cerebellar infarct • Cortical infarct • Hydrocephalus • Neoplasia • Metastatic lesions	• Electrolyte imbalance (Hypo and hyperglycemia, Hyponatremia, Hypercalcemia) • Endocrine (adrenal crisis, pituitary apoplexy, thyrotoxic crisis, myxedema coma) • Hepatic encephalopathy • High altitude cerebral edema	• Hypoglycemic agents • Opioids • Carbon monoxide • Methemoglobinemia • Sedatives • Toxic alcohols • Anticonvulsant • Anticholinergics • Psychiatric medications • Beta blockers • Salicylates • Neuroleptic malignant syndrome • Serotonin syndrome	• Locked in syndrome • Neuromuscular paralysis • Psychogenic unresponsiveness

*Treatment of coma i*s based on the three basic cause structural metabolic or toxins.

First: Coma from structural cause can be treated surgically targeted medication or mechanical ventilation. Neurosurgeon is involved for early intervention for intracranial hemorrhage, hydrocephalous.

Second: Coma due to metabolic-induced neuronal dysfunction, conditions like hypoglycemia, hyponatremia should be corrected.

Third: Toxin-induced neuronal dysfunction is managed by initiating the supportive care securing airway, adequate oxygenation, and ventilation; intravenous fluid, inotropes, and vasopressors if required and specific antidote if toxin is identified.

3. Discuss antiepileptic therapy in ED.

Primary management should aim at stabilization of airway, breathing, circulation and administration of medications to terminate the clinical and electrical seizure. Airway, breathing and circulation management is as described above. After stabilization of airway, breathing and circulation ABG analysis may be performed. Initial hyperpyrexia, acidosis, and hypertension may not be immediately treated as it usually subsides without any corrective measures. All the patients should get a blood glucose levels; serum calcium, magnesium, sodium, and potassium levels. If the patient is known epileptic on medication, then blood levels of antiepileptic medications must be performed. Based on history and clinical findings other investigations such as CT scan, lumbar puncture, blood toxicology panel may be performed. Therapy is applied in phase wise manner **(Table 7)**.

TABLE 7: Treatment summary for status epilepticus.

Immediate treatment (first 5–10 minutes)

1.	Monitoring of vitals	Airway, oxygen, cardiac monitor
2.	Securing IV lines	Two lines for blood samples and starting treatment
3.	To start IV fluids	• Fluid of choice is normal saline • To give 100 mg IV thiamine and 50 mL of 50% dextrose in patients with history of alcoholism
4.	First antiepileptic	• To give lorazepam/midazolam/diazepam IV • 0.1 mg/kg bolus dose of IV lorazepam in equal volume of diluent by slow IV push at ~2 mg/min
5.	Repeat dose if seizure persists	Repeat another half of the bolus dose if seizures are not controlled

Early treatment for next 10 minutes to 60 minutes

1.	Loading antiepileptic second-line IV agent	• Phenytoin: IV infusion 15 mg/kg @ 50 mg/min • (Fosphenytoin: IV infusion 15 mg PE/kg @ 100 mg PE/min) • Valproate: IV infusion 25 mg/kg at 3–6 mg/kg/min • Phenobarbital: IV infusion 10 mg/kg at a maximum rate of 100 mg/min • Levetiracetam 20 mg/kg bolus of over 15 minutes
2.	If seizure persists then two options	• Repeat half dose of any of the abovementioned antiepileptic drugs • To load with any of the other antiepileptic drug

Refractory status epilepticus (>60 minutes on going convulsions)

1.	Midazolam infusion (possible to avoid ventilator support)	• Loading: 0.2 mg/kg by slow IV bolus • Maintenance IV: 0.1–0.4 mg/kg/h • Maximum IV dose: 2.0–3.0 mg/kg/h
2.	Thiopental sodium	• Loading 3–5 mg/kg at 0.2–0.4 mg/kg/min • Maintenance IV dose: 3.0–5.0 mg/kg/h • Maximum IV dose: 5.0 mg/kg/h
3.	Propofol infusion	• Loading dose: 1–2 mg/kg at 10 mg/min • Maintenance IV dose: 2–10 mg/kg/h • Maximum IV dose: 15 mg/kg/h

Malignant/Super-refractory status epilepticus (seizures >24 hours)

1.	Magnesium infusion	• Loading: 2–6 g/h • Maintenance 3.5 mmol/L
2.	Hypothermia	• 32–35°C for <48 h • Endovascular cooling vs. external cooling
3.	Immunotherapy	• IV methylprednisolone 1 g/day × 5 days • IV immunoglobulins 0.4 g/kg/day × 5 days • Plasma exchange
4.	Ketogenic diet	• 1:1 or 1:4 ketogenic diet • To avoid glucose containing fluids
5.	Epilepsy surgery	Consider surgery in special circumstances with documented brain lesions responsible for status

Question 4

1. Enumerate the causes of acute onset dyspnea in adult patient based on severity and discuss investigations performed to establish the diagnosis.

Dyspnea or shortness of breath is one of the most common presenting symptoms to the ED. It has been observed to be reported in 50% of patients admitted in tertiary, acute care hospitals. It is one of the most dreaded symptoms to evaluate in ED. It needs to be worked up in matter of minutes as it may depict a potentially life-threatening event **(Table 8)**.

TABLE 8:	Common causes of acute onset dyspnea in ED.
Upper airway	Foreign body, laryngeal edema, laryngospasm, anaphylaxis, epiglottitis
Lower respiratory tract	• Acute asthma, acute exacerbation of chronic obstructive pulmonary disease (COPD), pulmonary embolism, pneumonia, pneumothorax • Massive pleural effusion, interstitial lung disease especially acute interstitial pneumonia, acute hypersensitivity pneumonitis, drug-induced lung disease • Acute aspiration acute respiratory distress syndrome (ARDS)
Cardiac	Acute coronary syndrome, cardiac tamponade, arrhythmias, valvular heart disease, heart failure with reduced ejection fraction
Others	• Metabolic acidosis, severe pain, myasthenic crisis, neuromuscular disorders such as Guillain–Barré syndrome, amniotic fluid embolism, fat embolism • Chest trauma, drug reaction, carbon monoxide poisoning • Anxiety and panic attacks

Investigations: Arterial blood gas, ECG, chest X-ray, high resolution computerized tomographic scans, spirometry.

2. Discuss noninvasive ventilation in ED-weaning protocol.

Weaning from nasal intermittent positive pressure ventilation (NIPPV) may be accomplished by progressively decreasing the amount of positive airway pressure, permitting the patient to be disconnected from the NIPPV for progressively longer durations, or a combination of both.

Noninvasive weaning (NIV) weaning can be attempted when all the following were concurrently met:
- Adequate oxygenation defined as arterial oxygen partial pressure to fraction of inspired oxygen ratio (PaO_2/FiO_2) >200 mm Hg during NIV with fraction of inspired oxygen (FiO_2) <0.5
- pH >7.35, RR <25 without use of respiratory accessory muscles
- Hemodynamic stability (assessed through heart rate and blood pressure)
- Kelly score ≤2

The weaning phase began when all the following criteria were reached after at least 1 hour of disconnection from NIV and by administering oxygen through a venturi mask with a FiO_2 titrated in order to maintain peripheral oxygen saturation (SpO_2) 88–92%:
- pH >7.35, RR <25 without use of respiratory accessory muscles
- Hemodynamic stability
- Kelly score ≤2

3. Suggest with justification initial ventilatory setting for invasive mechanical ventilator for COPD patient.

Initiate mechanical ventilation with the following initial settings for each mode:

Assist control mode—for patients in whom ACV is chosen as the initial mode of ventilation, use the following settings:
- Fraction of inspired oxygen (FiO_2) to maintain the oxygen saturation of hemoglobin (SO_2) >92%
- *Tidal volume:* 6–8 mL/kg
- *Ventilator rate:* 10–16 breaths/min (target minute ventilation 115 mL/kg)
- Positive end expiratory pressure (PEEP): 5–10 cmH_2O
- Inspiratory flow: 60 L/min. Aim I:E 1: 3 or more
- Trigger sensitivity: −1 to −2 cmH_2O when pressure triggering is used or 2 L/min when flow triggering is used.

Synchronous intermittent mandatory ventilation/pressure support ventilation: Usually less used for short-term ventilation. If chosen, use similar settings to ACV with the addition of pressure support (5–10 cmH_2O) for spontaneous breaths taken by the patient above the set rate. The pressure support can be subsequently increased as needed for patient comfort.

Pressure-limited ventilation: Although rarely chosen as an initial mode of ventilation. Set the inspiratory pressure to target a tidal volume of 4–8 mL/kg and an inspiratory: expiratory (I:E) ratio of no <1:3. The FiO_2, ventilator rate, applied PEEP, flow settings, and trigger sensitivity are similar to those of ACV.

Pressure support volume: Usually used as a weaning mode; titrate pressure support to keep respiratory rate <30/min.

Patients with COPD will often have higher than expected minute ventilation requirements and increased carbon dioxide retention, which typically improves over the patient's course.

Question 5

1. Discuss tricyclic antidepressant (TCA) poisoning.

Tricyclic antidepressant: Although their popularity has decreased in recent years, tricyclic antidepressants (TCAs) remain a frequent cause of drug exposure and overdose, in most cases requiring emergent medical care. TCAs are associated with more drug-related deaths than any other class of prescription medication.

Clinical features and diagnosis of tricyclic antidepressant toxicity: Tricyclic antidepressant at therapeutic dose of <1 mg/kg is not toxic. Ingestion of >10 mg/kg TCA is life-threatening. Geriatric and pediatric age group population and patient on cardiotoxic, sedative and antipsychotic drugs, patient with underlying heart and neurologic disease are at higher risk of developing TCA toxicity. Combination of four criteria: (1) History of TCA drug intake, (2) Clinical features, (3) Typical ECG findings, and (4) Positive urine drug screen for TCA are essential for diagnosis of TCA toxicity.

Antimuscarinic initial features: Dry mouth, mydriasis blurred vision, urinary retention, constipation, dizziness, and emesis, sinus tachycardia, most common dysrhythmia.

Mild-to-moderate toxicity: Drowsiness slurred speech ataxia altered mental status (e.g., agitation, confusion, lethargy, etc.), along with resting sinus tachycardia, dry mouth, mydriasis (pupil dilation), urinary retention fever.

Cardiac effects: Hypertension, tachycardia, orthostasis and hypotension, arrhythmias, ECG changes—prolonged QRS, QT, and PR interval.

CNS effects: Syncope, seizure, coma, myoclonus, hyperreflexia.

Pulmonary effect: Hypoventilation due to CNS depression.

GI effect: Decreased or absent bowel sound.

Investigations: Electrolyte, BUN, and creatinine levels, anion gap, complete blood cell count (CBC), blood alcohol level, arterial blood gases (ABGs) for evaluation of acidosis or hypoxia, ECG.

Treatment: Endotracheal intubation may be necessary for airway protection in comatose and with seizures.

Hypotension: Intravenous infusion of normal saline is indicated for CA-induced hypotension. For hypotension refractory to intravenous saline, vasopressors may be used.

Gastrointestinal decontamination: Activated charcoal can be considered.

Intravenous sodium bicarbonate

Lipid emulsion is sometimes considered.

2. Describe difference between neuroleptic malignant syndrome and serotonin syndrome.

Differentiating features of serotonin syndrome, neuroleptic malignant syndrome **(Table 9)**:

TABLE 9: Differentiating features serotonin syndrome and neuroleptic malignant syndrome.

Factors	Serotonin syndrome	Neuroleptic malignant syndrome
Causative medication	Serotonergic drugs	Dopamine antagonist
Physical examination	Hyperreflexia myoclonus ocular clonus	Severe rigidity hyporeflexia
Laboratory findings		Increased creatine kinase leukocytosis low serum iron
Course of illness	Symptoms seen within 24 hours	Slower in onset 1–2 weeks after starting/changing therapy resolves within 9–14 days of treatment
Treatment	Hydration sedation short acting antihypertensive	Withdrawal of culprit medication sedation cooling measures

3. Discuss organophosphorus poisoning drug therapies and treatment.

The initial treatment for a patient exposed to OP compounds must be directed at ensuring an adequate airway and ventilation, and at reversing excessive muscarinic effects. Seizures must be treated with standard anticonvulsants such as benzodiazepines or barbiturates.

Decontamination:
Procedure:
- Shower is preferable. Make the patient stand (if he is able to) under the shower, or seated in a chair.
- Wash with cold water for 5 minutes from head to toe using nongermicidal soap. Rinse hair well.
- Repeat the wash and rinse procedure with warm water.
- Repeat the wash and rinse procedure with hot water.

Treating personnel should protect themselves with water-impermeable gowns, masks with eye shields, and shoe covers.

Atropine: Atropine, a competitive antagonist of acetylcholine at the muscarinic postsynaptic membrane and in the CNS, will block the muscarinic manifestations of organophosphate poisoning.

Pralidoxime: This is a nucleophilic oxime which helps to regenerate acetylcholinesterase at muscarinic, nicotinic, and CNS sites.

Supportive measures: Maintain airway patency and oxygenation. Suction secretions. Endotracheal intubation and mechanical ventilation may be necessary. Monitor pulse oximetry or arterial blood gases to determine need for supplemental oxygen.

Prevention of further exposure: After the patient has recovered, he should not be re-exposed to organophosphates.

Question 6

1. Describe the approach to the management of a young adult with fever and jaundice. Also discuss the diagnostic algorithm.

Differential diagnosis of fever with jaundice is broad but knowledge of local disease epidemiology can point to the relevant differentials. Febrile jaundice usually occurs in the presence of parasitic infections (malaria, toxoplasmosis, and schistosomiasis), bacterial infections (typhoid, typhus, borreliosis, and leptospirosis) or viral infections (hepatitis and Lassa, Marburg, Ebola). The male presented with fever and jaundice possible causes are as in **Table 10**. Investigations should be aimed at confirming the diagnosis but it should only be correlated with the history and examination. The common investigations include CBC, renal function tests, liver function tests, chest X-ray, viral markers assay (HIV, HAV, HBV, HCV, HDV, HEV), USG of whole abdomen. Other tests may be carried out if required. Approach to the patient should be aimed at a proper history taking, clinical examination, and specific investigations. Patients should be admitted to an appropriate level of intensive care. Both supportive and specific antimalarial therapies are crucial for the patient's survival.

TABLE 10: Differential diagnosis for fever with jaundice.

Hepatic and biliary causes	• Acute cholangitis, acute cholecystitis • Acute pancreatitis • Primary sclerosing jaundice
Infections	• Malaria (plasmodium falciparum), viral hepatitis—B, C, D • Leptospirosis, dengue, yellow fever, brucellosis, rickettsia, cytomegalovirus, tuberculosis, Epstein–Barr virus, Amebic liver disease
Neoplasms	• Hodgkin's lymphoma, Chronic myeloid leukemia • Myelofibrosis
Inflammation	Septic thrombophlebitis
Hemolytic	Sickle cell crisis, Hemolytic uremic syndrome

2. Discuss malignant hyperthermia—clinical features and treatment pearls.

Malignant hyperthermia is a disease that causes a fast rise in body temperature and severe muscle contractions when someone receives general anesthesia with one or more of the following drugs—halothane, isoflurane, sevoflurane, desflurane or succinylcholine.

Signs and symptoms of malignant hyperthermia may vary and can occur during anesthesia or during recovery shortly after surgery. They can include: Severe muscle rigidity or spasms; rapid, shallow breathing and problems with low oxygen and high carbon dioxide; rapid heart rate; irregular heart rhythm; dangerously high body temperature; excessive sweating; patchy, irregular skin color (mottled skin).

Immediate treatment of malignant hyperthermia includes:

- *Medication:* A drug called dantrolene is used to treat the reaction by stopping the release of calcium into muscles. Other medications may be given to correct problems with a balance of the body's chemicals (metabolic imbalance) and treat complications.
- *Oxygen:* You may have oxygen through a face mask. In most cases, oxygen is given through a tube placed in the windpipe (trachea).
- *Body cooling:* Ice packs, cooling blankets, a fan with cool mist and chilled IV fluids may be used to help reduce body temperature.
- *Extra fluids:* You may also get extra fluids through an IV line.
- *Supportive care:* You may need to stay in the hospital in intensive care for a day or two to monitor your temperature, blood pressure, heart rate, breathing, and response to the treatment. Several laboratory tests will be done frequently to check the extent of any muscle breakdown and possible kidney damage. A stay in the hospital is usually needed until laboratory test results start to return to a standard range. With treatment, malignant hyperthermia usually resolves within a few days.

3. Explain postexposure prophylaxis (PEP) of needle stick injury from human immunodeficiency virus (HIV) positive patients for emergency care providers.

The decision to start PEP is made on the basis of degree of exposure to HIV and the HIV status of the source from whom the exposure/infection has occurred.

Basic regimen: Zidovudine (AZT)—600 mg in divided doses (300 mg/twice a day or 200 mg/thrice a day for 4 weeks + Lamivudine (3TC) - 150 mg twice a day for 4 weeks).

Expanded regimen: 4 weeks therapy, Basic regimen (+ Indinavir—800 mg/thrice a day, or any other protease inhibitor).

How to follow him up: PEP should be started, as early as possible, after an exposure. It has been seen that PEP started after 72 hours of exposure is of no use and hence is not recommended. The optimal course of PEP is not unknown, but 4 weeks of drug therapy appear to provide protection against HIV. If the HIV test is found to be positive at any time within 12 weeks, the healthcare worker (HCW) should be referred to a physician for treatment.

Question 7

1. Describe clinical features and management of sickle cell crisis.

Clinical Features

Vaso-occlusive crisis (VOC): Patients present with moderate to severe pain, which has variable intensity and frequency. Young children can have severe pain and swelling of both hands and feet (dactylitis).

Splenic sequestration crisis: Patients with SCD have spleen infarction before the end of childhood. The spleen is affected due to its narrow vessels and its role as a key player in the lymphoreticular system. Splenic sequestration crisis causes acute, painful enlargement of the spleen due to intrasplenic trapping of red cells.

Aplastic crisis: SC presents with sudden pallor and weakness confirmed by rapidly dropping hemoglobin levels that are accompanied by reticulocytopenia.

Acute chest syndrome (ACS): The presenting symptoms and signs include fever, cough, tachypnea, chest pain, hypoxia, wheeze, respiratory distress, and even failure. Any pulmonary infiltrate on chest radiography accompanied by abnormal lung findings should raise the suspicion of ACS.

Hemolytic crisis: An acute drop in hemoglobin level marks this crisis. It is common in patients with coexistent glucose-6-phosphate dehydrogenase (G6PD) deficiency.

Others: Femoral/humeral head osteonecrosis due to vaso-occlusion along with increased pressure from increased erythrocyte marrow, priapism, proliferative retinopathy, and renal complications are often due to vaso-occlusion.

General Management

Bed rest, fluids—oral or IV depending on hydration status, 5% dextrose in half normal saline, oxygen—if hypoxia present (<92%), encourage deep breathing, incentive spirometry, hydroxyurea (10–30 mg/kg/day)—helps by increasing fetal hemoglobin (HbF).

Pain management: Use analgesics as appropriate to the degree of pain, paracetamol, oral or IV for mild pain, non-steroidal anti-inflammatory drugs (NSAIDs) for moderate pain (if no renal insufficiency), opioids for moderate to severe pain—titrated doses (morphine 0.1 mg/kg every 15–30 min), intranasal fentanyl 2 µg/kg, especially in children.

Adjuvant therapy: Antibiotics—empirical broad-spectrum antibiotics, blood transfusion—exchange transfusion more advantageous, surgery—splenectomy, *consider* anxiolytic antiemetic medication to prevent constipation.

Specific Treatment

Aplastic crisis: Bone marrow suppression is often self-limited, but patients with SCD may require packet red blood cell (PRBC) transfusion is indicated if HB drops >2 g/dL from baseline.

Splenic sequestration: Initially, fluid resuscitate if patients are in shock to bridge to transfusion, as fluids may help the spleen release sequestered RBCs. Splenectomy is not routinely indicated.

Hemolysis: This condition is often self-limited. PRBC should be performed if transfusion is required, though often it is not. Rule out precipitating pathology.

Acute chest syndrome: Aggressive pain treatment can be required to reduce splinting and increase tidal volume. Anti-inflammatories may be used, though with caution bronchodilators are indicated if wheezing is present. Supplemental oxygen is recommended only if patients are hypoxic. Administer antibiotics to cover for infection.

Vaso-occlusive pain crisis: Pain crisis is a common reason for a visit to the ED; opioid medications are preferred; morphine 0.1 mg/kg every 15–30 minutes. Supplemental oxygen is only needed if patients are hypoxic. IV hydration is not routinely needed. If indicated, oral hydration is preferred. Gentle IV hydration can be used if indicated. Avoid boluses if possible.

2. Discuss ED physician role in the management of febrile neutropenia.

Febrile neutropenia (FN) is defined as "single oral temperature of >38.3°C (>101°F) or a temperature of >38.0°C (>100.4°F) sustained for >1 hour and an absolute neutrophil count (ANC) of <500 cells/mm^3 or expected to fall to <500 cells/mm^3 in next 48 hours".

Initial assessment includes targeted history, physical examination with emphasis on hydration, oral cavity, oropharynx, skin including any indwelling catheter, lungs, abdomen, perianal area and mental status. CBC, creatinine, electrolytes, liver function test, blood culture (two set), culture and stain samples from suspected site of infection, imaging studies if any site suspected.

Outpatient management may be considered in low-risk patient who resides close to the hospital, can come for frequent clinic visits and has a 24 hours care giver.

Inpatient management includes broad-spectrum antibiotics guided by patient's history and examination, allergies and culture data of the institution should be started within 60 minutes of presentation. Infectious Diseases Society of America (IDSA) recommends: Cefepime 2 g/8 hourly, ceftazidime 2 g/8 hourly, piperacillin tazobactam 4.5 g/6 hourly, meropenem 1 g/8 hourly and imipenem cilastatin 500 mg/6 hourly. Aminoglycoside, fluoroquinolones may be added in patients with complicated presentation.

3. Explain the blood component therapy in anticoagulant-induced upper GI bleeding in ED.

Treatment options for anticoagulants-induced upper GI bleeding include administration of FFP consists of the fluid portion of human blood frozen within 8 hours after collection. FFP is widely available, contains vitamin K-dependent clotting factors and has been the standard of care for urgent reversal of warfarin coagulopathy for years in the absence of RCTs. The recommended dose is an IV infusion of 15 mL/kg, corresponding to about 3–4 units of plasma (one unit = 250 mL) in the average adult weighing 70 kg. Time to effect of FFP is 10 minutes, but it takes a few hours for partial reversal of INR and at least 9 hours for complete reversal (i.e., INR <1.5)

Prothrombin Complex Concentrates (PCC) are pharmacological products that contain lyophilized inactivated concentrates of factors II, IX, and X, with variable amounts of factor VII, derived from the cryoprecipitate supernatant of large plasma pools after at least one viral inactivation step to minimize the risk of pathogen transmission. Variations in factor VII concentrations among available PCCs have led to classify them as either three- or four-factor complexes (3F-PCC or 4F-PCC, respectively). The PCCs are standardized according to their factor IX content and they are administered IV, usually at the dose of 25–50 IU of factor IX/kg, depending on baseline INR.

Recombinant activated factor VIIa (rFVIIa) is a biotechnology product that is structurally similar to the native FVIIa and enables hemostasis by activating the extrinsic pathway. Evidences are limited and so are not routinely used.

Question 8

1. Explain various pain assessment scores in children.

Though there are various pain assessment scores in children but we will discuss about the most commonly used ones. They are *Wong–Baker Pain Rating Scale* **(Fig. 1)** and FLACC scale **(Fig. 2)**.

Wong–Baker Pain Rating Scale: This scale for pain assessment based on the facial expressions, most commonly used one as it is simpler and easy to use. FLACC scale is a more specific pain score for children taking into consideration things specific to children.

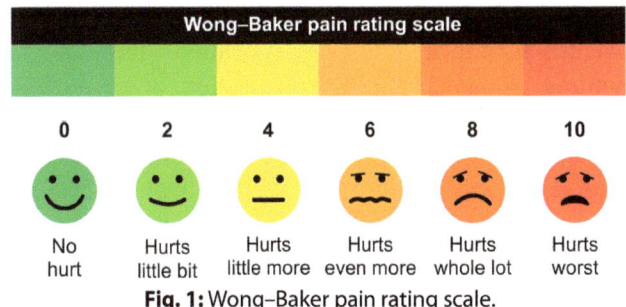

Fig. 1: Wong–Baker pain rating scale.

FLACC scale		0	1	2
1	Face	No particular expression or smile	Occasional grimace or frown, withdrawn, disinterested	Frequent to constant frown, clenched jaw, quivering chin
2	Legs	Normal position or relaxed	Uneasy, restless, tense	Kicking, or legs drawn up
3	Activity	Lying quietly, normal position, moves easily	Squirming, shifting back and forth, tense	Arched, rigid or jerking
4	Cry	No crying (awake or asleep)	Moans or whimpers; occasional complaint	Crying steadily, screams or sobs, frequent complaints
5	Consolability	Content, relaxed	Reassured by occasional touching, hugging or being talked to, distractible	Difficult to console or comfort

Fig. 2: FLACC scale.

2. Discuss procedural sedation and analgesia for reduction of hip dislocation in a known hypertensive adult on regular antihypertensive.

Procedural sedation should be carefully managed for hypertensive patients. The typical drugs used for procedural sedation and analgesia are combination of **propofol and ketamine known as ketofol**. Propofol induces hypotension, has rapid onset and shorter duration of action and is indicated in orthopedic reduction but does not provide analgesia. Propofol in combination with ketamine known as ketofol is the ideal drug for sedation and analgesia in this hypertensive patient for reduction of hip dislocation as ketamine adds analgesic properties. Its onset of action takes <1 minute and effectiveness last <10 minutes. The dose for procedural sedation of ketofol is 0.5 mg propofol + 0.5 mg ketamine. Though there are other drugs that can be used in this patient but this combination provides the best efficacy and so is the drug of choice.

3. Describe femoral nerve block and intercostal nerve block.

Femoral block indications: The femoral block aims to anesthetize the femoral nerve (and may also block the obturator and lateral femoral cutaneous nerves) through anesthetic spread beneath the fascia iliac. It provides analgesia for hip fractures or dislocations, femoral shaft fractures, patellar fracture or dislocation, and anesthesia for anterior thigh or patellar laceration repairs or abscess drainage. A femoral nerve block (FNB) results in anesthesia of the skin and muscles of the anterior thigh and most of the femur and knee joint, as well as the skin on the medial aspect of the leg below the knee joint.

Intercostal nerve block (ICNB) is a nerve block which temporarily or permanently interrupts the flow of signals along an intercostal nerve, usually performed to relieve pain. Successful intercostal nerve block results in the deposition of local anesthetic in the intercostal sulcus outside of the parietal pleura. Correct placement will result in ipsilateral numbness of the individual intercostal levels that have been blocked. Usually, the block level is determined by the number of blocks performed and is limited to the dermatome of the intercostal nerves which have been targeted.

Ultrasound guidance may decrease the chance of intravascular injection, pneumothorax, and allows injection closer to the midline than anatomic landmarks. The individual ribs to be blocked should be marked out as with the landmark technique. The ultrasound probe is then placed in a sagittal plane about 4 cm lateral to the spinous process. The ribs are visualized as a shadow while the pleura and lung are visualized anterior to the intercostal space. The needle can then be inserted in or out of a plane to the transducer and advanced until the tip is just below the inferior border of the rib. After negative aspiration, 3–5 mL of local anesthetic is injected, and the pleura should be visualized being pushed away.

Question 9

1. Discuss approach to acute onset bullous lesions.

A bullous lesion refers to fluid filled blisters on the skin. There are many causes of bullous lesions but among them some of the most common are—pemphigus, bullous pemphigoid, epidermolytic hyperkeratosis (bullous ichthyosis), toxic shock syndrome, bullous scabies, insect and arachnid bites, thermal trauma, bullous varicella, juvenile dermatitis herpetiformis, erythema multiforme with bullae. Here there is a summary of the most common bullous lesions and their differentiation **(Table 11)**.

When to consider further evaluation or treatment: Skin biopsy strongly recommended in atypical Staphylococcal scalded skin syndrome (SSSS) or Stevens–Johnson syndrome (SJS), all TEN and persistent or refractory disease. Patients with suspected SSSS, SJS, and toxic epidermal necrolysis (TEN) need close monitoring for other organ system involvement and life-threatening complications. Complicated SSSS, SJS, and all TEN should be managed in a burn unit.

Investigations: Although clinical findings and history paves the way for the diagnosis but certain tests are done to confirm the diagnosis. The tests include: Both direct immunofluorescence and immunoserology (IIF SSS) tests should be performed for diagnosis of the bullous and nonbullous variants of pemphigoid, and the BP180 NC16A enzyme-linked immunosorbent assay is recommended as an add-on test for disease activity monitoring.

Treatment: Topical and parenteral steroids remain the mainstay of treatment for bullous lesions along with immunosuppressants and general management.

TABLE 11: Differentiation between pemphigus vulgaris and bullous pemphigoid.

	Pemphigus vulgaris	Bullous pemphigoid
Age	Middle aged	Elderly
Clinical features	Monomorphic lesions	Polymorphic lesions
Blisters	Flaccid blisters, ruptures easily	Tense blisters
Content of blisters	Fluid filled	Often hemorrhagic
Mucosal involvement	Common	Rare
Nikolsky sign	Positive	Negative
Tzanck smear	Acantholysis	No acantholysis

2. Explain the approach to acute onset erythematous rash in children.

Childhood rashes are common and are not usually a cause for concern. Most rashes are harmless and disappear without the need for treatment. The most common causes of rashes in children are: Cellulitis chickenpox eczema erythema multiforme, hand, foot and mouth disease, impetigo, keratosis pilaris ("chicken skin"), measles, molluscum contagiosum, pityriasis rosea, prickly heat psoriasis, ringworm, scabies, scarlet fever, slapped cheek syndrome, urticaria (hives), meningitis.

As in cases of an adult the childhood rashes need to be diagnosed based on the history and clinical presentation **(Table 12)** along with the pattern of the rashes **(Table 13)**. It is important to determine the type of lesions, such as macules, papules, vesicles, plaques, or pustules. Other important characteristics include location and distribution, arrangement, shape, color, and presence or absence of scale **(Table 14)**. A table to differentiate the rashes would be helpful.

Treatment: Most of the diseases in children with rashes are self-limiting and do not require specific medications. So the mainstay of treatment aims at:
- Avoiding irritants to the skin
- Cleaning the skin properly
- Treating the symptoms
- In severe cases supportive treatment with broad spectrum antibiotics.

TABLE 12: Classification of skin lesion according to clinical presentation.

Vesiculobullous skin lesion	Pustular skin lesion	Papular skin lesion
• Impetigo • Scalded skin syndrome • Herpes simplex virus • Eczema herpeticum • Erythema multiforme • Stevens–Johnson syndrome and toxic epidermal necrolysis • Varicella (chickenpox) • Insect bites and stings (e.g., mosquitoes, bees), burn wounds (second degree)	• Infantile acne • Neonatal pustulosis • Secondarily infected vesiculobullous rash, acute generalized exanthematous pustulosis	• Scabies urticaria/serum sickness • Keratosis pilaris • Papular acrodermatitis • Molluscum contagiosum • Plane warts • Streptococcal infection (scarlet fever) • Rubella (German measles) • Measles (rubeola)

TABLE 13: Pediatric patient assessment with skin lesions/skin rashes.

Initial assessment of the rash	Is there any fluid-filled vesicles? Is the rash raised (papular) or flat (macular)? Is the rash red? Is the rash scaly? Is the rash itchy? When did the rash start? Where did the rash start, and how did it spread?
History: What is the past medical and drug history?	Did the patient present with other symptoms (e.g., fever, headache)? Has the patient been exposed to new topical applications (e.g., soap, lotions)? Has the patient ingested any unfamiliar foods? Has the patient had close contact with someone else with the same symptoms? Has the patient travelled recently?
General examination	If a systemic illness is expected, refer to a medical practitioner for further management
Examination of the skin	Examine the whole skin, even if the rash seems localized. Ensure that the patient is comfortable, with a close caregiver nearby. A rash resulting from a topical application will be present in a specific area (e.g., under arms, nappy area). A rash resulting from a systemic cause will be generalized and symmetrical. Systemic illness may also present in the mouth (e.g., syphilis, drug reactions like Stevens–Johnson syndrome)

TABLE 14: Differentiating red skin lesions/rashes.

Red rashes with epidermal breakage	Eczematous rashes atopic dermatitis (eczema)
Red rashes with without epidermal breakage	• Papulosquamous rashes (red and scaly) • Seborrhoeic dermatitis • Psoriasis • Tinea corporis • Pityriasis rosea
Red rashes with blanching	• Erythematous rashes (red and blanching) • Fever and exanthem • Erythema infectiosum • Roseola infantum • Kawasaki disease
Red rashes without blanching	• Purpuric rashes • Enterovirus infection • Septicemia • Leukemia • Henoch–Schönlein purpura • Idiopathic thrombocytopenic purpura (ITP), vasomotor straining • Child abuse • Trauma

3. Discuss panic disorder—presentation and treatment.

Panic attack is a brief period of extreme distress, anxiety, or fear that begins suddenly and is accompanied by physical or emotional symptoms. Panic disorder involves spontaneous panic attacks that occur repeatedly, worry about the future attacks and changes in behavior to avoid situations that are associated with the attack.

Presentation: Panic disorder is characterized by many somatic and cognitive symptoms. The following are characteristics of a panic attack which can occur at any time and generally last around 10 minutes. Following symptoms must be present to meet the diagnostic criteria of panic disorder. The symptoms of panic disorder have physical, behavioral, and cognitive effects:

Physical: Tachycardia, palpitations, shortness of breath, sweating or chills, chest pain, increased respiration rate, increased blood pressure, increased muscle tension, irritability, decreased sex drive, dizziness, nausea, diarrhea, muscle tension.

Behavioral: Sleep disturbance, difficulty with memory or concentration, apprehension, irritability, hyper-alertness, uncertainty.

Cognitive: Fear of losing one's mind, fear of losing control, sense of terror, fear of dying.

Medical Management

Medical management is usually led by a psychologist and includes a combination of the following:

Psychoeducation: Educating the patient about the disorder so they can develop an understanding and acceptance of their diagnosis; offering resources to facilitate their understanding.

Lifestyle changes: Avoiding stimulants such as caffeine, or other substances and medication that will hinder recovery, regular moderate exercise, stress management, cognitive behavioral therapy—breathing/relaxation exercises.

Cognitive restructuring: Working with patient to identify inaccurate cognitions and replacing them with realistic idea. Reintroducing the patient to feared stimuli to test his/her anxiety control, progress as tolerated to more challenging feared stimuli, hypnosis.

Pharmacological management: Antidepressants called selective serotonin reuptake inhibitors (SSRIs) are the first-line of treatment and most commonly used medications to treat panic disorder. Some of the common SSRIs used to treat panic disorder include: Fluoxetine, sertraline, paroxetine, fluvoxamine, citalopram, and escitalopram. Benzodiazepines may be used if SSRIs do not help. This is a form of antianxiety medication which provides rapid relief of symptoms, e.g., alprazolam, lorazepam.

4. Explain the approach to a patient with narrow complex tachycardia.

Electrocardiographic findings: Supraventricular tachycardias (SVTs) present with narrow complex tachycardia with QRS duration of <120 ms. Few cases of SVT cases can have a QRS duration of >120 ms **(Flowchart 1)**.

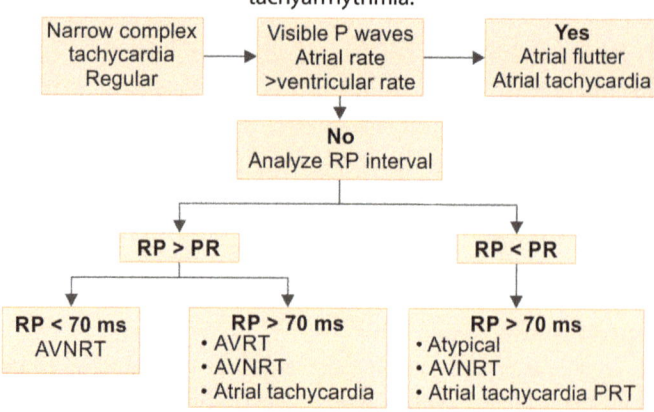

Flowchart 1: Electrocardiographic approach to narrow complex tachyarrhythmia.

The first approach in approaching a patient with narrow complex tachycardia should involve the following: The immediate response to an adult patient with tachycardia and a palpable pulse is to:
- Maintain an open airway
- Assist breathing if necessary
- Apply monitors to assess cardiac rhythm, blood pressure, and blood oxygenation
- Provide supplement oxygen to maintain O_2 saturation between 94 and 99%

Once the initial assessment is complete, follow the below mentioned protocol **(Flowchart 2)**.

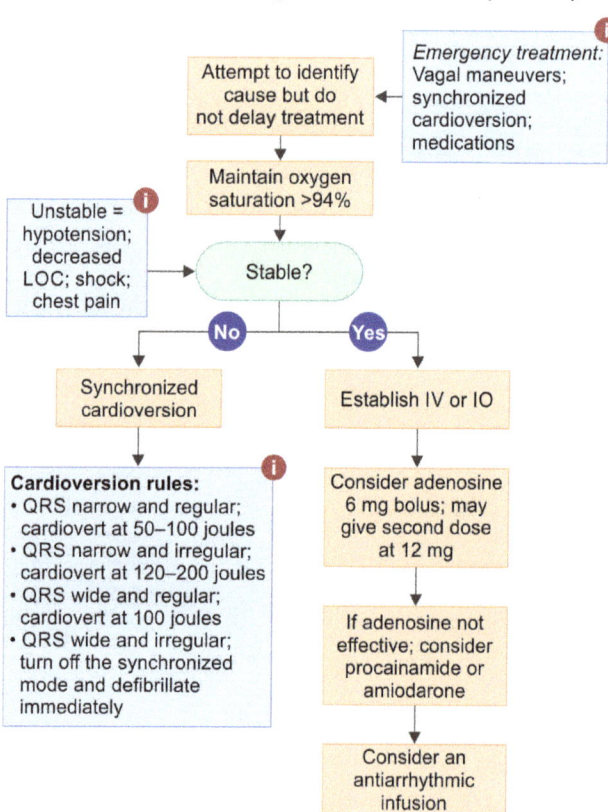

Flowchart 2: Approch to management of narrow complex tachycardia.

Question 10

1. Discuss delta gap and its clinical implications.

Delta ratio/gap is a formula used to assess raised anion gap acidosis and whether mixed acid base disorder is present or not. It is calculated as delta gap = difference of measured anion gap and normal anion gap/difference of normal HCO_3 and measured HCO_3.

Clinical implications of delta ratio value
- <0.4—Normal anion gap metabolic acidosis
- 0.4-0.8—Mixed-normal anion gap + High anion gap metabolic acidosis
- 0.8-2—Pure high anion gap acidosis
- >2—Mixed-high anion gap acidosis + Metabolic alkalosis

2. Explain the metabolic alkalosis—causes, clinical presentations, and management.

The causes of metabolic alkalosis can be summarized in **(Table 15)**.

TABLE 15: Causes of metabolic alkalosis.

Chloride sensitive	Chloride resistant	Miscellaneous
• Gastrointestinal: Vomiting, gastric drainage, chloride diarrhea, villous adenoma • Renal: Diuretics posthypercapnic • Low chloride intake • Cystic fibrosis	*Increased mineralocorticoid activity:* Primary/secondary hyperaldosteronism, Cushing's syndrome, Bartter's syndrome Severe hypokalemia	• Massive blood transfusion • Acetate containing colloids • Alkali therapy • *Hypercalcemia:* Milk alkali syndrome, bone metastatic

Clinical presentations: Metabolic alkalosis may not show any symptoms. People with this type of alkalosis more often complain of the underlying conditions that are causing it. These can include: Vomiting, diarrhea, and swelling in the lower legs (peripheral edema) fatigue. Severe cases of metabolic alkalosis can cause agitation disorientation seizures coma. The severe symptoms are most common when the alkalosis is caused by chronic liver disease.

Treatment: As with other acid–base disorders, correction of metabolic alkalosis is never complete until the underlying disorder is treated. When ventilation is controlled, any respiratory component contributing to alkalemia should be corrected by decreasing minute ventilation to normalize $PaCO_2$. The treatment of choice for chloride-sensitive metabolic alkalosis is administration of IV saline (NaCl) and potassium (KCl). H2-blocker therapy is useful when excessive loss of gastric fluid is a factor. Acetazolamide may also be useful in edematous patients. Alkalosis associated with primary increase in mineralocorticoid activity readily responds to aldosterone antagonists (spironolactone); when arterial blood pH is >7.60, treatment with IV hydrochloric acid (0.1 mol/L), ammonium chloride (0.1 mol/L), arginine hydrochloride, or hemodialysis should be considered.

3. Discuss the clinical features and management of hypercalcemia.

Hypercalcemia can be classified into mild hypercalcemia: 10.5–11.9 mg/dL; moderate hypercalcemia: 12.0–13.9 mg/dL; hypercalcemic crisis: 14.0–16.0 mg/dL.

Clinical Features

Everyone might not have signs or symptoms if your hypercalcemia is mild. More severe cases produce signs and symptoms related to the parts of your body affected by the high calcium levels in your blood. Examples include—excessive thirst and frequent urination, nausea, vomiting and constipation, bone pain and muscle weakness, confusion, lethargy and fatigue. It can also cause depression, palpitations and fainting, indications of cardiac arrhythmia, and other heart problems.

ECG features of hypercalcemia include: T wave flattening or inversion, mild prolongation of the QRS and PR intervals, ST elevation presence of J wave at the end of the QRS complex.

Management

Intravenous fluids and diuretics: Extremely high calcium levels in medical emergency need hospitalization for treatment with IV fluids and diuretics to promptly lower the calcium level to prevent arrhythmia and nervous system problems.

Calcitonin controls calcium levels in the blood. Mild nausea might be a side effect.

Bisphosphonates: Intravenous osteoporosis drugs, which can quickly lower calcium levels, are often used to treat hypercalcemia due to cancer. Risks associated with this treatment include breakdown (osteonecrosis) of the jaw and certain types of thigh fractures.

Prednisone: If your hypercalcemia is caused by high levels of vitamin D, short-term use of steroid pills such as prednisone is usually helpful.

Surgical procedures for problems associated with overactive parathyroid glands.

4. Briefly discuss clinical importance of osmolal gap for emergency physician.

The "osmolal gap" represents osmoles which are unaccounted for by sodium salts, glucose, and urea. Osmolal gap = Measured osmolality – Calculated osmolality.

In normal individuals, the osmolal gap is <10 mOsm/kg water.

In the event a significant osmolal gap is detected, the following causes should be considered:

Ethylene glycol ingestion, methanol ingestion, ethanol or isopropyl alcohol ingestion, end-stage renal disease without regular dialysis, ketoacidosis (diabetic or alcoholic), lactic acidosis, formaldehyde ingestion, paraldehyde ingestion, diethyl ether ingestion, infusion of nonconductive glycine, sorbitol, or mannitol solutions, severe hyperproteinemia, severe hyperlipidemia. Emergency physician can make a provisional diagnosis of the condition of the patient calculating the osmolar gap. So, it is a useful tool in emergency to come to a diagnosis.

SUGGESTED READING

1. Richhariya D, Sharma B. Textbook of Emergency Medicine including Intensive Care and Trauma, 2nd edition. New Delhi: Jaypee Brothers Medical Publishers (P) Ltd; 2022. pp. 20, 435, 453. (Question 1).
2. Richhariya D, Sharma B. Textbook of Emergency Medicine including Intensive Care and Trauma, 2nd edition. New Delhi: Jaypee Brothers Medical Publishers (P) Ltd; 2022. pp. 743-51. (Question 2).
3. Richhariya D, Sharma B. Textbook of Emergency Medicine including Intensive Care and Trauma, 2nd edition. New Delhi: Jaypee Brothers Medical Publishers (P) Ltd; 2022. pp. 833, 845, 850. (Question 3).
4. Richhariya D, Sharma B. Textbook of Emergency Medicine including Intensive Care and Trauma, 2nd edition. New Delhi: Jaypee Brothers Medical Publishers (P) Ltd; 2022. pp. 255, 570, 589. (Question 4).
5. Richhariya D, Sharma B. Textbook of Emergency Medicine including Intensive Care and Trauma, 2nd edition. New Delhi: Jaypee Brothers Medical Publishers (P) Ltd; 2022. pp. 1404, 1425. (Question 5).
6. Richhariya D, Sharma B. Textbook of Emergency Medicine including Intensive Care and Trauma, 2nd edition. New Delhi: Jaypee Brothers Medical Publishers (P) Ltd; 2022. p. 1373. (Question 6).
7. Richhariya D, Sharma B. Textbook of Emergency Medicine including Intensive Care and Trauma, 2nd edition. New Delhi: Jaypee Brothers Medical Publishers (P) Ltd; 2022. pp. 973, 987, 997. (Question 7).
8. Richhariya D, Sharma B. Textbook of Emergency Medicine including Intensive Care and Trauma, 2nd edition. New Delhi: Jaypee Brothers Medical Publishers (P) Ltd; 2022. pp. 351, 357, 389. (Question 8).
9. Richhariya D, Sharma B. Textbook of Emergency Medicine including Intensive Care and Trauma, 2nd edition. New Delhi: Jaypee Brothers Medical Publishers (P) Ltd; 2022. pp. 1015, 1053, 1221. (Question 9).
10. Richhariya D, Sharma B. Textbook of Emergency Medicine including Intensive Care and Trauma, 2nd edition. New Delhi: Jaypee Brothers Medical Publishers (P) Ltd; 2022. p. 305. (Question 10).

Emergency Medicine Paper 28

Egala VSSN Murthy

Question 1

1. Describe RUSH VTI protocol and compare original RUSH protocol with pearls and pitfalls.

Rapid ultrasound for shock and hypotension and velocity time integral (RUSH-VTI): Rapid ultrasound for shock and hypotension (RUSH) examination, which is a comprehensive assessment protocol performed with ultrasound that provides valuable information on why the patient is in shock. However, while the RUSH examination points out the causes of hypotension, it does not direct management. Addition of velocity-time integral (VTI) to the standard RUSH protocol cannot only be used to predict a patient's response to fluids ("fluid responsiveness"), but it can also guide resuscitation with the administration of fluids or inotropes. The goal of resuscitation in shock is to increase stroke volume. The VTI is a surrogate for stroke volume. Measuring left ventricular outflow tract (LVOT) diameter in emergent situations can be technically difficult and errors are magnified due to the squaring of the diameter in the equation. An easier and more accurate alternative is to only measure the LVOT VTI. A normal LVOT VTI is between 18 and 22 cm for heart rates between 55 and 95 beats/minute **(Table 1)**.

2. Discuss the differences in planning resuscitation for cardiogenic septic and obstructive shock in emergency department (ED).

It is estimated that fewer than half of hypotensive patients will increase their stroke volume as a response to fluids. Emergency physician can find out these patients by measuring the LVOT VTI (or the V_{max}) prior to and after a fluid challenge (small fluid bolus or passive leg raising). An increase of >15% would indicate fluid responsiveness. Simply, stroke volume (SV) can be increased with fluids or with inotropes. Fluid responsiveness is defined by an increase in SV of >15% after a fluid bolus. Contractile reserve is defined as an increase in SV of >20% after administration of inotropes. The concept of measuring stroke volume pre- and post-intervention (fluid bolus, inotropes or other interventions) has been shown to be more important than static measurements. A simplified VTI algorithm in the management of different types of shock is depicted in **Flowchart 1**.

TABLE 1: HIMAP version of RUSH examination.

View	Important questions	Probe position for RUSH examination
H = Heart	• Is there any pericardial effusion? • What is global ventricular function? • Is there RV strain? • What is base line LVOT-VTI?	
I = IVC	IVC-Collapsed/Full	
M = Morison's pouch in right upper quadrant	Aneurysm/Dissection	
A = Aorta	Is there any pneumothorax?	
P = Pulmonary		

(IVC: inferior vena cava; LVOT-VTI: left ventricular outflow tract and velocity time integral; RUSH: rapid ultrasound for shock and hypotension)

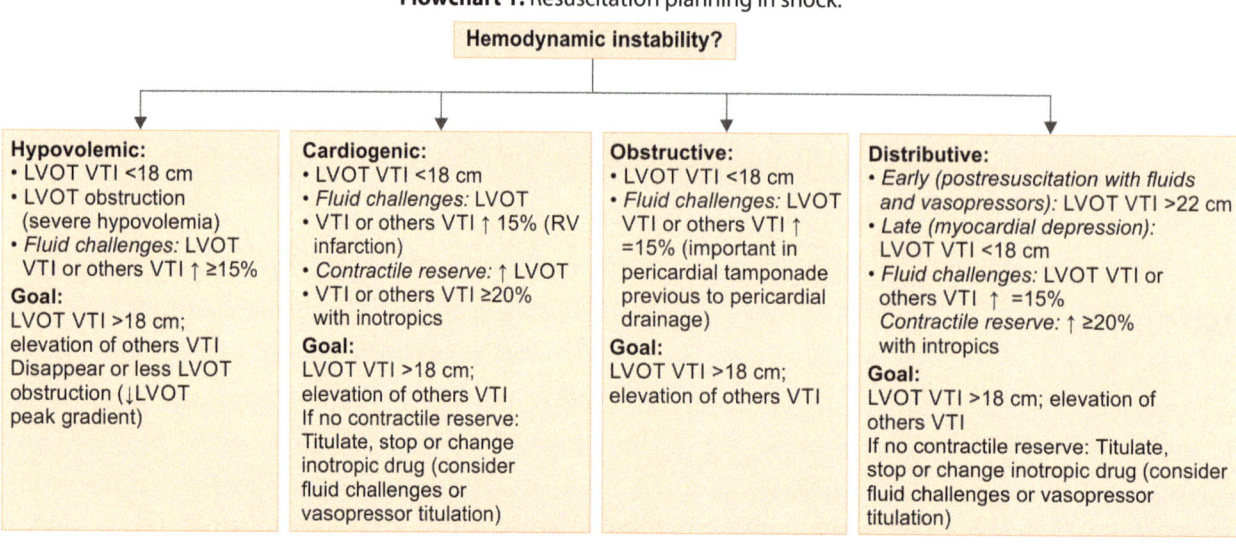

Flowchart 1: Resuscitation planning in shock.

(LVOT-VTI: rapid ultrasound for shock and hypotension and velocity time integral)

Question 2

1. Discuss the recent advances in equipment for emergency airway management.

A video laryngoscope with a hyper angulated blade shape provides superior laryngeal views without excessive cervical spine movement. It also has higher intubation success rates as compared to the conventional direct laryngoscope (DL). The intubating laryngeal mask airway (I-LMA) is another device which helps to minimize cervical spine movement during intubation than DL. Different types of supraglottic airways are commercially available. Some of the important ones are described here:

I-Gel: The I-Gel has a soft, gel-like cuff that seals the perilaryngeal structures without inflation which limits tissue compression caused by large cuffed devices. Lubricate the gel-like cuff prior to insertion, and advance the device into the posterior pharynx until resistance is met and the lips align with the lip line on the I-Gel. Complications of I-Gel include laryngospasm and sore throat; rarely vasovagal asystole and glottic hematoma. The I-Gel is available in various sizes for patients from 2 to >90 kg.

King Laryngeal Tube (King LT): The King LT is a single lumen tube with a proximal cuff that seals the posterior oropharynx while a distal cuff occludes the esophagus. It is placed blindly into the oropharynx until the lip aligns with the device lip line. The balloon is then inflated to a pressure of 60 cmH$_2$O. Tongue engorgement is a complication of this tube since the proximal balloon can impair venous drainage of the tongue which can be overcome by removing the tube. It is available in several sizes depending on the patient's height: 4–5 feet, size 3 (yellow); 5–6 feet, size 4 (red); and >6 feet, size 5 (purple).

Laryngeal Mask Airway (LMA): The LMA is a supraglottic airway (SGA) placed blindly through the mouth by occluding the structures around the larynx. The LMA consists of a single cuff inflated with 20–30 mL of air. To insert the LMA, place a gloved index finger into the oropharynx to guide the device into the oropharynx and position the cuff around the larynx. The LMA is useful when the vocal cords cannot be visualized during intubation attempts. There are various models, including an intubating LMA, that allow an endotracheal tube to be passed through the lumen.

2. Describe failed airway algorithm in emergency.

A failed airway can be considered when any of the following conditions is met:
- Oxygen saturation is maintained during or after one or more failed laryngoscopic attempts or
- Three failed attempts of orotracheal intubation by an experienced specialist, even when oxygen saturation can be maintained.

Cannot intubate, cannot oxygenate: Airway must be secured immediately (no time to evaluate). Avoid any further rescue attempt and the airway must be secured immediately to maintain oxygen saturation by balloon mitral valvotomy (BMV) or with an esophagogastroduodenoscopy (EGD).

Cannot intubate, can oxygenate: Various rescue options can be executed (time to evaluate) because the patient is oxygenated.

Airway management failure can be avoided by identifying and anticipating patient with difficult for intubation.

Question 3

Describe the recent advances in assessment and management of trauma.

1. Discuss newer technique devices and agents for achieving hemostasis.

Resuscitative endovascular balloon occlusion of the aorta (REBOA) has recently come up as a minimally invasive alternative to open aortic cross-clamping in the management of nonresponsive category of polytrauma patients. It will help in controlling noncompressible hemorrhage arising below the diaphragm. It is being used in both blunt and penetrating abdominal trauma. The use of REBOA provides for temporary hemorrhage control and improved hemodynamics until definitive surgical/endovascular control of hemorrhage achieved.

Mechanical: Direct pressure sutures staples ligating clips gauge sponges.

Thermal: Electrocautery, laser.

Chemical: Pharmacotherapy, topical hemostat (collagens cellulose gelatins), and topical sealants.

2. Explain the result of CRASH-3 trial.

According to CRASH-3 trial, tranexamic acid is safe in patients with traumatic brain injury and that treatment within 3 hours of injury reduces head injury-related death.

Role of tranexamic acid: Tranexamic acid is an antifibrinolytic agent that reduces blood loss after surgery and may reduce blood loss after traumatic injury. It prevents cleavage of plasmin and degradation of fibrin. As early as possible after injury, with administration of tranexamic acid, within 1 hour of injury decrease relative risk from bleeding by 32% and within 1–3 hours by 21%. Administration of tranexamic acid >3 hours after injury is less effective and potentially harmful; tranexamic acid must be given before transfer/arrival to a trauma center in order to meet the time requirement of early administration. The dose is 1 g intravenous (IV) bolus over 10 minutes, followed by 1 g IV over 8 hours.

3. What is chain of survival in trauma hemorrhagic shock?

Chain of survival for patients with severe hemorrhage: The chain starts with primary prevention and prehospital interventions. Once the patient arrives at the hospital, early recognition and resuscitation, achievement of definitive hemostasis, and subsequent actions, all factors responsible for outcome **(Fig. 1)**.

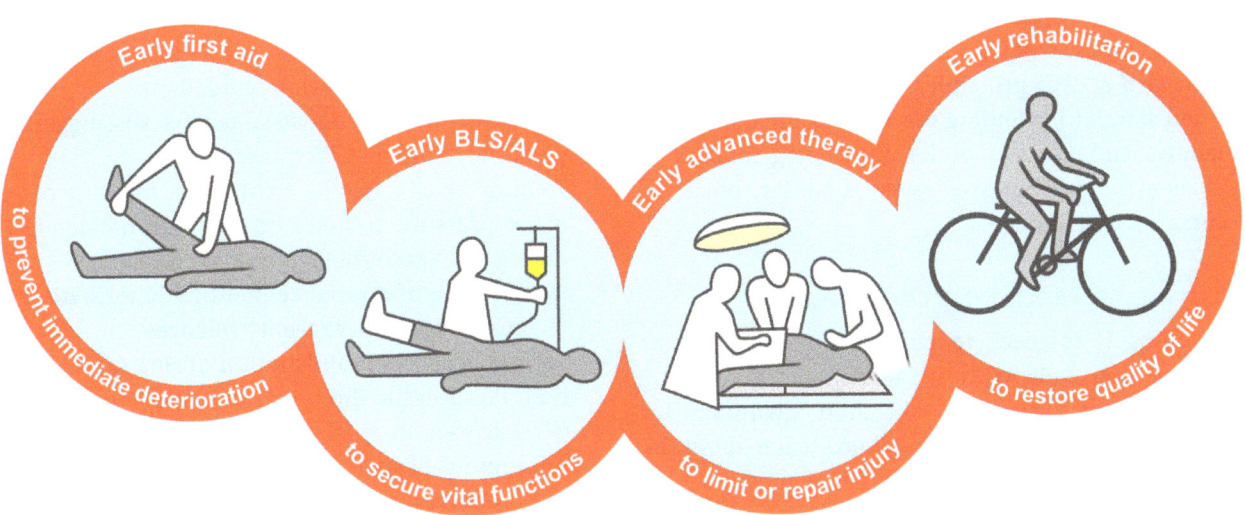

Fig. 1: Chain of survival in trauma.

Question 4

1. Discuss ROC curve and its significance in statistical analysis.

There is a pair of diagnostic sensitivity and specificity values for every individual cut-off. To construct a ROC graph **(Fig. 2)**, we plot these pairs of values on the graph with the 1-specificity on the x-axis and sensitivity on the y-axis. The shape of ROC curve and the area under the curve (AUC) help us estimate how high the discriminative power of a test is. The area under the curve can have any value between 0 and 1 and it is a good indicator of the goodness of the test. The perfect diagnostic test has an AUC 1.0, whereas a nondiscriminating test has an area 0.5 **(Fig. 2)**.

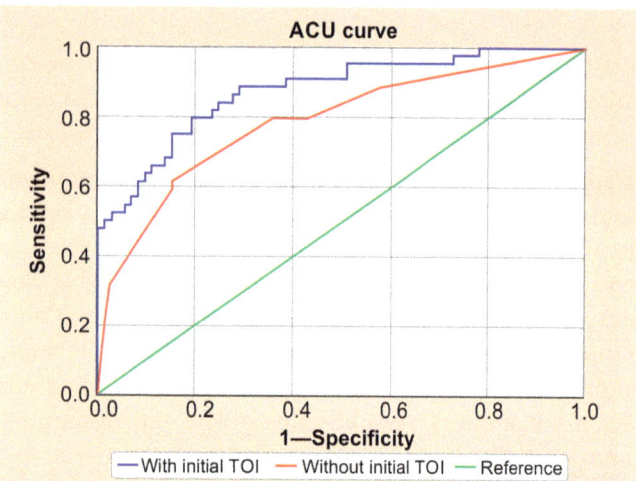

Fig. 2: ROC curve.

2. Describe CONSORT guidelines.

The CONSORT guidelines are a checklist which provides scientifically proven recommendations for reporting randomized controlled trials. Researchers hope to increase the openness and precision of reporting so that readers can evaluate the trial's validity and understand its conclusions. Every trial's process, from conception to the results analysis, is governed by these principles. The CONSORT standards are widely utilized in the medical profession and are regarded as the standard for reporting randomized clinical studies. The fields of psychology and education also accept principles like these. As with any established standard, adopting these raises the bar for the thoroughness and precision of the study being conducted. In conclusion, the guidelines offer suggestions for enhancing the accuracy of trial findings.

3. Discuss microteaching techniques.

Microteaching is to teach teachers the techniques for learning teaching skills. With this teaching, real teaching situations are put forward to take their advantage for developing skills and getting deeper knowledge about the art of teaching and how to teach. The types of microteaching are: The skill of introduction, the skill of explaining, the skill of questioning, the skill of demonstration, the skill of illustrating, the skill of reinforcement, the skill of stimulus variation, and the skill of blackboard writing.

4. Explain the odds ratio and relative risk.

The odds ratio is a statistical measure used to quantify the association between two binary variables. It is the ratio of the odds of an event occurring in one group to the odds of the same event occurring in another group. In other words, it tells us how much more or less likely it is for an outcome to occur in one group compared to another group.

In statistics, *the likelihood ratio* is a measure of the strength of evidence provided by the data in favor of one statistical hypothesis over another. It is defined as the ratio of the likelihoods of two different hypotheses, given the same observed data. The likelihood ratio is often used in hypothesis testing, model selection, and parameter estimation.

Question 5

1. What are the recent advances in cardiopulmonary resuscitation?

The American Heart Association (AHA) guidelines for adult, pediatric, neonatal, and resuscitation are revised in year 2020. These guidelines are helpful for the resuscitation providers and instructors during cardiac arrest resuscitation and also result in changes in resuscitation training and practice. The changes in the 2020 AHA guidelines for cardiopulmonary resuscitation (CPR) summarize here:

- Easy to remember resuscitation scenarios, algorithms, and visual aids guidance for basic life support (BLS) and advanced cardiovascular life support (ACLS) are developed.
- Re-emphasis is given on the importance of early initiation of CPR by lay rescuers.
- Early epinephrine administration has been reaffirmed, with emphasis like previous guidelines.
- Use of real-time audio-visual feedback is suggested as a means to maintain CPR quality.
- To improve CPR quality, continuous measure of arterial blood pressure and end tidal carbon dioxide ($ETCO_2$) during ACLS resuscitation is emphasized.
- Routine use of double sequential defibrillation is not recommended as per recent evidences.
- For medication administration during ACLS resuscitation, IV access is the preferred route but intraosseous (IO) access is acceptable if IV access is not available.
- After return of spontaneous circulation (ROSC), patient care requires close attention to oxygenation, blood pressure control, evaluation for percutaneous coronary intervention, targeted temperature management, and multimodal neuroprognostication.
- Postcardiac arrest recovery is long and continues process after the initial hospitalization, patients should have formal assessment and support for their physical, cognitive, and psychosocial needs.
- Debriefing after resuscitation for lay rescuers, EMS providers, and hospital-based healthcare workers is beneficial to support their mental health and well-being.

- Management of cardiac arrest in pregnancy focuses on maternal resuscitation and improves the chances of successful resuscitation of the mother with preparation for early perimortem cesarean delivery if necessary to save the infant.

The changes in algorithms and other performance aids are:
- A sixth link, recovery, is added to the resuscitation—chains of survival.
- The emphasis is given on the role of early epinephrine administration for patients with nonshockable rhythms in the universal Adult Cardiac Arrest Algorithm (modified now).
- Two new algorithms for opioid-associated emergency have been added for lay rescuers and trained rescuers.
- The Postcardiac Arrest Care Algorithm was updated to emphasize the need to prevent hyperoxia, hypoxemia, and hypotension.
- In postcardiac arrest care section new diagram is added to guide and inform neuroprognostication.
- A new algorithm has been added to address cardiac arrest in pregnancy.

2. Discuss the recent advances in management of stroke.

Until recently, recombinant tissue plasminogen activator (r-tPA) was the only acute ischemic stroke treatment. However, only 3–9% of patients with ischemic stroke actually receive r-tPA, in part because of the limited time window for treatment. In 2008, the ECASS-3 trial extended the window for r-tPA eligibility from 3 to 4.5 hours after symptom onset, with additional exclusion criteria, which increased r-tPA utilization by as much as 20% in some centers. In 2015, the introduction of advanced endovascular treatment approaches further expanded this treatment window in select patients to up to 7 hours from symptom onset. Since 2015, there have been five prospective randomized clinical trials showing efficacy of endovascular thrombectomy in addition to standard management, typically r-tPA, in improving outcomes of acute ischemic stroke patients with proximal internal carotid artery (ICA) or middle cerebral artery (MCA) occlusions, moderate to severe stroke severity, and presenting within 12 hours of symptom onset. About 15–25% of all ischemic strokes occur during sleep, without the patient knowing the exact time of symptom onset, often making the last known normal time >6 hours before time of presentation. As a result, these wake-up stroke (WUS) patients are excluded from r-tPA treatment and often mechanical thrombectomy as well. Currently, the WAKE-UP and EXTEND trials are underway to further investigate this approach in a larger cohort of patients with WUS.

Question 6

1. Discuss the clinical features and management of geriatric trauma.

Older patients are more vulnerable to trauma due to the combination of comorbid health conditions, prescribed medications, and frailty which increases the chances of subsequent complications, including infections, pneumonia, venous thromboembolism, and multisystem organ failure. Mortality after trauma increases with age but chronologic age is less important in trauma than frailty. Leading cause of traumatic death in the elderly is due to traumatic brain injury. The brain shrinks with increase in age and more susceptible to tearing and bleeding from the shearing forces in trauma as decreasing brain volume causes stretching of the bridging veins. Elderly patients with congestive heart failure (CHF) and those on warfarin or b-blockers have diminished cardiac reserve and are at higher risk of poor outcomes after trauma. Impairment of respiratory muscle mechanics occurs due to increase in chest wall rigidity and worsening kyphosis, and when associated with a weak diaphragm may lead to decreased fraction of expiratory volume in 1 second (FEV1) and decreased vital capacity, and result in an overall decline in respiratory reserve.

Liver and kidney disease: Ischemic, reperfusion injuries, and the risk of hemorrhage are very high with underlying renal, hepatic disease with cirrhosis.

In all unstable elderly patients with trauma aggressive resuscitation should be initiated. All elderly should be considered unstable if they present with persistently abnormal vital signs or not responsive to resuscitation efforts, and those who have evidence of active hemorrhage or deteriorating mental status. Apparently stable geriatric trauma patient should be thoroughly evaluated for occult life-threatening injuries. In elderly patients with trauma abnormal values of serum lactate level and base deficit indicate impending deterioration and may predict mortality. After initial resuscitation, persistently abnormal values of serum lactate and base deficit values should be repeated. Hemodynamic monitoring in elderly patients with trauma is essential. Ultrasonography and echocardiography widely replaced the use of pulmonary artery catheters. Even slight changes in hemodynamic (heart rate blood pressure) in geriatric trauma may signify occult injury and should be investigated thoroughly.

2. What is Good Samaritan law?

The Good Samaritan law is a bill passed by the Supreme Court of India on March 26, 2016. It helped protect individuals who helped accident victims from legal interventions.

Later, it was included in the draft of the Motor Vehicle Act, 2019. A Good Samaritan is exempted from all kinds of civil and criminal liabilities that arise from any act done by him/her to save the life.

3. Explain the factors and mitigation strategy of violence in ED.

There could be situation factors contributing to patients becoming difficult. With an open access to ED patients tend to walk in to ED even for conditions which are not actual medical emergencies. It becomes important to have a robust triage system to attend to such patients and be able to communicate with patients appropriately, e.g., a person coming into hospital for a fall from his bike last evening and having sustained grazed abrasion of his knees, wanting to get dressing done before he goes to his work. Though it is a priority for the patient, it has to be explained that he would be seen in timely order depending on other acuity in department where patients needing more urgent medical attention would be given priority. It is not uncommon to see patients and family members attending to ED seeking advice on wide spectrum of issues. Some of them unrelated to ED, e.g., when will a consultant be available? And when they do not get a reply, they tend to get angry. We need to realize that their anger is form of helplessness as they are not able to find the answer for their question. It would be better if we could spend few minutes in having a sensible discussion with such patients rather than trying to answer a complaint from an irate patient. In organizations where there is need identified it would be productive to have a patient relations personnel to help in smooth journey of patients. As the saying goes "a stitch in time saves nine".

Question 7

1. Explain HINTS test.

HINTS examination: It is a screening tool for distinguishing a central cause of vertigo from an acute peripheral vestibulopathy (APV), such as benign paroxysmal positional vertigo or vestibular neuritis and is particularly useful in an ED setting **(Table 2)**. If the HINTS examination is entirely consistent with peripheral vertigo (positive head impulse test, unidirectional and horizontal nystagmus, negative test of skew), then, it is 100% sensitive and 96% specific for a peripheral cause of vertigo. However, it must be kept in mind that all findings must be present for the HINTS examination to be invoked. If, e.g., the patient has horizontal rightward nystagmus with right gaze and no skew, but has no findings on impulse test, you cannot invoke the HINTS examination to clear the patient.

2. What is white cerebellar sign?

"White cerebellar sign" is a classic yet uncommon radiological finding. This sign is encountered when there is a diffuse decrease in the density of the supratentorial brain parenchyma, with relatively increased attenuation of the cerebellum. This sign indicates irreversible brain damage and has a very poor prognosis.

3. Discuss drawer test.

The anterior drawer test: It identifies the tears of the anterior cruciate ligament (ACL). The test is performed with the patient in a supine position, hip flexed at 45°, and knee flexed at 90°. While stabilizing the patient's foot, the examiner places his or her thumbs over the joint line while pulling the tibia forward. The thumbs are used to palpate for any translation of the tibia relative to the femur. A positive test result is defined as greater anterior translation of the tibia relative to the femur as compared with the other knee.

Posterior drawer test: It assesses for posterior cruciate ligament (PCL) injury. The posterior drawer test can be accomplished with the patient's knee flexed at 90° and the foot stabilized by the examiner. A smooth backward force is applied to the tibia. Posterior displacement of the tibia >5 mm, or a soft end point, indicates injury to the PCL.

TABLE 2: Distinguishing features between peripheral and central causes.

Feature	Peripheral	Central
Nystagmus	Commonly combined (horizontal and torsional), Inhibited by fixation of eyes on to object, does not change direction with gaze to other side	Purely vertical, horizontal, or torsional, not inhibited by fixation of eyes on object, may change direction with gaze toward fast phase of nystagmus
Imbalance	Mild to moderate, generally able to walk	Severe, not able to walk or stand sometimes
Nausea, vomiting	Commonly severe	Varies
Hearing loss, tinnitus	Common	Rare
Neurological (no auditory)	Rare	Common
Latency followed by provocative maneuver	Up to few seconds	Up to 5 seconds

4. Explain Ottawa knee and ankle rules.

The Ottawa knee rules are a set of rules used to help physicians determine whether an X-ray of the knee is needed. They state that an X-ray is required only in patients who have an acute knee injury with one or more of the following:
- Aged 55 years or over
- Tenderness at the head of the fibula
- Isolated tenderness of the patella
- Inability to flex knee to 90°
- Inability to bear weight (defined as an inability to take four steps, i.e., two steps on each leg, regardless of limping) immediately and at presentation.

The Ottawa ankle rules indicate that a radiograph is indicated if any of the following is positive:
- Tenderness along the posterior medial or lateral malleoli
- Base of the 5th metatarsal, navicular
- If the patient is unable to bear weight for four steps following the injury.

Question 8

1. What is ultrasound-guided CPR?

The POCUS-CA (point-of-care ultrasound in cardiac arrest) is a diagnostic tool in the intensive care unit and ED setting **(Fig. 3)**. The literature indicates that in the patient in a cardiorespiratory arrest it can provide information of the etiology of the arrest in patients with nondefibrillable rhythms, assess the quality of compressions during CPR, and define prognosis of survival according to specific findings and, thus, assist the clinician in decision-making during resuscitation. The point of care ultrasound in cardiac arrest (POCUS-CA) conducted by a trained clinician allows the evaluation of the quality of the compressions, the quick diagnosis of reversible causes of arrest with nondefibrillable rhythms, the monitoring interventions, and its response to treatment. It also provides prognostic information regarding the possibility of an ROSC and survival.

2. Discuss ultrasound-guided triage.

Lung ultrasound (US) is proven a reliable tool in diagnosing lung inflammatory processes—the results are immediate and the examination is safe, repeatable, and cheap. Lung parenchymal alterations can be observed at the onset, and a disposable probe cover can ensure a clean procedure. Severe acute respiratory syndrome coronavirus 2 (SARS-CoV-2) infection, symptoms from fever, dry cough, fatigue, and lymphopenia to viral pneumonia with acute respiratory distress syndrome (ARDS). US examinations are easily performed at the point of care, which can be the patient's bedside or even outside the hospital. All these qualities make it a precious tool in clinical practice, optimal to assist clinicians even in initial patient triage. Early literature suggests that patients with confirmed coronavirus disease-2019 (COVID-19) pneumonia demonstrate typical lung imaging features, including pleural line irregularities, B lines, and multifocal consolidations. Early use of lung US is used in Italy in COVID-19 patients, for early diagnoses and appropriate management. Every "field hospitals" (tent) equipped with US scanner to avoid contact between infected patients and noninfected ones, permit early diagnosis outside the hospital, effectively implementing a "US triage." Limitations for the implementation of US triage are the lack of specific protocols and operator experience, which influences the validity of test results.

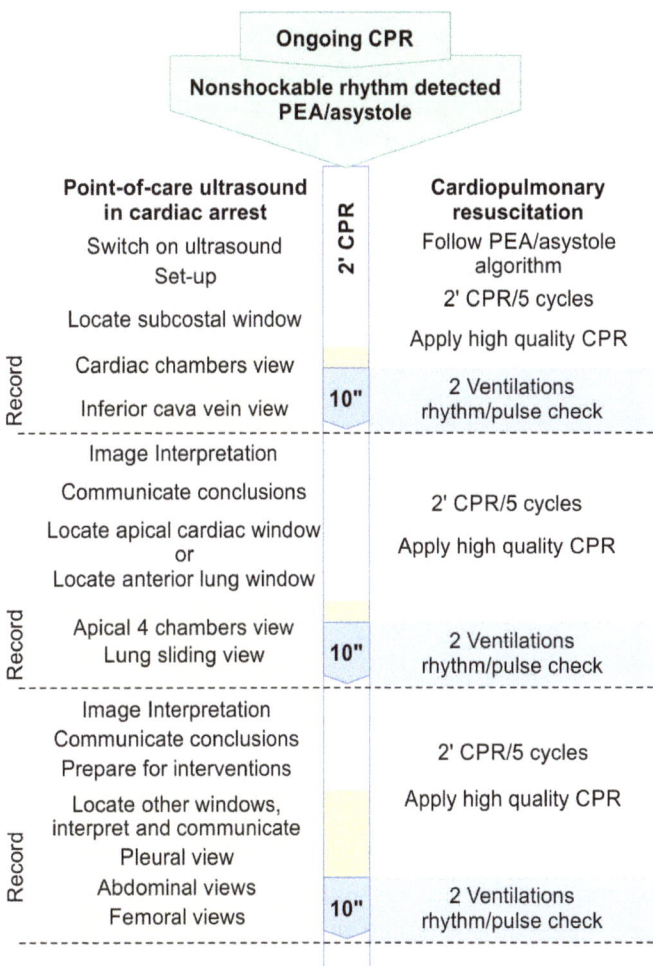

Fig. 3: Point-of-care ultrasound in cardiac arrest.

3. Discuss pediatric emergency ultrasound protocol.

Point-of-care ultrasonography (POCUS) is defined as ultrasonography brought to the patient and performed by the clinician in real time. With this technique, ultrasound (US) images can be obtained immediately and the physician can correlate real-time images with the patient's presenting signs and symptoms. POCUS is easily repeatable if the patient's conditions change, it can be used by various specialties in different situations and may be broadly divided into diagnostic and procedural applications. The premise of a POCUS examination is a focused examination in answer to a specific clinical question. Use of POCUS can alter workflow, increase the financial burden, and incorrect interpretations by untrained users can pose significant risks to patients. However, when POCUS is used as an extension of the physical examination, its benefits are immense, and can provide important information and guidance in management of patient.

4. What is water bath technique of ultrasound?

By submerging the patient's extremity in the water bath, the need for ultrasound gel or contact between the ultrasound transducer and the patient's skin is reduced, thus eliminating discomfort and distortion of the superficial tissue. Using water also avoids compression of these superficial structures. Sonographic examination of painful extremity pathology such as abscesses or lacerations involving the hand or foot can be possible **(Fig. 4)**.

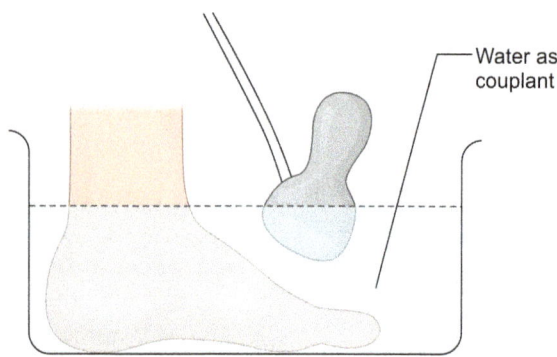

Fig. 4: Water bath technique of ultrasound.

Question 9

1. Discuss the role of telemedicine in emergency care.

Equipping ED treatment rooms with cameras, monitors, and high-speed internet invites new opportunities for remote consultation with specialists around the world. This technology empowers small rural hospitals to partner with sophisticated centers of excellence, no matter how far from the facility, to provide patients with a higher standard of care. Some EDs incorporate smart TVs in the examination rooms connected to the facility picture archiving and communication system so that imaging data can be pulled up in a patient room as an aid for discussions. In the future, touchscreen tablets outside every examination room door will function as both a room sign as well as a tool for medical staff to bring up patient data prior to entering the room—similar to having a paper chart mounted next to the door but more secure and capable of generating additional information. Additionally, Wi-Fi connected equipment, both in and outside of the hospital, allows for patient data to be securely collected and transmitted to physicians for evaluation and tracking. For example, systems currently exist in which a patient may upload glucometer readings or stethoscope sounds directly to their EMR for physicians to review.

2. Explain simulation as teaching tool in emergency.

Simulation is defined as "A technique that creates a situation or environment to allow persons to experience a representation of a real event for the purpose of practice, learning, evaluation, testing, or to gain an understanding of systems or human actions" as per healthcare simulation dictionary. Simulation-based education (SBE) became popular in emergency medicine (EM) in the last 20–25 years. SBE is one of the key components of the emergency medicine training curriculum in many countries. Simulation-based education plays a vital role in developing competencies in the EM trainees by providing them opportunities to become proficient in high-frequency high-risk situations and procedures, as well as low-frequency high-risk circumstances. This type of education also provides the trainees with a conducive and safe learning environment to practice and learn from their mistakes. SBE in recent years has proved to enhance not only the technical skills of the trainees but also the nontechnical skills of the trainees such as interprofessional teamwork, crisis resource management, communication, systems-based practice, and professionalism. In addition to the acquisition of knowledge, simulation in health care can be used of other purposes such as process testing, identification of latent safety threats, verification of systems-based practices, equipment validation, and research and development.

3. What are the tactical casualty combat care (TCCC) guidelines?

Tactical combat casualty care principles: TCCC was the first set of battlefield trauma care guidelines. It was the result of the Naval Special Warfare biomedical research program when it was realized that the most common cause of preventable death amongst injured service personnel was external hemorrhage, but that the use of tourniquets was actively discouraged. The resulting set of guidance was put together comprising a phased approach to care on the battlefield as laid out in **Table 3**.

TABLE 3: Phases of tactical casualty combat care.

Phase	Tactical situation	Aims
Care under fire	Personnel engaged in combat with ongoing threat	• Return fire and take cover—superior firepower prevents further wounds/casualties • Direct casualty to self-aid and continue combat or take cover as able • If able, stop life-threatening hemorrhage or place in recovery position if airway or consciousness impaired
Tactical field care	No longer engaged in hostile situation.	• Field triage • Disarm casualty with altered mental status—preventing further injury/casualties • Structured assessment using acronym MARCH (M: Massive hemorrhage; A: Airway; R: Respiration; C: Circulation; H: Hypothermia/Head Injury) • Perform secondary survey and treat other wounds if able
Tactical evacuation	Transportation available to higher level of medical care	As per tactical field care, however increased resources may mean better ability to treat and monitor certain conditions, e.g., traumatic brain injury

Question 10

1. Discuss quality improvement research in ED.

Institutions need to adapt appropriate quality indicators in emergency department like: Door to triage time, door to doctor time, door to needle time in stroke thrombolysis, pain score assessment, investigation return time, nurse/patient ratio, patient satisfaction level, time taken for discharge, mortality (adjusted), length of stay, left without been seen by doctor, pain assessment/reassessment, safety—patient falls, medication error, failed intubation rate, incident reporting, and hand hygiene compliance.

The ED is considered particularly high risk for adverse events (AE): 60% of ED patients experienced medication error. Various studies suggest that prevalence of AE related to ED is increasing and most of them are preventable. About 60% of ED patients experienced medication error. An adverse event is defined as "an injury caused by medical management rather than by the underlying disease or condition of the patient". Appropriate mock assessments periodically and audits are a must to ensure the policies and processes and implemented at the ground level.

2. Explain the communication skills in ED.

Communication skills are required in every profession and every work that one does **(Fig. 5)**. But here we are talking about communication being a very different kind of a skill set. It includes being able to communicate happiness about the delivery of a child or safety of the patient. It includes communicating about taking up the next course of action for patients about admission/surgery/follow up, etc. It could be about breaking bad news about death, bad outcomes, or the actual patient condition that most of the times people are not prepared to listen and accept. The preparation for any such conversation is completely different from one another. Some relatives/family members/patients can understand the situation/outcome, some are irate, some unhappy, and some angry. Emergency physician has obviously to deal with all types of these especially when such things happen in the middle of the night or odd hours and when there is less dependency on others in the hospital.

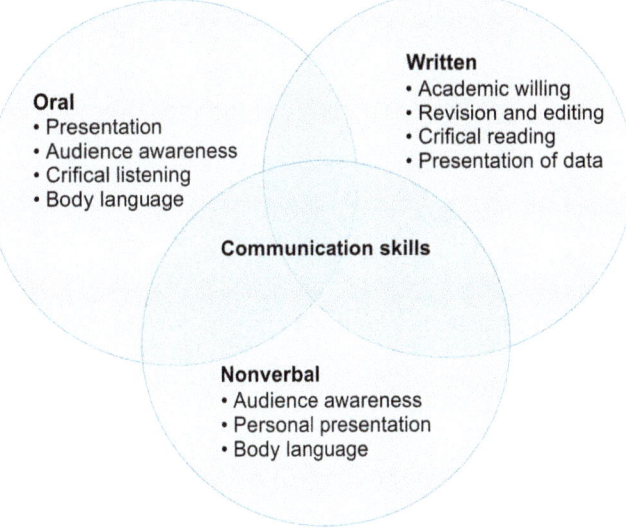

Fig. 5: Components of the communication skills.

3. What are the common errors in emergency and patient safety issues—medicolegal issues?

Five common emergency room errors are:
- *Diagnostic errors:* Including misdiagnosis and failure to diagnose.
- *Triage errors:* Patients who require immediate medical care are forced to wait behind patients with less-urgent conditions.
- *Medication errors:* Including providing the wrong medication, wrong dose, or failing to check for drug allergies or unsafe drug interactions.
- *Communication errors:* Such as discharge instructions that do not provide the necessary information for patients to properly manage their own care.
- *Failure to order* or correctly interpret diagnostic tests.

Legal issues in ED are:
- Consent
- Patient confidentiality
- Competence
- Documentation
- Medical error
- Medicolegal reports
- Duty of care transfer of responsibility
- Leaving against advice
- Leaving without being seen
- Refusing treatment.

■ SUGGESTED READING

1. Richhariya D, Sharma B. Textbook of Emergency Medicine including Intensive Care and Trauma, 2nd edition. New Delhi: Jaypee Brothers Medical Publishers (P) Ltd; 2022. pp. 365-72. (Question 1).
2. Richhariya D, Sharma B. Textbook of Emergency Medicine including Intensive Care and Trauma, 2nd edition. New Delhi: Jaypee Brothers Medical Publishers (P) Ltd; 2022. pp. 205, 216. (Question 2).
3. Richhariya D, Sharma B. Textbook of Emergency Medicine including Intensive Care and Trauma, 2nd edition. New Delhi: Jaypee Brothers Medical Publishers (P) Ltd; 2022. pp. 1533, 1594-5. (Question 3).
4. Richhariya D, Sharma B. Textbook of Emergency Medicine including Intensive Care and Trauma, 2nd edition. New Delhi: Jaypee Brothers Medical Publishers (P) Ltd; 2022. pp. 80-90. (Question 4).
5. Richhariya D, Sharma B. Textbook of Emergency Medicine including Intensive Care and Trauma, 2nd edition. New Delhi: Jaypee Brothers Medical Publishers (P) Ltd; 2022. p. 227. (Question 5).
6. Richhariya D, Sharma B. Textbook of Emergency Medicine including Intensive Care and Trauma, 2nd edition. New Delhi: Jaypee Brothers Medical Publishers (P) Ltd; 2022. pp. 120-22, 1637-40. (Question 6).
7. Richhariya D, Sharma B. Textbook of Emergency Medicine including Intensive Care and Trauma, 2nd edition. New Delhi: Jaypee Brothers Medical Publishers (P) Ltd; 2022. pp. 806, 1617. (Question 7).
8. Richhariya D, Sharma B. Textbook of Emergency Medicine including Intensive Care and Trauma, 2nd edition. New Delhi: Jaypee Brothers Medical Publishers (P) Ltd; 2022. p. 365. (Question 8).
9. Richhariya D, Sharma B. Textbook of Emergency Medicine including Intensive Care and Trauma, 2nd edition. New Delhi: Jaypee Brothers Medical Publishers (P) Ltd; 2022. pp. 101, 109, 195. (Question 9).
10. Richhariya D, Sharma B. Textbook of Emergency Medicine including Intensive Care and Trauma, 2nd edition. New Delhi: Jaypee Brothers Medical Publishers (P) Ltd; 2022. pp. 2, 50, 132. (Question 10).

Emergency Medicine Paper 29

Noel Fernando

Question 1

1. Illustrate the counter-current mechanism of urine acidification.

The counter-current mechanism is an important process that occurs in the kidneys to help maintain the proper pH balance of the body by regulating the acidity of urine. Urine acidification is one example of this process. The counter-current mechanism involves the interaction of two parallel loops of the nephron, known as the ascending and descending limbs of the loop of Henle. The descending limb of the loop of Henle is permeable to water, but not to solutes such as ions. As the fluid in the descending limb moves into the more concentrated medulla, it loses water but retains solutes, resulting in more concentrated urine (Fig. 1).

- Meanwhile, the ascending limb of the loop of Henle actively transports solutes such as sodium and chloride out of the urine, but not water. This results in the urine becoming less concentrated as it moves up the ascending limb.
- The two limbs of the loop of Henle form a counter-current system, with the fluid in the descending limb moving in the opposite direction to the fluid in the ascending limb. This helps to establish a concentration gradient in the medulla, which is important for urine acidification.
- In the distal tubules of the nephron, hydrogen ions (H^+) are secreted into the urine and exchanged for sodium ions (Na^+) in a process known as antiport. This is facilitated by the enzyme carbonic anhydrase, which helps to convert carbon dioxide (CO_2) and water (H_2O) into bicarbonate (HCO_3^-) and hydrogen ions (H^+).
- The exchange of hydrogen ions for sodium ions in the distal tubules creates a concentration gradient in the medulla, with higher concentrations of hydrogen ions in the more distal portions of the tubules. As the concentrated urine flows down the collecting ducts, water is reabsorbed, further concentrating the urine and increasing its acidity.

Overall, the counter-current mechanism plays an important role in urine acidification by establishing a concentration gradient in the medulla and facilitating the secretion of hydrogen ions into the urine, which helps to maintain the proper pH balance of the body.

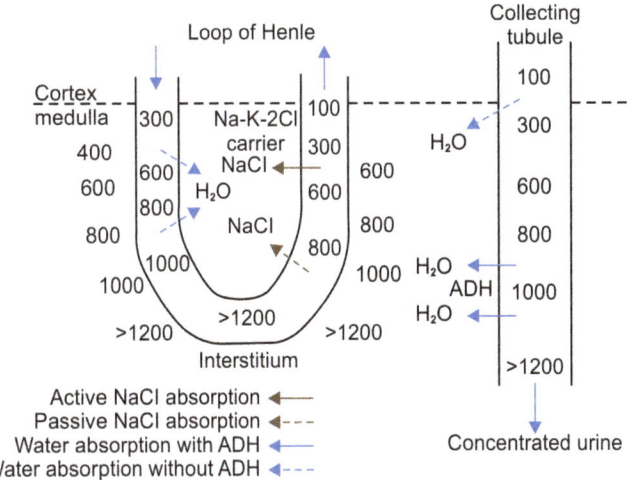

Fig. 1: Counter current mechanism.

2. Discuss various methods to provide renal replacement therapy.

Renal replacement therapy (RRT) describes the support provided to the failing kidneys with the primary objective of fluid and solute removal. RRT does not replace endocrine or cardiovascular functions of kidney. Basic principles RRT rely on passage of blood through a semi-permeable membrane to achieve solute and fluid removal. This happens by two standard methods and combinations of these.

Hemofiltration:
- Operates on the basis of convection.
- The hydrostatic pressure gradient drives water, across a semi-permeable membrane; solvent drag carries low molecular weight solutes (<5,000 Daltons) through the membrane in the same direction as the water; the resultant fluid is described as ultrafiltrate.
- The ultrafiltrate is discarded; a buffered, electrolyte fluid is administered post-filter to replace the ultrafiltrate.
- The volume of replaced fluid can be adjusted; the volume of replacement fluid relative to ultrafiltrate determines the net fluid balance.

Hemodialysis:
- Operates on the basis of diffusion (i.e., movement of solutes down a concentration gradient).
- Blood and dialysate fluid are separated by a semi-permeable membrane and flow past each other in opposite directions (counter-current flow).
- Dialysate is a fluid containing electrolytes, and a buffer—usually bicarbonate or lactate (bicarbonate is increasingly preferred in critically ill patients).
- Solutes move from blood to dialysate; buffer moves from dialysate to blood.
- Fluid removal can be achieved by ultrafiltration, i.e., by increasing the pressure across the membrane (transmembrane pressure) with fluid moving from the blood to the dialysate compartment. In a pure hemodialysis mode, this filtration component does not contribute significantly to solute removal.

Hemodiafiltration:
- Combines the principles of filtration and dialysis.
- Differs from hemodialysis in that the filtration component is increased beyond the point required for fluid removal alone and, therefore, solute drag contributes to solute clearance.
- The dialysis component tends to remove smaller solutes (<500 Daltons; urea, creatinine, electrolytes, and lithium); filtration is more effective in the removal of middle-sized (500–5,000 Daltons; large drugs, e.g., vancomycin) and large (>5,000 Daltons; cytokines, complement) solutes.

Continuous renal replacement therapy (CRRT):
- This is the most widely used RRT modality in modern critical care and includes the following sub-type
  - Continuous veno-venous hemofiltration (CVVH/CVVHF)
  - Continuous veno-venous hemodialysis (CVVHD)
  - Continuous veno-venous hemodiafiltration (CVVHDF)
- Typically, blood flows of 100–200 mL/minute are required.
- CVVHDF has the theoretical advantage of increased solute clearance; however, there is no good-quality evidence currently that it improves outcomes in terms of survival.
- The requirement for dialysate provision in CVVHDF may relatively increase costs.
- Requirement for anticoagulation.

Intermittent hemodialysis (IHD):
- IHD uses high blood flow rates (e.g., 400 mL/minute) against a counter-current flow of dialysate across the membrane—this leads to rapid solute clearance.
- High dialysate flows lead to high filtrate volumes.
- Sessions typically last for 3–5 hours at a time.
- The US ATN study showed no difference in outcome comparing a high-intensity (six sessions/week) regimen compared to a low-intensity (three sessions/week) regimen in hemodynamically stable critically ill patients with AKI.

Slow low efficiency dialysis (SLED):
- This newer hybrid mode of RRT combines low blood and dialysate flows over an extended period of 6–12 hours.
- It can be achieved using standard IHD equipment, while having the cardiovascular stability and solute removal advantages of CRRT.
- Its intermittent nature means that patients can be mobile in-between sessions, potentially facilitating investigations and rehabilitation.

Slow continuous ultrafiltration (SCUF):
- Utilizes filtration principle, removing up to 2 liters of fluid per hour.
- No replacement fluid is, however, used making this a simpler, less intensive form of RRT, suitable for patients in whom fluid overload is the only indication.

3. What are the emergency complications in a patient with renal transplant?

Renal transplant patients can be very complicated to manage because of the underlying pathology necessitating the transplant. They are prone to have unique postoperative complications due to the intake of vast array of immunosuppressants. They range from side effects of potent immunosuppressive drugs or from drug interactions, renal tract problems, respiratory infections, fever, postsurgical complications, cardiovascular, gastrointestinal, neurologic, endocrine and electrolyte imbalance.

Rejection: In general, a single kidney is transplanted in the right or left lower quadrant of the abdomen. Living donor transplants function immediately, while 30% of cadaver transplants undergo delayed graft function due to prolonged cold ischemic preservation. The renal transplant recipient will now require long-term immunosuppression to prevent rejection. The current regimen is based on a triple therapy approach that includes cyclosporine-microemulsion or tacrolimus, mycophenolate mofetil or azathioprine and corticosteroids. Antilymphocyte antibodies are also widely used with the triple therapy regimen. Due to the invent of the current potent immunosuppressive regimens it has led to less rejection, there is a greater incidence of medication-related problems.

Renal failure: Renal failure in transplant patients is uniquely caused by rejection.

Two common causes of acute renal failure are acute cyclosporine or tacrolimus nephrotoxicity and acute rejection. Elevated blood levels of cyclosporine or tacrolimus favor nephrotoxicity. The ideal time to draw a drug level is 1–3 hours before a dose is scheduled, making these levels unreliable at times in the ED. Renal transplant recipients that present with fever and allograft tenderness and increased creatinine make acute rejection the likely diagnosis.

Infections: Urinary tract infections occur in <10% of patients in the first posttransplant year and are similar to that in the general population. Therefore, the most common pathogen to cause urinary tract infections in renal transplant recipients is *E. (Escherichia) coli*. Remember, to avoid aminoglycosides, a nephrotoxic agent, when treating urinary tract infections. Pneumonia is the most common pulmonary infection in renal transplant recipients presenting to the ED. Nonopportunistic infections occur in the first month posttransplant, followed by opportunistic infections in the first year and community-acquired respiratory infections afterward. Macrolides should be avoided in the treatment of pneumonia. The macrolides inhibit the hepatic enzyme system that metabolizes the immunosuppressants.

Fever: It is a common problem in renal transplant patients. Immunosuppressed patients are susceptible to opportunistic infections which can progress to be fulminant, however, they are uncommon in the first posttransplant month.

The highest incidence of opportunistic infections occurs between the second- and sixth-month posttransplant. Opportunistic infections vary geographically; therefore, it is important that ED physicians understand what pathogens are prevalent in renal transplant patients at their institution and provide appropriate treatment. Cytomegalovirus (CMV) disease is an opportunistic infection common in renal transplant patients and with no variation in geographic prevalence. A renal transplant patient presenting 2 months after kidney transplant with high fever, elevated liver function tests and leukopenia likely has CMV disease. CMV is diagnosed with polymerase chain reaction (PCR) and most commonly presents between 1 and 6 months posttransplant. Patients presenting with a fever in the first year after transplant generally will require admission.

Surgical complications: Acute occlusion of the transplant renal artery or vein, peritransplant hematoma, urinary leak, lymphocele, obstructive uropathy, bleeding.

Cardiovascular complications: Arrhythmias is more common in renal transplant patients. The risk of cardiovascular disease is threefold to fivefold higher in renal transplant recipients compared with the general population. If diltiazem, verapamil or amiodarone is used beware of the immunosuppressive agents, cyclosporine, tacrolimus or sirolimus. The antiarrhythmic agents inhibit the hepatic P-450 enzyme system, subsequently, elevating the immunosuppressive levels.

Hypertensive emergencies: It can be treated with parenteral or oral antihypertensives.

Gastrointestinal disorders are common and their severity may be blunted by immunosuppressants, therefore radiologic studies are required.

Neurologic complications can result from side effects of immunosuppressive drugs, opportunistic infections or malignancy. Headaches in the renal transplant patient warrant a lumbar puncture and imaging studies of the brain.

Hematological problems: Anemia, leukopenia, and thrombocytopenia may be caused by immunosuppressants, antibiotics, antivirals, or corticosteroids. Corticosteroids can also cause osteoporosis, avascular necrosis or tendon rupture affecting the Achilles or quadriceps. Osteoporosis tends to affect the feet for unclear reasons. Cyclosporine and tacrolimus cause hyperkalemia and hypomagnesemia. The abovementioned immunosuppressants along with corticosteroids can cause de novo diabetes in 5–20% of renal transplant recipients. Lastly the combination of anemia, thrombocytopenia, and acute renal failure suggests hemolytic uremic syndrome.

The renal transplant recipient is prone to a number of complications. Hence, it is important that emergency physicians understand these complexities, including drug interactions, and make sure to effectively communicate with the transplant physician.

Question 2

1. Discuss pathophysiology of diabetic ketoacidosis.

Diabetic ketoacidosis (DKA) is an acute metabolic complication of diabetes caused by absolute or relative insulin deficiency. It commonly occurs in patients with type I diabetes. But also occurs in some patients with type II diabetes, often seen in Afro-Caribbean or Hispanic origin, commonly known as ketosis-prone type II diabetes.

- Insulin deficiency (absolute or relative) is accompanied by an increase in counterregulatory hormones (glucagon, cortisol, growth hormone, and adrenaline) leading to enhanced hepatic gluconeogenesis and glycogenolysis, leading to severe hyperglycemia.

- Enhanced lipolysis increases serum-free fatty acids, which are metabolized to ketones and cause a metabolic acidosis.
- Fluid depletion occurs via osmotic diuresis due to hyperglycemia, vomiting, and ultimately a reduced oral intake due to a reduced level of consciousness.

2. Explain diagnostic criteria for diabetic ketoacidosis.

- Ketonemia (>3 mmol/L) or significant ketonuria (>2+ on urine dipstick)
- Blood glucose >11 mmol/L or known diabetes mellitus
- Bicarbonate <15 mmol/L and/or venous pH <7.3.

3. What are the complications of diabetic ketoacidosis?

Hypokalemia and hyperkalemia: Due to profound acidosis the intracellular potassium is excreted into the intravascular compartment causing hyperkalemia. In contrary when the insulin infusion is started, it moves the potassium from intravascular compartment to intracellular compartment causing hypokalemia.

Hypoglycemia: It is a very common complication during the latter part of treatment, as insulin infusion causes significant hypoglycemia. We need a close monitoring to avoid this complication, hence the guideline advises to start a glucose infusion once the sugar level drops down to 14 mmol/L.

Cerebral edema and pulmonary edema: It is very common to have these complications. Due to high volume of intravenous fluid administration, fluid overload happens resulting in cerebral edema and pulmonary edema. Cerebral edema results in raised intracranial pressure eventually resulting in loss of airway reflexes which leads to aspiration.

Aspiration pneumonia:
Thromboembolism: In diabetic patients, vascular endothelial integrity, which provides the primary defense against thrombus, is impaired. Fibrinogen is high in diabetics at the level of factor VII, factor VIII, factor XI, factor XII, kallikrein and vWF, and these coagulation factors increase the activation and adhesion of the thrombocytes, as well as blood viscosity. Low levels of protein C in diabetic patients increase the tendency to coagulation. An increased level of plasminogen activator inhibitor factor-1 leads to impairment in fibrinolysis in these patients. In addition, the levels of some factors increasing thrombocyte aggregation were found to be higher in diabetic patients.

According to a study in DKA, the activity of protein C decreased considerably and the levels of fibrinogen, homocysteine and vWF increased; however, these factors recovered with DKA therapy. Changes in the turbulence of blood flow induced by hypovolemia caused by the effect of hyperglycemia and DKA can increase the thrombocyte aggregation and adhesion and lead to impaired endothelial integrity. In our patient, DKA may have triggered thrombosis by hypercoagulability and its effect of increasing stasis.

Question 3

1. Discuss anatomy and physiology of neuromuscular junction.

The neuromuscular junction (NMJ) **(Fig. 2)** is a specialized synapse between a motor neuron and a muscle fiber. This junction is responsible for the transmission of nerve impulses from the motor neuron to the muscle fiber, which results in muscle contraction. The anatomy and physiology of the neuromuscular junction can be divided into three main components—the presynaptic terminal, the synaptic cleft, and the postsynaptic membrane.

Presynaptic terminal: The presynaptic terminal is located at the end of the motor neuron and contains numerous synaptic vesicles. These vesicles store acetylcholine (ACh), which is the neurotransmitter that is released into the synaptic cleft to activate the muscle fiber. The presynaptic terminal also contains voltage-gated calcium channels that open in response to an action potential, allowing calcium ions to enter the cell and trigger the release of ACh.

Synaptic Cleft: The synaptic cleft is the narrow gap between the presynaptic terminal and the postsynaptic membrane. It is filled with a gel-like substance called the basal lamina, which contains various proteins and enzymes that help to maintain the structure and function of the NMJ. The basal lamina also contains the enzyme acetylcholinesterase (AChE), which breaks down ACh to terminate its action and prevent continuous muscle contraction.

Postsynaptic membrane: The postsynaptic membrane is the specialized region of the muscle fiber that is located directly opposite the presynaptic terminal. It contains numerous folds called junctional folds, which increase the surface area available for ACh receptors. The postsynaptic membrane also contains voltage-gated ion channels that open in response to ACh binding, allowing sodium ions to enter the cell and generate an action potential that triggers muscle contraction.

Overall, the neuromuscular junction is a complex and highly specialized structure that allows for the precise control of muscle contraction by the nervous system. Dysfunction of the NMJ can lead to various neuromuscular disorders, such as myasthenia gravis, which is characterized by muscle weakness and fatigue due to impaired neurotransmission at the NMJ.

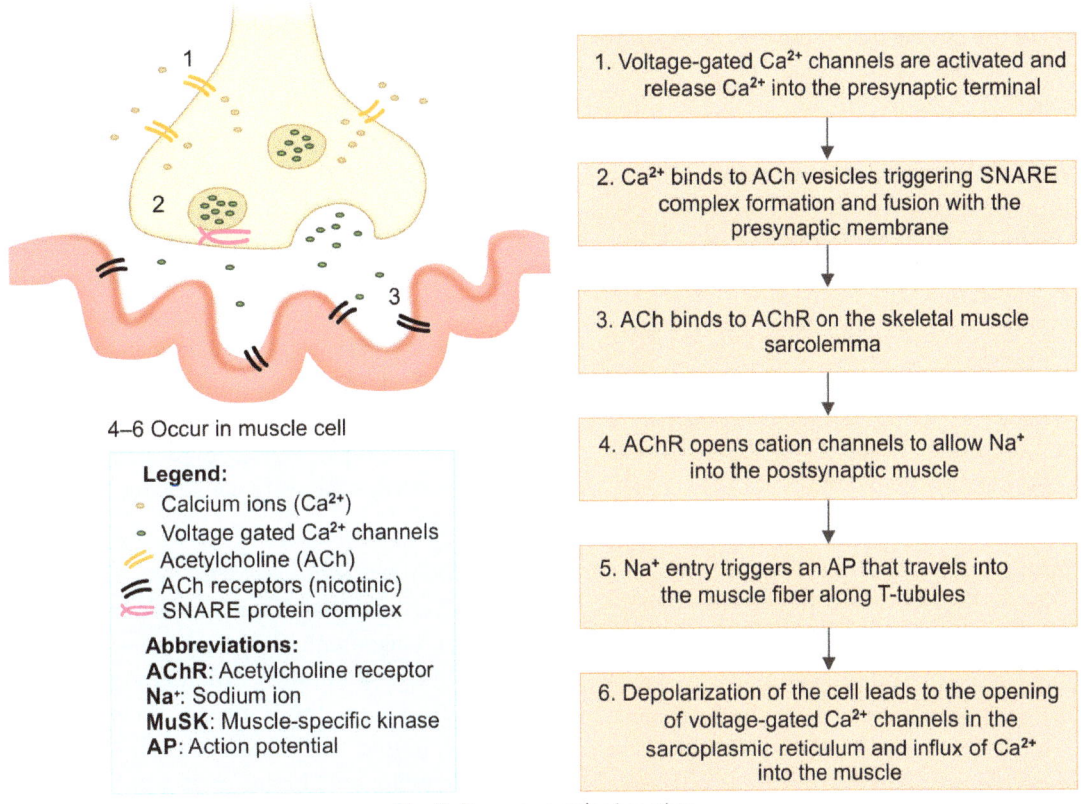

Fig. 2: Neuromuscular junction.

2. Enumerate differential diagnosis of acute onset of quadriparesis.

The differential diagnosis of this picture is potentially broad, encompassing myelopathies, polyneuropathies, neuromuscular transmission disorders, and myopathies, although many of these possibilities are rapidly excluded on the basis of the clinical features **(Table 1)**.

3. Discuss management of myasthenic crisis.

Myasthenic crisis is a life-threatening exacerbation of myasthenia gravis that is defined as worsening of myasthenic weakness requires due to weakness of respiratory muscles and bulbar (oropharyngeal) muscle weakness. This results in upper airway obstruction or severe dysphagia with potential aspiration, intubation, and ventilatory support are necessary for these group of patients.

Myasthenic crisis may be the initial manifestation of myasthenia gravis in about 15–20% of patients.

Diagnosis of a myasthenic crisis requires two components:

Careful cardiopulmonary evaluation with exclusion of other active processes:
- Thorough history, chest X-ray, EKG, and lung ultrasonography.
- Imaging (e.g., CT angiography to exclude PE).

Evidence of worsening muscular weakness:
- History and physical examination may be helpful (e.g., patient reports increasing limb weakness and this is confirmed on examination).
- Respiratory function assessment: Forced vital capacity (FVC) should be measured if the patient is not extremely dyspneic. Forced vital capacity should be reduced in order to make a diagnosis of myasthenic crisis.

Treatment strategies: Early ABCDE assessment and optimizing them appropriately.
- *Noninvasive ventilation:* Noninvasive ventilation (NIV) may be used on patient groups who have mild respiratory distress and expected to improve quickly. Most importantly they have a good cough and able to protect the airway. It is often used as an early therapy, prior to the

development of severe hypercapnia or acidosis, to prevent atelectasis and to relieve early mild respiratory muscle weakness. Evidence supports avoidance of prolonged use of NIV (e.g., days) and suggest that failure to respond to NIV early in the course of its application might be an indication for invasive mechanical ventilation. NIV is not appropriate in patients who are unable to achieve a satisfactory interface or are unable to cooperate. In these situation plan for early elective intubation.

TABLE 1: Differential diagnosis of acute onset flaccid quadriparesis.

Myelopathies	Infection
• Compressive myelopathy • Transverse myelitis • Brainstem encephalitis • Necrotizing myelopathy	• Poliomyelitis • Enterovirus • Flaviviruses

Neuropathies: Primary	Neuropathies: Secondary

• Guillain–Barré syndrome variants:
  – Acute inflammatory demyelinating polyneuropathy
  – Acute motor axonal neuropathy
  – Acute motor and sensory axonal neuropathy
  – Miller–Fisher syndrome
	• Metabolic: Diabetes, uremia, porphyria
	• Infection: Lyme disease, diphtheria, HIV, hepatitis C
	• Drugs/toxins: Alcohol, organophosphates, heavy metals (arsenic, thallium, gold)
	• Autoimmune: Vasculitis neuropathy, with or without connective tissue disorder
	• Malignant: Para neoplasia
	• Others: Critical illness polyneuropathy

Neuromuscular junction transmission disorder	Myopathies
• Myasthenia gravis • Lambert–Eaton myasthenic syndrome • Botulism • Venom: Snake, sea urchin	• Acute inflammatory myopathies *Others* • Conversion disorder/factitious disorder • Brainstem infarction (locked-in syndrome)

- **Invasive ventilation:** Invasive ventilation with positive pressure ventilation should be considered electively rather than as an emergent response to precipitous respiratory collapse. This allows clearance of secretions for patients in whom a prolonged course of crisis is anticipated.

    The threshold for elective intubation should be low if serial measurements demonstrate one or both of the following:
    - VC falls below 15-20 mL/kg
    - MIP is less negative than −25 to −30 cmH$_2$O (i.e., between 0 and −30 cmH$_2$O)

    Additional indications for mechanical ventilation include clinical signs of respiratory distress, progressive respiratory acidosis despite therapy, and inadequate secretion clearance (e.g., recurrent episodes of acute hypoxemia due to mucus plugging).

    For intubation, both a sedative and a neuromuscular blocking agent should be coadministered. Due to the relative paucity of acetylcholine receptors in myasthenia gravis, there is a relative resistance to succinylcholine, necessitating higher doses, and a relative sensitivity to nondepolarizing neuromuscular blockers, necessitating lower doses. Hence a nondepolarizing agent such as rocuronium is commonly used.

- **Supportive respiratory therapies:** Meticulous attention to pulmonary toilet is required for patients with myasthenic crisis due to ineffective cough mechanism. Evidence suggests that "aggressive" respiratory treatment that consisted of the use of suction, intermittent positive pressure breathing or bronchodilator treatments, sighs, and chest physiotherapy appeared to decrease the risk of prolonged respiratory complications.

Specific treatment
- *Inhibition of antibody synthesis:*
    - *Steroids:* High dose steroids are used as first line of management. They may cause a transient worsening of the symptoms, which is a rare complication. The dose of prednisolone is 1–1.5 mg/kg/day.
    - *Immunosuppressants:* The immunosuppressants play a major role in group of patients where steroids are contraindicated. The most common drugs used are mycophenolate or azathioprine. You can also use them as steroid-sparing agents, to decrease the steroid dose. Rituximab, cyclophosphamide, pulsed steroids if first-line therapy does not work. Thymectomy is viewed as definitive, but should wait until the patient is stable.
- *Protection of neuromuscular junction:*
    - *Eculizumab* is an option in severe and refractory cases. This is an antibody to the terminal C5 complement molecule, and it should prevent the formation of the membrane attack complex which is what damages the neuromuscular junction.

Restoration of neuromuscular transmission:
- Acetylcholinesterase inhibitors such as pyridostigmine could be started fairly early, but will probably have little effect in the initial stages of the crisis. They will become more important as the time comes to wean the patient from the ventilator. Pyridostigmine is usually given as 240–480 mg/day in several divided doses.

Autoantibodies removal: Antibody removal plays a prime role in the management of myasthenic crisis. The following strategies are commonly used. There is no difference in the

outcome between these strategies, depending upon the local hospital policy and resource availability, anyone of the following strategies used.
- Plasma exchange—usually five exchanges required, every second day.
- IV immunoglobulin—2 g/kg over 2 days. The mechanism of action is unknown. A single dose of 1 g/kg is probably equally effective but can be used as a 5-day course.

Question 4

1. Describe the physiology of lung volume and capacities.

Definition: Lung volumes refer to the volume of gas in the lungs at a given time during the respiratory cycle. Lung capacities are derived from a summation of different lung volumes **(Fig. 3)**. The average total lung capacity of an adult human male is about 6 liters of air. Lung volumes measurement is an integral part of pulmonary function test. These volumes tend to vary, depending on the depth of respiration, ethnicity, gender, age, body composition and in certain respiratory diseases. A number of the lung volumes can be measured by spirometry-tidal volume, inspiratory reserve volume, and expiratory reserve volume. However, measurement of residual volume, functional residual capacity, and total lung capacity is through body plethysmography, nitrogen washout, and helium dilution technique.

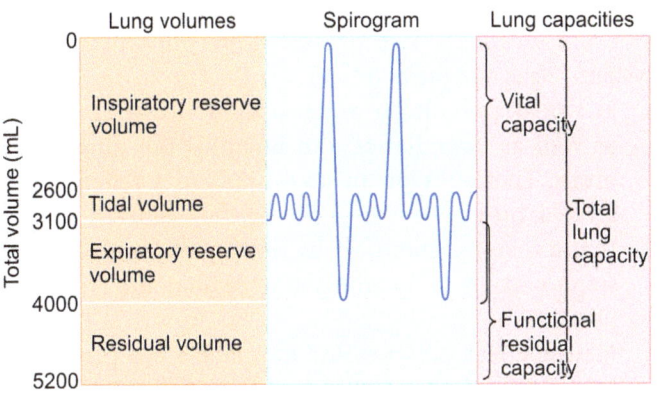

Fig. 3: Lung volume and capacities.

Lung volumes:
Tidal volume (TV): It is the amount of air that can be inhaled or exhaled during one respiratory cycle. This reflects the functions of the respiratory centers, respiratory muscles, and the mechanics of the lung and chest wall. The normal adult value is 10% of vital capacity (VC), approximately 300–500 mL (6–8 mL/kg); but can increase up to 50% of VC on exercise.

Inspiratory reserve volume (IRV): It is the amount of air that can be forcibly inhaled after a normal tidal volume. IRV is usually kept in reserve, but is used during deep breathing. The normal adult value is 1,900–3,300 mL.

Expiratory reserve volume (ERV): It is the volume of air that can be exhaled forcibly after exhalation of normal tidal volume. The normal adult value is 700–1,200 mL. ERV is reduced with obesity, ascites or after upper abdominal surgery.

Residual volume (RV): It is the volume of air remaining in the lungs after maximal exhalation. Normal adult value is averaged at 1,200 mL (20–25 mL/kg). It is indirectly measured from summation of FRC and ERV and cannot be measured by spirometry. In obstructive lung diseases with features of incomplete emptying of the lungs and air trapping, RV may be significantly high. The RV can also be expressed as a percentage of total lung capacity and values in excess of 140% significantly increase the risks of barotrauma, pneumothorax, infection and reduced venous return due to high intrathoracic pressures as noticed in patients with high RV who require surgery and mechanical ventilation thus needs high perioperative inflation pressures.

Lung capacities:
Inspiratory capacity (IC): It is the maximum volume of air that can be inhaled following a resting state. It is calculated from the sum of inspiratory reserve volume and tidal volume. IC = IRV + TV.

Total lung capacity (TLC): It is the maximum volume of air the lungs can accommodate or sum of all volume compartments or volume of air in lungs after maximum inspiration. The normal value is about 6,000 mL (4–6 L). TLC is calculated by summation of the four primary lung volumes (TV, IRV, ERV, and RV).

Total lung capacity may be increased in patients with obstructive defects such as emphysema and decreased in patients with restrictive abnormalities including chest wall abnormalities and kyphoscoliosis.

Vital capacity (VC): It is the total amount of air exhaled after maximal inhalation. The value is about 4,800 mL and it varies according to age and body size. It is calculated by summing tidal volume, inspiratory reserve volume, and expiratory reserve volume. VC = TV + IRV + ERV.

Vital capacity indicates ability to breathe deeply and cough, reflecting inspiratory and expiratory muscle strength. VC should be three times greater than TV for effective cough. VC is sometimes reduced in obstructive disorders and always in restrictive disorders.

Function residual capacity (FRC): It is the amount of air remaining in the lungs at the end of a normal exhalation. It is calculated by adding together residual and expiratory reserve volumes. The normal value is about 1,800–2,200 mL. FRC = RV + ERV.

Function residual capacity does not rely on effort and highlights the resting position when inner and outer elastic recoils are balanced. FRC is reduced in restrictive disorders. The ratio of FRC to TLC is an index of hyperinflation. In chronic obstructive pulmonary disease, FRC ranges up to 80% of TLC.

2. Discuss initial ventilator management in patients with respiratory acidosis.

Invasive mechanical ventilation is an intervention that is frequently used in acutely ill patients requiring either respiratory support or airway protection. The ventilator allows gas exchange to be maintained while other treatments are given to improve the clinical condition. Evidence clearly supports that noninvasive ventilation has improved outcomes with hypercapnic respiratory failure. When noninvasive ventilation fails or contraindicated, then it is time to step up to invasive ventilation.

Ventilator management
- The initial ventilator setting can vary greatly depending on the cause for intubation. As we are focusing on hypercapnic respiratory failure such as COPD, asthma. The most common ventilator mode to use in a newly intubated patient is assist control mode (AC). The AC mode provides good comfort and easy control of some of the most important physiologic parameters. It is started with a FiO_2 of 100% and titrated down guided by pulse oximetry or ABG, depending on the case.
- Low-tidal volume ventilation has been shown to be lung protective not only in ARDS but in other types of diseases. Starting the patient on a low-tidal volume (6–8 mL/kg of ideal body weight) will reduce the incidence of ventilator-induced lung injury (VILI). Always use a lung-protective strategy as there are not many advantages for higher tidal volumes and they will increase shear stress in the alveoli and may induce lung injury.
- Initial RR should be comfortable for the patient 10–12 bpm should suffice. A very important caveat on this is for patients with severe metabolic acidosis. For these patients, the minute ventilation should at least be matched to their preintubation ventilation as failure to do so will worsen acidosis and can precipitate complications such as cardiac arrest.
- Flow should be initiated at or above 60 L/minute to prevent auto-PEEP.
- Start with a low PEEP of 5 cmH_2O and titrate up as tolerated by the patient to the goal for oxygenation. Pay close attention to blood pressure and patient comfort while doing this.
- An ABG should be obtained 30 minutes after intubation and changes to the ventilator settings should be made in accordance with ABG findings.
- Peak and plateau pressures should be checked on the ventilator to assure there are no problems with airway resistance or alveolar pressure in order to prevent ventilator-induced lung injury.
- Attention should be given to the volume curves in the ventilator display as a reading showing that the curve is not coming back to zero at the time of exhalation is indicative of incomplete exhalation and development of auto-PEEP and correction should be made immediately.

Troubleshooting the ventilator: The most common corrections that have to be done with the ventilator are to solve hypoxemia and hypercapnia or hyperventilation:

Hypoxia: Oxygenation depends on the FiO_2 and the PEEP. To correct for hypoxia increasing any of these parameters should raise the oxygenation.

Hypercapnia: To modify CO_2 content in blood one needs to modify alveolar ventilation. To do this, the tidal volume or the respiratory rate may be tampered with. Raising the rate or the tidal volume, will increase ventilation and decrease CO_2.

Elevated pressures: Two pressures are important in the system—peak and plateau.
- The peak pressure is a measure of airway resistance as well as compliance and includes the tubing and bronchial tree. Plateau pressures are a reflection of alveolar pressure and thus of lung compliance.
- If there is an increase in peak pressure, the first step to take is to do an inspiratory hold and check the plateau.
- Elevated peak pressure and normal plateau pressure—high airway resistance and normal compliance. Possible causes are:
  - *Kinked ET tube:* The solution is to unkink the tube; use a bite lock if the patient is biting on the tube,
  - *Mucus plug:* The solution is to suction the patient,
  - *Bronchospasm:* The solution is to give bronchodilators.
- Elevated peak and elevated plateau: Compliance problems possible causes include:
  - *Mainstem intubation:* The solution is to retract the ET tube. For diagnosis, you will find a patient with

unilateral breath sounds and a dull contralateral lung (atelectatic lung).
- *Pneumothorax:* Diagnosis will be made by hearing breath sounds unilaterally and finding a hyperresonant contralateral lung. In intubated patients, placement of a chest tube is imperative as the positive pressure will only worsen the pneumothorax.
- *Atelectasis:* Initial management consists of chest percussions and recruitment maneuvers. Bronchoscopy may be used in resistant cases.
- *Pulmonary edema:* Diuresis, inotropes, high PEEP.
- *ARDS:* Use low-tidal volume, high PEEP ventilation.

Dynamic hyperinflation or auto-PEEP: This is a process in which some of the inhaled air is not fully exhaled at the end of the respiratory cycle. The accumulation of trapped air will increase pulmonary pressures and cause barotrauma and hypotension. The patient will be difficult to ventilate. To prevent and resolve auto-PEEP, enough time should be given for the air to leave the lungs during exhalation. The goal in management is to decrease the inspiratory to expiratory ratio, this can be achieved by decreasing respiratory rate, decreasing tidal volume (higher volume will require a longer time to leave the lungs), and increasing inspiratory flow (if the air is delivered quickly the inspiratory time is less and the expiratory time will be longer at any given respiratory rate). If auto-PEEP is severe causing hypotension, disconnecting the patient from the ventilator and letting time for all the air to be exhaled may be a life-saving measure. For a full description of the management of auto-PEEP please review the article titled "Positive End-Expiratory Pressure (PEEP)."

Another common problem found in mechanically ventilated patients is patient-ventilator dys-synchrony, usually termed as the patient "fighting the ventilator". Important causes include hypoxia, auto-PEEP, not satisfying the patient's oxygenation or ventilation demands, pain, and discomfort. After ruling out important causes such as pneumothorax or atelectasis, patient comfort should be considered and proper sedation and analgesia should be assured. Consider changing the ventilator mode as some patients may respond better to different modes of ventilation.

3. Explain the initial ventilator management in patients with metabolic acidosis.

Physiological response for metabolic acidosis: The compensatory mechanism for a metabolic acidosis is hyperventilation to decrease the arterial pCO_2. This hyperventilation was first described by Kussmaul in patients with diabetic ketoacidosis in 1874. The metabolic acidosis is detected by both the peripheral and central chemoreceptors and the respiratory center is stimulated. The initial stimulation of the central chemoreceptors is due to small increases in brain interstitial fluid (H^+). The subsequent increase in ventilation causes a fall in arterial pCO_2 which inhibits the ventilatory response. The maximal compensation happens in 12–24 hours, but in situations where the patient is critically ill or poor respiratory drive then the artificial ventilatory strategies should be used.

The expected pCO_2 at maximal compensation can be calculated from a simple formula

Expected pCO_2 = 1.5 [actual (HCO_3) + 8 mm Hg (units: mmols/L for (HCO_3), and mm Hg for pCO_2].

The limiting value of compensation is the lowest level to which the pCO_2 can fall—this is typically 8–10 mm Hg, though lower values are occasionally seen. When intubating these patients, careful attention should be paid to their preintubation minute ventilation. If this ventilation is not provided when starting mechanical support, pH will drop further possibly precipitating cardiac arrest. Once you calculate the target $PaCO_2$ level should be then set up the minute ventilation according to a rough calculation as **Table 2**, gives a rough estimate of what your patient's minute ventilation should be and this will usually be a good starting point for setting up my ventilator. However, 20–30 minutes after intubation always get a blood gas to check my acid-base status, specifically checking the pH (Goal >7.25 – <7.45). Readjust the minute ventilation set on the ventilator to achieve target CO_2.

Goal minute ventilation = [$PaCO_2$ (from blood gas) × minute ventilation (set on ventilator)]/[desired CO_2 (calculated from Winters' equation)]

Avoid excessive hyperventilation which can worsen the underlying metabolic acidosis.

TABLE 2: Target PCO_2 in metabolic acidosis.

Target CO_2	Minute ventilation
40 mm Hg	6–8 L
30 mm Hg	12–14 L
20 mm Hg	18–20 L

Question 5

1. Describe the pathophysiology of COVID-19 infection in humans.

Coronavirus disease-2019 (COVID-19) is a respiratory illness caused by the severe acute respiratory syndrome coronavirus 2 (SARS-CoV-2) virus. The virus primarily spreads through respiratory droplets when an infected person coughs, sneezes, or talks. The virus can also spread by touching a surface contaminated with the virus and then touching the mouth, nose, or eyes. Incubation period—median incubation period is 4–5 days; symptoms develop between 2 and 7 days in 75% of cases, after 14 days in <1% of cases.

- Once the SARS-CoV-2 virus enters the body, it infects the respiratory epithelial cells in the upper respiratory tract, including the nasal cavity, pharynx, and larynx. The virus binds to the angiotensin-converting enzyme 2 (ACE2) receptor on the surface of these cells; it allows the virus to enter the cell and start replicating.
- The virus then spreads to the lower respiratory tract, including the bronchioles and alveoli, where it can cause severe lung damage. In response to the viral infection, the body's immune system is activated, leading to the production of proinflammatory cytokines, which can cause a cytokine storm.
- The cytokine storm can cause significant lung damage and respiratory distress, leading to acute respiratory distress syndrome (ARDS), a severe and life-threatening complication. The virus can also cause damage to other organs, including the heart, liver, and kidneys.
- In severe cases, the virus can lead to a condition called sepsis, where the body's immune system overreacts and attacks its own tissues and organs. This can lead to multiple organ failure and, in some cases, death.
- The severity of COVID-19 infection can vary widely from mild flu-like symptoms to severe illness requiring hospitalization and intensive care. Older adults and people with underlying health conditions, such as diabetes, heart disease, and respiratory conditions, are at increased risk of developing severe illness and complications from COVID-19.

Pathogenesis: Coronaviruses express transmembrane glycoproteins ("spike" proteins) which allow the virus to attach to and gain entry to the target cell.

- Spike proteins on SARS-CoV-2 share many similarities with those of SARS-CoV and bind to surface ACE2 receptors.
  - Angiotensin converting enzyme 2 is expressed predominantly on type II pneumocytes but also on upper respiratory tract epithelial cells and small intestine enterocytes.
  - The SARS-CoV-2 spike protein appears to bind ACE2 with higher affinity than SARS-CoV, which may account for its greater transmissibility.
  - Other cofactors are likely required, including transmembrane serine protease 2 (TMPRSS2).
- Viral RNA replication occurs within the target cell, utilizing RNA-dependent RNA polymerase (RdRp).

2. Discuss awake proning in ARDS.

Recent reports in COVID-19 acute respiratory distress syndrome (C-ARDS) have shown that awake, self-proning improves oxygenation in this group of patients **(Flowchart 1)**.

Proning has been widely studied mainly in intubated ARDS patients and has shown improvement in oxygenation and reduced mortality in patients on invasive ventilation, in large randomized trials. However, with increasing clinical experience of treating COVID-19 patients, self-proning of conscious, awake, non-intubated patients with C-ARDS has shown profound improvement in oxygenation, leading to delay and even avoiding intubation and invasive ventilation altogether.

Physiological benefits with proning: Patients in a supine position have compromised pulmonary function, due to
- Atelectasis of the dorsal alveoli.
- Over-inflation of ventral alveoli due to increased respiratory drive.
- Ventilation-perfusion mismatch.

Mechanisms for improved oxygenation after awake proning:
- More uniform distribution of tidal volume and end-expiratory lung volume, thus reducing the cyclical opening and closing of alveoli (reduced atelectasis).
- Recruitment of areas in the posterior part of the lung, thus improving compliance, and decreasing the shunt.
- Decreased lung deformation (increased homogeneity) and lungs are less compressed in prone, thereby increased ventilation.
- Dorsal lung regions have a higher density of blood vessels (which is independent of gravity). Proning improves the ventilation in these nondependent lung fields, thereby improving the ventilation–perfusion (V:Q) matching.
- Increased perfusion toward the anterior alveoli; improving the V:Q ratio.
- The chest wall compliance reduces, as the anterior part of the chest is now facing the bed surface, reducing the regional lung stress and potentially decreasing the possibility of patient self-inflicted lung injury (p-SILI). Contraction of muscular diaphragm exerts a more uniform distribution of stress.
- Better secretion drainage.

Flowchart 1: Algorithm for awake proning in COVID-19 conscious respiratory failure patients.

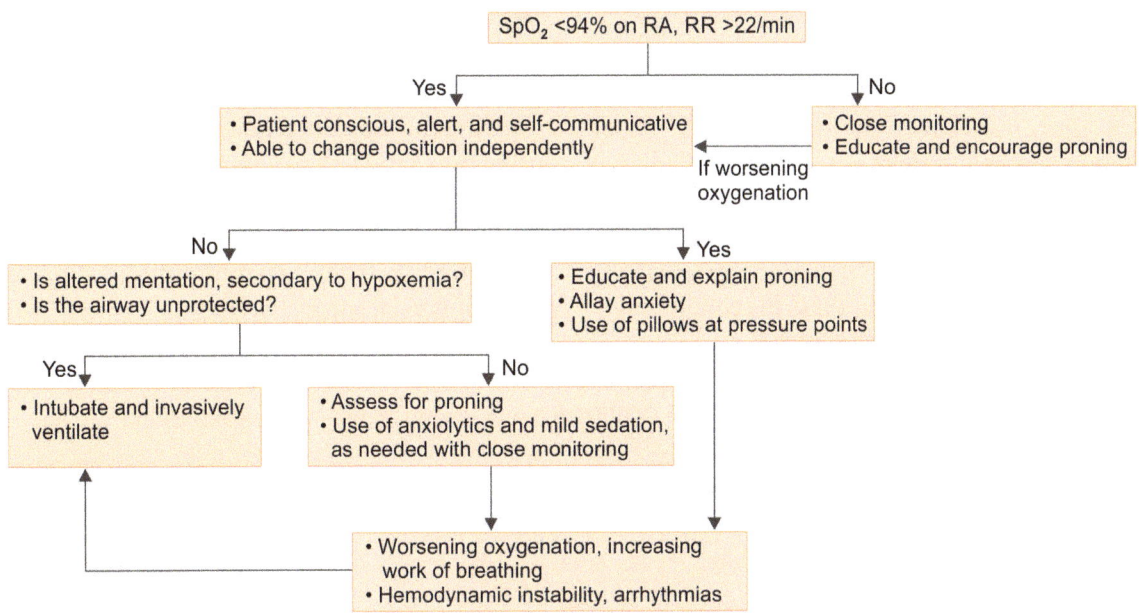

3. What is single breath count in emergency care?

Single breath count test: Single breath count test is a good bedside measurement of respiratory function which can be performed quickly and without additional equipment.

To perform, ask patient to count out loud after maximal inspiration. Ability to reach 50 indicates normal respiratory function. Single breath count of <15 typically correlates with low forced vital capacity (FVC) and respiratory muscle weakness.

Single-breath counting is very easy to perform in children, seems to correlate well with standard measures of pulmonary function, and shows promise for measuring asthma severity in children. It may reflect both restrictive and obstructive diseases and might be useful to demonstrate improvement with acute asthma treatment. Further work to define the range of reference SBC values (as a function of age and/or body size) and an evaluation of the utility of single breath count (SBC) in an ED population of acute asthmatics is underway.

4. How will you prepare your emergency department triage during the COVID-19 pandemic?

During the COVID-19 pandemic, emergency triage preparation is critical to ensure that limited resources are used effectively and patients receive the best possible care. Preparing the emergency department triage for a COVID-19 pandemic requires careful planning and coordination to ensure the safety of patients and healthcare workers **(Flowchart 2)**.

Here are some steps that can be taken:

Develop a triage protocol: A clear triage protocol should be developed that outlines the steps to be taken when a patient presents with COVID-19 symptoms. The protocol should include screening questions to identify potential cases, isolation procedures, and referral pathways.

Establish a designated COVID-19 area: A separate area should be designated for COVID-19 patients to reduce the risk of exposure to other patients and healthcare workers. This area should have adequate ventilation, negative pressure rooms, and personal protective equipment (PPE) available for staff.

Train staff on COVID-19 protocols: All staff should be trained on the triage protocol and infection prevention measures, including proper use of PPE, hand hygiene, and cleaning and disinfection procedures.

Screen patients before arrival: Patients should be screened for COVID-19 symptoms before arriving at the emergency department. This can be done through a telephone screening or a questionnaire.

Implement social distancing measures: Social distancing measures should be implemented in the waiting room and triage area to reduce the risk of transmission. This may include limiting the number of patients in the waiting room, spacing out chairs, and providing masks.

Monitor and adjust protocols as needed: The triage protocol should be monitored and adjusted as needed based on the evolving situation and guidance from public health authorities.

Communicate with patients: Patients should be informed of the triage protocol and any changes to emergency department procedures related to COVID-19. Clear communication can help reduce anxiety and ensure that patients receive appropriate care.

Plan for surge capacity: Develop a plan for how to handle a surge in patients. This may include repurposing areas of the hospital for triage or expanding triage into the community.

Monitor and adapt: Continuously monitor and evaluate the triage process to identify areas for improvement. Adapt the protocol as needed based on new information or changes in the situation.

It is important to remember that emergency triage during the COVID-19 pandemic is a complex and evolving situation. It is essential to stay up-to-date on the latest guidance and recommendations from public health authorities and be prepared to adjust protocols and procedures as needed.

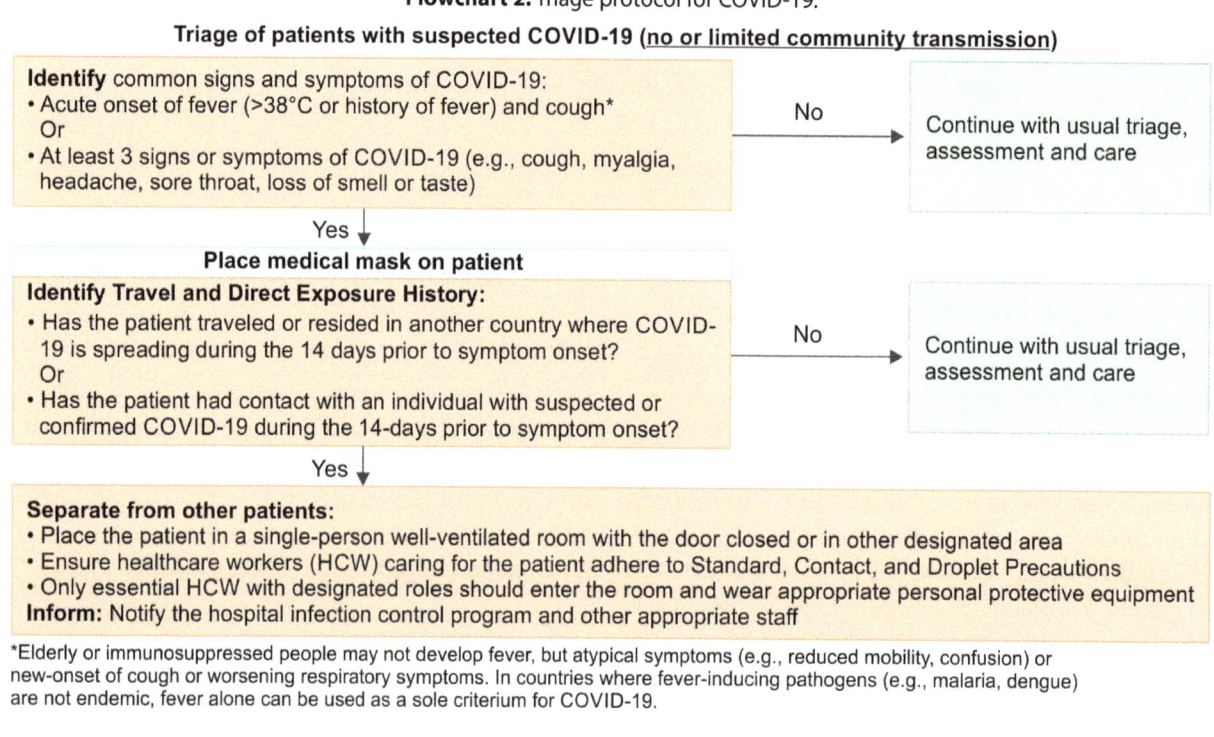

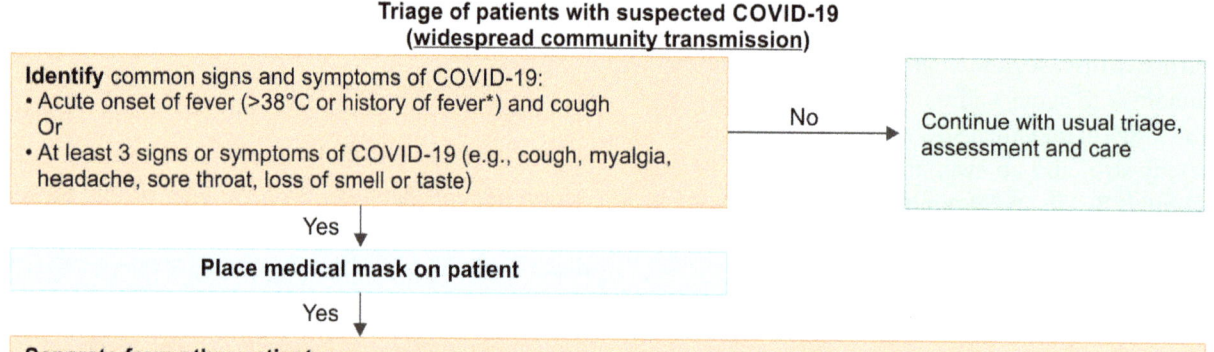

Flowchart 2: Triage protocol for COVID-19.

Question 6

1. Describe the rotator cuff injuries.

The rotator cuff is a group of muscles in the shoulder that allow a wide range of movement while maintaining the stability of the glenohumeral joint. The rotator cuff **(Fig. 4)** includes the following muscles: Subscapularis infraspinatus, teres minor supraspinatus. A helpful mnemonic to remember these muscles is "SITS". The glenohumeral joint is a ball and socket joint and comprises a large spherical humeral head and a small glenoid cavity. This anatomy makes the joint highly mobile, however, really unstable. Stabilization in the shoulder is provided collectively by the noncontractile tissue of the glenohumeral joint (static stabilizers) such as the capsule, the labrum, the negative intraarticular pressure, and the glenohumeral ligaments; and the contractile tissues (dynamic stabilizers) such as the rotator cuff muscles and the long head of the biceps brachii.

Rotator cuff syndrome: Rotator cuff syndrome (RCS) describes a spectrum of clinical pathology ranging from minor injuries such as acute rotator cuff tendinitis to advanced/chronic rotator cuff tendinopathy and degenerative conditions. Rotator cuff injuries represent a common cause of shoulder pain. The rotator cuff tendons, particularly the supraspinatus tendon, are uniquely susceptible to the compressive forces of subacromial impingement. Improper athletic technique, poor posture, poor conditioning, and failure of the subacromial bursa to protect the supporting tendons result in a progressive injury from acute inflammation, to calcification, to degenerative thinning, and finally to a tendon tear.

Treatment for RCS: Evidence suggests that conservative treatment with NSAIDs, and most importantly, physical therapy, should be the first attempt at therapy. Limit overhead activities and use ice packs or heating pads as supportive measures. Proper physical therapy effectively treats most patients without subacromial decompression. Subacromial injection with steroids showed a short-term benefit in some trials and may improve a patient's compliance with physical therapy. Surgical treatment with arthroscopy is done in cases of both acute and chronic full-thickness tears since delay can result in significant muscle atrophy, tendon retraction, and poorer surgical results.

Rotator cuff (RC) tendonitis/tendinosis: Acute or chronic tendinopathic conditions that result from a vulnerable environment for the RC secondary to repetitive eccentric forces and predisposing anatomical/mechanical risk factors.

Shoulder impingement: A clinical term often used non-specifically to describe patients experiencing pain/symptoms with overhead activities. It is best to subdivide shoulder impingement into internal and external conditions.

Internal impingement: Common in overhead-throwing athletes such as baseball pitchers and javelin throwers. Impingement occurs at the posterior/lateral articular side of the cuff as it abuts the posterior/superior glenoid rim and labrum when the shoulder is in maximum abduction and external rotation (i.e., the "late cocking" phase of throwing). The term "thrower's shoulder" refers to a common set of anatomic adaptive changes that occur over time in this subset of athletes. These adaptive changes include but are not limited to increased humeral retroversion and posterior capsular tightness.

Glenohumeral internal rotation deficit (GIRD) is a condition resulting from these anatomic adaptations, and GIRD is known to predispose the thrower's shoulder to internal impingement.

External impingement: External impingement (EI) encompasses etiologies of external compressive sources (i.e., the acromion), leading to subacromial bursitis and bursal-sided injuries to the RC.

Partial- versus full-thickness rotator cuff tears: Etiologies and underlying causes are known to be multifactorial. Degeneration, impingement, and tension overload due to trauma may all lead to rotator cuff tears. Most often, the tears initially begin as partial tears of the supraspinatus tendon. Eventually, they can progress to full-thickness tears including all four of the rotator cuff muscles.

It primarily presents in middle-aged to older patients. Repetitive overhead activities are commonly the reason for younger athletes.

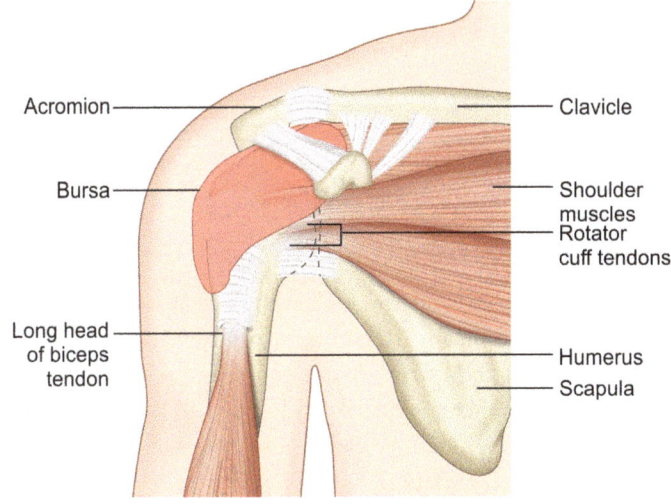

Fig. 4: Rotator cuff shoulder.

2. Draw the anatomy of brachial plexus.

The brachial plexus passes from the neck to the axilla and supplies the upper limb. It is formed from the ventral rami of the 5th–8th cervical nerves and the ascending part of the ventral ramus of the first thoracic nerve.

Anatomy: The brachial plexus **(Fig. 5)** is divided into roots, trunks, divisions, cords, and branches. There are five "terminal" branches and numerous other "preterminal" or "collateral" branches that leave the plexus at various points along its length.

- *The five roots* are the five anterior rami of the lower four cervical and first thoracic nerve roots (C5-C8, T1) after they have given off their segmental supply to the muscles of the neck. These roots merge to form three trunks:
  1. Upper trunk (C5–C6)
  2. Middle trunk (C7)
  3. Lower trunk (C8, T1)
- *Each trunk* then splits into anterior and posterior divisions, to form six divisions. The anterior/posterior divisions innervate flexor groups versus extensor groups:
  - Anterior divisions of the upper, middle, and lower trunks
  - Posterior divisions of the upper, middle, and lower trunks
- These six divisions will regroup to become the three cords. The cords are named by their position to the axillary artery.
  1. The posterior cord is formed from the three posterior divisions of the trunks (C5–C8, T1)
  2. The lateral cord is the anterior divisions from the upper and middle trunks (C5–C7)
  3. The medial cord is simply a continuation of the anterior division of the lower trunk (C8, T1)
  4. The *lateral cord* extends into the musculoskeletal nerve and the lateral root of the median nerve.
  5. The *posterior cord* extends into the radial nerve and axillary nerve.
  6. The *medial cord* extends into the ulnar nerve and the medial root of the median nerve.

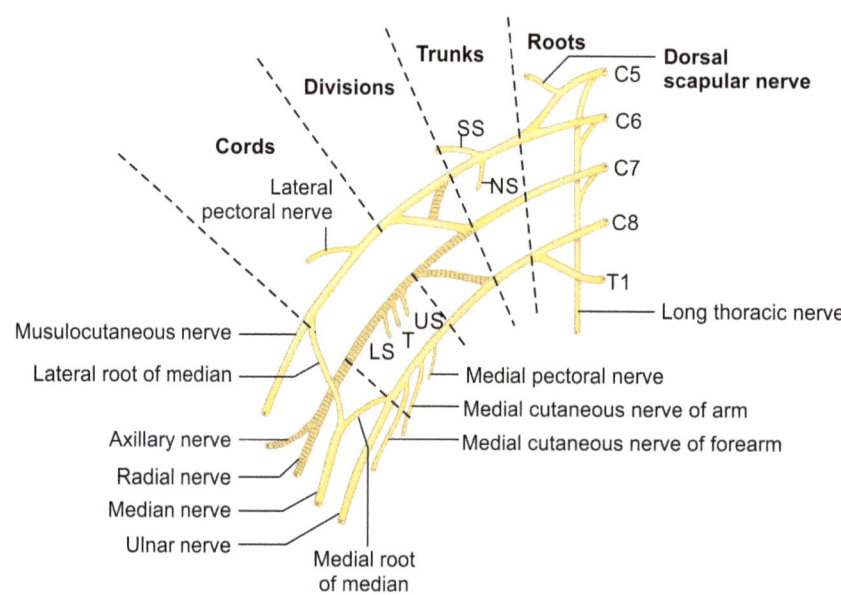

Fig. 5: Brachial plexus. (LS: lower subscapular nerve; NS: nerve to subclavius; SS: suprascapular nerve; T: thoracodorsal nerve: US: upper subscapular nerve)

3. Discuss clinical presentation of brachial plexus injuries.

Brachial plexus injuries are caused by damage to brachial plexus nerves, typically from trauma, tumors, inflammation, pressure, athletic injuries, or being excessively stretched. Some brachial plexus injuries can happen to babies during birth. *Erb's palsy* refers to numbness and paralysis of the upper brachial plexus. *Klumpke palsy* (also known as *Klumpke's palsy*) refers to loss of sensation in the wrist and hand and paralysis of the lower brachial plexus. A rare syndrome called *Parsonage-Turner syndrome*, or *brachial plexitis*, causes inflammation of the brachial plexus without any obvious shoulder injury.

Symptoms: Loss of sensation, arm weakness, sudden pain in the shoulder/arm, paralysis of arm.

Types of brachial plexus injuries are:
Neuropraxia: The mildest form of nerve damage which causes interruption in nerve signaling.

Neuroma: The nerve is torn and healed but the scar tissue puts pressure on the injured nerve preventing the nerve conduction.

Rupture: The nerve is torn but not torn from spinal cord.

Avulsion: This is the most severe type of nerve injury in which the nerve is torn from the spinal cord.

Incomplete avulsion injury has minimal chances for recovery.

Upper-trunk palsy injury: Upper-trunk palsy occurs with falls and road traffic accidents during which the angle between the shoulder and the neck forcibly widens, such as when a fall forces the shoulder down and the head to the opposite side. Patients with upper-trunk palsies are unable to use the shoulder to raise the arm away from the body, have weakness in the arm, and may be unable to bend the arm at the elbow. There may be loss of sensation in the shoulder, outside of the arm, and thumb. A severe upper-trunk injury may paralyze the shoulder muscles (deltoid muscle and rotator cuff), as well as the muscle in the upper arm (biceps). It is usually called as waiter tip's hand.

Lower-trunk palsy injury: Lower-trunk palsy occurs when the injury causes the angle between the arm and the chest wall forcibly widens. This may damage the lower nerves and the lower trunks.

Patients with a lower-trunk palsy will typically maintain shoulder and elbow strength, but will lose hand function. Over a period of time, this will cause the fingers to contract into a claw position, and the patient will not be able to perform fine motor tasks. Patients also typically have hand numbness in at least the ring finger and small finger.

Pan-plexus palsy injury: Pan-plexus palsy may occur if the force of the injury is extreme. In pan-plexus palsy, all levels of the nerves and trunk are damaged. This results in complete paralysis of the arm and hand.

Treatment: Pain control, physiotherapy, surgical Repair—early surgical repair has good outcome. Late surgeries have lower success rate. Recovery and rehabilitation take a long time.

Question 7

1. Discuss physiology of thermoregulation.

Heat regulation in the body is a complex process that involves multiple physiological systems working together to maintain the internal body temperature within a narrow range. The body's normal temperature is around 98.6°F (37°C), and any deviation from this range can have significant effects on the body's function. The main purpose of thermoregulation is to keep the enzyme systems of the body working properly. The part of the brain responsible for thermoregulation is called the hypothalamus. It receives information about the temperature status from some specialized nerve cells called thermoreceptors. The primary mechanisms by which the body regulates heat include:

Thermoregulatory center: The hypothalamus, located in the brain, acts as the body's thermostat and is responsible for monitoring the internal temperature and initiating responses to maintain the temperature within the desired range.

Sweating: The body's primary means of cooling is through the evaporation of sweat from the skin surface. Sweat is produced by sweat glands, which are activated by the sympathetic nervous system in response to elevated body temperature.

Vasodilation: Blood vessels in the skin dilate in response to elevated body temperature, allowing more blood to flow to the skin surface, where heat can be dissipated to the environment.

Shivering: When the body's internal temperature drops below the desired range, muscles throughout the body may contract rapidly, producing heat and raising the internal temperature.

Hormonal responses: Hormones such as adrenaline and thyroid hormone can affect metabolic rate and heat production in response to changing temperatures.

Together, these mechanisms work to maintain the body's internal temperature within a narrow range despite changes in the external environment. When the body is exposed to extreme temperatures, however, these mechanisms may become overwhelmed, leading to conditions such as heat exhaustion and heat stroke, or hypothermia if the body temperature falls too low.

2. Write a note on "Heat Stroke".

Heat-related illness is a spectrum of conditions progressing from heat exhaustion, heat injury, to life-threatening heat stroke. Heat stroke is a clinical constellation of symptoms that include a severe elevation in body temperature which typically, but not always, is >40°C. Also, there must be clinical signs of central nervous system dysfunction that may include ataxia, delirium, or seizures, in the setting of exposure to hot weather or strenuous physical exertion.

Risk factors include environmental variables, medications, drug use, and other medical comorbidities.

Clinical features: It is important to differentiate where the patient is on the heat illness continuum.

The signs and symptoms of heat exhaustion may present similarly include cramping, fatigue, dizziness, nausea, vomiting, and headache. If progression to end-organ damage occurs it then becomes heat injury. Finally, neurologic alteration distinguishes heat stroke from heat injury.

There are two forms of heat stroke, classic, and exertional. Classic heat stroke typically affects elderly individuals with chronic medical conditions while exertional heat stroke affects otherwise healthy people who engage in strenuous exercise in hot or humid weather.

Diagnosis: The workup of patients presenting with possible heat stroke should include vital signs—monitoring body temperature and rectal temperature.

Laboratory studies: Blood investigations such as CBC, CMP, PT/PTT, blood gasses, serum CPK, and urine myoglobin, toxicology screen, ECG, CXR. Elderly patients have polypharmacy which has to consider in atypical presentation.

Classic versus exertional heat stroke: In classical heat stroke, respiratory alkalosis predominates, whereas exertional heat stroke may also have concomitant lactic acidosis. Electrolyte derangements are variable between the two etiologies, but commonly in exertional heat stroke hypocalcemia, hyperphosphatemia, and hyperkalemia reflect muscle breakdown that occurs. Rhabdomyolysis is more common in exertional than classical heat stroke, with a higher elevation of CPK markers reported. In classic heat stroke, AST and ALT elevations are the most common laboratory abnormalities reported. Associated kidney injury, liver manifestations, and other end-organ damage may also occur in either presentation. Consequences of hyperthermia are:

Cardiovascular: Diversion of blood to peripheries in an attempt to cool leads to a reduction in the perfusion of other organs; reduced splanchnic blood flow with relative visceral ischemia; translocation of gut bacteria and SIRS response. Reduced cerebral perfusion contributes to CNS depression. Direct thermal injury to endothelium leads to activation of the clotting system and disseminated intravascular coagulation. Vasodilation occurs in an attempt to regulate temperature and as a consequence of the SIRS. Response may result in hypotension.

Renal: Fluid and electrolyte disturbance secondary to sweating, rhabdomyolysis, acute kidney injury.

Hematological: Disseminated intravascular coagulation.

Neurological: Altered mental state, permanent neurological injury in survivors (rarely).

Treatment: Management of heat stroke includes ensuring adequate airway protection, breathing, and circulation. After ABC's, rapid cooling becomes the mainstay of treatment with ancillary management in response to other end-organ damage.

Cooling methods: A core temperature of <39° should be sought.

Passive cooling: Move patient to cooler area, loosen clothing and insulate patient from the warm ground, keep the environment cool.

Cold water immersion (CWI): Optimum field treatment, rapid conductive heat loss due to the high thermal conductivity of water, enhanced by ice-cold water, impractical in the critically ill patient, cooling rate 0.2°/minute.

Evaporative cooling: Second-line of method for cooling, spray water over the skin to provide interface with environmental air, provide cool air over the patient, cooling rate 0.04–0.08°/minute.

Other modalities: Ice packs to groins, axilla, cold intravenous fluids, unsuitable as monotherapy—initiate while preparing other methods, active temperature management systems—e.g., intravascular cooling systems, extracorporeal circuits—renal replacement therapy, ECMO, and cardiopulmonary bypass will contribute to normalization in temperature. Body cavity lavage—relatively understudied as a cooling, rather than warming, strategy.

Pharmacotherapy

Antipyretics: Theoretical benefit in inhibition of prostaglandins and reduction in hypothalamic set point. Medications such as paracetamol, ibuprofen, and aspirin can be used.

Dantrolene: Theoretical benefit in inhibiting calcium release from sarcoplasmic reticulum and preventing muscle rigidity and heat production, presently indicated to treat malignant hyperthermia and neuroleptic malignant syndrome, no benefit in cooling or outcome demonstrated in a randomized controlled trial in heatstroke patients.

A small study suggested that high-dose benzodiazepine may blunt the shivering reflex and decrease oxygen consumption, therefore providing a theoretical benefit to patients. The problem is that heat stroke patients may be unable to compensate through mechanisms such as shivering. Therefore the universal use of benzodiazepines is not recommended but could be tailored to the shivering, agitated patient.

Question 8

1. Discuss antiplatelet drugs.

Antiplatelets can be classified based on the mechanism of action as follows:

- *Platelet aggregation inhibitors:*
  - Aspirin and related cyclooxygenase inhibitors
  - Oral thienopyridines such as clopidogrel, ticagrelor, ticlopidine, and prasugrel
- *Glycoprotein platelet inhibitors* (e.g., abciximab, eptifibatide, tirofiban)
- *Protease-activated receptor-1 antagonists* (e.g., vorapaxar)
- *Miscellaneous* [e.g., dipyridamole—a nucleoside transport inhibitor and phosphodiesterase type 3 (PDE3) inhibitor, cilostazol—also a PDE3 inhibitor]
- *Aspirin is the most commonly used oral antiplatelet drug*: It works by irreversibly inhibiting the cyclooxygenase enzyme (COX) activity in the prostaglandin synthesis pathway (PGH2). This prostaglandin is a precursor of thromboxane A2 (TXA2) and PGI2. Thromboxane A2 works by inducing platelet aggregation and vasoconstriction, and mediated by COX-1 enzyme, while PGI2 works by inhibiting platelet aggregation and induces vasodilation, and is mediated by COX-2. Low-dose aspirin (75–150 mg) can induce complete or near-complete inhibition of COX-1, thus inhibiting the production of TXA2, while larger doses are required to inhibit COX-2.
- *Oral thienopyridines* selectively inhibit adenosine diphosphate-induced (ADP-induced) platelet aggregation. These drugs are converted into the active drug with the help of the hepatic CYP450 system that can irreversibly inhibit the platelet P2Y12 receptor. Prasugrel is the most potent of all three drugs, has a rapid onset of action, and is superior to clopidogrel in patients undergoing coronary stenting. Ticlopidine has fallen out of favor because of bone marrow toxicity. Cangrelor is a new intravenous, reversible P2Y12 receptor antagonist and has a rapid onset of action. It achieves a significant degree of platelet inhibition compared with clopidogrel.
- *Glycoprotein platelet inhibitors* work by inhibiting glycoprotein IIb/IIIa (GpIIb-IIIa) receptors on platelets, thus decreasing platelet aggregation, and most commonly used in ACS. These drugs are only available in an intravenous form and are therefore used as short-term therapy.
- *Dipyridamole* has antiplatelet and vasodilating properties and inhibits platelet cyclic nucleotide phosphodiesterase. This enzyme is responsible for the degradation of adenosine monophosphate (AMP) to 5'AMP, which increases intraplatelet cyclic AMP accumulation and inhibits platelet aggregation. It also blocks the uptake of adenosine by the platelets, which also increases cyclic AMP.
- Cilostazol is also reported to have vasodilatory, antiplatelet properties, and antiproliferative effects. It also reduces smooth muscle cell hyperproliferation and intimal hyperplasia after an injury to the endothelium.

2. Explain high insulin euglycemic therapy.

High-dose insulin euglycemic therapy (HIET) is primarily used in the therapy of severe *calcium channel blocker toxicity*. HIET can also be used for severe beta blocker toxicity and potentially other toxicities/presentations requiring inotropic support.

Mechanism of action: The mechanism of action is simple because this method of treatment supports the "metabolic hunger" of the heart, which is caused by the calcium channel blockers or beta-blockers toxicity, which has a direct cardiotoxic effect. Poisoning with calcium channel blockers alone leads to several metabolic effects that must be emphasized:
- Hyperinsulinemia (insulin release is dependent on calcium uptake into the pancreatic beta cells via L-type calcium channels)
- Insulin resistance, which is caused by the toxicity of calcium channel blockers.
- Calcium channel blockers also impair the cardiac myocyte adaptive response of shifting from using free fatty acids, their favored "resting state" energy substrate, to carbohydrates, due to:
  - Impaired uptake of glucose and free fatty acids by cardiac myocytes
  - Inhibition of calcium-dependent mitochondrial activity required for glucose catabolism

Effects of Insulin:
- Increases the uptake of glucose and lactate into myocardial cells.
- Improves myocardial function without the need to increase oxygen demand.
- Increases pyruvate dehydrogenase activity, which improves lactate oxidation and the "cleansing" of cytosols from glycolysis by-products that may affect calcium turnover and lead to diastolic dysfunction.
- Improves myocardial contraction due to greater glucose availability.
- Increases the activity of calcium-dependent ATPase in the sarcoplasmic reticulum.
- Increases the concentration of calcium in the cytoplasm.
- Improves calcium inflow into mitochondria.

Treatment protocols
- Begin the treatment with an insulin bolus at a dose of 1 unit/kg intravenously (IV). If the glucose level is <11.1 mmol/L, administer 25 g of glucose intravenously (IV).

- Next, start to administer insulin as a continuous infusion at a dose of 0.5–1 unit/kg/hour (in adults this does is usually between 35 and 100 units/hour). It is recommended that insulin be administrated via an infusion pump to a separate intravenous route. If the response after 20 minutes is not adequate, the insulin dose should be increased by 0.5 unit/kg/hour every 15 minutes up to a maximum dose of 5 units/kg/hour.

Monitor: Glucose—every 20 minutes for first hour, then every 1 hour; potassium—replace only if <2.5 mmol/L; *therapeutic end points*—heartrate >60/minute; QRS <120 ms; improved BP (systolic BP >90 mm Hg), adequate urine output, improved mentation. Resolution of academia—therapy is weaned after the withdrawal of other vasopressors, as cardiotoxicity resolves.

3. Discuss intravenous lipid therapy.

Intravenous lipid emulsion is a sterile emulsion of soybean oil in water, used in parenteral nutrition. It is the current recommended antidote in the resuscitation of patients with refractory cardiac arrest induced by local anesthetics that are resistant to standard protocols. It may also have a role when standard therapy has failed in the arrest of a propranolol, tricyclic antidepressant, and verapamil overdose (needs further study).

Mechanism of action: The precise mechanism of action is unknown.

The early "lipid sink" theory by Weinberg et al. suggested that a lipid compartment gets created in the blood into which the lipophilic bupivacaine may dissolve, thereby removing bupivacaine from the aqueous plasma circulation. By binding bupivacaine to this "lipid sink," there would be a reduction in its free concentration available to organs sensitive to the effects of local anesthetics, such as the heart and brain.

The lipid compartment has multiple scavenging mechanisms like
- Removes the local anesthetic from high blood flow, sensitive organs (i.e., heart and brain), then
- Redistributes to muscles for storage and the liver for detoxification.

Lipid directly increases cardiac contractility, which improves cardiac output and increases preload through simple volume expansion. Contractility and vascular tone improve only when the local anesthetic concentration in the heart falls below sodium channel blocking thresholds. These cardiovascular benefits improve blood pressure and cardiac output.

The cardioprotective effects of lipid help to mitigate the ischemia-reperfusion injury at the cellular level.

Administration dosage formulations and dose: The most common formulation available 20% intravenous lipid emulsion preparations. The most prevalent formulations have 100% long-chain fatty acids derived from soybean oil. The formulations with 100% long-chain fatty acids contain linoleic acid (53%), oleic acid (24%), palmitic acid (11%), alpha-linolenic acid (8%), and stearic acid (4%). ILE is also available in 20% soybean oil and 80% olive oil combination.

For patients >70 kg, a rapid 100 mL bolus of 20% lipid emulsion followed by another 200–250 mL infusion over 15–20 minutes is the recommended course.

For patients <70 kg, a rapid 1.5 mL/kg (of lean body weight) bolus of 20% lipid emulsion followed by a 0.25 mL/kg/minute infusion should start. The same bolus dose is repeatable, along with doubling the infusion rate if cardiovascular instability continues. The recommended dosing limit is approximately 12 mL/kg.

Propofol which is reconstituted in 10% lipid emulsion, is not an acceptable therapy for Local anesthetic systemic toxicity. As large volume of the drug would be needed and it has significant cardio depressant effect worsening hemodynamic instability.

Adverse effects, early effects: Allergic reaction, lipid embolus, hyperlipidemia, hypercoagulability, and irritation.

Late effects: Transient rise in liver function test, hepatomegaly, splenomegaly, thrombocytopenia, acute pancreatitis, reduced immune response, impaired pulmonary gas exchange. However, the adverse effects induced by lipid emulsion are mild and transient.

Recent studies support the use of lipid therapy for various lipophilic drug overdoses.

Contraindications: Severe egg allergy, lipid storage disorders, impaired lipid metabolism.

Even though there is list of adverse effects and contraindications, its benefit outweighs the risk.

Monitoring: Close cardiac monitoring, allergic reactions monitoring, blood test monitoring (look for signs and symptoms of acute pancreatitis, acute cholecystitis): Triglyceride levels, lipase levels, liver enzymes, bilirubin levels.

Toxicity: Hypertriglyceridemia, acute pancreatitis, lipid embolus, ECMO/dialysis machine obstruction, fat overload syndrome in severe cases—severe metabolic acidosis and lactic acidosis.

Question 9

1. Explain calcium hemostasis.

Calcium hemostasis refers to the regulation of calcium levels in the body (**Fig. 6**), which is essential for maintaining healthy bones, muscles, and nerves, as well as proper blood clotting. There are three main players in calcium hemostasis—the parathyroid glands, the kidneys, and the bones. The parathyroid glands release parathyroid hormone (PTH) in response to low calcium, low phosphate and decreased vitamin D levels. PTH stimulates the release of calcium from bones into the bloodstream, increases the absorption of calcium in the intestines, and decreases the excretion of calcium by the kidneys.

- Hypercalcemia and raised vitamin D levels switch off PTH release via negative feedback.
- Hypomagnesemia prevents PTH release and therefore may cause hypocalcemia.
- Vitamin D promotes calcium and phosphate absorption from the gastrointestinal (GI) tract.
- Calcitonin produced by the thyroid decreases calcium levels.

The kidneys play a crucial role in calcium hemostasis by filtering and reabsorbing calcium in the blood. They also produce an active form of vitamin D, which helps the body absorb calcium from the intestines.

The bones store 99% of the body's calcium, and they release it into the bloodstream when calcium levels are low. Bone stores of calcium buffer the serum changes. They also produce osteocalcin, a hormone that helps regulate insulin secretion, glucose metabolism, and energy expenditure.

Overall, calcium hemostasis is a complex process that involves the coordination of several organs and hormones to maintain the right balance of calcium in the body.

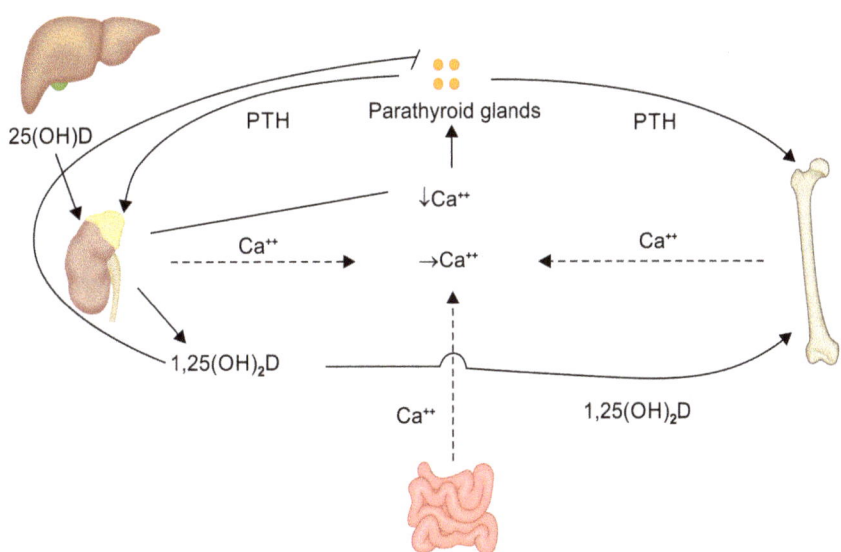

Fig. 6: Calcium hemostasis.

2. What are the causes of hypocalcemia?

- Hypoparathyroidism (congenital, autoimmune, after thyroid or parathyroid surgery)
- Vitamin D deficiency (decreased intake, malabsorption or failure of synthesis or activation)
- Inadequate dietary calcium
- Renal disease
- Hypomagnesemia (consider PPI-associated hypomagnesemia)
- Drugs (e.g., phenytoin, bisphosphonates, rifampicin, chemotherapy, blood transfusion, contrast dye)
- Hyperphosphatemia
- Respiratory alkalosis (increased albumin binding, relative fall in free ionized calcium)
- Acute pancreatitis (free fatty acids chelate calcium)
- *Malignancy:* Osteoblastic metastases (e.g., breast cancer, prostate cancer), tumor lysis syndrome (following chemotherapy).

3. Discuss the clinical features of hypocalcemia.

Neuromuscular: Hypocalcemia can lead to muscle cramps, tetany, carpopedal spasms, and twitching (Chvostek sign). These symptoms can be localized to certain muscle groups or can be more generalized throughout the body.

Cardiac: Bradycardia, hypotension, arrhythmias, palpitations, and even cardiac arrest in severe cases.

Bones: Decreased bone density, osteoporosis, and increased risk of fractures.

Dermatological: Dry skin, hair loss, and brittle nails.

Neurological: Mental state changes such as confusion, irritability, and even seizures.

Gastrointestinal symptoms: Dehydration, abdominal pain, diarrhea, and vomiting.

4. Describe treatment of hypocalcemia.

Any underlying cause of hypocalcemia should be investigated and corrected. Low magnesium levels should be corrected first. Without replenishing magnesium first any increase in calcium will be transient, therefore magnesium 2 g intravenously should be given if there is concurrent hypomagnesemia. The following investigations should be sent for further evaluation and management of hypocalcemia according to algorithm (**Flowchart 3**).

- Serum calcium and albumin—calcium may be spuriously low if the albumin is low. Therefore, corrected calcium should always be checked.
- Renal function
- Amylase
- Creatine kinase
- Magnesium
- Phosphate.
- ECG; hypocalcemia can lead to prolonged PT and QT, inverted T waves, and AV block.

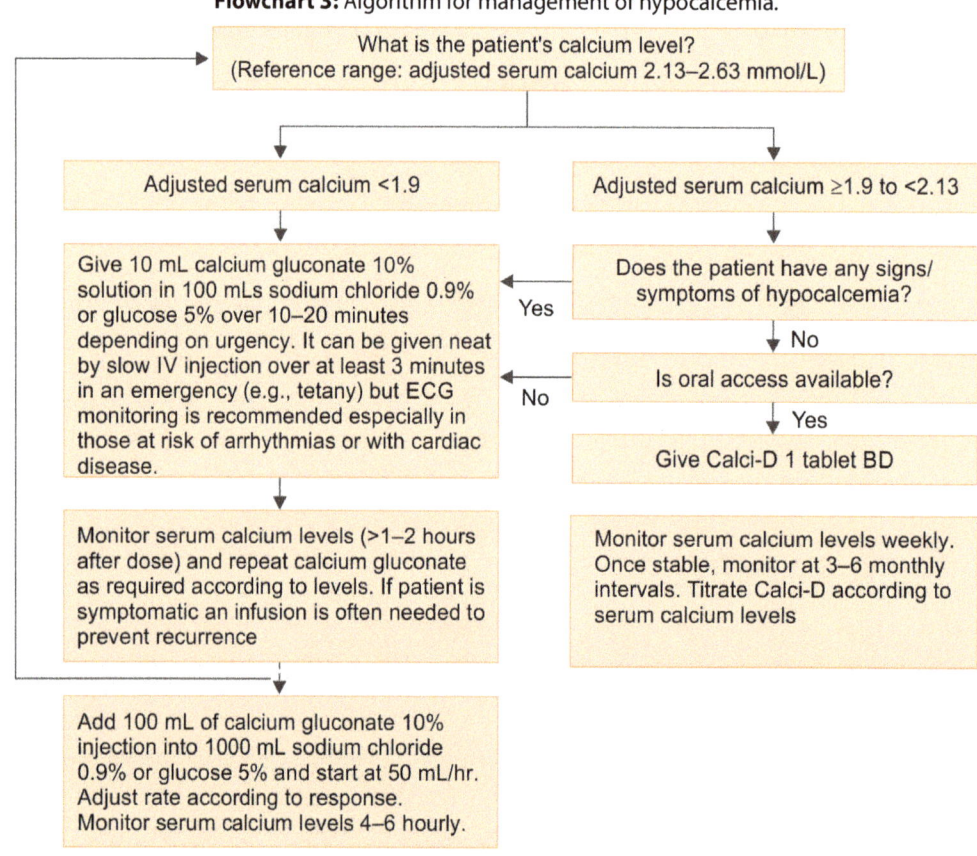

Flowchart 3: Algorithm for management of hypocalcemia.

Question 10

1. Discuss pathophysiology of heart failure.

Heart failure is a clinical syndrome characterized by typical symptoms (e.g., dyspnea, ankle swelling, fatigue) that may be accompanied by signs (e.g., elevated jugular venous pressure, pulmonary crackles, peripheral edema) caused by a structural and/or functional cardiac abnormality, leading to a reduced cardiac output and/or elevated intracardiac pressures at rest or during stress.

Classification—based on ejection fraction:
- Heart failure with reduced ejection fraction (HFrEF, EF <40%)
- Heart failure with preserved ejection fraction (HFpEF, EF >50%)
- Heart failure with mid-range ejection fraction (HFmrEF, EF 40–49%).

No evidence-based therapy to improve outcome can be offered for patients with preserved EF.

Reduced EF patients are usually symptomatic and require medical/surgical intervention.

The main structural alteration in with heart failure reduced EF is eccentric remodeling accompanied with chamber dilatation leading to volume overload. Heart failure with preserved EF shows impaired ventricular relaxation and/or filling, increased ventricular stiffness and thus elevated filling pressure accompanied by pressure overload often leading to backward failure.

Heart failure may be also classified according to the affected circulatory system (right–sided; left- sided) **(Table 3)** or the underlying pathophysiological factor leading to cardiac dysfunction (pressure-induced: Aortic stenosis, hypertension; volume-induced: ASD, VSD, mitral regurgitation). Excessive preload, excessive afterload or pump failure may lead to low output heart failure. High-output failure results from a mismatch of cardiac output (stroke volume, heart rate) and circulatory oxygen demand (e.g., high heart rate in anemia).

Pathophysiology of heart failure: The pathophysiology of heart failure involves changes in both the structure and function of the heart **(Flowchart 4)**. These changes can occur in the left, right, or both ventricles and can lead to symptoms such as shortness of breath, fatigue, and fluid accumulation.

One of the key mechanisms underlying heart failure is impaired contractility of the heart muscle. The causes are multifactorial as explained above. As a result, the heart is unable to pump blood effectively, leading to a reduction in cardiac output. Another important factor in heart failure is increased afterload, which refers to the resistance the heart must overcome to eject blood from the ventricles. Increased afterload can result from hypertension or stenosis of the aortic or pulmonary valves, and can lead to hypertrophy of the heart muscle. In addition, heart failure is often associated with neurohormonal activation, particularly of the renin-angiotensin-aldosterone system (RAAS) and sympathetic nervous system. Activation of these systems can lead to vasoconstriction, fluid retention, and increased heart rate, all of which can exacerbate heart failure. As the heart failure progresses, it can lead to changes in the structure of the heart, including ventricular dilation and hypertrophy, as well as fibrosis and remodeling of the extracellular matrix. These changes can further impair cardiac function and contribute to the progression of heart failure.

TABLE 3: Predominant clinical situations for left-sided and right-sided heart failure.

Left-sided heart failure	Right-sided heart failure
Coronary artery disease	Coronary artery disease (right ventricle myocardial infarction)
Hypertension	Chronic obstructive pulmonary disease
Myocarditis	Pulmonary hypertension
Heart valve disease	Pulmonary valve stenosis
Cardiomyopathy	• Pulmonary embolism • Tricuspid regurgitation • Pneumothorax • Pericardial effusion

(COPD: chronic obstructive pulmonary disease)

Flowchart 4: Pathophysiology of heart failure.

(ANP: A-type natriuretic peptide; BNP: B-type natriuretic peptide; RAAS: renin angiotensin aldosterone system; SNS: sympathetic nervous system)

2. Explain the biomarkers in diagnosis of heart failure.

Biomarkers are measurable substances in the body that can indicate the presence or severity of a disease. In the diagnosis of heart failure, several biomarkers have been identified that can aid in the diagnosis and management of the condition.

Pathophysiology: During HF, cardiomyocyte damage and restructuring leads to active and passive release of cardiomyocyte specific biomarkers. After an event of myocardial infarction, the cardiomyocytes are destroyed and fibrosis occurs. HF activates inflammatory pathways which also release other biomarkers, representative of systemic inflammation.

The following are the list of biomarkers useful in diagnosis of heart failure:

Brain natriuretic peptide (BNP) and N-terminal pro-BNP (NT-proBNP): These are hormones produced by the heart in response to increased pressure and volume, and are commonly used as diagnostic and prognostic markers for heart failure. Elevated levels of BNP and NT-proBNP are indicative of heart failure. Multiple studies support the use of NT-Pro BNP over BNP due to long half-life times, and increased diagnostic accuracy in ruling out the disease. NT-proBNP level >400 pg/mL is diagnostic of heart failure.

NT-Pro ANP (MR-proANP): The physiologic activity of ANP is similar to BNP, ANP acts by binding to NPR-A in cardiac atria, kidney, adrenal glands, and vascular smooth muscle cells, causing an increase in renal sodium excretion. This results in decreased extracellular fluid volume and blood volume, thereby improving cardiac ejection fraction and reduction of blood pressure. In healthy individuals, plasma levels of ANP are ~20 pg/mL and it rises 10–100 times in HF patients. It is difficult to measure the bioactive form of ANP due to its short half-life (2 minutes) and although the N-terminal prohormone form of ANP (NT-proANP) is more chemically stable, it is easily degraded. Therefore, mid-region of NT-proANP (MR-proANP) which is less susceptible to proteolytic degradation is used in clinical assessment.

Cardiac myosin binding protein C: As a circulating biomarker, cMyBP-C has first been assessed as a highly sensitive marker for myocardial injury and recent studies provide evidence that cMyBP-C could outperform cTn in the early detection of MI. Reasons for cMyBP-C's earlier detectability in the circulation could be its higher abundance in cardiomyocytes compared to cTn and, more importantly, an ischemia-induced shedding of cleaved N-terminal fragments of cMyBP-C. cMyBP-C is an important regulatory protein of the cardiac contractile complex. As a biomarker, there is convincing data on its promising potential to be clinically used to improve early rule-in and rule-out of MI. With respect to HF prognostication further trials are warranted to validate the prognostic and diagnostic ability of cMyBP-C.

Troponin: It is a protein found in cardiac muscle cells and is released into the bloodstream following damage to the heart muscle, such as during a myocardial infarction. Elevated levels of troponin can indicate heart failure or other cardiac conditions.

Heart type fatty acid binding protein: hFABP as a biomarker for CVD, not primarily focusing on MI such as cTn and cMyBP-C. Instead, circulating hFABP may well be a marker of cardiomyocyte-specific metabolic disorders as they occur not only during but also before the onset of HF, thus making hFABP a promising candidate biomarker for very early stages of subclinical HF, and for HF prognostication. On the other hand, currently available data is limited to a low number of trials and large-scale validation is needed in order to gain more information on its potential for clinical implementation.

C-reactive protein (CRP): CRP is a marker of inflammation and can be elevated in heart failure as a result of increased stress on the heart such as pericarditis, infective endocarditis.

Galectin-3: Galectin-3 is a protein involved in fibrosis, and elevated levels of galectin-3 have been associated with the development and progression of heart failure. The tissue of origin remains a matter of debate and thus its lack of cardiac specificity seems to be reflected by a limited prognostic value when compared with more established biomarkers such as NT-proBNP.

Growth differentiation factor (GDF): HF causes release of GDF15, whereas the specific tissue of origin is not completely determined. Instead, the utility of GDF15 must be taken as marker for systemic causes or effects of HF. Whether GDF15 allows for specific HF-related prognostication remains matter of debate. We can speculate that in patients with other causes of systemic inflammatory processes, GDF15 may lose its HF-specific prognostic value. Nevertheless, results from clinical trials suggest a promising role of GDF15 as a biomarker in HF prognostication. In this respect, further investigations and validations remain to be undertaken.

Soluble suppression of tumorigenicity 2 (ST2): ST2 is a protein involved in cardiac remodeling and fibrosis. Elevated levels of ST2 have been associated with increased mortality in heart failure patients.

Myocardial fibrosis markers: These include collagen peptides, matrix metalloproteinases (MMPs), and tissue inhibitors of MMPs (TIMPs), and can be elevated in heart failure patients with myocardial fibrosis.

Of all these biomarkers, NT-proBNP is most commonly used in clinical practice. These biomarkers can aid in the diagnosis and management of heart failure, as well as help to predict outcomes and guide treatment decisions. However, it is important to note that no single biomarker is definitive for the diagnosis of heart failure, and its interpretation should be considered in the context of other clinical and diagnostic information.

3. Discuss management of sympathetic crashing acute pulmonary edema.

This is a form of cardiogenic pulmonary edema SCAPE (sympathetic crashing acute pulmonary edema) and FOSPE (fluid overload subacute pulmonary edema) **(Table 4)**.

TABLE 4: Forms of cardiogenic pulmonary edema.

	SCAPE (sympathetic crashing acute pulmonary edema)	FOSPE (fluid overload subacute pulmonary edema)
Also known as	Flash pulmonary edema hypertensive cardiogenic pulmonary edema, hypertensive acute pulmonary edema, acute pulmonary edema	Congestive heart failure, decompensated heart failure
Acuity	Occurs rapidly	Gradual onset
Critically ill	Yes	Usually not
Key physiologic problem	Excessive overload, fluid shifts to lung	Fluid overload
Volume status	May be euvolemic hypovolemic or hypervolemic	Hypervolemic
Blood pressure	Hypertensive	May be hypotensive normotensive or hypotensive
Key therapeutic intervention	CPAP BIPAP Nitroglycerine	Volume removal (diuresis)
Systemic congestion	Often absent (patient often have preserved right ventricular function)	Ascites and /peripheral edema commonly seen

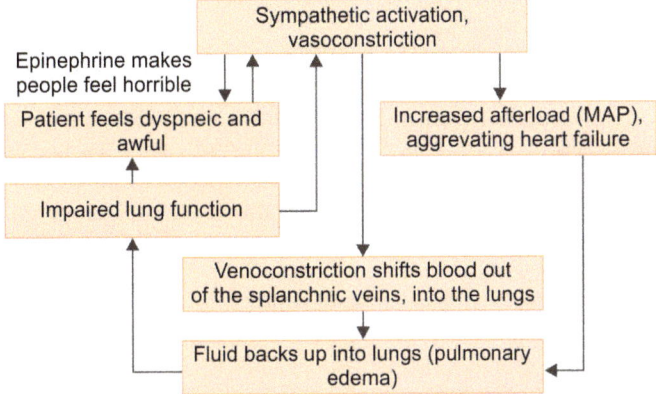

Flowchart 5: Physiology of sympathetic crashing acute pulmonary edema (vicious spiral of SCAPE).

SCAPE (sympathetic crashing acute pulmonary edema) is the extreme end of the spectrum of acute pulmonary edema. The patients have an abrupt redistribution of fluid in the lungs **(Flowchart 5)**, and when treated promptly and effectively, these patients will rapidly recover. Rapid volume distribution associated with sympathetic surge causes rapid progression of dyspnea to life-threatening pulmonary edema. These patients are too unstable and orthopneic to lie down for performing a 12-lead ECG at the time of arrival. Cardiac sensitive troponin is the elevated insignificant proportion of patients with heart failure and is associated with increased mortality. Bedside, screening echocardiography during the acute presentation would reveal preserved ejection fraction, suggesting that underlying mechanism is worsening of diastolic dysfunction.

Management: SCAPE is not a diagnostic dilemma. Early recognition and prompt initiation of treatment is the key to preventing morbidity and mortality. Immediate ED management of severe pulmonary edema has its impact on subsequent clinical course, rates of invasive mechanical ventilation, and rates of intensive care unit (ICU) admissions. Various options for initial treatment include NTG, NIV, diuretics, and morphine **(Flowchart 6)**.

Invasive ventilation: Intubation and use of invasive mechanical ventilation can be avoided if high-dose NTG and NIV are rapidly initiated in the emergency room. When a patient presents late with impending respiratory fatigue or without spontaneous breathing efforts, then the attending physician should proceed with intubation.

Noninvasive ventilation: Two commonly used forms of NIV are bi-level positive airway pressure (BiPAP) and continuous positive airway pressure (CPAP). NIV provides oxygenation, opens the flooded alveoli, and decreases dead space ventilation. It decreases preload and afterload, thereby decreasing cardiac oxygen demand workload. In addition, BiPAP also decreases the work of breathing during inspiration in severely orthopneic patients with SCAPE. NIV is associated with decreased rates of invasive mechanical ventilation and decreased mortality in patients with cardiogenic pulmonary edema, thereby decreasing the rates of associated complications. NIV interfaces include nasal and oronasal masks. Both are associated with similar improvements in gas exchange and avoidance of intubation.

Nitrates: Nitrates have a beneficial effect in acute heart failure syndrome (AHFS) by causing preload reduction, thereby decreasing the cardiac workload. They can be used sublingual until an intravenous access is gained. Initial intravenous dose of NTG in patients with cardiogenic pulmonary edema is 10–20 µg/minute infusion with gradual up-titration. Nitrates cause only venodilatation in these dose ranges, with higher doses required to cause arteriodilatation. Nitrates can cause hypotension, especially in volume-depleted patients and should be avoided in hypotensive patients.

However, the use of nitrates in SCAPE differs from that of other varieties of AHFS. A feasible method of use of high-dose nitrates is thus followed in patients with SCAPE. An initial "bolus" dose of 500–1,000 µg given over 2 minutes can be safely used. This is followed by high-dose infusion at 100 µg/minute with rapid up-titration till there is a clinical improvement, the usual target systolic BP being 140 mm Hg. Then, the infusion rate is sharply reduced and slowly discontinued as patient's condition allows.

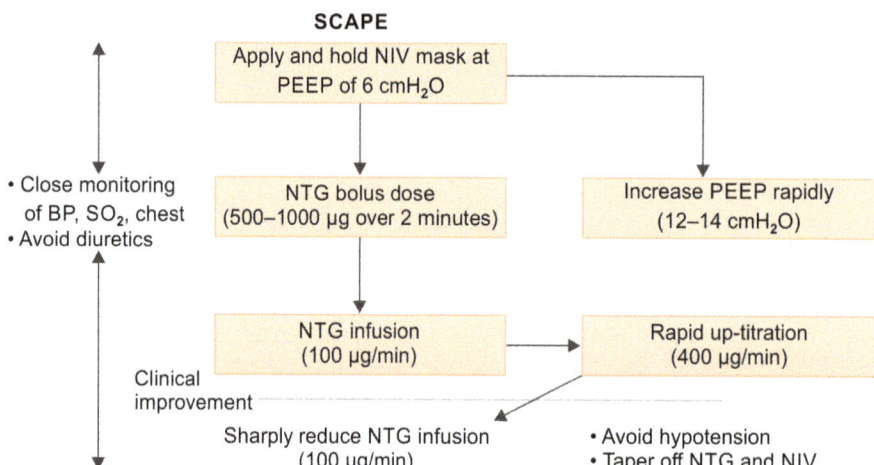

Flowchart 6: Suggested algorithm for sympathetic crashing acute pulmonary edema.

Morphine: It has long been used as an initial agent for the treatment of cardiogenic pulmonary edema. It causes venodilatation, thereby decreasing preload, it decreases anxiety and pain, thereby decreasing the myocardial oxygen demand and hence has potential benefit during AHFS. However, morphine can cause respiratory depression, which may lead to worsened hypoxia and respiratory arrest.

Diuretics: Loop diuretics such as furosemide have been primarily used in the management of acute pulmonary edema. The diuretic effect of furosemide starts in 30 minutes and peaks in 1.5 hours. However, despite its popularity, there is only poor evidence supporting its current use in SCAPE patients.

■ SUGGESTED READING

1. Bartfield JM, Ushkow BS, Rosen JM, Dylong K. Single breath counting in the assessment of pulmonary function. Ann Emerg Med. 1994;24:256-9. (Question 5).
2. Cooper MS, Gittoes NJL. Diagnosis and management of hypocalcaemia. BMJ. 2008;336(7656):1298-1302. (Question 9).
3. Goltzman D. (2014). Treatment of hypocalcaemia. [online] Available from: https://www.uptodate.com/contents/treatment-of-hypocalcemia [Last accessed June, 2023]. (Question 9).
4. Johnson EO, Vekris M, Demesticha T, Soucacos PN. Neuroanatomy of the brachial plexus: normal and variant anatomy of its formation. Surg Radiol Anat. 2010;32(3):291-7. (Question 6).
5. Mégarbane B, Bhalla A, Lavergne V. Evidence-based recommendations on the use of intravenous lipid emulsion therapy in poisoning. Clin Toxicol (Phila). 2016;54(10):899-923. (Question 8).
6. National Institutes of Health (NIH). (2021). COVID-19 Treatment Guidelines. [online] Available from: https://www.covid19treatmentguidelines.nih.gov/ [Last accessed June, 2023]. (Question 5).
7. NHS. How is acute hypocalcaemia treated in adults? UKMI Medicines Q&As 373.3 prepared 9th April 2014. [online]

Available from: https://www.evidence.nhs.uk/search?q=%22How+is+acute+hypocalcaemia+treated+in+adults%22 [Last accessed June, 2023]. (Question 9).

8. Richhariya D, Sharma B. Textbook of Emergency Medicine including Intensive Care and Trauma, 2nd edition. New Delhi: Jaypee Brothers Medical Publishers (P) Ltd; 2022. pp. 757, 791-5. (Question 1).

9. Richhariya D, Sharma B. Textbook of Emergency Medicine including Intensive Care and Trauma, 2nd edition. New Delhi: Jaypee Brothers Medical Publishers (P) Ltd; 2022. pp. 871-6. (Question 2).

10. Richhariya D, Sharma B. Textbook of Emergency Medicine including Intensive Care and Trauma, 2nd edition. New Delhi: Jaypee Brothers Medical Publishers (P) Ltd; 2022. pp. 838-43. (Question 3).

11. Richhariya D, Sharma B. Textbook of Emergency Medicine including Intensive Care and Trauma, 2nd edition. New Delhi: Jaypee Brothers Medical Publishers (P) Ltd; 2022. pp. 266-88, 580. (Question 4).

12. Richhariya D, Sharma B. Textbook of Emergency Medicine including Intensive Care and Trauma, 2nd edition. New Delhi: Jaypee Brothers Medical Publishers (P) Ltd; 2022. pp. 621-31. (Question 5).

13. Richhariya D, Sharma B. Textbook of Emergency Medicine including Intensive Care and Trauma, 2nd edition. New Delhi: Jaypee Brothers Medical Publishers (P) Ltd; 2022. pp. 1692-96. (Question 7).

14. Richhariya D, Sharma B. Textbook of Emergency Medicine including Intensive Care and Trauma, 2nd edition. New Delhi: Jaypee Brothers Medical Publishers (P) Ltd; 2022. pp. 538, 1457-58. (Question 8).

15. Richhariya D, Sharma B. Textbook of Emergency Medicine including Intensive Care and Trauma, 2nd edition. New Delhi: Jaypee Brothers Medical Publishers (P) Ltd; 2022. p. 316. (Question 9).

16. Richhariya D, Sharma B. Textbook of Emergency Medicine including Intensive Care and Trauma, 2nd edition. New Delhi: Jaypee Brothers Medical Publishers (P) Ltd; 2022. pp. 468-72. (Question 10).

17. Ushkow BS, Bartfield JM, Reicho PR, Raccio-Robak N. Single-breath counting for the assessment of bronchospastic patients in the ED. Am J of Emerg Med. 1998;16:100-1. (Question 5).

18. Vosloo M, Keough N, De Beer MA. The clinical anatomy of the insertion of the rotator cuff tendons. Eur J Orthop Surg Traumatol. 2017;27(3):359-66. (Question 6).

19. World Health Organization. (2021). Clinical management of COVID-19. [online] Available from: https://www.who.int/teams/health-care-readiness/covid-19 [Last accessed June, 2023]. (Question 5).

Emergency Medicine Paper 30

Noel Fernando

Question 1

1. Discuss hyperemesis gravidarum.

Nausea and vomiting in pregnancy (NVP) is a rather frequent symptom occurring in 70-80% women. NVP is one of the commonest reasons for hospitalization in pregnancy and negatively affects the quality of life. In most pregnant women the condition is self-limiting, yet, in a few, symptoms may persist throughout the duration of pregnancy. *Hyperemesis gravidarum (HG)* is a rare but severe form of NVP reported in 0.3-3.6% pregnancies and an obstetric emergency. Other causes of severe nausea and vomiting should be excluded before coming to the diagnosis of HG. HG, the severe form of NVP, is marked by a triad of severe protracted nausea and vomiting associated with weight loss >5% prepregnancy weight, dehydration, and electrolyte imbalances. Severe untreated forms may present with malnutrition, dehydration, neuropathies, Wernicke's encephalopathy, coma, and death. Serious maternal complications may also occur due to Mallory-Weiss tears and esophageal rupture, splenic avulsion, and pneumothorax associated with excessive vomiting.

Excessive vomiting results from emetogenic effects of human chorionic gonadotropin (hCG) the pathogenesis of which is largely unknown. There are no marked changes in the organ systems other than features of dehydration and malnutrition in severe cases. Some cases of HG may develop Wernicke's encephalopathy due to vitamin B_1 deficiency. Many oral antiemetics are safe for use in NVP **(Table 1)**. Women not responding to single medication may be given combination of different drugs. Parenteral route may be preferable for those with persistent NVP/HG. For the cases needing inpatient management, initial assessment should include ABCDE (airway, breathing, circulation, disability, exposure) and fluid resuscitation should be guided by degree of shock. Initial resuscitation should be done with crystalloids containing sodium and chloride with supplementation of potassium. Proton pump inhibitors or H_2 antagonists may be added to relieve gastritis or esophagitis. Intravenous antiemetics can be gradually replaced with oral medication once fluid therapy is weaned off. Thromboprophylaxis with low molecular weight heparin is indicated in admitted patients unless contraindicated.

TABLE 1: Antiemetics recommended for use in pregnancy.

First line	• Cyclizine 50 mg PO, IM or IV 8 hourly • Prochlorperazine 5–10 mg 6–8 hourly PO; 12.5 mg 8 hourly IM/IV; 25 mg PR daily promethazine 12.5–25 mg 4–8 hourly PO, IM, IV or PR • Chlorpromazine 10–25 mg 4–6 hourly PO, IV or IM; or 50–100 mg 6–8 hourly PR
Second line	• Metoclopramide 5–10 mg 8 hourly PO, IV or IM (maximum 5 days' duration); Domperidone 10 mg 8 hourly PO; 30–60 mg 8 hourly PR • Ondansetron 4–8 mg 6–8 hourly PO; 8 mg over 15 minutes 12 hourly IV
Third line	*Corticosteroids:* Hydrocortisone 100 mg twice daily IV; once clinical improvement occurs, convert to prednisolone 40–50 mg daily PO, dose gradually tapered until the lowest maintenance dose that controls the symptoms is reached

(IM: intramuscular; IV: intravenous; PO: by mouth; PR: by rectum)

Multidisciplinary team management with nutritionist, endocrinologist, and gastroenterologist should be used when enteral or parenteral treatment is required. As a last resort, in patients not responding to any treatment modality and with remitting severe symptoms, termination of pregnancy may be considered.

2. Explain the diagnosis of thromboembolism in pregnancy.

3. Discuss treatment of thromboembolic disease in pregnancy.

- Women who are pregnant or in the postpartum period have a fourfold to fivefold increased risk of thromboembolism compared with nonpregnant women. Approximately 80% of thromboembolic events in pregnancy are venous. The main reason for the increased risk of venous thromboembolism (VTE) in pregnancy is hypercoagulability. The hypercoagulability of pregnancy, which has likely evolved to protect women from the bleeding challenges of miscarriage and childbirth, is present as early as the first trimester and so is the increased risk of VTE. Among pregnant and postpartum women, the left lower extremity is the most common site of DVT (82%). Anatomic reasons (compression of the left common iliac vein by the right common iliac artery which is accentuated by the enlarging uterus) have been postulated. The signs and symptoms of VTE are nonspecific and common in pregnancy. Diagnosis of VTE by physical examination is frequently inaccurate, even though one study found that 80% of pregnant women with DVT experience pain and swelling of the lower extremity.

- *Management* (**Flowchart 1**): If pulmonary imaging is required, ventilation perfusion scanning is usually the preferred initial test to detect pulmonary embolism within pregnancy. Treatment should be commenced on clinical suspicion and not be withheld until an objective diagnosis is obtained. The mainstay of treatment for pulmonary thromboembolism in pregnancy is anticoagulation with low molecular weight heparin for a minimum of 3 months in total duration and until at least 6 weeks postnatal. Low molecular weight heparin is safe, effective and has a low associated bleeding risk.

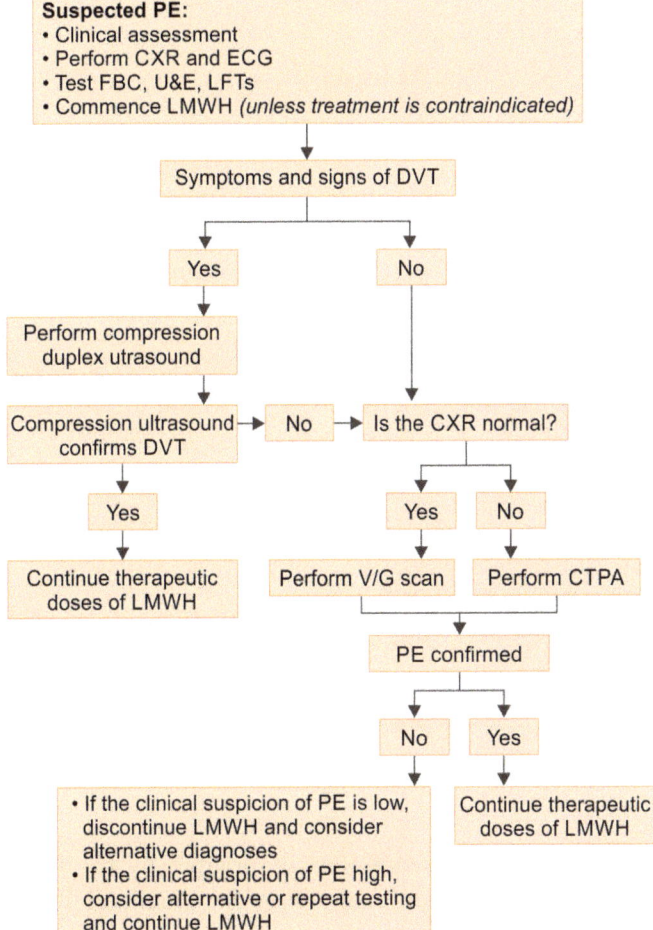

Flowchart 1: Management of DVT in pregnant.

Reproduced with permission from: Royal College of Obstetricians and Gynecologists. Thromboembolic Disease in Pregnancy and the Puerperium: Acute Management. Green-top Guideline No. 37b. London: RCOG; 2015.

(CTPA: CT-pulmonary angiography; CXR: chest X-ray; DVT: deep vein thrombosis; ECG: electrocardiograph; FBC: full blood count; LFTs; liver function tests; LMWH: low molecular weight heparin; PE: pulmonary embolism; U&E: urine examination)

Question 2

1. Discuss management of septic arthritis of knee joint in emergency department.

Diagnosis and differential diagnosis: A through history and physical examination are essential of diagnosis, but in diagnostic evaluation include blood tests (CBC, ESR, and CRP), analysis and culture of joint fluid, sometime sputum, spinal fluid, and urine tests. Imaging such as X-ray, CT scan, ultrasonography, and MRI is helpful for diagnosing septic arthritis. Usually a sample of joint fluid (joint aspiration) is essential. Synovial fluid (**Table 2**) should be submitted for cell count with differential, gram stain and microbiological (aerobic and anaerobic) culture. The higher the synovial WBC count, the greater the chances of septic arthritis. Multiple sets of blood tests and cultures also should be obtained when hematogenous septic arthritis is suspected to improve the chances of identifying a causative microorganism. Imaging helps well such as plain radiography of the infected joint may reveal joint destruction. CT and MRI help in evaluation of septic arthritis also and ultrasonography is done to identify accumulations of fluid or collections of pus (abscesses). Differential diagnosis for septic arthritis is rheumatic arthritis, Reiter's syndrome, psoriatic arthritis, ankylosing spondylitis, osteoarthritis.

Therapy: Successful treatment depends on antibiotics, antifungal drugs, removal of the pus, splinting of the joint, followed by physical therapy. Empiric antibiotics for nongonococcal septic arthritis usually involve the use of intravenous vancomycin directed against gram-positive organisms especially if there is a suspicion of methicillin-resistant *Staphylococcus aureus* (MRSA) based on community and institutional data.

2. What are the compartments of leg?

The lower leg subdivides into four compartments which are the anterior, lateral, superficial posterior, and deep posterior compartments (**Fig. 1**):

1. *Anterior compartment:* Tibialis anterior, extensor muscles of the foot, and fibularis (peroneus) tertius muscles. The anterior tibial artery and deep fibular (peroneal) nerve supply the anterior compartment.
2. *Lateral compartment:* Fibularis (peroneus) longus and fibularis (peroneus) brevis muscles. The superficial fibular (peroneal) nerve and branches from the anterior tibial artery supply these muscles.

TABLE 2: Synovial fluid analysis.					
Characteristics	**Normal**	**Noninflammatory**	**Inflammatory**	**Septic**	**Traumatic**
Color	Colorless	Yellow	Yellow	Yellow	Red
Appearance	Clear	Clear	Cloudy	Cloudy	Cloudy
WBC/mL	<200	<2,000	2,000–100,000	>100,000	
% PMNs	<25	<25	>50	>95	
Crystals	None	None	May be present	None	None
Cultures	Negative	Negative	Negative	Positive	Negative
Conditions		Trauma, osteoarthritis, viral infections	Inflammatory arthritis such as RA, spondyloarthritis, SLE, acute rheumatic fever, reactive arthritis, crystal induced arthritis	Bacterial arthritis, tubercular arthritis	Fractures, Coagulopathies

(PMNs: polymorphonuclear neutrophils; WBC: white blood cells)

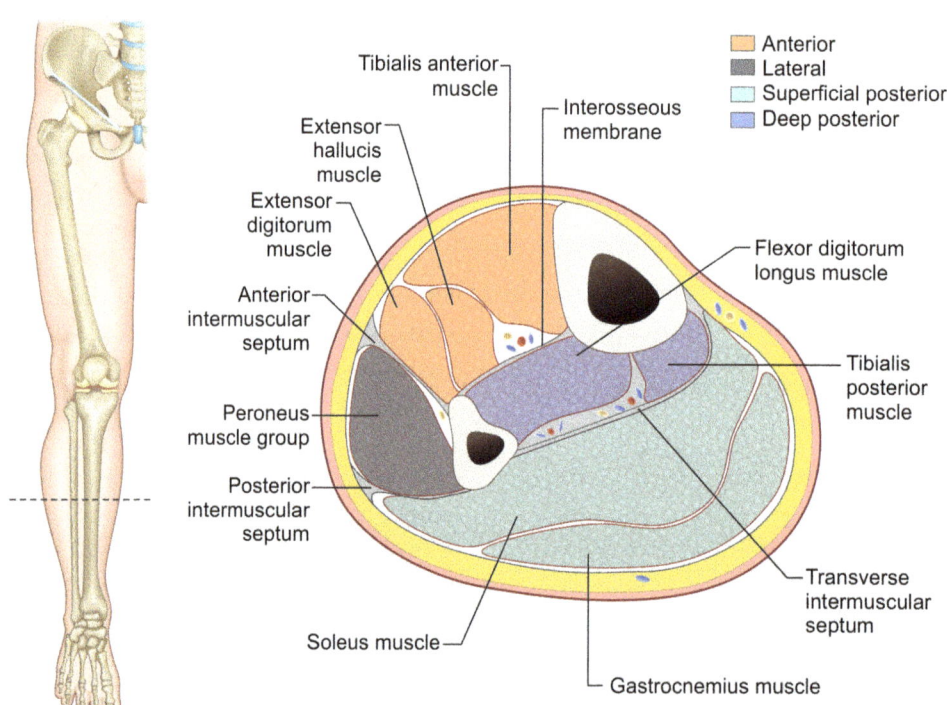

Fig. 1: Compartments of legs.

3. *Superficial posterior compartment:* Gastrocnemius, soleus, and plantaris muscles. Tibial nerve branches supply these muscles. The arteries that supply these muscles descend from the popliteal artery. The sural arteries (medial, lateral) supply the gastrocnemius. The soleus is variably supplied by the popliteal artery, posterior tibial artery, and fibular (peroneal) artery.
4. *Deep posterior compartment:* Tibialis posterior, flexor muscles of the foot, and popliteus muscles. The deep posterior compartment is innervated by the tibial nerve and supplied by the posterior tibial and fibular (peroneal) arteries.

3. Discuss high pressure hand injuries.

High-pressure injection (HPI) injuries of the hand occur when the hand comes into contact with the nozzle of a high-pressure injecting system such as a paint gun or air compressor. The material injected can traverse from the hand to the forearm and upper arm. This injury commonly occurs in male construction workers. In a HPI injury, the puncture wound is small and not distinct; pain and local swelling is minimal until hours later. Compartment syndrome is increased tissue pressure within a closed fascial space, resulting in tissue ischemia.

Clinical presentation: Pain, swelling of the affected hand. Physical examination shows a puncture wound, neurovascular compromise, and compartment syndrome.

Diagnosis: Raised inflammatory markers and X-ray identify radiopaque substances. CT and MRI help for soft tissue assessment.

Nonoperative management: Tetanus prophylaxis, parenteral antibiotics, limb elevation, early mobilization, monitoring for compartment syndrome. A total of 50% of injuries treated nonoperatively will ultimately require an operation. Delayed surgical management associated with higher reoperation rates and postoperative complications

Operative management: Irrigation and debridement, foreign body removal, and broad-spectrum antibiotics.

Indications: Most cases require immediate surgical debridement outcomes. Higher rates of amputation are seen when surgery is delayed >10 hours after injury; 48% of finger injuries require amputation.

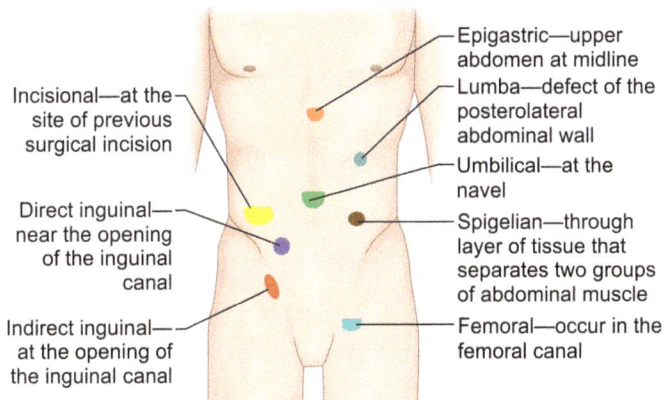

Fig. 2: Anatomical sites of hernias.

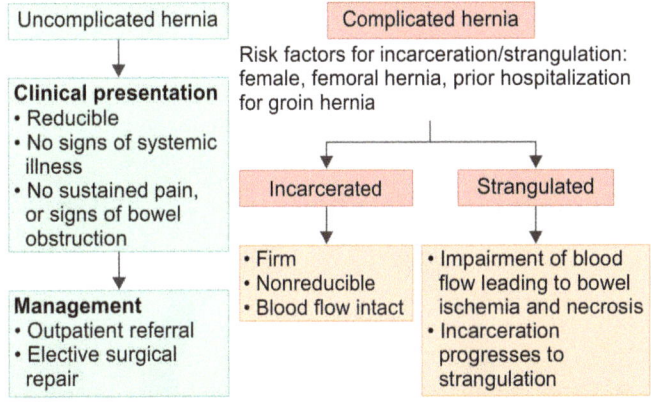

Flowchart 2: Clinical features of uncomplicated and complicated hernia.

Question 3

1. Discuss anatomical and clinical features of various uncomplicated hernias.

Internal hernias protrude within the body, while external hernias protrude through to the outside of the body **(Fig. 2)**. Reducible hernia refers to when the protruding tissue can be moved back to its original site using simple manipulation, while an irreducible hernia cannot be moved back. In a direct hernia, the peritoneal sac enters the inguinal canal directly via a defect or weakness in the posterior wall of the inguinal canal, usually the transversus abdominis. It usually protrudes directly to the abdominal wall but may exit through the external inguinal ring. Impulses on coughing or sneezing and easy reducibility are the main features of uncomplicated hernias **(Flowchart 2)**.

2. Explain the evaluation and management of obstructed hernia.

If the contents of the hernia become trapped in the weak point in the abdominal wall, the contents can obstruct the bowel, leading to severe pain, nausea, vomiting, and the inability to have a bowel movement or pass gas.

Strangulation: An incarcerated hernia can cut off blood flow to part of your intestine. An obstructed hernia is one in which the lumen of the herniated part of intestine is obstructed whereas a strangulated hernias one in which the blood supply of the hernia contents is compromised, thus, leading to ischemia. Hernias can also form intra-abdominally by twisting of the mesentery or from a lead point such as adhesions. These internal hernias can also lead to strangulated bowel, which is a surgical emergency. Approach to obstructed hernia is summarized in **Flowchart 3**.

3. Discuss ED evaluation and management of intestinal obstruction.

Bowel obstruction is defined as the impairment of passage of intestinal content. It is classified according to a couple of characteristics that are the site of obstruction, the degree of obstruction, and the presence of irrigation impairment (ischemia). The site of obstruction in general terms are the small bowel and the large bowel, which have an additional sub-classification, which can be extrinsic or intrinsic (intraluminal and intramural). ED evaluation management of intestinal obstruction is given in **Figure 3**.

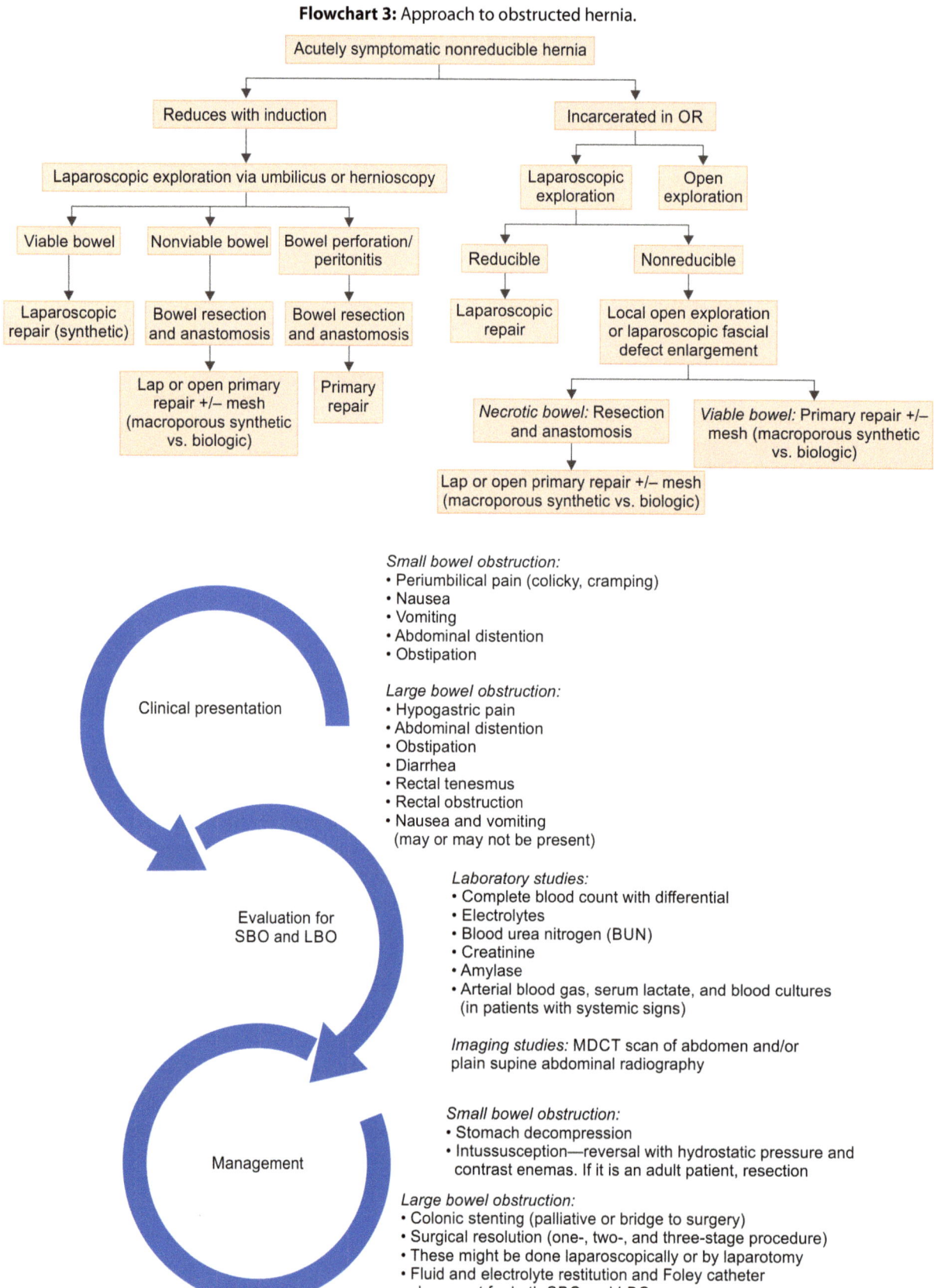

Fig. 3: Summary, evaluation, and management of bowel obstruction. (LBO: large-bowel obstruction; MDCT: multidetector computed tomography; SBO: small bowel obstruction)

Question 4

1. Write a short note on "examination of a victim of sexual assault in ED".

Following are the common injuries:
a. *Head:* Blow on head or head injury due to fall.
b. *Neck:* Gripping of throat.
c. Injuries on cheeks, lips, breast, and chest.
d. Generalized bruises, lacerations, contusions, bite marks, and nail marks.
e. The marks of rope knots on the wrists and ankles.

The examiner should strive to ascertain the following:
a. Whether these marks are of injuries or self-inflicted.
b. Apparent development of victim's body.
c. Amount of resistance offered.
d. Corroboration with statement of victim.

Examination of nails: Scraping from the nails beds constitutes important evidence. Tags of epithelium, hairs, piece of clothes, bloodstains are important to collect.

Gait: The victim's gait must be made a note. If consent is available, the victim's blood should be collected for grouping. This will help in ascertaining whether bloodstains are of the victim or assailant. A second examination after 48 hours may reveal deep bruises, which may not be evident at the first examination.

Examination of genitals: A gynecological examination should be conducted in lithotomy position and in good light. The history of last menstrual period must be asked for to differentiate menstruation from bleeding due to injuries.

2. Explain the role of contraception in a victim of rape.

Emergency contraception can stop pregnancy before it starts. Emergency contraception is a safe way to prevent unintentional pregnancy due to unprotected sex, contraceptives failure, rupture, slippage condom or diaphragm forgotten, oral pills or following sexual assault. Rape resulting in unintended pregnancies causes mental, social burden to the women, and society as a whole.

History of last menstrual period, length of cycle, and time since last unprotected intercourse, any history of chronic illness should be recorded. Physical examination is not generally required but perform urine pregnancy test if pregnancy is suspected. Follow up after the use of emergency contraceptive, if menstruation occurs within 7 days or expected periods, counsel and encourage for regular methods. If no menstruation occurs within 7 days or expected periods, perform urine pregnancy test, if negative wait for one more week and if positive counseling, No serious side effects of emergency contraceptive, only mild, resolves within 24 hours. Mild side effects are nausea, vomiting, mild headache, mild tenderness in breast, dizziness, fatigue, and delay in menstruation.

Types of emergency contraceptive pills are discussed here:
Ulipristal: It is more effective than progestin only or combined pill in preventing the unprotected pregnancy, approved in 2010 and can be taken up to 120 hours after unprotected intercourse.

Progestin-only: Progestin levonorgestrel 1.5 mg single dose or 750 µg 12 hours apart in 2 doses, can be taken up to 72 hours.

Combined pill: It contains both estrogen and progestin in higher dose and delays the ovulation most effective within 3 days of unprotected intercourse.

Question 5

Write short notes on the following:
1. Anatomy of wrist joint.
2. Radiological features of normal wrist joint.

The human hand has 27 bones—the carpals or wrist account for eight; the metacarpals or palm contain five; the remaining 14 are digital bones—fingers and thumb. The palm has five bones known as metacarpal bones, one to each of the five digits. These metacarpals have a head, a shaft, and a base. Joints of the hand include carpometacarpal joints found between the carpals and the metacarpals; the intermetacarpal joints among the metacarpals themselves; the metacarpophalangeal joints between the metacarpals and the proximal phalanges; and finally, the interphalangeal joints found between the proximal phalanges. Radiology of wrist joint is shown in **Figure 4**.

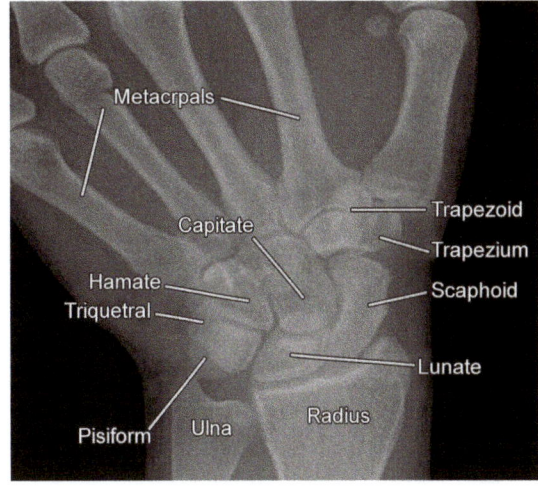

Fig. 4: Radiology of wrist joint.

3. Perilunate dislocation.

Lunate/*perilunate dislocations* are high energy injuries to the wrist associated with neurological injury and poor functional outcomes. Perilunate and lunate dislocations result when great force is applied to a hyperextended wrist. They usually result from a fall on an outstretched hand or occur in a motor vehicle crash. Perilunate dislocations are more common than lunate dislocations. Perilunate dislocation and perilunate fracture dislocation are injuries that involve traumatic rupture of the radioscaphocapitate (RSC) ligament, the scapholunate interosseous (SLI) ligament, and the lunotriquetral interosseous (LTI) ligament (**Figs. 5A and B**). Around 60% of perilunate dislocations are associated with a scaphoid fracture which is then termed a transscaphoid perilunate dislocation. The other types are perilunate, transradial styloid, and transscaphoid and transcapitate perilunar.

The surgical treatment of choice is open reduction and ligamentous repair with percutaneous pin fixation. In most settings, however, if a distal radial styloid fracture or a carpal bone fracture accompanies the perilunate dislocation, internal fixation is preferred. Complications include post-traumatic arthrosis, median nerve dysfunction, complex regional pain syndrome, tendon problems, and carpal instability. Despite appropriate treatment, loss of wrist motion and grip strength, as well as persistent pain, is common.

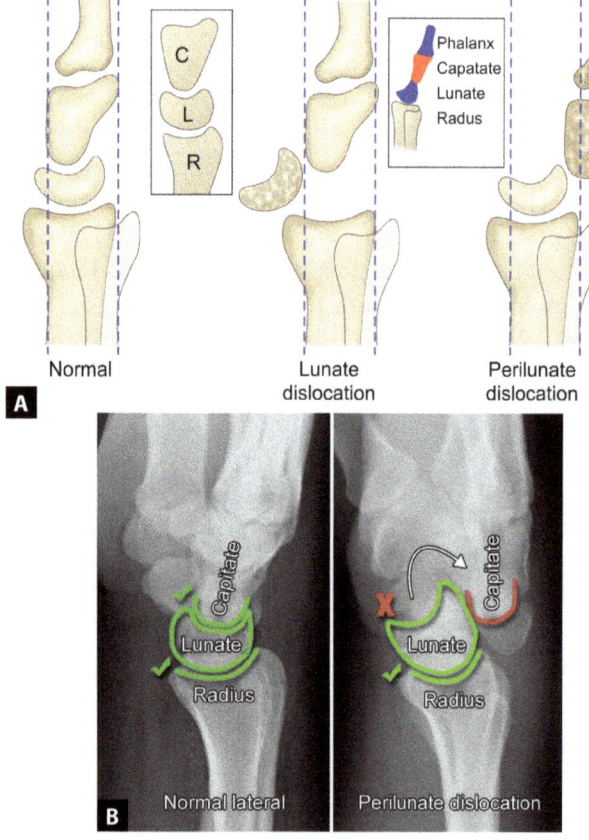

Figs. 5A and B: Perilunate dislocation.

Question 6

1. Describe normal anatomy of eye with diagram.

The eye is a fluid-filled sphere enclosed by three layers of tissue **(Fig. 6)**. Most of the outer layer is composed of a tough white fibrous tissue, the sclera. At the front of the eye, however, this opaque outer layer is transformed into the cornea, a specialized transparent tissue that permits light rays to enter the eye. The middle layer of tissue includes three distinct but continuous structures—(1) the iris, (2) the ciliary body, and (3) the choroid.

- The iris is the colored portion of the eye that can be seen through the cornea. It contains two sets of muscles with opposing actions, which allow the size of the pupil (the opening in its center) to be adjusted under neural control.
- The ciliary body is a ring of tissue that encircles the lens and includes a muscular component that is important for adjusting the refractive power of the lens, and a vascular component (the so-called ciliary processes) that produces the fluid that fills the front of the eye.
- The choroid is composed of a rich capillary bed that serves as the main source of blood supply for the photoreceptors of the retina. Only the innermost layer of the eye, the retina, contains neurons that are sensitive to light and are capable of transmitting visual signals to central targets.

There are two chambers of eye.

Anterior chamber: The anterior chamber, the space between the lens and the cornea, is filled with aqueous humor, a clear, watery liquid that supplies nutrients to these structures as well as to the lens. Aqueous humor is produced by the ciliary processes in the posterior chamber (the region between the lens and the iris) and flows into the anterior chamber through the pupil. A specialized meshwork of cells that lie at the junction of the iris and the cornea is responsible for its uptake. Under normal conditions, the rates of aqueous humor production and uptake are in equilibrium, ensuring a constant intraocular pressure. Abnormally high levels of intraocular pressure, which occurs in glaucoma, can reduce the blood supply to the eye and eventually damage retinal neurons.

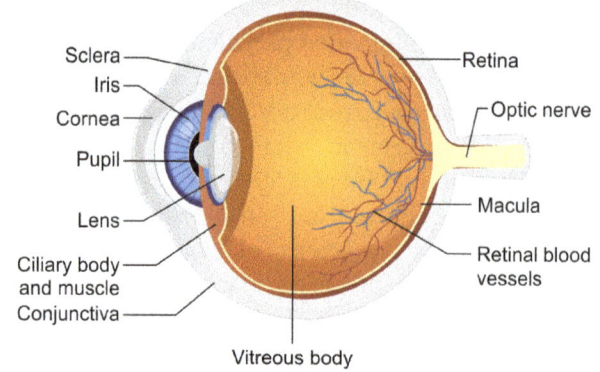

Fig. 6: Normal anatomy of eye.

Posterior chamber: The space between the back of the lens and the surface of the retina is filled with a thick, gelatinous substance called the vitreous humor, which accounts for about 80% of the volume of the eye. In addition to maintaining the shape of the eye, the vitreous humor contains phagocytic cells that remove blood and other debris that might otherwise interfere with light transmission. The housekeeping abilities of the vitreous humor are limited, however, as a large number of middle-aged and elderly individuals with vitreal "floaters" will attest. Floaters are collections of debris too large for phagocytic consumption that therefore remain to cast annoying shadows on the retina; they typically arise when the aging vitreous membrane pulls away from the overly long eyeball of myopic individuals.

2. Discuss orbital cellulitis.

Orbital cellulitis most commonly refers to an acute spread of infection into the eye socket from either extension from periorbital structures (most commonly the adjacent ethmoid or frontal sinuses (90%), skin, dacryocystitis, dental infection, intracranial infection), exogenous causes (trauma, foreign bodies, postsurgical), intraorbital infection (endophthalmitis, dacryoadenitis), or from spread through the blood (bacteremia with septic emboli). Periorbital cellulitis tends to be a less severe disease than orbital cellulitis. It involves the eyelids and soft tissues anterior to the orbital septum. Infection usually starts following an upper respiratory tract infection, external ocular infection, or following trauma to the eyelids. The most common organisms are *Staphylococci* and *Streptococci*. *Orbital cellulitis:* It is an extension of sinus infection into orbit or traumatic inoculation.

- *Bacteria: Streptococcus* (S.) *pneumoniae, Haemophilus* (H.) *influenzae, Catarrhalis, Staphylococcus aureus, Streptococcus* (S.) *pyogenes, Bacteroides.*
- Seen as erythema and swelling around eye, suspect if eyelid or periorbital inflammation is accompanied by any—ptosis, impaired extra ocular movements, pain with eye movement, chemosis, afferent papillary defect.
- *Signs that distinguish orbital from periorbital cellulitis are:* Loss of vision (due to optic nerve compression) ophthalmoplegia, painful eye movements, proptosis, chemosis, and conjunctival edema; CT scan may be performed to look for evidence of abscess formation.
- Urgent ophthalmology referral. Oral antibiotics to complete 3 weeks course. Cefuroxime (50 mg/kg IV every 8 hours), ampicillin-sulbactam (50 mg/kg IV every 6 hours)
- If anaerobic infection suspected clindamycin 10 mg/kg every 6 hours
- Inpatient management, possible surgical drainage. If visual acuity reduces, an afferent pupillary defect develops, or if antibiotics fail to improve symptoms.
- Complications of orbital cellulitis are visual loss, septicemia, cavernous sinus thrombosis, central retinal artery occlusion, optic neuritis, osteomyelitis, meningitis, orbital abscess, and endophthalmitis.

3. Explain the treatment of blunt eye trauma in ED.

Blunt injury to the eye can lead to various intrinsic eye injuries. Blunt trauma can result in open and closed globe injuries. The closed globe injuries are further classified as contusion and lamellar lacerations. Open globe injuries can be laceration and globe rupture. Globe rupture and retrobulbar hematoma are two emergent entities that are of importance. Blunt eye trauma can be due to coup, countercoup, and anteroposterior compression or horizontal tissue expansion. The mode of injury can be a direct blow to the eyeball or accidental blunt trauma. The traumatic lesions of blunt eye trauma are classified as closed globe injury, globe rupture, and extraocular lesions. Blunt trauma can result in contusions, abrasions, lacerations, internal hemorrhage, bone fractures, as well as death.

Anterior globe rupture: Usually masked by subconjunctival hemorrhage. The most common site of rupture is old surgical wounds such as cataract and keratoplasty. *The posterior globe rupture* can be the site of recti muscle insertion, where the sclera is the thinnest.

Retrobulbar hematoma: This may lead to orbital compartment syndrome and blindness. Delaying the treatment causes optic nerve ischemia and can lose the vision within few hours. Reduced visual acuity, reduced eye movements, proptosis are the markers of retrobulbar hematoma. There may be an afferent pupillary defect. Signs of raised intraocular pressure such as pain, photophobia are seen in extreme cases.

Ophthalmoscopic examination: It shows lens dislocation, hyphema, vitreous, subhyaloid, or retinal hemorrhage. Sometimes retinal edema ("commotio retinae") may be seen as white patches with diffuse margins on the posterior pole of the eye. Staining of the cornea reveals—corneal abrasion; investigation X-ray—to rule out orbital or facial fractures; CT facial bones is more sensitive in ruling out orbital/facial fractures.

Management: For minor eye injuries, treatment may include: *cold compresses*—icepacks reduce swelling and relieve pain. *Eye flushing:* Flush chemicals and other irritants with clean water for about 15 minutes. If bleeding use a dressing, apply firm direct pressure with gloved hand to the injured area. Continue to hold the pressure until the bleeding stops. If there are multiple wounds, apply pressure dressings to the worst injuries first, and then to the lesser bleeding injuries. It is an eye threatening emergency. Urgent lateral canthotomy and cantholysis should be done immediately at ED.

Question 7

1. Discuss splint immobilizers in ED for upper extremity injuries.

Padding in a cast or splint is a balance between protecting the soft tissues and maintaining immobilization **(Table 3)**. Under padding will result in skin breakdown or frank ulceration. Over padding may lead to loosen cast or splint and poor support. Reduction of fracture and splinting is recommended to reduce pain, blood loss and to prevent injury to surrounding structure. Reduction of fracture is helpful in re-establishing anatomic alignment, promote fracture healing, local hematoma works as a medium for callus formation, which then bridges together the two ends of the fractured bone.

TABLE 3: Common orthopedic injury and splinting procedure in emergency department.

Injury	Orthopedic procedure/spilt
Distal phalanx fracture of the hand	Finger protector splint
Boxer's fracture	Ulnar gutter splint
Metacarpal fracture	Radial or ulnar gutter splint
Scaphoid fracture	Thumb spica splint
Carpal fracture	Dorsal splint of the forearm
Radius and ulna fracture	Sugar-tong splint
Elbow dislocation	Posterior long arm (elbow) splint
Supracondylar fracture of the humerus	Posterior long arm (elbow) splint
Proximal humerus fracture	Coaptation splint, sling, and swathe
Shoulder dislocation	Shoulder immobilizer or sling and swathe
Metatarsal fracture	Posterior short leg (posterior ankle) splint
Ankle sprain	Posterior short leg (posterior ankle) splint
Ankle dislocation	Trilaminar ankle splint
Distal tibia/fibula fracture	Trilaminar ankle splint
Knee dislocation	Knee immobilizer or knee splint
Patellar dislocation	Knee immobilizer or knee splint

Crammer wire/malleable splints: Crammer wire is made up from malleable aluminum wires attached to a strong but flexible aluminum rod. Splint can bend easily at any angle. Main purpose is to keep upper or lower limb in desired position and preoperative management of patient for immobilization; available in various size ranging from width of 2″, 4″, 5″, 6″ and length of 12″, 18″, 24″. *Malleable splints:* Temporary methods for upper and lower limb immobilization; reusable, waterproof, lightweight. Made up off malleable aluminum with foam and padding, fastens in place with tape or strap, can be cut by household scissors.

2. What are the complications of fracture-dislocation and their ED management?

Complications of fracture-dislocation are summarized in **Table 4**. Many fractures cause blood vessel damage. Pulmonary embolism is the most common severe complication of serious fractures of the hip or pelvis; and other complications are compartment syndrome, infections, joint problems, and short limb osteonecrosis. The most common complications of dislocations are damage to the bones and tissues around joint, including muscle strains, ligament, and tendon sprains nerve damage.

Early complications include wound healing problems, shock, compartment syndrome, fat embolism, thromboembolism (pulmonary embolism), deep vein thrombosis, disseminated intravascular coagulopathy, and infection.

Delayed complications include osteomyelitis, delayed union, malunion, nonunion, avascular necrosis of bone, reaction to internal fixation devices, complex regional pain syndrome, and heterotrophic ossification can occur at a later stage in the healing process.

Immobilize fracture—use broad bandages (where possible) to prevent movement at joints above and below the fracture. Support the limb, carefully passing bandages under the natural hollows of the body.

3. Discuss dislocation of femoral head.

The femoral head is pushed either backward (posterior dislocation) out of the socket, or forward (anterior dislocation) **(Fig. 7)**. In approximately 90% of hip dislocation patients, the femur is pushed out of the socket in a backward direction called a posterior dislocation. Motor vehicle collisions are the most common cause of traumatic hip dislocations. The dislocation often occurs when the knee hits the dashboard in a collision. This force drives the thigh backwards, which drives the ball head of the femur out of the hip socket.

TABLE 4: Complications of fracture-dislocation and their ED management.

Complications	Description	Signs and symptoms	Interventions
Early complications			
Shock	Hypovolemic or traumatic shock resulting from hemorrhage	Cool, clammy skin or sweating, moist skin confusion	Management includes restoration of blood volume and circulation, relieving the patient's pain, providing adequate splinting
Rhabdomyolysis	Crush injury usually occurs in the very acute phase (around 1–3 days) postinjury	Significant muscle pain, swelling, fever, vomiting, coffee colored urine	Management includes fluid resuscitation and the management of associated renal failure
Compartment syndrome	*Risk factors:* Tibial or forearm fractures, high-energy wrist fractures, crush injuries	Pain out of proportion to the associated injury, pain on passive movement of the muscles of the involved compartments, severe swelling, neurovascular changes - 5Ps	• Remove any cast, splint of circumferential dressing and elevate limb to heart level • May require emergency fasciotomy
Fat embolism	*Risk factors:* Long bone fractures pelvic fractures, multiple fractures, crush injuries	Hypoxia, tachypnea, tachycardia, pyrexia	Administer oxygen, intensive care management
Pulmonary embolism	*Risk factors:* Serious limb injury surgery, Prolonged bed rest	• Pyrexia dyspnea and/or Tachypnea hemoptysis • Tachycardia • Hypotension • Lightheaded/Dizzy • Syncope cyanosis	• Administer oxygen • Intensive care management
Deep vein thrombosis	*Risk factors:* Reduced skeletal muscle contractions, bed rest. Lower limb fractures, pelvic fractures	Swollen, hard, painful limb tender to touch heat discoloration	Specialist referral
Disseminated intravascular coagulation (DIC)	Bleeding disorders with diverse causes, including massive tissue trauma	Ecchymoses, unexpected bleeding after surgery, bleeding from mucous membranes, venepuncture sites, gastrointestinal and urinary tracts	May require plasma, red blood cell and platelet transfusion and anticoagulant medication to prevent blood clotting
Infections	*Risk factors:* Open fractures, internal fixation, surgical wound	Increasing pain, heat redness, swelling, green or cloudy oozing/discharge, tenderness	Antibiotic therapy must be appropriate and adequate for prevention and treatment of infection
Late complications			
Osteomyelitis	An acute or chronic inflammatory process involving the bone and its structures secondary to infection with pyogenic organisms including bacteria (mostly *Staphylococcus*), fungi, and mycobacteria	Fever, lethargy, malaise or irritability in children, pain, swelling, redness, warm sensation over an area of bone, loss of range of movement	Specialist opinion
Delayed union	Occurs when the bone does not heal at a normal rate for the location and type of fracture. Delayed union may be associated with distraction of bone fragments, systemic or local infection, poor nutrition, or comorbidity	Discomfort, pain, reduced function in affected area	Orthopedic opinion
Malunion	Occurs when bone heals but not in the right position	Discomfort, pain, deformity reduced function in affected area swelling	Orthopedic opinion
Nonunion	Results from failure of the ends of a fractured bone to unite	Discomfort, pain, continued movement at fracture site beyond expected, healing times reduced function in affected area swelling	Orthopedic opinion
Complex regional pain syndrome	Abnormally severe pain and reduced function that develops following injury	Continuing pain, edema, changes in skin blood flow, reduced range of movement in the region of pain	Orthopedic opinion

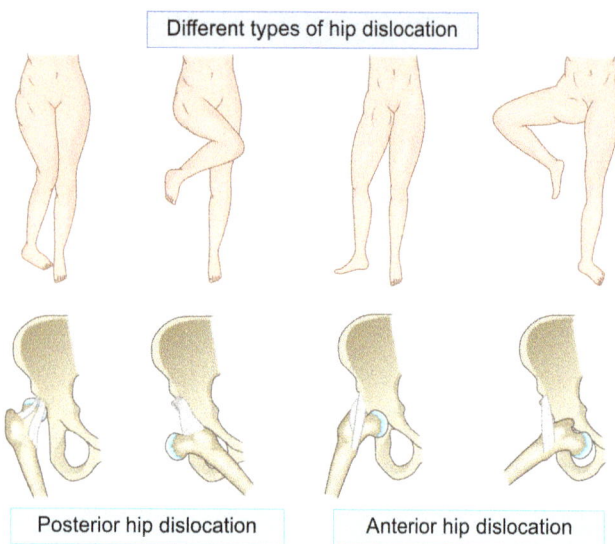

Fig. 7: Femoral head dislocation.

Grades of dislocation:
Type I: Simple dislocation without a fracture.

Type II: Dislocation with one or more rim fragments but with sufficient socket to ensure stability after reduction.

Type III: Dislocation with fracture of the rim producing gross instability.

Type IV: Dislocation with fracture of the head or neck of the femur.

Adequate sedation is required for reduction without further injury to articular surface. Hip dislocations can be either anterior or posterior, with posterior being most common. Reduction maneuvers, regardless of dislocation, involve axial traction in line of deformity. Maximal two attempts to be done. An assistant can help placing his/her hands-on pelvis and providing counter-traction.
Allis maneuver: It involves axial traction with gradual hip flexion combined with alternating internal and external rotation. Always look for ipsilateral knee injuries for intra-articular fracture **(Fig. 8)**.

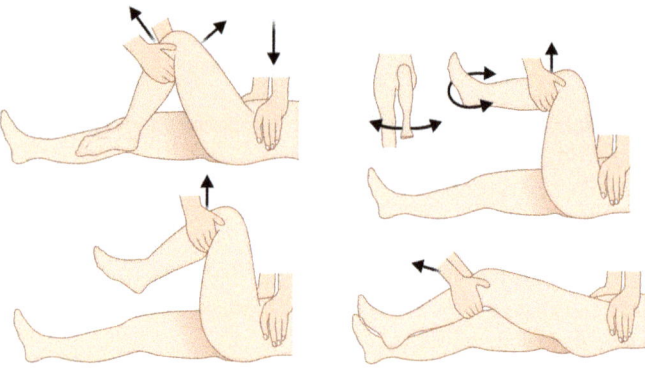

Fig. 8: Allis maneuver.

Question 8

Write briefly on the following:
1. NEXUS C-spine rule.
2. Canadian C-spine rule.

NEXUS (National Emergency X-Radiography Utilization Study) criteria and Canadian C-spine rule are followed in a trauma patient.

NEXUS criteria:
a. Absence of midline cervical tenderness.
b. Normal level of alertness and conscious level.
c. No evidence of intoxication.
d. Absence of focal neurologic deficit.
e. Absence of painful distracting injury.

Cervical spine imaging is not needed in patients who lack any one of the above five clinical criteria.

Canadian cervical spine rule for radiography: Cervical imaging is not required who meet these three criteria. Canadian rule consists of three assessments, which are asked in sequential order. To proceed to the next assessment, the answer to the previous assessment must be "Yes." If the answer to any assessments is "No," then imaging is immediately performed.

Assessment 1: There are no high-risk factors that mandate radiography.

Assessment 2: There are low risk factors that allow a safe assessment of range of motion.

Assessment 3: The patient is able to rotate his/her neck 45° to the left and to the right, regardless of the pain.

3. Ottawa knee rule.
4. Ottawa ankle rule.

The Ottawa knee rules are a set of rules used to help physicians determine whether an X-ray of the knee is needed. They state that an X-ray is required only in patients who have an acute knee injury with one or more of the following:
- Aged 55 years or over
- Tenderness at the head of the fibula
- Isolated tenderness of the patella
- Inability to flex knee to 90°
- Inability to bear weight (defined as an inability to take four steps, i.e., two steps on each leg, regardless of limping) immediately and at presentation.

The Ottawa ankle rules indicate that a radiograph is indicated if any of the following is positive:
- Tenderness along the posterior medial or lateral malleoli,
- Base of the 5th metatarsal, navicular or

If the patient is unable to bear weight for four steps following the injury.

Question 9

1. Discuss approach to acute pain in ear.

Acute pain in the ear can be caused by a variety of conditions, such as otitis media (middle ear infection), otitis externa (swimmer's ear), eardrum rupture, or a foreign body in the ear canal **(Table 5)**. Here is a general approach to evaluating and managing acute pain in the ear:

a. *Take a thorough history:* Ask the patient about the onset and duration of symptoms, any recent illnesses, previous ear problems, allergies, and medications.

b. *Perform a physical examination:* Inspect the outer ear and ear canal for signs of inflammation, discharge, or foreign bodies. Use an otoscope to examine the eardrum for signs of perforation, fluid, or redness.

c. *Consider the severity of pain:* Ear pain can range from mild discomfort to severe pain. Severe pain, especially if accompanied by fever, may indicate a more serious infection that requires immediate medical attention.

d. *Manage the pain:* Acetaminophen or ibuprofen can be used to relieve pain and reduce fever. If the pain is severe, a topical anesthetic such as benzocaine can be applied to the ear canal. However, topical anesthetics should be used with caution as they can cause allergic reactions or skin irritation.

e. *Treat the underlying condition:* Antibiotics may be necessary if the ear pain is caused by a bacterial infection, such as otitis media or otitis externa. However, antibiotics are not always necessary, and viral infections do not respond to antibiotics. In the case of a foreign body in the ear canal, removal may be necessary.

f. *Follow-up:* Patients with severe or persistent symptoms, signs of complications (such as hearing loss or facial weakness), or those who do not respond to initial treatment should be referred to an otolaryngologist for further evaluation.

It is important to note that this is a general approach and the specific management will depend on the individual patient's clinical presentation and medical history.

TABLE 5: Common causes of acute pain in ear.

Primary otalgia	Secondary otalgia
Infectious causes: • Acute or chronic otitis media • Acute otitis externa • Bullous otitis externa or myringitis • Auricular perichondritis • Herpes zoster oticus, Ramsay Hunt syndrome • Malignant otitis externa *Mechanical causes:* • Eustachian tube dysfunction • Cerumen impaction • Barotrauma • Hematoma of pinna *Inflammatory causes:* • Chondrodermatitis nodularis helicis • Wegener granulomatosis (with associated serous otitis media) *Neoplastic causes:* • Squamous cell carcinoma • Basal cell carcinoma • Melanoma • Cholesteatoma	• *Head:* Temporal arteritis • *Sinuses:* Sinusitis, nasal polyps • *TM joint:* TM joint disease, bruxism • *Salivary glands:* Sialadenitis (infection of salivary gland duct), sialolithiasis (salivary duct stones), salivary gland tumor • *Oral cavity:* Dental caries or other dental pathology, squamous cell carcinoma of the tongue • *Thyroid:* Thyroiditis, thyroid carcinoma • *Lymph node:* Lymphadenopathy, lymph node malignancies • *Neuralgia:* Trigeminal, glossopharyngeal, geniculate, sphenopalatine, vagal, and occipital neuralgia • *Pharynx:* Pharyngitis, oropharyngeal carcinoma, nasopharyngeal carcinoma, tonsillitis, post-tonsillectomy pain, peritonsillar abscess • *Larynx:* Laryngitis, vocal cord dysfunction, laryngeal carcinoma • *Musculoskeletal:* Myofascial pain, torticollis, cervical disc degeneration, cervical radiculopathy

2. Explain the assessment and management of acute onset vertigo.

Vertigo is a common, distressing presentation in general practice and constitutes approximately 54% of cases of dizziness. Classically, vertigo presents as a sensation of movement of the environment around the patient. Often patients describe a "spinning" sensation of either their body or their surroundings. This sensation can be confused with dizziness, which is a nonspecific term, so an adequate history is required to differentiate this symptom. Dizziness can be classified into four groups:

- Vertigo (spinning sensation)
- Disequilibrium (feeling of imbalance)
- Light-headedness (sensation of giddiness)
- Presyncope (sensation of feeling faint).

Vertigo can be classified as central or peripheral on the basis of vestibular symptom pathology **(Table 6)**. Vestibular symptoms originating from pathology in the cerebellum or brain stem are classified into the central type. Conversely, symptoms arising in the inner ear or from the vestibular nerve are classified as peripheral.

TABLE 6: Causes of vertigo based on origin.

Peripheral	Central
Benign positional vertigo	*Infection:* Meningitis, brain abscess
Labyrinthitis/neuronitis	Post-traumatic
Ménière's disease	Subclavian steal syndrome
Otitis media	Vertebrobasilar insufficiency
Wax or FB in the ear	Stroke
Acoustic neuroma	MS

Physical examination: A physical examination can assist in differentiating between central and peripheral subtypes of vertigo. Examination should involve the following:

Ear examination: An otoscopic examination should be performed to visualize the tympanic membranes for any vesicles that can be seen in a Herpes zoster infection or retraction pockets as seen in cholesteatoma. Vertigo triggered by pushing on the tragus or with the Valsalva maneuver is seen in a perilymphatic fistula. A hearing assessment should be performed.

Neurological examination: Initially, a focused neurological examination including gait, balance, and coordination needs to be performed. A gait and balance assessment (Romberg's sign and the heel-toe test), and examination for cerebellar signs can exclude central causes.

Eye examination: Eyes need to be examined for nystagmus and papilledema. Nystagmus is quick, jerky, involuntary movements of the eye. Vertical nystagmus is only seen if the cause is central. Nystagmus due to central causes may be horizontal, rotational or vertical, and does not disappear on fixing the gaze. Nystagmus in the peripheral type disappears with fixation of the gaze.

Cardiovascular examination: Pulse, blood pressure, heart rate, and rhythm should be checked. Carotid examination to identify bruits [in the case of a cerebrovascular accident (CVA)] is necessary. Further imaging to rule out CVA can be performed if this is clinically suspected.

Benign paroxysmal positional vertigo (BPPV): It is the most common cause of vertigo in clinical practice. It is caused by an accumulation of calcium crystals in the posterior semicircular canal. These crystals affect the movement of the endolymph in the semicircular canals, which causes vertigo. The classic symptoms of BPPV are brief episodes of vertigo, associated with nausea and nystagmus. The episodes of vertigo are triggered by rapid changes in the position of the head. Symptoms can last for weeks and recur after remission. Nystagmus seen in BPPV has a rotational nature. The Dix–Hallpike maneuver is used to diagnose BPPV. In contrast, the Epley maneuver can be used to treat BPPV. This procedure is performed in an attempt to dislodge the otoliths from the semicircular canals. It has a 77% success rate on the initial attempt and 100% on further attempts.

Acute labyrinthitis: The inner ear is composed of the bony and the membranous labyrinth. Acute labyrinthitis is inflammation of this labyrinth. It presents with vertigo and hearing loss, preceded by a viral infection. Middle ear infections can spread to the inner ear and cause labyrinthitis. The duration of symptoms ranges from days to weeks. Hearing loss is the main distinguishing factor between labyrinthitis and BPPV. Typically, no treatment is required for labyrinthitis. However, if suppurative labyrinthitis is suspected, the patient should be referred to the emergency department for drainage of otitis media.

Vestibular neuronitis (VN): It is caused by inflammation of the vestibular nerve. This inflammation precedes a viral upper respiratory tract infection (URTI) or herpes zoster infection and is caused by immune-mediated sequelae following the viral illness. It is commonly seen in middle-aged adults of both sexes. VN often occurs in epidemics during outbreaks of respiratory infections. The main characteristic of VN is an acute onset of vertigo without hearing loss or tinnitus. Similarly, to BPPV, symptoms of vertigo are aggravated by a change in the position of the head. Loss of balance is more prominent in VN, compared with other causes of vertigo, and patients may commonly present with falls. Initially, the vertigo is severe, lasts for 2–3 days and is followed by gradual recovery, which may take 2–6 weeks. Bed rest and antiemetics can be used in the first 24–72 hours. Patients can be reassured that symptoms will improve with time.

Investigations: Blood tests are not routinely ordered for patients presenting with vertigo. However, it is recommended that glucose levels of all patients with vertigo should be checked. Radiological tests including computed tomography (CT), magnetic resonance imaging (MRI) or magnetic resonance angiography (MRA) are indicated if:
- The examination is not consistent with a peripheral lesion.
- Prominent risk factors for CVA are present.
- Neurological signs and symptoms are present, or
- Symptoms of vertigo are accompanied by a headache.

In these cases, referral to a neurologist is recommended.

Treatment: Treatment is tailored to the specific causes of vertigo. Antiemetic medications such as betahistine are used for symptomatic management of acute vertigo. These medications should not be used long term. Patients should be warned about the side effects of drowsiness, dry mouth, and blurred vision. Benzodiazepines are not indicated and should be avoided because of their addictive nature. Lifestyle changes including salt restriction and avoiding alcohol and coffee are recommended. Assessment and management of the patient's risk of falls are important in vertigo. Sometimes the cause may be unclear, in which case refer to the medical/ENT team as appropriate.

3. Discuss malignant otitis externa.

Malignant otitis externa is a serious and potentially life-threatening infection that affects the external ear canal and adjacent structures. It is usually caused by a bacterial infection, most commonly *Pseudomonas aeruginosa*. Other organisms may be responsible are *Aspergillus fumigatus*, *Proteus mirabilis*, *Proteus* spp., *Klebsiella* spp., and *Staphylococci*. Also, it typically occurs in older adults with underlying medical conditions such as diabetes or immunosuppression.

Pathogenesis: The infection can spread, causing bony erosions and invasion of distant tissue, using the fascial planes and venous sinuses, with the involvement of the skull base and the surrounding tissue leading to cranial nerve and intracranial structures invasion. When the infection reaches the temporal bone through the fissure of Santorini, it invades the stylomastoid and the jugular foramina, containing the facial, glossopharyngeal, vagal, and accessory nerves.

Clinical presentation: Unremitting pain Purulent ear discharge Systemic illness Hearing loss Granulation tissue in the ear canal Possible facial nerve palsy.

Diagnosis: Blood investigations, white blood cell count, erythrocyte sedimentation rate and C-reactive protein, blood glucose, culture and sensitivities from the external auditory canal. Biopsy of the external auditory canal should be obtained to exclude other causes, such as malignancy or cholesteatoma. Computerized tomography detects bony erosions, demineralization, and destruction of bony cortex of mastoid. MRI is superior to CT with detecting anatomical locations and invasion of soft-tissue components, also better in evaluating intracranial complications. Gallium-67 tumor imaging (Ga-67) is a useful tool to monitor the resolution of the disease. The affected area usually shows increased uptake. Technetium (Tc-99) methylene diphosphate bone scanning; Tc99 is useful for the initial evaluation of the disease, but the test is not useful in assessing the prognosis of the disease, as it stays positive for a long period, even after the resolution of the infection. SPECT (single photon emission computed tomography), in addition to gallium-67 scan, is the investigation of choice to assess the progress of the disease.

Management: Antibiotic therapy—the treatment depends on the administration of systemic antimicrobial therapy with antipseudomonal activity. Although most cases are caused by *Pseudomonas aeruginosa*, other organisms have been identified as a cause of malignant otitis externa, and therefore the antibiotic management should be according to the isolated organism.

Hyperbaric oxygen therapy: Although it has been widely used in the treatment of malignant otitis externa (MOE), many studies showed no added benefit for using it as an adjuvant for medical or/and surgical therapy.

Surgical therapy: Surgical management is reserved for the patients in whom medical therapy has failed to cure the disease. Surgical therapy includes local debridement, removal of bony sequestrum, and abscess drainage.

Question 10

1. Discuss acute mesenteric ischemia.

Acute mesenteric ischemia (AMI) is a condition due to a sudden decline in blood flow through the mesenteric vessels. Without appropriate and timely treatment, necrosis of the small and large intestine results, leading to sepsis and potentially death. Due to the difficulty of diagnosis and the rapid progression, the condition is life-threatening if not identified and treated early. Diagnosis is difficult because symptoms are not specific, and the index of suspicion has to be high. Mortality rates for AMI range between 60 and 80%. AMI is classified as either occlusive or nonocclusive mesenteric ischemia (NOMI). Occlusive mesenteric arterial ischemia (OMI) is subdivided into acute thromboembolism and acute thrombosis.

Etiology: Embolic patients commonly have a positive medical history of cardiovascular diseases including recent myocardial infarction, congestive heart failure, and atrial fibrillation. Causes include peripheral arterial emboli, cardiac emboli, and an atheromatous plaque that ruptured or dislodged after surgery.

The typical thrombotic patient experiences a history of postprandial abdominal pain, leading to food avoidance and weight loss. The causes include atheromatous vascular disease (e.g., atherosclerosis, aortic aneurysm, and aortic dissection) and decreased cardiac output due to a secondary cause (e.g., dehydration, myocardial infarction, congestive heart failure).

The NOMI patient is typically critically ill, presents with several severe comorbidities, and is hemodynamically unstable. The causes include drugs that reduce blood flow (e.g., vasopressors and ergotamine), hypotension from severe medical conditions (e.g., myocardial infarction, sepsis, CHF, and renal disease), and patients that recently received major surgery (e.g., cardiac and abdominal surgery).

Pathophysiology: An acute mesenteric arterial embolism is often cardiogenic in origin and primarily affects the superior mesenteric artery (SMA). Preceding events include atrial tachyarrhythmia, congestive heart failure, myocardial ischemia or infarction, cardiomyopathy, and ventricular aneurysm, which results in thrombus formation that later embolizes to cause ischemia. Patients with acute mesenteric arterial thrombosis commonly have a preexisting atherosclerotic disease. Vasospasm in the SMA often accompanies NOMI secondary to cardiac failure, peripheral hypoxemia, or reperfusion injury.

Clinical presentation: Usually presents with severe abdominal pain not relating to physical examination (most commonly left upper quadrant). History of bowel emptying with severe pain, diarrhea, abdominal distension, bloody stool, NOMI—slow progressive abdominal pain.

Investigation: Biomarkers for mesenteric ischemia are nonspecific elevated lactate levels.

CT abdominal angiography is the preferred method of imaging for all types of acute mesenteric ischemia.

Management: Initial medical treatment focuses on fluid resuscitation and correcting electrolyte imbalances. Avoid vasopressors and alpha-adrenergic agents, which may cause vasospasm. Broad-spectrum antibiotics should be given before surgery to avoid abdominal sepsis if the necrotic bowel is resected. Early surgical exploration is required to assess the level of ischemia and spread of necrosis. Revascularization of the bowel is the primary goal of surgery and excision of necrotic bowel is necessary. Depending on the vessel occlusion type and location, open or endovascular surgical interventions are indicated in treating occlusive mesenteric arterial ischemia. As NOMI is secondary to vasospasm rather than occlusion, treatment is medically focused and relies upon reversing the underlying cause of the low-flow state. Catheter-directed papaverine (phosphodiesterase inhibitor) delivered by a side-hole catheter or thrombolysis catheter is an interventional option.

2. Describe various scoring systems in acute pancreatitis.

Once a diagnosis of acute pancreatitis is established, one should quickly work on two lines first, to assess severity so that you can triage the patient and decide whether to send him to ICU or Ward. Secondly one should try to establish the cause as quickly as possible because some of the etiologies such as common bile duct (CBD) stone and hypertriglyceridemia would need early intervention. The most important aspect of managing an acute pancreatitis patient is assessment of severity. It is always a challenge to talk to the relatives about severity of an attack and the likely outcome, i.e., the prognosis. There are various scales available to assess the severity such as Ranson's, Imrie's, APACHE II, etc., but easiest at bedside is to use BISAP scoring **(Table 7)**. Radiologic severity assessment score is CT severity score **(Table 8)**. Entire exercise of assessment is to know which patients have organ failure because the outcome depends on number of organs involved.

Atlanta criteria 2012 revision:
- *Mild acute pancreatitis:* No organ failure, no local or systemic complications
- Moderately severe acute pancreatitis, transient organ failure (<48 hours) and/or local or systemic complications without persistent organ failure
- *Severe acute pancreatitis:* Persistent organ failure (>48 hours)—single organ or multiorgan

TABLE 7: BISAP score (bedside index of severity of acute pancreatitis).

Blood urea nitrogen (BUN)	BUN >25 mg/dL (8.9 mmol/L)	(1 point)
Impaired mental status	Abnormal mental status with a Glasgow Coma Score <15	(1 point)
SIRS	Evidence of SIRS (systemic inflammatory response syndrome)	(1 point)
Age	Age >60 years old	(1 point)
Pleural effusion	Imaging study reveals pleural effusion	(1 point)

Score: 0–2 points: Lower mortality (<2%), 3–5 points: Higher mortality (>15%)

TABLE 8: CT findings and grading of acute pancreatitis (CT severity index [CTSI]).

Grading based upon findings on unenhanced CT

Grade	Findings	Score
A	Normal pancreas—normal size, sharply defined, smooth contour, homogeneous enhancement, retroperitoneal peripancreatic fat without enhancement	0
B	Focal or diffuse enlargement of the pancreas, contour may show irregularity, enhancement may be inhomogeneous but there is no peripancreatic inflammation	1
C	Peripancreatic inflammation with intrinsic pancreatic abnormalities	2
D	Intrapancreatic or extra pancreatic fluid collections	3
E	Two or more large collections of gas in the pancreas or retroperitoneum	4

Necrosis score based upon contrast-enhanced CT

Necrosis (%)	Score
0	0
<33	2
33–50	4
≥50	6

CT severity index equals unenhanced CT score plus necrosis score: Maximum = 10, ≥6 = severe disease.

The APACHE II score: The Acute Physiology and Chronic Health Examination (APACHE) II score was originally developed for critically ill patients in intensive care units (ICUs). Some limitations of the APACHE II score are—it is complex and cumbersome to use, it does not differentiate between interstitial and necrotizing pancreatitis, and it does not differentiate between sterile and infected necrosis. Finally, it has a poor predictive value at 24 hours.

Defining features of systemic inflammatory response syndrome (SIRS) are mentioned below:
1. Temperature >38.3°C or <36.0°C
2. Heart rate of >90 beats/minute
3. Respiratory rate of >20 breaths/minute or $PaCO_2$ of <32 mm Hg
4. WBC count of >12,000 cells/mm^3, <4,000 cells/mm^3, or >10% immature (band) forms.

The Harmless Acute Pancreatitis Score (HAPS) rules out "severe" pancreatitis and need for admission for acute pancreatitis based on three clinical values—peritonitis, creatinine, and hematocrit.

If the above criteria are normal (score of 0), the patient likely does not need ICU admission.

3. Discuss abdominal aortic aneurysm.

The aorta is the most common site of an aneurysm in the abdominal cavity and anteroposterior diameter of >3.0 cm is classified as an aneurysm. Most abdominal aortic aneurysms (AAAs) occur in the infrarenal region. Most aneurysms are fusiform (not saccular), entire circumference and all layers of the vessel are involved. The mean diameter of the infrarenal aorta is 1.66–2.16 cm in older women and 1.99–2.39 cm in older men. The most important complication of AAA is rupture, which occurs almost exclusively in aneurysms >4 cm. The most important risk factors are smoking, family history of AAA, increasing age, and history of atherosclerotic disease. For clinically significant aneurysms (>3.9 cm), the pathophysiology of AAA development and subsequent rupture is incompletely understood at this time. The aortic wall is made up of three layers—the intima, media, and adventitia. Within the media and adventitia, elastin and collagen are the most important components for maintaining the mechanical integrity of the vessel wall. Elastin is highly concentrated in the medial layer, whereas collagen is concentrated in the adventitia. Damage to and loss of elastin fibers and an associated reduction in the density of smooth muscle cells seem to be integral to the early development of AAA, whereas collagen degradation in the adventitia might be the most important factor in rupture.

Any older patient presenting to the ED with the clinical findings of abdominal pain, back pain, and shock, ruptured or leaking AAA should be suspected, but these symptoms and signs presentation are variable. Abdominal pain or back pain is prominent feature in patients with a ruptured AAA. AAA mostly ruptured, into the retroperitoneal space, remaining rupturing into intraperitoneal, IVC or duodenum. Most patients presenting to the ED are unaware with this vascular emergency. The early management of patients with suspected unstable AAA, either leaking or ruptured, should focus on rapid diagnosis and early definitive treatment. The presence of known risk factors for the disease (such as male gender, advanced age, and a history of smoking) in association with acute abdominal or back pain should raise the suspicion for an unstable AAA. Pulsatile mass on abdominal palpation has sensitivity ranging from 44 to 97%.

Most useful tool in the diagnostic evaluation of AAA in emergency department is bedside ultrasonography. Ultrasound is a highly accurate test, with a sensitivity and specificity approaching 100% in detecting AAA for emergency physicians. Ultrasound can also detect free fluid in the abdomen, associated with a free intraperitoneal rupture. Sonography does not reliably differentiate between ruptured and asymptomatic aneurysms because hemorrhage most frequently occurs into the retroperitoneal tissues, where ultrasound assessment is limited. CT is useful imaging modality for newly diagnosed AAA asymptomatic patients to define the anatomic details of the aneurysm; it should not be considered as the initial test of choice for patients with suspected ruptured AAA and instable patient. CT is helpful where ultrasound is technically limited or cannot distinguish between a symptomatic or incidental AAA. For those with a suspected ruptured AAA, aggressive resuscitation is priority, along with diagnostic measures, and consultation with vascular surgeon should occur simultaneously. Judicious fluid and blood replacement should begin for patients in shock, with large-bore, intravenous lines in place—once underlying disorder is an arterial rupture and hemorrhage is confirmed, vascular surgeon should be involved for surgical repair. For patients with an aneurysm >5.4 cm, referral should be made to vascular surgery. For those between 4.0 and 5.4 cm, surveillance with ultrasound is recommended every 6–12 months and, for those <4.0 cm, every 2–3 years is probably sufficient.

SUGGESTED READING

1. Richhariya D, Sharma B. Textbook of Emergency Medicine including Intensive Care and Trauma, 2nd edition. New Delhi: Jaypee Brothers Medical Publishers (P) Ltd; 2022. p. 1079. (Question 1).

2. Richhariya D, Sharma B. Textbook of Emergency Medicine including Intensive Care and Trauma, 2nd edition. New Delhi: Jaypee Brothers Medical Publishers (P) Ltd; 2022. p. 1359. (Question 2).
3. Moore KL, Dalley AF, Agur AM. Clinically Oriented Anatomy. 7th edition. Philadelphia, PA: Lippincott Williams and Wilkins; 2014. pp. 583-9. (Question 2).
4. Lewis HG, Clarke P, Kneafsey B, Brennen MD. A 10-year review of high-pressure injection injuries to the hand. J Hand Surg Br. 1998;23(4):479-81. (Question 2).
5. Richhariya D, Sharma B. Textbook of Emergency Medicine including Intensive Care and Trauma, 2nd edition. New Delhi: Jaypee Brothers Medical Publishers (P) Ltd; 2022. p. 698. (Question 3).
6. Richhariya D, Sharma B. Textbook of Emergency Medicine including Intensive Care and Trauma, 2nd edition. New Delhi: Jaypee Brothers Medical Publishers (P) Ltd; 2022. p. 141. (Question 4).
7. Richhariya D, Sharma B. Textbook of Emergency Medicine including Intensive Care and Trauma, 2nd edition. New Delhi: Jaypee Brothers Medical Publishers (P) Ltd; 2022. p. 1607. (Question 5).
8. Richhariya D, Sharma B. Textbook of Emergency Medicine including Intensive Care and Trauma, 2nd edition. New Delhi: Jaypee Brothers Medical Publishers (P) Ltd; 2022. p. 900. (Question 6).
9. Richhariya D, Sharma B. Textbook of Emergency Medicine including Intensive Care and Trauma, 2nd edition. New Delhi: Jaypee Brothers Medical Publishers (P) Ltd; 2022. p. 1624. (Question 7).
10. Richhariya D, Sharma B. Textbook of Emergency Medicine including Intensive Care and Trauma, 2nd edition. New Delhi: Jaypee Brothers Medical Publishers (P) Ltd; 2022. pp. 1570-1. (Question 8).
11. Richhariya D, Sharma B. Textbook of Emergency Medicine including Intensive Care and Trauma, 2nd edition. New Delhi: Jaypee Brothers Medical Publishers (P) Ltd; 2022. pp. 802, 908. (Question 9).
12. Richhariya D, Sharma B. Textbook of Emergency Medicine including Intensive Care and Trauma, 2nd edition. New Delhi: Jaypee Brothers Medical Publishers (P) Ltd; 2022. pp. 670, 717-22. (Question 10).

Emergency Medicine Paper 31

Devendra Richhariya

Question 1

1. Discuss pathogenesis of methanol poisoning.

Methylated spirit is very cheap and frequently available; hence it is easily adulterated and used as country liquor—among poor people who cannot afford ethyl alcohol for their drink. Methanol itself is less toxic agent. It becomes highly toxic when it is mixed with ethyl alcohol as it is adulterated. The rate of oxidation is very slow, only about 15% of that of ethyl alcohol. When taken with ethyl alcohol, it is metabolized only after complete metabolization of ethyl alcohol. In course of oxidation, formaldehyde and finally formic acid are formed which are highly toxic. Ethyl alcohol is preferentially metabolized by alcohol dehydrogenase resulting in reduced methanol toxicity.

2. Explain the clinical features of methanol poisoning.

Central nervous system (CNS) toxicity: It depresses CNS causing headache, dizziness, vertigo, dyspnea, cyanosis, cardiac depression, and muscular weakness. It is less respiratory depressant than ethyl alcohol, but its delayed effects are very dangerous which includes optic nerve atrophy resulting in complete blindness. The delayed toxicity may take 6–72 hours, (usually 12–24 hours) to develop.

Ocular toxicity: It is a delayed feature, which includes blurring of vision, which gradually leads to total or partial blindness. On examination pupillary dilatation, retinal edema, and hyperemia of the optic disc may be found. A total of 20% of the victims become totally blind, others have different form of visual disabilities.

Renal toxicity: There may be scanty micturition, which is acidic and contains acetone and format; sometimes there may be total anuria.

Gastrointestinal (GIT) toxicity: It includes nausea and abdominal pain. About 40% of the methanol users have high amylase level.

Respiratory toxicity: There may be dyspnea, respiratory distress and death is usually due to respiratory failure.

3. Discuss management of methanol poisoning.

The intoxicated person must be hospitalized and kept under close observation, even after initial recovery. He must be treated by an ophthalmologist for his visual problems. Initial managements are:

No evidence of effectivity of stomach wash although advocated. Oxygen inhalation and artificial respiration in moderate cases. In severe case patient should be intubated and mechanical respiration should be given. Circulation should be maintained by giving fluids and sympathomimetics. Maintaining fluid electrolyte balance should combat dehydration. Acidosis should be controlled by infusing sodium bicarbonate. Renal failure should be monitored carefully. Sedation can be given cautiously to prevent delirium and restlessness. Eyes should be protected from light and should be under regular observation.

Ethyl alcohol therapy is given to delay the absorption and metabolism and thus to prevent damaging effect of methanol:

In methanol poisoning start folinic acid 1 mg/kg (maximum dose is 50 mg)—repeat every 4 hourly, protect against ocular toxicity. Both alcohol (ethanol and methanol) metabolized by alcohol dehydrogenase so primary treatment is blocking this enzyme. **Fomepizole** also known as 4-methylpyrazole can be used alone or with hemodialysis to treat methanol and ethylene glycol poisoning. Dose 15 mg/kg loading then 10 mg/kg every 12 hourly (total 4 doses) till serum ethanol is <20 mg/dL. In case of dialysis 4 hourly doses are required as it is dialyzable. Studies highlighted greater safety of fomepizole than ethanol (alternative) in the treatment of methanol poisoning.

The (alternate) antidote for methanol poisoning is ethanol. Absolute alcohol is suitable for intravenous (IV) use. Ethanol is given orally or IV to maintain a blood ethanol level of 100–150 mg/dL. This will block methanol metabolism. In mild poisoning, oral ethanol is adequate. Give 10% ethanol 7.5 mL/kg IV, over 30–60 minutes, as a loading dose. The recommended maintenance dose for non-drinkers is 10% ethanol 1 mL/kg/h IV. For chronic ethanol drinkers, the maintenance dose is 10% ethanol 1.96 mL/kg/h IV. If the patient is undergoing hemodialysis, the maintenance dose is 3 mL/kg/h. (A solution of about 10% ethanol can be made by mixing 60 mL of absolute alcohol suitable for IV use in 500 mL of 5% dextrose).

Ethanol can be administered orally if the IV preparation is not available. Concentrations <20% are preferred to avoid gastric irritation. A loading dose of 95% ethanol, 0.8 mL/kg followed by 0.1 mL/kg/h can be given. If the patient is undergoing hemodialysis, increase the dose up to 0.2 mL/kg/h and administer via a nasogastric; tube. For chronic ethanol drinkers, the maintenance dose is 0.2 mL/kg/h. The alcohol should be diluted in water or fruit juice.

If no alcohol is available in the hospital, give arrack (gin or whisky) 1.8 mL/kg as a loading dose, and 0.2 mL/kg/h as maintenance dose orally, after diluted with water or fruit juice. If the patient is undergoing hemodialysis, the maintenance dose is 0.7 mL/kg/h. Dose should be loading with 50 g of 50% ethyl alcohol (e.g., 125 mL of gin, whisky, or vodka) orally followed by further oral dose for 3–4 days or an IV infusion of 10–12 g ethanol/h, to achieve a blood concentration of about 500–1,000 mg/L.

Ethanol should be given until methanol is undetected in the blood. A serum ethanol level of 100 mg/dL is essential to achieve the best countereffect of methanol. The above regimes should be maintained for 2–3 days, unless contraindicated for any reason, or until plasma methanol concentration is <20 mg/dL. Blood ethanol level should be monitored hourly initially, and at longer intervals thereafter, depending on the facilities available. As prolonged ethanol administration can cause hypoglycemia, especially in children, determine blood glucose levels and give glucose orally or 5% or 50% dextrose IV. If convulsions are present give diazepam 5–10 mg IV (pediatric dose: 0.2 mg/kg). Repeat if necessary.

Hemodialysis is effective in removing the absorbed poison and its metabolites. Indication for dialysis: (1) If ingest >30 g methanol, (2) Develop metabolic acidosis (pH 7.1 rise in creatinine) or mental, visual or fundoscopic abnormalities attributable to methanol, (3) Has a blood methanol concentration >500 mg/L. Hemodialysis is more effective than peritoneal dialysis. If dialysis is used, increased quantities of ethanol (17–22 g/h) must be administered.

Question 2

1. Discuss pathophysiology and management of smoke inhalation.
2. What is the clinical utility of hyperbaric oxygen?

Pathophysiology: Fire-related smoke inhalation is the major cause for carbon monoxide (CO) poisoning. Other potential sources of CO are poorly functioning heating systems, improperly vented fuel-burning equipment (kerosene heaters, charcoal grills, camping stoves, gasoline-powered generators) and motor vehicles working in poorly ventilated areas (e.g., ice rinks, warehouses, parking garages); methylene chloride (dichloromethane), an industrial solvent, and a component of paint remover. Inhaled or ingested methylene chloride is converted to CO by the liver, can also cause CO toxicity in the absence of ambient CO. CO diffuses very rapidly across the pulmonary capillary membrane and binds to the iron moiety of heme with around 240 times more affinity of oxygen. Once CO binds to the heme, an allosteric change occurs that greatly reduces the ability of the other three oxygen binding sites to release oxygen to peripheral tissues. This leads to a leftward shift of the oxyhemoglobin dissociation curve, and impairment in tissue oxygen delivery. CO also reduces the peripheral oxygen utilization. Around 10–15% of CO is extravascular and bound to molecules such as myoglobin, cytochromes, and nicotinamide adenine dinucleotide phosphate (NADPH) reductase, leads to an impairment of oxidative phosphorylation at the mitochondrial level.

Mild to moderate CO-toxicity: Patients present with headache (the most common presenting symptom), nausea, and dizziness, malaise. Patients may also present with symptoms ranging from mild confusion to coma. Some may have a "cherry red" appearance of the lips.

Severe CO toxicity: It can present with neurologic symptoms such as seizures, syncope, or coma, and also cardiovascular manifestations such as myocardial ischemia, ventricular arrhythmias, and lung problems such as breathlessness, pulmonary edema, and metabolic disorder such as profound lactic acidosis.

Delayed neuropsychiatric syndrome: Nearly 40% of patients with severe CO toxicity, a syndrome of delayed neurologic sequelae (DNS) can arise after apparent recovery within a year. The development of DNS poorly correlates with COHb levels, although majority of cases are associated with loss of consciousness during acute intoxication. Clinical features of this syndrome are variable degrees of cognitive deficits, personality changes, movement disorders, and focal neurologic deficits, DNS normally occur within 20 days of CO toxicity, and may persist for a year or longer.

The diagnosis of CO poisoning is based upon high carboxyhemoglobin level measured by CO-oximetry of an arterial blood gas (ABG) sample.

Management: Take care airway breathing and circulation.

High-flow oxygen and hyperbaric oxygen: The half-life of CO for a patient is breathing room air is about 250–320 minutes, for a patient breathing high-flow oxygen via a nonrebreathing face mask is about 90 minutes and with 100% hyperbaric oxygen is about 30 minutes. Indications for hyperbaric oxygen (HBO) are as follows:

- CO level >25%
- CO level >20% in pregnant patient
- Loss of consciousness or low Glasgow Coma Scale (GCS)
- Severe metabolic acidosis (pH <7.1)
- Evidence of end-organ damage (e.g., ECG changes, chest pain, or altered mental status).

Hyperbaric oxygen therapy (HBO): This treatment involves exposing patients to 100% O_2 under supra-atmospheric conditions. This leads to a reduction in the half-life of COHb, from about 90 minutes on 100% normobaric oxygen to about 30 minutes during HBO. The amount of oxygen dissolved in the blood also rises from around 0.3–6.0 mL/dL, which substantially increases the release of non-hemoglobin-bound O_2 to the tissues. HBO treatment may be beneficial in preventing the late neurocognitive deficits associated with severe CO toxicity.

Comatose patients, or those with low GCS, should be intubated and mechanically ventilated using 100% oxygen. In smoke inhalation patients (who may suffer from both cyanide and carbon monoxide poisoning) hydroxocobalamin should be given. The dose of hydroxocobalamin is 70 mg/kg given as intravenously (IV).

Question 3

1. Discuss acute mountain sickness (AMS).

Acute mountain sickness is a multisystem disorder with prominent neurological features characterized by headache and fatigue; anorexia, nausea, or vomiting; fatigue or weakness; dizziness or lightheadedness; or insomnia. Headache is the more common symptom. The diagnosis of AMS is clinical; no diagnostic modalities or physical findings can reliably confirm the diagnosis. Symptoms generally occur at elevations above 2,500 m (8,202 ft) but sometimes occur at as low as 2,000 m (6,562 ft). These nonspecific symptoms may easily be mistaken for a variety of other conditions, particularly in the setting of comorbid illness or the extremes of age. Symptoms of AMS typically develop 6–10 hours after ascent but could appear as earlier (i.e., 1 hour). Onset beyond 3 days at a given altitude, the absence of headache, or the lack of rapid response to oxygen or descent suggest other diagnoses. Subarachnoid hemorrhage, intracranial mass, migraine, dehydration, exhaustion, carbon monoxide exposure, substance abuse, and alcohol hangover, among others, are diagnoses that must be considered in the early evaluation of possible AMS.

2. Explain high-altitude pulmonary edema.

Leakage of the pulmonary blood gas barrier leads to accumulation of fluid in the lungs. In high altitude pulmonary vasoconstriction occurs and pulmonary hypertension occurs in all individuals. High altitude pulmonary edema should be differentiated from asthma, bronchitis, heart failure mucus plugging, myocardial infarction, pneumonia, pulmonary embolus.

Diagnosis: Manifestations of high-altitude pulmonary edema (HAPE) include—decreased exercise tolerance, a prolonged recovery period after exertion at altitude. Dyspnea, chest discomfort, and dry cough are frequent. In severe cases, the physical examination reveals tachycardia and tachypnea. Auscultation reveals rales, often asymmetrical in distribution, and usually found in the right mid-lung initially. Cyanosis and orthopnea may become prominent in severe cases. The electrocardiogram could report sinus tachycardia and may suggest acute pulmonary hypertension (i.e., right axis deviation, right bundle branch block, right ventricular hypertrophy by voltage, right atrial enlargement). Hemodynamic measurements reveal high pulmonary artery pressure and pulmonary vascular resistance, as well as low to normal pulmonary wedge pressures, cardiac output, and systemic arterial blood pressure.

Treatment: The treatment is based on—oxygen (4–6 L/min until improved, then 2–4 L/min to conserve supplies and maintain SaO_2 >90%); minimize exertion and keep patient warm; descend or evacuate at 500/1,000 m (1,640–3,281 ft) as soon as possible; if descent/O_2 unavailable, portable hyperbaric therapy may be lifesaving; consider nifedipine (10 mg PO, then 30 mg extended-release PO q 12–24 h) if no high-altitude cerebral edema (HACE); consider inhaled beta-agonists (salmeterol, 50 mcg inhaled per 12 h, or albuterol); consider expiratory positive airway pressure (EPAP) mask; dexamethasone only if HACE develops.

3. Discuss high-altitude cerebral edema.

Diagnosis: High-altitude cerebral edema is preceded in major case by symptoms of AMS and is considered the end stage of AMS. HACE can present 3–5 days after arrival to elevations as low as 2,750 m (9,022 ft) but is most commonly seen in remote environments well above this altitude, where the onset of symptoms may be much more abrupt over a period of hours. The diagnosis is clinical and based on altered sensorium and ataxia. Mental status changes may include irrational behavior that rapidly progresses to lethargy, obtundation, and coma. If untreated, death results from brain herniation.

Treatment: Immediate descent or evacuation at 1,000 m (3281 ft); oxygen to maintain SaO_2 >90%; dexamethasone (8 mg IV/IM/PO initially, then 4 mg/6 h). If descent is not an option, one may use a portable hyperbaric chamber and/or supplemental oxygen to temporize illness, but this should never replace or delay evaluation/descent when possible.

Question 4

1. Discuss approach to wide-complex tachycardia.

A wide QRS (duration exceeding 120 ms) during tachycardia suggests ventricular tachycardia (VT) or a supraventricular tachycardia (SVT) in specific scenarios. SVT with a concurrent bundle branch block or intraventricular conduction defect can produce wide-complex tachycardias despite a supraventricular origin.

Clinical approach of a patient with a wide complex tachycardia: QRS >120 ms in ECG are called wide complex tachycardia and are common in clinical practice. Wide QRS complex are seen in VT, SVT with aberrancy or bundle branch block (BBB) and SVT with antegrade conduction over an accessory pathway (pre-excited tachycardia). Drug toxicities and electrolyte imbalances are also presenting as QRS abnormalities.

Medical history and physical examination are very important and helpful in diagnosis. A history of angina, myocardial infarction, or congestive cardiac failure are strong indicators for the presence of VT. Young patients are more likely to have idiopathic VT. Hemodynamic tolerance for the arrhythmia is a poor guide to diagnosis as both SVT and VT can present with hemodynamic collapse. On the contrary, idiopathic VT's may be well tolerated hemodynamically.

Clinical examination of the patient can help in differentiating and categorizing these patients. Clinical signs of AV dissociation include "cannon A" waves in the jugular venous pulse, variability in the intensity of the first heart sound, and variability in arterial blood pressure. Vagal maneuvers that result in termination of tachycardia indicate the presence of SVT. However, these tests are not very reliable as a few VT's can also terminate with vagal maneuvers.

2. Explain endocarditis prophylaxis in ED.

Endocarditis prophylaxis: The American Hospital Association (AHA) recommends preprocedure antibiotic prophylaxis to the high-risk cardiac lesions. *High risk includes*—prosthetic valves, cyanotic congenital heart lesions (not repaired), transplants with valvopathy and previous history of endocarditis. The procedures for which antibiotic prophylaxis should be given include—dental work, procedures involving infected skin, subcutaneous and musculoskeletal tissue (e.g., abscess drainage). Antibiotic such as antistaphylococcal penicillin or cephalosporin should be used. If community-associated methicillin-resistant *Staphylococcus aureus* (CA-MRSA) is present in the community, vancomycin/clindamycin depending on local susceptibility patterns should be used. No prophylaxis is required for clean non-contaminated wounds.

For low-risk procedures, antibiotic prophylaxis is not required. Foley catheter insertion, endotracheal intubation, joint aspiration, arthroscopy, local anesthetic administration, etc., do not require prophylaxis.

Risk of infection from an emergency room (ER) procedure for patients with orthopedic implants is low. Only high-risk category, i.e., in first 2 years after joint replacement, previous implant infection, patients on immunosuppression, prophylaxis is indicated for procedures such as abscess drainage.

Question 5

1. Discuss peripheral blood smear examination.

A blood smear, peripheral blood smear or blood film is a thin layer of blood smeared on a glass microscope slide and then stained in such a way as to allow the various blood cells to be examined under microscope. A normal peripheral blood smear indicates the appropriate appearance of red blood cells, with a zone of central pallor occupying about 1/3 of the size of the red blood cells (RBC). A blood smear can be used to help diagnose or check on many conditions, such as anemia, jaundice, sickle cell disease, thrombocytopenia, malaria, glucose-6-phosphate dehydrogenase (G6PD) deficiency, and leukemia.

Diagnosis of malaria is based on clinical suspicion and laboratory confirmation of parasitemia, microscopic examination of peripheral blood smear (PBS). Confirmation is done by thin and thick film (more reliable when parasitemia is very low). Nothing found better than direct examination of smear, but it is time-consuming need infrastructure and single negative PBS cannot rule out malaria.

2. Explain autoimmune hemolytic anemia.

Autoimmune hemolytic anemia (AIHA) occurs when immune system mistakes RBCs as unwanted substances and body produces antibodies that destroy RBCs, which can lead to a low amount of RBCs (known as anemia). Acquired autoimmune hemolytic anemia resembles those of other anemias and may include fatigue, pale color, rapid heartbeat, shortness of breath, dark urine, chills, and backache. In severe cases, yellow skin color (jaundice) may be present and the spleen may be enlarged. Autoimmune hemolytic anemia as the cause is confirmed when blood tests detect increased amounts of certain antibodies, either attached to RBCs (direct antiglobulin or direct Coombs test) or in the liquid portion of the blood (indirect antiglobulin or indirect Coombs test). Steroids, such as hydrocortisone or prednisone, with rituximab are helpful in management **(Flowchart 1)**.

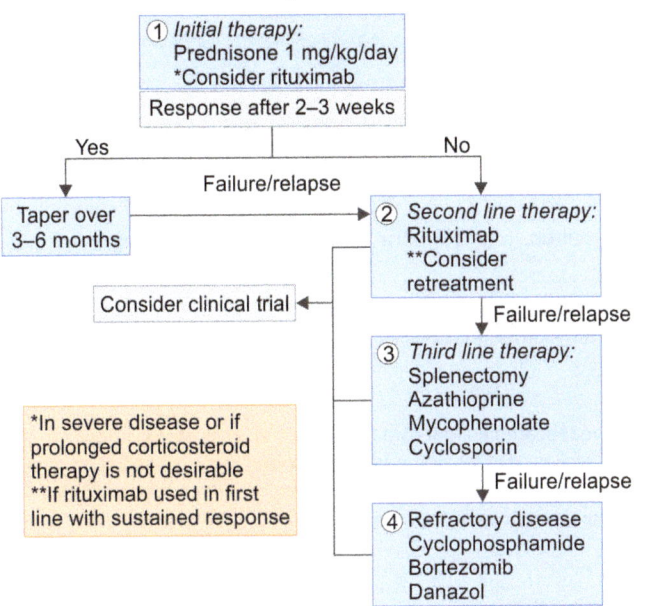

Flowchart 1: Approach to management of autoimmune hemolytic anemia.

Question 6

1. Discuss pathogenesis of rabies.

Pathogenesis of rabies: The live virus, once introduced through the epidermis or mucous membrane, multiplies and ascends centripetally up the peripheral nerves to the CNS resulting in generalized encephalomyelitis. Once the virus reaches the CNS, it multiplies exclusively in the gray matter and then spreads centrifugally along autonomic nerves to other tissues including salivary glands and cornea. The pathognomonic lesion is an intracytoplasmic eosinophilic inclusion body commonly known as Negri bodies. These Negri bodies are seen only with infection of "street virus" and not with "fixed virus". So far the virus has not been isolated from the blood of rabies patients and hence, the hematogenous route of spread is ruled out. In rabies, there is no initial viremia and the virus is not accessible to the normal immune mechanism of the body. The viremia or the stimulation of the normal immune mechanism is only during the end stages of the fatal disease therefore the role of naturally acquired infection is practically nonexistent.

2. Explain the clinical features of rabies.

Rabies in man is known as hydrophobia in general. *The disease can be divided into different stages:*

Prodromal stage: The disease begins with prodromal symptoms such as fever, headache, myalgia, sore throat and vomiting. There is pain and tingling or numbness at the site of bite in about 80% of cases. It is the most important complaint at this time and is related to the multiplication of virus at the local site. This stage may last for 3–4 days.

Stage of acute encephalitis: This stage is characterized by excessive motor activity and agitated behavior. There is widespread excitation and stimulation of nervous system involving the sensory, the motor, the sympathetic and mental systems. There are symptoms of confusion, hallucination, muscle spasms, and convulsions. There is exaggerated sensitivity to noise, light, touch or currents of air. Autonomic symptoms such as increased perspiration, salivation, lacrimation, pupillary dilatation, and hypotension are present. Hypoxia and hyperventilation progress to hypoventilation and repeated apnea.

Stage of brainstem dysfunction: Now the characteristic symptom of hydrophobia appears which is pathognomonic of rabies and is absent in animals. This fear of water is due to painful, violent, involuntary contraction of diaphragm, respiratory, laryngeal and pharyngeal muscles, initiated by swallowing of liquids. Progressively, even the sight, smell or sound of liquids can precipitate spasm of muscles of deglutition. More than 80% patients succumb to the disease during this stage. Death is due to respiratory arrest, convulsions or choking. Rest of the patients may progress to next stage.

Stage of paralysis: Paralytic symptoms can occur at any time during the course of illness. Now the muscle spasms cease and there is apathy, stupor, coma, and generalized flaccidity. Death occurs due to hypoxia or heart failure. Occasionally, rabies may present as Guillain-Barré type of ascending paralysis. This may be seen with bite of a vampire bat or in patients who have received postexposure prophylaxis against the disease.

Death: Once the symptoms develop, the disease is fatal and the patient dies within 2 weeks. There are no quarantine restrictions for a rabies patient. However, since the saliva, urine or tears, etc., may contain the virus, all the persons coming in contact should be immunized against rabies. Transmission from man to man, though uncommon is possible.

3. Discuss postexposure prophylaxis after dog bite.

Postexposure prophylaxis (PEP) for rabies: Human rabies is essentially a fatal disease once the clinical signs develop, although 100% preventable. Rabies PEP consists of thorough wound care along with administration of modern anti-rabies vaccine and rabies immunoglobulin. This is highly effective if carried out systematically and diligently. If a person has received preexposure prophylaxis (PrEP), then it eliminates the need for rabies immunoglobulin (RIG) in case of an exposure. The key to survival is administration of PEP as soon as possible. A patient with category III exposure needs thorough wound cleansing and a first dose of vaccine along with rabies immunoglobulin on the day of bite or day of reporting **(Table 1)**. The vaccination is done according to one of the World Health Organization (WHO) approved schedules to achieve a serum antibody titer of >0.5 IU/mL, which is considered acceptable according to WHO. In case of any confusion regarding exposure it is always better to give overtreatment rather than undertreatment for prevention of rabies.

TABLE 1: Postexposure prophylaxis in rabies.

Categories	Nature of contact	Recommended treatment	
		Unknown, sick, proven, wild animal	Healthy animal
I	Touching or feeding animals, licks on intact skin, no mucous membrane exposure	None	None
II	Nibbling of uncovered skin, minor scratches or abrasions without bleeding	Modern tissue culture, rabies vaccine	Modern tissue culture, rabies vaccine
III	Single or multiple transdermal bites or scratches, contamination of mucous membrane or broken skin with saliva from animal licks, exposure due to direct contact with bats	Modern tissue culture, rabies vaccine and rabies immunoglobulins (RIG)	Modern tissue culture, rabies vaccine and rabies immunoglobulins (RIG)

1. Start pre-exposure vaccination particularly in children and others likely to have repeated animal contact, and are at a risk of dog bites.
2. Start full treatment on first day and discontinue vaccine if animal is alive and well on day 10, or if it has been found rabies negative on reliable laboratory examination. Encourage patient to return for another dose of vaccine on day 21, so that a full preexposure series has been completed.
3. If there is significant delay in presentation or if the patient is immunosuppressed, it may appropriate to double the first dose of vaccine. Administration of two ampoules of vaccine, one in each arm, on day 0.

Question 7

1. Discuss etiology of community-acquired pneumonia.

Community-acquired pneumonia (CAP) is defined as an acute infection of the pulmonary parenchyma, contracted outside the hospital, with clinical symptoms of pneumonia along with the presence of an infiltrate on chest X-ray. The diagnosis of CAP requires that a patient should not be hospitalized or in a nursing home in the previous 14 days. *Streptococcus pneumoniae, Mycoplasma pneumoniae, Haemophilus influenzae, Chlamydophila* spp., and viruses are the most common pathogens implicated in the development of CAP.

2. Explain the clinical and radiological features in a patient with pneumonia.

Clinical features of pneumonia: For typical pneumonias, cough, fever, chest pain are the common presentation with which the patients come to the emergency department. Cough may be with expectoration whitish to greenish; rarely patients can have hemoptysis. Mucopurulent sputum is mostly found with bacterial pneumonia. Patients may present only with high grade sudden onset of fever, which is continuous, but many a times patients have already taken antipyretics for that. Chest pain can be pleuritic or dull aching in nature. Atypical presentation may also occur like poor oral uptake, nausea, vomiting, and diarrhea, change of mental status or disorientation. This is more common in elderly patients.

Radiologic features of typical pneumonia: Consolidation typical air bronchogram bronchopulmonary segment. May be lobar or multi-lobar infiltration not seen in perihilar region and localized centrally within the lobes and not toward the periphery. Any lobes can be affected.

Radiologic features of atypical pneumonia: Often reflects a primary infection before features of atypical pneumonia develops. This phase is also called occult pneumonia. Infiltration begins in peripheral region and spreads to periphery and not restricted to lobes. Lower lobes are predominantly affected. However other lobes are also involved. There may be ground glass opacities and interstitial shadow.

3. Discuss CURB-65 score.

Assessment of the severity of illness is important for diagnostic and treatment decisions for pneumonia. These assessments of illness by scoring system affect the decision between inpatient and outpatient treatment and ICU admission versus admission to a general ward.

Scoring systems: Two scoring systems can assist the emergency physician in the identification of patients who may be candidates for outpatient treatment: *CURB-65* is a severity of illness score, and the PSI (pneumonia severity index) is a prognostic model. *CURB-65* is a more simplified tool that uses five criteria to determine patients at lower risk for adverse events. These criteria are confusion; uremia [blood urea nitrogen (BUN) >7 mmol/L]; respiratory rate (>30); blood pressure (60 diastolic); age 65 years or greater. Direct admission to an ICU or high-level monitoring unit is recommended for patients with either of the major criteria or with three of the minor criteria. Major criteria are invasive mechanical ventilation or septic shock with the need for vasopressors.

4. Discuss outpatient antibiotic therapy for CAP (community-acquired pneumonia).

Initial empiric antimicrobial therapy for CAP outpatient
- *No comorbidities or risk factors for MRSA or pseudomonas aeruginosa*: Amoxicillin or doxycycline or macrolide (if local pneumococcal resistance is 25%).
- *With comorbidities:* Combination therapy with amoxicillin/clavulanate or cephalosporin and macrolide or doxycycline OR monotherapy with respiratory fluoroquinolone.

Question 8

1. Discuss etiology and assessment of a 25-year-old patient presenting with fever and altered sensorium.

Fever and CNS symptoms: Specific neurological diagnoses in a traveler are rare. Fever and headache are common symptoms and seen in systemic infections such as malaria, dengue and chikungunya infection and rickettsial diseases. Malaria and meningitis are the commonest treatable causes of fever and CNS symptoms and must always be excluded first. Cerebral malaria is caused by *Plasmodium falciparum* and can present with confusion, headache, seizures, or decreased consciousness. Any patient with neurological symptoms and a history of travel to a malaria endemic region should be considered to have cerebral malaria and investigated. Other causes of fever and encephalopathy include bacterial infections (typhoid, Lyme disease, leptospirosis) and human immunodeficiency virus (HIV) seroconversion.

Assessment: Examination should comprise an assessment of how unwell the patient is along with a meticulous examination to look for any localizing features which may point to a diagnosis such as jaundice, rash, skin lesions, lymphadenopathy, retinal or conjunctival changes, hepatosplenomegaly or neurological findings. The examination should include looking for genital lesions and a thorough examination for eschars (pointing to rickettsial infections) as these are often found in "hard to assess" places such as the natal cleft and under the breasts. Patients with respiratory distress, hypotension or shock, hemorrhage, confusion, meningism or other neurological findings should be urgently investigated. Even if an initial physical examination is unremarkable, it should be repeated if the diagnosis is unclear, as new findings may appear in due course of hospitalization that will help in the diagnostic process (such as skin lesions or a tender liver).

2. Explain the pathophysiology of cyanotic spells (Tet spells).

Also called as hyperpneic spells, hypoxic spells, anoxic, blue, Cyanotic or Tet spells are paroxysmal hypoxic events in a child due to decreased pulmonary blood flow and right to left shunting. They can occur in any heart condition involving ventricular septal defect (VSD) and a restriction to pulmonary blood flow. Increased contractility (due to catecholamines) and decreased right ventricular size (due to various factors) can trigger a reflex resulting in hyperventilation, some peripheral vasodilation without bradycardia, and this may initiate a spell (**Flowchart 2**). Place infants with hypercyanotic spells in the knee-chest position and give oxygen; sometimes, opioids (morphine or fentanyl), volume expansion, sodium bicarbonate, beta-blockers (propranolol or esmolol), or phenylephrine may help. Repair surgically at 2–6 months or earlier if symptoms are severe.

Flowchart 2: Pathophysiology of cyanotic spell.

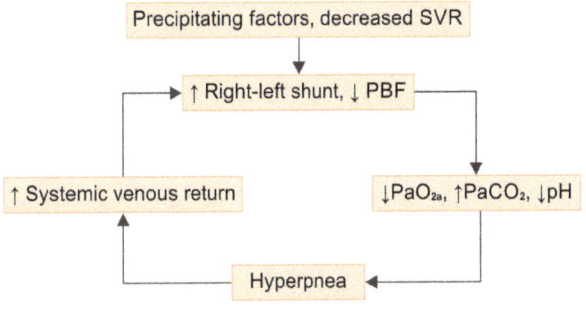

(SVR: systemic vascular resistance).

3. Discuss management of a child with cyanotic spell.

Management: The definitive diagnosis is readily established by detailed echocardiography. Prostaglandin E1 (PGE1; alprostadil) IV infusion to keep the PDA open (dose 10–60 ng/kg/min, if poor response saturations and acidosis not improving) the dose can be increased to maximum 300–400 ng/kg/min. Apnea is a common side effect of PGE1 so infusion should be started in ICU settings with ventilator support available. Flushing, diarrhea, and hypotension are other common side effects. Intravenous fluid for blood volume expansion 10 mL/kg 0.9% saline bolus, improve preload repeat until liver edge is palpable—enhance further opening of the PDA and pulmonary blood flow through the duct, correction of metabolic abnormalities, e.g., hypoglycemia, hypocalcemia, acidosis and sepsis. Oxygen to maintain the saturations 75–85% (do not give 100% oxygen by mask in patients with duct dependent lesions as high level of oxygen triggers closure of ductus arteriosus). Inotropes/vasopressors are required to maintain adequate systemic perfusion. If above measures are not helpful, intubation and ventilation with adequate sedation are required to improve oxygenation and minimize the metabolic demands.

Definitive management includes: For transposition of great vessels-arterial switch operation, total anomalous pulmonary venous connection—surgical rerouting of pulmonary veins, severe valvular pulmonary stenosis—balloon valvotomy and ductal stenting/Blalock–Taussig (BT) shunt for duct dependent pulmonary circulation.

Question 9

1. Give definition of delirium.

Delirium is defined as acute onset fluctuating changes in cognition, attention, and awareness, changes are rapid in onset within hours or day and usually reversible. Patient of delirium typically presents as inattention, disorganized thinking, perception disturbance, and altered conscious level (somnolent or agitated). Elderly group is at increased risk of mortality if delirium is missed in emergency department (ED).

2. Discuss etiology of acute delirium in ED.

- Elderly male
- Multiple comorbidities
- Advance form of comorbidities
- Previous episode of delirium
- Advance dementia
- Chronic kidney disease
- End stage liver disease
- Postoperative status like recent hip fracture
- Conditions like burn hypo albuminemia dehydration
- Malnutrition infection acquired immunodeficiency syndrome (AIDS)
- Multiple medications and dependence like benzodiazepine
- Alcohol abuse or withdrawal
- Socially neglected stressful people
- Visual or hearing problem
- Poor mobility terminally ill
- Prolong intensive care unit admission.

3. Explain the assessment of a patient with delirium.

Confusion assessment methods (CAM): First described by Inouye and colleagues in 1990 based on the *Diagnostic and Statistical Manual of Mental Disorders Revised 3rd edition revised* (DSMIIIR) criteria, helpful for non-psychiatric trained physician to diagnose delirium quickly and accurately. CAM consists of four components: 1. Acute onset mental status changes fluctuating course, 2. Inattention, 3. Disorganized thinking, and 4. Altered level of consciousness. First two components are mandatory and either of two from rest of the two necessary for diagnosis of delirium.

Taking history in these patients is difficult as patient is often confused and disoriented. In most of the patient history alone give the diagnostic clues so emergency physician should obtain the information through previous medical records, family members, and friends. History of fever, headache, suicidal tendency fall or trauma alcohol use or any substance abuse should be recorded. Elderly are more vulnerable for acute confusional state/delirium so emphasis should be given on their medication chart and recent changes done in medication doses. Appropriate laboratory and radiological test should be carried out to confirm the suspected conditions. Complete hemogram, kidney function test, liver function test, thyroid function test, arterial blood gases interpretation are the basic investigations. Electrocardiograph, cardiac enzyme should be performed urgently if any cardiac event is suspected. Chest X-ray will be helpful in identifying the lung pathology. CT head is not indicated in all cases of acute confusional states but more helpful in elderly group of patients, and/or on anticoagulation history of trauma immuno-compromised patient noncontract CT head is usually sufficient.

4. Discuss pharmacological restraint in an agitated patient in ED.

Physical or chemical restrains of patient are required whenever there is possibility of "self-harm" and agitated behavior dangerous to hospital staff. Close observation of patient is required to record changes in tone speech irritability, clinched jaw and fist for intervention at the right time. Physician must record the GCS before applying any measures for agitation control. Medications used for chemical restrain are haloperidol (antipsychotic agent)/lorazepam.

Few characteristic features of commonly used haloperidol and lorazepam:

Drug therapy: Haloperidol is commonly used first line medication for delirium. *Haloperidol is* given in 2–5 mg intramuscular. *Olanzapine:* 2.5–5 mg orally once a day; *Risperidone* 0.5 mg orally twice daily. *Quetiapine* 12.5–25 mg orally twice daily is used for hypoactive form of delirium. *Benzodiazepine*: Lorazepam 2 mg IV is also used commonly alone or with haloperidol, diazepam is the drug of choice when delirium is suspected due to alcohol withdrawal.

Question 10

1. Discuss Stevens–Johnson syndrome (SJS).

Stevens-Johnsons syndrome and toxic epidermal necrolysis (TEN) synonyms: Lyell syndrome, SJS, and TEN are blistering diseases of the skin. In 1922 Stevens and Johnson described a condition which was characterized by disseminated cutaneous eruption with central necrosis, febrile erosive stomatitis, and severe purulent conjunctivitis. Adverse reactions of drugs are the common causes of these complex conditions (SJS and TEN). Adverse drug reaction is the cause in about >80% of the TEN and 50% cases in SJS. Condition is associated with widespread erythema, necrosis and bullous detachment of extensive areas of epidermis. SJS is considered as erythema multiform major. Epidermal detachment in SJS is <10% while epidermal detachment in TEN is >30%. A total of 10–30% cases overlap between SJS and TEN. Diagnosis is mostly clinical.

Clinical presentation: The patient with SJS/TEN presents with fever, malaise, muscle, and joint pain with purpuric lesions which occur on the face, upper torso, and proximal limbs. Lesions gradually involve other body parts eventually turning into fluid-filled blisters. Hemorrhagic crust on lips is characteristic. Ocular manifestations include conjunctivitis, clouding, symblepharon, corneal erosions, and photophobia. Erosion can spread to GI tract and respiratory tract giving rise to symptoms such as dysphagia, diarrhea, pulmonary edema, and bronchopneumonia. Glomerulonephritis represents renal involvement.

Management: Indian Association of Dermatologist, Venerologist, and Leprologist (IADVL) consensus treatment guidelines for SJS/TEN *Immediate management:*
- Stop all drugs
- Fluid replacement
- Nutritional support
- Sterile Vaseline or paraffin gauze dressing
- Temperature regulation
- Antacids and analgesics
- Initiation of disease specific therapy—corticosteroids, cyclosporine, IV immunoglobulin, plasmapheresis
- Other drugs—cyclophosphamide, thalidomide, N-acetyl cysteine, pentoxifylline.

Continued management:
- Ophthalmic and oral care
- Pulmonary care
- Antibiotics.

2. Explain staphylococcal toxic shock syndrome.

Staphylococcal scalded skin syndrome, also known as Ritter disease is a disease characterized by denudation of the skin caused by exotoxin producing strains of the *Staphylococcus* species, typically from a distant site. It usually presents 48 hours after birth and is rare in children >6 years; commonly seen in infants and children due to exotoxin released by *Staphylococcus aureus* group 2 phage 71. Exotoxin is an epidermolytic toxin also called exfoliating toxin or epidermolysis.

Clinically, intense erythematous cutaneous eruptions occur following an upper respiratory tract infection or purulent conjunctivitis. Painful erosions appear when erythematous sheets of skin are shed which is referred to as potato chip desquamation. Patient should be admitted and treated promptly with antibiotics covering *Staphylococcus aureus*.

Staphylococcal scalded skin syndrome tends to appear abruptly with diffuse erythema and fever. The diagnosis can be confirmed by a *skin biopsy specimen*, which can be expedited by frozen section processing, as staphylococcal scalded skin syndrome should be distinguished from life-threatening toxic epidermal necrolysis.

■ SUGGESTED READING

1. Richhariya D, Sharma B. Textbook of Emergency Medicine including Intensive Care and Trauma, 2nd edition. New Delhi: Jaypee Brothers Medical Publishers (P) Ltd; 2022. pp. 1452-1554. (Question 1).

2. Richhariya D, Sharma B. Textbook of Emergency Medicine including Intensive Care and Trauma, 2nd edition. New Delhi: Jaypee Brothers Medical Publishers (P) Ltd; 2022. pp. 249, 1496-7. (Question 2).
3. Richhariya D, Sharma B. Textbook of Emergency Medicine including Intensive Care and Trauma, 2nd edition. New Delhi: Jaypee Brothers Medical Publishers (P) Ltd; 2022. pp. 1708-10. (Question 3).
4. Richhariya D, Sharma B. Textbook of Emergency Medicine including Intensive Care and Trauma, 2nd edition. New Delhi: Jaypee Brothers Medical Publishers (P) Ltd; 2022. pp. 478, 1230. (Question 4).
5. Richhariya D, Sharma B. Textbook of Emergency Medicine including Intensive Care and Trauma, 2nd edition. New Delhi: Jaypee Brothers Medical Publishers (P) Ltd; 2022. pp. 956, 1331. (Question 5).
6. Richhariya D, Sharma B. Textbook of Emergency Medicine including Intensive Care and Trauma, 2nd edition. New Delhi: Jaypee Brothers Medical Publishers (P) Ltd; 2022. pp. 1342-5. (Question 6).
7. Richhariya D, Sharma B. Textbook of Emergency Medicine including Intensive Care and Trauma, 2nd edition. New Delhi: Jaypee Brothers Medical Publishers (P) Ltd; 2022. pp. 592-600. (Question 7).
8. Richhariya D, Sharma B. Textbook of Emergency Medicine including Intensive Care and Trauma, 2nd edition. New Delhi: Jaypee Brothers Medical Publishers (P) Ltd; 2022. pp. 1190, 1299-1300. (Question 8).
9. Richhariya D, Sharma B. Textbook of Emergency Medicine including Intensive Care and Trauma, 2nd edition. New Delhi: Jaypee Brothers Medical Publishers (P) Ltd; 2022. Chapter 118, pp. 815-9. (Question 9).
10. Richhariya D, Sharma B. Textbook of Emergency Medicine including Intensive Care and Trauma, 2nd edition. New Delhi: Jaypee Brothers Medical Publishers (P) Ltd; 2022. pp. 1025-7. (Question 10).

Emergency Medicine Paper 32

Devendra Richhariya

Question 1

1. Discuss use of point-of-care ultrasound (POCUS) in coronavirus disease-2019 (COVID-19) infections.

Lung ultrasound (US) is proven a reliable tool in diagnosing lung inflammatory processes—the results are immediate and the examination is safe, repeatable, and cheap. Lung parenchymal alterations can be observed at the onset, and a disposable probe cover can ensure a clean procedure for severe acute respiratory syndrome coronavirus 2 (SARS-CoV-2) infections, symptoms from fever, dry cough, fatigue, and lymphopenia to viral pneumonia with acute respiratory distress syndrome (ARDS). US examinations are easily performed at the point of care, which can be the patient's bedside or even outside the hospital. All these qualities make it a precious tool in clinical practice, optimal to assist clinicians even in initial patient triage. Early literature suggests that patients with confirmed COVID-19 pneumonia demonstrate typical lung imaging features, including pleural line irregularities, B-lines, and multifocal consolidations. Early use of lung US is used in Italy in COVID-19 patients, for early diagnoses and appropriate management.

2. Discuss hydroxychloroquine use and COVID-19.

During initial phase of pandemic various repurposed drugs are used in combination or alone [*tab hydroxychloroquine (HCQ) 400 mg BD × 1 day followed by 200 mg BD × 9 days*] though their efficacy is not established: HCQ + azithromycin (in age <50 and no cardiac comorbidities) OR HCQ + doxycycline (in age >50 and no cardiac comorbidities).

3. Explain the uses of dexamethasone in COVID-19.

The UK RECOVERY TRIAL has demonstrated mortality benefit with low dose dexamethasone in COVID-19 patients requiring oxygen—strongly recommended therapy:
- Tab dexamethasone 6 mg/day orally for 10 days OR
- Intravenous (IV) dexamethasone 20 mg/day IV × 5 days followed by 10 mg/day IV × 5 days; titrate dose and duration to culmination of oxygen dependency. OR
- IV methylprednisolone 2 mg/kg IV total dose in three divided doses for 7 days followed by 1 mg/kg for 5 days and then 0.5 mg/kg for 5 days (preferably within 48 hours of admission or if oxygen requirement is increasing and if inflammatory markers are increased) OR
- IV hydrocortisone 50 mg IV 6 hourly × 7 days followed by 50 mg IV 12 hourly × 4 days followed by 50 mg IV 24 hourly × 3 days.

Question 2

1. Discuss sample size calculation for a research study in emergency department (ED).

"How big a sample do I require to get a reliable estimate and valid inference in my research study?" is one of the most frequently asked questions by researchers. For answering this question, the sample size should be determined on the basis of scientific statistical criteria, which take into account the objective of the study, outcome parameter, and study design along with certain assumptions. The criteria will vary according to whether the study design is observational or interventional/experimental and also whether the parameter is "a proportion" or an average.

2. Write briefly about Cox regression model.

A Cox model is a statistical technique that can be used for survival-time (time-to-event) outcomes on one or more predictors. The response variable is the hazard function $\lambda(t)$, which assesses the probability that the event of interest (in this case, death) occurred before t. Cox regression (or proportional hazards regression) is method for investigating the effect of several variables upon the time a specified event takes to happen. In the context of an outcome such as death this is known as Cox regression for survival analysis.

3. Discuss forest plot.

A forest plot is a graphical display of estimated results from a number of scientific studies addressing the same question. A forest plot is an essential tool to summarize information on individual studies, give a visual suggestion of the amount of study heterogeneity, and show the estimated common effect, all in one figure (**Fig. 1**).

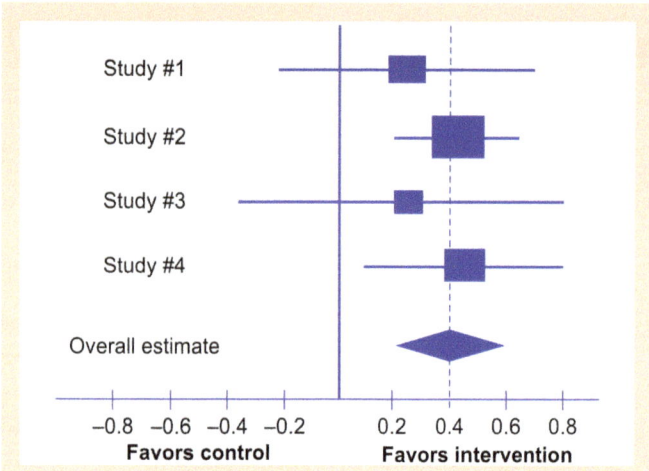

Fig. 1: Example of forest plot.

Question 3

1. Enumerate "Do not attempt resuscitation" guidelines by Indian Council of Medical Research (ICMR).

Do not attempt resuscitation guidelines: Cardiopulmonary resuscitation (CPR) is an emergency procedure performed in an attempt to revive patient suffering from cardiac and or respiratory arrest. In certain situation providing CPR is likely to increase the suffering of patient who has serious and terminal illness. Doctors and hospital are regularly faced ethical dilemma, to perform CPR or not. Do Not Attempt Resuscitation (DNAR) is an option that may be exercised by treating physician in such a situation in the best interest of the patient. DNAR relates to CPR only and its limited value in certain situation and not to other form of treatment. ICMR guidelines aim to guide treating physician and patient/surrogate in preserving dignity in death and avoid prolonged suffering to patient through non-beneficial CPR while continuing to provide other potentially curative and supportive care. Open communication and decision-making would enhance mutual trust and respect between treating physician and patient/surrogate.

- "Do not attempt resuscitation" would apply to a patient with a progressive debilitating, incurable, terminal illness where CPR would be inappropriate, non-beneficial, and likely to prolong the suffering of patient in the best judgment of treating physician. DNAR should be discussed with sensitivity. Compassionate care is important while applying this principle.
- DNAR is distinct from withdrawal or withholding of other life support treatment and advance directives do not come under the purview of this document.
- There should be adequate opportunity, time and space to discuss with the patient and family in private and facilitate clear understanding of DNAR and its implication. This should be done in anticipation of an impending cardiac arrest during current hospitalization.
- Teamwork and good communication are of crucial importance in decision-making. Combined decision may be taken with the help of another physician, psychologist or social worker, counsellor or hospital administration.
- DNAR form should be available in the language understood by patient/surrogate and treating physician. In case the patient/surrogate does/do not sign the DNAR form, same should be recorded.
- Hospital administration should make effort to sensitize their healthcare professional on all issues related to DNAR.

2. Discuss euthanasia.

The word "euthanasia" is derived from Greek word which means "a good death". In current world euthanasia has been defined as the bringing about a gentle and easy death for someone suffering from an incurable and painful disease or in an irreversible coma. Euthanasia may be classified on the basis of informed consent.

Voluntary euthanasia: Euthanasia is conducted with the consent of the patient. It is legal in Belgium, Luxembourg.

Non-voluntary euthanasia: Euthanasia conducted where the consent of the patient is unavailable, e.g., child euthanasia which is illegal worldwide.

Involuntary euthanasia: Euthanasia conducted against the will of the patient.

Passive and active euthanasia: Passive euthanasia involves act of omission which often involves withdrawing of life support measures such as artificial feeding, antibiotics which are necessary to continue the life.

Legal status of passive euthanasia in India: On 7th March 2011 Supreme Court of India legalized passive euthanasia by means of the withdrawal of life support to patient in permanent vegetative state. The decision was made as a part of the verdict in a case involving Aruna Shanbaug who has been in vegetative state for 37 years in King Edward Memorial Hospital. The high court rejected the active euthanasia by means of lethal medication (injection) and still illegal in India and most of the countries. In the absence of the law regulating euthanasia in India court stated its decision becomes the law of the land until Indian parliament enacts a suitable law.

Question 4

1. Explain discharge against medical advice from ED.

Discharge against the medical advice is a common problem, in which a patient chooses to leave the hospital before the treating physician recommends the discharge. Discharge against the medical advice is a problem for many physicians who treat hospitalized patient and expose the patient to risk of inadequately treated medical problem and result in need for readmission. Many physicians struggle with the desire to respect the patient's wishes to leave against the medical advice. In practice managing this issue presents more complications than simply identifying and prioritization.

Physician-patient communication, informed consent, and underlying psychiatric issues are relevant in practical management. Understanding why patient chooses to leave the hospital against the medical advice is important; interventions can be done earliest in high-risk patient to prevent morbidity and mortality.

Managing against medical advice (AMA) discharges: Informed consent is one of the important elements of care in patient who have decided to leave. An informed consent means that the patient has arrived at the decision in consultation with his/her physician and full understanding of risk, benefit, and alternatives of the decision. Informed consent in discharge planning can be straight forward if the steps are clear. Few questions should be included in evaluation form of a patient who is leaving against medical advice, e.g., does patient understand the admission, diagnosis, prognosis, risk, and benefits of leaving the hospital; is patient aware of alternative of treatment; can patient communicate choice; can patient articulate reason.

Follow-up: After discussion and discharge with his/her physician and made an informed decision to leave against the medical advice, the physician's responsibility is to ensure that the discharge is a safe and appropriate as possible, helping the patient to follow-up after discharge.

2. What are the medicolegal implications of a prisoner absconding from ED?

Absconding of a patient from ED is of great concern especially if patient is under trial or prisoner. As a result of absconding treatment and safety of these patients as well as safety of society is also under risk. Absconding is associated with increased risk of suicide, self-harm, homicide, and becoming missing from the society. Broadly, absconding has been defined as leaving the hospital without permission. This might be due to difference in the inpatient clinical profile and hospital environment. The common diagnosis in the absconding group is psychiatric and related disorder and substance use disorder, whenever prisoner admits in ED for treatment mostly accompanied by police force. Most of the events occur during daytime, because at that time many more people move around and visit, making less difficult to make way for exit. Increase in staffing security nursing care helps in improving the monitoring and observation of inpatient.

3. How to declare a patient "brought dead"?

In every hospital occasionally patient is brought to ED who are apparently dead- or dead-on arrival (DOA). Such cases may be natural death or unnatural death. Every doctor should be aware of the procedure to be followed in dead on arrival cases, because such cases have legal, ethical, and social ramification. Ethically and legally a doctor should immediately declare a person dead once the diagnosis of death can be clearly established. Legally the cause of death certificate has to be issued by the doctor in all natural deaths and after medicolegal autopsy in all unnatural death. Next to kin/relatives get the death certificate by municipality/corporation/panchayat.

Procedure to be followed in brought dead (dead on arrival): First and foremost all cases of brought dead should be documented clearly in death register or brought dead register, subsequently adequate history should be collected regarding event before death, related to disease, drug usage, injuries and perform complete examination of dead body. If there are injuries, poisoning, signs or suspicion of regarding the nature of death, case should be register as medicolegal case (MLC) and jurisdictional police must be informed. The body must not be handed over to relatives, dead body should be shifted to mortuary (or empty and safe room if no mortuary available), wait for the police to arrive and necessary action.

If there are no injuries or poisoning sign and looks like a case of natural death and it was treated in same hospital (any doctor of same hospital) then the cause of death certificate can be issued by hospital (after persuading all treatment notes, discharge summary, and case sheet) and dead body can be handed over to relatives for final rites.

If there are no injuries or poisoning signs and looks like natural death and if the case was not treated by any hospital or doctor, then the case has to be made medicolegal and jurisdictional police must be informed immediately. The body should not be handed over to relative and they should be informed that this is the only way to get legally a cause of death certificate.

In some hospital they issue only "Brought Dead Certificate" certifying mere confirmation of death but not the cause of death is unethical and illegal and misleading. This may lead to false statistics about disease and conditions.

Question 5

1. Discuss prerequisites before initiating clinical tests to declare a patient "brain dead".

Determination of brain death starts with documenting an irreversible and proximate cause for coma in a patient who is on invasive ventilator support with continued cardiac functions. A combination of clinical history of present illness, findings on clinical examination, radiologic imaging, and laboratory data is necessary to establish irreversibility and proximate causes. The patient's history and/or central nervous system (CNS) radiologic image findings should be suggestive of mechanism of brain injury that may completely stop brain functions. The range of these clinical states may include circulatory arrest with no cerebral perfusion to a penetrating injury to the skull or a severe CNS infection with global cerebral edema with tentorial herniation. The patient's clinical examination with no sedative agents should be that of comatose patient who is defined as having eyes closed and no appropriate interaction to external environment stimuli. Hypothermia, CNS depressants, and neuromuscular blocking (NMB) agents may obfuscate the clinical examination and need to be systematically excluded. Furthermore, severe electrolyte or endocrine abnormalities may also impact a patient's mental status and need to be corrected before the diagnosis of coma.

2. Explain the clinical tests required to be done to declare a patient "brain dead".

After some prerequisites, *three essential steps* are mandatory for its determination:
1. *Documentation of irreversible coma* due to a known proximate cause
2. *Documentation of absence of brain stem reflexes*
3. *Documentation of apnea—the apnea test.*

Diagnosis of brain death is performed by neurologic criteria based on current medical guidelines—clinical, laboratory values, and radiological findings. The examination shows that the patient's eyes are not held open voluntarily and that no movements are made to verbal or noxious stimuli. Standard point of noxious stimulation includes nail bed, supraorbital or temporomandibular pressure.

Documentation of coma:
- Absence of motor response to a standardized painful stimulus
- Beware of local spinal reflexes causing spontaneous or stimulus-related motor movements

Documentation of absence of brainstem reflexes:
- Brain stem reflexes are lost in rostral to caudal direction
- Reflexes in medulla oblongata are the last to cease

Documented tests:
- Absent pupillary reflexes (nerves—optic and oculomotor)
- Absent oculocephalic movement—doll's eye reflex (nerves—vestibular part of vestibulocochlear, oculomotor, and abducens)
- Absent oculovestibular reflex—cold calorie test (nerves—vestibular part of vestibulocochlear, trochlear, and abducens)
- Absent corneal reflex—(nerves—trigeminal and facial)
- Absent cough reflex—(nerves—glossopharyngeal and vagus).

3. Discuss care of patient who has been declared "brain dead" and is a potential organ donor.

"Care of the donor" is associated with "the care of multiple recipients." A brain-dead patient with potential organ donor requires the similar intensity of care in order to preserve organ perfusion and improved quality of grafts. Improved quality of care and titration of inotropes and fluids with the use of invasive lines is mandatory in intensive care.

Potential donor: Potential donor is one who becomes brain-dead due to catastrophic brain injury, and the physician and the family expressed intend to withdraw life support. The organ procurement organization initiates counselling the family by using "presumptive strategy" wherein grief counsellors establish the communication with the family and explain that organ donation is the natural thing in the interests of the potential donor as well as the pool of recipients.

Fluctuating donor hemodynamic complicates the declaration time of brain death from the time of diagnosis. When the time to organ retrieval from the diagnosis of brain death is longer the chances of hemodynamic instability are greater. Optimum donor care should be ensured in intensive care unit, in view of hormonal and inflammatory changes accompanying brain death to avoid graft dysfunction and chances of rejection. However, in the last two decades, outcomes have improved following transplant surgery due to increased awareness of donor management.

Question 6

1. Explain airway ultrasound in ED.

Airway ultrasound is a valuable, noninvasive, simple, and portable POCUS for evaluation of airway management even in anatomy distorted by pathology or trauma. Ultrasound enables us to identify important anatomy of the upper airway such as thyroid cartilage, epiglottis, cricoid cartilage, cricothyroid membrane, tracheal cartilages, and esophagus. Use of ultrasound is important in assessment of airway anatomy for difficult intubation, endotracheal tube (ETT), and laryngeal mask airways (LMA) placement and depth, assessment of airway size, ultrasound-guided invasive procedures such as percutaneous needle cricothyroidotomy and tracheostomy, prediction of postextubation stridor and left double-lumen bronchial tube size, and detecting upper airway pathologies.

2. Discuss Broselow tape.

The Broselow pediatric emergency tape is a color-coded tape measure **Figure 2A** that is used worldwide as a quick reference for pediatric emergencies. Included on this tape are precalculated emergency medications, airway and equipment sizes, and defibrillator shock doses.

The majority of critically ill children present with conditions that do not allow for conventional measurement of body weight. Therefore, it is recommended to utilize the length-based resuscitation (Broselow tape) **(Fig. 2B)** to guide the selection of appropriate medication dosage and equipment size.

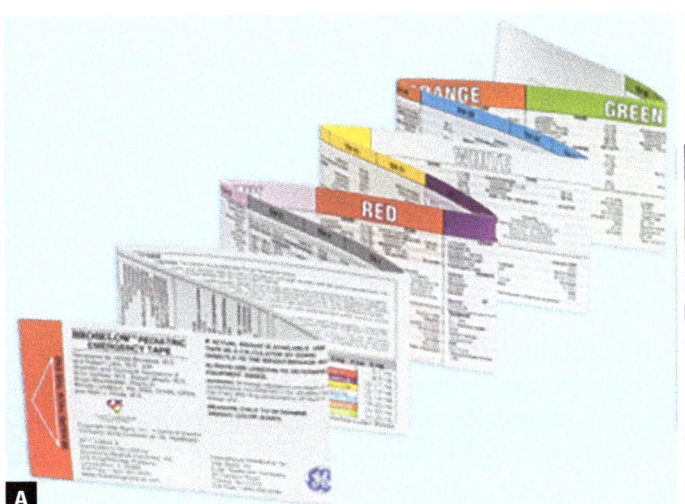
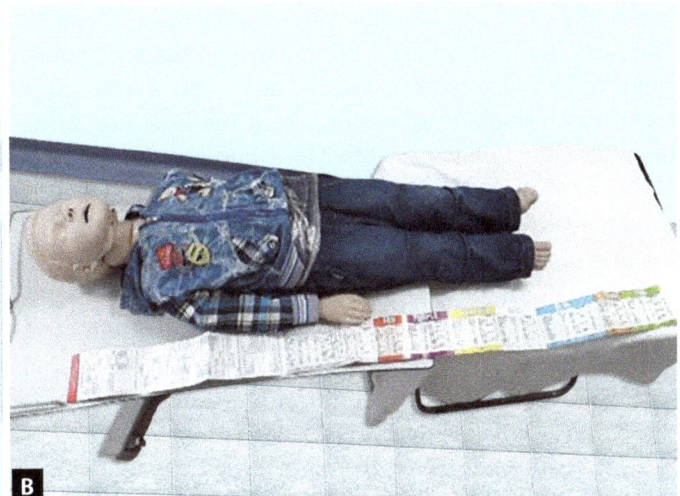

Figs. 2A and B: (A) Broselow pediatric emergency tape; (B) Use of Broselow tape.

3. Explain the nerve blocks in a trauma patient.

Pain is the most common presentation of patients seeking care in the ED. Safe and appropriate pain management is an important component of high quality and compassionate care. Ultrasound-guided nerve blocks have emerged as an important tool available to emergency clinicians as part of a multi-modal analgesic strategy. These nerve block techniques have similarly benefitted patients in the ED by relieving pain while reducing the need for adjunctive analgesics. In particular IV opioids, while commonly used, can lead to undesired and at times serious dose-related side effects, including respiratory depression, hypotension, and depressed consciousness. Furthermore, in patients with extensive injuries requiring procedural intervention, nerve blocks utilize less local anesthetic when compared to the potentially large volumes required for local infiltration, thus reducing the potential for toxicity. Unlike in the operating room, the goal of ED nerve blocks is not to provide full sensory and motor blockade, but rather to provide significant pain relief in conjunction with standard systemic analgesics, and reduce opioid-related adverse effects. Common nerve blocks are femoral blocks, popliteal sciatic blocks, posterior tibial nerve block, interscalene block of the brachial plexus, axillary block.

Considerations when choosing an anesthetic agent include onset, duration, operator comfort, and local availability. Lidocaine and bupivacaine are commonly available in ED settings. For less experienced operators, lidocaine may be preferred over bupivacaine, due to its more favorable safety profile in the event of unintentional injection into vasculature. **Table 1** reviews the recommended dosing, onset, and estimated duration of action of commonly used local anesthetics in the ED.

TABLE 1: Dosing, onset, and duration of action of commonly used local anesthetics.

Anesthetic	Maximum dose	Onset	Duration
Lidocaine 1% without epinephrine	4.5 mg/kg	Rapid	60–120 min
Lidocaine 1% with epinephrine	7 mg/kg	Rapid	90–180 min
Bupivacaine 0.5% without epinephrine	2.5 mg/kg	Slow	180–360 min
Bupivacaine 0.5% with epinephrine	3 mg/kg	Slow	300–480 min

Question 7

1. Discuss grief counseling.

Grief counseling refers to a specific form of therapy which focuses on general counseling with the goal of helping the individual grief and addresses personal loss in a healthy manner. Grief counseling is offered by psychologist, counsellor or by social worker. Specific task of grief counseling includes emotional expression about the loss, accepting the loss, adjusting the life after loss, coping with changes within oneself and the world after the loss. Typical feeling experienced by individual and addressed in grief counseling include sadness, anxiety, anger, loneliness, guilt, isolation, confusion or numbness.

Purpose of grief counseling is to help individual work through the feelings, thoughts, and memories associated with the loss of loved ones. Grief counseling generally directed toward positive adjustment following loss after the death of loved ones. Grief counseling helps individual cope with the pain associated with the loss, feel supported through the anxiety surrounding life changes that may follow the loss and develop strategies for seeking support and self-care.

2. Explain home isolation of a COVID-19 positive patient.

Criteria for home isolation COVID-19 mild cases (asymptomatic to mild symptoms, no oxygen therapy, no X-ray/CT findings, no rise of inflammatory markers, no risk factors): Mild upper or lower respiratory tract infection with mild symptoms—fever, cough, sore throat, nasal congestions, malaise, headache, loss of taste or smell. Mild gastrointestinal symptoms (nausea, vomiting diarrhea); clear sensorium, no oxygen dependency, no respiratory distress, room air SpO_2 >95%, no hypotension, and no multiorgan involvement.

General measures during home isolation include:
- Balanced diet
- Adequate sleep
- Breathing exercises
- Remain physically active
- Hot water gargles three times a day
- Positive mood and outlook
- In case of symptoms seek medical advice
- Monitor saturation with pulse oximeter
- Temperature monitoring and paracetamol as needed
- Multivitamins—*Zinc, Vitamin C, and Vitamin D.*

Immediate medical attention must be taken if serious signs or symptoms develop.

These could *include:*
- Difficulty in breathing, saturation <94%
- Persistent pain/pressure in the chest
- Mental confusion or inability to arouse
- Developing bluish discolorations of lips/face and
- As advised by treating medical officer.

Patient under home isolation will end home isolation after 17 days of onset of symptoms (or date of sampling, for presymptomatic cases) *and no fever for 10 days. There is no need for testing after the home isolation period is over.*

Question 8

1. Discuss fishbone analysis for quality improvement in ED.

The fishbone analysis (diagram) is a visual tool used to explore the factors that influence or cause a given outcome to help to understand the problem more clearly. Quality improvement tool is named by its inventor Kaoru Ishikawa and its resemblance to a fish skeleton. Constructing the fishbone diagram helps to understand the multiple causal factors of the particular problem and helps us to identify areas of further investigation **(Fig. 3)**.

How to draw fishbone diagram/analysis:
- First write single statement in a box that describes the problem.
- Then identify major relevant categories of causes (people, place, policies, and procedures). Draw these main causes (bones) of the large arrow.

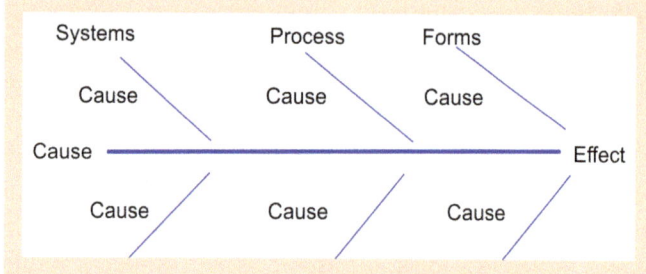

Fig. 3: Fishbone diagram.

- For each main cause (bone) consider factors contribute to it (minor causes). We can use brainstorming for this step.
- Continue analyzing fishbone diagram until every possible contributing cause and influence has been identified.

2. Discuss DAWN and DEFUSE-3 trials.

Recent success of DAWN and DEFUSE 3 trials has further extended the window for mechanical thrombectomy from 6 to 24 hours. These trials have also made it easier to manage patients presenting with wake-up strokes or unknown time of onset in the preceding 24 hours **(Table 2)**.

DAWN trial enrolled 206 patients with stroke onset between 6 and 24 hours. There was a 33% adjusted difference in functional outcome in favor of the intervention arm. The number needed to treat for one additional patient to achieve functional independence was 3. Likewise, in the DEFUSE-3 trial there was a 28% adjusted difference in functional outcome in favor of the intervention arm and therefore the number needed to treat for one additional patient to achieve functional independence was 3.6.

Mechanical thrombectomy is now strongly recommended for patients in whom large arteries within the brain are blocked.

TABLE 2: Characteristics of DAWN and DEFUSE-3 trials.

DAWN	DEFUSE-3 trials
Clinical inclusion criteria: Age 18 years, baseline NIHSS score 10, prestroke mRS <1	Clinical inclusion criteria: Age 18–90 years, baseline NIHSS score ≥6, prestroke mRS ≤2
Eligible 6–24 h after last seen well	Eligible 6–16 h after last seen well
Occlusion of intracranial ICA or proximal MCA	Occlusion of extracranial or intracranial ICA or proximal MCA
• Group A: >80 years, NIHSS ≥10; infarct volume ≤21 • Group B: <80 years, NIHSS ≥10; infarct volume ≤31 • Group C: <80 years, NIHSS ≥20; infarct volume ≤51	Infarct volume <70 mL + ratio of ischemic tissue to initial infarct volume of >1.8
CT or magnetic resonance-based imaging	CT or magnetic resonance-based imaging
Rapid software for image analysis	Rapid software for image analysis
Only Trevo (Stryker, Kalamazoo, MI, USA) device allowed for recanalization	All FDA-approved devices for recanalization allowed

(ICA: internal carotid artery; MCA: middle cerebral artery)

Question 9

1. Discuss Modified Early Warning Score (MEWS).

Modified Early Warning Score is based on blood pressure, heart rate, respiration, oxygen saturation, and alertness. In some triage scale urine output and pain score is also taken into consideration. Patient's clinical deterioration can be anticipated by this score and requirement of hospitalization can also be assessed. MEWS score uses basic equipment and simple parameter so it is easy to use by junior most staff also. MEWS is useful for triaging of medical emergencies but not for trauma patient triaging. MEWS score >5 is considered as risk of clinical deterioration and need of hospitalization. Components and scoring of MEWS are given in **Table 3**.

TABLE 3: Modified Early Warning Score (MEWS).

Vital signs	3	2	1	0	1	2	3
Systolic BP	<70	71–80	81–100			>200	
Heart rate		<40	41–50	51–100	101–110	111–129	>130
Respiratory rate		<9		9–14	15–20	21–29	>30
Temperature		<35		35–38.4		>38.5	
AVPU				Alert	React to voice	React to pain	No response

In some triaging system, urine output and pain score is also added in early warning score.
(AVPU: A–alert, V–response to voice, P–response to pain, U–unconscious)

2. Explain prehospital antibiotic therapy in suspected sepsis.

Sepsis has been recognized as one of the most leading causes of death in the past decades. Some studies have suggested that earlier initiation of antibiotics has shown positive outcomes in sepsis patients. The rapid administration of antibiotics for septic shock has demonstrated improved outcomes, preferably within 1 hour after arrival at the ED. Several retrospective studies showed that early antimicrobial therapy is associated with improved survival, and that any delay in administration of antibiotics after development of septic shock is associated with an increase in mortality.

3. Discuss vancomycin as an empiric treatment in sepsis.

Empiric antibiotic therapy is targeted at the suspected organism(s) and site(s) of infection and preferably administered within the first hour. One of the most common resistant strain bacteria that can cause sepsis is methicillin-resistant *Staphylococcus aureus* (MRSA). Vancomycin is the first-line therapy for treating sepsis infection caused by MRSA, but recently there have been some MRSA strains that are resistant to vancomycin therapy. A higher vancomycin target trough level is required for selected infections (i.e., sepsis, pneumonia, meningitis, osteomyelitis, and endocarditis) of 15–20 mg/L and 10–15 mg/L for less severe infections, respectively. For nonobese adult patients with normal renal function, a loading dose of 20–35 mg/kg (maximum dose: 3,000 mg) is recommended. For obese patients, a loading dose of 20–25 mg/kg using actual body weight, up to a maximum dose of 3,000 mg may be considered.

Question 10

1. Discuss evaluation and management of a neonate with fever.

One of the most common presenting complaints in pediatric age group is fever, which is associated with several illnesses. All types of fever can be divided into four main groups based on the etiology, i.e., infectious, inflammatory, neoplastic, and miscellaneous. Each of them shows certain characteristics, which can provide us clue about the underlying etiology; such as fever related to viral infections is typically associated with a slow declining fever with relatively shorter duration, which may be up to 1 week, whereas in a bacterial infection the fever gets subsided promptly after administration of proper antibiotics. Usually, the pathogens are eliminated once the antimicrobial therapy is employed, but still the fever may persist for few more days as a result of tissue injury and related inflammatory changes. Cause of very high-grade fever, i.e., higher than 105.8°F is usually associated with noninfectious cause, and most importantly due to central nervous system dysfunction. The pyrogens play a big role in inducing fever, by raising the hypothalamus temperature set point. These pyrogens may be endogenous and exogenous. Endogenous pyrogens are mainly cytokines such as interleukins 1 and 6 (IL 1, Il 6), tumor necrosis factor α (TNF-α), interferons β and γ. Many exotoxins such as drugs, malignancies, and inflammatory diseases can also produce fever by production of endogenous pyrogens. Changes in the heart rate from baseline are the most prominent clinical finding, and most of the patients have fever associated with tachycardia (increase in heart rate by 10, for each raise in temperature of 1.8°F). Disproportionately increase in heart rate is commonly seen in noninfectious conditions, or in infections in which toxins play role in clinical manifestation.

Full sepsis evaluation including complete blood count (CBC) with differential count, blood culture, urine culture, urinalysis (catheterized or suprapubic aspiration), lumbar puncture (cell count, glucose, protein, Gram stain, and culture) should be performed. Chest X-ray (CXR) is indicated if there are respiratory signs and symptoms.

Antipyresis includes use of both pharmacological and non-pharmacological approach. However, use of antipyretics may help to manage the child overall, but it does not appear to play any role in occurrence of febrile seizures. Antipyretic agents act upon the arachidonic acid pathway. The main action is to competitively bind on cyclooxygenase (COX) enzymes catalytic site competing with arachidonic acid, hence inhibiting production of prostaglandin E2.

2. Explain evaluation and management of a febrile infant between 1 and 12 months of age.

Yale observation scale (YOS) score is an objective scoring system based on child's alertness, playfulness, interaction with the environment, color, state of hydration, quality of cry and whether the child is consolable or not. In young infant (<8 weeks) YOS cannot be relied upon to determine the risk of serious bacterial infection (SBI). In this age group, a history of poor feeding, lethargy, irritability, moaning, increased sleepiness or difficulty in breathing, seizure or cyanotic episode is overly concerning for SBI. An infant with urinary tract infections (UTI) may only have a low-grade fever with vomiting or diarrhea. In young infant, physical examination may reveal mottled skin, pallor, bulging fontanelle, weak cry, grunting, tachypnea, tachycardia, and lethargy. Meningeal signs may not be present even in meningitis. In children >8 weeks of age, clinical impression is more reliable. A child with sepsis is usually not interested in surrounding and does not smile. Parents often report a change in child's behavior. Localizing signs are more reliable in older children (toddlers), like in case of meningitis the presence of nuchal rigidity and positive Kernig's or Brudzinski's signs. There are three common criteria (Boston criteria, Rochester criteria, and Philadelphia criteria) commonly used to determine if the patient is at low-risk or high-risk for SBI. These risk stratification rules are derived for febrile young infants and are not helpful in neonates. They all have following components in common for a patient to be in low-risk category:

- Patient must appear well
- No signs of focal infection on examination
- Peripheral white blood cells (WBC) count within a specific range
- No evidence of UTI on rapid urine testing.

Full sepsis evaluation including CBC with differential count, blood culture, urine culture, urinalysis (catheterized or suprapubic aspiration), lumbar puncture (cell count, glucose, protein, Gram stain, and culture) should be performed. CXR is indicated if there are respiratory signs and symptoms. Stool study is indicated if there is diarrhea. All cultures, including lumbar puncture, should be obtained before starting antibiotics unless the infant is in respiratory distress or shock. Any patient who appears ill or toxic (inconsolable, lethargic, tachypneic, has poor perfusion or grunting) should be admitted and treated for sepsis while entertaining other diagnoses such as congenital heart disease or metabolic conditions.

- Admit all patients
- IV ampicillin (<1 week: 100 mg/kg/day, div q12h; >1 week: 200 mg/kg/day, div q6h)
- IV cefotaxime (<1 week: 100 mg/kg/day, div q12h; 1–4 weeks: 150 mg/kg/day, div q8h)
- Gentamicin 2.5 mg/kg IV can be used instead of cefotaxime
- In case of suspected meningitis increase the dose of cefotaxime to 200 mg/kg/day div q6h
- Ceftriaxone is not recommended for this age group because of the concern of inducing unconjugated hyperbilirubinemia
- IV acyclovir if herpes simplex virus (HSV) infection is suspected; high-dose acyclovir (20 mg/kg IV) improves outcome in patients.

SUGGESTED READING

1. Richhariya D, Sharma B. Textbook of Emergency Medicine including Intensive Care and Trauma, 2nd edition. New Delhi: Jaypee Brothers Medical Publishers (P) Ltd; 2022. p. 626. (Question 1).
2. Richhariya D, Sharma B. Textbook of Emergency Medicine including Intensive Care and Trauma, 2nd edition. New Delhi: Jaypee Brothers Medical Publishers (P) Ltd; 2022. pp. 80-90. (Question 2).
3. Richhariya D, Sharma B. Textbook of Emergency Medicine including Intensive Care and Trauma, 2nd edition. New Delhi: Jaypee Brothers Medical Publishers (P) Ltd; 2022. pp. 131-6. (Question 3 and 4).
4. Richhariya D, Sharma B. Textbook of Emergency Medicine including Intensive Care and Trauma, 2nd edition. New Delhi: Jaypee Brothers Medical Publishers (P) Ltd; 2022. pp. 151-7. (Question 5).
5. Richhariya D, Sharma B. Textbook of Emergency Medicine including Intensive Care and Trauma, 2nd edition. New Delhi: Jaypee Brothers Medical Publishers (P) Ltd; 2022. pp. 365, 385-91, 1228. (Question 6).
6. Richhariya D, Sharma B. Textbook of Emergency Medicine including Intensive Care and Trauma, 2nd edition. New Delhi: Jaypee Brothers Medical Publishers (P) Ltd; 2022. pp. 136, 625. (Question 7).
7. Richhariya D, Sharma B. Textbook of Emergency Medicine including Intensive Care and Trauma, 2nd edition. New Delhi: Jaypee Brothers Medical Publishers (P) Ltd; 2022. pp. 53, 827. (Question 8).
8. Richhariya D, Sharma B. Textbook of Emergency Medicine including Intensive Care and Trauma, 2nd edition. New Delhi: Jaypee Brothers Medical Publishers (P) Ltd; 2022. pp. 42, 323. (Question 9).
9. Richhariya D, Sharma B. Textbook of Emergency Medicine including Intensive Care and Trauma, 2nd edition. New Delhi: Jaypee Brothers Medical Publishers (P) Ltd; 2022. pp. 1158-68. (Question 10).

Emergency Medicine Paper 33

Narendra Nath Jena, Subbulakshmi Dhanabal

Question 1

1. Discuss pathways of transmission of pain.

Pain receptors are free nerve endings, present in superficial layer of skin, arterial walls, joint surfaces, the flax, and tentorium in cranial vault. Pain can be elicited by stimuli such as mechanical, thermal, and chemicals pain stimuli. Fast pain elicited by mechanical and thermal stimuli, slow pain by all three types. Chemicals that excite chemical pain are bradykinin, serotonin, histamine, potassium ions, acetylcholine, and proteolytic enzymes. Prostaglandins and substance P enhance sensitivity of pain endings. Increase in sensitivity of pain receptors is called hyperalgesia. Slow pain is carried by C fibers and fast pain by A delta fibers. First order neurons of slow pain synapse in substantia gelatinosa in the dorsal horn of spinal cord **(Fig. 1)**. Second order neurons crossover to the opposite side and ascend in the anterolateral pathway. Tract carrying slow pain is also called paleospinothalamic tract and fast pain called neospinothalamic tract.

2. Explain local anesthetics drugs.

Drug therapy is the mainstay of pain management in emergency department. Knowledge of appropriate pharmacologic agents for managing the intensity of pain is the key. Ideal pharmacologic agent should be easy to administer with appropriate quality and safety measures **(Table 1)**.

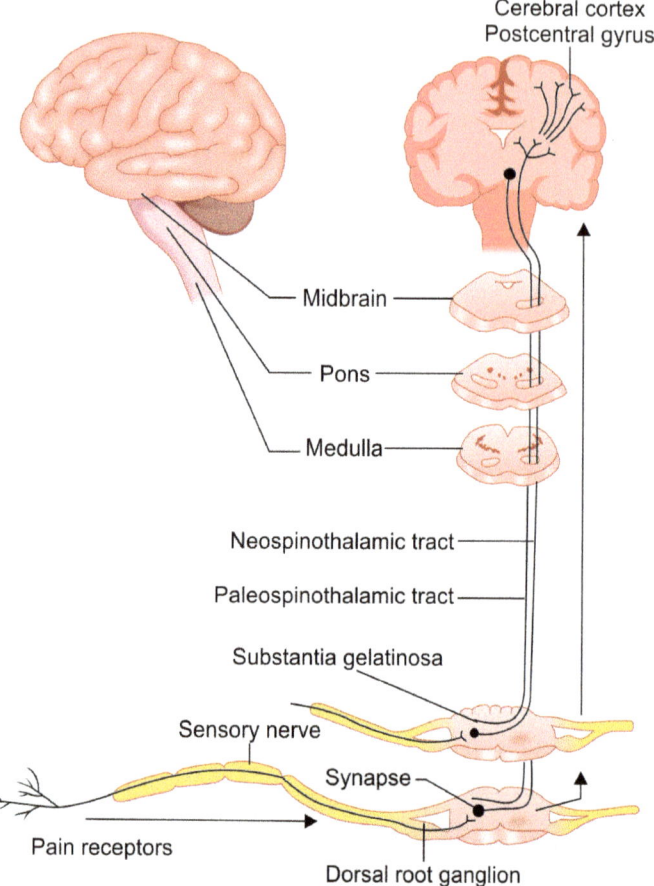

Fig. 1: Pathways of transmission of pain.

TABLE 1: Local anesthetic agents.

	Agents	Concentration for subdermal use	Concentration for regional anesthesia use	Onset (minute)	Comments
Amides	Bupivacaine	0.50–0.75%	0.25–0.50%	2–10 min	High lipid soluble and high protein binding
	Levobupivacaine	0.25%	0.50%	10–20 min	High lipid soluble and high protein binding
	Lidocaine	0.5–1.0%	1–2%	<1 min	Medium lipid soluble and medium protein binding
	Mepivacaine	0.5–1.0%	1–2%	3–20 min	Low lipid soluble and medium protein binding
	Prilocaine	4%	NA	5–6 min	Medium lipid soluble and medium protein binding
Esters	Procaine	0.25–0.50%	0.5–2.0%	5	Low lipid soluble and low protein binding
	Chloroprocaine	1–2%	1–2%	5–6	Low lipid soluble and low protein binding
	Tetracaine	NA	0.2–0.3%	6–7	High lipid soluble and high protein binding

3. Discuss hematoma block.

Hematoma block is a local anesthetic technique where the agent is injected directly into the fracture site. Anesthetizing the bones around a fracture allows for better analgesia while reducing them, most commonly used in reducing distal radius fractures. Lidocaine and bupivacaine are used in combination. Lignocaine without adrenaline, dosage is 4.5 mg/kg.

Question 2

1. Explain the physiology of temperature regulation.

Temperature is regulated by a balance of heat production and heat loss. The production is by product of metabolism, basal metabolic rate (BMR) of individual cells in the body, muscle activity, thyroxine, epinephrine, and thermogenesis effect of food. Heat loss is occurred by dissipation from deeper organs to skin, conduction from core to skin, and from skin to periphery. Rate of blood flow from core to skin increases the efficiency of heat conduction and this is in turn also controlled by sympathetic nervous system, by vasoconstriction of vessels. Regulation centers are present in the hypothalamus. Anterior hypothalamic-preoptic region has cold and heat sensitive neurons, this area when the body gets heated leads to profuse sweating and inhibits excess heat production. Posterior hypothalamus receives central and peripheral temperature sensations. Skin has both cold and heat receptors. Posterior hypothalamus combines signals from the body and anterior hypothalamic preoptic area to control temperature. Regulation is done by vasodilation or constriction and by decreasing or increasing thermogenesis. Dorsomedial portion of hypothalamus near the wall of third ventricle has primary motor center for shivering. Sympathetic chemical excitation is done adrenaline and noradrenaline by increasing cellular metabolism. This process is called non-shivering or chemical thermogenesis, and occurs by uncoupling of oxidative phosphorylation. Thyroxine also increases heat production. Regulation of internal body temperature is impaired in transaction of spinal cord.

2. Enumerate the methods of measuring the body temperature.

Body temperature is measured by using a device called the thermometer. Mercury thermometers were initially used, now only electronic ones are used. Now infrared (IR) thermometers have become popular; they are used to measure at different sites—oral, rectal, axilla, tympanic, and by skin. The average body temperature is 98.6°F (37°C). Rectal temperature is considered most accurate. Axillary temperature readings are about 0.5–1°F (0.3–0.6°C) lower than an oral temperature.

3. Discuss management of heat stroke.

Heat stroke is hyperthermia with neurological dysfunction due to failure of thermoregulatory system. Classic heatstroke is non-exertional and exertional heat stroke occurs from physical activity in hot conditions. Clinical features include neurological dysfunction, hyperthermia, and perspiration loss.

Maintain airway breathing and circulation, cardiac monitoring. Treatment of heat stroke involves rapid mechanical cooling along with resuscitation measures. The body temperature must be lowered quickly. The patient should be moved to a cool area which is either indoor or in a shade and clothing may need to be removed to promote passive clothing. Active cooling methods include immersion in cold water, or a hyperthermia vest can be applied. Cold compresses to the torso, head, neck, and groin will help in bringing the body core temperature down. A fan or dehumidifying air-conditioning unit may be used to aid in evaporation of the water.

Immersion should be avoided for an unconscious person, but if there is no alternative, the patients' head must be held above water. Dantrolene, a direct-acting paralytic which abolishes shuddering and is effective in many other forms of hyperthermia has no individual or additive effects to cooling in the context of heat stroke, showing a lack of endogenous thermogenic response to cold water immersion. Aggressive ice-water immersion is the gold standard for life-threatening heat stroke.

Adequate hydration is essential adjunct to cool the temperature. In mild cases of dehydration, adequate hydration can be achieved by drinking water, or isotonic sport drinks. In exercise- or heat-induced dehydration, an imbalance of electrolytes can occur and is exacerbated by overconsumption of water. Hyponatremia can be corrected by intake of hypertonic fluids. Absorption is rapid and complete in most people but in the event of confusion, impaired conscious level or if the patient is unable to tolerate oral fluid, then an intravenous (IV) rehydration and electrolyte replacement may be required. The person's condition should be reassessed at regular intervals including the vital signs to ensure stability.

Appropriate resuscitative measures are indicated with maintenance of fluid levels to prevent dehydration, monitoring of skin and core temperatures, removing the cause of hyperthermia, removal of clothes, active cooling to <40°. Antipyretics are of no use. Rhabdomyolysis prevention is done by maintaining a urine output >2–3 mL/kg/h, crystalloids infusion, IV mannitol or furosemide, and maintaining normal electrolyte levels.

Question 3

1. Explain the pathophysiology of acclimatization.

- Acclimatization occurs over days to weeks mainly in cellular and mitochondrial metabolism (**Flowchart 1**).
- Acute hypoxia causes rapid unconsciousness if hypoxia stress is sufficient, SaO_2 <65%.
- Acute response enables temporary homeostasis.
- Primary initial adaptation is through increased ventilation, modulated by the carotid body.
- With ascent, hyperventilation is attenuated by respiratory alkalosis.
- Renal excretion of bicarbonate occurs to compensate and pH returns to normal thus increasing ventilation, this process of maximizing ventilation is termed as ventilators acclimatization and takes 4–7 days at a given altitude.
- Serum erythropoietin levels increase resulting in increased red blood cells (RBCs) over days to weeks.
- This may, however, progress to chronic mountain polycythemia.
- Hypoxia shifts the oxyhemoglobin curve to right and respiratory alkalosis shifts the curve to left.
- Peripheral venoconstriction causes an increase in central blood volume resulting in diuresis.
- This along with respiratory alkalosis results in decreased plasma volume and the resulting hyperosmolarity occurs due to resetting of osmolar center of the brain.
- Hemoconcentration increases oxygen carrying capacity of blood.
- Stroke volume increases initially and increase in heart rate is required to maintain cardiac output.
- Pulmonary vasoconstriction occurs due to hypoxia, increasing resistance and arterial pressure, this mechanism on hyperactivity leads to high-altitude pulmonary edema.
- Cerebral blood flow increases brain oxygenation and increased blood volume may lead to high altitude cerebral edema.
- Exercise capacity is also drastically affected, due to inadequate oxygenation of muscle as a result of low driving pressure for oxygen diffusion.
- Frequent night time awakenings are common at high altitudes, driven by Cheyne–Stokes respiration.
- Limitations—even good acclimatizers cannot tolerate extreme altitudes for long, because of rapid deterioration of physiological functioning. Weight loss due to loss of fat and lean body mass is unavoidable.

Flowchart 1: Pathophysiologic changes in high-altitude illness.

2. What is the management of acute mountain sickness?

Acute mountain sickness (AMS) is a multisystem disorder with prominent neurological features characterized by headache, fatigue or weakness, anorexia, nausea or vomiting, dizziness or lightheadedness, and insomnia. Headache is the more common symptom. The diagnosis of AMS is clinical; no diagnostic modalities or physical findings can reliably confirm the diagnosis **(Table 2)**.

Treatment: Non-pharmacologic—first of all, the prevention is important: Avoid alcohol and sleeping medications. In case of mild AMS avoid further ascent until symptoms resolved. Acclimatization for 1–2 days at the same altitude is recommended. Hydration by water and reducing activity level could help the patient. In case of moderate or severe AMS the patient must descend at less altitude.

TABLE 2: Management of acute mountain sickness.

Mild AMS	• No further ascent • Descent to lower altitude or acclimatization at same altitude • Acetazolamide, 125–250 mg BD (increases rate of acclimatization) • Symptomatic treatment with antiemetics and analgesics
Moderate to severe AMS	• Immediate descent for worsening symptoms • Low flow O₂ • Acetazolamide, 250 mg BD and/or dexamethasone 8 mg PO, IM, IV then 4 mg QID • Hyperbaric therapy if patient cannot descend
High altitude cerebral edema	• Immediate descent or evacuation • O₂ 2–4 L/min or titration to SaO₂ >90% • Dexamethasone 8 mg PO, IM, IV then 4 mg QID • Hyperbaric therapy if patient cannot descend
High altitude pulmonary edema	• Immediate descent or evacuation • O₂ 4 L/min or titration to SaO₂ >90% • Nifedipine 30 mg PO BD, or tadalafil 10 mg PO BD if no oxygen or descent • Hyperbaric therapy if patient cannot descend • Measures to minimize exertions and maintain warmth • Dexamethasone if cerebral signs present, 4 mg PO QID
Periodic breathing/insomnia	Acetazolamide 62.5–125 mg PO at bedtime as needed

[AMS: acute mountain sickness; BD: bis in die (twice daily); IM: intramuscular; IV: intravenous; PO: per os (taken by mouth); QID: quater in die (four times a day)]

Pharmacologic: In case of mild AMS consider classical analgesics and antiemetics. In case of moderate or severe AMS consider dexamethasone (4 mg every 6 hours); and/or acetazolamide (250–500 mg per orally twice daily); if unable to descend, vigilant observation for deterioration; oxygen (1–2 L/min) and/or portable hyperbaric therapy (2–4 psi) for a few hours if available. The hospital care is based on the same recommendations.

3. Explain caisson sickness.

The original name for decompression sickness (DCS) is "caisson disease". Clinical manifestations of DCS are categorized as type 1 and type 2. Type 1 DCS manifestations are mild and musculoskeletal pain and mild cutaneous symptoms and type 2 clinical manifestations are more serious. Type 2 symptoms are divided into three categories—neurologic, inner ear, and cardiopulmonary. Neurologic symptoms include numbness, paresthesia or tingling, muscle weakness, impaired gait, physical coordination or bladder control, paralysis or change in mental status. Severe neurologic DCS symptoms usually appear within 10 minutes of surfacing and in 90% of cases symptoms will be present within the first 3 hours. In some cases, it can take up to 24 hours for symptoms to be noticed by the diver.

Decompression illness should be differentiated from the other conditions with similar symptom includes inner ear barotrauma; middle ear or maxillary sinus barotrauma; contaminated breathing gas, oxygen toxicity; musculoskeletal strains or trauma sustained before, during, or after a dive; seafood toxin ingestion; immersion pulmonary edema; water aspiration; and coincidental neurologic disorders, such as stroke. Hypoglycemia, thermal stress, and age-related conditions should also be considered. Medical or event history can provide important insights.

Management is by maintaining FiO₂ of 100%, cardiopulmonary resuscitation (CPR), isotonic fluid resuscitation, and hyperbaric therapy. There are several steps in decompression illness management: On-the-scene evaluation and first aid, transport, and definitive medical evaluation and treatment. Providing high partial pressure oxygen is the primary first aid measure for DCI. Inert gases from the lung will be eliminated by providing high oxygen concentration to the patient. Ischemic insults produced by bubble blockages can also be minimized by high oxygen partial pressure in the bloodstream. Sustained oxygen delivery can reduce or even eliminate symptoms. Various oxygen delivery systems are available at diving site such as continuous-flow oxygen systems, nonrebreather or pocket masks, however, such equipment delivers modest oxygen fractions.

Question 4

1. Discuss physiology of blood flow in the heart.

At the start of the cardiac cycle, **(Fig. 2)** toward the end of diastole, the whole of the heart is relaxed. The atrioventricular (AV) valves are open because the atrial pressure is still slightly greater than the ventricular pressure. The semilunar valves are closed, as the pressure in the pulmonary artery and aorta is greater than the ventricular pressures. The cycle starts when the sinoatrial node (SAN) initiates atrial systole **(Table 3)**.

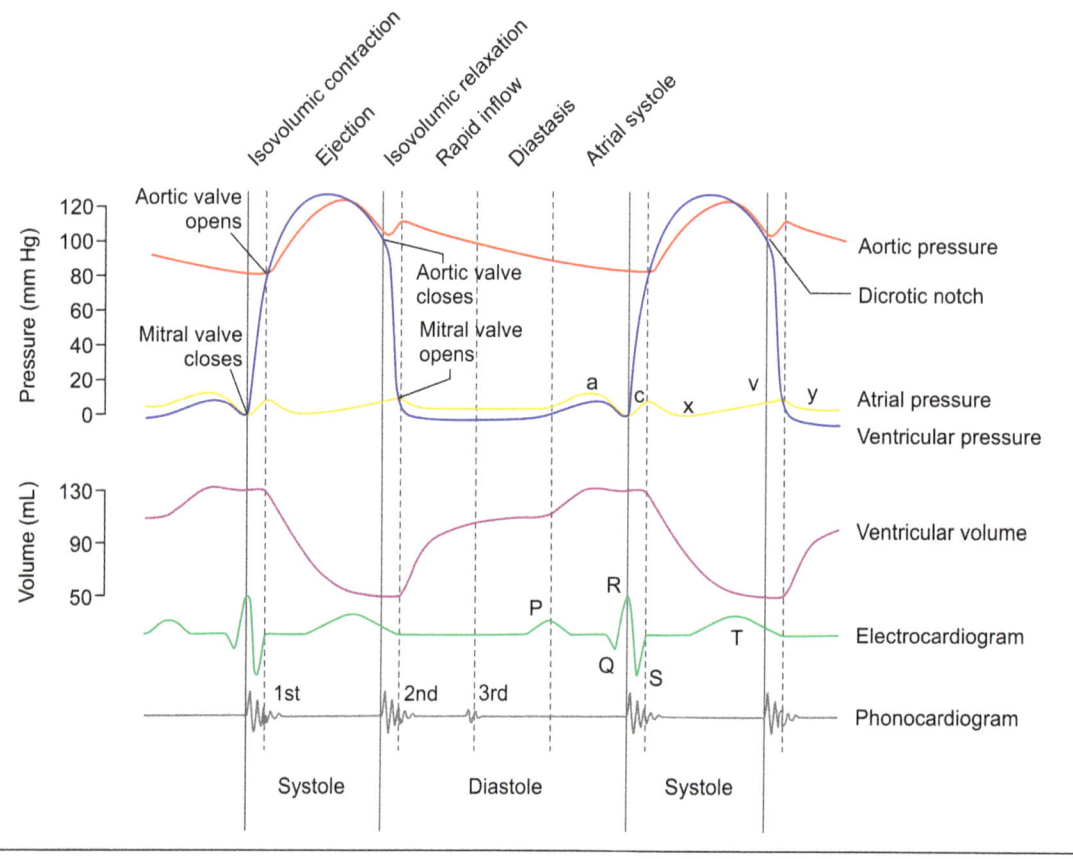

Fig. 2: Cardiac cycle.

TABLE 3: Cardiac cycle phases.

Cardiac cycle phase	Atrioventricular valves	Semilunar valves
Atrial systole	Open (atrial pressure > ventricular pressure)	Closed (arterial pressure > ventricular pressure)
Isovolumetric contraction	Closed (ventricular pressure > atrial pressure)	Closed (arterial pressure > ventricular pressure)
Ventricular ejection	Closed (ventricular pressure > atrial pressure)	Open (ventricular pressure > arterial pressure)
Isovolumetric relaxation	Closed (ventricular pressure > atrial pressure)	Closed (arterial pressure > ventricular pressure
Ventricular filling	Open (atrial pressure > ventricular pressure)	Closed (arterial pressure > ventricular pressure)

2. Explain POCUS in estimation of fluid volume in shock.

Rapid ultrasound in shock (RUSH) exam has gained popularity. This framework organizes the potential etiologies of shock into three broad, sonographically assessable systems that drive hemodynamics, simplified as **(Table 4)**:
a. *The Pump:* Cardiac function
b. *The Tank:* Intravascular volume status
c. *The Pipes:* Vascular emergencies in the venous and arterial system.

Careful evaluation of these components can enable clinicians to quickly identify the underlying etiology of shock in patients with undifferentiated hypotension and subsequently allow early initiation of the most appropriate treatment.

TABLE 4: POCUS in estimation of fluid volume in shock.

Pump	Tank	Pipes
• Estimate contractility of the heart to evaluate for cardiogenic shock and to determine ability to tolerate volume resuscitation • Identify the presence of pericardial effusion and tamponade • Evaluate for signs of right heart strain to indicate possible pulmonary embolism	• Determine the size and collapsibility of the inferior vena cava as a marker of volume status • Assess for the presence of free fluid in the peritoneum to indicate hypovolemic shock • Identify the presence of pneumothorax/tension pneumothorax • Evaluate the lung parenchyma for evidence of pulmonary edema associated with cardiogenic shock • Assess the costophrenic angles for evidence of pleural effusion/hemothorax	• Evaluate the thoracic and abdominal aorta for the presence of either an aneurysm (AAA) or dissection • Study the deep veins of the lower extremities to identify thrombus (DVT) when PE is a consideration

Question 5

1. Describe the anatomical characteristics of pediatric airway.

The pediatric airway is smaller in diameter and shorter in length than the adults. The young child's tongue is relatively larger in the oropharynx than the adults. The larynx in infants and young children is located more anteriorly compared with the adults **(Table 5)**.

2. How does pediatric airway differ from adult airway?

Differentiating features of pediatric and adult airway are as given in **Table 6**.

3. Enumerate steps of management of difficult pediatric airway.

A difficult airway as defined by the American Society of Anesthesiologists is difficulty with balloon mitral valvuloplasty (BMV), difficulty with tracheal intubation, or both. Other characteristics of the difficult airway include:

- More than two attempts at intubation with the same laryngoscopic blade,
- Need for a change in blade or use of intubation stylet, and
- Need for an alternative intubation technique or rescue.

The incidence of difficult pediatric airways in the emergency setting is not known, although the child who cannot be intubated and cannot be ventilated appears to be less common than the adult. As in adult patients, it is essential to anticipate difficult airway management in children in order to avoid the "cannot intubate, cannot ventilate" situation. Three questions will help guide management decisions:

1. Will I be able to bag-mask ventilate to maintain oxygenation?
2. Are laryngoscopy and intubation likely to be successful?
3. What rescue device, if needed, is most appropriate for this patient?

TABLE 5: Anatomical characteristics of pediatric airway.

Pediatric anatomy	Potential implications	Airway maneuvers
Large head and occiput	May push head forward, occluding airway	Shoulder roll should be used to align airway axes in infants
Large tongue	May occlude upper airway in sedated, obtunded, or paralyzed patient	Jaw thrust, chin lift, oral or nasopharyngeal airway
Floppy epiglottis	May obscure laryngeal view	Lifting the epiglottis directly with a straight blade, or potentially a curved blade may be necessary to visualize the glottis
Superior larynx and anterior cords	May make visualization of cords difficult	Shoulder roll may be required to align airway axes; video laryngoscopy may improve glottic view
Cricoid narrowing	Subglottic space is narrowest portion of the pediatric airway	Monitor cuff insufflation pressures in small children
Large adenoids and tonsils	May cause upper airway obstruction	Oral and nasal airway adjuncts may help; jaw thrust and chin lift are also likely to help
Small cricoid cartilage	Makes open cricothyrotomy technically difficult	Needle cricothyrotomy preferred in young children
Low gastroesophageal sphincter tone, relatively small lungs	Insufflation of stomach with bag-valve-mask ventilation or swallowed air can compromise respiratory status	Use proper bag-valve-mask ventilation technique; consider early placement of orogastric or nasogastric tube to deflate stomach when using positive pressure ventilation

TABLE 6: Difference between pediatric and adult airway.

Anatomical structure	Infant	Adult
Head	Larger prominent occiput resulting in sniffing position	Flat occiput
Tongue	Relatively larger	Relatively smaller
Larynx	Cephalad position, opposite C2 and C3 vertebrae	Opposite C4 to C6
Epiglottis	Omega shaped, soft	Flat, flexible
Vocal cords	Short, concave	Horizontal
Smallest diameter	Cricoid ring, below cords	Vocal cords
Cartilage	Soft, less calcified	Firm, calcified
Lower airway	Smaller, less developed	Larger, more cartilage

Emergent Pathway: Call for help. Call pediatric ENT. Pursue emergency oxygenation/ventilation options:

- Attempt "two-person two hand bag" mask ventilation
- Optimize jaw thrust/chin lift
- Consider oral and or nasal airway
- Insert laryngeal mask airways (LMA) or supraglottic device
- One quick attempt at direct laryngoscope by experienced operator
- Exclude laryngospasm and breath holding as possible etiology, treat accordingly.

If failed, consider awakening patient, emergency surgical airway, emergency cricothyrotomy, and rigid bronchoscopy by ENT.

Note: Surgical cricothyrotomy is contraindicated in children <10 years old because the cricothyroid membrane is too small. Therefore, in children <10 years of age, needle cricothyrotomy is the subglottic, invasive airway of choice.

Question 6

1. Discuss buffer systems, respiratory and renal regulation of acid-base balance.

Acid-base equilibrium is closely tied to fluid metabolism and electrolyte balance. A pH of 7.43–7.37 is required to maintain ideal homeostasis.

Acid-base physiology: CO_2 produced during metabolism combines with water (H_2O) in the blood to create carbonic acid (H_2CO_3), which dissociates into hydrogen ion (H^+) and bicarbonate (HCO_3^-). The H^+ binds with hemoglobin in red blood cells and is released with oxygenation in the alveoli, at which time the reaction is reversed by another form of carbonic anhydrase, creating water (H_2O), which is excreted by the kidneys, and CO_2 which gets exhaled.

Acid-base balance: It is maintained by chemical buffering, pulmonary activity, and renal activity.

Chemical buffering: Intracellular and extracellular buffers provide an immediate response to acid-base disturbances. An ideal buffer is made up of a weak acid and its conjugate base. The conjugate base can accept H^+ and the weak acid can relinquish it. The relationship between the pH of a buffer system and the concentration of its components is described by the Henderson–Hasselbalch equation:

$$pH = pK_a + \log[(\text{anion})/(\text{weak acid})]$$

where pK_a is the dissociation constant of the weak acid.

The most important extracellular buffer is the HCO_3^-/CO_2 system, described by the equation:

$$H^+ + HCO_3^- \leftrightarrow H_2CO_3 \leftrightarrow CO_2 + H_2O$$

An increase in H^+ drives the equation to the right and generates CO_2. CO_2 is controlled by alveolar ventilation while H^+ and HCO_3^- concentrations can be finely regulated by renal excretion. Other important chemical buffers include organic and inorganic phosphates and proteins such as hemoglobin and plasma proteins.

Pulmonary pH regulation: A decrease in pH leads to increases in tidal volume or respiratory rate thus facilitating elimination of CO_2. It is about 50–75% effective and takes minutes to hours to compensation.

Renal pH regulation: The kidneys control pH by adjusting the amount of HCO_3^- that is excreted or reabsorbed. HCO_3^- reabsorption occurs mostly in the proximal tubule and collecting tubule. The H_2O dissociates into H^+ and hydroxide (OH^-); in the presence of carbonic anhydrase, the OH^- combines with CO_2 to form HCO_3^-, which is transported back into the circulation. Acid is actively excreted into the proximal and distal tubules where it combines with urinary buffers such as phosphate (HPO_4^{-2}), creatinine, uric acid, and ammonia—to be excreted. The ammonia buffering system is especially important as the tubular cells actively regulate ammonia production in response to changes in acid load.

2. Describe the difference between arterial blood gas (ABG) and venous blood gas (VBG).

a. *pH:* The pH between a VBG and ABG correlates closely and accurately measures the severity of an acidosis. The average VBG pH is 0.03–0.04 less than the ABG pH values **(Table 7)**.

b. *pCO_2 and pO_2:* Venous and arterial measured values drastically differ as venous blood carries significant amount of CO_2 while arterial blood carries high levels of O_2.

c. *Bicarbonate:* The bicarbonate (HCO_3) correlates well between arterial and venous samples with a difference of 0.52–1.5 mmol/L.
d. *Lactate:* The lactate level correlates well between arterial and venous blood gases, with a mean difference of 0.02–0.08.
e. *Base deficit:* Arterial and venous base deficit values correlate and do not lead to clinically significant differences.

TABLE 7: Difference between arterial blood gas (ABG) and venous blood gas (VBG).

Parameters	ABG	VBG	Arteriovenous (A-V) difference
pH	7.35–7.45	7.31–7.41	~0.4
pCO_2 (kPa)	4.7–6.0	5.5–6.8	~0.6
pCO_2 (mm Hg)	35–45	41–51	~6
Bicarbonate (mmol/L)	22–28	23–29	~1
pO_2 (kPa)	10.6–13.3	4.0–5.3	~8.0
pO_2 (mm Hg)	80–100	30–40	~55
SO_2 (%)	>95	75	>20

3. Discuss acid-base disorders in trauma.

- In the trauma setting, acidosis is due to hypoperfusion secondary to hemorrhagic shock.
- Without oxygen supply, peripheral tissues switch to anaerobic metabolism, increasing the production of lactic acid.
- Impact on body's most vital functions such as control of ventilation, perfusion of pulmonary capillaries, diffusion across the alveolar membrane, and binding and unbinding of hemoglobin.
- Metabolic acidosis decreases cardiac contractility, even in cases of moderate metabolic acidosis (pH <7.20).
- Thereby decreasing cardiac contractility and by causing alterations in membrane polarization thus increasing arrhythmias.
- Acidosis also causes increased pulmonary vascular resistance, resulting in increased afterload on a right ventricle.
- Extreme acidosis leads to vasodilation refractory to common vasopressors and inotropes, requiring much higher doses.
- Acidosis in the hemorrhaging patient has its impact on hemostasis as it exacerbates the triad of acidosis, hypothermia, and coagulopathy.
- Management of extreme acidosis in trauma patients aims to improve tissue perfusion, buffering, respiratory elimination, and renal elimination.
- As the metabolic acidosis in trauma patients with hemorrhagic shock is due to decreased tissue perfusion, it can be improved by intravascular resuscitation along with control of hemorrhage and blood transfusion if required.
- Treatment of additional electrolyte abnormalities, like hyperkalemia is vital
- Rapid resuscitation of intravascular volume, maintenance of peripheral perfusion, and correction of coagulopathy are mainstream management.
- Administration of buffer, hyperventilation, and renal replacement therapy may also play a supporting role in the resuscitation of extreme acidosis in trauma.

Question 7

1. Explain the physiology of adrenal hormone secretion.

Adrenal gland is capsulated retroperitoneal organ divided *into two zones outer part known as adrenal cortex and outer adrenal medulla*. Adrenal cortex further subdivided into three zones—(1) *Zona fasciculata* which secrets glucocorticoid (cortisol). (2) *Zona reticularis* secrets the DHEA (dehydroepiandrosterone acetate) which is the intermediate metabolite for sex steroids androgen and estrogen. *Zona glomerulosa* secrets mineralocorticoids (aldosterone). (3) *Adrenal medulla* secretes catecholamines, epinephrine, and norepinephrine. Important functions of adrenal hormone are summarized in **Table 8**.

TABLE 8: Important functions of adrenal hormone.

System	Physiological response
Cardiovascular	Maintain cardiac contractility cardiac function and vascular tone thus provide cardiovascular stability
Endocrine	Inhibit insulin secretion, epinephrine synthesis
Inflammatory	Maintain inflammatory homeostasis, anti-inflammatory action of cortisol, reduce circulating leukocyte and cytokines response, eosinophils, and lymphocytes
Metabolic	• Gluconeogenesis lipolysis, muscle protein catabolism • Raise plasma glucose during stress
Renal	Increase in glomerular filtration rate

2. What is the management of adrenal crisis?

Adrenal crisis is endocrine emergency and should be considered in acutely unwell patient with profound unexplained circulatory shock. Severity depends on level of defect, primary or secondary etiology [hypothalamic-pituitary-adrenal (HPA) axis]. Initial diagnosis is completely based on clinical evaluation. Detailed history, physical examination, and investigation are helpful in evaluating the patient (subacute, chronic symptoms) in outpatient department but not very helpful in emergency department. High index of suspicious is important for diagnosis of adrenal crisis in emergency department. *Emergency physician should start the empiric treatment immediately even before receiving the confirmatory laboratory results.* One may not get classic laboratory results in acute adrenal failure like adrenal hemorrhage.

Confirmatory diagnostic testing: Patient with all forms of adrenal deficiency has low cortisol level. Low serum cortisol level and inadequate response to stimulation test confirm the diagnosis.

1. *First step* is early morning serum cortisol <3 µg/dL to confirm the adrenal deficiency while diagnosis is doubtful when cortisol level >15 µg/dL.
2. *Second step* is to find out if cortisol deficiency is due to adrenocorticotropic hormone (ACTH) or corticotropin-releasing hormone (CRH) deficiency, give 250 µg of synthetic ACTH (cosyntropin) and measure the serum cortisol if serum cortisol >8 µg within 30 minutes, considered normal response, and exclude primary adrenal deficiency, but basal corticotropin level is required to differentiate between primary and secondary adrenal deficiency. Corticotropin level is high in primary and low or normal in secondary adrenal deficiency. Insulin tolerance test is a test of choice for suspected secondary adrenal failure.
3. But in emergency department and in crisis situation both above method of diagnosis, early morning cortisol level and stimulation test are not practical, random serum cortisol level >34 µg/dL excludes the adrenal deficiency while random cortisol level below 15 µg/dL in patient with severe sepsis or shock suggestive of acute adrenal crisis.

Empiric treatment for adrenal crisis before confirm laboratory results:

- Hydrocortisone is drug of choice it has both glucocorticoid and mineralocorticoid properties.
- Empiric antibiotics can be started depending on underlying conditions.
- Fresh frozen plasm to reverse coagulopathy.
- Hyperkalemia should be corrected.
- Thyroxine supplementation requirement in primary HPA axis failure (clinical hypothyroidism).
- Correction of dehydration and hypoglycemia.
- Vasopressors.

Treatment of adrenal crisis **(Table 9)** condition is straight forward with parenteral administration of 100 mg of hydrocortisone intravenously as bolus along with correction of hypovolemia with 1,000 mL of isotonic saline within first 1 hour, followed by 50–100 mg hydrocortisone in 5% dextrose every 6 hourly intravenously or intramuscularly depending on age and body surface area. In case hydrocortisone is not at disposal, then any other synthetic glucocorticoid such as prednisolone can be used in proportionate doses.

Long-term hormone replacement therapy should be initiated once patient is recovered from crisis, IV steroid should be changed to oral preparation and prednisolone with longer half-life is required only once daily. Fludrocortisone (mineralocorticoid) is usually given in patient with primary adrenal failure. Androgen transdermal DHEA 25–50 mg is also added for primary adrenal failure.

TABLE 9: Treatment guidelines for acute adrenal crisis.

Fluid resuscitation	At least 2–3 L of normal saline to restore volume and normal sodium balance
Intravenous steroids	Intravenous hydrocortisone 100 mg bolus followed by 100 mg two or three times per day (300–400 mg daily is initial regimen)
Antibiotics	Broad spectrum antibiotics for febrile patient
Vasopressors	In case of refractory shock
Glucose	50% dextrose may be used if required
In stabilized patient	• Oral prednisolone fludrocortisone and androgen replacement • Patient education regarding steroid management during acute febrile illness (double the dose of steroid for 3 days) regular follow-up with physician

Question 8

1. Discuss physiology of hemostasis.

Physiology of hemostasis: The normal hemostatic system consists of a complex process that limits blood loss through the formation of a platelet (primary hemostasis) and the production of cross-linked fibrin (secondary hemostasis), which strengthens the platelet plug. These reactions are counterregulated by the fibrinolytic system **(Flowchart 2)**. Hemostasis is a process of balance between the coagulation and the fibrinolytic system. The coagulation system consists of two main components—primary and secondary hemostasis.

- *Primary hemostasis:* In a normal adult, when the vascular subendothelial surface is exposed due to injury to a vessel, platelets interact with the exposed collagen forming a platelet plug at the site of injury to arrest the initial site of ooze, with the help of von Willebrand factor which connects the platelet to the vascular subendothelium and fibrinogen that helps in binding of platelets together.

This process occurs within 20 seconds of injury and needs to be stabilized by secondary hemostasis.

- *Secondary hemostasis (coagulation cascade):* The secondary hemostasis consists of two different pathways named intrinsic and extrinsic pathway.

The intrinsic pathway begins by the activation of factor XII by the damaged vascular surface that further results in activation of factors XI, IX, and finally factor X. The extrinsic pathway is activated by the conversion of factor VII to its activated form, which directly helps in activation of factor X. These pathways finally merge at the point of factor X activation. Following the activation of the factor X, a common pathway is followed that results in formation of cross linked fibrin clot which on deposition stabilizes the primary homeostasis.

Fibrinolytic system: The fibrinolytic system limits the size of the fibrin clot. Plasminogen is synthesized in liver and is activated to form plasmin by tissue plasminogen activator which is released from the endothelial cells. Plasmin degrades fibrinogen and fibrin monomer into low-molecular weight fragments, thus limiting the clot size.

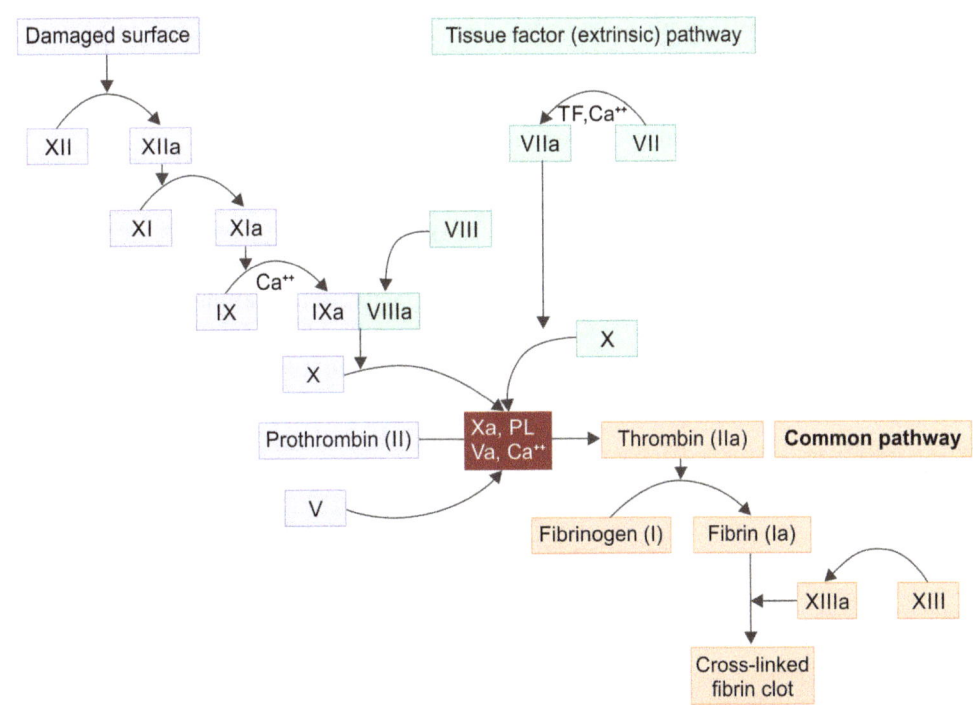

Flowchart 2: Physiology of hemostasis extrinsic and intrinsic pathways.

2. What are the tests of primary and secondary hemostasis?

Test for primary hemostasis:
Platelet count: Normal value 150–400,000/mm^3
Bleeding time: Normal range 2.5–10.0 min

Tests for secondary hemostasis:
Prothrombin time (PT) and international normalized ratio (INR): Normal value 11–13 s—prolonged in case of warfarin usage which inhibits production of vitamin K-dependent clotting factors and in case of liver disease and antibiotics such as moxalactam, cefoperazone, cefotaxime that inhibit vitamin K-dependent factors.

Activated partial thromboplastin time (aPTT): Normal range 22–34 s—prolonged due to heparin therapy, factor deficiencies.

Fibrinogen level: Normal range 200–400 mg/dL—reduced in case of DIC (disseminated intravascular coagulation); increased in case of inflammatory processes as it is an acute-phase reactant.

Thrombin clotting time normal range: 10–12 s—can be prolonged in case of low fibrinogen level, abnormal fibrinogen molecule (liver disease), heparin usage, FDP (fibrin degradation products), multiple myeloma.

3. What is von Willebrand disease?

Most common bleeding disorder can be congenital (heterogeneously inherited) or acquired [due to formation of auto antibodies against von Willebrand factor (vWF)]. von Willebrand disease occurs due to either decreased production of vWF (type 1) or production of abnormal vWF which is dysfunctional (type 2) or no production at all (type 3). Skin and mucosal bleed is the most common form of presentation.

Common lab abnormalities seen include prolonged bleeding time, low or normal vWF antigen, low vWF activity. It is difficult to distinguish between hemophilia A and von Willebrand disease due to the variability in vWF level.

Treatment can be non-transfusion and transfusion. Non-transfusion therapy includes usage of desmopressin as it induces the release of vWF from storage sites within the endothelium. It can cause 2-4-fold increase in vWF. The dose shall be repeated in 24 hours but the effectiveness is marked reduced due to depleted storage. Due to desmopressin's antidiuretic property, fluids to be restricted to prevent hyponatremia.

Transfusion therapy includes administration of recombinant vWF 40-50 IU/kg for minor bleed, 50-80 IU/kg for major bleed. Platelet transfusion can be tried in type 3 who do not respond to vWF products. Cryoprecipitates are reserved for life-threatening emergencies.

Question 9

1. Discuss physiology of urine formation.

About 180 L of fluid is filtered at the glomerulus. The filtrate is reabsorbed later by the different portions (four major sites) of the nephron while leaving 1.5 L of urine production to exit the body daily **(Fig. 3)**.

Site 1: *Proximal tubule* absorption of Na^+ K^+ Cl^- glucose, amino acid, urea, HCO_3^- and water secretion of creatinine and H^+. The sodium transport occurs mainly via:

a. Direct entry of sodium along the electrochemical gradient.
b. Transport of Na^+ and K^+ coupled to active reabsorption of glucose, amino acids and other anions.
c. Exchange with H^+. Hence K^+ is effectively reabsorbed in the proximal tubule, creating an isotonic fluid with marked change in the composition.

Site 2: *Ascending Loop of Henle-Absorption of Na Cl K^+* occurs via Na^+ K^+ ATPase at the basolateral membrane located in the medullary portion of Ascending limb of loop of Henle. Thus, accumulation of sodium in the medullary interstitium with no water absorption results in an osmotic gradient facilitating reabsorption of water from descending loop of Henle.

Site 3: *Cortical diluting segment of loop of Henle:* This portion of the nephron is not permeable to water hence Na^+ absorption occurs through Na^+ Cl^- symporter, thus diluting the fluid.

Site 4: *Distal tubule (DT) and collecting duct (CD)* reabsorption of sodium, urea and chloride along with water: Sodium gets actively reabsorbed with passive diffusion of Cl^- and secretion of K^+ and H^+. Sodium absorption in this segment is facilitated via amiloride sensitive sodium channel hence controlled by aldosterone. Thus, the blood that is filtered at the glomerulus as glomerular filtrate passes through proximal convoluted tubule, loop of Henle, distal convoluted tubule, collecting duct undergoes absorption and secretion at various segments to finally result in formation of urine.

2. What is the mechanism of action of various classes of diuretic drugs?

High efficacy diuretic these drugs: For example, sulphonyl derivatives most potent drugs are furosemide, bumetanide, torsemide. These drugs inhibit Na^+ K^+ $-2Cl^-$ cotransport inhibitors at the ascending loop of Henle hence called loop diuretics. They are very effective in management of edema, acute pulmonary edema, cerebral edema, hypertension, and hypercalcemia off malignancy.

Medium efficacy diuretics: Benzothiadiazides (thiazides) such as hydrochlorothiazide, benzthiazide, hydroflumethiazide, bendroflumethiazide**.** Thiazide such as chlorthalidone, metolazone, xipamide, indapamide, clopamide. These drugs act by inhibiting Na^+-Cl^- symport at the early distal convoluted tubule; predominantly used in edema, hypertension, diabetes insipidus, hypercalciuria.

Weak or adjunctive diuretic: Carbonic anhydrase inhibitors like acetazolamide inhibits are used mainly in glaucoma, epilepsy, acute mountain sickness, periodic paralysis and to alkalinize urine.

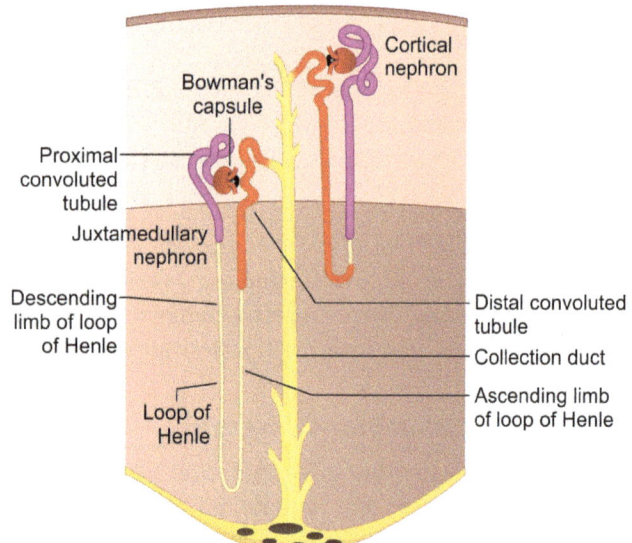

Fig. 3: Physiology of urine formation.

Potassium sparing diuretics: Aldosterone antagonist–spironolactone, eplerenone—inhibits renal epithelial sodium channels at the late distal convoluted tubule and at collecting duct. *Inhibitors of renal epithelial Na+ channel*—triamterene, amiloride—are used to counteract K⁺ loss due to thiazides and loop diuretics, edema, hypertension, congestive cardiac failure. *Osmotic diuretics* such as mannitol, isosorbide, and glycerol create an osmotic gradient and dilute luminal fluid at the proximal convoluted tubule, also increase the extracellular volume thus increasing the renal blood flow. Highly indicated in case of increased intracranial or intraocular tension, to maintain glomerular filtration rate, to counteract low plasma osmolarity.

3. What are the complications of diuretics?

Hypokalemia: Predominantly noted with thiazide and acetazolamide due to loss of potassium.

Acute saline depletion: Overuse of high efficacy drugs can result in excessive diuresis.

Dilutional hyponatremia: It occurs in patients with congestive cardiac failure especially with use of high efficacy agents. Kidney is unable to retain salt due to diuresis but able to retain water, hence causing dilutional hyponatremia.

Gastrointestinal (GI) disturbances: Nausea, vomiting, and diarrhea are common with all diuretics.

Central nervous system (CNS) disturbances: Headache, giddiness, weakness, paresthesia can occur in patients on thiazides and loop diuretics, mental confusion, drowsiness, ataxia can occur with spironolactone.

Allergic reaction: It can occur to any diuretic.

Hyperuricemia: Long-term, high dose of thiazides can cause increase in blood urate levels.

Magnesium depletion: Long-term use of thiazides and loop diuretics can cause magnesium loss resulting in cardiac arrhythmias.

Bone marrow depression: Rarely seen in patients using acetazolamide.

Hypocalcemia: It can be seen in high efficacy drugs on chronic intake.

Hearing loss: It occurs due to increased salt content of endolymph caused by use of high efficacy agents in patients with renal insufficiency.

Question 10

1. Discuss anticonvulsants.

Antiepileptic drug **(Table 10)** mainly acts on three different mechanisms:
- Prolongation of sodium channel inactivation
- Facilitation of gamma-aminobutyric acid (GABA) mediated Cl⁻ channel opening
- Inhibition of T type calcium current.

2. Explain anti-arrhythmic drugs.

There are four main classes of anti-arrhythmic drugs **(Table 11)**.

TABLE 10: Choice of antiepileptic drugs for specific type of seizures.

	Seizures			Epilepsies	
	Partial seizures and localization- related seizures	**Tonic-clonic**	**Generalized absence**	**Myoclonic**	**Atonic/tonic**
First-line drugs	• Carbamazepine • Phenytoin • Lamotrigine • Valproate • Oxcarbazepine	• Valproate • Lamotrigine • Phenytoin • Carbamazepine	• Ethosuximide • Valproate	• Valproate • Lamotrigine • Topiramate	• Valproate • Lamotrigine • Topiramate
Second-line drugs	• Primidone • Phenobarbital • Felbamate	• Topiramate • Primidone • Phenobarbital • Felbamate	• Topiramate • Lamotrigine • Clonazepam	• Primidone • Phenobarbital • Clonazepam • Ethosuximide • Felbamate	• Phenytoin • Phenobarbital • Primidone • Clonazepam • Felbamate
Add-on drugs	• Topiramate • Levetiracetam • Zonisamide • Gabapentin • Tiagabine	• Levetiracetam • Zonisamide	Zonisamide	• Levetiracetam • Zonisamide	• Levetiracetam • Zonisamide

- Decision regarding stopping the antiepileptic should be taken only after consulting the pediatric neurologist.
- Recurrence of seizure can occur when following abnormalities are present.
- Neurologic abnormalities, mental retardation, complex partial seizures, consistently abnormal electroencephalograms.

TABLE 11: Classification of anti-arrhythmic drugs.

	IA	IB	IC
Class I • Membrane stabilizing (Na channel blockers) • Class I A-Moderately prolong conduction • Class I B-Minimal effect on conduction • Class I C-Marked prolongation of conduction	• Quinidine • Procainamide • Disopyramide	• Lidocaine • Mexiletine	• Propafenone • Flecainide
Class II (Blockade of β-adrenergic receptors)	• Propranolol • Esmolol • Sotalol (class III properties also)		
Class III (Prolongation of repolarization)	• Amiodarone • Dronedarone • Dofetilide • Ibutilide		
Class IV (Calcium-channel blockers)	• Verapamil • Diltiazem		
Drugs for paroxysmal supraventricular tachycardia	• Adenosine • Digoxin		

SUGGESTED READING

1. Richhariya D, Sharma B. Textbook of Emergency Medicine including Intensive Care and Trauma, 2nd edition. New Delhi: Jaypee Brothers Medical Publishers (P) Ltd; 2022. pp. 355-56, 362. (Question 1).
2. Richhariya D, Sharma B. Textbook of Emergency Medicine including Intensive Care and Trauma, 2nd edition. New Delhi: Jaypee Brothers Medical Publishers (P) Ltd; 2022. pp. 1692-6. (Question 2).
3. Richhariya D, Sharma B. Textbook of Emergency Medicine including Intensive Care and Trauma, 2nd edition. New Delhi: Jaypee Brothers Medical Publishers (P) Ltd; 2022. pp. 1697-1700, 1708-11. (Question 3).
4. Richhariya D, Sharma B. Textbook of Emergency Medicine including Intensive Care and Trauma, 2nd edition. New Delhi: Jaypee Brothers Medical Publishers (P) Ltd; 2022. pp. 364-73. (Question 4).
5. Richhariya D, Sharma B. Textbook of Emergency Medicine including Intensive Care and Trauma, 2nd edition. New Delhi: Jaypee Brothers Medical Publishers (P) Ltd; 2022. pp. 1124-34. (Question 5).
6. Richhariya D, Sharma B. Textbook of Emergency Medicine including Intensive Care and Trauma, 2nd edition. New Delhi: Jaypee Brothers Medical Publishers (P) Ltd; 2022. pp. 304-10. (Question 6).
7. Richhariya D, Sharma B. Textbook of Emergency Medicine including Intensive Care and Trauma, 2nd edition. New Delhi: Jaypee Brothers Medical Publishers (P) Ltd; 2022. pp. 893-8. (Question 7).
8. Richhariya D, Sharma B. Textbook of Emergency Medicine including Intensive Care and Trauma, 2nd edition. New Delhi: Jaypee Brothers Medical Publishers (P) Ltd; 2022. pp. 536-40. (Question 8).
9. Richhariya D, Sharma B. Textbook of Emergency Medicine including Intensive Care and Trauma, 2nd edition. New Delhi: Jaypee Brothers Medical Publishers (P) Ltd; 2022. pp. 743-60. (Question 9).
10. Richhariya D, Sharma B. Textbook of Emergency Medicine including Intensive Care and Trauma, 2nd edition. New Delhi: Jaypee Brothers Medical Publishers (P) Ltd; 2022. pp. 836, 1213. (Question 10).
11. Richhariya D, Sharma B. Textbook of Emergency Medicine including Intensive Care and Trauma, 2nd edition. New Delhi: Jaypee Brothers Medical Publishers (P) Ltd; 2022. p. 480. (Question 10).

Emergency Medicine Paper 34

Subbulakshmi Dhanabal, Narendra Nath Jena

Question 1

1. Differentiate between neurogenic and spinal shock.

All these types of shocks are associated with tachycardia, whereas neurogenic shock is associated with bradycardia. The term "spinal shock" denotes the acute loss of motor, sensory and reflex functions below the level of injury and can be associated with neurogenic shock **(Table 1)**.

TABLE 1: Differentiate between neurogenic and spinal shock.

	Neurogenic shock	Spinal shock
Definition	Sudden loss of the sympathetic nervous system signals	Immediate temporary loss of total power, sensation, and reflex below the level of injury
Mechanism	Disruption of autonomic pathway → loss of sympathetic tone and vasodilation	Peripheral neuron becomes temporarily unresponsive to brain stimuli
BP	Hypotension	Hypotension
Pulse	Bradycardia	Bradycardia
Motor	Flaccid paralysis	Variable
Time	48–72 hours immediately	After spinal cord injury
Bulbocavernosus reflex	Absent	Variable

2. Explain the differences in children to be considered in treating spinal cord injury.

Acute spinal cord injury (SCI) occurs when spinal cord is damaged from an accident such as fall, sports injury, or during birth. SCI is a common cause of long-lasting disability and death in children. SCI is a medical emergency. Spine cord injury without radiographic abnormality is a unique pediatric entity, which is more common in thoracic spine region. The first treatment starts at the site of accident—keep the child as still as possible by using SPINE board for transportation. Flaccid paralysis with hypotension and relative bradycardia indicates neurogenic shock, in which early administration of vasopressors is indicated. Aggressive fluid management (not indicated) results in worsening of spinal cord edema. Corticosteroids are not recommended in children as they may increase the risk of infection and do not result in significant neurological outcomes.

Rehabilitation: It is most important to focus on maximizing the child's ability at home and in the community. We can encourage to strengthen his or her self-esteem and have independence.

Preventing muscle from wasting and contracture is a valid role in rehabilitation.

3. Discuss management of mild traumatic brain injury in the emergency room (ER).

The most common symptoms leading the patient to visit ER following a mild traumatic brain injury are headache, nausea and dizziness.

Headache: Post-traumatic headache is treated mostly with acetaminophen and non-steroidal anti-inflammatory drugs (NSAIDs) (ibuprofen and naproxen). Headache associated with migraine is treated using intravenous (IV) dopamine antagonist (metoclopramide, prochlorperazine, and chlorpromazine) and ketorolac. Prolonged or debilitating post-concussive headache—refer to a neurologist. Treatment may include gabapentin, valproic acid, topiramate, amitriptyline, carbamazepine, and cyproheptadine.

Nausea: Ondansetron is recommended for significant nausea and difficulty in tolerating liquids. Physical and cognitive rest should be considered. Patient must be kept in a well hydrated manner.

Dizziness: Concussion-associated dizziness mostly resolves with rest. It may also occur due to injury to vestibular system. In case of prolonged symptom, vestibular rehabilitation may be helpful.

Question 2

A 10-year-old boy presents to the ER with severe pain in his eye, watering, and photophobia. He says that he was hit in the eye while playing ball.

1. Discuss differential diagnosis of acute painful eye.

Mild pain:
- Blepharitis
- Dacryocystitis
- Superficial keratitis
- Preseptal cellulitis
- Episcleritis

Moderate pain:
- Corneal abrasion
- Corneal ulcer
- Corneal foreign body
- Chemical burns
- Endophthalmitis

Severe pain:
- Acute angle closure glaucoma
- Iritis/uveitis
- Scleritis
- Ultraviolet keratitis

Pain with movement:
- Orbital cellulitis

Eyelid pain:
- Chalazion
- Hordeolum.

2. What is the use of ultrasonography (USG) in ocular trauma?

Ultrasonography (USG) helps to detect wide variety of ocular pathologies from trauma such as dislocated lens, globe disruption, vitreous hemorrhage, hyphemia, retinal detachment orbital emphysema, retrobulbar hemorrhage. Suspected globe rupture is a relative contraindication to USG examination due to risk of extruding globe contents with direct pressure on and around the eye.

Globe rupture: Distortion of normal shape of globe, decrease in size of globe anterior chamber collapse, vitreous hemorrhage.

Lens dislocation: Highly reflective oval mass moving, independently of the surrounding, structure with eye movement.

Hyphema: Echoic structure of variable echogenicity, depending on age of bleed.

Retrobulbar hemorrhage: Echo lucent posterior to globe.

3. Describe the management of corneal abrasion in the ER.

Majority of the corneal abrasion heals spontaneously, so the primary aim is to relieve pain and prevent infection. Topical NSAIDs such as ketorolac and diclofenac relieve pain; topical tetracycline—1 drop hourly for 24 hours to prevent infection. Patching of the eye does not provide healing, but some patients feel better. Abrasions from fingernails, vegetable matter or contact lens should not be patched as it may increase the risk of infection. If abrasion is large and spasm is marked, consider topical cyclopentolate 1%—one drop 3 times a day along with topical antibiotics. Large and small abrasion in the central visual axis should be checked by ophthalmologist within 24 hours and 48-72 hours respectively.

4. Explain the management of chemical ocular injury in the ER.

The common chemical injuries to eye are alkali, acid, and cyanoacrylate (super glue). Alkali injuries tend to be more serious than acid injuries because they cause liquefactive necrosis that allows deep penetration into tissue. In case of acid injuries, it causes coagulative necrosis that acts as a barrier to further tissue penetration.

Treatment: Irrigation at the scene and continue in the ER. Instill topical anesthetic and continue irrigation for at least 30 minutes. Then check the pH by touching a strip of litmus paper to the inferior conjunctival fornix. If pH is >7.4, continue irrigation until pH remains neutral. Irrigation should be done using normal saline or isotonic solution by hand or through *Morgan lens*. After irrigation, perform eye examination and inspect facial skin and eyelids for burns. Evert the eyelids and remove any particulate matter with cotton. Document visual acuity and measure intraocular pressure; use slit lamp to evaluate corneal injury. The cornea may become cloudy with severe burns. Identify the chemical substance, note the pH (usually mentioned in the bottle), in case of pH <12 and >2, it does not cause serious injury, but duration of exposure increases the severity. Patient with chemosis/chemical conjunctivitis can apply erythromycin ointment 4 times a day.

Topical cyclopentolate 1%—one drop, 3 times a day to relieve pain.

Administer tetanus toxoid. Consider doxycycline 100 mg BD and topical corticosteroids to reduce corneal melting and corneal inflammation respectively.

In case of cyanoacrylate (super glue)—install generous amount of erythromycin ointment onto the eye and surrounding the eyelid—to moisture, lubricate, and antibiotic coverage.

Clumps of glue begin to loosen, remove only those pieces that are easily removable. Gentle traction may separate the lids. Glue will loose and become easier to remove in a few days.

Refer to ophthalmologist within 24 hours for complete removal.

Question 3

1. What are the infectious and noninfectious causes of sore throat?

Pain or a scratchy sensation in the throat, pain that worsens with swallowing or talking, difficulty swallowing, fever, cough—many conditions can cause a sore throat on one side, including tonsillitis, laryngitis, canker sores, and tooth infections **(Table 2)**.

TABLE 2: Infectious and noninfectious causes of sore throat.

Infectious cause		Noninfectious cause
Viral	Bacterial	• GERD
• Rhinovirus	• *Streptococcus pyogenes*	• Smoking
• Coronavirus	• *Fusobacterium necrophorum*	• Dry air
• Adenovirus		• Irritation (due to allergy)
• Herpes simplex virus	• *Streptococcus dysgalactiae*	• Inflammation
• Parainfluenza	• *Neisseria gonorrhoeae*	
• Influenza	• *Corynebacterium diphtheriae*	
• Respiratory syncytial virus	• *Arcanobacterium haemolyticum*	
• Coxsackie virus A	• *Chlamydia*	
• Epstein–Barr virus	• *Chlamydia pneumoniae*	
• Cytomegalovirus	• *Mycoplasma*	
• HIV type 1	• *Mycoplasma pneumoniae*	

(GERD: gastroesophageal reflux disease; HIV: human immunodeficiency virus)

2. Explain the red flag symptoms and signs of acute sore throat.

- Toxic appearance
- Shock
- Fever >2 weeks
- Duration of sore throat >2 weeks
- Trismus
- Drooling
- Cyanosis
- Hemorrhage
- Asymmetric tonsillar swelling
- Respiratory distress
- Suspicion of parapharyngeal space infection
- Suspicion of diphtheria
- Apnea
- Severe, unremitting pain
- "Hot potato" voice
- Chest or neck pain
- Weight loss.

3. Discuss risk stratification and investigation for sore throat.

Risk factors:
- Age: 3–15 years
- Exposure to tobacco smoke
- Allergies
- Exposure to chemical irritants
- Chronic sinus infection
- Close quarters
- Weakened immunity

Investigations:
- Complete blood count
- Throat swab for culture and sensitivity
- Rapid antigen diagnostic test.

4. What is the empirical management of patient with acute sore throat?

- *In case of viral infection (most common cause):* Symptomatic treatment—oral hydration, antipyretics, analgesics, rest, and IV fluids (if not tolerating orally).
- In case of bacterial infection [*Streptococcus*—group A beta-hemolytic streptococci (GABHS)]: Single dose IM benzathine penicillin G (1.2 million units), penicillin VK 500 mg BD × 10 days (or amoxicillin 500 mg).
- First generation cephalosporin or clindamycin (if penicillin allergy or resistant).
- Single dose PO or IM dexamethasone (in immunocompromised).

Question 4

1. Discuss open pneumothorax.

It is also referred to as a *communicating pneumothorax*, associated with a defect in the chest wall. More common in combat injuries, but is also seen with civilian gunshot wounds. Air can sometimes be heard flowing loudly in and out of the defect, prompting the term "sucking chest wound". The loss of chest wall integrity causes the involved lung to paradoxically collapse on inspiration and expand slightly on expiration, forcing air in and out of the wound. Immediate treatment involves placing an occlusive dressing over the wound (three-sided occlusive dressing) **(Fig. 1)**, which helps convert the injury to a closed pneumothorax. One side of the dressing should be left untapped to prevent conversion of the injury to a tension pneumothorax.

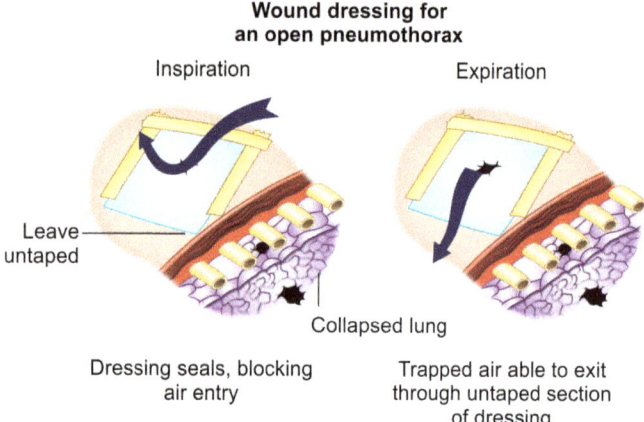

Fig. 1: Three-sided occlusive dressing.

2. Describe rib fractures.

The most common bony injuries in chest trauma are rib fractures. It is a painful injury, heals slowly, closely associated with mortality and morbidity. Principle diagnostic goal with clinically suspected rib fractures is detection of significant complications such as hemopneumothorax, pulmonary contusion, intra-abdominal injuries and major vessel injuries. Perform serial chest imaging to evaluate for developing pneumothorax; presence of rib fractures in any patient with localized pain and tenderness over one or more ribs after chest trauma. It takes great force to fracture the 1st and 2nd, such fractures may lead to blunt myocardial injury, bronchial tears, and major vessel injury. Multiple rib fractures, middle (5th–8th) and lower (9th–12th) with unexplained hypotension is a result of intra-abdominal bleeding mainly from liver or spleen. Consider doing CT scan or USG of abdomen with middle or lower segment rib fractures. A total of 50% of rib fractures are not apparent on conventional radiograph, furthermore injuries to cartilaginous portion may never be appreciated. US remains a promising diagnostic tool for rib fractures and cartilaginous injuries.

Treatment: Do not immobilize chest wall with tape or binder. For mild to moderate pain—use adequate analgesics with combination of opioids, benzodiazepines, topical lidocaine patch, and NSAIDs. For severe pain, intercostal nerve block or serratus anterior plane block using long acting bupivacaine can be used. Epidural analgesics may be a better choice than IV opioids. In complications such as pneumothorax (moderate to severe), tension pneumothorax, hemopneumothorax—needle decompression followed by intercostal drainage tube can be placed.

Complications: Pain due to rib fractures can greatly interfere with ventilation, leading to splinting, and atelectasis. Prolong the time for weaning from ventilator support. Patient will have difficulty coughing and adequately clearing the secretions, especially elderly and preexisting pulmonary pathology, such patients need observation for 24–48 hours.

Flail chest: Segmental fractures of three or more adjacent ribs anteriorly or laterally often result in an unstable chest wall physiology known as flail chest. This injury is characterized by a paradoxical inward movement of the involved chest wall segment during spontaneous inspiration and outward movement during expiration (**Fig. 2**).

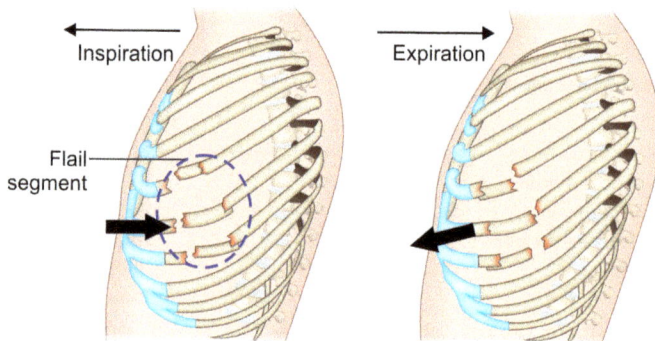

Fig. 2: Flail chest.

3. Explain the role of ultrasound in the ER in chest trauma.

Point of care ultrasonography (POCUS) can quickly diagnose pneumothorax, hemothorax, and pericardial tamponade as part of the extended focused assessment with sonography in trauma (FAST) examination. In trained hands, US has greater sensitivity and equal specificity for detecting hemothorax in patients with chest trauma compared with chest radiography. Likewise, the sensitivity of US for detecting pneumothorax approaches 92%, with near 100% specificity (as compared with 50–80% sensitivity and 90% specificity for chest radiographs); thus, US appears to have greater "diagnostic performance" than clinical examination and chest radiograph together. US in the ED can detect occult pneumothorax as accurately as CT. In addition, US has also been found helpful for describing small, medium, or large pneumothorax with good agreement with CT.

Question 5

A 28-year-old female presents to the ER with vaginal bleeding. She has lost about 200–250 mL of blood. She has had a normal vaginal delivery about 48 hours prior to the presentation.

1. What are the causes of postpartum hemorrhage?

The causes of postpartum hemorrhage are called the four Ts (tone, trauma, tissue, and thrombin) **(Table 3)**.

TABLE 3: Causes of postpartum hemorrhage.

Primary postpartum hemorrhage	Secondary postpartum hemorrhage
• Uterine atony • Retained placental fragments • Lower genital tract laceration • Uterine rupture • Uterine inversion • Hereditary coagulopathy	• Failure of uterine lining to sub involute • Retained placental tissue • Genital tract wounds • Uterogenital infections

2. Enumerate the risk factors of postpartum hemorrhage.

Conditions that may increase the risk for postpartum hemorrhage include the following:
- Placental abruption—the early detachment of the placenta from the uterus
- Placenta previa
- Overdistended uterus
- Multiple pregnancy
- Gestational hypertension or preeclampsia
- Having many previous births
- Prolonged labor
- Infection

3. Discuss investigation and management of postpartum hemorrhage.

Investigation: Complete blood count (hemoglobin and hematocrit), coagulation profile, blood grouping and typing, Urine analysis, blood culture, ultrasound for viewing uterus.

Management: The initial resuscitative steps include aggressive fluid and blood resuscitation while identifying and treating the underlying cause.

Treating the underlying cause
Tone: Perform bimanual uterine massage. Drugs to improve uterine tone are oxytocin 20 units in 1 L NS (or 10 units IM), misoprostol 1,000 µg PR/PO once methylergonovine 0.2 mg IM/IV/PO carboprost 250 µg IM every 15–90 minutes.

Trauma: Examine for cervical, vaginal or perineal laceration or hematoma. Repair laceration. Incise, drain and appropriately ligate bleeding vessel causing a hematoma. Correct uterine inversion with manual replacement. Uterine rupture requires surgery.

Tissue: Inspect the placenta for missing fragments, if a portion is absent, manually evacuate the uterine cavity. Invasive placentation may require hysterectomy. Consider a balloon tamponade with either uterine-specific balloon device (Bakri or Rusch) or an adaptation of Foley catheter or condom as a temporizing measure.

Thrombin: Consider DIC in the setting of severe preeclampsia, sepsis, placental abruption, shock or intrauterine fetal demise. Replace coagulation factors.

4. What are the complications of postpartum hemorrhage?

- Hypovolemic/hemorrhagic shock
- Cerebral anoxia
- Renal failure
- Anemia
- Puerperal sepsis
- Sheehan's syndrome—hypopituitarism.

Question 6

1. Discuss causes of acute low back pain.

- *Intrinsic lesions:*
  - Multiple sclerosis
  - Spinal stenosis
  - Transverse myelitis
  - Syringomyelia
  - HIV myelopathy
  - Surfers myelopathy
  - Vertebral osteomyelitis
- *Extrinsic lesions:*
  - Epidural hematoma
  - Epidural abscess
  - Discitis
  - Disc herniation
  - Neoplasm.

2. Explain the red flag symptoms in back pain.

- Trauma
- Saddle anesthesia
- Fever
- Midline bony spinal tenderness
- Unexplained weight loss
- Bladder deficit
- Neurological deficit
- History of intravenous drug
- History of recent instrumentation.

3. Discuss cauda equina syndrome.

It is a condition with back pain with associated neurologic deficits, perianal sensory loss, fecal incontinence or urinary incontinence with or without retention, and sciatica in one or both legs.

Etiology: Herniated disc, tumor abscess, a history of malignancy and a rapid progression of neurologic symptoms, especially bilateral symptoms, increase the likelihood of compression.

Depending on the level of compression and the amount and area of the spinal cord or cauda equina that is compressed.

Common findings: Urinary retention PVRU >100 mL, weakness or stiffness in the lower extremities, paresthesia or sensory deficits, gait difficulty, and abnormal results on straight leg raise testing. The most common sensory deficit occurs over the buttocks, posterosuperior thighs, and perineal regions and is commonly called saddle anesthesia. Anal sphincter tone is decreased in 60–80% of cases.

Investigation: MRI localized to the lumbosacral spine, CT myelogram.

The presence of cord compression is an indication for urgent consultation with a spine surgeon for decompression and/or radiation therapy for a tumor mass, determined by MRI findings.

Question 7

1. Discuss clinical presentation of acute limb ischemia.

Clinical presentations of acute limb ischemia are given as below **(Table 4)**:

TABLE 4: Clinical presentations of acute limb ischemia.

Symptoms and signs	6 Ps	Pressure measurements
• Rest pain • Ulcer • Gangrene	• Pain • Pale • Pulseless • Paresthesia • Paralysis	• Pedal pressure • Great toe pressure • Ankle brachial index • Toe brachial index

2. Explain the Rutherford criteria for acute limb ischemia.

The classification is objective (grade 0, no obvious ischemia; grade 1, mild ischemia; grade 2, moderate ischemia; grade 3, severe ischemia) **(Table 5)**.

TABLE 5: Rutherford criteria of limb ischemia.

Grade	Category	Sensory loss	Motor deficit	Prognosis	Doppler arterial	Venous
I	Viable	None	None	No immediate threat	Audible	Audible
IIA	Marginally threatened	None or minimal toes	None	Salvable if promptly treated	Inaudible	Audible
IIB	Immediately threatened	More than toes	Mild, moderate	Salvable if promptly revascularized	Inaudible	Audible
III	Irreversible	Profound, anesthetic	Profound, paralysis	Amputation	Inaudible	Inaudible

3. Enumerate differential diagnosis of acute limb ischemia.

- Trauma
- Dissection
- Arteries
- Hypercoagulable state
- Popliteal entrapment
- Popliteal adventitial cyst
- Compartment syndrome.

4. Discuss ER management of acute limb ischemia.

Appropriate analgesia: As with any painful condition there is no rationale to withhold analgesia to facilitate assessment.

Appropriate anticoagulants: Eighty-units/kg bolus intravenous (IV) heparin (unfractionated) should be given immediately to all patients with acute limb ischemia; even when they are likely to be undergoing surgery or angiography. This is to prevent propagation of thrombosis. In patients in whom definitive treatment is deferred an intravenous heparin infusion (18U/kg/hour) should be prescribed or can be started on therapeutic low molecular weight heparin (LMWH).

Appropriate IV fluids: Patients with acute limb ischemia are often dehydrated. These patients are likely to be undergoing surgery or be given iodinated contrast that will be a further renal insult. Reperfusion of ischemic tissue releases toxic metabolites, potassium, creatinine kinase, and myoglobin, which can further damage the kidneys. Administration of potassium should be avoided. Aggressive rehydration should be initiated unless coexistent cardiac conditions are limiting.

Expert consultation: Refer to a vascular specialist urgently. Any delay risks jeopardizing the limb, particularly if there is sensorimotor impairment or compartment syndrome.

Simple measures to improve vascularity: Keep the foot dependent; avoid pressure over the heal and extremes of temperature; maximize tissue oxygenation; correct hypotension; and treat if any associated cardiac conditions present.

Question 8

A 58-year-old male presents to ER with distended abdomen, vomiting, and constipation for 2 days. You suspect bowel obstruction.

1. Discuss common causes of bowel obstruction.

Mechanical:
- Adhesions
- Fecal impaction
- Hernia
- Intussusception
- Trauma
- Tumor
- Volvulus
- Functional
- Inflammation
- Neurological disorders
- Medication.

2. What are the key features of bowel obstruction?

The four cardinal symptoms of bowel obstruction are pain, vomiting, obstipation/absolute constipation, and distention **(Table 6)**.

TABLE 6: Key features of bowel obstruction.

Site	Vomiting	Pain	Distension	Bowel sound
Pylorus or duodenum (11%)	High volume	Minimal	Mild	Succession
Small intestine (48%)	Moderate to severe	Colicky	Moderate	Hyperactive
Large intestine (37%)	Late effect minimum	Colicky	Severe	Borborygmi

3. Explain ER management of patient with bowel obstruction.

- IV fluids isotonic saline and electrolyte replacement.
- Foley catheterization should be inserted to monitor the patient's urine output if the patient is unstable or septic.
- Nasogastric tube insertion will allow for bowel decompression to relieve distention proximal to the obstruction and help control emesis, allow for accurate assessment of intake and output, and lower the risk of aspiration.
- Stable patients with partial or low-grade obstruction resolve with nasogastric tube decompression and supportive measures.
- Patients who present with reducible hernias will require nonemergent surgical intervention to prevent future recurrence.
- Nonreducible or strangulated hernias require emergency surgical intervention.
- Chronic disease states such as Crohn's disease and malignancy require initial supportive measures and longer periods of nonoperative management.

Question 9

A 28-year-old man presents to the ED with severe pain in the left lower leg following crush injury 2 days ago. The left lower leg is edematous and red. Crepitus is present.

1. Describe anatomy and pathophysiology of compartment syndrome.

Anatomy: The lower leg consists of four compartments—anterior, lateral, superficial posterior, and deep posterior **(Table 7)**.

Pathophysiology of compartment syndrome: Compartment syndrome develops when the pressure within an osteofascial compartment exceeds that of arterial pressure resulting in reduced or absent blood flow. The muscle becomes ischemic and edematous further increasing compartment pressures. Ultimately ischemia can lead to muscle necrosis. A high index of suspicion is required to identify early compartment syndrome. The only initial feature may be pain out of proportion to the injury.

The pathophysiology of compartment syndrome includes:
- External compressive force or internal expanding force
- Osteofascial compartment pressure > arterial pressure
- Reduced or absent blood flow
- Muscle ischemia and edema
- Muscle necrosis, ischemic contractures, neurological deficit, infection, rhabdomyolysis, renal failure, possible amputation, and death.

TABLE 7: The lower leg consists of four compartments.

Structure	Anterior	Lateral	Superficial posterior	Deep posterior
Muscles	• Tibialis anterior muscle • Extensor hallucis longus • Extensor digitorum longus • Peroneus tertius	• Peroneus longus • Peroneus brevis	• Gastrocnemius • Soleus • Plantaris	• Tibialis posterior • Flexor hallucis longus • Flexor digitorum longus
Vessels	• Anterior tibial artery • Anterior tibial veins			• Peroneal artery • Peroneal vein • Posterior tibial artery • Posterior tibial vein
Nerves	Deep peroneal nerve	Common peroneal nerve		Tibial nerve

1. Discuss clinical assessment of the above patient.

- Look if arm held in an abducted and external rotation position.
- Loss of normal contour of the deltoid and acromion prominent posteriorly and laterally.
- Humeral head palpable anteriorly.
- Check for range of movements.
- Palpable fullness below the coracoid process and toward the axilla.
- Possible damage to rotator cuff musculature and bone.
- Vascular injuries may result from traction of the axillary blood vessels, resulting in a reduced pulse pressure or a transient coolness in the hands.
- Look for peripheral nerve injuries.

2. Discuss investigations in above case.

X-ray of shoulder joint:
- Anterior dislocation—the humeral head lies below the coracoid on the AP view, the Y-view shows the humeral head anterior to the glenoid.
- In the axial view a lesion is often seen in dislocation, known as a Hill-Sachs deformity. This always occurs in recurrent dislocations.
  - The tear that occurs to the lower part of anterior labrum is called Bankart lesion. Sometimes a tear develops in the upper labrum, often referred to as superior labral anteroposterior tear (or SLAP lesion) this occurs often due to sports injury and not dislocation.
- Posterior dislocation—the humeral head may appear to have the contour of a "light bulb" rather than a "walking stick". The Y-view shows the humeral head lying posteriorly.

CT and/MRI for assessment of soft tissue injury.

2. Explain investigation of compartment syndrome.

- *Blood investigations:* Serum creatine phosphokinase (normal—130 IU, acute compartment syndrome—1,000–5,000 IU, Crush syndrome >100,000 IU).
  Renal function tests, white blood cell count, serum potassium, serum glutamic oxaloacetic transaminase (SGOT), and lactate dehydrogenase (LDH).

Urine for myoglobin:
- *Imaging* X-ray CT angiogram Doppler
- *Intracompartmental pressure measurement* may be helpful if the diagnosis is uncertain. If the difference between the intracompartmental and diastolic pressure is <30 mm Hg, then a fasciotomy is required.

3. Enumerate the treatment of compartment syndrome.

- Remove all tight envelopes
  - Remove the dressings
  - Remove cotton wrappings, casts or splints
- Intravenous analgesics for pain
- Avoid any nerve blocks which may mask symptoms
- Place the extremity at heart level. Do not elevate as that leads to a decrease in arterial circulation
- Fluid management for management of dehydration
- In the case of leg injury, immobilize in slight plantar flexion to decrease posterior compartmental pressure
- Fasciotomy
- Excision of dead muscle tissue and possible amputation.

Question 10

A 24-year-old wrestler had injury to his right shoulder while wrestling. He comes to the ER with pain in his shoulder and restricted shoulder movement. He has two episodes of shoulder dislocations in the past.

3. Explain the management of anterior shoulder dislocation.

Management consists of pain management and implementations of dislocation reduction technique.

External rotation: With the patient supine, slowly adduct the dislocated arm against the patient's side.

Flex the elbow to 90°. Hold the patient's wrist and slowly externally rotate the arm while held adduction and flexed at 90°.

Milch technique: With the patient supine, the arm is externally rotated and then abducted over the patient's head while maintaining external rotation. Gentle force can be applied over the humeral head by the operators thumb in the axilla.

Kocher's technique: Flex the elbow to 90° and apply downward traction in line with the humerus. Externally rotate the shoulder to bring the humeral head forward. Pull the elbow across the patient's body adducting the shoulder and then internally rotate the arm. This maneuver has a higher rate of axillary nerve damage than other techniques.

- Arm sling immobilization for 3 weeks
- Surgical repair in recurrent joint instability.

SUGGESTED READING

1. Richhariya D, Sharma B. Textbook of Emergency Medicine including Intensive Care and Trauma, 2nd edition. New Delhi: Jaypee Brothers Medical Publishers (P) Ltd; 2022. pp. 1570-8. (Question 1).
2. Richhariya D, Sharma B. Textbook of Emergency Medicine including Intensive Care and Trauma, 2nd edition. New Delhi: Jaypee Brothers Medical Publishers (P) Ltd; 2022. pp. 899-906. (Question 2).
3. Richhariya D, Sharma B. Textbook of Emergency Medicine including Intensive Care and Trauma, 2nd edition. New Delhi: Jaypee Brothers Medical Publishers (P) Ltd; 2022. pp. 929-33. (Question 3).
4. Richhariya D, Sharma B. Textbook of Emergency Medicine including Intensive Care and Trauma, 2nd edition. New Delhi: Jaypee Brothers Medical Publishers (P) Ltd; 2022. pp. 1580-5. (Question 4).
5. Richhariya D, Sharma B. Textbook of Emergency Medicine including Intensive Care and Trauma, 2nd edition. New Delhi: Jaypee Brothers Medical Publishers (P) Ltd; 2022. p. 1113. (Question 5).
6. Richhariya D, Sharma B. Textbook of Emergency Medicine including Intensive Care and Trauma, 2nd edition. New Delhi: Jaypee Brothers Medical Publishers (P) Ltd; 2022. pp. 1040-2. (Question 6).
7. Richhariya D, Sharma B. Textbook of Emergency Medicine including Intensive Care and Trauma, 2nd edition. New Delhi: Jaypee Brothers Medical Publishers (P) Ltd; 2022. pp. 547-50. (Question 7).
8. Richhariya D, Sharma B. Textbook of Emergency Medicine including Intensive Care and Trauma, 2nd edition. New Delhi: Jaypee Brothers Medical Publishers (P) Ltd; 2022. pp. 694-8. (Question 8).
9. Richhariya D, Sharma B. Textbook of Emergency Medicine including Intensive Care and Trauma, 2nd edition. New Delhi: Jaypee Brothers Medical Publishers (P) Ltd; 2022. pp. 1671-3. (Question 9).
10. Richhariya D, Sharma B. Textbook of Emergency Medicine including Intensive Care and Trauma, 2nd edition. New Delhi: Jaypee Brothers Medical Publishers (P) Ltd; 2022. p. 1630. (Question 10).

Emergency Medicine Paper 35

Devendra Richhariya

Question 1

A 42-year-old male presents to the emergency room (ER) with fever and shortness of breath for 2 days. He is tachypneic, hypoxic, and hypotensive.

1. Enumerate differential diagnosis of noninfectious causes of fever.

Noninfectious etiologies of *fever* or hyperthermia **(Table 1)** include autoimmune diseases, trauma, inflammatory conditions, environmental stressors, giant cell (temporal) arteritis, Adult still's disease (juvenile rheumatoid arthritis), systemic lupus erythematosus (SLE), periarteritis nodosa/microscopic polyangiitis (PAN/MPA), rheumatoid arthritis (RA), antiphospholipid syndrome (APS), gout, and pseudogout.

2. Discuss echocardiography in pulmonary embolism (PE).

Abnormalities are present in approximately 30–40% of patients with PE. Transthoracic echocardiography (TTE) is noninvasive, and rapidly available at the bedside, but lacks the sensitivity of transesophageal echocardiogram (TEE). TEE has greater sensitivity and diagnostic ability than TTE, but is invasive, of limited availability, often requires procedural sedation, and is unable to accurately detect peripheral PE. Echocardiography is most useful in patients with contraindications to other imaging modalities, hemodynamically unstable patients who cannot be transported outside the emergency department (ED), or in patients with suspected massive PE to justify thrombolytics. Echocardiographic findings of PE are shown in **Figure 1**.

TABLE 1: Noninfectious etiologies of fever.

Important cause	Other causes
• Acalculous cholecystitis	• Burn
• Adrenal insufficiency	• Acute respiratory distress syndrome (late)
• Benign postoperative fever	• Drug overdose
• Drug fever	• Drug withdrawal
• Pancreatitis	• Gout
• Thyroid storm	• Heat stroke
• Transfusion reaction	• Intracranial hemorrhage
	• Malignant hyperthermia
	• Myocardial infarction
	• Seizure
	• Serotonin syndrome
	• Thromboembolic disease
	• Vasculitis

3. Describe an approach to a patient with suspected PE and with hemodynamic instability.

Systemic anticoagulation is the mainstay of the treatment for venous thromboembolism (DVT + PE). Unfractionated heparin and low molecular weight heparin (LMWH) are the two most common options. LMWH is preferred over unfractionated heparin as per recent data. Early administration of heparin is recommended but no study found morbidity or mortality benefits if heparin is administered early and prior to imaging. Other measures such as placing the affected limb at neutral level, removal of tight clothing, dressing, and cast are equally important. Vascular consultation and catheter-directed thrombolysis should be arranged. Systemic thrombolysis is another option with alteplase 50–100 mg infusion over 4 hours. The management of PE will be dealt under following headings. The initial management starts with resuscitation of PE patient **(Box 1)**.

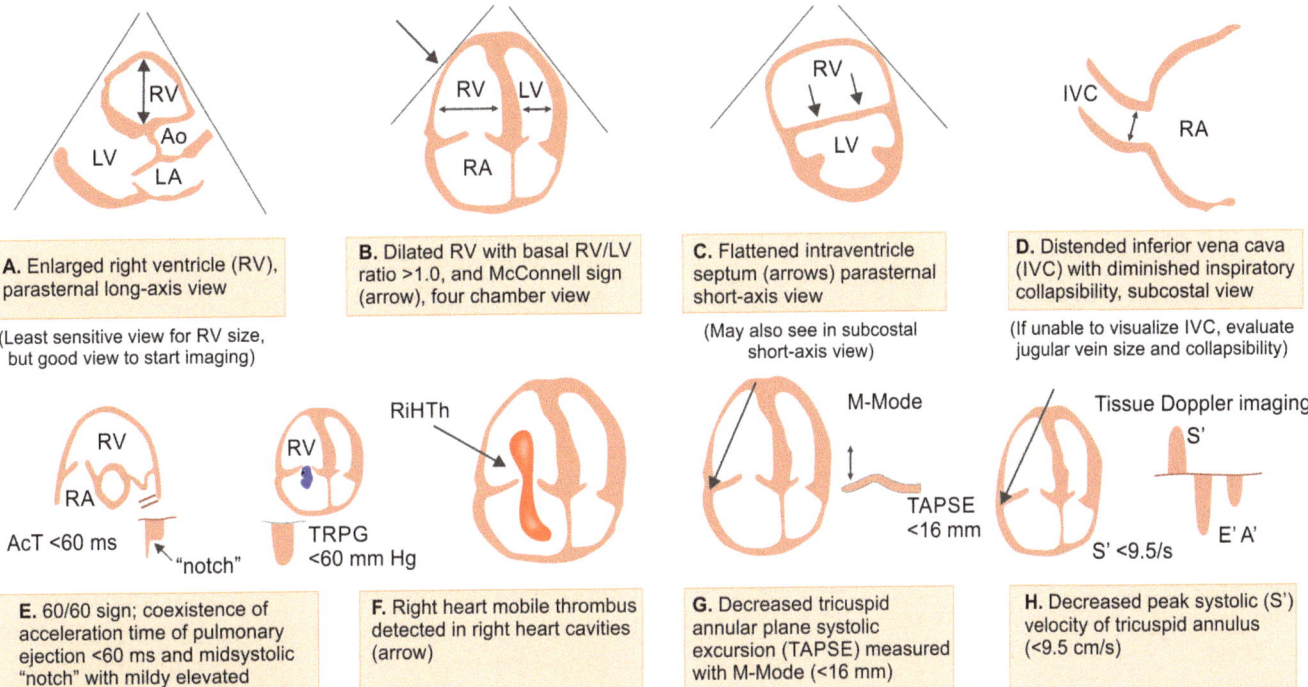

Fig. 1: Echocardiographic assessment of right ventricle in pulmonary embolism—*whenever feasible evaluate right ventricles in several views A–D.* (LV: left ventricular; RA: right atria; TRPG: tricuspid regurgitation peak gradient)

BOX 1: Important points to remember during resuscitation of pulmonary embolism patient.

- Use high-flow nasal cannula for hypoxemic failure.
- Add inhaled pulmonary vasodilators, whenever possible.
- First thrombolytics, then intubation.
- Define criteria of intubation—depressed mental status or respiratory exhaustion.
- *Intubation pearls:*
  - Before intubation, try to increase the systolic blood pressure 130–140 mm, usually with an epinephrine infusion.
  - Be prepared with push-dose epinephrine to support the blood pressure after intubation. Have a low threshold for using this for hypotension or worsening bradycardia.
  - Consider getting inhaled pulmonary vasopressors at the bedside and ready to be given through the ventilator circuit as soon as the patient is intubated. Administration of a milrinone dose through the endotracheal tube may also be utilized, if this is available.
  - Use meticulous preoxygenation and apneic oxygenation, paired with intubation by the most experienced operator present.
  - Use sedatives that are hemodynamically stable (e.g., ketamine).
  - Avoid over-vigorous bag ventilation, which will cause excessive intrathoracic pressures.
  - Pay extreme attention to the patient's hemodynamics and oxygenation in the first 10 minutes after intubation, as this is when they are most likely to arrest.
- Epinephrine due to its beta agonist action is the first line vasopressor. Helps in pulmonary vasodilatations as well. Vasopressin as second-line drug—systemic vasoconstriction with pulmonary vasodilatation.
- Nitric oxide and epoprostanol—comparable results. High FiO_2 is a poor man's pulmonary vasodilator.
- Try to limit ABG punctures. These may be the sites of bleeding when urgent thrombolysis is done.
- Similar caution has to be taken for central venous cannulation—single puncture, experienced physician.
- Intubation and positive pressure ventilation increases peripheral vascular resistance. Avoid or delay intubation.
- Fluid boluses—very small, guided by US massive PE are not a fluid depleted state. Expect the IVC to be full. If not, suspect another diagnosis.

(ABG: arterial blood gas; IVC: inferior vena cava; PE: pulmonary embolism)

Question 2

An 18-year-old female presents to the ER with history of ingestion of 20 tablets of paracetamol (each of 500 mg) about 3 hours back. She is hemodynamically stable and has no comorbidities.

1. What are the minimal toxic doses of paracetamol in adults and children?

Acetaminophen is rapidly absorbed mainly in the small intestine with peak plasma concentrations reaching within 1 hour and complete absorption within 4–5 hours of ingestion. Therapeutic dose of acetaminophen is 10–15 mg/kg/dose in children (up to a maximum of 75 mg/kg/day) and 325–1,000 mg/dose in adults every 4–6 hourly (not to exceed 4,000 mg/day). Therapeutic concentration ranges between 10 and 20 µg/mL. Elimination half-life is usually 2–4 hours. Toxicity occurs usually after a single dose of ≥150 mg/kg or in multiple staggered doses.

2. Discuss pathophysiology of paracetamol toxicity.

At therapeutic dose, around 90% of acetaminophen is metabolized in the liver and around 2–3% is excreted unchanged in urine. Rest of the metabolism takes place via cytochrome P450 oxidase pathway and gets converted to a toxic metabolite N-acetyl-p-benzoquinonimine (NAPQI). This NAPQI gets conjugated with glutathione to form nontoxic metabolites which are excreted in urine. In case of overdoses, the glucuronide and sulfates get saturated and more of NAPQI is produced. With depletion of glutathione stores in liver due to excess of NAPQI, the concentration of toxic metabolite NAPQI increases leading to liver damage and hepatic necrosis. Patients taking substances or medications that induce the cytochrome P450 system (alcohol, anticonvulsant or antituberculous drugs) or those with glutathione depletion (poor nutrition, alcoholics, and acquired immunodeficiency syndrome patients) are at increased risk of hepatic toxicity.

3. What are the signs and symptoms of paracetamol overdose?

The clinical features of acetaminophen toxicity have been divided into four stages **(Table 2)**.

4. Discuss the investigations for the above-mentioned patient in the ER.

a. Serum acetaminophen concentration—should be obtained 4 hours after ingestion.
b. Liver function tests (LFT)—may not be abnormal until >18 hours after the overdose. Alanine aminotransferase (ALT) and aspartate aminotransferase (AST) are the most sensitive markers of liver damage.
c. International normalized ratio (INR)—is a very sensitive marker of liver damage and the best prognostic parameter.
d. Renal function—creatinine is a useful prognostic marker and a low urea may suggest malnutrition and therefore glutathione depletion.
e. Blood sugar levels—to look for hypoglycemia.
f. Blood gas analysis—to check for acid-base disturbances. Metabolic acidosis, if present, is a poor prognostic sign.

5. Describe briefly the treatment of the patient in the ER.

The timing of the overdose decides the treatment to be followed in case of acetaminophen toxicity **(Table 3)**. Paracetamol treatment nomogram (**Rumack–Matthew nomogram**) should be used to interpret the measured serum paracetamol levels. N-acetylcysteine (NAC) should be continued if (any one of the following):

a. Paracetamol level is on or above treatment line between 4 and 15 hours after single ingestion.
b. Serum paracetamol is still detectable 15 hours after single ingestion.
c. Serum paracetamol is detectable 4 hours after uncertain time of ingestion.
d. INR >1.3
e. ALT >53 IU/L.

TABLE 2: Clinical features of acetaminophen toxicity.

Stages	Time course	Clinical manifestations	Laboratory abnormalities
Stage 1	<24 hours	Asymptomatic or anorexia, nausea, vomiting	Hypokalemia
Stage 2	2–3 days	• Improvement in anorexia, nausea, and vomiting • Abdominal pain, hepatic tenderness, jaundice	Elevated serum transaminases, elevated bilirubin and prolonged prothrombin time if severe
Stage 3	3–4 days	• Recurrence of anorexia, nausea, and vomiting • Encephalopathy, anuria, jaundice	Hepatic failure, metabolic acidosis, coagulopathy, renal failure, pancreatitis
Stage 4	>4 days	Clinical improvement and recovery (7–8 days) or deterioration to multiorgan failure and death	Improvement and resolution or continued deterioration

TABLE 3: Management of acetaminophen poisoning according to timing.

Timing	Total dose	Investigation	Management
Single ingestion <1 h	>150 mg/kg	Delay blood sampling until 4 hours post-ingestion	Activated charcoal (50 g orally), IV antiemetic, admit for observation while sampling awaited at 4 hours
Single ingestion >1 h but <4 h	>150 mg/kg	Delay blood sampling until 4 hours post-ingestion	Activated charcoal (50 g orally), IV antiemetic, admit for observation while sampling awaited at 4 hours
Single ingestion >4 h but <8 h	<150 mg/kg	Blood sampling for serum paracetamol level	If the result is expected to be available before 8 hours of ingestion, treatment should be guided by the result
	>150 mg/kg	Blood sampling for serum paracetamol level	If the result is not expected to be available before 8 hours, NAC should be started immediately without waiting for result
Single ingestion 8–24 h	<150 mg/kg	Blood sampling for serum paracetamol level	Treatment should be guided by the result
	>150 mg/kg	Blood sampling for serum paracetamol level	NAC should be started immediately without waiting for result
Single ingestion >24 h	>150 mg/kg	Blood sampling for serum paracetamol level	NAC should be started immediately without waiting for result
Timing unclear or ingestion is staggered		Blood sampling for serum paracetamol level	Treatment should be started immediately without waiting for result

(IV: intravenous; NAC: N-acetylcysteine)

Question 3

A 70-year-old male comes to ER with history of giddiness and nausea since morning. He has a pulse rate of 48/min. His ECG shows irregular pacing.

1. What are the indications for permanent pacing in adults?

The most common indications for permanent pacemaker implantation are sinus node dysfunction (SND) and high-grade atrioventricular (AV) block.

Indications:
a. Sick sinus syndrome
b. Symptomatic sinus bradycardia
c. Tachycardia bradycardia syndrome
d. Atrial fibrillation with SND
e. Compete AV block
f. Prolonged QT syndrome
g. Cardiac resynchronization therapy with biventricular pacing
h. Cardiomyopathy (hypertrophic/dilated).

2. Enumerate five letter pacemaker code.

Pacemakers are devices that detect the electrical activity of the heart and stimulate it to contract at a faster rate.
Letter 1: Chamber that is paced (A = atria, V = ventricles, D = dual-chamber).
Letter 2: Chamber that is sensed (A = atria, V = ventricles, D = dual-chamber, 0 = none).
Letter 3: Response to a sensed event (T = triggered, I = inhibited, D = dual - T and I, R = reverse).
Letter 4: Programmability (P = simple, M = multiprogrammable, R = rate adaptive, 0 = none)
Letter 5: Antitachycardia functions (P = pacing, S = shock, D = dual-shock and pace)

3. Describe the causes of pacemaker malfunction.

The main causes of pacemaker failure are lead dislodgment, low output, lead maturation, and lead or pacer failure (fibrosis, fracture, low pacing voltage, or elevated myocardial pacing thresholds).

4. Define pacemaker syndrome.

Pacemaker syndrome is most commonly seen in the setting of a single chamber device with ventricular sensing and pacing lead. Since there is no atrial sensing lead to guide the ventricle, the ventricle contracts at the programmed rate regardless of the timing of atrial contraction. Symptoms include exercise intolerance, dyspnea, cough, chest discomfort, abdominal distention, nausea, fatigue and tiredness, dizziness, syncope or presyncope, and hypotension. This constellation of symptoms is referred to as "pacemaker syndrome" and is a result of loss of AV synchrony.

5. What are the advanced cardiac life support interventions in patient with pacemaker?

Cardiopulmonary resuscitation (CPR) chest compressions may be performed as usual. If resuscitation efforts are successful, the implanted device should be interrogated to assess its function. If the implanted device delivers a shock during CPR, the responder may feel a tingling sensation on the patient's body surface. However, the shocks delivered by the implanted defibrillator will not pose a danger to the person administering CPR. The unpleasant tingling sensation can be prevented by wearing gloves during CPR.

Question 4

A 27-year-old male presents to the ER with a high-grade fever, headache, and retro-orbital pain and joint pains for 2 days. He has a heart rate of 102/min, BP 100/76 mm Hg, and SpO_2 96% on room air. He also complains of nausea and abdominal pain. You suspect dengue. Discuss:

1. Phases in dengue.

Dengue fever has an acute and sudden onset. It comprises of three phases—febrile, critical, and recovery.

Febrile phase: It lasts for 2–7 days with development of high-grade fever suddenly. It is accompanied by facial flushing, skin erythema, generalized body ache, myalgia, retro-orbital pain, arthralgia, rash, and hemorrhagic manifestations such as petechiae and mucosal membrane bleeding and headache.

Critical phase: At 3–7th day from onset of symptoms, there is an increased permeability of capillaries along with raised hematocrit levels. There is a drop in temperature of fever between 37.5 and 38°C and less. The leakage from capillaries is predominant and usually lasts for 24–48 hours. Once the patient has crossed the 24–48 hours critical phase, the physiological response involves a gradual reabsorption of fluid from extravascular compartment in the next 48–72 hours. Patient's condition improves, appetite returns to normal, gastrointestinal (GI) symptoms resolve and diuresis ensues.

2. Severe dengue.

Severe dengue: The clinical features are progressively life-threatening with a prolonged critical phase. Depending upon the condition of patient and progression of symptoms, the presence of one or more of the following is defined as severe dengue:
a. Plasma leak from capillaries in to extravascular compartment—rise in hematocrit count that may progress to shock.
b. Signs of respiratory distress secondary to fluid overload.
c. Fluid overload in pulmonary or GI system—pleural effusion/ascites.
d. Signs of bleeding due to thrombocytopenia.
e. Decreased adequate perfusion leading to severe organ impairment.

3. Laboratory investigations in dengue.

Investigations:
a. *Complete blood count with peripheral smear:* Hematocrit count is evaluated at the initial hours of febrile phase to maintain as baseline, in order to compare with in subsequent testing. Increased level of hematocrit count with parallel decrease in platelet levels is an early indication of critical phase of dengue fever.
b. *Additional tests:* Arterial blood gas analysis in cases of sudden on breathlessness, dyspnea on exertion, chest discomfort, desaturation status, LFT, random blood glucose, serum electrolytes, serum urea, serum creatinine, bicarbonate levels, lactate count, cardiac enzymes, urine routine and examination.
c. *Radiological studies:* Chest X-ray, ultrasound abdomen/computed tomography (CT) abdomen.

4. Management of the abovementioned patient in the ER.

Patient requiring hospital admission and intervention: The patients in need of in-hospital management for close observation and approach to critical phase.

An initial hematocrit level must be obtained before starting fluid therapy: Start with isotonic fluid solutions such as 0.9% saline, Ringer's lactate or Hartmann's solution at 5–7 mL/kg/hour for first 1–2 hours. Then reduce it at a rate of 3–5 mL/kg/hour for next 2–4 hours, further maintain at 2–3 mL/kg/hour or less according to clinical response of the patient. Reassess hydration status of patient every half hourly in order to rule out early signs of pleural effusion or fluid overload. Repeat hematocrit level and watch for increase in levels despite fluid therapy. If the hematocrit level remains the same with minimal increase, continue with same rate at 2–3 mL/kg/hour for next 2–4 hours. In case of increased hematocrit levels rapidly, increase the rate of fluid administration to 5–10 mL/kg/hour for 1–2 hours. Repeat the hematocrit levels every 2 hourly and adjust the rate of fluid therapy accordingly.

Maintenance fluid can be calculated using the Holliday-Segar formula: A total of 4 mL/kg/hour for first 10 kg body weight + 2 mL/kg/hour for next 10 kg body weight + 1 mL/kg/hour for subsequent body weight.

Question 5

A 46-year-old male presents to the ER with uneasiness, severe headache, and a blood pressure (BP) of 230/128 mm Hg. Comment briefly on the following:
1. Hypertension and hypertensive emergency.

2. Treatment (including therapy goals) of hypertensive emergency in acute ischemic stroke for thrombolysis.
3. Treatment (including therapy goals) of hypertensive emergency in aortic dissection.
4. Treatment (including therapy goals) of hypertensive emergency in intracerebral bleed.
5. Treatment (including therapy goals) of hypertensive emergency in eclampsia/preeclampsia.

In adults, hypertension is defined as a systolic blood pressure (BP) equal to or over 140 mm Hg, or a diastolic BP equal to or over 90 mm Hg according to European, Indian, and UK standards. The American Heart Association uses a definition of BP >130/80 mm Hg instead **(Table 4)**.

Clinical presentation of hypertensive emergencies in ED is associated with different diseases and they manifest in various forms such as pulmonary edema, myocardial ischemia, aortic dissection, preeclampsia, hypertensive encephalopathy. So, in each subset of presentation the choice of antihypertensive agent is different **(Table 5)**. The target BP goals in hypertensive emergencies of varied etiology are also different **(Table 6)**.

TABLE 4: Grading of hypertension in adults.

Grading	Systolic (mm Hg)		Diastolic (mm Hg)
Mild	140–159	and/or	90–99
Moderate	160–179	and/or	100–109
Severe	≥180	and/or	≥110
Hypertensive urgency	Severe hypertension *without* acute organ failure		
Hypertensive emergency	Severe hypertension *with* evidence of acute target organ failure		

For a child, refer to standardized tables of blood pressure for diagnosis.

TABLE 5: Choice of pharmacological agent in hypertensive emergency according to presentation.

Condition	Preferred drugs	Drugs to avoid
Acute pulmonary edema/heart failure	Fenoldopam/nitroprusside + nitroglycerin (up to 60 µg/min) + loop diuretic	Hydralazine, β-blockers
Myocardial ischemia and infarction	Labetalol/esmolol + nitroglycerin (up to 200 µg/min) +/− Nicardipine/fenoldopam if BP uncontrolled or poorly controlled	Hydralazine, minoxidil, diazoxide, nitroprusside
Hypertensive encephalopathy	Labetalol/nicardipine/fenoldopam	Beta blockers, methyldopa, clonidine, diazoxide, hydralazine, nitroglycerin
Acute aortic dissection	Labetalol or nicardipine + esmolol or nitroprusside + esmolol/ IV metoprolol	Hydralazine, minoxidil
Preeclampsia, eclampsia	Labetalol/nicardipine	Diuretics, angiotensin-converting enzymes
Acute renal failure, microangiopathic anemia	Fenoldopam/nicardipine	
Intracerebral hemorrhage	Nimodipine (oral)/nicardipine/labetalol/ nitroprusside/enalaprilat	Beta blockers, methyldopa, clonidine, diazoxide, hydralazine, nitroglycerin
Hyperadrenergic states/sympathetic overdrive	Phentolamine/nitroprusside/labetalol/nicardipine/verapamil. Alternatively, fenoldopam +/− a benzodiazepine (in cocaine overdose)	Beta blockers (in cocaine overdose)

TABLE 6: Target BP goals for specific emergencies.

Conditions	Target BP goals
Hypertensive encephalopathy	MAP lowered by maximum 20% or to DBP 100–110 mm Hg within first hour then gradual reduction in BP to normal range over 48–72 h
Ischemic stroke	MAP lowered no >15%–20%, DBP not <100–110 mm Hg in first 24 hours (thrombolytic protocols in stroke may allow slightly more aggressive management)
Intracerebral hemorrhage	MAP lowered by 20–25%
Hypertensive retinopathy	MAP lowered by 20–25%
Left ventricular failure	MAP to 60–100 mm Hg
Aortic dissection	SBP 100–120 mm Hg
Acute renal insufficiency	MAP lowered by 20–25%
Pregnancy-induced hypertension	SBP 130–150 mm Hg, DBP 80–100 mm Hg

(DBP: diastolic blood pressure; MAP: mean arterial pressure; SBP: systolic blood pressure)

Question 6

A 20-year-old male presents to the ER with complaints of lower limb weakness for 2 days.

1. Discuss the critical and emergent causes of neuromuscular weakness.

Neuromuscular diseases affect the function of muscles due to problems with the nerves and muscles in your body. The most common sign of these diseases is muscle weakness. The two common causes of severe neuromuscular weakness are myasthenia gravis and the Guillain-Barré syndrome.

2. What are the non-neurologic causes of weakness?

Metabolic causes: Hypokalemia, hyperkalemia, hypophosphatemia, and thiamine deficiency.

Muscle disorders: Infection, viral myositis, inflammatory myopathy—polymyositis, dermatomyositis.

3. How would you assess a hemodynamically stable patient for a neural/muscular cause of weakness?

Medical history and neurological examination should be focused on the onset, progression, pattern, and severity of muscle weakness as well as cranial nerves testing and tests for autonomic dysfunction. Associated non-neurological features such as fever, rash or other skin lesions, etc., should also be noted (**Flowcharts 1A to D**).

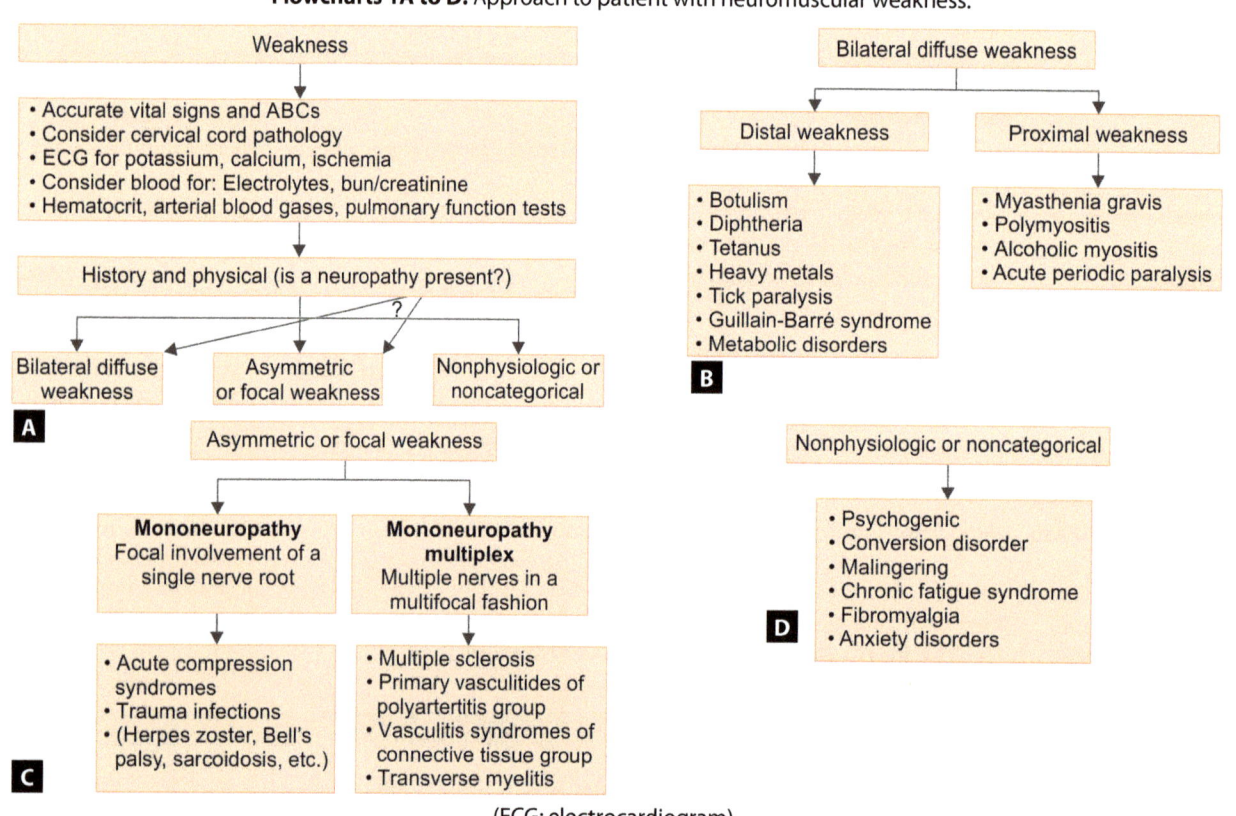

Flowcharts 1A to D: Approach to patient with neuromuscular weakness.

(ECG: electrocardiogram)

Question 7

A 46-year-old female presents to the ER with jaundice, fever with chills and right upper quadrant pain for 2 days.

1. What could be the differential diagnosis in the above case?

Biliary: Cholecystitis, cholangitis, cholelithiasis.

Colic: Colitis, diverticulitis, ileitis, retrocecal appendicitis, perforated duodenal ulcer.

Hepatic: Abscess, hepatitis, masses, hepatic congestion.

Pulmonary: Pneumonia, PE.

Renal: Nephrolithiasis, pyelonephritis.

2. Discuss the management (investigations and treatment) of the abovementioned patient in the ER.

Blood tests in abdominal pain should be focused according to clinical evaluation, keeping in mind that specificity and diagnostic accuracy are low. For example, a *positive likelihood ratio* (LR+) of acute appendicitis with WBC >10,000/mm^3 is only 1:59, while with WBC >15,000/mm^3 is 4:5.

Among laboratory tests it is important to include glucose, electrolytes, creatinine, and LFT. A dangerous approach is to rely on "normal" blood test rather than to clinical evidence and avoid observation and re-evaluation.

Arterial blood gas analysis is essential for critically ill patients with abdominal pain—metabolic acidosis and hyperlactatemia, if combined with high levels of creatine phosphokinase and creatinine, must create the suspicion of a systemic involvement, a widespread and advanced pathologic process.

Role of abdominal X-ray: A standing chest radiograph remains the primary investigation of choice for the detection of free intraperitoneal gas, and may detect lower lobar pneumonia. Plain abdominal radiography should be used selectively in the event of suspected intestinal obstruction or perforation.

Role of US and CT: Abdominal, contrast enhancement CT scan is the examination with the highest specificity and sensitivity, but bedside ultrasound is now considered the first diagnostic approach in the ED.

Correct analgesia facilitates clinical evaluation because it makes the patient better and more collaborative to examination, thus reducing possible complications, increasing the sensitivity of instrumental investigations, without altering the objective framework. **Flowchart 2** summarizes the management of abdominal pain.

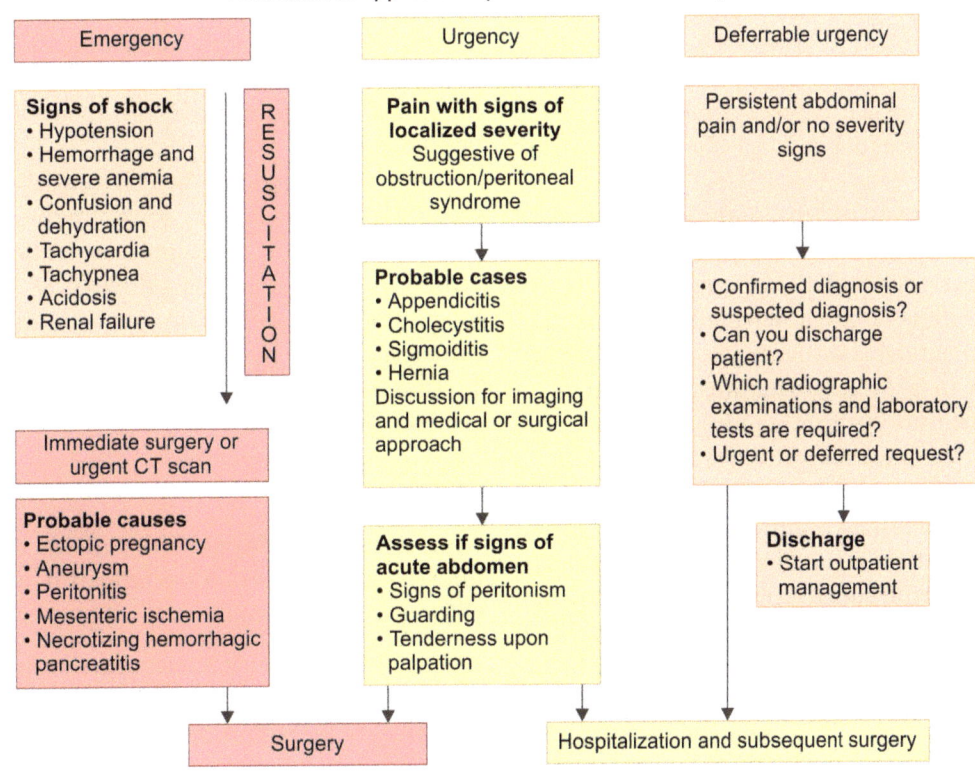

Flowchart 2: Approach to patient with abdominal pain.

Question 8

A 57-year-old patient, a known case of chronic renal disease on regular dialysis—thrice a week, presents to the ER from the dialysis unit with hypotension.

1. Discuss key elements of history of the hemodialysis patient in the ER.

Emergency physician frequently attends the patients who are chronically receiving renal replacement therapy (RRT) and should be prepared for complications related to chronic kidney disease (CKD)/end-stage renal disease (ESRD) and related to these procedures. So, it is worthy to discuss RRT including peritoneal dialysis (PD) and hemodialysis (HD). Infections, bleeding, complications related to volume management and electrolyte abnormalities are common in patients on RRT. When patients fail to get their RRT as scheduled, complications related to fluid management and electrolyte are become more problematic. Among patients with ESRD, infections due to sepsis are the leading cause of mortality. It is also important to note that a percentage of patients with ESRD on RRT proceed to renal transplantation. It is important for the emergency physician to take immediate corrective action in worsening renal function with renal transplant patient that may be caused by any of the insults that can cause acute kidney injury (AKI) and that early identification of the cause and rapid treatment are crucial in the patient with only a single functioning kidney.

2. Explain the differential diagnosis of peridialytic hypotension.

Hypotension: Most frequent complication observed during hemodialysis is *Low* BP occurring in 50% of patient. During hemodialysis average 1–3 L of fluid is removed over a 4-hour session, but 2 L/h fluid removal is possible. During ultrafiltration, normal BP maintenance is depending on cardiovascular compensatory mechanisms and refilling of the vascular space by fluid shifts from the interstitial and intracellular compartments. Most common cause of intradialytic hypotension is excessive ultrafiltration due to underestimation of the patient's ideal blood volume (dry weight).

Differential diagnosis of intradialytic hypotension includes myocardial dysfunction from ischemia, hypoxia, arrhythmias, and early pericardial tamponade. Other causes contribute to hypotension are abnormalities of vascular tone from sepsis or antihypertensive medications. Measures should be taken to prevent intradialytic hypotension are improving nutrition, performing ultrafiltration before dialysis, and increasing the sodium concentration of the dialysate solution, all these measures enhance the vascular refilling. The timing of intradialytic hypotension is often helpful in formulating a differential diagnosis. The causes of hypotension during early phase of dialysis session are preexisting hypovolemia, predialysis fluid losses, GI bleeding, sepsis, vomiting, diarrhea, or decreased intake of salt and water. Blood loss can occur from blood tubing or hemodialyzer filter leaks. If hypotension occurs at the end of dialysis, mostly cause is excessive ultrafiltration, but pericardial or cardiac disease can also precipitate hypotension at the end of dialysis. Orthostatic hypotension, tachycardia, dizziness, and syncope may occur due to hypotension during hemodialysis.

3. Write a short note on disequilibrium syndrome.

Dialysis disequilibrium: It is a clinical syndrome occurring at the end of dialysis when large solute clearances occur during hemodialysis and is characterized by nausea, vomiting, and hypertension, which can progress to seizure, coma, and death. Patient's first dialysis session or during hypercatabolic states are the conditions when this clinical syndrome occurs most. Dialysis disequilibrium may occur due to osmolar imbalance between the brain and the blood resulting cerebral edema, limiting solute clearance when initiating hemodialysis is a preventive measure. This condition can be managed by stopping dialysis and administering 5 mL of 10–23% sodium chloride or mannitol 0.25 g/kg IV to increase serum osmolality.

Question 9

A 42-year-old male was carrying out repair works on an electric pole when he suffered an electrical injury. He presented to the ER with burns on anterior abdominal wall.

1. Discuss clinical features of electrical injury.

Cardiovascular system: Ventricular fibrillation—most common changes in cardiac activity include sinus tachycardia, supraventricular tachycardia, and atrial fibrillation.

Clinical presentation involves either direct impact on respiratory center leading to respiratory arrest or due to suffocation attributed to the contraction of respiratory muscles involved in the pathway of electric current. Respiratory failure initially presents due to underlying cardiac arrest.

Due to vascular damage, kidneys are at high risk for ischemic injury. Muscular contraction is caused by tetany producing rhabdomyolysis, orthopedic injuries, and necrosis of muscles.

Compartment syndrome: The patients with high voltage injuries are more prone to compartment syndrome even with a contact <1 second.

Vascular injury: Electric current passing through extremities may cause spasm in peripheral arteries, thrombosis and/or aneurysm formation. Extensive injury to vascular system may lead to rhabdomyolysis or compartment syndrome.

2. Explain the ED management of a patient with electrical injuries.

Intervention should initiate with securing airway, maintaining breathing, and adequate circulation at the earliest. Administration of oxygen and ventilation should be started immediately in a patient with signs of apnea.

Establish IV access and give isotonic fluids to maintain urine output at 1–1.5 mL/kg/h. Obtain an ECG and place the patient on cardiac monitoring. *According to Parkland formula, it is ideal to raise fluid requirement by two times on the basis of burnt surface area.* Fluid requirement should be calculated from the time of burn. Establishment of an isotonic balanced crystalloid such as Ringer's lactate solution for fluid resuscitation is necessary. Keep a note of the urine output on an hourly basis and maintain an output between 0.5 and 1 mL/kg/hour in the initial 24 hours.

For correction in serum electrolyte imbalances: Start sodium bicarbonate at 1–2 mEq/kg. In cases of high voltage injuries and larger extent of burns, one is likely to develop severe acidosis and myoglobinuria. Hence an initial bolus of fluids should be administered following a correction by sodium bicarbonate.

In order to increase osmotic dieresis, patient should be started on mannitol at 1 g/kg of body weight. Maintain a urine output at 2–3 mL/kg/hour, at a urinary pH above 6.5. Sodium bicarbonate alkalizes the urine; therefore, it causes myoglobin to be more soluble.

For better pain control it is advisable to start a short-acting opioid such as fentanyl (1 µg/kg IV), as a continuous infusion and is more easily titratable. In case airway is not secured, it is vital to intubate the patient. Superficial and deep burns need cleaning and dressing under aseptic conditions, along with antibiotic coverage.

Question 10

A 27-year-old is brought to the ER by his parents. He is very agitated and combative.

1. Discuss an approach to a patient with acute agitation in the ER.

Initial assessment of the agitated patient should prioritize safety, with adequate screening of the patient for weapons, interview conducted in a room that allows privacy without compromising security, easily accessible entry and exit points for the provider and readily available personnel and protocols for appropriate restraint and intervention, as necessary. Despite the fact that agitated patients present unique challenges that include violence toward healthcare professionals, most physicians tend not to receive formalized training in managing these high-risk individuals.

The causes of agitation may be metabolic, ranging from electrolyte abnormalities, abnormal glucose levels and hypoxia to disorders of thyroid hormones and nutritional deficiencies (e.g., Wernicke's encephalopathy). Infectious causes, shock, thermal dysregulation, intracranial injury or abnormality and toxins can all manifest as agitation. Psychiatric causes of agitation can include psychosis, schizophrenia, delusions, and personality disorders. It is, therefore, essential to keep broad differential diagnosis in mind when dealing with agitated patients, as most of the abovementioned conditions will likely require rapid identification and timely management for reversal of symptoms.

2. Explain the restraints in the ER.

The ED physician should consider the use of verbal de-escalation tactics first when the situation allows, and the patient appears to be receptive and cooperative. These include communicating with the patient in a calm, concise, respectful manner while avoiding provocative statements, threats, and condescension. If verbal techniques fail to manage the patient's agitation, the use of restraint should be considered. Typically, chemical restraint is preferable to physical restraint, but these may be used in combination as appropriate for the severely combative patient.

Pharmacologic options traditionally incorporate antipsychotic agents and benzodiazepines. Classically, first-generation (typical) antipsychotics such as haloperidol (2.5–5 mg IM/IV) are used. However, second-generation (atypical) antipsychotics, such as olanzapine (10 mg IM or 5–10 mg PO) have been shown in recent studies to perform better with lower rates of adverse events compared to first-generation antipsychotics. Commonly used benzodiazepines include lorazepam (2–4 mg IM/IV) and midazolam (2.5–5 mg IM/IV). All medication used to control agitation should aim to calm, not sedate the patient, and can be titrated up to achieve the desired effect.

Physical restraint, when applied, should be done so in a systematic, team-based approach with coverage of five points (four limbs and head) and avoidance of prone positioning. In any form of restraint, post-restraint monitoring and evaluation should be implemented to assess for any adverse effects from the intervention to the patient and progression of patient condition.

■ SUGGESTED READING

1. Richhariya D, Sharma B. Textbook of Emergency Medicine including Intensive Care and Trauma, 2nd edition. New Delhi: Jaypee Brothers Medical Publishers (P) Ltd; 2022. p. 526. (Question 1).
2. Richhariya D, Sharma B. Textbook of Emergency Medicine including Intensive Care and Trauma, 2nd edition. New Delhi: Jaypee Brothers Medical Publishers (P) Ltd; 2022. p. 1467. (Question 2).
3. Richhariya D, Sharma B. Textbook of Emergency Medicine including Intensive Care and Trauma, 2nd edition. New Delhi: Jaypee Brothers Medical Publishers (P) Ltd; 2022. p. 497. (Question 3).

4. Richhariya D, Sharma B. Textbook of Emergency Medicine including Intensive Care and Trauma, 2nd edition. New Delhi: Jaypee Brothers Medical Publishers (P) Ltd; 2022. p. 1321. (Question 4).
5. Richhariya D, Sharma B. Textbook of Emergency Medicine including Intensive Care and Trauma, 2nd edition. New Delhi: Jaypee Brothers Medical Publishers (P) Ltd; 2022. p. 513. (Question 5).
6. Richhariya D, Sharma B. Textbook of Emergency Medicine including Intensive Care and Trauma, 2nd edition. New Delhi: Jaypee Brothers Medical Publishers (P) Ltd; 2022. p. 838. (Question 6).
7. Richhariya D, Sharma B. Textbook of Emergency Medicine including Intensive Care and Trauma, 2nd edition. New Delhi: Jaypee Brothers Medical Publishers (P) Ltd; 2022. p. 634. (Question 7).
8. Richhariya D, Sharma B. Textbook of Emergency Medicine including Intensive Care and Trauma, 2nd edition. New Delhi: Jaypee Brothers Medical Publishers (P) Ltd; 2022. pp. 756-9. (Question 8).
9. Richhariya D, Sharma B. Textbook of Emergency Medicine including Intensive Care and Trauma, 2nd edition. New Delhi: Jaypee Brothers Medical Publishers (P) Ltd; 2022. pp. 1713-8. (Question 9).
10. Richhariya D, Sharma B. Textbook of Emergency Medicine including Intensive Care and Trauma, 2nd edition. New Delhi: Jaypee Brothers Medical Publishers (P) Ltd; 2022. p. 1050. (Question 10).

Emergency Medicine Paper 36

Nandha Kumar Selvam

Question 1

1. Explain the causes of emergency department (ED) crowding.

The causes of ED crowding are classified under five categories:

1. *Health system level:*
- Decreased national inpatient capacity.
- Post-pandemic urge of hospitals in "return to normal" scenario.
- Inadequate hospital inpatient capacity leading to poor management of patients flow.
- Lack of wider primary care facility and underinsurance end up in hospitalizations from acute deterioration of chronic diseases.
- Long-term hospital occupancy due to lack of post-discharge healthcare facilities.
- Lack of psychiatric units has made ED a default location for most of the acutely decompensated psychiatric patients.

2. *Hospital factors:*
- Hospital with high inpatient census.
- Lack of leadership alignment and priority at all levels of hospital administrations.
- Hospitals functioning capacity mismatch with ED that functions 24 × 7.
- Lack of primary and after-hours care options increasing hospitalization.
- Lack of inpatient nursing capacity due to illness further decreasing hospital functioning capacity.
- Infection control impact on space and patient dwell time.

3. *Emergency department input factors:*
- Emergency department surges in volume occur, particularly the day following weekends and holidays.
- Inability of PCPs to see patients in timely manner results in possibly unnecessary ED visits.
- Both primary care providers/physicians (PCPs) and specialists send patients to ED for further workup while waiting for rooms or operation theater.
- Inequitable queuing of ED admission to accommodate high revenue generating patients coming on outpatient department (OPD) basis.

4. *Emergency department throughput issues:*
- Increased complexity of ED patients demands resources.
- Availability of time intensive technology in ED increases patients' evaluation time.
- Laboratory, radiology, consultant delays
- ED nursing shortage and turnover
- ED documentation requirements have paradoxical negative impact on physician and nurse efficiency.
- Multiple simultaneous provider distractions, i.e., referral calls, non-beneficial laboratory calls, etc.

5. *Emergency department output factors:*
- High hospital census or operational inefficiency prevents bed availability.
- Inefficient transfer process from ED to inpatient units.
- Inpatient discharges often occur very late in the day; by then, the ED is backed up.
- Hectic hospital rounds block admission availability
- Inpatient bed informal set-asides (blocking).
- Failure to address end-of-life care.

2. Discuss the measures to deal with ED crowding taken under three categories.

1. *Emergency department input:*
- Establish urgent care center to slow down the ED case flows.
- Triage low acuity patients out and maintain separate zone for their treatment.
- Extend primary care hours or availability so that admission due to worsening of chronic diseases will come down.
- Ambulance diversion but has impact over patients outcome.

Focusing attention on ways to decrease lower-acuity ED visits diverts administrative energy from addressing the real issue—excessive boarding functionally decreases ED size. It is important to underscore that diverting low-acuity patients to alternate sites does not decrease admission demand or impact boarding. It should be noted that many ED-based solutions do significantly to improve ED operations and patient flow within the ED, but most do not address boarding and crowding. Thus, meaningful solutions are at the institutional level.

2. *Emergency department throughput:*
- Physicians at triage indirectly reduces ED length of stay and prevent patients being without seen or identify higher acuity patients.
- Bedside registration, implementing fast-track and improving ancillary turnaround times.
- Increasing ED staffing along with ED in design and beds.
- Establishing inpatient unit to manage ED boarding patients.
- Availability of after-care clinics with evening hours within 48 hours of ED discharges.
- Discharge nursing calls and discharge lounges.

Maintaining ED morale among nursing is paramount. Burnout and poor morale lead to nurse callouts, often leaving holes in the schedule and forcing nurses to become inefficient and overextended or further decreasing the functional size of the department by needing to close ED beds.

3. *Emergency department output (hospital-based solutions):*
- Availability of inpatient ancillary services off-hours (evenings and weekends)
- Availability of procedures and consults throughout the entire week.
- Synchronizing inpatient discharge with admission demand.
- Temporary boarding on inpatient hallways.
- Stop elective surgeries/procedures and transfers.
- Centralized bed control and allocation by the management.
- After-care appointments made within 48 hours of discharge.
- Admitting service (MD, nurses, or both) providing care for the admitted patient in the ED may reduce the hospital length of stay.

Core solutions and key actions:
- Emergency department crowding must be acknowledged as a serious patient safety issue by medical leadership, regulators, payers, and legislators.
- Addressing crowding must become a top institutional priority with visible, committed leadership, and aligned incentives.
- Hospitals should budget inpatient occupancy <85%.
- While <2 hours of boarding should be the benchmark, adherence to 4 hours for 90% of admitted patients should be the minimum universal standard for all institutions.

Question 2

1. What is Florali trial? Discuss.

- This trial is a multicenter randomized controlled open label trail recorded from 23 intensive care units (ICUs) in France and Belgium. It compared various effects of HFNC (high flow nasal cannula) with standard non-rebreather (NRB) mask and non-invasive ventilation in patients with acute hypoxemic respiratory failure **(Table 1)**.
- *Inclusion criteria:* Adult ≥ 18 years, no history of chronic respiratory failure and acute hypoxemic respiratory failure with RR >25 per minute, P/F ≤300 mm Hg, $PaCO_2$ ≤45 mm Hg.
- *Outcomes:* Primary outcomes are intubation rates within 28 days of enrollment while secondary outcomes are ICU mortality, 90 days mortality, and ventilator free days up to 28 days.
- *Results:* Through enrollment over 2 years, the final study population for analysis was 310 patients. Baseline characteristics were similar between groups and the common cause of acute hypoxemic respiratory failure was community-acquired pneumonia. Regarding patient comfort, the reported discomfort was reduced in high flow nasal cannula (HFNC) group as compared to the other two groups.
- Lastly, there was no difference in serious adverse events between the three groups.
- *Conclusion:* In adult pneumonia patients with acute hypoxemic respiratory failure, HFNC shown to be associated with decreased ICU and 90 days mortality and may lead to decreased intubation rates, all while increasing patients comfort and decreasing dyspnea as compared to NRB mask and bilevel positive airway pressure non-invasive ventilation (BiPAP NIV).

TABLE 1: Florali trial.

Oxygen delivery system	Heated and humidified high flow nasal cannula (n = 106)	Standard NRB mask (n = 94)	Non-invasive ventilation, i.e., BiPAP (n = 110)
Intubation rates within 28 days	38%	47% OR = 1.45 (0.83 – 2.55)	50% OR = 1.65 (0.96 – 2.84)
ICU mortality	11%	19% OR = 1.85 (0.84 – 4.09)	25% OR = 2.55 (1.21 – 5.35)
90 days mortality	12%	23% OR = 2.01 (1.01 – 3.99)	28% OR = 2.50 (1.31 – 4.78)
Ventilator free days up to 28 days	24 ± 8	22 ± 10	19 ± 12

(BiPAP: bilevel positive airway pressure; ICU: intensive care unit; NRB: non-rebreather)

2. Explain the airway management in coronavirus disease-2019 (COVID-19) disease.

In COVID patients, rapid viral transmission within hospitals has been documented and remains a major concern. Medical procedures are likely to aerosolize patient sputum and thus significantly increase the risk of exposing healthcare workers to respiratory pathogens. Avoiding emergent intubation and preparing with personal protective equipment (PPE) and powered air-purifying respirators (PAPR) would be essential in protecting healthcare workers. COVID-19 airway response team with specialized training in airway management should be involved in the care of this patient population. Current recommendations are as follows:

Pre-intubation protocols:
- Any kind of airway management should be better planned in negative pressure environment.
- Patient must have functioning intravenous (IV) cannula and monitor basic physiological parameters.
- Appropriate airway equipment such as suction, laryngoscopes with different sized blades, bougie, laryngeal mask airway (LMA) should be readily kept available.
- Airway trolley with essential medications should be placed at the entry of room to minimize exposure.
- High efficiency particulate filter (≥0.3 μm) has to be connected immediately after placing ET tube.
- Appropriately assigning roles to all the personnel.
- Optimize hemodynamics with inotropes or vasopressor prior to induction.

Protocols during intubation:
- Preoxygenate with proper protection strategy but avoid bag-mask ventilation
- Consider video laryngoscope for initial attempt and have low threshold for surgical airway even with unsuccessful two attempts.
- Minimize time to cuff inflation and connection to ventilator circuit.
- Using lidocaine and avoiding fentanyl to minimize coughing.
- Use longer acting paralytic agents like rocuronium.

Post-intubation protocols:
- Proper containment of all equipment that contacted patient airway
- Appropriately replace outer gloves and contaminated PPE
- Maintain adequate sedation and paralysis to minimize dys-synchrony
- Maintain lung protective ventilator settings such as low tidal volumes (4–6 mL/kg), positive end-expiratory pressure (PEEP) of 8–10 cmH$_2$O, plateau pressure of ≤30 cmH$_2$O, and target SpO$_2$ of 90–95%.

Extubation protocols:
- Minimize the number of personnel during extubation and assign roles
- Check for cuff leak and give prolonged spontaneous breathing trial to ensure successful extubation
- Discontinue circuit flow prior to extubation and minimize time between extubation and covering of patients airway with a mask
- Prepare for possible reintubation or surgical airway equipment in case of extubation failure
- Prepare with post-extubation oxygen support plan with HFNC or BiPAP or continuous positive airway pressure (CPAP).
- Contain and properly dispose any airway equipment

Question 3

A 12-year-old boy weighing 49 kg presents to the emergency room (ER) with abdominal pain, nausea, and vomiting for 2 days. The blood glucometer gives a "high" reading. He is acidotic with a pH of 7.15 and bicarbonate of 8 mmol/L. The blood ketones come as 4 mmol/L. You diagnose him as diabetic ketoacidosis.

1. Discuss the fluid management in diabetic ketoacidosis (DKA).

- Calculate fluid deficit and it is often 5–10% of the body weight which is 50–100 mL/kg.
- Start with isotonic crystalloid at 15–20 mL/kg/h in case child is in shock.
- Once vital signs have stabilized, resist the desire to correct the fluid deficit too rapidly to avoid hyperosmolar state, pulmonary edema, and cerebral edema.
- After achieving normotension, fluid can be given at the rate of 250–500 mL/h.
- When blood sugar falls to 250 mg/dL, fluid should be changed to 5% dextrose in 0.45% saline and infuse at the rate of 150–250 mL/h.
- Safe method for fluid replacement is 50% given in first 8 hours and rest given over next 16–24 hours.

2. Explain the insulin therapy in DKA.

- Insulin therapy has to be initiated as soon as the fluid management been started as only insulin can correct ketoacidosis.
- Avoid giving bolus insulin and initiate infusion at the rate of 0.1 units of regular insulin per kg per hour.

- Monitor parameters such as pH, bicarbonate, blood glucose, and urine output.
- Target glucose reduction per hour could be 50–100 mg/dL but shall double the insulin infusion if the improvement in pH is too low (<0.03/h).
- When blood glucose reaches 250 mg/dL and ketoacidosis about to resolve (pH >7.3 or bicarbonate >15 mEq/L), give basal insulin dose via subcutaneous route, taper the insulin infusion to 0.02–0.05 unit/kg/h along with dextrose saline infusion and continue for few hours.

3. Discuss the role of bicarbonate.
- Bicarbonate is often indicated only in critically ill patients with pH <7.0 and unstable hemodynamic from poor cardiac contractility.
- More than benefits, it has been associated with dreadful complications such as cerebral edema, volume overload, hypernatremia, and paradoxical central nervous system (CNS) acidosis.
- Corrections should be avoided if pH is >7.1 or serum bicarbonate >10 mEq/L.

4. Enumerate the investigations and monitoring.
- Check random blood sugar and serum electrolytes (sodium, potassium, calcium, magnesium, phosphate).
- Send venous blood gas analysis to know acid base status, anion gap, and lactate level.
- Check acetone level preferably from urine sample but serum acetone is often available bedside.
- Other routine studies are complete blood count, creatinine, and urine complete analysis.
- Parameters to be monitored during DKA evaluation and management are:
  - Check serum glucose level every hour
  - Monitor pH, bicarbonate, anion gap, electrolytes by doing blood gas analysis every 2 hours.
  - Among all, serum sodium, potassium, and osmolality are the critical values to be monitored.
  - Average potassium deficit is 3–5 mEq/kg and initial serum level is usually normal or high in case of DKA. If initial levels are low, it is dangerous and requires potassium supplementation once the urine output is established.
  - In case of hyperosmolarity, avoid rapid fluid replacement to prevent cerebral edema.
  - Continuous cardiac monitor to watch QTc prolongation.

5. What are the complications of DKA?
- Dehydration
- Shock/hypotension
- Hypo/Hyperkalemia
- Hypoglycemia
- Aspiration pneumonia
- Sepsis
- Acute tubular necrosis
- Hypercoagubility leading to MI stroke and DVT
- Cerebral edema

Question 4

A 2-year-old boy presents to the ER with high-grade fever and is unable to bear weight on his right leg for 1 day. There is no history of fall or trauma. He had sore throat about 3–4 days back. The child cries during movement of the right leg. His knee appears to be normal. Vaccination is complete as per schedule. There is no history suggestive of any significant medical illness.

1. What is the likely differential diagnosis in the above case?
- Septic arthritis
- Osteomyelitis
- Transient synovitis
- Reactive or toxic synovitis
- Gonococcal arthritis
- Acute rheumatic fever
- Juvenile idiopathic arthritis
- Poststreptococcal reactive arthritis

2. What are the Kocher's criteria?
- Criteria to diagnose septic arthritis and differentiate from transient synovitis in children
- It is applicable to all joints such as hip (most common), knee, and ankle joint
- Criteria and each criterion carries 1 point:
  - Non-weight bearing on affected side
  - Erythrocyte sedimentation rate (ESR) >40 mm/h
  - Fever >38.5°C
  - White blood cells >12,000 cells/mm^3
- Scores and likelihood of septic arthritis
  - 1–3%
  - 2–40%
  - 3–93%
  - 4–99%

3. What investigations would you ask for?
- Complete blood count, ESR, and C-reactive protein (CRP).
- Blood cultures and throat cultures.
- Arthrocentesis should be planned immediately.

- Joint fluid to be analyzed for cell count, gram stain, culture, and polymerase chain reaction (PCR) studies.
- Evaluate for other sources of infection such as urinary and skin infection.
- Imaging with plain radiography, ultrasonography (USG), computed tomography (CT), and magnetic resonance imaging (MRI) can aid in diagnosis.

4. What would be the treatment for this child in the ED?

- Treatment should be initiated as early as possible as prognosis depends on the length of time between symptom onset and treatment initiation.
- Immediate arthrocentesis followed by rapid IV antibiotics administration.
- If orthopedic care seems to be delayed, initiate IV empirical antibiotics.
- Initial IV antibiotic therapies for acute suppurative arthritis are:
  - *Staphylococcus aureus:* Vancomycin 10 mg/kg every 6–8 hours (or) clindamycin 10 mg/kg every 6–8 hours.
  - *Streptococcus species:* Clindamycin 10 mg/kg every 6–8 hours (and) cefotaxime 50 mg/kg every 6–8 hours (or) ceftriaxone 50 mg/kg every 12 hours
  - *Gram-negative bacilli and Haemophilus influenzae*: Cefotaxime 50 mg/kg every 8 hours (or) ceftriaxone 50 mg/kg every 12 hours
  - *Unknown:* Vancomycin (or) clindamycin (and) cefotaxime (or) ceftriaxone.

Question 5

1. Discuss the levels of evidence in biomedical research.

Critically-appraised individual articles and synopses include as below **(Fig. 1)**:

Filtered evidence:
Level I: Evidence from a systematic review of all relevant randomized controlled trials.
Level II: Evidence from a meta-analysis of all relevant randomized controlled trials.
Level III: Evidence from evidence summaries developed from systematic reviews.
Level IV: Evidence from guidelines developed from systematic reviews.
Level V: Evidence from meta-syntheses of a group of descriptive or qualitative studies.
Level VI: Evidence from evidence summaries of individual studies.

Level VII: Evidence from one properly designed randomized controlled trial.

Unfiltered evidence:
Level VIII: Evidence from nonrandomized controlled clinical trials, nonrandomized clinical trials, cohort studies, case series, case reports, and individual qualitative studies.

Level IX: Evidence from opinion of authorities and/or reports of expert committee.

Two things to remember:
1. Studies in which randomization occurs represent a higher level of evidence than those in which subject selection is not random.
2. Controlled studies carry a higher level of evidence than those in which control groups are not used.

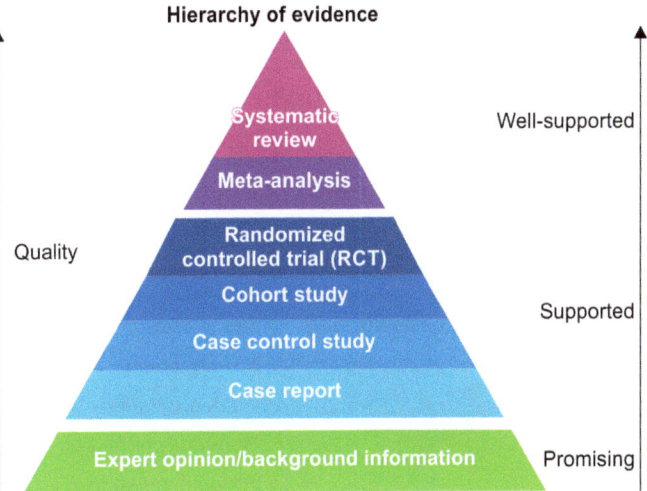

Fig. 1: Levels of evidence in biomedical research.

2. What is linear correlation coefficient?

The linear correlation coefficient, also known as Pearson's correlation coefficient or Pearson's r, is a value that reflects the strength and direction of the linear relationship between two variables, x and y. This value is calculated by finding the ratio of the covariance between the two variables and the product of their standard deviations. It is a normalized measurement of covariances where the result (value of r) always lies between −1 and 1).

Pearson's correlation coefficient makes certain assumptions. If even one of these assumptions is not met, the test cannot be accurately conducted and an alternative correlation test should be used instead.
- The sample is selected randomly and is representative of the target population.
- Both the variables are measured on a continuous scale; the interval or ratio scale.

- The data contains paired samples and therefore each subject has both *x* and *y* variable values.
- There must be independence of observations; values of variables between subjects should have no relationship.
- There is a linear association between the variables.
- There are no outliers present in the data.
- The *x* and *y* variables follow an (approximately) normal distribution.

Types of correlations: The correlation coefficient is reflected by Pearson's *r*. The value of *r* can range between –1 and 1, where:
- Positive values indicate a positive correlation (0 < *r* 1)
- Negative values indicate a negative correlation (–1*r* < 1)
- A value of 0 indicates no correlation (*r* = 0)

Pearson's *r* can be calculated using the following formula:

$$r = \frac{n(\Sigma xy) - (\Sigma x)(\Sigma y)}{\sqrt{[n\Sigma x^2 - (\Sigma x)^2][n\Sigma y^2 - (\Sigma y)^2]}}$$

The following **Table 2** reflects broad cut-offs that can be used to interpret strength, the value of *r*, whether negative or positive:

TABLE 2: Correlation coefficient.

Value of r (correlation coefficient)	Interpretation
0.00–0.10	No correlation
0.10–0.39	Weak correlation
0.40–0.69	Moderate correlation
0.70–0.89	Strong correlation
0.90–1.00	Very strong correlation

Question 6

A 1-year-old child presents to the ED with history of fever, abdominal pain, vomiting, and bloody diarrhea for 1 day.

1. Discuss the differential diagnosis of bloody diarrhea in children.

- Inflammatory bowel disease
- Intussusception
- Pseudomembranous colitis
- Hemolytic uremic syndrome
- Parasitic infections
- Bacterial infections
  - *Salmonella* species
  - *Shigella* species
  - *Campylobacter* species
  - Shiga toxin producing *Escherichia coli* (*E. coli*)

2. What investigations would you ask for?

- Complete blood count
- C-reactive protein
- Serum glucose
- Serum electrolytes
- Urine complete analysis
- Serum blood urea nitrogen (BUN) and creatinine
- Rapid stool test to detect fecal lactoferrin
- Stool culture or rectal swabs
- Ultrasound abdomen has a diagnostic role.

3. How would you treat a child with sepsis in the ER?

- If a child presenting with a signs and symptoms of sepsis or shock, look hard for the source of infections.
- Record initial vital parameters as it is main tool to follow up with the improvement or deterioration of the child in ED.
- Send lactate early and draw blood/urine for culture/sensitivity study as soon as suspecting sepsis in child.
- Initiate broad-spectrum antibiotics as early as possible for any case of sepsis or septic shock.
- Infuse normal saline or ringer lactate solution at 20 mL/kg over 5–30 minutes as an initial bolus to child with sepsis or septic shock. Aim for 60–100 mL/kg in the first hour.
- If shock persisting, an additional 20 mL/kg can be infused over 20–30 minutes following the initial bolus.
- After initial volume expansion, use 5% dextrose in 0.9% normal saline as a maintenance fluid replacement.
- Monitor the response by measuring lactate, vital signs, clinical appearance, urine output, or shock index.
- Do not delay vasopressor when blood pressure does not respond to initial bolus of crystalloids.

Question 7

You are the ED consultant on floor. You are called in that one of the relatives is having a heated argument with one of the ER resident doctor.

1. Discuss the factors leading to difficult physician patient interaction.

Emergency department is the crucial place for the medical encounter and high-pressure conditions turn up the heat on the patient physician interaction.
- *Life-threatening illnesses* are more likely to be the scenario in any ED, hence decisions must be made quickly in all aspects such as evaluating patients, giving treatment

orders, discussing with patient/relatives about their clinical status and following up with patient response to the given treatment.

- *Patient's physical distress and fear* push them to extremes of behavior and that will happen soon when they are not addressed properly at earliest.
- *Personalities of individual patient and physician* and the range of personal, social, and professional expectations that each brings to the interaction always have the potential to turn the medical encounter into a difficult one.
- Not only is the patient *unfamiliar to the physician*, but members of this patient group may also be non-compliant, perhaps because of psychiatric illness or distress, perhaps because of substance dependence, denial, or inability to pay for routine medical care and prescription drugs. When acute illness eclipses the reason for the patient's neglect of proper medical care, he/she presents in the ED, often with many slight to severe, untreated health problems.
- *Patients may have been brought to the hospital against their wishes*, by friends, family members, an emergency response team, or police. If so, they may be hostile, combative, or abusive and attempt to refuse treatment or to leave the hospital.
- *Ethnic, cultural, and language differences* may present barriers to good communication.

2. Analyze the ED preparedness and prevention of violence.

Physician's first intervention is to assure the patient in a non-threatening way that, regardless of the circumstances, his or her health is the physician's primary concern. Often physicians must maintain control of their own emotions, responding to patient anger and even abuse calmly.

Physician must determine, almost simultaneously:
- Whether the patient is likely to pose a threat of harm to him- or herself or to others.
- Whether or not a medical emergency or need exists? Whether the patient is in physical distress? Intoxicated? Psychotic? Attempting to get a prescription for narcotics?
- Whether the patient is competent to accept or refuse treatment? If not, whether someone is present who can speak as the patient's surrogate?

Answers to these questions determine how the encounter proceeds:
- If a medical need is present and the patient is not combative or hostile and is competent to discuss and give consent for treatment or refusal for treatment, the encounter resembles a traditional acute medical intervention.
- If medical need is present and the patient is highly combative with frankly compromised mental status, he or she can be restrained or sedated so that the need can be assessed and treatment can proceed. The physician may ask security personnel or police to detain or control the patient.

Determining decision-making competency of the patient often avoids difficult patient physician interaction and knowing guidelines to determine that competency by a physician is something important to run a peaceful environment.

Future education programs on physician-patient communication in the ED should focus on strengthening physicians' ability to communicate with patients in a more open way. They should adopt socioemotional-oriented communication skills, expressing respect and kindness, and allowing patients to briefly describe their symptoms and participate in the treatment process to achieve physician-patient consensus.

Question 8

1. Discuss the updated recommendations from 2020 American Heart Association (AHA) pediatric advanced and basic life support guidelines.

High-quality cardiopulmonary resuscitation (CPR) is the foundation of resuscitation. New data reaffirm the key components of high-quality CPR—providing adequate chest compression rate and depth, minimizing interruptions in CPR, allowing full chest recoil between compressions, and avoiding excessive ventilation.

- A respiratory rate of 20–30 breaths per minute is new for infants and children who are (a) receiving CPR with an advanced airway in place or (b) receiving rescue breathing and have a pulse.
- For patients with non-shockable rhythms, the earlier epinephrine is administered after CPR initiation, the more likely the patient is to survive.
- Using a cuffed endotracheal tube decreases the need for endotracheal tube changes.
- The routine use of cricoid pressure does not reduce the risk of regurgitation during bag-mask ventilation and may impede intubation success.
- For out-of-hospital cardiac arrest, bag-mask ventilation results in the same resuscitation outcomes as advanced airway interventions such as endotracheal intubation.
- Resuscitation does not end with return of spontaneous circulation (ROSC). Excellent postcardiac arrest care is critically important to achieving the best patient

outcomes. For children who do not regain consciousness after ROSC, this care includes targeted temperature management and continuous electroencephalography monitoring. The prevention and/or treatment of hypotension, hyperoxia or hypoxia, and hypercapnia or hypocapnia are important.

- After discharge from the hospital, cardiac arrest survivors can have physical, cognitive, and emotional challenges and may need ongoing therapies and interventions.
- Naloxone can reverse respiratory arrest due to opioid overdose, but there is no evidence that it benefits patients in cardiac arrest.
- Fluid resuscitation in sepsis is based on patient response and requires frequent reassessment. Balanced crystalloid, unbalanced crystalloid, and colloid fluids are all acceptable for sepsis resuscitation. Epinephrine or norepinephrine infusions are used for fluid-refractory septic shock.

2. Discuss neuroprognostication after cardiac arrest in adults.

Hypoxic brain injury is the leading cause of morbidity and mortality in survivors of out of hospital cardiac arrest. It accounts for a smaller but significant portion of poor outcomes after resuscitation from in-hospital cardiac arrest. Accurate neurological prognostication is important to avoid inappropriate withdrawal of life-sustaining treatment in patients who may achieve meaningful neurologic recovery with life-sustaining treatment. Neuroprognostication relies on interpreting the results of diagnostic tests and correlating those results with outcome. Many of the tests considered are subject to error due to the effects of medications, organ dysfunction, and temperature. A false positive test for poor neurologic outcome could lead to inappropriate withdrawal of life support from a patient who otherwise might have recovered. General considerations in patients who remain comatose after cardiac arrest:

- Neuroprognostication should involve a multimodal approach and not be based on any single finding.
- Neuroprognostication should be delayed until adequate time has passed to avoid any false positive or false negative results due to underlying organ dysfunction or temperature.
- Teams should have regular and transparent multi-disciplinary discussions with surrogates about the anticipated time course for neuroprognostication.
- It is reasonable to perform multimodal neuroprognostication at a minimum of 72 hours after achieving normothermia, though individual prognostic tests may be obtained earlier than this.

Question 9

A 78-year-old female comes to the ER after a slip and fall. She is in severe pain and has fracture of the femur neck. She has diabetes mellitus, hypertension, and chronic obstructive pulmonary disease (COPD). Pain is persistent even after intravenous analgesics that can be offered. You decide to do a fascia iliaca block for pain relief.

1. Discuss the anatomy of fascia iliaca.

Anatomy: The fascia iliaca compartment is a potential space lying between the fascia iliaca anteriorly and the iliacus and psoas muscles (iliopsoas) posteriorly. The fascia iliaca attaches to the iliac crest laterally and to the fascia overlying the psoas muscle medially. It lies posteriorly to the external iliac vessels and anteriorly to the nerves of the lumbar plexus. More distally, the fascia iliaca invests the femoral nerve and passes posterior to the femoral artery and vein which lie within the lacuna vasorum. Here, femoral nerve descends through the fibers of psoas major before passing distally between iliaca and psoas muscles. Lateral cutaneous nerve of thigh passes deep to fascia iliaca before leaving the fascial plane around the level of the inguinal ligament. Obturator nerve penetrates through the fascia iliaca compartment, passes posterior to the common iliac artery before reaching the obturator foramen. Since the proximal end of anatomical course of all three nerves lies within fascia iliaca compartment, placement of local anesthesia beneath the fascia iliaca results in anesthesia of all the three nerves. *Fascia iliaca block* (**Fig. 2**) aims to block the femoral nerve, obturator nerve, and lateral cutaneous nerve of thigh simultaneously. In real-time practice, it is safer than femoral block and lumbar plexus block.

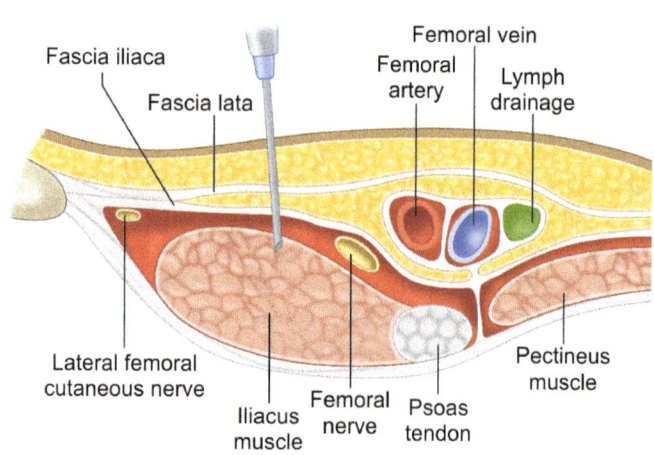

Fig. 2: Fascia iliaca block.

2. Explain the indications, contraindications, and complications of fascia iliaca block for pain relief.

Indications:
- Pre-, peri-, and postoperative analgesia after fractured neck of femur
- Hip and knee surgery, above knee amputation
- Application of plaster cast to femoral fracture in pediatric patients

Contraindications:
- Previous femoral bypass surgery
- Patient refusal and allergy to local anesthesia
- Infection at the block site
- Relative contraindications include patients with coagulopathy, peripheral neuropathy, or neurological conditions.

Complications:
- Block failure
- Hematoma
- Neuropraxia
- Local anesthetics systemic toxicity
- Quadriceps weakness
- Perforation of peritoneal cavity contents and bladder puncture.

3. Give a brief description of various approaches to the fascia iliaca block.

Landmark-guided approach: Anterior superior iliac spine, inguinal ligament, and pubic tubercle are the anatomical landmarks and line connecting the anterior superior iliac spine and pubic tubercle are divided into thirds. Patient positioned supine; injection is performed at a point 1 cm caudal to junction of lateral one-third and medial two-third of the inguinal ligament with femoral pulse being felt 1.5 cm medial to the point of injection.

Ultrasonography-guided infra-inguinal approach: Using high frequency linear probe placed transversely, identify femoral artery at the inguinal crease and lateral to that at the depth 2–4 cm, iliopsoas muscle with overlying fascia iliaca will be identified with hyperechoic femoral nerve lying between them. Probe may be tilted cranially and caudally until optimal images of the femoral nerve and fascia iliaca are obtained. Following skin disinfection and local anesthesia infiltration, needle has to be introduced using in plane technique with the aim of placing the needle tip beneath fascia iliaca around the lateral third of the inguinal line. Correct needle placement is confirmed by separation of the fascia iliaca from the iliopsoas muscle with local anesthesia spreading toward the femoral nerve medially and the iliac crest laterally.

Ultrasonography-guided supra-inguinal approach: In this approach, placing high frequency linear probe sagittal, obtain an image of ilium and iliaca muscle. The femoral artery is seen by moving the probe inferiorly and medially along the inguinal ligament. The probe is then moved laterally and superiorly along the inguinal ligament toward the anterior superior iliac spine to lie lateral to the femoral nerve. The deep circumflex artery is identified superficial to the fascia iliaca and 1–2 cm cephalad to the inguinal ligament, and this provides a further landmark for needle placement. The needle is inserted 2–4 cm caudad to the inguinal ligament aiming ultimately to be beneath the fascia iliaca cephalad to the inguinal ligament. Local anesthesia spread should be seen between the fascia iliaca and iliacus muscle and into the iliac fossa.

4. Enumerate the drugs used with doses.

- Long-acting local anesthetics agents are preferred to provide extended analgesia.
- Hence preferred drugs are ropivacaine and levobupivacaine.
- Approximately 30–40 mL of local anesthesia is required.
- Dosing should not exceed the safe limits to avoid systemic toxicity.

Question 10

A 56-year-old diabetic, hypertensive, and with ischemic heart disease presents to ER with type I respiratory failure, hypotension, and severe acidosis. He has pneumonia and appears to be confused. You decide to intubate this sick acidotic patient.

1. Discuss the salient features of intubation a sick acidotic patient in ER.

Any patients with physiological derangement pose a significant challenge in airway management as equivalent as anatomical derangements. Physiological derangements such as right **ventricular** failure, excess **oxygen** consumption, **low** BP/oxygen saturation/volume status, and severe metabolic **acidosis** (pneumonic- **V.O.L.A**) are leading to physiologically difficult airway by posing high risk for cardiopulmonary collapse and even cardiac arrest during or immediately after airway management.

Here, the above case has the combination of hypoxemia, hypotension, and acidosis, which is a significant challenge for airway management and even lead to cardiac arrest.

But airway management in such cases is essential to prevent further worsening of clinical conditions of the patient. There are certain ways to mitigate this physiological perturbation while managing airway:
- Right ventricular failure has to be managed by reducing afterload using pulmonary vasodilator. Avoidance of acidosis, hypercapnia, hypoxia through proper preoxygenation, apnea oxygenation, careful fluid administration, and vasopressor.
- Excessive oxygen consumption correcting anemia if exists.
- Low oxygen saturation can be managed by upright position, awake intubation, noninvasive positive pressure ventilation (NIPPV)/CPAP, apnea oxygenation and using anxiolysis/analgesia.
- Low BP/volume can be managed with crystalloids resuscitation, inotropes, vasopressor, hemodynamically neutral drugs for intubation.
- In severe acidosis, often avoid intubation as it suppresses the compensatory hyperventilation and worsens acidosis. But still intubation would be beneficial if done with maintenance of spontaneous respiration during intubation. Always treat underlying cause, minimize apnea time, and awake intubation.

In hemodynamically unstable patients, pre-intubation resuscitation with fluids, vasopressor or inotropes has to done before airway management. In case of failure of those measures, careful choice of induction agents is essential to ensure hemodynamic stability during intubation.

In patients with severe metabolic acidosis, whose high-minute ventilation requirement may not be met by the mechanical ventilator, intubation should be avoided or delayed, as long it is reasonable despite a critically low pH. In these cases, noninvasive positive pressure ventilation—measuring the patient's respiratory rate and tidal volumes—may provide an accurate estimate of the patient's intrinsic minute ventilation and adequately support hyperventilation until treatment of the underlying metabolic acidosis is initiated.

Post-intubation, a ventilator setting that allows the patient to maintain their own excessive minute ventilation should be selected so that their respiratory compensation can be sustained. Compensatory hyperventilation puts these patients at high risk of developing relative hypoventilation, flow starvation, patient-ventilator dys-synchrony, and further deteriorating acidosis. Therefore, emphasis is on to optimize patient-ventilator synchrony and maintain high minute ventilation, especially in the spontaneously breathing patient.

2. Discuss ketamine versus etomidate as an induction agent in this patient.

This critically ill patient with hypotension, hypoxemia, and metabolic acidosis poses a great challenge for airway management as there is a high chance for post-intubation hypotension and worsening of acidosis which could even lead to cardiac arrest. Hypotension prior to intubation and during intubation is major risk factors for complications such as cardiopulmonary arrest, longer ICU stays, and increased mortality. If this patient failed to be optimized hemodynamically with crystalloids or vasopressor resuscitation prior to intubation, stable induction agents should be used to prevent physiological perturbations along with inotropes or vasopressor infusions. *Choice of induction agents is etomidate or ketamine.*

Etomidate is a non-benzodiazepine sedative with shorter duration of action and minimal histamine release. It protects from myocardial and cerebral ischemia as it can maintain neutral BP. It does not blunt the sympathetic response to intubation and can cause cortisol inhibition. This drug does not require dose reduction in case of hypotension.

Ketamine is a dissociative agent that provides analgesia unlike etomidate and has amnestic effect. Ketamine preserves respiratory drive and causes bronchial smooth muscle relaxation, hence suitable during awake intubation or status asthmaticus patient. Through its sympathomimetic properties and catecholamine release, it increases heart rate and BP. Due to this particular mechanism, it is useful in hypotensive and hypovolemic patients. If patient found to have acute ischemic cardiac event, ketamine cannot be used.

In this patient, induction agent of choice would be ketamine as it maintains the BP along with preservation of respiratory drive during the intubation.

■ SUGGESTED READING

1. Richhariya D, Sharma B. Textbook of Emergency Medicine including Intensive Care and Trauma, 2nd edition. New Delhi: Jaypee Brothers Medical Publishers (P) Ltd; 2022. pp. 114-8. (Question 1).
2. Richhariya D, Sharma B. Textbook of Emergency Medicine including Intensive Care and Trauma, 2nd edition. New Delhi: Jaypee Brothers Medical Publishers (P) Ltd; 2022. p. 216. (Question 2).
3. Richhariya D, Sharma B. Textbook of Emergency Medicine including Intensive Care and Trauma, 2nd edition. New Delhi: Jaypee Brothers Medical Publishers (P) Ltd; 2022. pp. 871-6. (Question 3).

4. Richhariya D, Sharma B. Textbook of Emergency Medicine including Intensive Care and Trauma, 2nd edition. New Delhi: Jaypee Brothers Medical Publishers (P) Ltd; 2022. pp. 1159-68. (Question 4).
5. Richhariya D, Sharma B. Textbook of Emergency Medicine including Intensive Care and Trauma, 2nd edition. New Delhi: Jaypee Brothers Medical Publishers (P) Ltd; 2022. pp. 80-90. (Question 5).
6. Richhariya D, Sharma B. Textbook of Emergency Medicine including Intensive Care and Trauma, 2nd edition. New Delhi: Jaypee Brothers Medical Publishers (P) Ltd; 2022. pp. 1178-80. (Question 6).
7. Richhariya D, Sharma B. Textbook of Emergency Medicine including Intensive Care and Trauma, 2nd edition. New Delhi: Jaypee Brothers Medical Publishers (P) Ltd; 2022. pp. 119-22. (Question 7).
8. Richhariya D, Sharma B. Textbook of Emergency Medicine including Intensive Care and Trauma, 2nd edition. New Delhi: Jaypee Brothers Medical Publishers (P) Ltd; 2022. pp. 227, 239. (Question 8).
9. Richhariya D, Sharma B. Textbook of Emergency Medicine including Intensive Care and Trauma, 2nd edition. New Delhi: Jaypee Brothers Medical Publishers (P) Ltd; 2022. p. 387. (Question 9).
10. Richhariya D, Sharma B. Textbook of Emergency Medicine including Intensive Care and Trauma, 2nd edition. New Delhi: Jaypee Brothers Medical Publishers (P) Ltd; 2022. p. 213. (Question 10).

Emergency Medicine Paper 37

Devendra Richhariya

Question 1

1. Draw and describe the cerebrospinal fluid production, flow, and normal findings on examination.

Cerebrospinal fluid (CSF) produced in the lateral ventricles **(Fig. 1A)** travels through the interventricular foramina to the third ventricle, through the cerebral aqueduct to the fourth ventricle, and then through the median aperture (also known as the foramen of Magendie) into the subarachnoid space at the base of the brain **(Fig. 1B)**.

2. Discuss CSF findings of bacterial, viral, and tubercular meningitis.

Normal findings of CSF and changes in meningitis are given in **Table 1**.

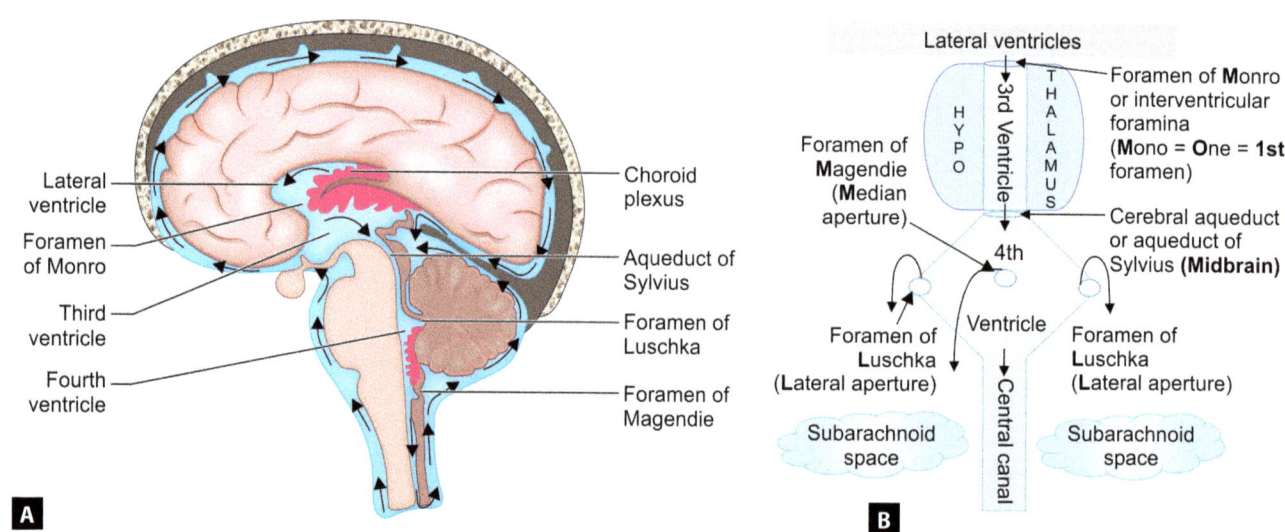

Figs. 1A and B: (A) CSF production; (B) CSF flow. (CSF: cerebrospinal fluid)

TABLE 1: Cerebrospinal fluid (CSF) findings in different types of meningitis.

	Normal	Bacterial	Viral	Fungal	Tubercular
Opening pressure (cm CSF)	<170 mm	>300	200	300	Raised
Appearance	Clear	Turbid/ purulent	Clear	Clear	Clear
CSF WBC (cells/µL)	<5	1,000–5,000	5–1,000	5–100	5–100
Predominant cells	None	Neutrophil	Lymphocytes	Lymphocytes	Lymphocytes
CSF protein	28–32 mg/dL	Raised	Normal–mildly raised	Markedly raised	Raised
CSF glucose (mg/dL)	45	Very low	Normal/slightly low	Very low	Low
CSF plasma: glucose ratio	0.66	Very low	Normal/slightly low	Very low	Low
CSF lactates	Normal	>35 mg/dL	Normal	>25 mg/dL	
% of PMNs	0	>80%	1–50%	1–50%	<30%

(CSF: cerebrospinal fluid; PMN: polymorphonuclear leukocytes; WBC: white blood cell)

3. Describe the differences between encephalitis and meningitis.

Encephalitis is the pathologic diagnosis, but clinically it signifies inflammation of the brain parenchyma. It is associated with broad differential diagnosis, and its possible causes are categorized into infectious (viral, bacterial, or parasitic), postinfectious, and noninfectious (metabolic, toxic, autoimmune, or paraneoplastic).

Meningitis is a clinical syndrome characterized by inflammation of membranes of the brain or spinal cord. The classic triad of *fever, altered mental status*, and *neck stiffness* is seen in <50% of patients with meningitis. At least two of four symptoms of fever, altered mental status, neck stiffness, and headache will be present in 95% of patients. Associated symptoms are genitourinary complaints, rash, and cough.

Question 2

1. Draw a normal conduction system of heart.

The cardiac conduction system is made up of five elements (Fig. 2):
1. Sinoatrial (SA) node
2. Atrioventricular (AV) node
3. Bundle of His
4. Left and right bundle branches
5. Purkinje fibers

2. Describe cardiac cellular electrophysiology.

Cardiac cellular electrophysiology (Fig. 3): The action potential (AP) is the fundamental electrophysiologic event in cardiac cells. The coordinated flux of ions into and out of the cardiac cell forms the basis for cardiac depolarization and repolarization.

Steps in cardiac electrophysiology: Resting (phase 4), upstroke (phase 0), early repolarization (phase 1), plateau (phase 2), and final repolarization (phase 3) are the five phases of the AP.

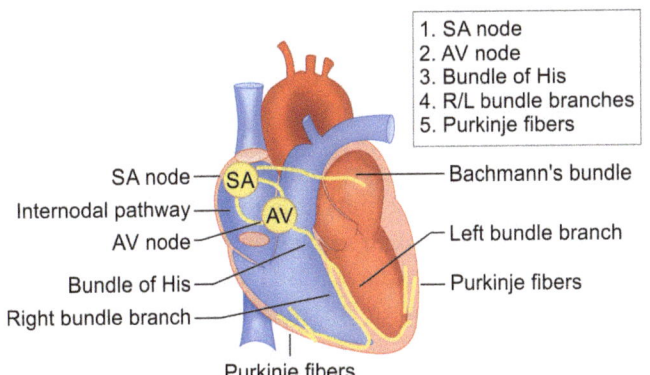

Fig. 2: Cardiac conduction system.

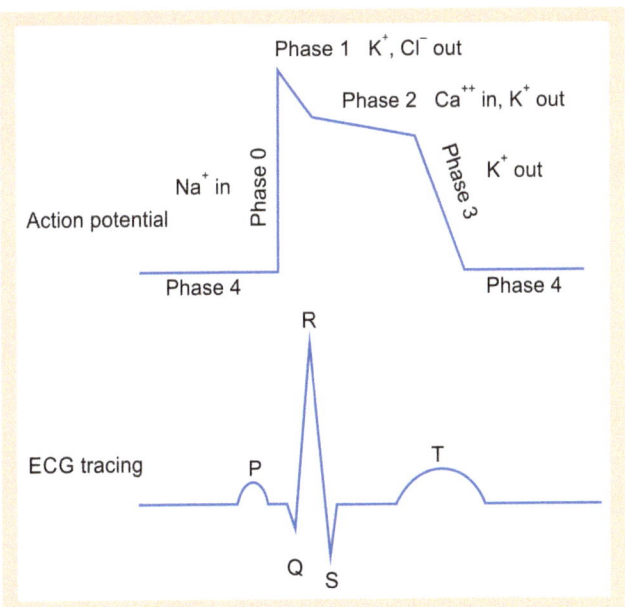

Fig. 3: Cardiac cellular electrophysiology.

3. Discuss various mechanisms of dysrhythmia.

Arrhythmogenic mechanisms with regard to the basic mechanisms of cardiac arrhythmia can be distinguished on two levels: cellular and tissue levels. Mechanisms acting at the cellular level comprise automaticity and triggered activity. The latter has been shown to be related to afterdepolarizations in the membrane potential. However, reentry-based arrhythmia is generated at the tissue level. It is observed most frequently and, therefore, it represents the main topic of this study. Yet, as found in experiments, afterdepolarizations can be decisively involved in the re-entry process (Fig. 4).

Automaticity: It is the ability to generate a spontaneous action potential. All cardiac cells can display this property, but, in a normal heart, most do not. Depending on the location within the heart, therefore, automaticity may be classified as either normal or abnormal. Cardiac cells with normal automaticity are called pacemaker cells. The dominant pacemaker of the heart is normally the sinus node, but there also exist cells capable of spontaneous diastolic depolarization, such as specialized fibers of the atria, AV junction, and the His–Purkinje system. These secondary pacemakers lie dormant (latent) until the sinus node activity is removed, allowing the latent pacemaker's rhythm to become visible.

Triggered rhythms: These are known to be caused by after-depolarizations, which are oscillations in the membrane potential following an AP. One mechanism by which triggered activity causes arrhythmia is observed when the afterdepolarization (of either type) is large enough to reach the threshold potential. The resulting action potential is called a triggered AP. An arrhythmia is induced when impulse initiation shifts from the sinus node to the triggered focus. For this to happen, the rate of triggered impulses must be faster than the rate of the sinus node.

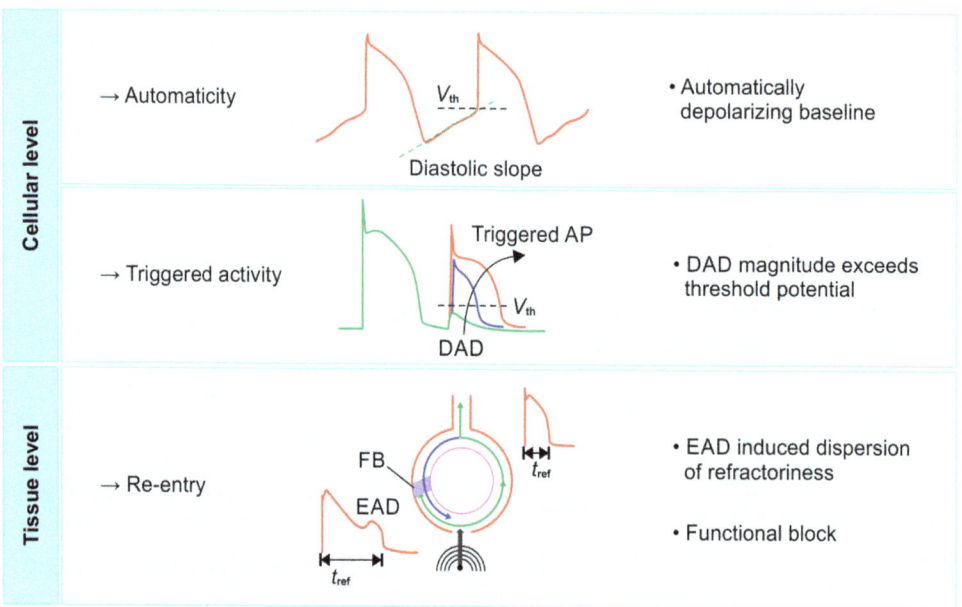

Fig. 4: Mechanisms of cardiac arrhythmias. (AP: action potential; DAD: delayed afterdepolarization; EAD: early afterdepolarization; t_{ref}: reference travel; V_{th}: threshold potential)

Question 3

1. Discuss the pathophysiology of bronchial asthma.

Pathophysiologic hallmark of asthma: Airways are abnormally filled with eosinophil lymphocytes, mast cells macrophages, and myofibroblasts; furthermore, diameter of airways is reduced due to contraction of smooth muscles, vascular congestions, bronchial wall edema, and thick secretions. *Pathophysiologic changes lead to airflow obstruction and give rise to various clinical manifestations*: Increased work of breathing, increased airway pressure, decreased expiratory flow rates, hemodynamic instability, ventilation–perfusion mismatch, hypoxemia, hypercarbia, and ventilatory failure due to respiratory muscle fatigue. Continuous airway inflammation and prolonged bronchospasm lead to permanent airway remodeling, fibrosis hyperplasia, hypertrophy of smooth muscle cells, mucous gland hyperplasia and hypersecretion, and angiogenesis; all these changes lead to irreversible loss of lung functions. Stimulus or triggers for acute asthma are acute respiratory viral infections (most common 40–80%) pollution, indoor agents such as dust, occupational exposures, vapors, gases, aspirin, β-blockers, and nonsteroidal anti-inflammatory drugs (NSAIDs). Cold air exposure, hormonal changes during menstruation, and pregnancy-related emotional stress can also give rise to acute asthma.

2. Discuss clinical and laboratory (blood gas and pulmonary functions) parameters in a patient with severe asthma.

Typically, asthma presents with dyspnea, wheezing, and cough. Physical examination includes vital signs (tachycardia and tachypnea) and chest findings (wheezing). Clinical examination findings help us to identify the associated comorbid illnesses such as pneumonia, pneumothorax, and upper airway obstruction. Condition such as foreign body in airway generally mimic the acute severe asthma and fail to respond to therapy and revisit ED and labeled as: refractory asthma".

Arterial blood gas (ABG) is a routine practice in emergency for patients with asthma and chronic obstructive pulmonary disease (COPD). Though oxygen saturation (SO_2) is very sensitive and noninvasive, ABG is more accurate for hypercarbia and hypoxemia status. Sometimes, the venous sample may also demonstrate the CO_2 retention and can be used as a surrogate to avoid the painful procedure of arterial puncture.

Interpretation of pulmonary function test (PFT) **(Fig. 5)** is done by comparing the measured value with the reference values of a normal, healthy, and nonsmoking person. Severe asthma had prominent air trapping, evident as reduced forced vital capacity (FVC) over the entire range of forced expiratory volume in 1 second (FEV_1)/FVC. This pattern was confirmed with measures of residual lung volume/total lung capacity (TLC) in a subgroup. In contrast, nonsevere asthma did not exhibit prominent air trapping, even at FEV_1/FVC <75% predicted.

3. How would you teach a patient regarding the use of metered-dose inhalers?

A metered-dose inhaler (MDI) is a handheld device filled with medicine that must be breathed into the lungs (inhaled) **(Fig. 6)**.

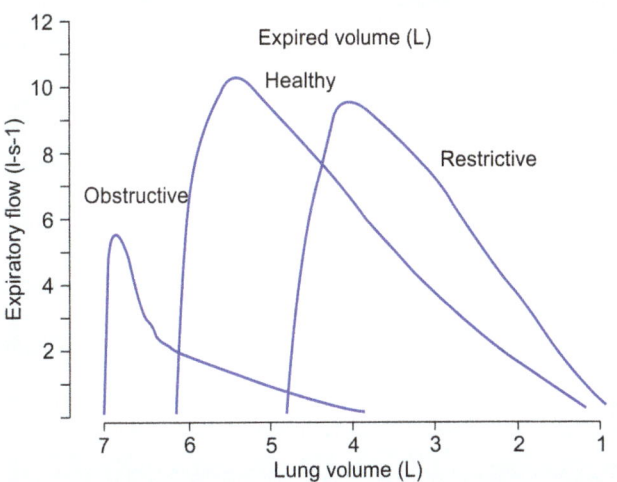

Fig. 5: Abnormal spirometry (abnormal restrictive and obstructive airflow pattern in volume–flow curve and volume–time curve).

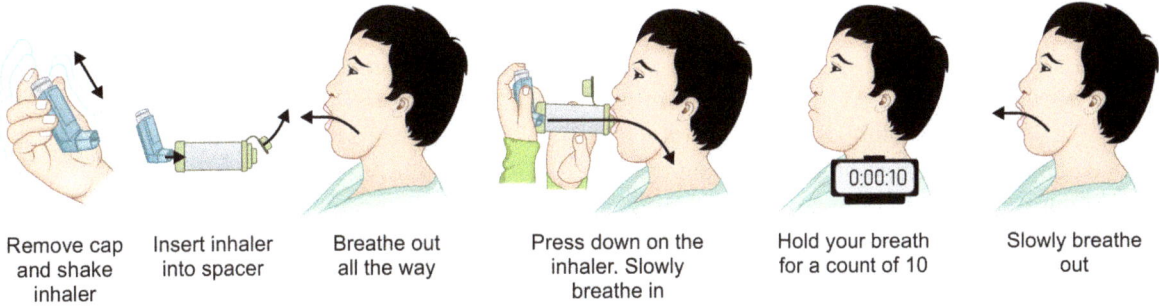

Fig. 6: Steps to use a metered-dose inhaler.

Question 4

1. Draw and describe the functional unit of a kidney.

The functional unit of a kidney is called the nephron. It comprises a coiled renal tubule and a vascular network of peritubular capillaries. The tubule consists of different regions, each with their own important function. Each kidney contributes to the total glomerular filtration rate (GFR) through its approximately 1 million nephrons **(Fig. 7)**. The volume of fluid filtered per unit time is termed GFR and can be calculated by measuring any steady-state concentration of chemical in the in-blood plasma and is freely filtered by the kidney but is neither secreted nor absorbed in the kidney [GFR—(urine concentration flow)/plasma concentration]. Structural and functional changes within the kidney occur with progressive damage to nephrons. Initially, the kidney tries to maintain GFR with the remaining healthy nephrons through hyperfiltration and compensatory hypertrophy of nephron, and normal clearance of plasma solutes is maintained by the kidney. If risk factors cannot be removed or physiologic insult to nephron persists and damaged nephrons cannot recover, renal reserve may be exhausted permanently. Decline in GFR, leading ultimately to oliguria, decreased urine output (UOP), or anuria, the absence of urine formation, and finally renal injury and/or renal failure occur.

2. Discuss the evaluation of renal functions.

Four important steps in the renal function: (a) Glomeruli receive blood flow delivered through circulation, (b) an ultrafiltrate is formed in the glomeruli and then delivered to the renal tubules, (c) renal tubules reabsorbed the solutes and/or water, and (d) tubular fluid (now urine) exits the tubules, draining to the renal pelvis, the ureters, and the bladder, and urine is then expelled via the urethra. Any process that interferes with any of the above four structures or steps involved in this process causes renal disease. Rapid decline in renal function gives rise to acute kidney injury (AKI), and progressive decline/insult of renal function during months or years resulting in chronic kidney disease (CKD).

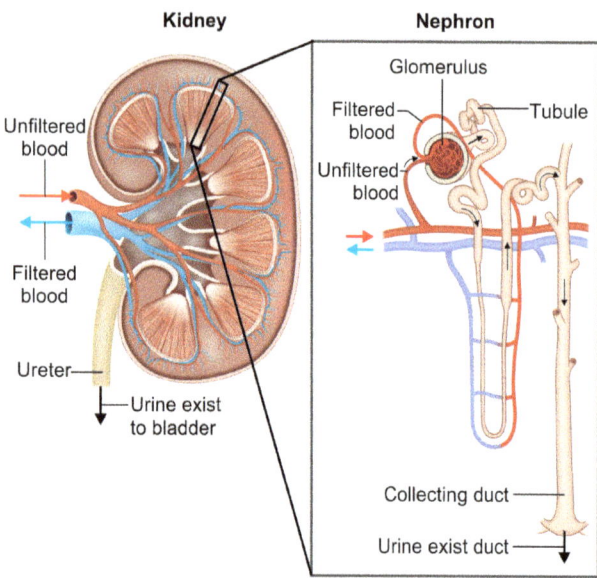

Fig. 7: Nephron: Basic unit of kidney.

TABLE 2: Urine analysis findings in acute tubular necrosis, prerenal azotemia, and hepatorenal syndrome.

Parameter	Acute tubular necrosis	Prerenal azotemia	Hepatorenal syndrome
Sediments	Granular cast ±	None	None
Osmolality	Same as plasma	Greater than plasma	Greater than plasma
Urine sodium	≥20 mmol/L	≤10 mmol/L	≤10 mmol/L
Urine output	Variable	Fluid responsive	Nonfluid responsive
Prognosis	Recovery	Recovery	Poor

3. Describe urinary findings of acute tubular necrosis.

Acute tubular necrosis (ATN): It is the most common intrarenal cause of acute renal failure. Many causes of ATN are transient ischemic episodes, toxic injury to kidney, heavy metals, myoglobinuria, and rhabdomyolisis and contrast exposure. *Urine analysis—iso-osmolar* osmolar (osmolality 300–400) urinary Na > 20 FeNa >1%. Muddy brown cast is nonspecific but sensitive **(Table 2)**.

Question 5

1. Explain the organization of a hospital disaster plan.

Establishing the emergency operation center (EOC): EOC serves as central command post during a disaster, generally established outside the ED. It should be large enough for key people and support staff. It should be located in a safe area.

How to activate and when to activate incident command center (ICS) **(Table 3)**:
a. Determine who will activate the ICS
b. Notifying the hospital personnel
c. Briefing all core members regarding assignments and clear immediate direction
d. Activation of ICS should be announced using standardized codes, such as "Disaster Code"

TABLE 3: Overall responsibilities of the head of incident command center.

Logistic (provide support)	Planning (prepare action plan)	Finance (cost accounting and procurement)	Operations (direct tactical action)
Responsible for acquisition and maintenance of facilities, services, personnel, equipment, and materials	• Collect, analyze, and display information • Prepare incident action plan • Maintain situation and resource status • Maintain incident documentation • Prepare demobilization • Promote continuity of operations	• Monitors incident costs • Maintains financial records • Administers procurement contracts	Carry out the medical objective to the best of their ability
Other important command staff			
Public information officer	Safety officer	Liaison officer	
Provides information to the news media, serves as the central point for information dissemination	Monitors the facility and anticipates, detects, and corrects unsafe situations	Function as an incident contact person for representatives from other assisting and cooperating agencies	

2. Discuss the pathophysiology of blast injuries.

There are four main types of blast effects as shown in **Figure 8**. A primary injury is caused by a direct effect of blast wave overpressure on tissue. Primary blast injury mostly affects air-filled structures such as the lungs, ears, and gastrointestinal (GI) tract, by the following mechanisms: spalling, shearing, and implosion. Spalling is the displacement and fragmentation of a dense medium into a less dense medium. Shearing is the stress caused by the blast wave traveling through different tissue densities at different velocities. Implosion is where the less dense material is displaced into denser material. A secondary blast injury is due to collateral damage from flying objects and sharps. Tertiary blast injury results from the victim being propelled through the air and striking stationary objects. A quaternary blast injury is a result of burns, smoke inhalation, or chemical agent release.

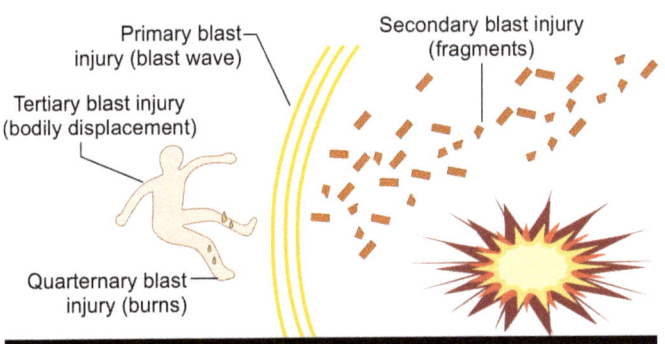

Fig. 8: Pathophysiology of bomb blast.

Question 6

1. Discuss the physiology of temperature regulation to cold exposure.
2. Discuss the pathophysiological aspects of hypothermia.

Thermoregulation is the process by which an organism maintains its internal body temperature within a certain range, despite changes in external conditions. For the human body, it ranges between 36.5 and 37.5°C. The main purpose of thermoregulation is to keep the enzyme systems of the body working properly **(Flowchart 1)**.

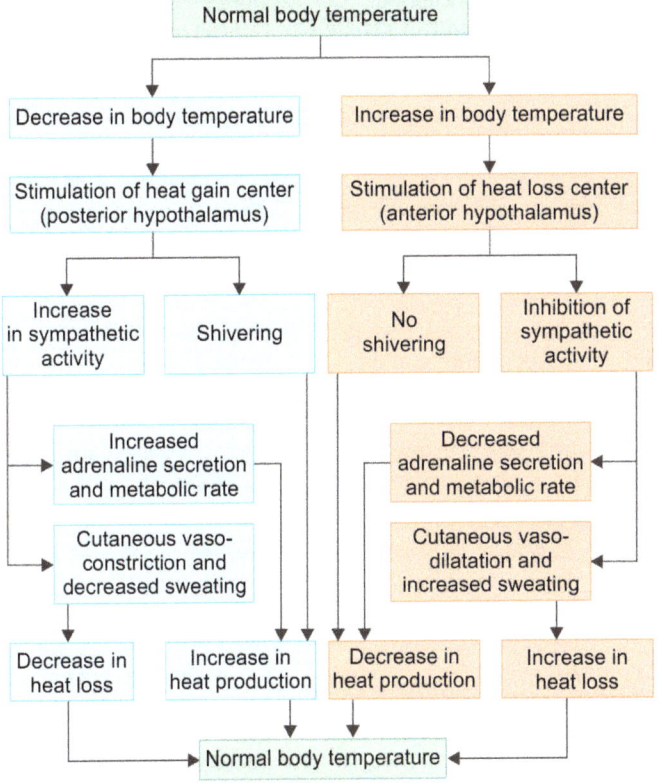

Flowchart 1: Pathophysiology of temperature regulation.

3. Discuss the targeted temperature management in the ED.

Studies suggest that after achieving return of spontaneous circulation (ROSC) (period of global cerebral hypoxia–ischemia), mild induced hypothermia is used as a neuroprotective and outcome improving measure. Mild-induced hypothermia suppresses the many pathological processes leading to delayed cell death, including apoptosis (programmed cell death). Hypothermia reduces the release of excitatory amino acids and free radicals and decreases the cerebral metabolic rate for oxygen ($CMRO_2$) by about 6% for each 1°C reduction in core temperature. Hypothermia reduces the inflammatory response associated with the postcardiac arrest syndrome. The previous term therapeutic hypothermia is replaced by the new term "targeted temperature management (TTM)". Several treatment recommendations on TTM by "The Advanced Life Support Task Force of the International Liaison Committee on Resuscitation (ILCOR)": TTM are indicated for adults after out-of-hospital cardiac arrest (OHCA) with an initial shockable/nonshockable rhythm or any other initial rhythm who remain unresponsive after ROSC. Temperature is maintained between 32 and 36°C with the temperature control monitoring system. The minimum duration of TTM should be at least 24 hours. Following the TTM trial, many intensive care clinicians elected to use 36°C as the target temperature for postcardiac arrest temperature control. There are several advantages of selecting a target temperature of 36°C as compared to a target temperature of 33°C: vasopressor support is reduced to minimum with lower lactate levels, the rewarming phase is shorter, and chances of rebound hyperthermia after rewarming are less.

Question 7

1. Draw the oxygen–hemoglobin dissociation curve and discuss the factors affecting it.

Oxyhemoglobin dissociation curve: Oxygen in blood depends on hemoglobin concentration and SO_2. Partial pressure of oxygen (PO_2) is the driving force for the oxygen molecule to bind with hemoglobin so the oxyhemoglobin dissociation curve shows SO_2 at any given PO_2 (generally, we can say that the higher the PO_2, the higher the SO_2). But the curve is not linear; the *flat part of the curve* shows that PO_2 has little effect on SO_2 over this range while the *steep part of the curve* shows that even a small change in PO_2 makes a significant change in SO_2 over this range **(Fig. 9)**.

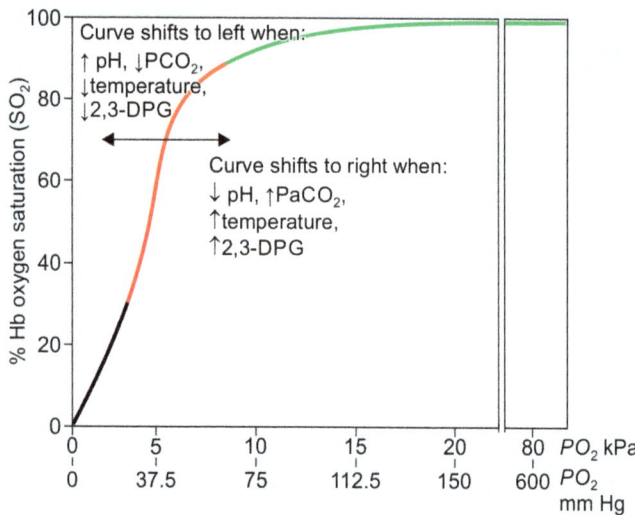

Fig. 9: Oxyhemoglobin dissociation curve. The curve defines the relationship between PO_2 and the percentage saturation of hemoglobin with oxygen (SO_2). (2,3-DPG: 2,3-diphosphoglycerate)
Note: The sigmoid shape—it is relatively flat when PO_2 is >80 mm Hg (10.6 kPa) but steep when PO_2 falls <60 mm Hg (8 kPa).

2. Describe the rationale, indications, and complications of various methods of oxygen delivery.

Oxygen delivery devices can be classified on the basis of their design. There are three basic designs available: (a) Low-flow system, (b) reservoir, and (c) high-flow system, while the fourth available design is enclosure. So, the physician should be able to choose the appropriate oxygen delivery system on the basis of two important questions: How much oxygen can be delivered by system and whether the fraction of inspired oxygen (FiO_2) delivered remain fixed or can be altered according to the patient's requirement? On the basis of FiO_2 delivered, the system can be further divided into low (<35%), moderate (35–65%), and high (>70%) oxygen concentration delivery devices. FiO_2 delivered depends on *patient factors* (inspiratory flow rate, tidal volume, respiratory rate, and presence of a respiratory pause) and *device factors* (volume of the mask, tightness of fit, oxygen concentration, and air vent size). Characteristics of various low- and high-flow oxygen devices are summarized in **Table 4**.

TABLE 4: Oxygen delivery devices and their characteristics.

Methods	Amount of O₂ flow/FiO₂	Precaution	Advantages	Disadvantages
Low-flow oxygen therapy				
Nasal cannula	• Low flow (1–6 L/min) • FiO₂ 24–44%	• To check whether both prongs are in the patient's nostrils • In patient with chronic lung disease to deliver 2–3 L/min	• Patient able to talk and eat • Can be used in home setting • Well tolerated • Inexpensive	• May cause irritation to nasal mucosa • May cause epistaxis
Simple face mask	• Low flow (5–10 L/min) • FiO₂ 35–50%	• Frequently check placement of mask • Check for claustrophobia • CO₂ retention may occur unless flow rate < 2 L/min or minute ventilation is high	Can provide increased oxygen demand for a limited period of time	• Tight seal required • Difficult to keep mask over mouth and nose • Oxygen wasting • Uncomfortable for patient while speaking or eating • Problematic with RT in situ
Partial rebreather mask	Minimum 10 L/min 40–70%	• Reservoir bag should be two-thirds filled during inspiration • Reservoir bag should be free of kinks	Patient can inhale room air through openings in mask if oxygen supply is briefly interrupted	Tight seal required (eating and talking are difficult)
Nonrebreathing mask	• Minimum 10 L/min (prevent bag collapse on inspiration) • FiO₂ 60–80%	• Maintain flow rate so that the reservoir bag collapses only slightly during inspiration • Check whether valves are functioning properly	• Delivers highest possible oxygen concentration • Suitable for a spontaneously breathing patient with severe hypoxemia	• Not useful for long-term therapy • Malfunction can cause CO₂ retention • Feeling of suffocation • Expensive
High-flow oxygen therapy				
Air entrainment mask (AEM) venturi system	• Variable flow can be set • FiO₂ 24–50% • Fixed system	• FiO₂ varies with back pressure • Different colored vents are used for achieving different FiO₂	• Easy to apply disposable low-cost system • Precise FiO₂ can be achieved	• Only to be used in adult • FiO₂ >40% • Not sure whether FiO₂ varies with back pressure
High-flow oxygen cannula system	Flow rate up to 50 L/min or more FiO₂ 35–90%	FiO₂ is ensured but system dependent	Wide range of FiO₂, relative/absolute humidity can be used in adult, children, and infants	• FiO₂ depends on system input and patient breathing pattern • Infection risk

Question 8

1. Explain the basic physics of point-of-care ultrasound and its clinical application.

Two basic principles need to be understood regarding how ultrasound is generated and an image is formed. The first is the *piezoelectric effect*, which explains how ultrasound is generated from ceramic crystals in the transducer. An electric current passes through a cable to the transducer and is applied to the crystals, causing them to deform and vibrate. This vibration produces the ultrasound beam. The frequency of the ultrasound waves produced is predetermined by the crystals in the transducer. The second key principle is the *pulse-echo principle*, which explains how the image is generated. Ultrasound waves are produced in pulses, not continuously, because the same crystals are used to generate and receive sound waves, and they cannot do both at the same time. In the time between the pulses, the ultrasound beam enters the patient and is bounced or reflected back to the transducer. These reflected sound waves, or echoes, cause the crystals in the transducer to deform again and produce an electrical signal that is then converted into an image displayed on the monitor. The transducer generally emits ultrasound only 1% of the time; the rest of the time is spent receiving the returning echoes.

2. Describe the utility of M mode in point-of-care ultrasound.

M mode or "motion" mode is a form of ultrasound imaging that is of high clinical utility in the ED. It can be used in a variety of situations to evaluate motion and timing and can document tissue movement in a still image when the recording of a video clip is not feasible.

3. Enumerate five artifacts pertaining to lung ultrasound.

1. Reverberation artifact
2. Acoustic shadowing
3. Acoustic enhancement
4. Bayonet artifact
5. Resolution artifacts

Question 9

1. Discuss the pathophysiology of traumatic shock.

Pathophysiology of traumatic hemorrhagic shock is described in **Flowchart 2**.

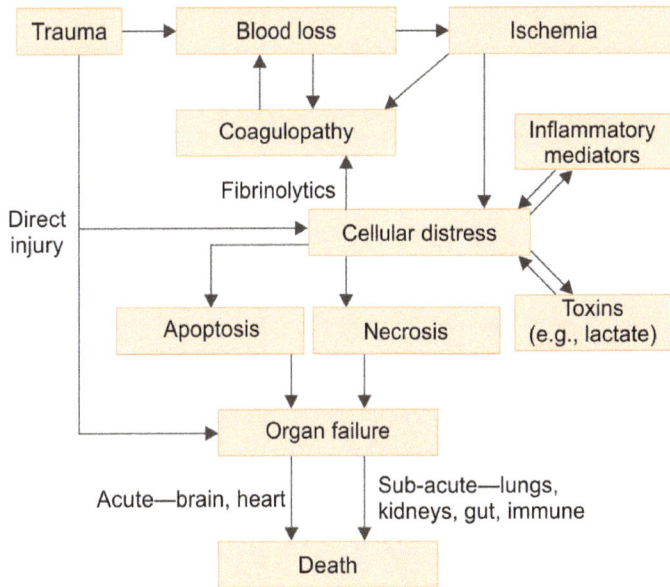

Flowchart 2: Pathophysiology of hemorrhagic shock.

2. What is the interpretation of various components of waveform produced by thromboelastography?

Thromboelastography (TEG) is a noninvasive test that quantitatively measures the ability of whole blood to form a clot. TEG is used to assess viscoelastic changes in clotting whole blood under low shear conditions after adding a specific coagulation activator (**Figs. 10A and B**).

- TEG is a technique used for the characterization and quantification of the status of a patient's coagulation state.
- It can be used to measure hemostasis by studying the strength and elasticity of the clot and how quickly the clot breaks up.
- It can be viewed in real time and management decisions about blood products can be tailored based on the patient's clinical state.

Question 10

1. Discuss the colloids versus crystalloids in the management of hypovolemic shock.

Intravenous fluids are administered to virtually all acutely ill patients. The choice of fluid should be individualized based on the ongoing disease process, acid–base status, and electrolyte requirement. Thorough knowledge about intravenous fluids and their judicious use in the ED can improve patient outcomes.

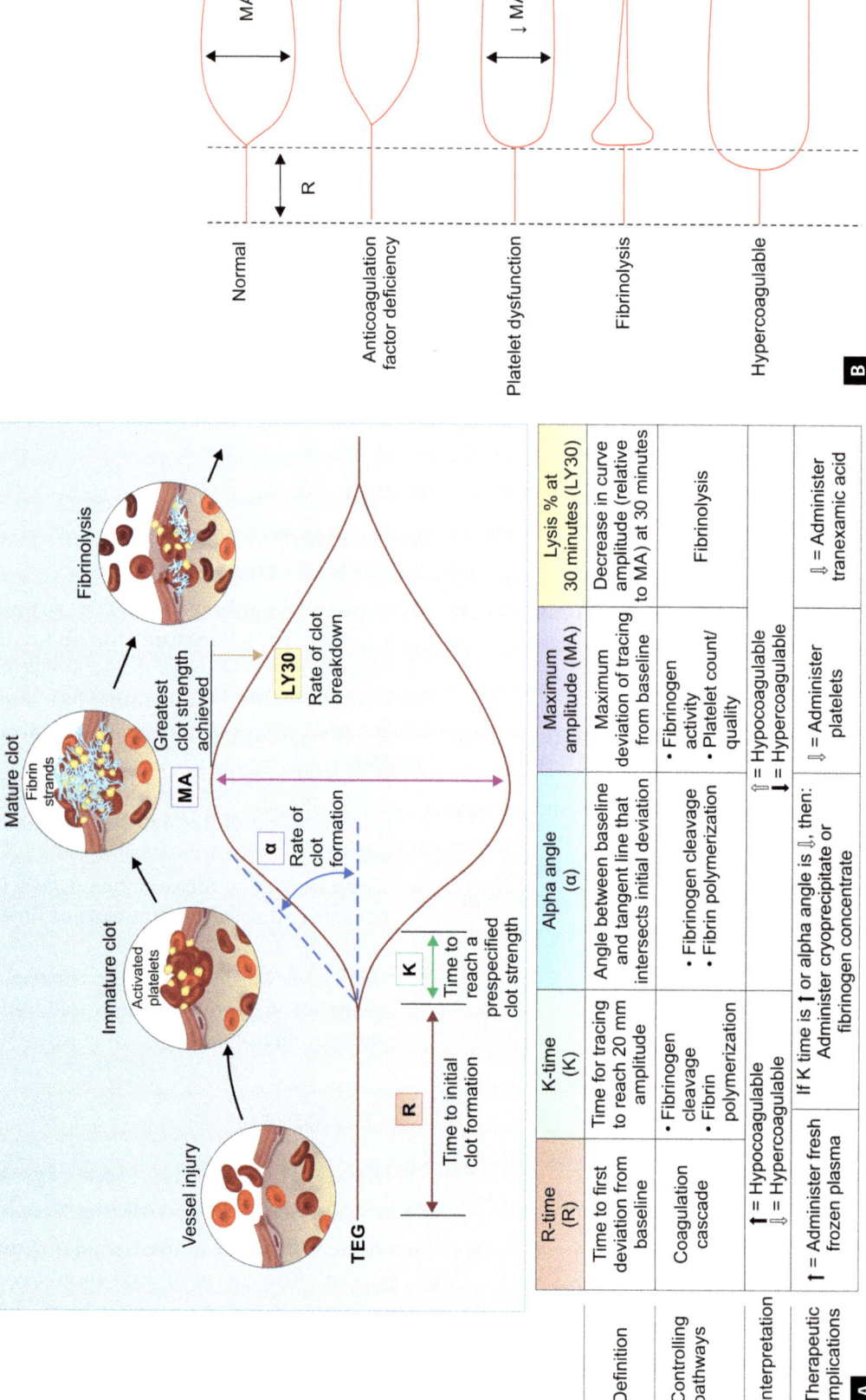

Figs. 10A and B: Thromboelastography (TEG).

Crystalloids are the oldest form of intravenous fluids. They are basically simple solutions of electrolytes and/or sugars in water. They include isotonic solutions primarily used in resuscitation and hypotonic solutions used as maintenance fluid therapy. The most popular crystalloid in clinical practice, 0.9% saline, contains 154 mmol/L of sodium and chloride each. Thus, the concentrations of both sodium (plasma sodium ~ 140 mmol/L) and chloride (plasma chloride ~ 100 mmol/L) are much higher than in plasma, resulting in a strong ion difference (SID) of 0. SID is the difference between the predominantly positive charge (sodium) and negative charge (chloride) in plasma. The normal SID of plasma is about 40. Any decrease in SID produces acidosis and conversely any increase produces alkalosis. Infusion of large volumes of 0.9% saline leads to higher chloride concentrations in plasma and a decrease in SID. This decrease in SID (and hence bicarbonate) leads to hyperchloremic acidosis.

Balanced crystalloids which are also known as "physiological solutions" have a chemical composition approximating that of extracellular fluid. These solutions employ metabolizable anions such as lactate, acetate, gluconate, or maleate to maintain electroneutrality, as bicarbonate is unstable in plastic. They have concentrations of chloride similar to plasma and hence are devoid of harmful hyperchloremic metabolic acidosis.

Colloids unlike crystalloids consist of large molecules and are believed to stay in the intravascular space for longer duration before leaking into the interstitium. They are used as resuscitation fluids in the ED, for critically ill, and during surgery. In the past, it was thought that colloids are three to four times more effective than crystalloids in restoring the intravascular volume. This, however, was not substantiated in several recent trials, which suggested that only marginally lesser volume of colloids is required to produce similar hemodynamic effect when compared to crystalloids.

2. Explain the etiopathogenesis of metabolic alkalosis.

Metabolic alkalosis may not show any symptoms. People with this type of alkalosis more often complain of the underlying conditions that are causing it. These can include vomiting, diarrhea, swelling in the lower legs (peripheral edema), and fatigue. Severe cases of metabolic alkalosis can cause agitation, disorientation, seizures, and coma. The severe symptoms are most common when the alkalosis is caused by chronic liver disease. The causes of metabolic alkalosis are summarized in **Table 5**.

TABLE 5: Causes of metabolic alkalosis.

Chloride sensitive	Chloride resistant	Miscellaneous
Gastrointestinal: Vomiting, gastric drainage, chloride diarrhea, and villous adenoma *Renal:* • Diuretics • Posthypercapnic • Low chloride intake • Cystic fibrosis	• Increased mineralocorticoid activity: Primary/secondary hyperaldosteronism • Cushing's syndrome • Bartter syndrome • Severe hypokalemia	• Massive blood transfusion • Acetate-containing colloids • Alkali therapy • Hypercalcemia: Milk alkali syndrome • Bone metastatic

3. Explain SID.

The Stewart or strong ion approach to acid–base disturbances has gained acceptance among many intensivists because of perceived weaknesses of the traditional approach in the evaluation of patients with critical illnesses. As per Stewart approach, dissociation (and pH) is governed by laws of physical chemistry. *Law of conservation of mass*: Amount of substance in a solution remains constant unless added or removed or generated or destroyed by chemical reaction. *Law of conservation of electric charge*: Sum of all cations always equals sum of all anions. *Law of mass action*: Dissociation equilibrium of all incompletely dissociated substances must be satisfied at all times. According to this approach, HCO_3^- is a dependent variable.

Three mathematically *independent* determinants of blood pH are:

a. SID
   $SID = ([Na^-] + [K^-] + [Ca^{2+}] + [Mg^{+2}]) - ([Cl^-]) = [HCO_3^-] + [A^-]$
   $SIDa = ([Na^+] + [K^+] + [Ca^{2+}] + [Mg^{2+}]) - ([Cl^-])$
   $SIDe = [HCO_3^-] + [A^-]$
   Total charges contributed by all nonbicarbonate buffers, primarily albumin, phosphate, and, in whole blood, hemoglobin. *Normal SID is 40–42.*
b. Total weak acid buffers (A TOT) = Total $[A^-]$ and its weak acid $([A^-] + [HA])$
c. PCO_2
   Strong anion gap (SIG) = Apparent SID (SIDa) – effective SID (SIDe). It is due to unmeasured anions. It represents standard base excess (SBE).
   i. *Metabolic acidosis*: Decrease in SID by addition of strong anions
   ii. *Metabolic alkalosis*: Increase in SID by additions of strong cations (with weak anions)

The Stewart approach is much more cumbersome and may be more prone to error, given its dependence upon multiple measurements of different variables. When measurements obtained from automated blood chemistry devices are used to calculate the *SIG*, the results can also vary substantially depending upon which device is used. Therefore, the traditional approach in the analysis of all acid–base disturbances is preferred. Moreover, if serum albumin concentration is considered in the traditional analysis of acid–base disturbances, the Stewart approach is nonsuperior over the traditional Schwartz–Bartter approach to acid–base disturbances.

SUGGESTED READING

1. Richhariya D, Sharma B. Textbook of Emergency Medicine including Intensive Care and Trauma, 2nd edition. New Delhi: Jaypee Brothers Medical Publishers (P) Ltd; 2022. p. 845. (Question 1).
2. Richhariya D, Sharma D. Textbook of Emergency Medicine including Intensive Care and Trauma, 2nd edition. New Delhi: Jaypee Brothers Medical Publishers (P) Ltd; 2022. pp. 473-80. (Question 2).
3. Richhariya D, Sharma B. Textbook of Emergency Medicine including Intensive Care and Trauma, 2nd edition. New Delhi: Jaypee Brothers Medical Publishers (P) Ltd; 2022. pp. 575-82. (Question 3).
4. Richhariya D, Sharma B. Textbook of Emergency Medicine including Intensive Care and Trauma, 2nd edition. New Delhi: Jaypee Brothers Medical Publishers (P) Ltd; 2022. pp. 743-52. (Question 4).
5. Richhariya D, Sharma B. Textbook of Emergency Medicine including Intensive Care and Trauma, 2nd edition. New Delhi: Jaypee Brothers Medical Publishers (P) Ltd; 2022. pp. 172-9. (Question 5).
6. Richhariya D, Sharma B. Textbook of Emergency Medicine including Intensive Care and Trauma, 2nd edition. New Delhi: Jaypee Brothers Medical Publishers (P) Ltd; 2022. p. 1686. (Question 6).
7. Richhariya D, Sharma B. Textbook of Emergency Medicine including Intensive Care and Trauma, 2nd edition. New Delhi: Jaypee Brothers Medical Publishers (P) Ltd; 2022. pp. 242-8. (Question 7).
8. Richhariya D, Sharma B. Textbook of Emergency Medicine including Intensive Care and Trauma, 2nd edition. New Delhi: Jaypee Brothers Medical Publishers (P) Ltd; 2022. pp. 365-73. (Question 8).
9. Richhariya D, Sharma B. Textbook of Emergency Medicine including Intensive Care and Trauma, 2nd edition. New Delhi: Jaypee Brothers Medical Publishers (P) Ltd; 2022. p. 1536. (Question 9).
10. Richhariya D, Sharma B. Textbook of Emergency Medicine including Intensive Care and Trauma, 2nd edition. New Delhi: Jaypee Brothers Medical Publishers (P) Ltd; 2022. p. 305. (Question 10).

Emergency Medicine Paper 38

Devendra Richhariya

Question 1

A 35-year-old male, unrestrained driver with history of road traffic crash presents to the emergency department (ED) with grade IV hemorrhagic shock.

1. How will you manage this patient?

Class IV hemorrhagic shock (severe) is defined as per Advanced Trauma Life Support (ATLS) 10th edition: >40% blood loss (2,000 mL); decrease in Glasgow Coma Scale (GCS), blood pressure, pulse pressure, capillary refill and urine output; pulse rate >140 beats per minute; confused; lethargic; and base deficit ≤10 mEq/L; class IV hemorrhagic shock needs to activate massive transfusion protocol as well.

Resuscitation and initial stabilization are the key to management in any patient coming to the ED. Primary survey is done by following the ABCDE (airway, breathing, circulation, disability, exposure) approach.

Airway: Maintain airway. Take spinal precautions by applying a cervical collar. In case of severe injury with a GCS of <8, the patient requires intubation. Use of short-acting induction agents that have limited effect on blood pressure or intracranial pressure (ICP) is recommended. Maintain inline cervical spine stabilization during intubation.

Breathing: Maintain oxygenation and use capnometry to control partial pressure of carbon dioxide (PCO_2) and avoid hyperventilation. Prolonged (>6 hours) hypocapnia causes cerebral vasoconstriction and worsens cerebral ischemia. Keep oxygen saturation >90%, partial pressure of arterial oxygen (PaO_2) >60 mm Hg, and PCO_2 at 35–45 mm Hg.

Circulation: Provide aggressive fluid resuscitation to prevent hypotension and secondary brain injury, identify the bleeding source, and perform immediate hemorrhage control.

During resuscitation of hemorrhagic shock, volume infusion in the face of continued blood loss results in dilutional coagulopathy and hypothermia, while the transient elevation in blood pressure contributes to further bleeding from wounds and vessels. Permissive hypotension, therefore, can facilitate an environment that optimizes coagulation, albeit at the potential expense of optimal tissue perfusion pressure, until repair restores the integrity of the system. Permissive hypotension is the act of maintaining a blood pressure lower than physiologic levels in a patient who has suffered from hemorrhagic blood loss.

If the bleeding in trauma patients is unlikely or difficult to be controlled quickly, immediate transfusion of blood components in a 1:1:1 ratio of RBC, fresh frozen plasma (FFP), and platelets should be considered. In simple terms, if the emergency team recognizes that the patient will require four or more units of RBCs in 1 hour (or more than 10 units in 24 hours), they should start transfusing 1 unit of RBC 1 Unit of FFP, and 6 units of random donor platelets (RDP) [or 1 unit of single donor apheresis platelets (SDP) as 1 unit of SDP (apheresis platelets) is equivalent to 6 units of RDP]. Hypothermia must be controlled during transfusions with the help of inline warmers. Studies supporting a newer approach of 1:1:1 blood component transfusion state that the Assessment of Blood Consumption (*ABC*) score in trauma was developed to assist clinicians in discerning when massive transfusion would be required to resuscitate trauma patients. Hemorrhage is the most common cause of early death in trauma patients. Massive transfusion protocols (MTPs) have been designed to accelerate the release of blood products but can result in waste if activated inappropriately. The Assessment of Blood Consumption (ABC) Score **(Table 1)** has become a widely accepted score for MTP activation.

TABLE 1: Assessment of blood consumption (ABC) score.

Components	Points
Penetrating injury	1
FAST positive	1
Heart rate >100 beats/min	1
Systolic BP <90 mm Hg	1

(BP: blood pressure; FAST: focused assessment with sonography in trauma; MTP: massive transfusion protocol)
Note: Trigger for massive blood transfusion protocol ≥2 (accuracy of prediction of MTP 75%).

2. What are the key considerations of managing pediatric, geriatric, and pregnant patients with traumatic hemorrhagic shock?

a. It is important to recognize that in infants <1-year-old and in children 1–5 years old, the stroke volume is relatively fixed, and therefore cardiac output is much more dependent on heart rate than it is in older children of 6–10 years old or in adults. Hypotension and a heart rate at <100 beats per minute in an injured child are signs of impending vascular collapse. The nurse clinician must be knowledgeable about the normal pediatric vital sign parameters and anticipate the following assessment priorities:
   i. Older people are more likely to take anticoagulants, which are medications that help prevent blood clots. This means that if they go into hypovolemic shock, which then develops into hemorrhagic shock, they are at a higher risk of serious complications and even death.
   ii. Recognition of hemorrhage in obstetric patients is complicated by the normal physiological changes that occur during pregnancy. Mean blood pressure usually decreases 4–6 weeks after conception, primarily due to maternal systemic vasodilation and, to a lesser extent, from the high-flow, low-resistance circuit in the uteroplacental circulation. Later in pregnancy, during the second trimester, blood pressure tends to increase to normal levels. In addition to hemodynamic changes in vascular tone and resistance, circulating blood volume increases by as much as 40–50% above nonpregnant volumes, further confounding the diagnosis of acute hemorrhage.

Question 2

A 65-year-old nonhelmeted, two-wheeler rider with road traffic crash presents to the ED with noisy breathing, moaning and groaning, and withdrawal to painful stimuli.

1. Discuss the management with important pearls and pitfalls in this case.

The patient is a case of head trauma. Hence, as per ATLS, we will approach the patient with ABCDE.

Airway: We will give supplemental oxygen to the patient, look for any foreign body or secretions to be suctioned out, provide definitive airway, and put cervical collar to prevent cervical injury.

Breathing: Look for any deviation of trachea, distended neck vessels, and any asymmetrical chest rise to rule out pneumothorax, flail chest, etc. Obtain chest X-ray imaging.

Circulation: Two large-bore cannulas, intravenous fluids, and 1 L warm isotonic fluid are given to the patient. Call for blood in case of transfusion required.

Disability: Assess level of consciousness and pupillary reflexes along with plantar reflexes. Act accordingly.

Exposure: Preserve hypothermia.

Head trauma leads to brain parenchymal injury which is termed traumatic brain injury (TBI). TBI is defined as any disruption in the function of brain due to external force. TBIs are caused due to falls, road traffic accident, blunt head injury, assault, blast injury, and sometime child abuse. Ability of autoregulation and maintenance of cerebral blood flow are disrupted when any TBI occurs. Cerebral vasoconstriction occurs due to hypertension, alkalosis, and hypocarbia and cerebral vasodilation occurs due to hypotension, acidosis, and hypercarbia. After TBI, increase in intracranial blood volume (due to vasodilatation) causes brain swelling. This is the compensatory mechanism of brain to maintain optimal cerebral blood flow in view of damaging brain tissue. Secondary to TBI, various devastating intracranial and extracranial events occur such as severe intracranial hypertension, seizures, cerebral edema, hypotension, hypoxia, anemia, and hyper- and hypocapnia. These devastating events determine the final outcome in the patient after TBI. Hypotension and hypoxia clearly worsen the patient outcome. In short, pathophysiology of TBI involves alteration in cerebral blood flow, parenchymal injury, cerebral edema, ICP, and herniation.

2. Describe the clinical and radiologic features of raised ICP.

a. *Symptoms:* Headache, vomiting, disorientation, and lethargy
b. *Signs:* Depressed level of consciousness (lethargy, stupor, and coma), hypertension (with or without bradycardia), papilledema, sixth cranial nerve palsy, and Cushing triad (hypertension, bradycardia, and irregular respiration)
c. *Radiological features:* CT/MRI of small ventricles and basal cisterns, loss of distinction between gray and white matter, and homogeneous appearance of parenchyma
d. Prominent subarachnoid space around the optic nerves (~45%)
e. Vertical tortuosity of the optic nerves (~40%)
f. Papilledema, flattening of the posterior sclera (~80%), and intraocular protrusion of the optic nerve head
g. Enhancement of the preplaminar (intraocular) optic nerves (~50%)

3. Discuss the New Orleans Criteria versus Canadian CT head rule.

The New Orleans Criteria (NOC) and Canadian CT Head Rule (CCHR) are previously developed clinical decision rules to guide CT use for patients with minor head injury and with GCS of 13–15 for the CCHR and a score of 15 for the NOC **(Table 2)**.

TABLE 2: New Orleans versus Canadian CT head rule.

	New Orleans criteria	Canadian CT head rules
CT if any criteria present	• Headache • Vomiting (any) • Age >60 years • Drug or alcohol intoxication • Seizure • Trauma visible above clavicles • Short-term memory deficits	• Dangerous mechanism of injury • Vomiting ≥2 times • Patient >65 years • GCS score <15, 2 hours postinjury • Any sign of basal skull fracture • Possible open or depressed skull fracture • Amnesia for events 30 minutes before injury
Need for neurosurgical intervention	• *Sensitivity:* 99–100% • *Specificity:* 10–20%	• *Sensitivity:* 99–100% • *Specificity:* 36–76%
Clinically significant intracranial injury	• *Sensitivity:* 95–100% • *Specificity:* 10–33%	• *Sensitivity:* 80–100% • *Specificity:* 35–50%

(GCS: Glasgow Coma Scale)

Question 3

1. List the differential diagnosis and management of acute loss of vision in the ED.

The different causes of painless loss of vision are:
a. Central retinal artery occlusion
b. Central retinal vein occlusion
c. Acute ischemic optic neuropathy
d. Vitreous hemorrhage
e. Amaurosis fugax
f. Transient ischemic attack
g. Retinal detachment

The various causes of painful loss of vision are:
a. Acute angle-closure glaucoma
b. Optic neuritis
c. Giant cell arteritis
d. Uveitis

2. Discuss topical ophthalmologic medications in the ED.

a. Applying medication to the skin or mucous membranes allows it to enter the body from there. Medication applied in this way is known as topical medication. It can also be used to treat pain or other problems in specific parts of the body. Topical medication can also be used to nourish the skin and protect it from harm.
b. Ophthalmic topical drugs are indicated for several diseases of the anterior segment of the eye; acute states such as conjunctivitis, keratitis, and iritis; or chronic conditions, such as dry eye and glaucoma **(Table 3)**.

TABLE 3: Topical ophthalmic medication.

Classification	Examples (available as ophthalmic solution, suspension, or ointment)	Indications
Antibacterials	0.5–1% chloramphenicol, 0.3 and 0.5% gentamicin, 0.3% ciprofloxacin, 1% fusidic acid, 0.3% levofloxacin, 0.3% ofloxacin, 0.3% lomefloxacin, 0.3% norfloxacin, moxifloxacin, 10% sulfacetamide sodium	Dacryocystitis, conjunctivitis, cataract, ophthalmia neonatorum, keratitis, blepharitis
Antivirals	Acyclovir, idoxuridine, vidarabine, trifluridine, ganciclovir	Viral infection, e.g., dendritic corneal ulcers, keratitis, keratoconjunctivitis sicca
Corticosteroids	0.1% Betamethasone, dexamethasone, prednisolone acetate and phosphate, fluorometholone, hydrocortisone, loteprednol, rimexolone	Keratoconjunctivitis sicca, uveitis, episcleritis, scleritis
Mast cell stabilizers	Lodoxamide, sodium cromoglycate, nedocromil, pemirolast, ketotifen, olopadine	Keratoconjunctivitis sicca, conjunctivitis
Anti-inflammatory agents	Diclofenac sodium, flurbiprofen, ketorolac	Inflammation and allergic conjunctivitis
Antihistamines	Antazoline, emedastine, levocabastine	Conjunctivitis

Question 4

1. Draw and explain arterial blood supply to medial wall of nose.

Nasal mucosa has a very rich blood supply from internal carotid artery (ICA) and external carotid artery (ECA). Kiesselbach plexus (Little's area) is situated anteriorly and formed by anterior and posterior ethmoidal arteries (branches of ICA), sphenopalatine, and branches of internal maxillary artery (branches of ECA). Posteriorly nasal mucosa gets blood supply from the posterior branch of the sphenopalatine artery **(Fig. 1)**. Pathology behind epistaxis is erosion of mucosa and rupture of superficial arteries or veins. Nearly 90% of patients present with anterior epistaxis from Little's area. Rest 10% patients present with posterior epistaxis that is more serious than anterior and more commonly seen in old age patients with comorbidities.

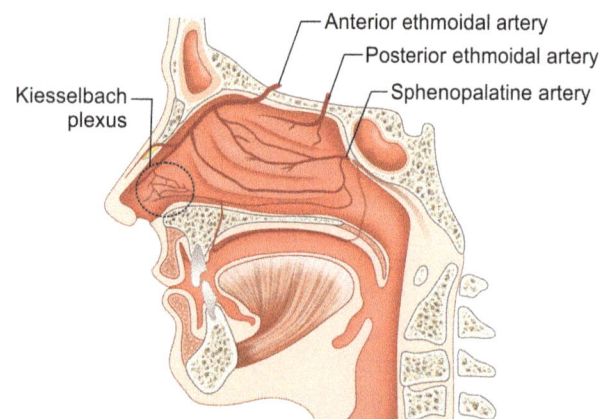

Fig. 1: *Nasal anatomy:* Arterial blood supply to the medial wall of nose.

2. Describe the management of epistaxis.

a. *History:* For stable patients, nasal and systemic history are important. Specific questions regarding duration, severity, frequency, location, laterality, precipitating factors of epistaxis, and methods used to stop epistaxis need to be asked. Past medical history, use of medication (especially aspirin, warfarin, nonsteroidal anti-inflammatory drugs (NSAIDs), heparin, ticlopidine, and dipyridamole), and family history should be documented.

b. *Physical examination:* Check vitals of patient. Make the patient stable if any abnormality is observed. Nasal examination requires nasal examination instruments including nasal speculum, adequate illumination, proper suction and topical medicines, cauterization, and ready packing material.

c. *Topical vasoconstrictor:* It (0.05% oxymetazoline) is beneficial in hemorrhage control and localizing bleeding point. Clots should be suctioned out for better examination. The nasal floor should be parallel to room floor. Tilted head would restrict visualization to the anterior and upper part of nasal cavity only. Nasal speculum is used for internal examination.

d. *Posterior epistaxis:* It should be suspected in constant posterior pharyngeal trickling even after placing anterior packing; epistaxis from both nares and location of bleed cannot be visualized from anterior examination. Fiberoptic endoscopy by an experienced consultant is an advanced option for better visualization of nasal cavity and nasopharynx. Throat examination would complete examination in patients with epistaxis. Trickling of blood on the posterior pharyngeal wall would indicate posterior epistaxis and ongoing bleeding.

e. *Blood investigations:* These are not routinely indicated in single infrequent cases. For recurrent bleeding or a patient with other comorbidities, few routing blood tests can be done, i.e., complete blood count (CBC), PT-INR (prothrombin time—international normalized ratio), activated partial thromboplastin time (aPTT), liver function tests, etc. CT scan or MRI is indicated to evaluate surgical anatomy or local pathology. Angiography is rarely required.

f. *Treatment:* The first stage of treatment is to maintain hemodynamic instability. Hypotension or hypertension should be managed accordingly. Local treatment of epistaxis is divided into *surgical* or *nonsurgical management.* The aim of management is to identify and control the source of bleeding. There are various methods to control bleeding.
   i. Manual hemostasis
   ii. Cauterization
   iii. *Nasal packing:* Anterior and posterior nasal packing
   iv. Surgical treatment

3. Discuss the approach to the management of a foreign body in nose.

Nasal foreign bodies are more likely to be found in the right side of the nose. Children who insert foreign objects into their nose are often brought by caregivers or parents who witnessed the insertion. Therefore, a significant number of nasal foreign bodies are brought due to an observed or suspected history of insertion, within 24 hours of the incident, and with no clinical symptoms secondary to the foreign body. However, as time passes, patients are more likely to manifest with nasal pain, unilateral nasal discharge, and epistaxis and, less frequently, with features of surrounding cellulitis or even meningitis.

Radiography is seldom useful in the evaluation of nasal foreign bodies since substances such as wood or plastic are unlikely to be easily visualized. While button batteries and magnets can be visualized on plain X-rays, these foreign bodies carry a risk of corrosion and necrosis to the surrounding tissue and, as such, expeditious removal takes priority over pursuing identification through radiography, especially if the object is visible on direct examination. If, however, only suspicion of a nasal foreign body is maintained, a plain radiograph may be useful to rule out the presence of a foreign body that may otherwise result in significant morbidity if missed.

As with any foreign body removal, the first attempt is most likely to be successful, with subsequent attempts associated with increasing complications. Therefore, preparation is key and centers around optimization, visualization, and examination of each nostril and nasal cavity, especially when mechanical removal is planned. A head lamp or stand lamp, with or without adjuncts such as nasal speculums can be used to enhance the visual field.

Positive-pressure method: This method generally employs the concept of introduction of positive pressure through an alternate orifice such as the mouth or nostril opposite to the affected side in order to push the foreign body outward from its impacted region.

Mechanical extraction: Similar to aural foreign bodies, various instruments can be used to grasp or anchor behind the nasal foreign body under direct visualization, including alligator forceps, Katz extractors, wax curettes, and right-angle hooks, with care taken not to push the foreign object further into the nasal cavity during manipulation. Bonding to the object using glue at the end of a cotton tip, similar to the technique described for foreign bodies in the ear, is also sometimes used.

Question 5

1. What is the approach to acute pelvic pain in a woman?

The female pelvis comprises organs of the reproductive system: vagina, uterus, fallopian tubes, and ovaries; urinary system: ureters and urinary bladder; gastrointestinal system: sigmoid colon and rectum; as well as components of the musculoskeletal system. Acute pelvic pain can originate from the reproductive organs or from any structures that lie next to or pass through the pelvis. The pelvic organ nerve innervation is from T9–L1 and S2–S4 spinal nerves. Pain may be initiated by inflammation, distention, or ischemia of an organ or by spillage of blood, pus, or other material into the pelvis. The dull aching or the visceral pain is a result of the overlap of afferent innervation supplying the pelvic organs and the appendix, ureters, and colon, making their precise localization difficult. On the other hand, sharp stabbing-like pain results when the afferent nerves in the parietal peritoneum adjacent to an affected organ are stimulated. Further characteristics of pelvic pain along with features and differential diagnoses are given in **Table 4**.

2. Briefly discuss differential diagnoses of vaginal bleeding in a nonpregnant adolescent.

Females of different age groups with vaginal bleeding present to the ED and the emergency physician should be aware of causes related to their age. A large number of females who present with bleeding in emergency are in the reproductive age group.

Adolescent: Anovulatory cycle (hypothalamic–pituitary–ovarian axis immaturity), pregnancy exogenous hormones/oral contraceptives (OCP) coagulopathy, and pelvic infections

Reproductive: Pregnancy, anovulatory cycle [polycystic ovary syndrome (PCOS)], exogenous hormones/OCP leiomyoma, and cervical/endometrial polyps

Life-threatening causes: Acute heavy menstrual bleeding, genitourinary trauma, uterine arteriovenous malformation (AVM)

Acronym for abnormal uterine bleeding: PALM-COEIN: Polyp, adenomyosis, leiomyoma, malignancy, and hyperplasia (structural causes). Coagulopathy, ovulatory dysfunction, endometrial causes, iatrogenic causes not yet classified (nonstructural causes)

3. Discuss the diagnostic algorithm of vaginal bleeding in a woman with <20-week pregnancy.

Possible causes of bleeding:
a. Placenta previa
b. Placental abruption
c. Vasa previa
d. Premature or term labor
e. Genitourinary lesion or laceration
f. Genitourinary infection

Emergency department management includes:
a. Maternal stabilization
b. Electronic fetal monitoring (cardiotocodynamometry) to identify fetal distress
c. Emergency obstetrician consultation
d. Place two large-bore IV lines
e. Obtain CBC, coagulation panel, fibrin degradation product, cross-match maternal blood
f. Administer anti-D Ig IM if the mother is Rh negative.
g. Transvaginal scan for retroplacental clot
h. Immediate delivery indicated.

TABLE 4: Characteristics of acute pelvic pain with corresponding features and differential diagnoses.

Characteristics of pain	Features	Differential diagnoses
Site of pain	Right lower quadrant of the abdomen	Acute appendicitis, pyelonephritis, ectopic pregnancy, ovarian cyst or torsion, ureteric colic, inguinal hernia, mittelschmerz, and musculoskeletal pain
	Left lower quadrant of the abdomen	Diverticulitis, ectopic pregnancy, ovarian cyst or torsion, pyelonephritis, ureteric colic, perirectal abscess, inguinal hernia, mittelschmerz, and musculoskeletal pain
	Lower abdomen	Cystitis, bowel obstruction, inflammatory bowel disease, dysmenorrhea, ectopic pregnancy, uterine perforation or myomas, abortion, PID, endometritis, ovarian hyperstimulation syndrome, placental abruption, ovarian vein thrombosis, incarcerated/strangulated hernia, displaced intrauterine device, somatization disorder, and musculoskeletal pain
Onset of pain	Acute	Vascular, obstructive, viscus perforation causes
	Subacute	Inflammatory causes
	Chronic	Malignancy, inflammatory causes
Character of pain	Tearing-like	Dissection of aorta or its branches
	Stabbing-like	Irritation of parietal peritoneum
	Colicky	Obstruction of tubular organ, smooth muscle spasms, e.g., ureteric colic
	Dull	Visceral pain
Radiation of pain	Loin to groin	Nephrolithiasis
	Migration of pain from umbilicus to right lower abdomen	Acute appendicitis
	Radiation to back	Aortic dissection, PID, cystitis
Associating factors of pain	Hypotension or signs of shock	Ruptured ectopic pregnancy, leaking aortic aneurysm, aortic dissection
	Fever	Acute appendicitis, PID, pyelonephritis
	Diarrhea, nausea, vomiting, anorexia	Gastrointestinal pathology
	Vaginal bleeding or discharge, dyspareunia, cervical motion tenderness	STI, PID, TOA
	Vaginal bleeding	Placental abruption, miscarriage, mittelschmerz
	Urinary frequency or hesitancy, hematuria	Nephrolithiasis, UTI
	Pressure-like feeling in perineum	Uterine prolapse
Time course or pattern of the pain	Mid-cycle vaginal bleeding	Mittelschmerz
	During and postcoital pain	PID, gynecological malignancy
	Infertility treatment	OHSS, ovarian torsion
	Urogenital procedure or surgery	Wound infection or sepsis, venous thrombosis, venous thrombophlebitis, thermal injury
	Trauma	Sexual assault, intimate partner violence, female genital mutilation
Aggravating factors	Change in posture	Musculoskeletal pain
	Menstruation	Endometriosis, adenomyosis
	Dyspareunia	PID, TOA
	Bouncy movements like jumping or travelling over bumpy road	Peritonitis
Relieving factors	Laying still	Peritonitis, musculoskeletal pain
	Passage of urine	Acute urinary retention
Severity	Mild discomfort	PID, UTI, mesenteric ischemia, hernia
	Moderate pain	Peritonitis, aortic aneurysmal leak or dissection, appendicitis, ovarian or adnexal cyst, miscarriage, placental abruption, strangulated or incarcerated hernia, and musculoskeletal pain
	Uncontrollable	Ovarian or adnexal torsion, ureteric colic, labor pain

(OHSS: ovarian hyperstimulation syndrome; PID: pelvic inflammatory disease; STI: sexually transmitted infections; TOA: tubo-ovarian abscess; UTI: urinary tract infection)

Question 6

A 10-year-old presents with history of FOOSH, severe pain and swelling at elbow.

1. What should be the clinical, diagnostic, and management approach to the child?

FOOSH is the nickname for an injury caused by having *"fallen onto an outstretched hand."* These injuries are among the most common injuries affecting the hands and wrists that occur when trying to break a fall. Treatment of a FOOSH injury depends on its severity. The severity of FOOSH injuries can vary greatly depending on various factors. The complex anatomy of the wrist, hand, and elbow often leads to confusion and misdiagnosis of FOOSH injuries; the high prevalence of these injuries makes it imperative for urgent care providers to be proficient in diagnosis and management. Adequate treatment, follow-up, and patient education are essential to minimize the risk for long-term complications.

Medical history and Physical examination should focus on the following:
a. *How injury occurred:* High impact, light impact, sporting event, car accident, etc.
b. Any previous falls, surgery, or previous fractures
c. Medications or illness which predisposes a patient to musculoskeletal injuries
d. *Location of pain:* Ulnar, radial, volar, dorsal, elbow, or hand

The *inspection*, which is taking place throughout the entire history, should focus on key identifiers regarding FOOSH. These include edema, ecchymosis, abrasions, lacerations, visible deformities, erythema, guarding, facial expressions of the patient, and visible signs of distress or pain.

After the inspection period, evaluate the patient's ability regarding range of motion. There is conflicting research on performing motion on patients with injuries, as it can in some instances lead to adverse outcomes. Rather, simply asking the patient to demonstrate range of motion can aid in assessing severity and guide your next steps.

Examination, diagnosis, and management: When examining a FOOSH injury (or any orthopedic injury), palpate with a purpose. It is inherent in our role as urgent care clinicians to distinguish among injuries which need immediate stabilization, injuries which need immediate consultation, and injuries that need prompt, but not immediate, follow-up. It is important to consider all differentials, as it is common for more than one injury to be present after a FOOSH.

2. Enumerate complications which can develop in the child.

Wrist injuries typically occur when a child falls, landing on their hand with their arm extended. The resulting force can cause serious damage to the bones, ligaments, and tendons in the hand and wrist. Complications include avascular necrosis of scaphoid, scapholunate advance collapse (SLAC), and scaphoid nonadvanced collapse (SNAC) of wrist, as well as avascular necrosis and chronic pain. These can lead to significant morbidity and decreased quality of life.

3. Enumerate the injuries which can happen due to fall on an outstretched hand.

Various fractures caused by FOOSH are distal radius fracture, radial or ulnar styloid fracture, radial head fracture, scapholunate tear, scaphoid fracture, distal radioulnar joint fracture, hamate fracture, synovitis, cellulitis, bruise, or clavicle or shoulder injury.

4. Discuss the Salter–Harris classification of fractures.

Salter–Harris classification: Fracture line to the physis and prognosis for growth disturbance **(Table 5 and Fig. 2)**

TABLE 5: Salter–Harris classification of fractures.

Type	Characteristics
I	Separation through the physis usually through the area of hypertrophic and degenerating cell columns
II	Fracture through a portion of the physis that extends through the metaphysis
III	Fracture through a portion of the physis that extends through the epiphysis and into the joint
IV	Fracture across the metaphysis, physis, and epiphysis
V	Crush injury to physis

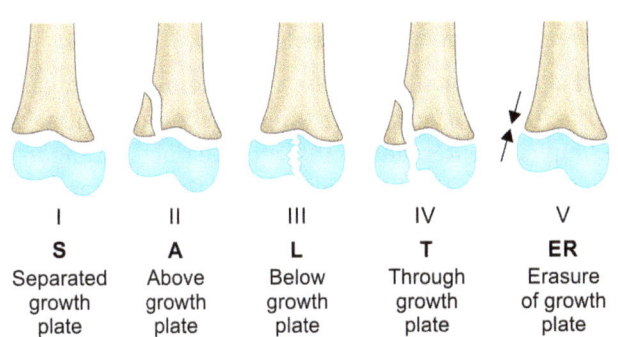

Fig. 2: Salter–Harris fracture types I–V.

Question 7

1. Describe the radiological features on X-ray and ultrasound in a patient with acute abdominal pain.

Role of abdominal X-ray: A standing chest radiograph remains the primary investigation of choice for the detection of free intraperitoneal gas and may detect lower lobar pneumonia. Plain abdominal radiography should be used selectively in the event of suspected intestinal obstruction or perforation. In several studies, the use of abdominal X-ray as the first diagnostic step for abdominal pain has shown a very low diagnostic power, being significant only for intestinal obstruction. In this situation, the sensitivity of abdominal X-ray is 65–90% while specificity is 50–80%. Therefore, even if the CT scan sensitivity and specificity are higher, in the suspicion of intestinal obstruction the abdominal X-ray is a first-level test. Ingestion of a foreign body is another indication for abdominal X-ray, which allows to evaluate the shape, size, and position in order to establish the subsequent procedures. Several studies have shown a higher sensitivity of ultrasound in the suspicion of hollow organ perforation (ultrasound 90% vs. abdominal X-ray 70%). The only limit is the operator skill.

Role of ultrasound and CT: In most cases, the ultrasound abdominal examination is sufficient to diagnose diseases of the upper right abdominal quadrant (cholecystitis and cholangitis) and to diagnose renal colic, urinary tract infections, and ectopic pregnancy. It is also fundamental in the diagnosis of aortic syndrome and in diagnosing perforation and intestinal obstruction. If the ultrasound examination is negative or nondiagnostic but the clinical presentation is persistently altered, it is necessary to perform an abdominal CT scan, generally with the contrast medium, except that there are absolute contraindications (history of anaphylactic shock or severe renal impairment). In the literature, it is shown that by using this method of approach (CT execution to patients with nonconclusive ultrasound), it is possible to reduce the number of CT scan to <50%.

2. Discuss Meckel's diverticulum.

Meckel's diverticulum is the most common congenital anomaly of the gastrointestinal tract. It results from incomplete obliteration of the vitelline duct leading to the formation of a true diverticulum of the small intestine. Meckel's diverticula are uncommon and often clinically silent, particularly in the adult. Meckel diverticulum occurs in about 2% of the population, is about 2 inches in length, is usually located within 2 feet of the ileocecal valve, and usually presents before 2 years of age (rule of 2).

Meckel's diverticulum presents with painless bleeding per rectum. It can also cause intussusceptions and intestinal obstruction. Painless bleeding from the heterotrophic gastric mucosa of Meckel's diverticulum is diagnosed by a technetium scan. If the diagnosis is still in doubt, ultrasound and CT scan should be done. The choice of treatment is surgical resection of Meckel's diverticulum and an anastomosis of the small bowel.

3. What is modified Alvarado score?

In patients who present to the ED with abdominal pain, the most common diagnosis suspected is appendicitis which requires surgery. History, physical examination, and laboratory evaluation included in the initial ED evaluation although no single laboratory value can rule-in or rule-out the diagnosis of appendicitis. Risk scores and imaging scoring systems are included in the evaluation of patients with suspected appendicitis. Alvarado score, also known by its mnemonic, MANTRELS score, is commonly used in addition to the history, physical, and laboratory values. Eight predictive factors are used in Alvarado score **(Table 6)** given a point value of 1 or 2 based on diagnostic weight.

TABLE 6: Patient selection for treatment of appendicitis in observation unit.

Diagnosis is considered based on history, physical examination, and laboratory values.

Alvarado score/MANTRELS score: Used to risk stratify suspected patients.

Suspected appendicitis patient with:
a. Negative or indeterminate initial imaging results
b. Diagnostic uncertainty and lower risk scoring

Nonoperative treatment of appendicitis should not be considered in the emergency department observation unit (EDOU).

Alvarado scoring system for appendicitis

Characteristics			Points
Symptoms	Nausea and/or vomiting		1
	Anorexia		1
	Migration of pain to right lower quadrant		1
Signs	Tenderness in right lower quadrant		2
	Rebound		1
	Temperature > 37.3°C (99.1°F)		1
Laboratory tests White blood cell count	>10,000/dL		2
	Left shift		1
Score	Risk	Management	
1–4	Low risk	• Observation • Serial clinical reassessment and laboratory studies	
5–6	Intermediate risk	Repeat risk assessment with Alvarado score	
7–10	High risk	• Admission • Contrast-enhanced CT abdomen	

Question 8

1. Discuss differential diagnoses of acute-onset joint pain.

Injury, infection, inflammatory process, or acute exacerbation of a chronic arthritis can give rise to acute joint pain **(Table 7)**. History of recurrent acute pain could be due to chronic arthritis. Joint pain is often exacerbated by both active and passive motion of the joint and can also occur at rest, as seen in acute inflamed joint (inflammatory or infective arthritis). If muscles or tendons are actively or passively moved, then periarticular pain can be exacerbated, commonly seen with overuse conditions.

Number of joints involved: Bursitis/tendinitis or any periarticular problem usually involves a single joint. Arthritis should be differentiated into monoarticular (septic and gouty arthritis), oligoarticular [juvenile idiopathic arthritis (JIA), sarcoidosis, seronegative spondyloarthritis], or polyarticular [acute: viral arthritis, or gonococcemia; chronic rheumatoid arthritis, systemic lupus erythematosus (SLE), psoriatic arthritis, or dermatomyositis].

2. Discuss the synovial fluid examination findings of various causes of acute arthritis.

Synovial fluid analysis **(Table 8)** is a very useful test to march toward diagnosis, especially in case of septic arthritis and crystal arthritis or to differentiate between inflammatory and infective arthritis; it is also used in a case of joint effusion if there is diagnostic dilemma. These can be done through arthrocentesis. Synovial fluid analysis includes routine such as cell count and differential, sugar or glucose testing, and microscopic assessment such as Gram stain and bacterial culture. Also, crystal analysis should be done. Gram stain and cultures should be sent to a microbiology laboratory once aspirated. Crystal analysis is performed using polarizing microscopy, with monosodium urate crystals in gout appearing as needle-shaped crystals that are negatively birefringent. In contrast, calcium pyrophosphate crystals in pseudogout appear as polymorphic (often rhomboid) positively birefringent crystals.

3. Discuss the initial approach to acute-onset monoarticular arthritis.

Joint pain is one of the most common presentations in an emergency ward. Thorough initial assessment always helps to differentiate and characterize joint pain. Detailed clinical history and physical examination **(Flowchart 1)** may help in evaluating whether the patient has articular or periarticular disease.

TABLE 7: Differential diagnosis of acute-onset joint pain.

Monoarticular	Polyarticular	Periarticular
• Gout	• Acute rheumatic fever (ARF)	• Bursitis
• Hemarthrosis	• Drug-induced arthritis	• Cellulitis
• Osteoarthritis	• Gonococcal arthritis	• Tendonitis
• Pseudogout	• Immune complex	
• Septic arthritis	• Lyme disease	
• Trauma	• Reiter's syndrome	
	• Rheumatoid arthritis (RA)	
	• Seronegative spondyloarthropathies	
	• Systemic lupus erythematosus (SLE)	
	• Viral arthritis	

TABLE 8: Synovial fluid analysis.

Characteristics	Normal	Noninflammatory	Inflammatory	Septic	Traumatic
Color	Colorless	Yellow	Yellow	Yellow	Red
Appearance	Clear	Clear	Cloudy	Cloudy	Cloudy
WBC/mL	<200	<2,000	2,000–100,000	>100,000	
% PMNs	<25	<25	>50	>95	
Crystals	None	None	May be present	None	None
Cultures	Negative	Negative	Negative	Positive	Negative
Conditions		Trauma, osteoarthritis, viral infections	Inflammatory arthritis such as RA, spondyloarthritis, SLE, acute rheumatic fever, reactive arthritis, crystal-induced arthritis	Bacterial arthritis, tubercular arthritis	Fractures, coagulopathies

(PMNs: polymorphonuclear leukocytes; RA: rheumatoid arthritis; SLE: systemic lupus erythematosus; WBC: white blood cell)

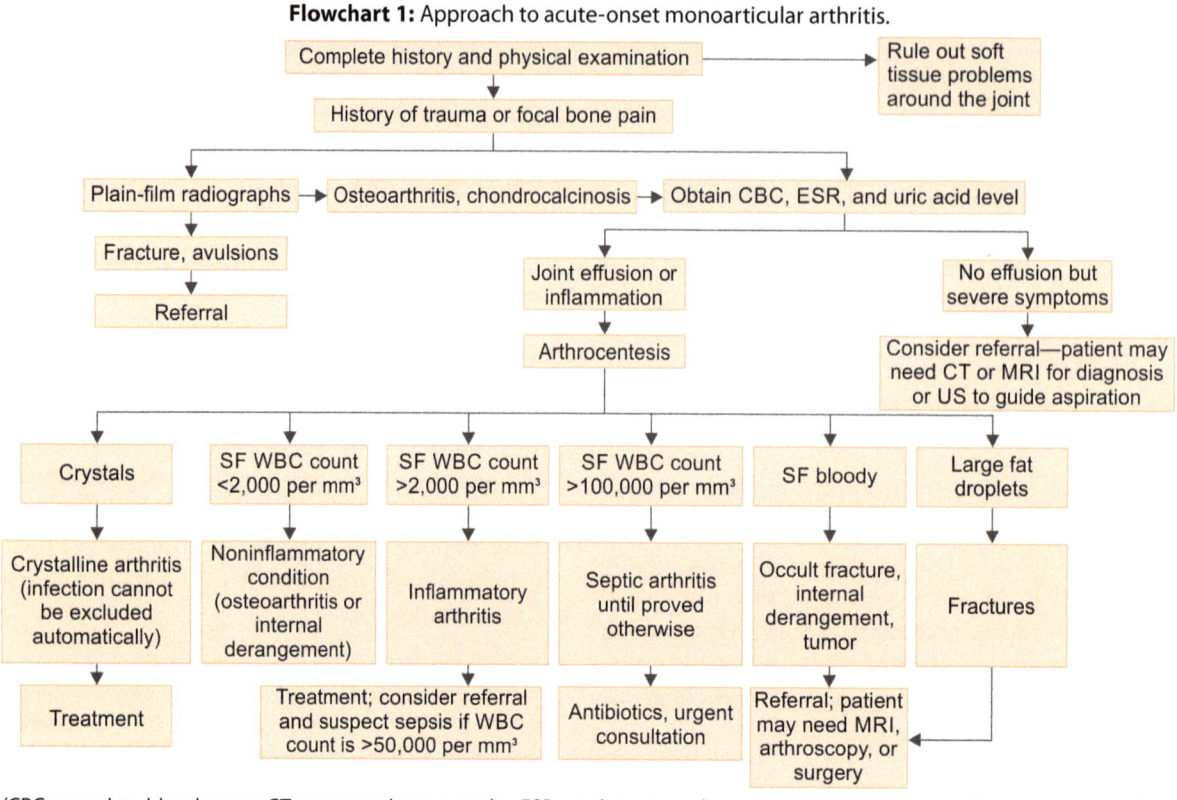

Flowchart 1: Approach to acute-onset monoarticular arthritis.

(CBC: complete blood count; CT: computed tomography; ESR: erythrocyte sedimentation rate; MRI: magnetic resonance imaging; SF: synovial fluid; US: ultrasound; WBC: white blood cell)

Question 9

1. Draw and discuss the nerve supply of urinary bladder.

The urinary bladder is innervated by three sets of peripheral nerves: (1) pelvic parasympathetic nerves, which arise at the sacral level of the spinal cord, excite the bladder, and relax the urethra; (2) lumbar sympathetic nerves, which inhibit the bladder body and excite the bladder base and urethra; and (3) pudendal nerves. Neurological control is complex, with the bladder receiving input from both the autonomic and somatic arms of the nervous system **(Fig. 3)**.

Sympathetic—hypogastric nerve (T12–L2): It causes relaxation of the detrusor muscle, promoting urine retention.

Parasympathetic—pelvic nerve (S2–S4): Increased signals from this nerve cause contraction of the detrusor muscle, stimulating micturition.

Somatic—pudendal nerve (S2–S4): It innervates the external urethral sphincter, providing voluntary control over micturition.

In addition to the efferent nerves supplying the bladder, there are *sensory (afferent) nerves* that report to the brain. They are found in the bladder wall and signal the need to urinate when the bladder becomes full.

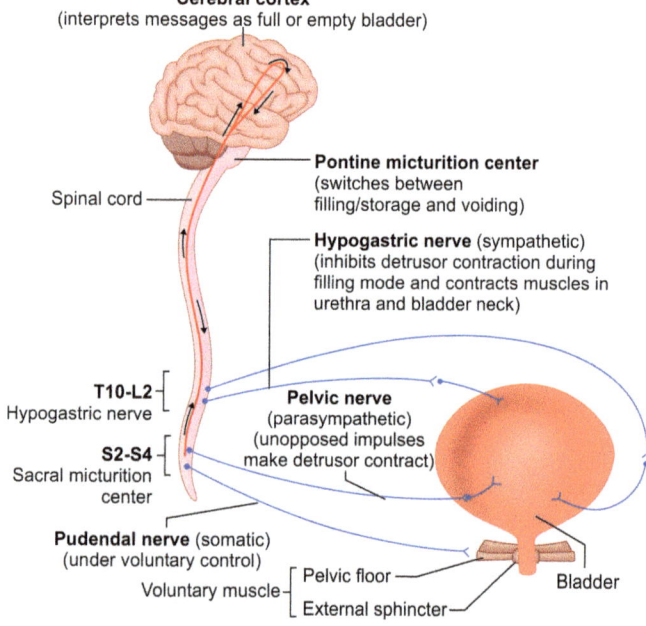

Fig. 3: Nerve supply of urinary bladder.

2. Discuss the approach to a patient with acute retention of urine.

Detailed history, physical examination, and diagnostic testing can help determine the etiology of urinary retention **(Flowchart 2)**.

3. Discuss the approach to a patient with hematuria.

Hematuria can be caused by various underlying pathological conditions or diseases. Age and location of pathology in urinary tract are the main determinants of the causes of hematuria. In the initial evaluation of hematuria, several questions should always be asked. Approach to patient with hematuria as shown in **Flowchart 3**.

Flowchart 2: Approach to a patient with acute retention of urine.

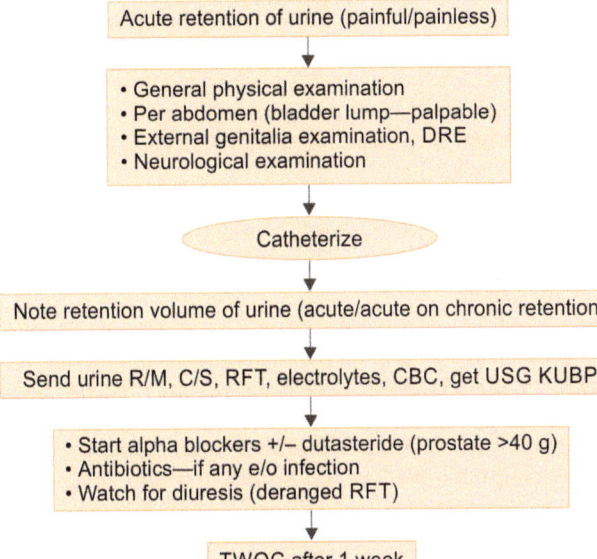

(CBC: complete blood count; C/S: culture and sensitivity; DRE: digital rectal examination; RFT: renal function test; R/M: routine microscopy; TWOC: trial without catheter; USG KUBP: ultrasound kidney, ureter, bladder, and prostate)

Flowchart 3: Approach to a patient with hematuria.

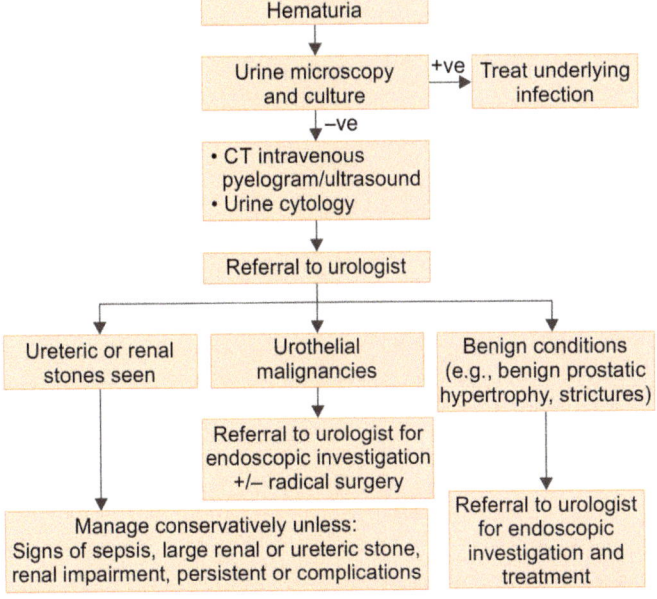

Question 10

1. Draw and discuss a diagram of rotator cuff muscles of shoulders along with their functions.

Rotator cuff muscles surround the proximal humerus and move the arm in different directions. Four muscles form the rotator cuff (**Fig. 4**). These muscles are:

a. *Supraspinatus muscle:* It arises from supraspinatus fossa on dorsal scapula, attaches to superior facet on greater tuberosity of humerus, and abducts the arm.
b. *Infraspinatus muscle:* It arises from infraspinous fossa on dorsal aspect of scapula, attaches to middle facet of greater tuberosity of humerus, and externally rotates the arm.
c. *Teres minor:* It arises from superior part of lateral border of scapula, attaches to inferior facet of greater tuberosity of humerus, and externally rotates the arm.
d. *Subscapularis:* It arises from ventral surface of scapula, attaches to lesser tuberosity of humerus, and internally rotates the arm.

2. Discuss the risk factors for rotator cuff injury.

There are two main causes of rotator cuff tears: *Injury and degeneration*. An injury to the rotator cuff, such as a tear, may happen suddenly when falling on an outstretched hand. It may also develop over time due to repetitive activities. Rotator cuff tears may also happen due to aging, with degeneration of the tissues. Repetitive overhead activity or prolonged bouts of heavy lifting can irritate or damage the tendon. The rotator cuff can also be injured in a single incident during falls or accidents.

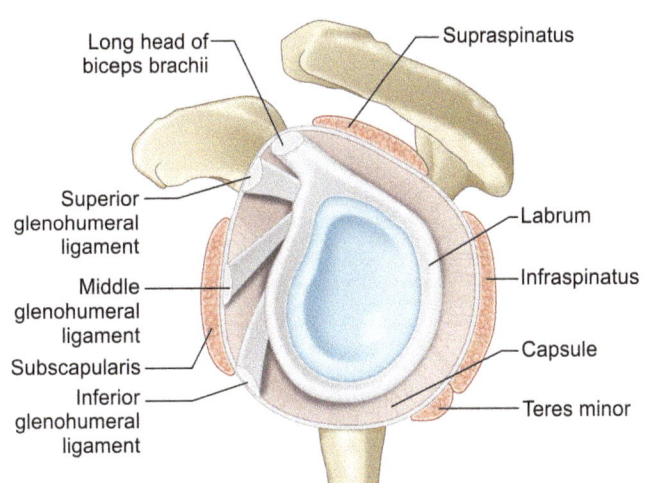

Fig. 4: Rotator cuff muscles of shoulders.

3. Discuss the clinical assessment of rotator cuff injury.

Examination findings in rotator cuff injury:

Drop arm test (supraspinatus muscle): Ask the patient to lower the arm slowly from abduction.

Positive result—immediate drop of the arm accompanied by pain.

External rotation lag test (infraspinatus and supraspinatus):

Examiner passively rotates the patient arm in external rotation.

Positive result—patient unable to maintain the position of full external rotation.

Internal rotation lag test (subscapularis): Hand of affected arm is lifted off of back by examiner and ask to maintain position.

Positive result—unable to maintain position.

4. Discuss the imaging in a patient with rotator cuff injury.

X-ray: It does not show rotator cuff tear but helps to visualize the bone spurs or other potential causes of pain such as arthritis.

Ultrasound: This test helps to produce images of structures, particularly soft tissues such as muscle and tendons. It helps to assess these structures during movement.

MRI: It helps in displaying all structures in great detail.

■ SUGGESTED READING

1. Richhariya D, Sharma B. Textbook of Emergency Medicine including Intensive Care and Trauma, 2nd edition. New Delhi: Jaypee Brothers Medical Publishers (P) Ltd; 2022. pp. 1533-8. (Question 1).
2. Richhariya D, Sharma B. Textbook of Emergency Medicine including Intensive Care and Trauma, 2nd edition. New Delhi: Jaypee Brothers Medical Publishers (P) Ltd; 2022. p. 1561. (Question 2).
3. Richhariya D, Sharma B. Textbook of Emergency Medicine including Intensive Care and Trauma, 2nd edition. New Delhi: Jaypee Brothers Medical Publishers (P) Ltd; 2022. p. 900. (Question 3).
4. Richhariya D, Sharma B. Textbook of Emergency Medicine including Intensive Care and Trauma, 2nd edition. New Delhi: Jaypee Brothers Medical Publishers (P) Ltd; 2022. pp. 915, 947. (Question 4).
5. Richhariya D, Sharma B. Textbook of Emergency Medicine including Intensive Care and Trauma, 2nd edition. New Delhi: Jaypee Brothers Medical Publishers (P) Ltd; 2022. pp. 1059, 1067, and 1095. (Question 5).
6. Richhariya D, Sharma B. Textbook of Emergency Medicine including Intensive Care and Trauma, 2nd edition. New Delhi: Jaypee Brothers Medical Publishers (P) Ltd; 2022. p. 1615. (Question 6).
7. Richhariya D, Sharma B. Textbook of Emergency Medicine including Intensive Care and Trauma, 2nd edition. New Delhi: Jaypee Brothers Medical Publishers (P) Ltd; 2022. pp. 25, 638, and 1240. (Question 7).
8. Richhariya D, Sharma B. Textbook of Emergency Medicine including Intensive Care and Trauma, 2nd edition. New Delhi: Jaypee Brothers Medical Publishers (P) Ltd; 2022. pp. 1033-46. (Question 8).
9. Richhariya D, Sharma B. Textbook of Emergency Medicine including Intensive Care and Trauma, 2nd edition. New Delhi: Jaypee Brothers Medical Publishers (P) Ltd; 2022. pp. 735, 742. (Question 9).
10. Richhariya D, Sharma B. Textbook of Emergency Medicine including Intensive Care and Trauma, 2nd edition. New Delhi: Jaypee Brothers Medical Publishers (P) Ltd; 2022. p. 1604. (Question 10).

Emergency Medicine Paper 39

Devendra Richhariya

Question 1

A 55-year-old presents to the emergency department (ED) with sudden onset of transient loss of consciousness (TLOC).

1. Discuss briefly the differential diagnosis in this case.

It is very important to identify life-threatening etiologies such as acute coronary syndrome (ACS), aortic dissection, leaking abdominal aortic aneurysm (AAA), subarachnoid hemorrhage (SAH), ruptured ectopic pregnancy, and gastrointestinal (GI) bleed which may present as syncope in about 15% of cases. Missed diagnosis in these conditions can lead to medicolegal action in patients presenting as syncope. The physician evaluating a patient with TLOC should be alert to the possibility of this disease in addition to cardiovascular diagnosis of ominous significance.

a. *Cardiac syncope:* Cardiac causes which are associated with syncope include arrhythmia, ischemia, structural/valvular abnormalities (e.g., aortic stenosis), cardiac tamponade, and pacemaker malfunction. Bradycardia and tachycardia are the second most common reason of syncope after reflex syncope.
b. *Hemorrhage:* Large blood loss because of acute severe bleeding can manifest as syncope. Important potential causes include trauma, GI bleed, leaking AAA, ruptured ovarian cyst, ectopic pregnancy rupture, and ruptured spleen.
c. *Massive pulmonary embolism:* Hemodynamically significant pulmonary embolism is an uncommon but well documented cause of syncope.
d. *Subarachnoid hemorrhage:* Patients presenting with syncope following a headache require evaluation for a possible SAH.

2. Discuss the key physical examination findings and diagnostic algorithm of syncope.

There are two main objectives for evaluation of a patient with syncope in the ED:
a. To identify the syncope so that an effective specific treatment strategy can be given
b. To assess the prognosis in view of death, severe adverse events, and syncope recurrence.

During ED evaluation, though the differential diagnosis of syncope is extensive, the main focus remains on the treatment of the underlying cause when syncope is obvious. However, the cause of syncope often remains unclear. The first challenge during evaluation of syncope is to differentiate it from seizure. Epilepsy, stroke, and head trauma may present with TLOC and syncope-like situations. Taking careful history alone can narrow down the diagnosis. History of previous seizure, head injury, tongue bite, the presence of a tonic-clonic activity, abnormal posturing, incontinence of bowel or bladder, missed antiepileptic medication, and postictal confusion gives clue about seizure. Syncope is associated with sweating or nausea and rapid return of orientation upon awakening. Supine and upright blood pressure (BP) and a 12-lead electrocardiograph (ECG), followed by additional testing in selected patient subgroups, including carotid sinus massage, echocardiography, ECG monitoring, and tilt table testing help in diagnosis. Coronary angiography or CT angiography and electrophysiology (EP) study are also recommended.

3. Discuss the ED disposition of a patient with syncope.

Syncope is a common, disabling, and often challenging symptom. It can cause fall and injury and can be the warning sign before sudden cardiac death. Differentiation of syncope from other causes of TLOC such as seizure **(Table 1)** and "syncope mimics" (pseudoseizure, nonsyncopal TLOC, and psychological disorder) is very important for an emergency physician while evaluating such type of patient.

TABLE 1: Differentiation of syncope caused by neurally mediated hypotension, arrhythmias, seizures, and psychogenic causes.

	Neurally mediated hypotension	Arrhythmia	Seizures	Psychogenic
Demographics and clinical settings	• Female > male • Younger age (<55 years) • >2 episodes • Standing • Warm room • Emotional upset	• Male >female • Older age groups • Fewer episodes (<3) • During exertion or supine position • Family history of sudden death	• Younger age <45 years • Any setting	• Female > male • Younger age • Occurs in the presence of gathering, often many episodes in a day, no identifiable trigger
Premonitory symptoms	Longer duration >5 seconds with palpitation, blurred vision, nausea, warmth, diaphoresis, light-headedness	• Shorter duration (<6 seconds) • Palpitation less common	Sudden onset or brief aura	Usually absent
Observation during events	Pallor, diaphoresis, dilated pupil, slow pulse, low BP, incontinence may occur, brief clonic movement may occur	Blue not pale, incontinence can occur, brief clonic movement can occur	Blue face, no pallor frothing from mouth, prolonged syncope, tongue bite, eye deviation, incontinence more likely, increase in heart rate and BP	Normal color, no diaphoresis, eye closed, normal heartrate and BP, no incontinence, prolonged duration
Residual symptoms	Common, prolonged fatigue common, oriented	• Uncommon • Unless prolonged unconsciousness, oriented	Common, aching muscle, disoriented fatigue, headache, slow recovery	Uncommon, oriented

(BP: blood pressure)

Question 2

A 20-year-old person presents with recurrent seizures and altered sensorium for 8 hours. While evaluating in the ED, he develops a generalized tonic-clonic seizure.

1. How will you rapidly assess and manage the patient?

Stabilization phase (0-5 minutes seizure activity):

Airway: Consider nasopharyngeal airway, suction.

Breathing: Supplement oxygen

Circulation: Secure intravenous access. Check blood glucose levels. If sugar level <60 mg/dL, start intravenous dextrose (D50W) 50 mL.

Initial therapy phase (5-20 minutes): Benzodiazepines are the first therapy of choice:
a. 10 mg for >40 kg, 5 mg for 13-40 kg of intramuscular midazolam single dose, OR
b. 0.1 mg/kg/dose, maximum: 4 mg/dose of intravenous lorazepam, may repeat dose once, OR
c. 0.15-0.2 mg/kg/dose, maximum: 10 mg/dose intravenous diazepam, may repeat dose once.

If none of the above benzodiazepines is available, any one of the following may be administered.
a. 15 mg/kg/dose of intravenous phenobarbital single dose, OR
b. Intranasal midazolam and buccal midazolam, OR
c. 0.2-0.5 mg/kg, maximum: 20 mg/dose of rectal diazepam single dose

Second therapy phase (20-40 minutes): At this point, a response to the therapy administered in the previous phase should be evident. If there is a lack of response, the following can be administered as a single dose:
a. 20 mg PE/kg, maximum: 1,500 mg PE/dose of intravenous fosphenytoin single dose, OR
b. Intravenous levetiracetam 60 mg/kg, maximum: 4,500 mg/dose, single dose, OR
c. 40 mg/kg, maximum: 3,000 mg/dose of intravenous valproic acid, single dose.

If none of the options are available, a single dose of intravenous phenobarbital 15 mg/kg can be administered. Consider definitive airway protection by endotracheal intubation and mechanical ventilation.

Third therapy phase (40-60 minutes): If the seizure persists, repeat any drug of the second-line therapy or administer anesthetic doses of:
a. Thiopental 100-250 mg bolus with repeat bolus of 50 mg every 2-3 minutes till seizures are controlled followed by infusion of 3-5 mg/kg/h, OR
b. Propofol 2 mg/kg IV bolus followed by 5-10 mg/kg/h infusion, OR
c. Midazolam 0.1-0.3 mg/kg bolus followed by infusion at 0.05-0.4 mg/kg//h.

If the patient needs third-line therapy, then the airway must be protected by endotracheal intubation and mechanical ventilation. The patient should undergo continuous electroencephalography (EEG) monitoring.

2. Enumerate the causes of generalized status epilepticus.

a. *Drug-related:* Discontinuation of antiepileptic medications. Few drugs may lower the seizure threshold or increase clearance of antiepileptic medications such as isoniazid and erythromycin.
   Drug withdrawal: Alcohol, barbiturates, or opioid withdrawal.
b. *Infection:* Meningitis, encephalitis, brain abscess
c. Stroke
d. *Metabolic causes:* Electrolyte disturbances, hypoglycemia
e. Hypoxia
f. Central nervous system (CNS) tumors
g. Traumatic brain injury.

3. Describe the indication for a CT scan of head in a patient with seizure in the ED.

A CT scan is usually the first step for patients with new seizures, which ensures that there is no underlying hemorrhage or tumor. Most of these CT scans will be normal because there is no lesion, or if there is a lesion it may not be visible on a CT scan. The onset of seizures is seen before the age of 1 year or after the age of 20 years. There is evidence of focal seizures on history, examination, or EEG. Recommendation of CT head if there is neurological or neuropsychological deficit.

Question 3

A 60-year-old person presents with dizziness for 2 hours.

1. Discuss briefly the differential diagnosis of acute-onset dizziness.

Dizziness is an impairment in spatial perception and stability and can range from fleeting faintness to a severe balance disorder that makes normal functioning impossible **(Table 2)**.

Accordingly, dizziness can be classified into four groups:
1. Vertigo
2. Disequilibrium without vertigo
3. Presyncope or near faint
4. Psychological dizziness (associated with panic attacks and anxiety disorders).

The four most common vestibular diagnoses causing sudden-onset dizziness will be reviewed in detail. These are vestibular neuritis (VN) (or neuronitis), benign paroxysmal positional vertigo (BPPV), vestibular migraine (VM), and Ménière's disease.

2. Discuss the key differences between peripheral and central vertigo.

The most important feature in distinguishing between central and peripheral vertigo is the features of nystagmus **(Table 3)**. Centrally derived nystagmus is seen in brain and brain stem lesions. These may be in the horizontal plane, as in peripheral lesions, or in the form of vertical nystagmus. The most important point in diagnosis is history and physical examination. After a well-received history and physical examination, the diagnosis is largely approached.

TABLE 2: Causes of vertigo.

Peripheral	Central	Systemic/vertigo mimics
• BPPV	• Stroke/TIA	• Ototoxic drugs
• Labyrinthitis	• Epilepsy	• Anemia
• Ménière's disease	• Migraine	• Hypoglycemia
• Vestibular neuritis	• Brain tumors	• Dyselectrolytemia
• Perilymph fistula	• Multiple sclerosis	• Cardiac arrhythmias
• Acute otitis media	• Familial ataxia syndrome	• Aortic dissection
• Schwannoma	• Postconcussion syndrome	• Carbon monoxide poisoning
	• Meningitis/ encephalitis	• Adrenal insufficiency
		• Pulmonary embolism
		• Anxiety and panic attacks
		• Hyperventilation syndrome
		• Thiamine deficiency

(BPPV: benign paroxysmal positional vertigo; TIA: transient ischemic attack)

TABLE 3: Distinguishing features of peripheral and central causes of vertigo.

Feature	Peripheral	Central
Nystagmus	Commonly combined (horizontal and torsional), inhibited by fixation of eyes on to the object, does not change direction with gaze to other side	Purely vertical, horizontal or torsional, not inhibited by fixation of eyes on the object, may change direction with gaze toward fast phase of nystagmus
Imbalance	Mild to moderate, generally able to walk	Severe, not able to walk or stand sometimes
Nausea, vomiting	Commonly severe	Varies
Hearing loss, tinnitus	Common	Rare
Neurological (no auditory)	Rare	Common
Latency followed by provocative maneuver	Up to few seconds	Up to 5 seconds

In peripheral vertigo, the pathology is mostly in the temporal bone, especially in the labyrinth. Central pathologies are the reflection of pathologies in the area extending from the vestibular system to the brain. If a patient has a vertical nystagmus in the spontaneous gaze, that is, upward and downward, this always suggests a central lesion. In peripheral vertigo, auditory complaints, hearing loss, ringing, humming, and ear fullness may accompany the patient. Sometimes, as in VN, the patient may not have auditory findings. Auditory findings are not usually encountered in central vertigo. It is accompanied by remarkable findings such as vision loss, diplopia, coordination disorders, ataxia, and speech difficulties. Peripheral vertigo is usually described as spinning around, whereas in central vertigo, the feeling of instability and drunkenness is more prominent.

3. Discuss the management algorithm of acute-onset vertigo.

The most important points in diagnosis are history and physical examination (**Flowchart 1**). After a well-received history and physical examination, the diagnosis is largely approached. Bedside blood sugar should be checked while a medical history is taken from the patient and a physical examination is performed. Oral or IV glucose is given if the patient is hypoglycemic. ECG is taken to detect tachycardia, bradycardia, and dysrhythmia that may cause symptoms in the patient. Short PR, ischemia findings, prolonged QT interval, Wolf–Parkinson–White findings, and QRS width are investigated on ECG. The patient's arterial BP is measured and a pulse oximeter is inserted. The patient is monitored. The patient is examined with an otoscope. Bedside oculomotor examination provides important information for diagnosis. Oculomotor examination is done in two ways: dynamic and static. In static oculomotor examination, asymmetric eye movements and type of nystagmus are determined. In dynamic oculomotor examination, the oculomotor reflex is evaluated with the head impulse test and the head shaking test. Laboratory tests that should be requested for the patient are whole blood analysis, electrolytes, and β-hCG in women of childbearing age. If the physical examination findings support central pathologies or are suspicious, first, non-contrast brain tomography is taken. Diffusion-weighted MRI and MRI angiography are particularly important for detecting cerebrovascular disease of the brain stem and cerebellum.

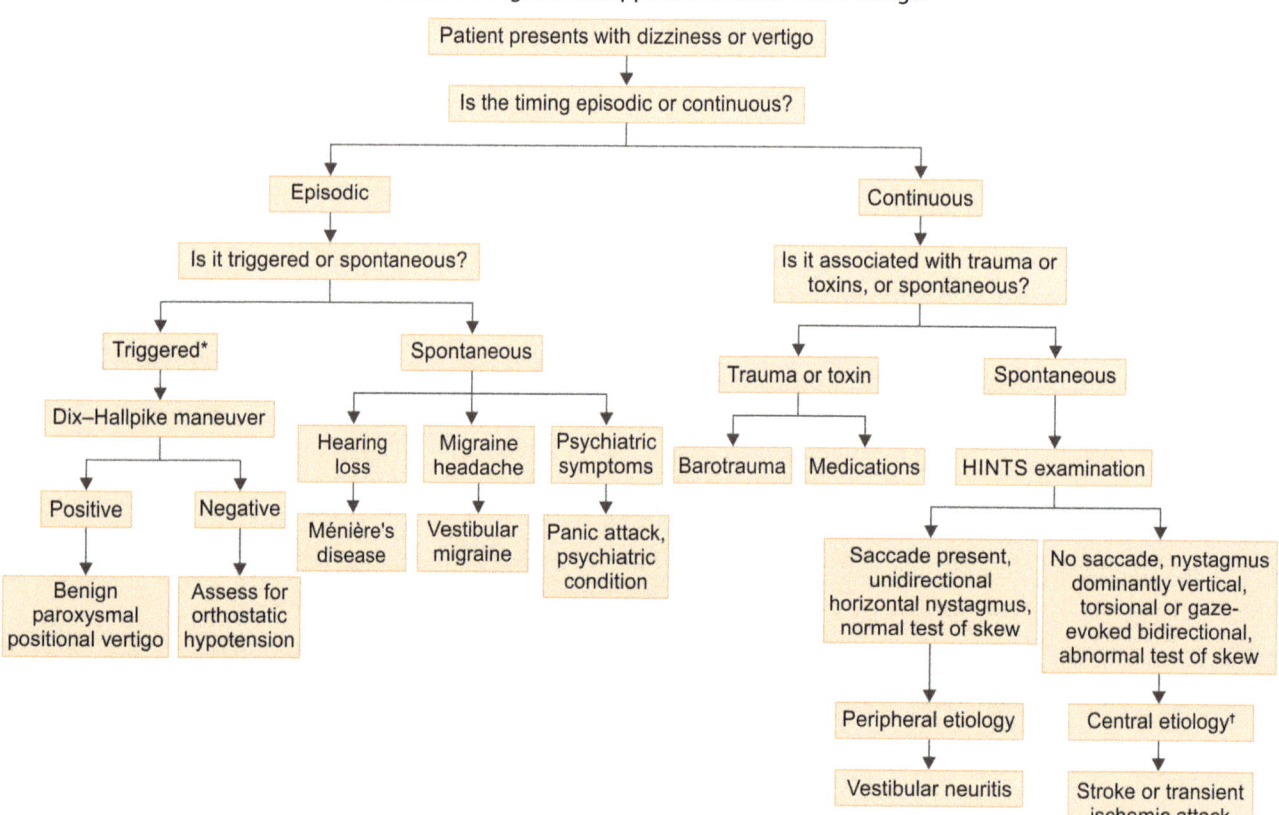

Flowchart 1: Algorithmic approach to acute-onset vertigo.

(HINTS: head impulse, nystagmus, and skew)
*Exacerbation of symptoms with movement does not aid in determining whether the etiology is peripheral versus central.
†Central causes can also occur with patterns triggered by movement.

Question 4

A 45-year-old person presents to the ED with history of hemoptysis for 1 day and develops massive hemoptysis in the ED.

1. Discuss the differential diagnosis of hemoptysis.

The most common causes of mild hemoptysis are bronchitis, bronchiectasis, bronchogenic carcinoma, and tuberculosis **(Table 4)**. About 20–40% of cases of minor hemoptysis are due to bronchitis and bronchiectasis, while bronchogenic and metastatic carcinomas account for 20% of the cases. However, in India, tuberculosis is the most common cause of mild to massive hemoptysis, where it can be seen in active disease or as its sequelae. In western part of the world, malignancies are the main cause of massive hemoptysis.

TABLE 4: Differential diagnosis of hemoptysis.

Airway diseases	Infections	Pulmonary vascular diseases	Others
Airway trauma, bronchitis, bronchiectasis, bullous emphysema, bronchovascular fistula, bronchial adenoma, bronchogenic carcinoma, metastatic cancer (to bronchus or trachea foreign body in airway)	Tuberculosis (active or cavitary), invasive mycetoma, bronchiectasis, cystic fibrosis, pneumonia (*Staphylococcus, Klebsiella, Legionella*), lung abscess, hydatid cyst	Congenital heart defects, congestive heart failure, mitral stenosis, tricuspid endocarditis, pulmonary arteriovenous malformation, pulmonary artery pseudoaneurysm, pulmonary embolism, pulmonary veno-occlusive disease, pulmonary hypertension	• *Drugs and toxins* (argemone alkaloid cocaine use) • *Pulmonary renal syndrome* (Wegner's granulomatosis, Goodpasture syndrome), immunologic lung disease, SLE • *Genetic defects of collagens* (Ehlers–Danlos syndrome) Bone marrow transplantation • *Disorders of coagulation* Anticoagulant and antiplatelet medications DIC, thrombocytopenia, liver disease, Von Willebrand's disease • *Iatrogenic* Bronchoscopy with endobronchial biopsy or TBLB or TBNA, pulmonary artery catheterization, airway stent • *Idiopathic* Idiopathic pulmonary hemosiderosis • *Trauma* Blunt trauma chest, penetrating lung injury • *Catamenial hemoptysis*

(DIC: disseminated intravascular coagulation; SLE: systemic lupus erythematosus; TBLB: transbronchial lung biopsy; TBNA: transbronchial needle aspiration)

2. How will you manage the patient?

History and physical examination are useful in localization of lesion in around 50% of cases **(Table 5)**. The initial approach to managing life-threatening hemoptysis involves resuscitation and protection of airway (ABC approach). The second step is directed at localizing the site and cause of bleeding and the final step is the application of definitive and specific treatments to prevent recurrent bleeding.

On the basis of history and physical and laboratory examination, specific therapy should be started to correct the cause because invasive therapeutic interventions do not help to control bleeding secondary to coagulopathies and immunologically mediated disorder such as Goodpasture syndrome. Specific therapies such as antibiotics, correction of coagulopathies with platelet, fresh frozen plasma (FFP), cryoprecipitates, blood transfusion, steroids, immunosuppressive therapies, or plasmapheresis are mandatory to control the precipitating factor. Vitamin K supplements and tranexamic acid are also used to control bleeding. Intravenous vasopressin has also been used, but caution is advised in patients with coexistent coronary artery disease or hypertension. Vasoconstriction of the bronchial artery may also hamper effective bronchial artery embolization (BAE) by obscuring the site of bleeding, leading to difficulties in cannulation of the artery. Recombinant activated factor VII (rFVIIa) has been used in hemoptysis with community-acquired pneumonia. Danazol or gonadotropin-releasing hormone (GRH) has been used in catamenial hemoptysis. Systemic antifungal agents have been tried in the management of hemoptysis related to mycetoma, but results are not satisfactory. However, percutaneous or direct bronchoscopic instillation of these drugs in the cavity has promising results. This technique is useful in cases of bleeding after failed BAE and in those who are not fit for surgery. Radiation therapy has been used in vascular tumor or mycetoma-related massive hemoptysis by necrosis of feeding vessel and vascular thrombosis due to perivascular edema.

TABLE 5: Evaluation (history and physical examination) of a patient with hemoptysis.

History	Probable diagnosis
Smoking, asbestos exposure	Bronchogenic carcinoma
Risk factors for aspiration (alcohol, swallowing disorder, altered sensorium, or diminished consciousness)	Lung abscess, pneumonia, FB aspiration
Recent chest trauma or procedure	Traumatic or iatrogenic lung injury
Previously diagnosed pulmonary, cardiac, or systemic disease	Important clue
Symptoms	
Hoarseness of voice	Bronchogenic carcinoma
Purulent sputum	Pneumonia, lung abscess, bronchiectasis, Bronchitis
PND/Orthopnea	MS/LVF
Dyspnea and pleuritic chest pain	• Pneumonia • Pulmonary embolism
Weight loss, night sweats, cough, fever	• Tuberculosis • Bronchogenic carcinoma
Signs	
Localized decreased breath sounds, Localized wheeze Stridor	• Bronchogenic carcinoma • FB aspiration • Tracheal tumor
Bronchial breath sounds	Pneumonia
Pleural rub	Pneumonia, Pulmonary embolism
Diastolic murmur	Mitral Stenosis
Clubbing	• Suppurative lung disease, bronchiectasis • Bronchogenic CA
S3 gallop	LVF
• Oral aphthous ulcers, genital ulcers, and uveitis • Saddle nose, rhinitis, and septal perforation	• Bechet's disease in which AVMs are present • Wegener's granulomatosis

(AVM: arteriovenous malformation; CA: carcinoma; FB: foreign body; MS: mitral stenosis; LVF: left ventricular failure; PND: paroxysmal nocturnal dyspnea; S3: third heart sound)

Question 5

A 35-year-old person, a known case of rheumatic heart disease, presents to the ED with profuse, watery diarrhea, dyspnea, and palpitation for 1 day. Cardiac monitor reveals atrial fibrillation with a heart rate of 180 beats/min. The BP is 80/50 mm Hg.

1. Discuss the clinical assessment and management in this case.

Atrial fibrillation in a rheumatic heart disease is under-recognized but is prevalent in many countries around the world. It causes significant morbidity and mortality, mainly in the young. The incidence of atrial fibrillation increases with severity of valvular stenosis. The respiratory tract infection is more commonly present in patients with atrial fibrillation as compared to patients without atrial fibrillation. In view of profuse diarrhea, point-of-care echocardiography is used to assess volume status and hemodynamic monitoring. Systemic embolization is present in a significant number of patients with rheumatic heart disease with atrial fibrillation. In this patient, dyspnea is present so he needs to be evaluated for embolization **(Flowchart 2)**.

Flowchart 2: Rheumatic heart disease and atrial fibrillation.

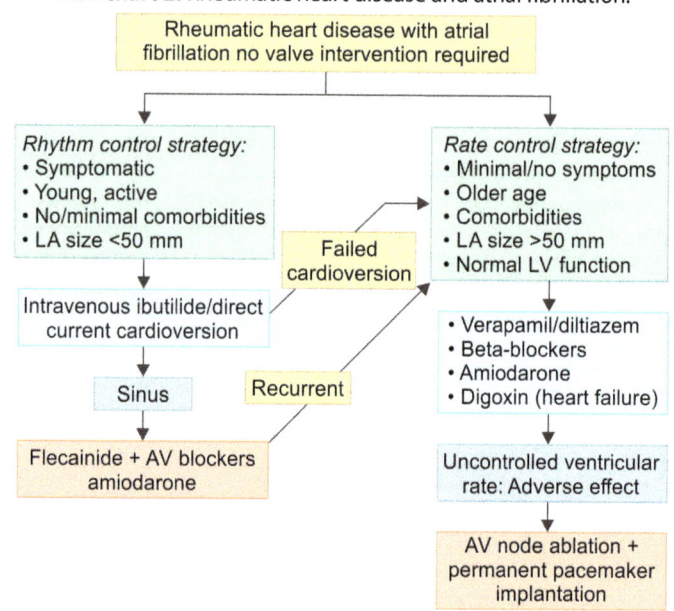

(AV: atrioventricular; LA: left atrial; LV: left ventricular)

2. Discuss the role of point-of-care ultrasound in this case.

Hypotension and shock are commonly encountered in the emergency room (ER). They can be cardiogenic in origin or may result from noncardiac causes such as hemorrhage, hypovolemia, or sepsis. As shock requires aggressive early intervention in order to prevent end-organ damage due to inadequate tissue perfusion, distinguishing cardiogenic shock from shock of other etiologies is extremely important. The *major advantage* of echocardiography is that it can quickly determine whether the shock is cardiogenic or noncardiogenic, apart from also providing plenty of hemodynamic information that is useful irrespective of the type of shock. A brief 2D echocardiographic examination itself can help in excluding common cardiac causes of hypotension such as extensive myocardial infarction (MI) with severe left ventricular (LV) systolic dysfunction, right ventricular (RV) infarction, mechanical complication of MI, nonischemic severe LV systolic dysfunction, pericardial effusion with tamponade, and massive pulmonary embolism.

Question 6

A young female patient presents with acute-onset tetanic spasms of hands and reduced urine output preceded by nausea and muscle weakness. The laboratory investigation shows a white blood cell (WBC) count of 2,50,000/μL.

1. Discuss the assessment and management of this patient.

Generally, features of hypocalcemia begin when the serum ionized calcium level drops below 2.5 mg/dL. The main symptoms and signs include extremity and facial paresthesia, Chvostek and Trousseau signs, muscle cramps, hyperreflexia, stridor, bronchospasm, carpopedal spasm, tetany, personality disorder, memory and concentration difficulties, seizure, cloudiness, extrapyramidal findings, and congestive heart failure. ECG findings include prolonged QT interval, QRS and ST changes mimicking ischemia, and ventricular arrhythmias.

Diagnostic evaluation: Serum albumin level, kidney functions, serum levels of other electrolytes, serum vitamin D level, parathyroid hormone (PTH) level, and serum phosphate level should be requested. All patients should have ECG. A high serum alkaline phosphatase level is important for secondary hypoparathyroidism or severe vitamin D deficiency. A high amylase level supports the diagnosis of pancreatitis as the underlying cause. The calcium level in urine should be checked. A low urinary calcium level indicates hypoparathyroidism and vitamin D deficiency.

Treatment of severe acute symptomatic hypocalcemia is urgent. If the patient has carpopedal spasm, tetany, convulsion, QG prolongation in ECG or if it is not symptomatic and if the patient's corrected calcium level is below 7.5 mg/dL, IV calcium gluconate is given. The patient is given IV 10–20 mL of 10% calcium gluconate in 100 mL of 5% dextrose or isotonic sodium chloride in 10 minutes. Afterward, IV infusion starts with 100 mL of 10% calcium gluconate in 1,000 mL of 5% dextrose or isotonic sodium chloride at a rate of 50 mL/h. The cardiac rhythm of the patient must be monitored during IV calcium infusion.

2. Describe Cairo–Bishop criteria.

Tumor lysis syndrome (TLS) refers to metabolic consequences resulting from sudden release of intracellular metabolites, nucleic acids, and proteins from tumor cells undergoing death spontaneously or posttreatment. It is divided into two groups, i.e., laboratory and clinical, based on the *Cairo-Bishop definitions*.

Laboratory TLS is defined as the presence of ≥2 of the following laboratory abnormalities: uric acid ≥8 mg/dL, potassium ≥6 mEq/L, phosphorus >4.5 mg/dL in adults (≥6.5 mg/dL in children), and calcium ≤7 mg/dL or 25% change in these laboratory values from the baseline, present 3 days before or 7 days after initiation of therapy.

Clinical TLS is defined as laboratory TLS accompanied with ≥1 of the following: Serum creatinine ≥1.5 times the upper limit of normal, seizure, cardiac dysrhythmia, or death.

The clinical manifestations noted are acute kidney injury, seizures, and cardiac dysrhythmias or cardiac arrest. Renal failure occurs due to the precipitation of uric acid within renal tubules. Phosphorus released from cells may combine with calcium and get precipitated in renal tubules and parenchyma also. Hyperkalemia causes cardiac dysrhythmias or cardiac arrest. Hypocalcemia may cause tetany and seizures and can lead to dysrhythmias. Hypovolemia can further precipitate renal failure.

Question 7

1. Briefly describe Indian scorpions of medical importance and their venoms.

Indian scorpion pathophysiology and complex venom: Phospholipase, acetylcholinesterase, hyaluronidase, serotonin, and neurotoxins.

Mode of action: Neurotoxins bind reversibly to voltage-gated ion channels (sodium, calcium, and potassium) and keep them in an open state. They affect somatic and autonomic nervous systems (autonomic storm—primary cause of morbidity and mortality). Hyperkalemia, hyperglycemia, and increased secretion of renin and aldosterone are characteristic of the Indian red scorpion.

2. What are the clinical features of a sting by a venomous scorpion?

Clinical presentation: Pain, erythema, induration, wheal, paresthesia, and hyperesthesia are the local features

Systemic features: Allergic—urticaria, wheeze, and angioedema

Autonomic: Sympathetic—tachycardia, hyperthermia, hypertension, profuse sweating, and urinary retention; Parasympathetic—bradycardia, hypotension, urination, hypersalivation, bronchospasm, and priapism. Cardiovascular—hypertension, tachycardia, cardiogenic shock, and arrhythmias; Gastrointestinal—nausea, vomiting, diarrhea, and abdominal pain

Neurological: Cranial nerves:—nystagmus, miosis/mydriasis, and tongue fasciculations; *Peripheral*—spasticity, clonus, brisk reflexes, and ascending paralysis; *Central*—respiratory failure, coma, and stroke.

Rare: Disseminated intravascular coagulation (DIC), pulmonary edema, rhabdomyolysis, and renal failure

3. Explain the management of a patient stung by a venomous scorpion.

Management: First aid—paracetamol (pain relief); airway maintenance and ventilation; *Anaphylaxis*—adrenaline, chlorpheniramine, and hydrocortisone. *Hospital*—airway, breathing, and circulation. Local anesthesia should be given for severe pain. Hourly monitoring—temperature, pulse, BP, respiratory rate, and oxygen saturation. ECG monitoring—cardiac arrhythmias. Arterial blood gas (ABG) and serum electrolytes (potassium, magnesium, and calcium). Scorpion antivenom—systemic envenomation. Tetanus prophylaxis should be given. Fluid imbalance correction (crystalloids). Benzodiazepines should be administered for delirium and agitation.

Bawaskar's protocol: 0-4 hours: Scorpion antivenom + prazocin; *4-6 hours:* Prazocin; *6-10 hours:* Prazocin + dobutamine + BiPAP; *10-12 hours:* Scorpion antivenom + sodium nitroprusside/nitroglycerine + BiPAP; *>12 hours:* Dobutamine.

Preventive measures: Clear debris and rubbish from areas of work and rest. Use insect repellants. Inspect shoes and clothes for scorpions. Use flashlight when walking in dark places.

Question 8

1. Discuss the physiology of thyroid hormone production.

Thyroid hormones are made by the thyroid gland. The thyroid gland makes and releases two types of thyroid hormones: thyroxine (T4) and triiodothyronine (T3). The thyroid gland and the pituitary gland work together **(Flowchart 3)**. Thyroid hormone changes are a common feature in emergency patients with no known thyroid dysfunction. A decrease in T3 is frequently observed with normal levels of free T4 (fT4) and thyroid-stimulating hormone (TSH), a condition known as euthyroid sick syndrome (ESS), non-thyroidal illness syndrome (NTIS), or low T3 syndrome. Interpretation of thyroid function test is given in **Table 6**.

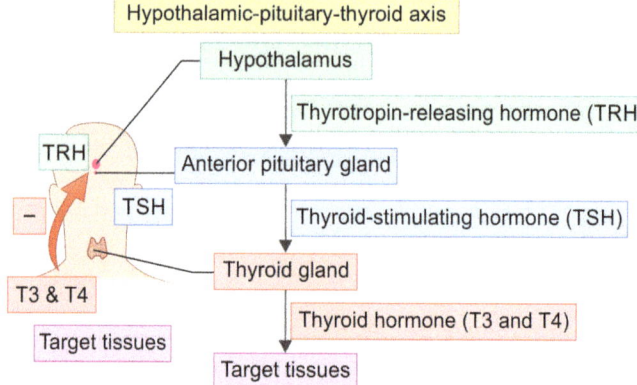

Flowchart 3: Physiology of thyroid hormone production.

(T3: triiodothyronine; T4: thyroxine)

TABLE 6: Interpretation of thyroid function test.

TSH	Free T4	Free T3	Interpretation
Normal	Normal	Normal	None
Low	High	High	Hyperthyroidism
Low	Normal	Normal	Subclinical hyperthyroidism
Low	Normal	High	T3 toxicosis
Low	High	Normal	Thyroiditis, T4 ingestion, hyperthyroidism in older adults, comorbid conditions
Low	Low	Low	Euthyroid sick syndrome, central hypothyroidism
High	Normal	Normal	Subclinical hypothyroidism, recovery from a euthyroid sick syndrome

(T3: triiodothyronine; T4: thyroxine; TSH: thyroid-stimulating hormone)

2. Discuss the Burch–Wartofsky point scale for thyroid storm.

The Burch–Wartofsky point scale (BWPS) **(Table 7)** is a quantitative diagnostic tool based on three major observations in patients with thyroid storm: (1) Continuum of end-organ dysfunction, (2) high variability of symptoms and signs between patients, and (3) high mortality associated with missed diagnosis.

3. Discuss the management of a patient with thyroid storm.

Thyroid storm is an unrecognized, undertreated, life-threatening form of severe thyrotoxicosis. It is rare and mostly an acute reaction to thyroid and non-thyroid surgery, trauma infections, contrast media, amiodarone, or after delivery in preexisting hyperthyroidism. Other risk factors are acute coronary syndrome, pulmonary embolism, and diabetic ketoacidosis.

TABLE 7: Burch–Wartofsky point scale.

Temperature (°F)		Cardiovascular dysfunction	
99–99.9	5	Tachycardia (beats/min)	
100–100.9	10	99–109	5
101–101.9	15	110–119	10
102–102.9	20	120–129	15
103–103.9	25	130–139	20
≥104.0	30	≥140	25
		Atrial fibrillation	10
Central nervous system effects		**Heart failure**	
Absent	0	Mild (pedal edema)	5
Mild (agitation)	10	Moderate (bibasilar rales)	10
Moderate (delirium, psychosis, extreme lethargy)	20	Severe (pulmonary edema)	15
Severe (seizure, coma)	30		
Gastrointestinal–hepatic dysfunction		**Precipitant history**	
Moderate (diarrhea, nausea/vomiting, abdominal pain)	10	Positive	0
Severe (unexplained jaundice)	20	Negative	10

Total: <25: storm unlikely; 25–45: impending storm; >45: thyroid storm.
Source: Burch HB, Wartofsky L. Life-threatening thyrotoxicosis. Thyroid storm. Endocrinol Metab Clin North Am. 1993;22(2):263-77.

Prompt recognitions and treatment are warranted as mortality is almost 100%. Causes of mortality in a patient of thyroid storm are sepsis multi-organ failure, congestive heart failure arrhythmias, and DIC. *Clinical features* of thyroid storm typically include hyperpyrexia, out-of-proportion tachycardia, and altered mental status (agitation, delirium, and coma) along with a clinical picture of hyperthyroidism. *Classic features* of thyroid storm include fever, marked tachycardia, heart failure, tremor, nausea and vomiting, diarrhea, dehydration, restlessness, extreme agitation, and delirium or coma. Fever is typical and may be higher than 105.8°F (41°C).

Thyroid function test: Usual findings include elevated T3, T4, and fT4 levels; increased T3 resin uptake; suppressed TSH levels; and an elevated 24-hour iodine uptake. Management of thyroid storm is summarized in **Table 8**.

TABLE 8: Management of thyroid storm.

β adrenergic blockers	Propranolol 60–80 mg orally every 4 hours (IV 0.5–1.0 mg as test dose, then repeat 1–2 mg every 15 minutes till desired effect, then 1–2 mg every 3 hours), or metoprolol 25–50 mg orally every 6 hours, or esmolol 50–100 μg/kg/min infusion
Inhibition of thyroid hormone synthesis	Propylthiouracil 500–1,000 mg loading, then 250 mg every 4 hours or methimazole 60–80 mg/day
Inhibition of thyroid hormone release	Saturated potassium iodide solution (50 mg/drops) 1–2 drops orally or per rectally or Lugol's solution (8 mg iodide/drops) 5–7 drops
Corticosteroid	Hydrocortisone 300 mg IV, then 100 mg every 8 hours
Treatment of underlying precipitant	Empirical antibiotics
Supportive measures	Volume resuscitation, cooling blankets, fan, ice packs/lavage
Others	Lorazepam, diazepam

Question 9

1. Explain the modified Lynch algorithm for erythematous rash.

2. Explain the modified Lynch algorithm for life-threatening rash.

The modified Lynch algorithm provides a systematic approach to the diagnosis of rashes by providing a number of questions and branching points to narrow down the differential diagnosis of important and life-threatening rashes for the emergency physician.

Major groups of dermatologic emergencies include vesiculobullous disorder **(Table 9)** and drug reaction, infections, autoimmune disorders, inflammatory cutaneous disorders, and environmental disorders.

Vesiculobullous disorders are:
a. Erythema multiforme (EM) major
b. *Stevens–Johnson syndrome (SJS):* It is considered to be a severe form of EM.
c. *Toxic epidermal necrolysis (TEN):* It is considered to be a more severe form of SJS.
d. Generalized bullous fixed drug eruption
e. Pemphigus vulgaris
f. Bullous pemphigoid
g. DRESS (drug rash with eosinophilia and systemic symptoms) syndrome.

3. What is staphylococcal scalded skin syndrome?

Staphylococcal scalded skin syndrome, also known as Ritter disease, is a disease characterized by denudation of the skin caused by exotoxin-producing strains of the *Staphylococcus* species, typically from a distant site. It usually presents 48 hours after birth and is rare in children older than 6 years.

It is commonly seen in infants and children due to exotoxin released by *Staphylococcus aureus* group 2 phage 71. Exotoxin is an epidermolytic toxin, also called exfoliating toxin or epidermolysin.

TABLE 9: Differentiation between EM, SJS/TEN, and bullous fixed drug eruption.

	EM	SJS/TEN	Generalized bullous fixed drug eruption
Lesion pattern	Typical target lesion present	Flat/atypical target lesion present	Absence of target lesions/bullous lesions with surrounding rim of erythema
Mucosal involvement	Yes	Yes	Yes/no
Distribution	Mainly acral involvement/limbs	Widespread	Widespread
Blister/erosions	Yes, at the center of target lesions	• Yes • <10%: SJS; • 10–30%: SJS/TEN overlap; • >30%: TEN	Yes
Recurrence history	Occasional	Rare	Common
Prognosis	Excellent	Mortality depends on risk factors (SCORTEN)	Generally favorable if <20% body surface area is involved

(EM: erythema multiforme; SCORTEN: score of toxic epidermal necrosis; SJS: Stevens–Johnson syndrome; TEN: toxic epidermal necrolysis)

Clinically, intense erythematous cutaneous eruptions occur following an upper respiratory tract infection or purulent conjunctivitis. Painful erosions appear when erythematous sheets of skin are shed which is referred to as potato chip desquamation. The patient should be admitted and treated promptly with antibiotics covering *S. aureus*.

Staphylococcal scalded skin syndrome tends to appear abruptly with diffuse erythema and fever. The diagnosis can be confirmed by a *skin biopsy specimen*, which can be expedited by frozen section processing, as staphylococcal scalded skin syndrome should be distinguished from life-threatening toxic epidermal necrolysis.

Question 10

A 16-year-old boy presents to the ED with breathlessness, palpitation, sweating, and tremors. On examination, Chvostek's sign and Trousseau's signs are present.

1. Classify anxiety disorders as per DSM-5.

Anxiety is a normal emotion that healthy people feel at times. If a person feels a disproportionate amount of anxiety or for prolonged periods of time, then there may be an underlying anxiety disorder. Anxiety disorders can affect 20% of adults at some point in their lives and can vary from specific phobias (7–9%), social anxiety (7%), panic disorder (3%), and generalized anxiety disorder (3%). A panic attack is an abrupt period of fear and discomfort associated with physical and cognitive symptoms. The DSM-5 (Diagnostic and Statistical Manual of Mental Disorders, fifth edition) criteria for diagnosing panic disorder are as follows: Four or more of the following symptoms:

a. Palpitations, pounding heart, or accelerated heart rate
b. Sweating
c. Trembling/shaking
d. Shortness of breath/feeling of smothering
e. Feeling of choking
f. Chest pain or discomfort
g. Nausea/abdominal distress
h. Feeling dizzy, unsteady, lightheaded, or faint
i. Chills/heat sensations
j. Paresthesia (numbness or tingling sensations)
k. Derealization (feeling of unreality) or depersonalization (being detached from oneself)
l. Fear of losing control/going crazy
m. Fear of dying

2. Discuss the assessment and management of this case in the ED. How will you differentiate an organic anxiety disorder from a primary anxiety disorder?

General approach to panic disorders: Take a thorough history about the precipitants and situation leading to the symptoms. Pay special consideration to alcohol and drug use (both prescribed and illicit). Take a full social and past social history to help determine if there are any elements in the patient's life that may have led to their current state of mind.

It is also important to pay attention to stimulant use including caffeine and nicotine (tea, coffee, and tobacco usage) as excessive use of these can exacerbate anxiety states.

There are many significant medical conditions that can present with anxiety symptoms and one must try and exclude these as the cause of symptoms **(Table 10)**.

TABLE 10: Common medical conditions that can present with anxiety or as an anxiety disorder.

Cardiac	• Acute coronary syndromes (MI and angina) • Cardiac dysrhythmias • Congestive cardiac failure
Respiratory	• Pulmonary embolus • Asthma and COPD exacerbations • Hypoxia/hypercapnia
Endocrine	• Hyperthyroidism • Hypoglycemia • Pheochromocytoma • Hypoparathyroidism
Neurological	• TIAs and stroke • Seizure disorders/postictal state • Head injury/intracranial bleeding
Environmental	• Alcohol intoxication and withdrawal • Drug abuse/intoxication and acute withdrawal • Carbon monoxide poisoning

Treatment for anxiety disorders: Significant anxiety can sometimes manifest as acute agitation. In these patients, proceed with cautious verbal and environmental de-escalation strategies as described earlier, with use of medical or physical restraint as appropriate to the circumstance.

Specialized treatment with selective serotonin reuptake inhibitors (SSRIs) and serotonin and norepinephrine reuptake inhibitors (SNRIs) should be initiated by doctors experienced in their use, and hence the patients should be referred to psychiatric services. Benzodiazepines must be prescribed with caution due to risks of addiction and dependence. It may be appropriate to use them in short, minimal dosed prescriptions from the ED to allow patients to bridge the gap till they can be seen and assessed by psychiatric services. Other treatment modalities including counselling, psychotherapy, and cognitive-behavioral therapy (CBT) have been shown to improve symptoms. Often a combination of medication, counseling, and CBT is needed for long-term treatment success.

Most patients with anxiety disorder can be discharged from the ED with arrangements for outpatient follow-up. However, patients with suicidal or homicidal ideation, severe depressive symptoms, or psychosis require inpatient care.

SUGGESTED READING

1. Richhariya D, Sharma B. Textbook of Emergency Medicine including Intensive Care and Trauma, 2nd edition. New Delhi: Jaypee Brothers Medical Publishers (P) Ltd; 2022. pp. 415-20. (Question 1).
2. Richhariya D, Sharma B. Textbook of Emergency Medicine including Intensive Care and Trauma, 2nd edition. New Delhi: Jaypee Brothers Medical Publishers (P) Ltd; 2022. p. 835. (Question 2).
3. Richhariya D, Sharma B. Textbook of Emergency Medicine including Intensive Care and Trauma, 2nd edition. New Delhi: Jaypee Brothers Medical Publishers (P) Ltd; 2022. pp. 801-13. (Question 3).
4. Richhariya D, Sharma B. Textbook of Emergency Medicine including Intensive Care and Trauma, 2nd edition. New Delhi: Jaypee Brothers Medical Publishers (P) Ltd; 2022. pp. 556-61. (Question 4).
5. Richhariya D, Sharma B. Textbook of Emergency Medicine including Intensive Care and Trauma, 2nd edition. New Delhi: Jaypee Brothers Medical Publishers (P) Ltd; 2022. p. 490. (Question 5).
6. Richhariya D, Sharma B. Textbook of Emergency Medicine including Intensive Care and Trauma, 2nd edition. New Delhi: Jaypee Brothers Medical Publishers (P) Ltd; 2022. p. 971. (Question 6).
7. Richhariya D, Sharma B. Textbook of Emergency Medicine including Intensive Care and Trauma, 2nd edition. New Delhi: Jaypee Brothers Medical Publishers (P) Ltd; 2022. p. 1736. (Question 7).
8. Richhariya D, a Sharma B. Textbook of Emergency Medicine including Intensive Care and Trauma, 2nd edition. New Delhi: Jaypee Brothers Medical Publishers (P) Ltd; 2022. p. 891. (Question 8).
9. Richhariya D, Sharma B. Textbook of Emergency Medicine including Intensive Care and Trauma, 2nd edition. New Delhi: Jaypee Brothers Medical Publishers (P) Ltd; 2022. p. 1027. (Question 9).
10. Richhariya D, Sharma B. Textbook of Emergency Medicine including Intensive Care and Trauma, 2nd edition. New Delhi: Jaypee Brothers Medical Publishers (P) Ltd; 2022. p. 1053. (Question 10).

Emergency Medicine Paper 40

Constatine AU

Question 1

A 1-year-old female is brought to the emergency room (ER) with a history of falling off of beds. The baby is crying and inconsolable.

1. Describe the important anatomical and physiological aspects that must be considered while managing such a patient.

While caring for this child, it is crucial to remember that she is only 1 year old and not an adult.

General

- Smaller body mass.
- Energy imparts from falling objects.
- Contusion or impact results in greater force as per unit of body area.
- The child's defense system is still maturing, making it less effective against illnesses, and their physiological reserve is limited.
- Children have less fat and less connective tissues to protect their internal organs; the internal organs lie close to one another; hence, a high frequency of multiple injuries in pediatric populations.
- The ratio of body surface area to body mass is higher and hypothermia may develop quickly.
- At 1 year old, children's bones are more fragile than adults because the sutures of the skull bones are not fully fused; meaning the clinical presentation of increased intracranial pressure might be delayed or subtle.

Airway and Breathing

- Compared to an adult, a kid's airway is much narrower and more easily obstructed.
- With a relatively large head, the neck is naturally flexed. Consider, putting padding/towels behind body to keep the neutral position, provided that it is safe to do so.
- The soft tissues of an infant's oral cavity are relatively small compared to those in the oropharynx. Hence, the assessment of the larynx may be difficult.
- Both the larynx and vocal cords are located more cephalad and anterior than in adults. Hence, the airway acquires a more acute angle.
- The epiglottis is long and stiff.
- Short trachea, hence, there is a higher risk of intubation into right mainstem bronchus.
- In children, the tidal volume, dead space, and pumping capacity of the heart are smaller. In addition, children's physiological reserve to fight against trauma is less than that in adults. Therefore, deterioration may occur suddenly and rapidly.

Circulation

- Due to heightened sympathetic nerve activity, children's heart rates are higher than adults', which may raise their risk of cardiac dysrhythmias.
- Smaller total blood volume, hence, the reserve is less. In turn, the circulatory system may failure rapidly.

Disability

- For neurological reasons, the child may react more intensely to pain by crying.
- *Head injury:*
  - Open fontanelles and sutures, hence, they have higher ability to tolerate higher intracranial pressure.
  - More prone to secondary brain injury in childhood.
  - If bulging fontanelles or suture diastases is present, severe brain injury is assumed.
  - When a computed tomography (CT) scan (brain or body) is necessary, the radiation-dose must be kept "as low as reasonably achievable" (ALARA).

2. Discuss the PECARN versus CHALICE rules.

Both the PECARN and the CHALICE are clinical rules that gauge the severity of head injuries in children. The PECARN aims to exclude the use of CT scans of the brain, whereas the CHALICE aims to identify the children who need a CT scan of the brain. Both rules were derived from high-quality methods, but their study populations were different. Only the PECARN includes a version for children <2 years of age. With regards to this case, since the kid is only 1 year old, the PECARN rule is preferable.

3. Describe injuries that would suggest child abuse or non-accidental injury (NAI).

Acquiring inconsistent histories from different family members may point to child abuse or non-accidental injury (NAI). In addition, being under or over protective of the kid may sometimes be indicative of child abuse. Some findings that may suggest child abuse or NAI include the following:

General
- Multicolored bruises (i.e., resulting from different episodes)
- Evidence of numerous previous injuries (e.g., old scars or healed fractures).

Head
- Multiple subdural hematomas, especially ones without a fresh skull fracture
- Skull fractures seen in children <2 years of age
- Retinal hemorrhages
- Injuries to perioral area.

Trunk and Limbs
- Ruptured internal viscera without definite explanation
- Rib fractures seen in children <2 years of age
- Injuries located at the medical aspect of limbs
- Fractures of long bones in children <3 years of age
- Injuries to genital, perianal, or perioral areas.

Other Points to Look for
- Bizarre injuries (e.g., bites, cigarette burns, and rope marks)
- A second- or third-degree burn with sharp demarcation
- Unusual emotions or behaviors, such as fear, anxiety, withdrawal, anger, obsessive-compulsive behaviors, and interest in sexual topics.
  The doctor should ensure that the child is not being mistreated by watching for indicators of dread, anxiety, withdrawal, or violence. The child safety is of the highest priority. Err on the safe side. In case of doubt, seek advice from the seniors.

Question 2

A 5-year-old child presents with fever, respiratory distress, and drooling for 2 days. His oxygen saturation is 78%, blood pressure (BP) 110/70, and heart rate (HR) 110/min.

1. Discuss the differential diagnosis of this condition.

The child is in respiratory distress, if not respiratory failure. The differential diagnosis may include the following:

- *Respiratory tract in origin:*
  - Upper airway problem (e.g., foreign body obstruction, croup, acute epiglottitis, retropharyngeal abscess, anaphylaxis)
  - Lower airway problem (e.g., foreign body aspiration, asthma, bronchitis)
  - Lung parenchyma disease (e.g., pneumonia)
- *Nonrespiratory tract in origin:*
  - Problem with control of breathing—the central nervous system
  - Cardiac problem (e.g., cyanotic heart disease)
  - Renal disease
  - Mixed types.

2. Discuss the management of each differential diagnosis.

For all differential diagnoses, the general treatment is to provide oxygen and intravenous (IV) access and to perform a thorough physical examination of the patient. Investigations such as chest X-rays, total blood count, and tests on blood gas, sputum, urine, and serology are necessary. Specific treatment will be given depending on the findings.

First, upper airway obstruction may present with a roaring cough, hoarseness, and trouble breathing, which are all symptoms of croup, a viral infection that affects many children. Nebulized epinephrine, corticosteroids, and supportive care (e.g., keeping the child comfortable and hydrated) are all parts of the treatment strategy for such diagnoses.

Second, lower airway obstruction (e.g., asthma) may present with wheezing, coughing, and difficulty in breathing. Caring for children with such an obstruction includes giving them bronchodilators such as salbutamol and steroids (inhalation, oral, or IV).

Third, lung tissue diseases such as pneumonia are caused by bacteria or viruses. Fever and crepitations are common features. Patients are given antipyretics (e.g., paracetamol), antibiotics (e.g., amoxicillin/clavulanic acid), and other supportive care.

Fourth, for respiratory distress or failure that is caused by nonrespiratory systems, the general treatment involves administering oxygen and treating the underlying causes. For example, the medulla oblongata controls the breathing. Infection in the central nervous system or drug overdose may result in a loss of breathing control. Usually, the child breathes slowly or even suffers from apnea, and intubation may be needed. This child will require intensive care unit (ICU) care.

Question 3

1. What are Duckett Jones criteria?

Rheumatic illness is diagnosed using the Jones criteria:
a. In a child with clinical manifestations suggestive of streptococcal pharyngitis, there should be evidence of group A streptococcal infection (GAS), including elevated or rising antistreptococcal antibody titers (e.g., antistreptolysin O, anti-DNase B), a positive throat culture, or a positive rapid antigen test.
b. The modified Jones criteria are divided into major criteria and minor criteria. Children between 5 and 15 years of age are regarded as the high-risk population.
   i. *Major criteria:* Carditis, chorea, erythema marginatum, arthritis in low-risk-populations; polyarthritis in high-risk populations and subcutaneous nodules.
   ii. *Minor criteria:* Polyarthralgia in low-risk populations, monoarthralgia in high-risk populations; elevated erythrocyte sedimentation rate [erythrocyte sedimentation rate (ESR): >60 mm/h in low-risk populations, >30 in high-risk populations] or C-reactive protein (>3.0 mg/dL), fever (equal or >38.5°C), and prolonged PR interval on an electrocardiogram (ECG).

Diagnosis: Two major or one major and two minor manifestations with evidence of GAS, suggesting an acute rheumatic fever.

2. Discuss the pathophysiology of acute rheumatic fevers.

A streptococcal infection triggers an immunological response that results in an inflammatory illness known as acute rheumatic fever (ARF). This illness causes inflammation of the brain, skin, joints, heart, and body. In addition, the body's connective tissue is targeted by a rise in antibodies, which harms the heart valves and other organs, potentially leading to fever, rash, joint inflammation, and heart problems. Children are most frequently affected by ARF, which typically develops 14–28 days following a streptococcal infection.

3. Explain the management of a patient with an acute rheumatic fever.

Patients with ARF should be treated by evaluating their health and creating a treatment plan with four aims. The first aim is to minimize the inflammatory effects on the heart and joints. The second aim is to treat the GAS infection (usually the pharynx). The third aim is to provide symptomatic relief. The fourth aim is to start secondary prophylaxis, generally with nonsteroid anti-inflammatory drugs, corticosteroids, aspirin, Penicillin VK, sulfonamides, or erythromycin.

Question 4

A 4-week-old baby presents with projectile non-bilious vomiting with preserved appetite and visible peristalsis. The baby is severely dehydrated.

1. How will you rapidly assess and stabilize the patient?

The history suggested the child was at risk of dehydration. The physical examination may provide more evidence to support such a concern. Checking the general alertness, anterior fontanelle, sunken eyeballs, mucous membrane, skin turgor, pulse rate, respiration rate, and capillary refill time are necessary. It may be difficult to measure blood pressure in this child. It is essential to monitor the patient's vital signs after starting a line for IV fluids. The usual rule of thumb is to administer IV bolus 20 mL/kg stat dose, the actual rate should be adjusted according to the clinical progress. A blood sample is required to test acid–base and electrolyte balance. While rehydrating, use isotonic fluids and implant a nasogastric tube if needed. Doctors may also use other care methods, such as antiemetic medication, if necessary. The person's response to treatment must be closely monitored.

2. What is your likely diagnosis and how will you confirm the diagnosis?

Likely to be infantile hypertrophic pyloric stenosis (IHPS) and the following features may be present:
- *Physical findings:*
  - Right upper quadrant "olive-like" mass
    - Most easily palpated after a period of vomiting or on an empty stomach
  - Visible peristalsis from left to right
  - Scaphoid abdomen (sign of malnutrition)
  - Succussion splash
- *Blood:* Hypochloremia and metabolic alkalosis (+ hypokalemia if the patient is in a later stage), secondary to repeated vomiting.
  - *Ultrasound:* Thickened pylorus, "target" sign on transverse view, cervix sign on longitudinal view
  - *Abdominal X-ray:* Distended gastric bubble
  - *Barium study:* String sign/beak sign.

3. Discuss the differential diagnosis of recurrent vomiting in infancy, childhood, and adolescence.

In addition to the causes from the gastrointestinal (GI) tract, other systems are capable of causing recurrent vomiting. Here are some possible differential diagnoses:

- Gastrointestinal tract:
  - Infantile hypertrophic pyloric stenosis (IHPS)
  - Volvulus
  - Intussusception
  - Intestinal atresia
  - Malrotation
  - Necrotizing enterocolitis
  - Inflammatory/infection [e.g., urinary tract infection (UTI), GI infection]
  - Gastroesophageal reflux
  - Intestinal obstruction
  - Cystic fibrosis
  - Pancreatitis
- Non-GI tract:
  - Metabolic causes [e.g., diabetic ketoacidosis (DKA)]
  - Autoimmune disorders
  - Endocrinopathies
  - Lactose allergy
  - Central nervous system (CNS) causes (e.g., head injury/possible child abuse)
  - Intoxication
  - Migraines
  - Functional abdominal pain
  - Mental disorders.

TABLE 1: Clinical features of various degrees of dehydration in the child.

Clinical signs	Mild dehydration 3–5%	Moderate dehydration 6–10%	Severe dehydration >10%
Physical examination			
Mental status	Normal	Listless or irritable	Lethargic, comatose
Thirst	Slight	Moderate	Severe
Anterior fontanel	Flat	Sunken	Sunken
Eyes	Normal	Sunken	Deeply sunken
Skin turgor	Normal	Decreased	Decreased
Mucus membrane	Normal	Dry	Dry
Pulse quality	Normal	Normal then decreased	Decreased to thready
Measurement			
Capillary refill	<2 second	Prolonged	Prolonged
Blood pressure	Normal	Normal	Normal then decreased
Heart rate	Normal	Increased	Increased
Respiratory rate	Normal	Tachypnea	Tachypnea
Urine output	Decreased	Moderately decreased	Oliguria or anuria
Weight loss	3–5%	6–9%	>10%

Question 5

A 2-year-old child presents with passage of watery stool for 1 day.

1. Discuss the composition of oral rehydration solution.

People with low moisture can be revived with an oral rehydration salt (ORS) solution consisting of sugar, salt, and electrolytes, which is frequently consumed in a liquid form. The World Health Organization (WHO) recommends using an ORS containing the following ingredients: 3.5 g of sodium chloride, 2.5 g of trisodium citrate dihydrate, 20 g of glucose, and 1 L of filtered water. Regular doses of a small amount of this solution (e.g., 1–2 tablespoons every few minutes) are advised. If the child is still dehydrated, ORS should be given until the dehydration has been corrected and the patient can handle more substantial food and beverages.

2. Describe the clinical features of various degrees of dehydration in the child.

In general, dehydration categorizes as mild (3–5% weight loss), moderate (6–10% weight loss), and severe (>10% of weight loss) **(Table 1)**.

3. Discuss the principles of management if the child is severely dehydrated.

Quick and forceful rehydration is essential if the child is critically exhausted. Hypertonic saline or Ringer's lactate are good examples of IV fluids to use for this reason. The total volume and rate at which fluids should be given will be determined by several criteria, including the severity of dehydration and any underlying medical conditions. The doctor should check the child for electrolyte imbalances and other problems, such as trauma, which should be monitored closely. In addition, the root cause should be addressed. Oral rehydration therapy can be started if the baby can handle it.

Question 6

1. Explain the forensic evaluation of bullet wounds.

Generally, a forensic investigation of a gunshot wound requires a comprehensive examination of the projectile, the entrance wound, the exit wound, and the environment of the crime. The following are the main points to consider:

- Police, or the legal attorney, should be present during the patient's examination and treatment to preserve the chain of evidence.
- All of the patient's clothes, belongings, and fragments must be retained, labeled, and passed on to the police.
- And any missile fragments police must be present for safety purposes.
- Photos may be taken by the police during the patient management. Consider the issue of consent.
- *History:*
  - Number of shots heard
  - Type of gun used
  - Distance between the patient and the firing gun
  - Blood loss on scene
- *Initial management of injuries involving a penetrated extremity:*
  - Hemorrhage control
  - Pain control
  - Tetanus prophylaxis and wound management
  - Consideration of antibiotics
  - Obtain an X-ray or a CT scan for the following scenarios:
    - An open fracture
    - Joint penetration
    - Suspected radio-opaque foreign body
- *Entry wound features:*
  - Muzzle imprint (redness matching the shape of the barrel)
  - Abrasion ring (roundish, irregular, inverted, burnt wound edge)
  - Powder tattoo
  - Gunpowder burn
  - Soot
  - Smaller and more regular invagination
- *Exit wound features:*
  - Large
  - Irregular margin
  - Eversion
  - Explosive
  - Split flaps
- Cut around, not through, bullet holes when removing a patient's clothing
- Use plastic-covered instruments to remove bullets
  - Direct contact of the bullet with metallic objects (e.g., probes, forceps, or scalpel blades) may cause scratches or other marks on the surface of a bullet, which may interfere with the forensic examination.
  - The surface of a bullet may be examined for striation (i.e., tiny scratches on the surface created by the rifling of the gun's barrel)
  - If in doubt, consult the expert before the procedure for safety purpose.
- Not all bullets need to be removed.
- *Indications for bullet removal:*
  - Pressure area around the bullet is painful for the patient
  - Bulging skin that causes cosmetic distress
  - Located in a joint space
  - Located in the globe of the eye
  - Located in a vessel lumen, causing ischemia or increasing risk of embolization
  - Impinging on a nerve and causing pain
  - Abscess formation.
  - Required for forensic investigation, with the consent of the patient and surgeon when no harm or unnecessary pain is expected.
  - Documented elevated lead levels, usually in children and occurring several months after injury (extremely rare).

2. How will you assess the age of a laceration wound across a thigh?

The age of a laceration can be estimated by studying its physical traits and by checking for infection, necrotic tissue, serosanguinous discharge, and inflammation at the wound site. It is essential to record the wound's length and width and to monitor for granulation tissue or epithelialization as healing indicators. Clinical photos should be taken with the patient's consent. In addition, one may better understand a wound's age by examining the sensitivity and inflammation around the area. It is important to look at the wound's color to see if it is fresh or old and red or yellow and to document scab formation after approximately 24 hours and when a wound has become infected. After 24 hours, epithelium begins to grow at the edges of a wound. Epithelialization of small clean wounds may be completed in 4–5 days. After 36 hours, puss may be seen around the site. The wound's age can also be determined by investigating [with polymerase chain reaction (PCR)] messenger ribonucleic acid (mRNA) levels of inflammatory cytokines, and wound-healing factors.

3. Discuss POCSO Act.

In 2012, the Protection of Children from Sexual Offences (POCSO) Act was enacted in India to shield young people from sexually harmful activities such as sexual abuse, sexual harassment, and pornography. This Act protects minors (defined as any individual under the age of 18) from sexual assault, sexual harassment, and exploitation, including using a child for pornographic purposes. The article lays forth processes to report, investigate, and try such offenses. Furthermore, it mandates the creation of Special Courts to prosecute cases involving crimes against minors and to ensure their safety throughout the trial.

Question 7

1. Explain handing over and taking over patient care during shift change in the emergency department (ED).

Patients must be safely transferred in the ED during a shift change. The departing clinician should communicate pertinent information about the patient's condition to the physician taking over including any important laboratory or imaging results and the patient's diagnosis, therapy, and care plan. The physician taking over must thoroughly review this data, share any concerns, and follow up if necessary. In complicated cases, the hand-over process should involve the nurses because their input is always important. If possible, the departing physician should introduce the physician taking over to the patients and their relatives. Moreover, the departing physician should be ready to answer any questions, despite being off duty. Patients who undergo this procedure are more likely to receive safe, high-quality care inside the ED.

2. Discuss preparing a duty roster for ED residents.

In principle, sufficient and appropriately-skilled staff must be scheduled for each shift to provide appropriate patient care and to satisfy the service demand. The rosters must conform to relevant regulatory laws and policies (e.g., antidiscrimination, work health, and safety legislation) and must be fair (e.g., the number of working hours should be the same). Furthermore, the roster must ensure there is enough supervision from the seniors. House-rules, such as applications for leave (e.g., priority leaves such as examination leave) and resolutions for conflicts concerning dates, must be established between the management and the team. These house-rules must be open, respected by all stack-holders, and regularly reviewed.

One method is to use regular and nonregular cycles. First, the regular service demand must be decided. For example, the Day (AM) Shift needs four residents, the Evening (PM) Shift needs another four, and the Night (N) Shift needs two. Due to leaves, >10 residents are needed to fulfill the roster. In other words, about 15 residents are needed to fit this 10-resident cycle. A total of 10 out of 15 will be allocated to the regular cycle: AM1, AM2, AM3, AM4, Rest 1, Rest 2; PM1, PM2; N1 and N2. The remaining five will be allocated to the non-regular-cycle and they will fill in the rest days and annual leaves of regular cycle. They may also serve as reserve in case of sick leave, urgent leave, and a sudden surge in service demand. Usually, newcomers and those who arranged long leaves are allocated to the nonregular cycle. Some departments may use rostering-software to draft the roster, which can accommodate individual duty and leave requests and keep track of working hours easily.

The draft-roster will then be reviewed by the management and the residents' representatives. Adjustment is allowed; after all, we are all human and make mistakes. The revised draft should then be sent to all residents. Further adjustments may be allowed before a certain deadline, when the final version is released. It must be noted that service demand and resident-need are dynamic; hence, the roster may be dynamic to a certain extent. House-rules for when, how, who, and under what situations someone can request a change in the roster must be established. Changes must be recorded because they may affect the number of service hours for individual residents. Compensation or adjustment should be administered as soon as possible, typically in the coming month, to preserve fairness.

It is essential to keep all of the residents and stakeholders apprised of any changes to the roster, which should be displayed in a highly trafficked location of an ED.

3. What are the common medical errors in ED?

Misdiagnosis, medication administration errors, failure to diagnose, delayed treatment, wrong-site surgery, and insufficient follow-up are all common causes of patient harm in urgent care. Additionally, mistakes in documentation, miscommunication, lack of informed consent, and inability to spot indicators of abuse are all potential problems. Patient tracking, provider communication, and triage can all contribute to a medical mistake.

4. Discus communication skills during resuscitation.

Communication between medical staff, patients, and family members is crucial during resuscitation.

With the patient: Depending on the clinical presentation, the patient may be unconscious, making communication difficult. For conscious patients, always update and explain the clinical problems, potential progress, and advantages and disadvantages of a treatment. Consent should be sought for invasive procedures. Never assume that a nonresponding patient is unconscious.

Among healthcare providers: Communication between healthcare personnel is crucial for providing high-quality care and ensuring patient safety and emotional well-being. All messages must be clear and specific (i.e., who, what, and how) and the roles must be clearly listed. Healthcare providers should also use closed-loop communication and must show mutual respect, regardless of rank or duty. Benefitting patients is the focus of healthcare. Like the crew-resource management, it does not matter who is right; what matters is; what is right. Knowledge sharing, constructive intervention, summarization, regular-review, and time-outs are some beneficial skills. Each team member should know his or her own limit.

With the relatives: With regard to the relatives, attentively listening and focusing on setting realistic goals are all hallmarks of clear communication. Be kind but firm; never offer false hope. It must be noted that relatives might be emotional and even be violent. To ensure staff safety, if possible, always be accompanied by a nurse or a social worker and sometimes security guards. Healthcare providers should also be sensitive to and accommodating of cultural and linguistic diversity.

Question 8

1. What are CONSORT guidelines?

The CONSORT guidelines are a checklist which provides scientifically proven recommendations for reporting randomized controlled trials. Researchers hope to increase the openness and precision of reporting so that readers can evaluate the trial's validity and understand its conclusions. Every trial's process, from conception to the results analysis, is governed by these principles. The CONSORT standards are widely utilized in the medical profession and are regarded as the standard for reporting randomized clinical studies. The fields of psychology and education also accept principles like these. As with any established standard, adopting these raises the bar for the thoroughness and precision of the study being conducted. In conclusion, the guidelines offer suggestions for enhancing the accuracy of trial findings.

2. Explain parametric versus nonparametric statistical tests.

Parametric tests use the sample's mean and standard deviation to calculate the population as a whole, assuming that the data are typically distributed. Nonparametric tests do not assume a specific distribution and instead employ rankings and other statistics to calculate based on the information. Information that does not fit the average distribution profile necessitates nonparametric examinations.

3. Discus type II error with an example.

Whenever a test fails to identify a genuinely present effect, this is known as a type II mistake. Occasionally, medical tests might give misleading/false negative results, even when the patient has the ailment that they are screened for. A lady with breast cancer obtaining a cancer-free screening report is a typical example.

4. Discuss likelihood ratio with an example.

The likelihood ratio (LR) is a tool that uses the sensitivity and specificity to look at a test result. It has two versions:
- *Positive LR: (sensitivity)/(1-specificity)*—the bigger the positive LR, the higher the chance of a positive test result is true positive, i.e., the person has a high chance of having the target condition or disease.
- *Negative LR: (1-sensitivity)/(specificity)*—the smaller the negative LR, the higher the chance of a negative test result is true negative, i.e., the person has a high chance of not having the target condition or disease.
- An LR of one means the test result does not tell whether the disease is present or not.

A positive human immunodeficiency virus (HIV) test, for instance, the positive LR is used. The bigger the positive LR, the higher is the chance that the person has HIV.

On the other hand, if the HIV test is negative, the negative LR is used. The smaller the negative LR, the higher is the chance that the person does not have HIV.

Question 9

1. Explain the simulation training for emergency physicians in resource-constraint setting.

Simulation training has been invaluable for medical doctors working in areas with little materials. It was an excellent way for doctors to hone their skills in a risk-free setting before encountering an actual emergency. In additional to hard-core clinical skills like resuscitation, effective communication, debridement, conflict-management, etc., may be used in simulation. Efficient emergency care relies heavily on effective communication and teamwork, which can be improved through training sessions. The performance may be video-taped and the participants may comment on their own performance. This is a kind of active learning.

2. Discuss the role of telemedicine in emergency care.

Whenever it comes to giving immediate medical attention, telemedicine is invaluable. Telemedicine ranges from simple consultation over the phone (audio-only) to real-time face-to-face consultation. To go to the extreme, surgical procedure may be carried out via high-tech sophisticated communication technology and robots.

Technology facilitates remote patient monitoring and communication with doctors, which can contribute to quicker and more precise diagnoses. Consequently, telehealth enables patients to receive timely care. It may also aid in delivering remote consultation and guidance for managing specific disorders, including stroke and intensive care. Furthermore, medical records can be accessed remotely, streamlining the process of sharing patient information. In conclusion, telemedicine has excellent potential to improve access to quality and timely emergency care.

In the past, telemedicine usually involved only between healthcare providers. A junior doctor may phone up the senior and ask for advice. Nowadays, doctors may offer consultation to patients directly. The Covid Pandemic added much momentum to this practice. It has an additional benefit on infection control. The Covid patient stays at home. Consultations with doctors or nurses are conducted over the internet with real-time-video. Drugs and sick leave are sent to the patient's home. In other words, the patient is home-quarantined. The chance of spreading the disease to the community is reduced.

3. Explain the flipped classroom concept and its relevance to emergency medicine.

The phrase "flipped classroom" refers to a method of blended learning. It is one of the subtypes of the rotation model of blended learning. The other three subtypes are: (1) station rotation, (2) lab rotation, and (3) individual rotation. Flipped classroom is the most commonly used subtype.

The flipped classroom subtype may be delivered in various ways. Precourse materials are distributed to the students, who are expected to read the materials. In some settings, paper or online quizzes are included. In addition, the pre-course module may include scenarios or cases.

When the students and teachers meet, they discuss or drill on scenarios or cases. Traditional lecturing on theory is avoided as much as possible, which allows for more in-depth conversations and opportunities for student engagement. Interactions and conceptual development are utilized to facilitate students' learning by deepening understanding, strengthening relationships, and making learning meaningful. Evidence has shown that the benefits of flipped learning include the development of skills such as collaboration, communication, creativity, critical thinking, and self-directed learning.

The flipped classroom model has been implemented in emergency medicine, where it allows students to get a foundational understanding of a medical topic outside of class and apply that knowledge in class through exercises such as case studies and simulations. The advanced cardiac life support (ACLS) and the pediatric advance life support (PALS) of the American Heart Association and the advanced trauma life support (ATLS) of the American College of Surgeons are typical examples.

This model allows students to take what they have learned and apply it in a real-world context. Learners will be better equipped to engage in active learning and understanding and may apply their skills and knowledge in their day-to-day duties. The flipped classroom model also permits more targeted instruction, since teachers can focus on meeting the needs of their students and giving them more constructive comments during class sessions.

Question 10

Briefly describe the study design, strengths, weaknesses, and conclusions of the following trials.

1. CRASH-III Trial

Tranexamic acid (TXA) was investigated in a 2013 multicenter randomized controlled experiment known as the CRASH-III study to determine its effect on mortality in trauma patients. Total mortality among trauma patients was shown to be lowered by 9% thanks to TXA. Although this research had some excellent points, it also had significant flaws, such as the fact that it was not blinded and had a small sample size. However, scientists concluded that TXA could be a valuable treatment for trauma patients.

2. RECOVERY Trial

Nearly 11,000 individuals participated in the RECOVERY study, a randomized controlled experiment that assessed the efficacy of therapy with coronavirus disease-2019 (COVID-19) patients. Minimal improvement in patient outcomes was observed when dexamethasone was combined with hydroxychloroquine. The large number of participants and randomization in the study gave credibility to the results. However, its shortcomings lie in its inability to assess the treatment's efficacy in less severe cases. In severe COVID-19 cases, the trial found that standard therapies such as dexamethasone and hydroxychloroquine did not improve patient outcomes.

3. DEFUSE-3 Trial

The DEFUSE-3 study compared acute heart stroke treatment options between endovascular therapy and medical management. Its large sample size, blinding, and randomization were all in its favor. However, the lack of a control group and the study's narrow applicability were its drawbacks. The authors concluded that patients with acute ischemic stroke who had endovascular therapy had better functional outcomes than the other participants.

4. WOMAN Trial

Women experiencing postpartum hemorrhages were tested with TXA in a randomized controlled experiment called WOMAN to see if it would help reduce the risk of mortality. The study's strengths lie in its substantial sample size and inclusion of a placebo control group for evaluation. However, the blinding process is complicated, and the data was collected retroactively, both of which are limitations. The analysis revealed that women experiencing postpartum hemorrhage who took TXA had a lower risk of dying from their condition.

ACKNOWLEDGMENTS

Special thanks to Dr Gary Chu, Dr Stephen Yeung, and Dr Keung-Kit Chan for their valuable advice.

SUGGESTED READING

1. Richhariya D, Sharma B. Textbook of Emergency Medicine including Intensive Care and Trauma, 2nd edition. New Delhi: Jaypee Brothers Medical Publishers (P) Ltd; 2022. pp. 1124-34. (Question 1).
2. Richhariya D, Sharma B. Textbook of Emergency Medicine including Intensive Care and Trauma, 2nd edition. New Delhi: Jaypee Brothers Medical Publishers (P) Ltd; 2022. pp. 1185-9. (Question 2).
3. Richhariya D, Sharma B. Textbook of Emergency Medicine including Intensive Care and Trauma, 2nd edition. New Delhi: Jaypee Brothers Medical Publishers (P) Ltd; 2022. pp. 1190-1200. (Question 3).
4. Richhariya D, Sharma B. Textbook of Emergency Medicine including Intensive Care and Trauma, 2nd edition. New Delhi: Jaypee Brothers Medical Publishers (P) Ltd; 2022. pp. 1178-80. (Questions 4 and 5).
5. Richhariya D, Sharma B. Textbook of Emergency Medicine including Intensive Care and Trauma, 2nd edition. New Delhi: Jaypee Brothers Medical Publishers (P) Ltd; 2022. pp. 124-30. (Question 6).
6. Richhariya D, Sharma B. Textbook of Emergency Medicine including Intensive Care and Trauma, 2nd edition. New Delhi: Jaypee Brothers Medical Publishers (P) Ltd; 2022. pp. 49-54. (Question 7).
7. Richhariya D, Sharma B. Textbook of Emergency Medicine including Intensive Care and Trauma, 2nd edition. New Delhi: Jaypee Brothers Medical Publishers (P) Ltd; 2022. pp. 80-90. (Question 8).
8. Richhariya D, Sharma B. Textbook of Emergency Medicine including Intensive Care and Trauma, 2nd edition. New Delhi: Jaypee Brothers Medical Publishers (P) Ltd; 2022. pp. 108-112. (Question 9).
9. Walls RM, Hockberger RS, Gausche-Hill M. Rosen's Emergency Medicine: Concepts and Clinical Practice. 9th edition. Philadelphia, PA: Elsevier; 2018. pp. 1-2. (Question 10).
10. Richhariya D, Sharma B. Textbook of Emergency Medicine including Intensive Care and Trauma, 2nd edition. New Delhi: Jaypee Brothers Medical Publishers (P) Ltd; 2022. (Question 10).

Emergency Medicine Paper 41

Devendra Richhariya

Question 1

1. Draw and describe an anatomical diagram of aortic arch and its branches.

The aortic arch is the segment of the aorta that helps to distribute blood to the head and upper extremities via the brachiocephalic trunk and the left common carotid and the left subclavian arteries. The aortic arch also plays a role in blood pressure homeostasis via baroreceptors found within the walls of the aortic arch (**Fig. 1**).

2. What are the steps in cannulation of the right subclavian vein in the emergency room (ER)?

Subclavian vein catheter insertion is a good choice for long term as this allows the patient to move the neck freely. Supraclavicular and infraclavicular approaches (**Figs. 2A and B**) are the two traditional approaches used for subclavian vein catheterization. The supraclavicular approach provides a good sonographic visualization. Both approaches are associated with risk of developing pneumothorax. Insertion of a central venous access, whether it is being used for a short or a long period of time, is a common procedure, which is often undertaken by emergency physicians, intensivists, and anesthetists.

The associated morbidities include punctured arteries for almost 10% of cases and hemothorax or pneumothorax for about 3% of cases.[1,2] These complications can be serious or even fatal.[2]

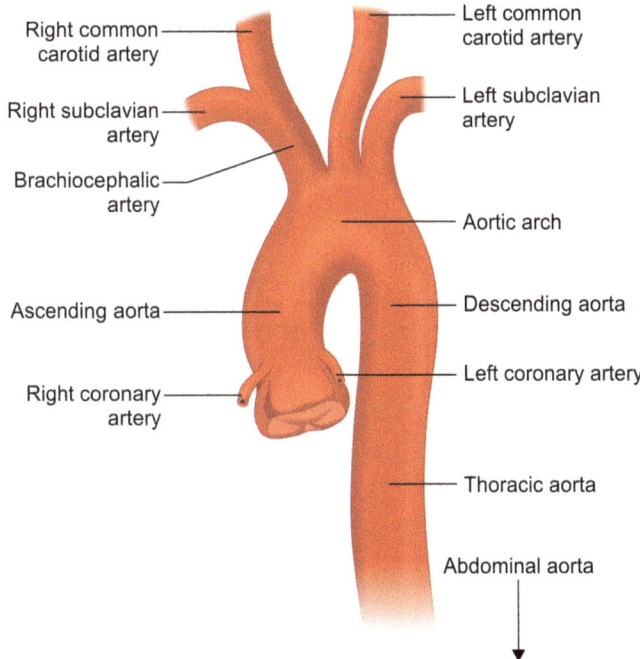

Fig. 1: Anatomical diagram of aortic arch and its branches.

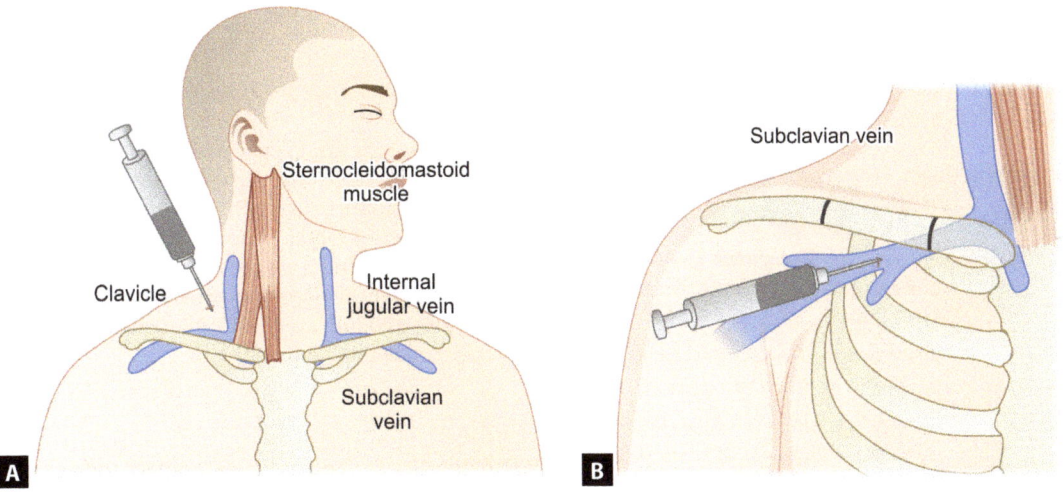

Figs. 2A and B: (A) Supraclavicular approach; (B) Infraclavicular approach to subclavian vein.

Question 2

1. Discuss the physiological principles of respiration.

Pulmonary gas exchange is transfer of oxygen from atmosphere to blood and tissue (oxygenation) and carbon dioxide from blood to atmosphere. The gas exchange takes place between alveoli and capillaries as they are in close contact (alveolar-capillary membrane) and thus O_2 and CO_2 are able to diffuse **(Figs. 3A and B)**. Carbon dioxide elimination (from bloodstream to alveoli) is very efficient and uncomplicated and depends on *alveolar ventilation* (total air transported from alveoli to atmosphere). Ventilation is regulated by the respiratory center situated in brainstem. Oxygenation is more complex than carbon dioxide elimination. Almost all oxygen molecules are attached to hemoglobin, so the amount of oxygen in blood depends on the hemoglobin concentration in blood and saturation of hemoglobin with oxygen (SO_2).

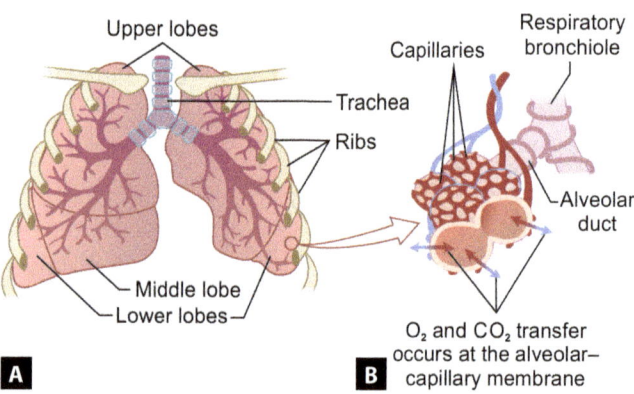

Figs. 3A and B: (A) Normal lung; (B) Pulmonary gas exchange.

2. Discuss the diagnosis of acute respiratory distress syndrome in emergency.

Acute respiratory distress syndrome (ARDS), which is a common cause of type I respiratory failure has been redefined **(Table 1)**.

TABLE 1: Berlin definition (2012) of acute respiratory distress syndrome.	
Timing	Within 1 week of known clinical insult or new or worsening respiratory symptoms
Chest imaging	Bilateral opacities on chest radiograph or chest computed tomographic scan
Origin of edema	Respiratory failure not fully explained by cardiac failure or fluid overload
Contd...	

Contd...

Oxygenation	
Mild	PaO_2/FiO_2 ratio 200–300 mm Hg with PEEP or CPAP ≥5 cmH_2O
Moderate	PaO_2/FiO_2 ratio 101–200 mm Hg with PEEP ≥5 cmH_2O
Severe	PaO_2/FiO_2 ratio ≤100 mm Hg with PEEP ≥5 cmH_2O

(CPAP: continuous positive airway pressure; FiO_2: fraction of inspired oxygen; PaO_2: partial pressure of arterial oxygen; PEEP: positive end-expiratory pressure)

Question 3

1. What are the endocrine changes frequently seen in sepsis?

Endocrinopathy during sepsis can manifest as hyperglycemia and insulin resistance or as insufficient production of either adrenal corticosteroids or vasopressin **(Fig. 4)**.

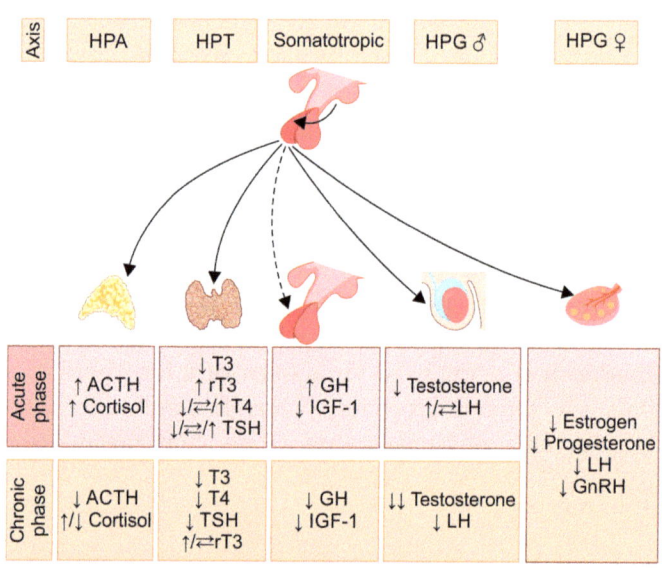

Fig. 4: Hormonal changes in sepsis: Differences between acute and chronic phases.
Symbols: ↑—increase, ↓—decrease, – normal, ♂—male, ♀—female.
[ACTH: adrenocorticotropic hormone (corticotropin); GH: growth hormone (somatropin); GnRH: gonadotropin releasing hormone (gonadoliberin); HPA: hypothalamic–pituitary–adrenal; HPG: hypothalamic–pituitary–gonadal; HPT: hypothalamic–pituitary–thyroid; IGF-1: insulin-like growth factor 1; LH: luteinizing hormone; rT3: reverse triiodothyronine; T3: triiodothyronine; T4: thyroxine; TSH: thyroid stimulating hormone]

2. Discuss the diagnosis of sepsis in the ER.

The definition of sepsis evolved over the years and presently sepsis-3 (2016) define sepsis as a "life-threatening organ dysfunction caused by dysregulated host response to infection." whereas septic shock is recognized as "a subset of sepsis in which underlying circulatory and cellular metabolic abnormalities are profound enough to substantially increase mortality."

In the present definition of sepsis, the authors emphasized that the previous distinction of sepsis, severe sepsis, and septic shock is no longer relevant. An infection without organ dysfunction or hypotension or evidence of hypoperfusion does not warrant similar aggressive response and can simply be categorized as having an infection only and not "sepsis". Previous "severe sepsis" is now termed "sepsis". For standardization of organ dysfunction purpose, the task force promotes the use of quick sequential organ failure assessment (qSOFA) score **(Table 2)** for out of ICU settings and sequential organ failure assessment (SOFA) score for ICU settings. A screening tool for sepsis in the emergency department (ED) is given in **Table 3**.

TABLE 2: qSOFA score.

H	**H**ypotension: SBP ≤100 mm Hg
A	**A**ltered mental status (any GCS <15)
T	**T**achypnea: Respiratory rate ≥22 breaths/min

(GCS: Glasgow Coma Score; SBP: systolic blood pressure)

TABLE 3: Screening tool to rule in/out sepsis in the emergency department.

This is a simplified tool that can be used to screen patients for sepsis in the ED or in critical care unit

1. Obtain proper history for any potential source of infection	Lung infections, kidney infections such as urinary tract infection, infection lingering in the abdomen, meningitis and endocarditis, skin and soft-tissue infection, wound infection, catheter-related infections, and bloodstream infections	Yes/no
2. Search for signs and symptoms that would indicate	Fever >38.3°C or temperature <36°C, altered mental status with a GCS <15, heart rate >90 bpm (tachycardia), respiratory rate >20 bpm (tachypnea), leukocytosis or leukopenia (WBC count >12,000 µ/L or <4,000 µ/L, respectively)	Yes/no

- If both of the above are answered YES, suspicion of infection is present
- Laboratory investigations that should be ordered are complete blood count with differential, blood lactate, cultures, and basic metabolic panel. Ultrasound abdomen, CT scan, chest X-ray, amylase, lipase, arterial blood gas (ABG), and procalcitonin should be obtained according to the signs and symptoms and according to physician discretion

3. Whether the organ dysfunction criteria are present?	If suspicion of infection and organ dysfunction is present, the patient's condition is labeled as *septic shock* and should be entered into the protocol	Yes/no

Question 4

1. Discuss the physiology of cerebral circulation.

Cerebral blood flow (CBF) and autoregulation: The central nervous system (CNS) is enclosed in a bony vault. The CNS comprises brain parenchyma, cerebrospinal fluid, and blood. In normal physiology, these three elements are in homeostasis. The adult brain represents 2% of body weight. It receives 12–15% of the total cardiac output. This represents the high metabolic rate of brain parenchyma. CBF is 45–55 mL/100 g/min. Cerebral metabolic rate of oxygen is 3–3.5 mL/100 g/min. Intracranial pressure (ICP) (supine) is 8–12 mm Hg. Normal CBF is maintained by cerebral blood vessels by its constriction and dilatation ability under various physiological condition; this is called autoregulation. Factors affecting cerebral blood flow are temperature, seizures, partial pressure of carbon dioxide in arterial blood ($PaCO_2$), partial pressure of arterial oxygen (PaO_2), mean arterial pressure (MAP), and vasoactive agents. Normal functioning of brain depends upon the cerebral perfusion pressure (CPP) which is the difference between the MAP and ICP. *CPP = MAP − ICP*. CPP roughly denotes the CBF. CBF is maintained well when MAP is maintained between 60 and 150 mm Hg **(Fig. 5)**.

2. Discuss the diagnosis of cortical venous sinus thrombosis in ER.

Cortical vein thrombosis (CVT) occurs when a blood clot (thrombus) forms within the cortical vein system but does not involve the dural sinuses, such as the superior sagittal sinus and transverse sinus **(Fig. 6)**. Risk factors for adults include pregnancy and the first few weeks after delivery, problems with blood clotting for example, antiphospholipid syndrome, protein C and S deficiency, antithrombin III deficiency, lupus anticoagulant, or factor V Leiden mutation. Clinical manifestations can include headache, papilledema, visual loss, focal or generalized seizures, focal neurologic deficits, confusion, altered consciousness, and coma. Diagnostic algorithm for cortical vein thrombosis in ER is shown in **Flowchart 1**.

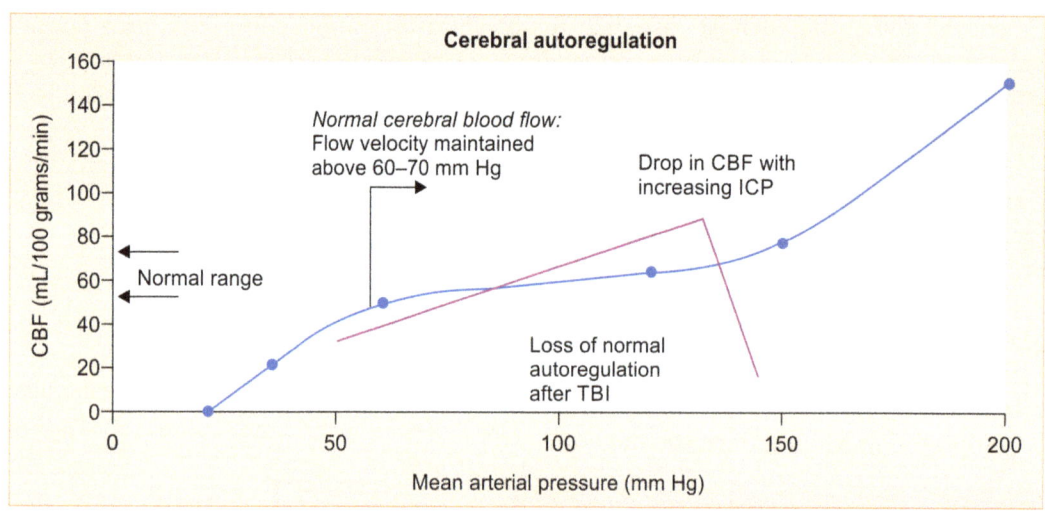

Fig. 5: Determinants of cerebral blood flow. (CBF: cerebral blood flow; ICP: intracranial pressure; TBI: traumatic brain injury)

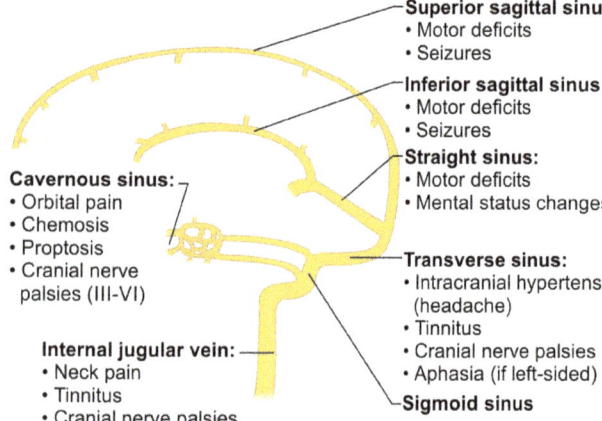

Fig. 6: Involved sinuses and presentation.

Flowchart 1: Algorithm for diagnosis of cortical vein thrombosis (CVT).

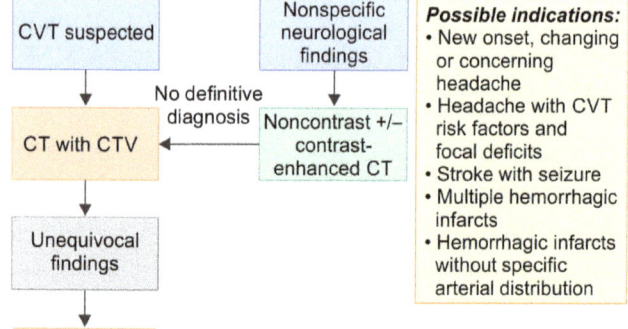

(CT: computed tomography; CTV: CT venography; MRI: magnetic resonance imaging; MRV: MR venography)

Question 5

1. Discuss the anatomy of intrinsic muscles of the hand.

Four muscle groups comprise the intrinsic hand. These are the thenar, hypothenar, interossei, and the lumbrical muscles.

The thenar muscle, or thenar eminence, is a collection of three muscles at the fleshy base of the thumb (first digit) on the palmar aspect that acts to exert movement about the thumb. The muscles of the hand are innervated by the *radial, median, and ulnar nerves*. The radial nerve innervates the finger extensors and the thumb abductor, that is, the muscles that extend at the wrist and metacarpophalangeal joints (knuckles) and abduct and extend the thumb. Action of various muscles of hand and their innervations are given in **Table 4**.

TABLE 4: Intrinsic muscles of hand.

Muscle	Action	Innervation
Thenar group		
Flexor pollicis brevis	Flexes thumb	Median nerve
Abductor pollicis brevis	Abducts thumb	
Opponens pollicis	Opposes thumb	
Hypothenar group		
Flexor digiti minimi	Flexes finger 5	Ulnar nerve
Abductor digiti minimi	Abducts finger 5	
Opponens digiti minimi	Opposition of finger 5	
Midpalmar group		
Lumbricals	Flexes 2nd–5th MP joints and extends 2nd–5th PIP and DIP joints	• Lateral 2 lumbricals: Median nerve • Medial 2 lumbricals: Ulnar nerve
Dorsal interossei	Abducts fingers 2–5	Ulnar nerve
Palmar interossei	Adducts fingers 2–5	
Adductor pollicis	Adducts thumb	

(DIP: distal interphalangeal; MP: metacarpophalangeal; PIP: proximal interphalangeal)

2. Discuss the clinical presentation of ulnar nerve injuries.

Symptoms of ulnar nerve entrapment and damage include **(Fig. 7)** claw hand, elbow pain (cubital tunnel syndrome), wrist pain (Guyon's canal syndrome), and numbness and tingling in the ring fingers.

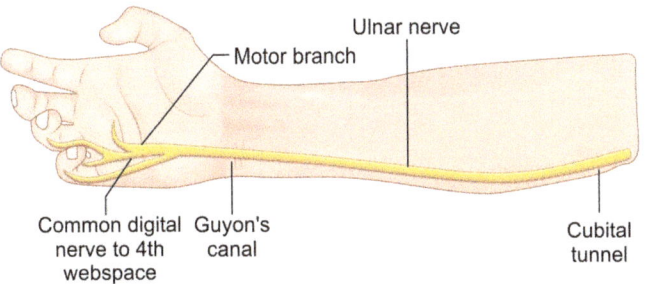

Fig. 7: Ulnar nerve injury: Clinical presentation.

Question 6

1. Discuss the physiology of regulation of intracerebral pressure.

Knowledge of the Monro–Kellie doctrine is essential to understand brain pathophysiology in injury. In 1783, Alexander Monro deduced that the cranium is a rigid box and is filled with the nearly incompressible brain and that its volume remains constant. In 1824, George Kellie confirmed Monro's observation. The doctrine states that any increase in the volume of the cranial contents raises the ICP and the increase in volume of a content occurs at the expense of the other two. The initial reaction is to reduce venous blood and CSF. When these compensatory mechanisms get exhausted, the pressure increases drastically, and brain herniation can occur **(Fig. 8)**.

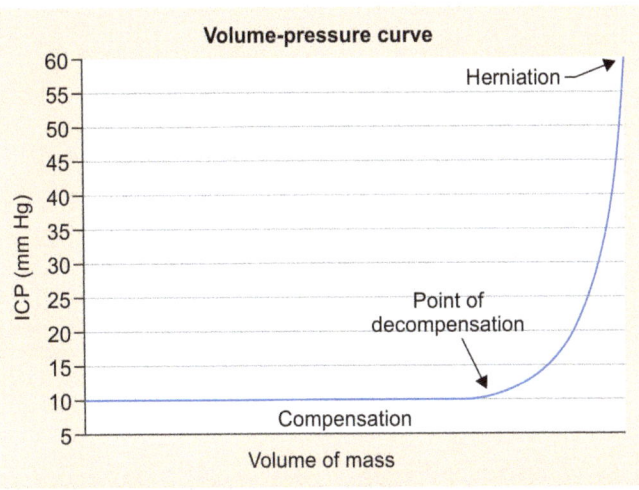

Fig. 8: Intracranial pressure (ICP) versus volume curve.

2. Discuss the clinical presentation and investigations of high-altitude cerebral edema.

High-altitude cerebral edema (HACE) is preceded in major case by symptoms of acute mountain sickness (AMS) and is considered the end stage of AMS. HACE can present 3–5 days after arrival to elevations as low as 2,750 m (9,022 ft) but is most commonly seen in remote environments well above this altitude, where the onset of symptoms may be much more abrupt over a period of hours. The diagnosis is clinical and based on altered sensorium and ataxia. Mental status changes may include irrational behavior that rapidly progresses to lethargy, obtundation, and coma. If untreated, death results from brain herniation.

Treatment: Immediate descent or evacuation at 1,000 m (3,281 ft), oxygen to maintain $SaO_2 > 90\%$, and dexamethasone (8 mg IV/IM/PO initially and then 4 mg per 6 hours). If descent is not an option, one may use a portable hyperbaric chamber and/or supplemental oxygen to temporize illness, but this should never replace or delay evaluation/descent when possible.

Question 7

1. Discuss the immunological response in SARS CoV-2 infection.

Progression of illness due to SARS CoV-2 (severe acute respiratory syndrome coronavirus 2) is classified into three categories: mild, moderate, and severe. Systemic inflammatory markers are elevated in moderately severe/severe categories. Inflammatory cytokines and biomarkers such as interleukin-2 (IL -2), IL-6, IL-7, granulocyte colony-stimulating factor, macrophage inflammatory protein 1α, tumor necrosis factor-α, C-reactive protein, ferritin, and D-dimer are significantly elevated in severe category patients. Troponin and N-terminal pro B-type natriuretic peptide can also be elevated. Severe COVID-19 patients are at a higher risk of thrombosis due to low blood flow (induced by both vasoconstriction and stasis) together with endothelial injury and hypercoagulability. SARS-CoV-2 aggression on the host cells through angiotensin-converting enzyme 2 (ACE2) receptors, the excessive immune response-induced cytokine storm, the local and systemic inflammatory response responsible for an endothelial damage, and a hypercoagulability state lead to both systemic and macro- and microthrombosis.

2. Discuss the management of vaccine-induced anaphylaxis.

Treatment of anaphylaxis

a. *Oxygenation:* It is done through face mask or endotracheal intubation, if needed. Mechanical ventilation is

indicated for severe bronchospasm, apnea, or cardiac arrest.
b. *Epinephrine:* It is a universally recommended drug. Intramuscular dose is 0.3–1 mL.
c. Intravenous dose 3–5 mL of 1:10,000 dilutions. *Mechanism of action*: It increases intracellular cyclic adenosine monophosphate (cAMP) levels in leukocytes and mast cells which inhibits the histamine release. It has beneficial effects on myocardial contractility and peripheral vascular tone and bronchial smooth muscle also.
d. *IV fluids and inotropes*: These are the treatment of choice. Norepinephrine infusion, methoxamine, phenylephrine, vasopressin, and methylene blue can be tried in refractory cases.
e. *Nebulization* with salbutamol is recommended in cases where bronchospasm is seen. Aminophylline 5–6 mg/kg IV is given over 30 minutes. Ketamine and magnesium sulfate can also be used in severe cases of asthma.

Question 8

1. Discuss the anatomy of coronary circulation.

The two main coronary arteries are the left main and the right coronary arteries **(Fig. 9)**.

Left main coronary artery (LMCA): It supplies blood to the left side of the heart muscle (the left ventricle and left atrium). LMCA divides into the following branches:
a. The left anterior descending artery branches off the left coronary artery and supplies blood to the front of the left side of the heart.
b. The circumflex artery branches off the left coronary artery and encircles the heart muscle. This artery supplies blood to the outer side and back of the heart.

Right coronary artery (RCA): It supplies blood to the right ventricle, the right atrium, and the sinoatrial (SA) and atrioventricular (AV) nodes, which regulate the heart rhythm. It divides into smaller branches, including the right posterior descending artery and the acute marginal artery. Together with the left anterior descending artery, RCA helps supply blood to the middle or septum of the heart.

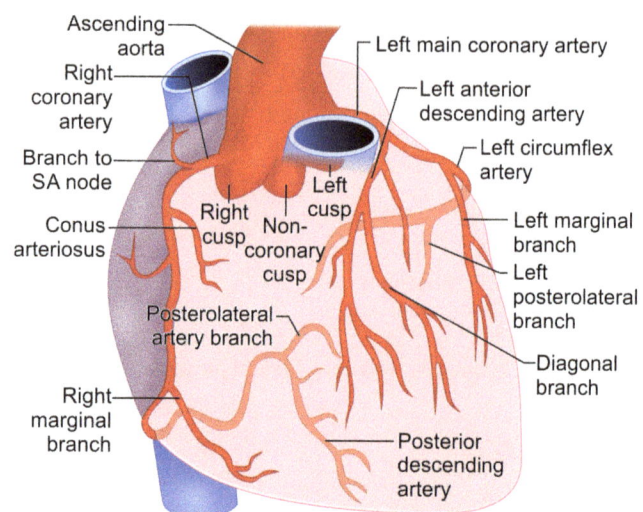

Fig. 9: Anatomy of coronary circulation. (SA: sinoatrial)

2. Explain Frank–Starling law and Poiseuille law application in ER.

The *Frank-Starling law* is the description of cardiac hemodynamic as it relates to myocyte stretch and contractility. This law states that the stroke volume of the left ventricle will increase as the left ventricular volume increases due to the myocyte stretch causing a more forceful systolic contraction **(Fig. 10A)**.

The *law of Poiseuille* states that the flow of liquid depends on variables such as the length of the tube (L), radius (r), pressure gradient (ΔP), and the viscosity of the fluid (η) in accordance with their relationship **(Fig. 10B)**:

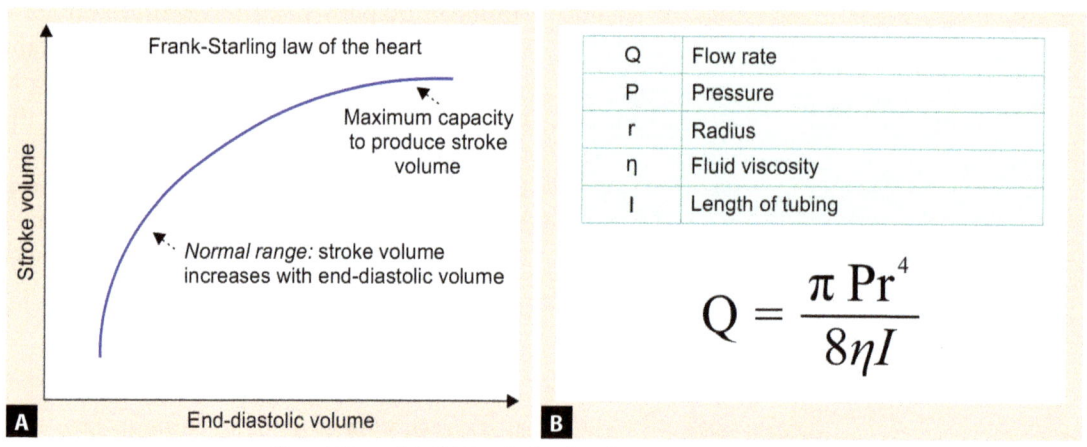

Figs. 10A and B: (A) Frank–Starling law; (B) Poiseuille law.

a. The change in diameter has the most drastic effect on the resistance.
b. The radius of the vessel is directly proportional to the flow of volume.
c. Minute changes in the radius can result in large changes in volume flow.
d. Poiseuille's law is used to find the flow rate of volume in the case of laminar flow.

Question 9

1. Discuss the physiology of sodium homeostasis.

Sodium is an important electrolyte mainly found in extracellular fluid, which helps maintain fluid balance, blood pressure, nerve impulse conduction, and muscle contraction. The human body tightly maintains serum [Na⁺] between 138 and 142 mEq/L despite what may be marked changes in daily intake depending on the person's diet. The sodium balance is the difference between the amount of Na absorbed by the gut and the amount excreted via urine, feces, and skin. Sodium balance in the body is closely linked to that of water and is finely maintained by the kidneys. Hyponatremia is a condition of excess water relative to Na⁺ and is defined as a serum [Na⁺] 100 mOsm/L H₂O with the exception of samples from patients with psychogenic polydipsia, which drives down urine osmolality below the typical minimum.

2. Discuss the causes of hyponatremia in elderly presentation to ER.

a. Diarrhea and vomiting
b. Diuretics (most common thiazides)
c. Chronic heart failure and cirrhosis
d. Nephrotic syndrome
e. Acute or chronic kidney disease
f. Syndrome of inappropriate antidiuretic hormone (SIADH)
g. Hypothyroidism
h. Glucocorticoid deficiency
i. Mineralocorticoid deficiency
j. Salt-losing nephropathies
k. Cerebral salt wasting

Question 10

1. Discuss the role of kidney in acid–base maintenance.

The kidneys play a major role in the regulation of acid–base balance by reabsorbing bicarbonate filtered by the glomeruli and excreting titratable acids and ammonia into the urine **(Fig. 11)**.

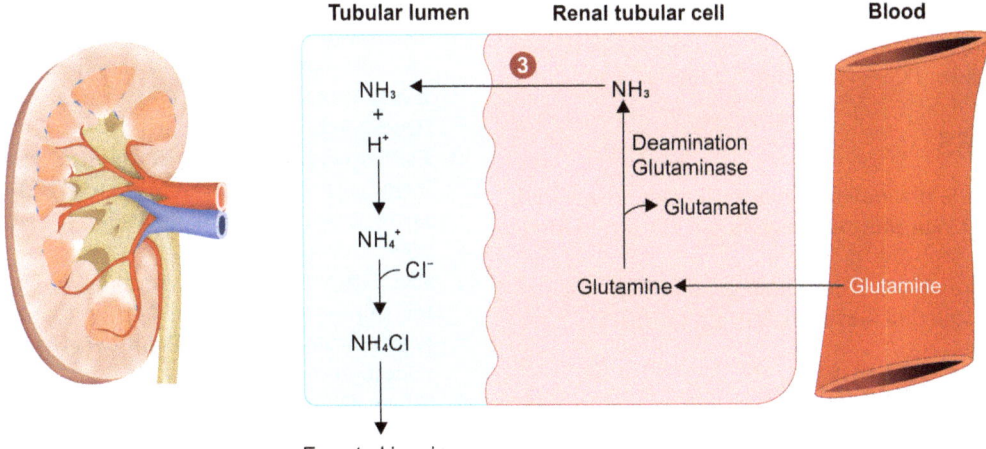

Fig. 11: Renal mechanism: Acid–base balance.

2. Discuss the acute kidney injury scoring system in ER.

Acute kidney injury (AKI) is a common presenting problem encountered in the ED associated with an increased risk of mortality and often progression to chronic kidney disease. A variety of definitions for AKI have been proposed in the literature. In 2012, the Kidney Disease: Improving Global Outcomes (KDIGO) group defined AKI based on the urine output and the serum creatinine (S. Cr) concentration. This definition is an increase in S. Cr of ≥0.3 mg/dL within 48 hours or an increase in S. Cr > 1.5 times baseline within 7 days or decreased urine output for 6 hours **(Table 5)**. Other classification systems of AKI, such as RIFLE (risk, injury, failure, loss, and end-stage) and Acute Kidney Injury Network (AKIN), can also be used, but as per studies all three criteria are effective tools for predicting mortality without significant differences among them, but the advantage of KDIGO is that it covers parameters in AKIN and RIFLE.

Acute kidney injury is defined as a sudden reduction in kidney function that is characterized by a diminished glomerular filtration rate (GFR) as manifested by an increased S. Cr or reduced urine output. AKI is further divided into three categories: (a) *Prerenal*, a kidney blood flow decrease; (b) *intrarenal*, or kidney parenchymal injury; and (c) *postrenal*, or urine flow obstruction.

TABLE 5: KDIGO guidelines for acute kidney injuries.

AKI Stage	Serum creatinine	Urine output
1	1.5–1.9 × baseline OR ≥0.3 mg/dL increase	<0.5 mL/kg/h for 6–12 hours
2	2.0–2.9 × baseline	<0.5 mL/kg/h for >12 hours
3	3.0 × baseline or initiation of renal replacement therapy	<0.3 mL/kg/h for ≥24 hours or anuria for ≥12 hours
RIFLE criteria		
AKI stage	Serum creatinine	Urine output
1	Increase in S. Cr ≥150% mg/dL	<0.5 mL/kg/h for 6–12 hours
2	Increase in S. Cr ≥ 200–300% mg/dL	<0.5 mL/kg/h for ≥12 hours
3	Increase in S. Cr 300% OR creatinine >4 mg/mL with acute increase 0.5 mg/dL or initiation of renal replacement therapy	<0.3 mL/kg/h for ≥24 hours or anuria for ≥12 hours

(KDIGO: Kidney disease: Improving global outcomes; RIFLE: risk, injury, failure, loss, and end-stage)
Source: Moore PK, Hsu RK, Liu KD. Management of acute kidney injury: core curriculum 2018. Am J Kidney Dis. 2018;72(1):136-48.

■ REFERENCES

1. Hrics P, Wilber S, Blanda MP, Gallo U. Ultrasound-assisted internal jugular vein catheterization in the ED. Am J Emerg Med. 1998;16(4):401-3.
2. Abboud PAC, Kendall JL. Ultrasound guidance for vascular access. Emerg Med Clin North Am. 2004;22(3):749-73.

■ SUGGESTED READING

1. Australasian Society of Clinical Immunology and Allergy. (2023). ASCIA Guidelines - Acute Management of Anaphylaxis. [online] Available from https://www.allergy.org.au/hp/papers/acute-management-of-anaphylaxis-guidelines. [Last accessed May,2023]. (Question 7).
2. Erwin J, Varacello M. Anatomy, Shoulder and Upper Limb, Wrist Joint. In: StatPearls [Internet]. Treasure Island, FL: StatPearls Publishing; 2023. (Question 5).
3. Richhariya D, Sharma B. Textbook of Emergency Medicine including Intensive Care and Trauma, 2nd edition. New Delhi: Jaypee Brothers Medical Publishers (P) Ltd; 2022. p. 1558. (Question 4).
4. Richhariya D, Sharma B. Textbook of Emergency Medicine including Intensive Care and Trauma, 2nd edition. New Delhi: Jaypee Brothers Medical Publishers (P) Ltd; 2022. p. 284. (Question 1).
5. Richhariya D, Sharma B. Textbook of Emergency Medicine including Intensive Care and Trauma, 2nd edition. New Delhi: Jaypee Brothers Medical Publishers (P) Ltd; 2022. pp. 1557, 1709. (Question 6).
6. Richhariya D, Sharma B. Textbook of Emergency Medicine including Intensive Care and Trauma, 2nd edition. New Delhi: Jaypee Brothers Medical Publishers (P) Ltd; 2022. pp. 302, 572. (Question 2).
7. Richhariya D, Sharma B. Textbook of Emergency Medicine including intensive Care and Trauma, 2nd edition. New Delhi: Jaypee Brothers Medical Publishers (P) Ltd; 2022. pp. 311-3. (Question 9).
8. Richhariya D, Sharma B. Textbook of Emergency Medicine including Intensive Care and Trauma, 2nd edition. New Delhi: Jaypee Brothers Medical Publishers (P) Ltd; 2022. pp. 320, 327. (Question 3).
9. Richhariya D, Sharma B. Textbook of Emergency Medicine including Intensive Care and Trauma, 2nd edition. New Delhi: Jaypee Brothers Medical Publishers (P) Ltd; 2022. pp. 453-5. (Question 8).
10. Richhariya D, Sharma B. Textbook of Emergency Medicine including Intensive Care and Trauma, 2nd edition. New Delhi: Jaypee Brothers Medical Publishers (P) Ltd; 2022. pp. 622-31. (Question 7).
11. Richhariya D, Sharma B. Textbook of Emergency Medicine including Intensive Care and Trauma, 2nd edition. New Delhi: Jaypee Brothers Medical Publishers (P) Ltd; 2022. pp. 743-5. (Question 10).
12. Whyte AF, Soar J, Dodd A, Hughes A, Sargant N, Turner PJ. Emergency treatment of anaphylaxis: concise clinical guidance. Clin Med (Lond). 2022;22(4):332-9. (Question 7).

Emergency Medicine Paper 42

Devendra Richhariya

Question 1

1. Discuss clinical presentation of hip fracture in emergency department (ED).

Clinical presentation of hip fracture (Garden classification **Fig. 1**) is summarized here:
a. Radiating pain to the knee.
b. Inability to bear weight.
c. Shortening or sideways rotation of the affected leg.
d. Increased pain in the hip during rotation of the leg.
e. Swelling on the side of the hip.

2. Give a plan for pain relief of a 75-year-old female, known hypertensive with previous history of percutaneous transluminal coronary angioplasty (PTCA), presently admitted with hip fracture.

Drug therapy is the mainstay of pain management in emergency department. Knowledge of appropriate pharmacologic agents for managing the intensity of pain is the key. Ideal pharmacologic agent should be easy to administer with appropriate quality and safety measures **(Table 1)**.

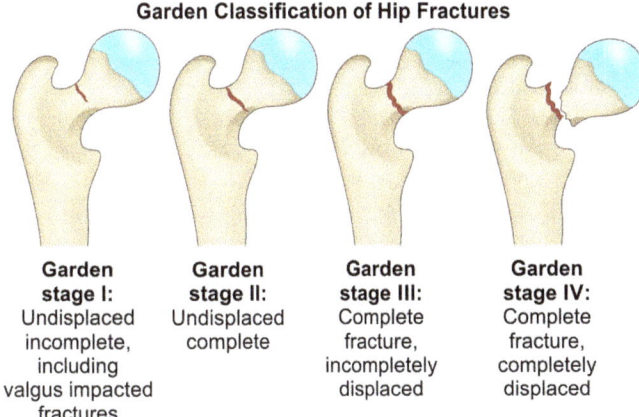

Fig. 1: Garden classification of hip fractures.

TABLE 1: Pharmacologic management of pain.		
Opioids analgesic therapy		
Drugs	**Initial dose for adult**	**Comments**
Morphine	2–6 mg intravenous (IV) 10 mg IM/SC	Nausea vomiting transient hypotension
Fentanyl	50–100 µg IV	Less CV depression than morphine
Meperidine (Pethidine)	25–50 mg IV 50–100 mg IM/SC	With MAO inhibitors may precipitate serotonin syndrome if taken within 14 days
Tramadol	50–100 mg in 100 mL NS IV over 30–45 minutes as infusion	CNS side effects are common
Opioid agonist-antagonist analgesic		
Butorphanol	1 mg IV or 2 mg IM every 4 hours	Sedation dizziness nausea
Pentazocine	30 mg IV/IM/SC every 4–6 hours	CNS side effects
Adjunctive medications with opioid		
Ondansetron	4–8 mg IV/PO	Can prolong QT interval
Prochlorperazine	5–10 mg IV/IM/PO	Can cause extrapyramidal reactions
Promethazine	25–50 mg IVIM	Can cause extrapyramidal reactions
Metoclopramide	5–10 mg IV/IM/PO	Can cause extrapyramidal reactions
Nonopioids analgesics		
Acetaminophen (paracetamol)	325–1000 mg PO every 4–6 hours >50 kg 1 g IV every 6 hourly <50 kg 15 mg/kg IV every 6 hourly	Liver dysfunction Maximum dose not >3 g/day

Contd…

Contd…

Drugs	Initial dose for adult	Comments
Aspirin (acetylsalicylic acid)	325–650 mg every 4 hourly	GI irritation, mucosal bleeding, platelet dysfunction, tinnitus, CNS toxicity
Ibuprofen (NSAIDs)	400–800 mg PO every 4–6 hourly	GI upset, platelet and renal dysfunction, bronchospasm
Naproxen (NSAIDs)	250–500 mg PO every 8–12 hours	GI upset, platelet and renal dysfunction, bronchospasm
Indomethacin (NSAIDs)	25–50 mg PO every 8 hourly	GI upset, platelet and renal dysfunction, bronchospasm

(CNS: central nervous system; MAO: monoamine oxidase; NSAIDs: non-steroidal anti-inflammatory drugs)

Question 2

1. Explain the causes of acute painful swelling in the right inguinal region in a young male.

Differential diagnosis of right inguinal region pain is given in **Table 2**.

TABLE 2: Differential diagnosis.

Children	Gastroenteritis, mesenteric enteritis, Meckel's diverticulitis, intussusception, Henoch-Schönlein purpura, lobar pneumonia
Adult	Regional enteritis, ureteric colic, perforated peptic ulcer, torsion of testis, pancreatitis, rectus sheath hematoma
Adult female	Pelvic inflammatory disease, pyelonephritis, ectopic pregnancy, torsion of ovarian cyst, endometriosis
Elderly	Diverticulitis, intestinal obstruction, colonic carcinoma, torsion appendix epiploic, mesenteric infarction, leaking aortic aneurysm

2. Throw light on "appendicitis—conservative or surgical debate".

Nonoperative or medical management: Appendicitis has long been a surgically treated disease, recently few studies of nonsurgical management dot the surgical literature. Based on higher rate of failure with antibiotics alone, nonoperative management of acute appendicitis has not been recommended. Nevertheless, antibiotic treatment may be a useful temporizing measure in environments with no surgical expertise. Intravenous antibiotics have been shown to reduce the incidence of postoperative wound infection and intra-abdominal abscess. Antibiotic should be administered 30 minutes prior to skin incision. As the typical flora of appendix resembles that of colon, a second-generation cephalosporin or a combination of antibiotics directed at gram negatives and anaerobes will suffice. In nonperforated appendicitis, a single preoperative dose, and in cases of perforation, an extended course of at least 5 days of antibiotics is advocated.

Operative management: Open or laparoscopic appendectomy—once the diagnosis of appendicitis is confirmed, the surgeon must decide whether to perform an open or laparoscopic appendectomy. Meta-analysis and systematic reviews have addressed the controversy. Based on the data available, one cannot convincingly recommend either open or laparoscopic appendectomy over the other. One situation in which laparoscopic appendectomy may be advisable is when diagnosis of appendicitis is in doubt.

Question 3

1. Discuss causes and clinical presentation of brachial artery injury.

Penetrating trauma is generally considered to be the most common cause of a vascular injury in the upper extremity. In addition to the usual types of blunt and penetrating injuries, supracondylar fractures or dislocation of the humerus may injure the brachial artery.

The following findings were considered to be signs of arterial injury—active bleeding, rapidly growing and pulsatile hematoma, pale and cold extremities, absent or very weak distal pulses, associated neurologic deficits, and associated injuries to bony and soft tissues.

Clinical presentation of penetrating vascular injury is classified in hard and soft signs of injury. This will allow physician to decide best management plan. Signs which are classified as hard signs, represent immediate intervention while signs which are classified as soft signs, represent diagnostic testing to better illicit the type of injury.

Hard signs:
a. External arterial bleeding
b. Rapidly expanding hematoma
c. Palpable thrill, audible bruit
d. Obvious arterial occlusion—pulseless, pallor, paresthesia, pain, paralysis

Soft signs:
a. History of arterial bleeding at the scene
b. Diminished unilateral distal pulse
c. Neurologic deficient
d. Proximity of penetrating wound to major artery
e. Small nonpulsatile hematoma

f. Abnormal flow—velocity waveform on Doppler ultrasound
g. Abnormal ankle—brachial pressure index (<0.9)

2. Explain the evaluation and management of dashboard injury.

Dashboard knee injuries are a common mechanism of trauma in seat-belted passengers involved in road-traffic accidents. They can cause a syndrome of knee pain arising from a spectrum of pathology including prepatellar soft-tissue lacerations and bruising to meniscal and ligament injuries as well as fractures. Dashboard injuries can cause simultaneous knee and hip injuries, usually PCL (posterior cruciate ligament) and posterior hip dislocation **(Fig. 2)**. The recommended treatment for partial tears or strains usually involves rest, icing, over-the-counter anti-inflammatory and pain medications, and physical therapy. The treatment should also include "rest, ice, compression, and elevation (RICE)". Stage II PCL injuries may require surgery, depending on the severity of the injury.

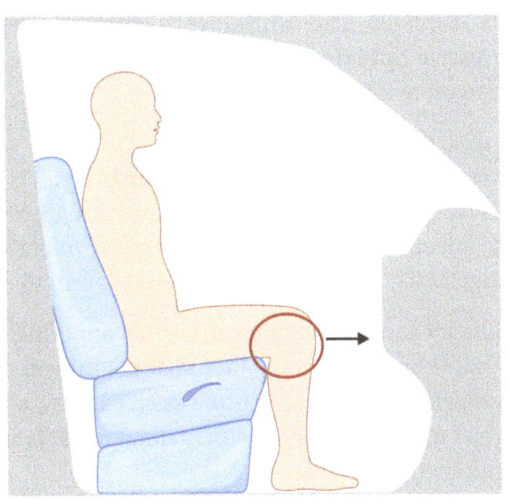
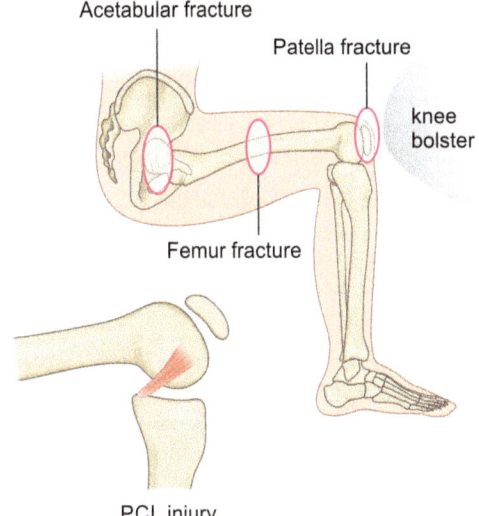

Fig. 2: Dashboard injury.

Question 4

1. What is hyperemesis gravidarum (HG)? Discuss its physiology and management in ED.

Nausea and vomiting in pregnancy (NVP) is a rather frequent symptom occurring in 70–80% women. NVP is one of the commonest reasons for hospitalization in pregnancy and negatively affect the quality of life. In most pregnant women, the condition is self-limiting, yet, in a few, symptoms may persist throughout the duration of pregnancy.

Hyperemesis gravidarum (HG) is a rare but severe form of NVP reported in 0.3–3.6% pregnancies and an obstetric emergency. Other causes of severe nausea and vomiting should be excluded before coming to the diagnosis of HG. HG, the severe form of NVP is marked by a triad of severe protracted nausea and vomiting associated with weight loss >5% pre-pregnancy weight, dehydration, and electrolyte imbalances. Severe untreated forms may present with malnutrition, dehydration, neuropathies, Wernicke's encephalopathy, coma, and death. Serious maternal complications may also occur due to Mallory–Weiss tears and esophageal rupture, splenic avulsion and pneumothorax associated with excessive vomiting.

Excessive vomiting results from emetogenic effects of human chorionic gonadotropin (hCG) the pathogenesis of which is largely unknown. There are no marked changes in the organ systems other than features of dehydration and malnutrition in severe cases. Some cases of HG may develop Wernicke's encephalopathy due to vitamin B_1 deficiency.

Many oral antiemetics are safe for use in NVP **(Table 3)**. Women not responding to single medication may be given combination of different drugs. Parenteral route may be preferable for those with persistent NVP/HG. For the cases needing inpatient management, initial assessment should include ABCDE (airway, breathing, circulation, disability, exposure) and fluid resuscitation should be guided by degree of shock. Initial resuscitation should be done with crystalloids containing sodium and chloride with supplementation of potassium. Proton pump inhibitors or H_2 antagonists may be added to relieve gastritis or esophagitis. Intravenous antiemetics can be gradually replaced with oral medication once fluid therapy is weaned off. Thromboprophylaxis with low molecular weight heparin is indicated in admitted patients unless contraindicated. Multidisciplinary team management with nutritionist, endocrinologist, and gastroenterologist should be used when enteral or parenteral treatment is required. As a last resort, in patients not responding to any treatment modality and with remitting severe symptoms, termination of pregnancy may be considered.

TABLE 3: Antiemetics recommended for use in pregnancy.

First line	• Cyclizine 50 mg PO, IM or IV 8 hourly • Prochlorperazine 5–10 mg 6–8 hourly PO; 12.5 mg 8 hourly IM/IV; 25 mg PR daily, promethazine 12.5–25 mg 4–8 hourly PO, IM, IV or PR • Chlorpromazine 10–25 mg 4–6 hourly PO, IV or IM; or 50–100 mg 6–8 hourly PR
Second line	• Metoclopramide 5–10 mg 8 hourly PO, IV or IM (maximum 5 days' duration) domperidone 10 mg 8 hourly PO; 30–60 mg 8 hourly PR • Ondansetron 4–8 mg 6–8 hourly PO; 8 mg over 15 minutes 12 hourly IV
Third line	*Corticosteroids:* Hydrocortisone 100 mg twice daily IV; once clinical improvement occurs, convert to prednisolone 40–50 mg daily PO, dose gradually tapered until the lowest maintenance dose that controls the symptoms is reached

(IM: intramuscular; IV: intravenous; PO: by mouth; PR: by rectum)

2. Discuss management of postpartum hemorrhage due to precipitous labor in ED.

Postpartum hemorrhage (also called PPH) is when a woman has heavy bleeding after giving birth. It is a serious condition. It usually happens within 1 day of giving birth, but it can happen up to 12 weeks after having a baby. The causes of postpartum hemorrhage are called the four Ts (tone, trauma, tissue, and thrombin) **(Table 4)**. The conditions that may increase the risk for postpartum hemorrhage include the following:
a. Placental abruption—the early detachment of the placenta from the uterus
b. Placenta previa
c. Overdistended uterus
d. Multiple pregnancy
e. Gestational hypertension or preeclampsia
f. Having many previous births
g. Prolonged labor
h. Infection

Investigations: Complete blood count (hemoglobin and hematocrit), coagulation profile, blood grouping and typing urine analysis, blood culture, ultrasound for viewing uterus.

TABLE 4: Causes of postpartum hemorrhage.

Primary postpartum hemorrhage	Secondary postpartum hemorrhage
• Uterine atony • Retained placental fragments • Lower genital tract laceration • Uterine rupture • Uterine inversion • Hereditary coagulopathy	• Failure of uterine lining to sub-involute • Retained placental tissue • Genital tract wounds • Uterogenital infections

Management: The initial resuscitative steps include aggressive fluid and blood resuscitation while identifying and treating the underlying cause.

Treating the underlying cause:
Tone: Perform bimanual uterine massage. The drugs to improve uterine tone are oxytocin 20 units in 1 L NS (or 10 units IM), misoprostol 1,000 µg PR/PO once, methylergonovine 0.2 mg IM/IV/PO, carboprost 250 µg IM every 15–90 minutes.

Trauma: Examine for cervical, vaginal or perineal laceration or hematoma. Repair laceration. Incise, drain and appropriately ligate bleeding vessel causing a hematoma. Correct uterine inversion with manual replacement. Uterine rupture requires surgery.

Tissue: Inspect the placenta for missing fragments, if a portion is absent, manually evacuate the uterine cavity. Invasive placentation may require hysterectomy. Consider a balloon tamponade with either uterine-specific balloon device or an adaptation of Foley catheter or condom as a temporizing measure.

Thrombin: Consider DIC in the setting of severe preeclampsia, sepsis, placental abruption, shock or intrauterine fetal demise. Replace coagulation factors.

Question 5

1. Discuss causes of temporomandibular joint (TMJ) dislocation and its management in ED.

Jaw (mandible) dislocation results due to the displacement of mandibular condyles from articular groove in temporal bone. Most of the dislocations can be managed and reduced in emergency department. The temporomandibular joint (TMJ) is formed by articular surface between the mandibular condyles and the temporal bone. It is lined by synovial membrane and acts by hinge as well as sliding mechanism. It is supported by various ligaments. Dislocation of mandible can happen in four positions—anterior, posterior, superior and lateral. Risk factors for mandibular dislocations are as following: Shallow mandibular fossa, dystonia, convulsions, hypermobility syndrome, and previous history of TMJ dislocation.

Before relocation of any joint, a plain X-ray must be done to rule out any fracture. Likewise, X-ray of mandible also must be done to rule out any mandible fracture especially in traumatic dislocation. Orthopantomogram is the view of choice in case of jaw dislocation. It is a panoramic view that is acquired with camera planning around the patient. CT scan is more sensitive in diagnosing mandibular dislocations and other abnormality, hence its use is increasing in traumatic dislocations. It is acceptable nowadays to do CT scan as initial imaging modality in traumatic mandibular pathologies.

In emergency department, initially assessment of ABCs (airway, breathing, circulations) is to be done primarily. If every sign and investigation is suggestive of isolated acute mandibular dislocation, then it is to be decided whether close reduction in emergency is appropriate or not. Maxillofacial surgeon opinion is required in complicated as well as chronic mandibular dislocations.

Classical technique: This is the most commonly used technique **(Fig. 3)**. While doing this maneuver physician stands in front of sitting patient and places gloved thumbs on inferior molars a deep as possible and fingers are curved beneath the body and angle of mandible. Backward and downward pressure is to be given through thumb and fingers with slight mouth opening. This helps to reposition condyles back into fossa by disengaging them from anterior eminences. Sometimes it is difficult as the strength of masseter contractions has to be overcome. A risk of fingers bitten or disease transmission is involved in such procedures.

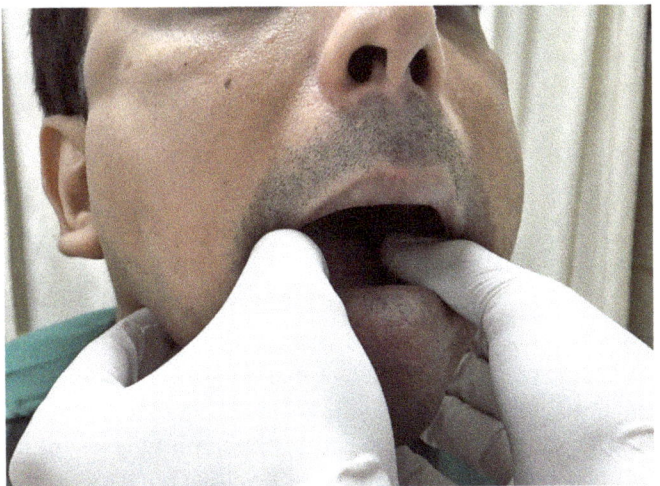

Fig. 3: Classic technique.

Recumbent approach: Standing behind the recumbent patient, physician places both thumb on inferior molars and gives downward and backward pressure until condyles reaches back to normal position **(Fig. 4)**.

Wrist pivot method: With same position as classical method, cephalad pressure on tip of mentum by thumb and caudal pressure on inferior molars by fingers, as shown in **Figure 5,** is to be given to reduce displaced mandible.

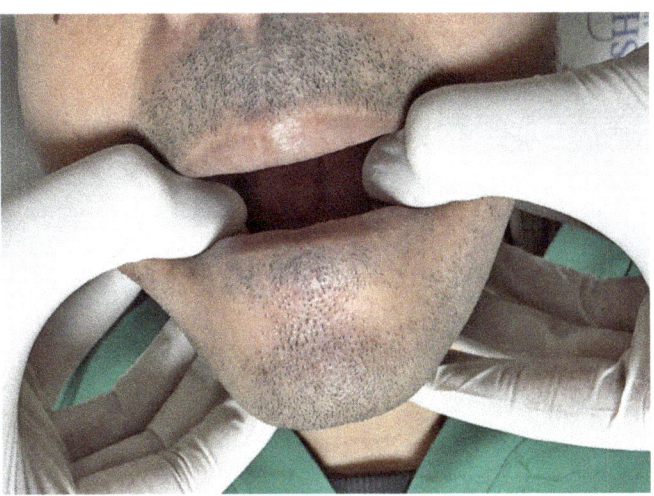

Fig. 4: Recumbent technique.

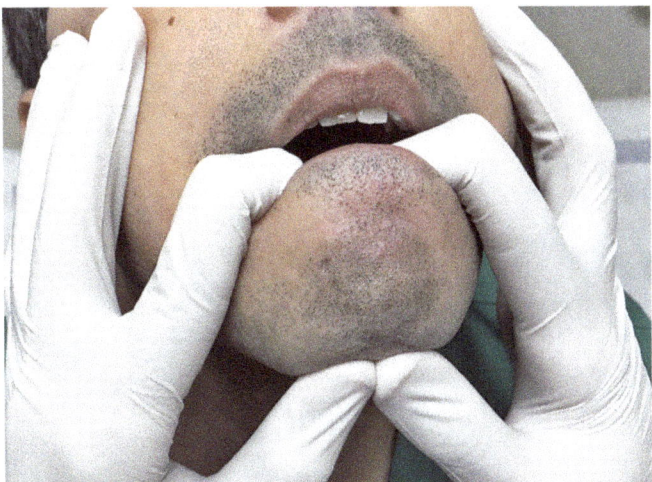

Fig. 5: Wrist pivot method.

2. Explain the management of periodontal abscess.

A periodontal abscess is described as a localized accumulation of pus within the gingival wall of a periodontal pocket. More prevalent in patients with previous periodontal pockets, it develops rapidly, destroying periodontal tissues and depicting clear symptoms **(Table 5)**.

TABLE 5: Periodontal abscess.	
\multicolumn{2}{l}{When a prolonged infection in tooth or in gingival tissue persists for a long time asymptomatically or there is sudden trauma to the tissue there is formation of abscess.}
Pathophysiology	Usually of sudden onset on marginal or interdental gingiva. Purulent exudates may be expressed
Clinical presentation	Localized, painful and rapidly expands
Red flags	Gingiva is fluctuant
History	Long-standing infection of tooth or gingival, forceful embedding of apple core, toothbrush into gingiva
Physical examination	Purulent exudate in 24–48 hours
Investigations	Radiographs OPG or IOPA are most commonly done and FNAC
Treatment	Removal of exudate under LA with an incision or opening the canal

(FNAC: fine needle aspiration cytology; IOPA: intraoral periapical; OPG: orthopantomogram)

Question 6

1. Discuss causes of acute onset diplopia and its management.

Causes include—cranial nerve palsies (from trauma, intracranial lesions, diabetes), extraocular muscle weakness (from cranial nerve palsy), exacerbates diplopia, direct trauma to the eye (orbital wall fractures causing mechanical restriction or entrapment of the extraocular muscles) **(Flowchart 1)**.

Management: First aim of management should be to identify and treat of the condition, where this is possible and to relieve patient symptoms. In children who rarely appreciate diplopia the aim will be to maintain the binocular vision thus to promote proper visual development. Thereafter period of observation of around 9–12 months is appropriate before any intervention as some palsies recover without need of surgery **(Flowchart 2)**.

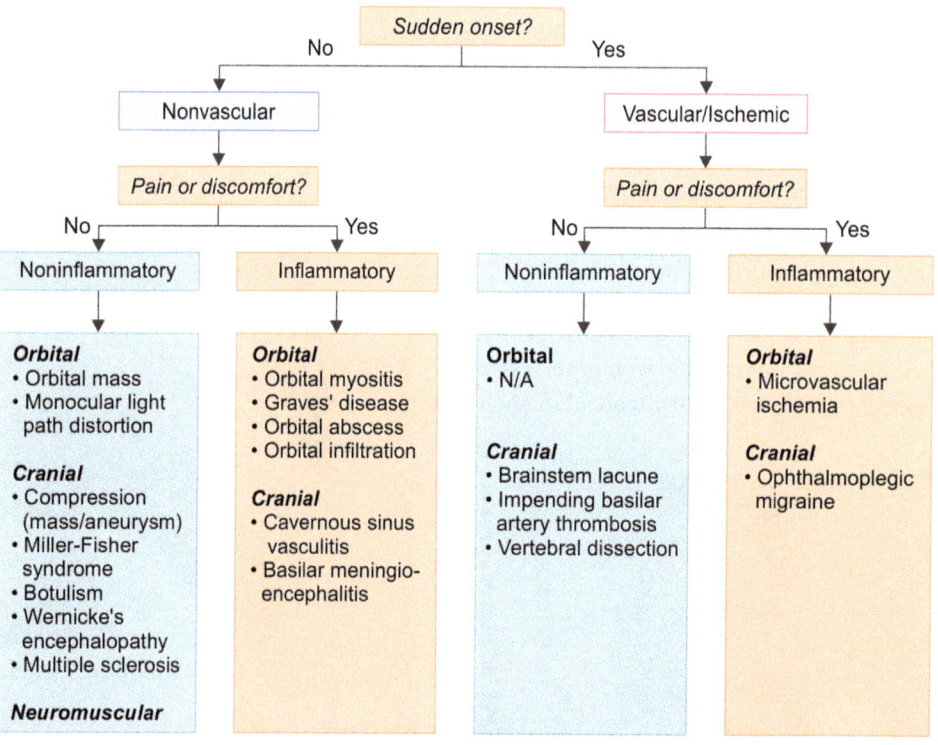

Flowchart 1: Causes of diplopia.

2. Explain the acute hematochezia and its management in ED.

Hematochezia refers to fresh red bleed per rectally and it signifies active upper gastrointestinal (UGI) bleed, distal large bowel or anorectal bleed.

Causes: Colonic bleed (95%), diverticular disease, ischemia, anorectal disease, neoplasia, inflammatory bowel disease, and radiation colitis.

The emergent treatment of the patient presenting with GI bleed is very important **(Flowchart 3)**. Initial rapid resuscitative measures should be promptly started

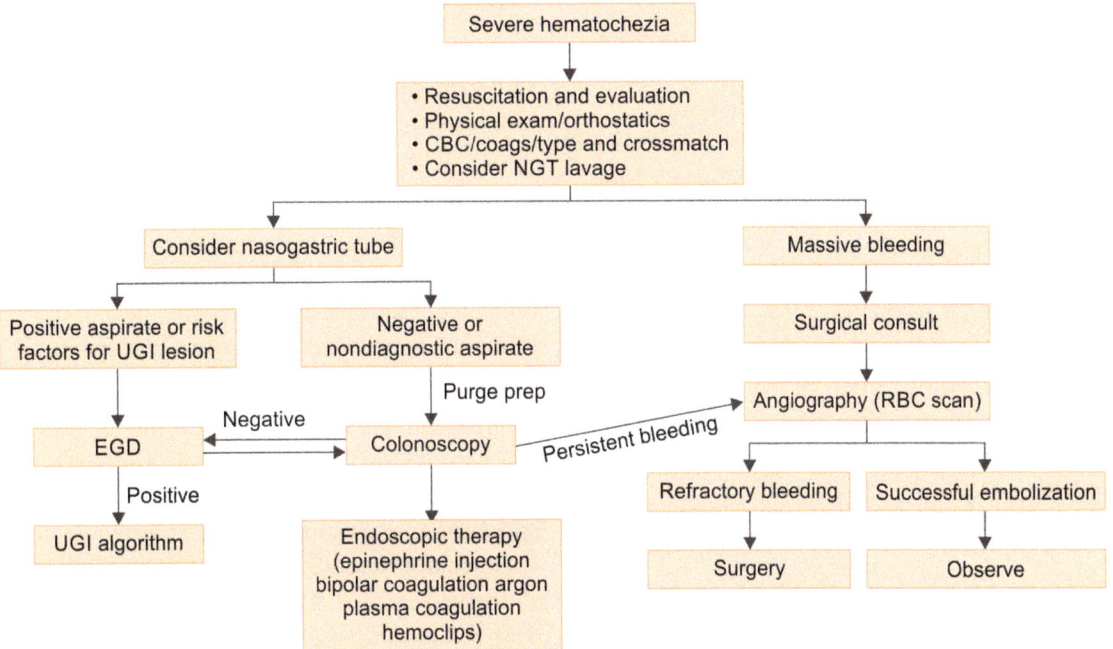

Flowchart 2: Approach to management of diplopia.

Flowchart 3: Approach to management of hematochezia.

in emergency which includes putting two large bore intravenous cannula and fluid resuscitation. Blood samples should be collected for complete blood counts, liver and renal function tests, coagulation profile, and blood grouping/crossmatching. Patients with massive upper GI bleed may need endotracheal intubation for airway protection.

Packed red blood cells (RBC) transfusion: Patients presenting with massive GI bleed should be given packed RBC in the emergency department only as rapid blood loss can result in vital organ hypoperfusion leading to multiorgan dysfunction. In euvolemic patients with upper GI hemorrhage, the PRBC transfusion should be planned to *target hemoglobin level of 7 g%*. Overzealous PRBC transfusion should be avoided as it may increase the risk of rebleed and transfusion-related complications.

In patient with lower GI bleed, the decision of PRBC transfusion should be individualized as no specific target hemoglobin level has been identified. Clinician should assess the hemodynamic status and transfusion-related untoward reactions before planning for PRBC transfusion.

Question 7

1. Write a note on "examination of an elderly female victim of physical assault in ED".

Any registered medical practitioner can conduct the examination and it is not mandatory for a gynecologist to examine such a case. If in case a female doctor is not available for examination, a male doctor should conduct the examination in the presence of a female attendant. In case of a minor/person with disability, his/her parent/guardian/

any other person with whom the survivor is comfortable may be present. *The Criminal Law Amendment Act, 2013, in Section 357C Criminal procedure code states that:* Both private and public health professionals are obligated to provide treatment and denial of treatment is punishable under Section 166 B IPC with imprisonment for a term which may extend to 1 year or with fine or with both. Thus, it is clear that every hospital should be equipped to handle such examination in quick and effective way to provide uniform and comprehensive healthcare services. In order to achieve this following may be considered:

a. Every hospital should have a standard operating procedure (SOP) for management of cases of sexual violence and these must be printed and available to all staff of the hospital.
b. The administrative guidelines regarding interdepartmental handling of such cases for examination and evidence collection should be clear to all the staff.
c. Administration should simultaneously help clinical staff to inform police and complete medicolegal procedures.
d. The hospital should have a uniform method of examination and evidence collection. A kit with required proforma along with the utilities such as nail cutters, syringes, and swabs can be kept ready for immediate use.

Health professionals need to maintain a clear and foolproof chain of custody of medical evidence collected and referring to appropriate agencies for further assistance (for example, legal support services, shelter services, etc.).

2. What are the steps in preparing the injury report?

Documentation: The collected samples for evidence are properly packed, sealed, and preserved in separate envelopes in the hospital till the time police are able to complete their paper work for dispatch to forensic lab test including DNA. A copy of all documentation (including that pertaining to medicolegal examination and treatment) must be provided to the survivor free of cost.

At the time of history taking, examination, and evidence collection any police personnel should not be present. The whole body must be examined for marks of violence. The victim should be requested to undress herself. A special attention should be given to the nature of the injuries.

Following are common injuries:
a. *Head:* Blow on head or head injury due to fall.
b. *Neck:* Gripping of throat.
c. Injuries on cheeks, lips, breast, and chest are common.
d. Generalized bruises, lacerations, contusions, bite marks, nail marks.
e. The marks of rope knots on the wrists and ankles.

The examiner should strive to ascertain following:
a. Whether these marks are of injuries or self-inflicted.
b. Apparent development of victim's body.
c. Amount of resistance offered.
d. Corroboration with statement of the victim.

Examination of nails: Scraping from the nails beds constitutes important evidence. Tags of epithelium, hairs, piece of clothes, and bloodstains are important to collect.

Gait: The victim's gait must be made a note. If consent is available, the victim's blood should be collected for grouping. This will help in ascertaining whether bloodstains are of the victim or assailant. A second examination after 48 hours may reveal deep bruises, which may not be evident at the first examination.

Examination of genitals: A gynecological examination should be conducted in lithotomy position and in good light. The history of last menstrual period must be asked for to differentiate menstruation from bleeding due to injuries.

Local signs of violence:

Pubic hair: Pubic hair may be combed for foreign hairs. Pubic hair matted due to seminal stains, blood or secretions may be cut and preserved. Stains of blood or semen from skin must be scraped bluntly and preserved.

Collection of vaginal secretions: Instillation of 15 mL of normal saline in posterior fornix and aspiration of contents can be collected and examined. A wet preparation when studied under microscope may reveal motile or nonmotile spermatozoa. Absence of spermatozoon does not mean absence of intercourse. Ziehl–Neelsen staining of another slide may reveal acid fast, rod-shaped organisms, which are *Smegma Bacilli*.

Evidence of venereal disease: The examiner should keep in mind the signs of various venereal diseases such as syphilis, gonorrhea, chancroid, etc.

Injuries: Hymen—especially in virgin victim examination of hymen is important. Signs of recent rupture of hymen are ragged edematous edges of the hymen and hemorrhage.

Examination of vagina: Distensibility of vagina should be noted in relation to number of fingers it admits. The character and extent of injury will vary in proportion to:
a. Disproportion of male and female organ.
b. Whether victim is virgin or not.
c. Extent of penetration.
d. Amount of force.

Lacerations of posterior fourchette are very commonly associated with forceful intercourse especially with a virgin. Finger penetration may lead to lateral vaginal wall tears.

Bruising and lacerations in the vagina also must be recorded properly. Absence of injuries may be due to inability of the survivor to offer resistance to the assailant because of intoxication or threats. Pictorial representation of these injuries can be very helpful for corroborative evidence.

Question 8

1. What is the role of POCUS in traumatic ocular injury?

Point-of-care ultrasonography (POCUS) helps to detect wide variety of ocular pathologies from trauma such as dislocated lens, globe disruption, vitreous hemorrhage, hyphemia, retinal detachment, orbital emphysema, retrobulbar hemorrhage. Suspected globe rupture is a relative contraindication to USG examination due to risk of extruding globe contents with direct pressure on and around the eye.

Globe rupture: Distortion of normal shape of globe, decrease in size of globe, anterior chamber collapse, and vitreous hemorrhage.

Lens dislocation: Highly reflective oval mass moving, independently of the surrounding, structure with eye movement.

Hyphema: Echoic structure of variable echogenicity, depending on age of bleed.

Retrobulbar hemorrhage: Echo lucent posterior to globe.

2. Discuss classification of shock in trauma.

The physiologic effects of hemorrhage are divided into four classes based on clinical signs, useful for estimating the acute blood loss. The following classification system is useful in emphasizing the early signs and pathophysiology of the shock state **(Table 6)**:

a. *Class I hemorrhage:* <15% blood volume loss (usually occurs in those donated 1 unit of blood)
b. *Class II hemorrhage:* 15-30% blood volume loss (uncomplicated mild hemorrhage for which crystalloid fluid resuscitation is required).
c. *Class III hemorrhage:* 31-40% blood volume loss (complicated moderate hemorrhagic state in which at least crystalloid infusion is required and also blood replacement).
d. *Class IV hemorrhage:* >40% blood volume loss (severe hemorrhage form in which patient will need aggressive resuscitative measures. Blood transfusion is required).

TABLE 6: Signs and symptoms of hemorrhage by class based on ATLS 2018 guidelines.

Parameter	Class I	Class II (Mild)	Class III (Moderate)	Class IV (Severe)
Approximate blood loos	<15%	15–30%	31–40%	>40%
Heart rate	↔	↔/↑	↑	↑/↑↑
Blood pressure	↔	↔	↔/↓	↓
Pulse pressure	↔	↓	↓	↓
Respiratory rate	↔	↔	↔/↑	↑
Urine output	↔	↔	↓	↓↓
Glasgow coma scale score	↔	↔	↓	↓
Base deficit	0 to –2 mEq/L	–2 to –6 mEq/L	–6 to –10 mEq/L	–10 mEq/L or less
Need for blood products	Monitor	Possible	Yes	Massive transfusion protocol

Question 9

1. Discuss inhalational injury management in ED.

Inhalation injuries cause formation of casts, reduction of available surfactant, increased airway resistance, and decreased pulmonary compliance. Patients require aggressive measures to keep airway free of mucus and other secretions, e.g., chest physiotherapy, airway suctioning, therapeutic serial bronchoscopies, and early aggressive ambulation. Bronchodilators that are useful in the treatment of inhalation injury include albuterol or levalbuterol for wheezing/bronchospasm and racemic epinephrine for stridor or retractions, typically administered every 4 hours **(Table 7)**.

2. Explain the ED management of a patient with suspected corneal injury.

Majority of the corneal abrasion heals spontaneously, so the primary aim is to relieve pain and prevent infection. Topical NSAIDs such as ketorolac and diclofenac relieve pain. Topical tetracycline—one drop hourly for 24 hours to prevent infection. Patching of the eye does not provide healing, but some patients feel better. Abrasions from fingernails, vegetable matter or contact lens should not be patched as it may increase the risk of infection. If abrasion is large and spasm is marked, consider topical cyclopentolate 1%—one drop—3 times a day along with topical antibiotics. Large and small abrasion in the central visual axis should be checked by ophthalmologist within 24 hours and 48-72 hours respectively.

TABLE 7: Smoke inhalation injury.

Injury subtype	Mechanism	Clinical consequences	Treatment
Upper airway Injury	Thermal burn from heat transfer	Airway edema and obstruction	• Titrate humidified oxygen to maintain saturation >90% if airway obstruction
Lower airway parenchyma	Chemical and particulate irritants	• Fibrin cast obstruct the airways • Inflammation • Ventilation perfusion mismatch • Atelectasis • Bronchospasm	• Definitive airway management • Bronchodilators • Fiber optic bronchoscopy to evaluate lower respiratory tract inhalation injury • Respiratory physiotherapy and mucolytics • Weaning ventilation • Extubation planning
Systemic cellular dysfunction due to carbon monoxide and cyanide exposure	Asphyxia and hypoxia	• Lactic acidosis • CNS insult • CVS insult	

(CNS: central nervous system; CVS: cardiovascular system)

The common chemical injury to eye is alkali, acid, and cyanoacrylate (super glue). Alkali injuries tend to be more serious than acid injuries because they cause liquefactive necrosis that allows deep penetration into tissue. In case of acid injuries, it causes coagulative necrosis that acts as a barrier to further tissue penetration.

Treatment: Irrigation at the scene and continue in the ER. Instill topical anesthetic and continue irrigation for at least 30 minutes. Patient with chemosis/chemical conjunctivitis apply erythromycin ointment—4 times a day.

Topical cyclopentolate 1%—one drop—3 times a day to relieve pain.

Administer tetanus toxoid. Consider doxycycline 100 mg BD and topical corticosteroids to reduce corneal melting and corneal inflammation respectively.

In case of cyanoacrylate (super glue): Install generous amount of erythromycin ointment onto the eye and surrounding the eyelid to moisture, lubricate, and antibiotic coverage.

Clumps of glue begin to loosen, remove only those pieces that are easily removable. Gentle traction may separate the lids. Glue will loose and become easier to remove in a few days.

Refer to ophthalmologist within 24 hours for complete removal.

Question 10

1. Discuss management of patient with life-threatening cervical spine injury.

Nonoperative management of spinal cord injury: Traditionally, all spinal cord injuries were treated nonoperatively with a spinal brace for a period of 6-8 weeks combined with bed rest. With advances in radiology and surgical techniques, many patients are being operated.

Operative intervention: Indication, principle, and timing of surgery—indications of operative interventions are: 1. Neurological deficit and 2. Unstable spine. The goals of surgery are: Decompression to relieve pressure, ensure adequately sized canal, and fix the vertebral column after aligning the bones. Surgery entails removal of the fragments in the canal thereby relieving cord pressure. Fixation is done with rods, plates, and screws to 1-2 levels above and below the fractured.

Timing of decompression: Studies showed improvement in neurology with two or greater grade improvement over 3-6 months after early, i.e., <24 hours decompression, the results have been better mainly in cervical spine injury.

Spinal instability: White and Panjabi described three subsystems for stability: Passive—spinal column; Active—spinal muscles and tendons; Control—neural feedback.

2. Discuss spinal cord syndromes.

Incomplete spinal cord syndrome (ISCS) occurs when lesions involve specific structural and/or functional anatomic regions of the cord, with some preservation of sensory and/or motor function below the lesion **(Fig. 6)**. The clinical presentation of the incomplete spinal cord syndromes is largely determined by the involvement of the three tracts—corticospinal tract, spinothalamic tract, and posterior column of the spinal cord. There are eight types of incomplete spinal cord syndromes based on clinical presentations: *1. Central cord syndrome; 2. Brown–Séquard syndrome (unilateral cord syndrome); 3. Anterior cord syndrome; 4. Posterior syndrome; 5. Caudal equine syndrome; 6. Conus medullaris syndrome; 7. Subacute combined degeneration myelopathy; and 8. Cruciate paralysis. Central cord syndrome occurs due to syringomyelia, anterior cord syndrome due to anterior spinal artery occlusion, and posterior cord syndrome due to posterior spinal artery occlusion.*

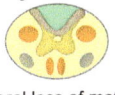

Fig. 6: Incomplete spinal cord syndromes.

SUGGESTED READING

1. Richhariya D, Sharma B. Textbook of Emergency Medicine including Intensive Care and Trauma, 2nd edition. New Delhi: Jaypee Brothers Medical Publishers (P) Ltd; 2022. pp. 355, 1615. (Question 1).
2. Richhariya D, Sharma B. Textbook of Emergency Medicine including Intensive Care and Trauma, 2nd edition. New Delhi: Jaypee Brothers Medical Publishers (P) Ltd; 2022. p. 702. (Question 2).
3. Richhariya D, Sharma B. Textbook of Emergency Medicine including Intensive Care and Trauma, 2nd edition. New Delhi: Jaypee Brothers Medical Publishers (P) Ltd; 2022. pp. 1603-14. (Question 3).
4. Richhariya D, Sharma B. Textbook of Emergency Medicine including Intensive Care and Trauma, 2nd edition. New Delhi: Jaypee Brothers Medical Publishers (P) Ltd; 2022. pp. 1079, 1112-3. (Question 4).
5. Richhariya D, Sharma B. Textbook of Emergency Medicine including Intensive Care and Trauma, 2nd edition. New Delhi: Jaypee Brothers Medical Publishers (P) Ltd; 2022. pp. 925, 938. (Question 5).
6. Richhariya D, Sharma B. Textbook of Emergency Medicine including Intensive Care and Trauma, 2nd edition. New Delhi: Jaypee Brothers Medical Publishers (P) Ltd; 2022. pp. 657, 900. (Question 6).
7. Richhariya D, Sharma B. Textbook of Emergency Medicine including Intensive Care and Trauma, 2nd edition. New Delhi: Jaypee Brothers Medical Publishers (P) Ltd; 2022. pp. 20, 138-41. (Question 7).
8. Richhariya D, Sharma B. Textbook of Emergency Medicine including Intensive Care and Trauma, 2nd edition. New Delhi: Jaypee Brothers Medical Publishers (P) Ltd; 2022. pp. 1533, 1555. (Question 8).
9. Richhariya D, Sharma B. Textbook of Emergency Medicine including Intensive Care and Trauma, 2nd edition. New Delhi: Jaypee Brothers Medical Publishers (P) Ltd; 2022. pp. 899-906. (Question 9).
10. Richhariya D, Sharma B. Textbook of Emergency Medicine including Intensive Care and Trauma, 2nd edition. New Delhi: Jaypee Brothers Medical Publishers (P) Ltd; 2022. pp. 1570-2. (Question 10).

Emergency Medicine Paper 43

Shweta Tyagi

Question 1

1. Discuss etiology and management of acute febrile illness.

It is the elevation in core body temperature exceeding the daily variation with a rise in hypothalamic set point. Normal temperature variation—at 6 AM, maximal normal body temperature is 37.2°C (98.9°F) while at 4 PM to 6 PM, maximal normal body temperature is 37.7°C (99.9°F). Normal circadian variation is 0.5°C or 1°F.

Fever of unknown origin (FUO): Fever of unknown origin has multiple origins. It was derived in 1961 by Petersdorf and Beeson as—duration of fever for at least 3 weeks, fever >38.3°C on several occasions, uncertain diagnosis despite of 1 week of investigations in hospital.

Hyperpyrexia: Body temperature >41.5°C or 106.7°F is termed as hyperpyrexia, usually seen in central nervous system (CNS) hemorrhages, heat stroke, neuroleptic malignant syndrome, serotonin syndrome, etc.

Fever with chills and rigors: Rise in hypothalamic set point → neurons in vasomotor center gets activated → cutaneous vessels of hands and feet vasoconstricts → shunting of blood away from periphery to the internal organs essentially decreases heat loss from the skin and the person may shiver violently. Once the higher temperature is reached, heat loss starts and cutaneous vessels dilate for dissipation of heat. Patient feels hot and sweating starts. The pathophysiology of fever is shown in **Flowchart 1**.

Etiology

It is broadly classified as:

Infectious Causes

Fever with chills and rigors is most suggestive of infection. *Viral* such as dengue, viral hepatitis, cytomegalovirus, Epstein–Barr virus, human immunodeficiency virus (HIV) infection, etc.; *bacterial* such as typhoid fever, tuberculosis, abscesses in any organ, infective endocarditis; *parasitic* causes such as malaria, amebiasis, toxoplasmosis; *unusual infections*—rickettsiosis, brucellosis, legionellosis, leptospirosis, Lyme disease; *fungal* infections.

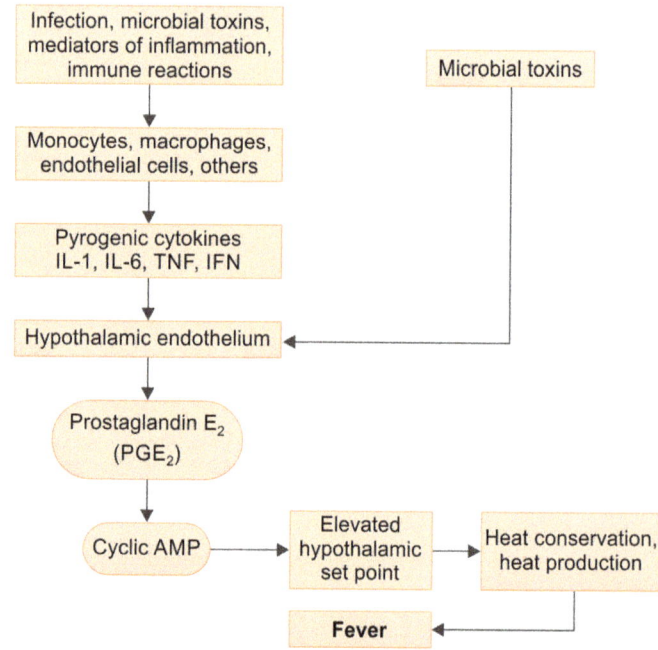

Flowchart 1: Pathophysiology of fever.

(IFN: interferon; IL: interleukin; PGE$_2$: prostaglandin; TNF: tumor necrosis factor; AMP: adensoine 5 monophosphate)

Tropical fever: It is also termed as monsoon fever, the fever which is seen in tropical and subtropical areas. Diseases to be considered are malaria, dengue, scrub typhus, rickettsiosis, leptospirosis, and enteric fever. Tropical fevers have very high morbidity and mortality rate. Symptoms overlap and it is difficult to differentiate at the time of presentation. Empiric therapy needs to be initiated at the time of onset. *HIT WIDE AND HIT EARLY.*

Noninfectious Inflammatory Causes

Autoimmune conditions: Mixed connective tissue disorders, systemic lupus erythematous, rheumatoid arthritis, relapsing polychondritis, polymyositis, antiphospholipid syndrome, ankylosing spondylitis, and sarcoidosis.

Vasculitis: Churg-Strauss syndrome, Takayasu arteritis, giant cell arteritis, allergic vasculitis.

Malignant conditions: Most commonly seen with malignancies of reticuloendothelial origin such as leukemia and lymphoma. Other causes such as multiple myeloma, plasmacytoma, myelodysplastic syndromes, renal cell carcinoma, malignant histiocytosis, aleukemic leukemia can also present only with FUO; solid tumors and metastasis from breast, colon, lung, and pancreas.

Thermoregulatory disorders: Central (brain tumor, encephalitis, stroke) and peripheral (exercise-induced hyperthermia, hyperthyroidism).

Less Common Causes

Factitious fever—artificially induced by the patient, e.g., intravenous injections by contaminated water, more common in young women working as health care professionals.

Drug fever is relatively a common condition but remains frequently undiagnosed. Usually associated with rash and eosinophilia (seen in 25% cases) but may not be always present. Drugs like barbiturates, antibiotics like carbapenems, cephalosporins, minocycline, nitrofurantoin, and vancomycin.

Evaluation

Importance of a good history, physical examination, and focused laboratory testing makes the diagnosis in majority of cases. *History* should be taken from the patient or from the person most familiar with the patient. Duration of fever, onset of fever, associated localizing sign and symptoms, significant weight loss, night sweats should be asked. Pattern of fever is important. Special focus should be on history of recent travel, exposure to pets, and intake of raw milk, immunosuppression, and drugs including antimicrobials, presence of skin rash, eschar, high risk behavior, and contact to a patient having tuberculosis.

History of presence of oral ulcers and joint pains. General and systemic examination in detail is must. Special focus should be on musculoskeletal system if diagnosis is uncertain. Hydration and perfusion status are also assessed. Presence of hemorrhagic manifestations, erythematous mottling of skin, facial flushing, signs of circulatory failure or vascular permeability, lymphadenopathy gives an idea of the illness.

Investigations

- *Routine:* Complete hemogram with differential, erythrocyte sedimentation rate (ESR), chest X-ray, liver function test (LFT), renal function test (RFT), specific investigations pertaining to tropical fever syndrome such as dengue serology, malarial antigen, Weil Felix, brucella serology, blood cultures, urine routine and microscopy, ultrasound abdomen.
- *Specific:* Sputum microscopy and culture, lactate dehydrogenase (LDH), tuberculin test, anti-nuclear antibodies (ANA), extractable nuclear antigen (ENA) profile, triglycerides, prostate specific antigen, ferritin levels, serum protein electrophoresis. Lumbar puncture and cerebrospinal fluid (CSF) analysis in clinically indicated cases.
- *Serological:* Epstein–Barr virus (EBV), polymerase chain reaction (PCR), cytomegalovirus (CMV), HIV
- *Radiological:* Contrast-enhanced computerized tomography (CECT) chest and abdomen, CECT brain/magnetic resonance imaging (MRI) brain
- *Transoesophageal echo* if indicated to look for infective endocarditis
- *Bone marrow aspiration and biopsy.*
- *Positron emission tomography-computed tomography (PET CT) scan of whole body, biopsy* of lymph nodes or any significant soft tissue swelling if other tests are elusive.

Treatment

- Main objective is to reduce the elevated hypothalamic set point and facilitate the heat loss from the body.
- Majority of fever are self-limiting, e.g., viral fever.
- Antipyretics are indicated in all kinds of fever for symptomatic relief.
- Cooling blankets have role in hyperpyrexia.
- Treat the underlying cause.
- Specific therapy of malaria to be started only when peripheral smear or rapid diagnostic test for malaria is positive. Empirical therapy is not indicated.
- Antibiotics in case of enteric fever (drug of choice—ceftriaxone).
- Empirical therapy for typhoid, scrub typhus, and leptospirosis is to be initiated at the earliest.
- Role of glucocorticoids, nonsteroidal anti-inflammatory drugs (NSAIDS), disease-modifying antirheumatic drugs (DMARDs), biological agents used in autoimmune conditions.

2. Explain inotropic support in patient with septic shock.

Inotropes are used to raise the cardiac contractility, cardiac output and mean arterial pressure (MAP). Dobutamine is an inotrope that causes vasodilation. It increases myocardial oxygen consumption like isoproterenol. *Dobutamine* is useful in severe, medically refractory heart failure, and cardiogenic shock. It is also useful in pharmacological cardiac stress testing. *Isoproterenol* also is an inotropic and chronotropic agent rather than a vasopressor. The drug high affinity for β-2 adrenergic receptor causes vasodilation and a decrease in MAP. Therefore, it is useful in hypotension due to bradycardia.

Dobutamine → 0.5–1 µg/kg/min, → 2–20 µg/kg/min, → 20–40 µg/kg/min; doses >20 µg/kg/min are not recommended in heart failure and should be reserved for salvage therapy.
a. Initial agent of choice in cardiogenic shock with low cardiac output and maintained blood pressure.
b. Add-on to norepinephrine for cardiac output augmentation in septic shock with myocardial dysfunction.
c. Increases cardiac contractility and rate; may cause hypotension and tachyarrhythmias.
d. Must be diluted; a usual concentration is 250 mg in 500 mL dextrose 5% in water (D5W) OR normal saline (NS) (0.5 mg/mL)

Milrinone: 0.125–0.75 µg/kg/min
a. Alternative for short-term cardiac output augmentation to maintain organ perfusion in cardiogenic shock refractory to other agents.
b. Increases cardiac contractility and heart rate at high doses; may cause peripheral vasodilation, hypotension and/or ventricular arrhythmias.
c. Renally cleared; dose adjustment in renal impairment needed.
d. Must be diluted; e.g., a usual concentration is 40 mg in 200 mL D5W (200 µg/mL).

Question 2

1. Discuss the pathophysiology and management of paraquat poisoning.

Highly toxic herbicide, common agent for self-harm in Asian countries (lethal in small amounts, cheap, available), leading single agent causing death from pesticide poisoning in many countries occurs sporadically elsewhere, >50% case fatality rate. Paraquat is rapidly but incompletely absorbed and then largely eliminated unchanged in urine within 12–24 hours.

Pathophysiology: Paraquat generates reactive oxygen species which cause cellular damage via lipid peroxidation, activation of nuclear factor kappa B (NF-κB), mitochondrial damage and apoptosis in many organs, actively taken up against a concentration gradient into lung tissue leading to pneumonitis and lung fibrosis. Paraquat also causes renal and liver injury.

Clinical features ulceration of the mucous membranes (paraquat tongue), esophageal perforation, nausea, sweating, vomiting, tremors, convulsions, pulmonary edema, cardiovascular collapse, renal failure (early), liver dysfunction with abnormal LFTs, acute alveolitis over 1–3 days followed by a secondary fibrosis (3–7 days) with death at up to 5 weeks. Ingestion of large amounts of liquid concentrate (>50–100 mL of 20% ion w/v) results in fulminant organ failure and death (hours to days). Ingestion of smaller quantities usually leads to toxicity in the two key target organs (kidneys and lungs) developing over the next 2–6 days (still >50% mortality).

Management:
- *Investigations* paraquat assay, sodium dithionite test on urine (if changes color to blue → confirms urine paraquat concentration >1 mg/L, indicates a very poor prognosis) complete blood count, LFT, lipase, coagulation profiles (multi-organ dysfunction) CT chest endoscopy.
- *If presenting within 4 hours of ingestion:* Airway breathing circulation of emergency management, administer single dose-activated charcoal/Fuller's earth 30%, 250 mL Q 4 hourly → until comes out in stools or activated charcoal, avoid giving oxygen (theoretically could induce oxygen free radical formation and subsequent injuries). Send urine for sodium dithionite test (a semiquantitative test which may help in prognosis. Lighter blue reaction indicates chances of survival/ingestion within few hours back). (Rest same as in presenting within 6 hours). Gastric lavage is contraindicated owing to corrosive nature of paraquat.
- *If presenting within 6 hours of ingestion:* Airway breathing circulation management in emergency, extracorporeal techniques such as hemoperfusion, hemodialysis may be tried. (Hemoperfusion > hemodialysis). Corticosteroids, N-acetylcysteine, vitamin C, vitamin E are theoretically useful drugs and may be tried on case-to-case basis.
- *Cases presenting late* or showing strong reaction with sodium dithionite test may be given supportive management/palliative care. Cases may deteriorate within a week of ingestion due to multiorgan damage, requiring ventilator support/hemodynamic support.

2. Discuss high flow oxygen therapy in emergency department (ED).

Oxygen support therapy should be given to the patients with acute hypoxic respiratory insufficiency in order to provide oxygenation of the tissues until the underlying pathology improves. Maximum flow rate of 15 L/min is produced by low flow and high flow conventional oxygen support systems and FiO_2 changes depending on the patient's peak inspiratory flow rate, respiratory pattern, the mask that is used, or the characteristics of the cannula. The inspiratory flow rate requirement of patients with respiratory insufficiency varies between 30 and 120 L/min. The inability to provide adequate airflow leads to discomfort in patients. High-flow nasal oxygen (HFNO) cannulas are able to delivered warmed and humidified air matching the body temperature with the regulated flow rates of 5–60 L/min, and oxygen delivery varies between 21 and 100%.

Studies show that physiological parameters are improved with HFNO treatment when compared to conventional oxygen systems. Although there are studies indicating successful applications in different patient groups, there are also studies indicating that it does not create any difference in clinical parameters, but patient comfort is better in HFNO when compared with standard oxygen therapy and noninvasive mechanical ventilation (NIMV).

Question 3

1. Explain the approach to a case of acute dysentery in an adult patient in ED.

Bacterial infections are by far the most common causes of dysentery. These infections include *Shigella*, *Campylobacter*, *Escherichia coli*, and *Salmonella* species of bacteria. The frequency of each pathogen varies considerably in different regions of the world.

While evaluating a patient at bedside it is more useful to ascertain whether it is small bowel diarrhea or large bowel diarrhea because that guides you to further evaluation and proper management. Frequency and volume are most important points in history. Voluminous stools 3–6 times a day are suggestive of small bowel origin while more frequent but scanty stools are suggestive of large bowel origin. Next are contents. Presence of blood/mucous suggests large bowel, i.e., colitis while profuse watery diarrhea suggests small bowel, i.e., enteritis. Crampy abdominal pain can be present in both but tenesmus points to a large bowel/rectal origin. A detailed history will go a long way in providing clue to the cause of diarrhea and one can manage.

Physical examination: Goal of the physical examination is to assess the patient's degree of dehydration. Generally ill appearance, dry mucous membranes, delayed capillary refill time, increased heart rate, and abnormal orthostatic vital signs can be helpful in identifying more severe dehydration. Fever is more suggestive of inflammatory diarrhea. The abdominal examination is important to assess for pain and acute abdominal processes. A rectal examination may be helpful in assessing for blood, rectal tenderness, and stool consistency.

Investigations: Hardly any investigations are required in routine cases. Stool routine and culture may be advised if there is suspicion of invasive diarrhea based on presence of fever and blood in stools. Hemogram and RFT must be done if patient is dehydrated. A film for malarial parasite may be handy if there is high fever with chills as sometimes malaria can present as diarrhea (algid malaria).

Treatment: Mainstay of treatment of acute diarrhea is restoring/maintaining fluid and electrolyte balance.

2. Describe the role of biomarkers in cardiac ischemia.

Cardiac markers for diagnosis and risk stratification: Timing of cardiac markers—in patients with symptoms consistent with acute coronary syndrome (ACS):

- Immediately send blood samples for cardiac troponin I (cTnI) or cardiac troponin T (cTnT)
- Reassess cTnI or cTnT 3–6 hours after symptom onset
- *After 6 hours:* If initial and serial cTn values are normal, and/or patient has electrocardiogram (ECG) changes, and/or patient is in immediate/high risk category
- *Day 3 or 4:* In patients with myocardial infarction (MI) to assess infarct size.

An increased cTn suggests myocardial cell injury but does not throw light on cause of the injury as cTn values increase in many other cardiac/noncardiac causes. Imaging techniques such as angiography are used to find the cause and actual site of injury.

Role of other cardiac markers in ACS diagnosis: Other cardiac markers include creatinine kinase (CK), myoglobin, and B-type natriuretic peptide (BNP). The sensitivity and specificity of CK levels for cardiac damage are lower compared to other markers as raised CK levels are usually associated with many noncardiac conditions as well. CK myocardial isoenzyme (CK-MB) is useful for early diagnosis of acute MI. Unlike CK level, CK-MB is more specific to cardiac injury but it cannot help in ascertaining infarct size; however, it is useful in detecting early reinfarction. CK-MB and myoglobin are not required if contemporary troponin assays are being performed as they do not add any additional diagnostic value. BNP or N-terminal (NT)-pro hormone BNP (NT–pro-BNP) is sometimes done in patients with suspected ACS to assess risk and as a prognostic marker.

Question 4

1. Discuss etiology, evaluation, and management of an elderly patient with acute delirium.

Delirium is defined as acute onset fluctuating changes in cognition, attention, and awareness, changes are rapid in onset within hours or day and usually reversible. Patient of delirium typically presents as inattention, disorganized thinking, perception disturbance, and altered conscious level (somnolent or agitated). Elderly group is increased risk of mortality if delirium is missed in emergency department.

Confusion assessment methods (CAM): First described by Inouye and colleagues in 1990 based on the *Diagnostic and Statistical Manual of Mental Disorders Revised 3rd edition* (DSMIIIR) criteria, helpful for nonpsychiatric-trained physician to diagnose delirium quickly and accurately. CAM consists of four components:
a. Acute onset mental status changes fluctuating course
b. Inattention
c. Disorganized thinking and
d. Altered level of consciousness. First two components are mandatory and either of two from rest of two necessary for diagnosis of delirium.

Diagnosis: Delirium is a clinical diagnosis, so thorough history and physical examination is a must for the diagnosis. Compared to the patient's baseline, acute onset of attention deficits and cognitive abnormalities, fluctuating in course is virtually diagnostic of delirium.

Screening tools: Delirium triage screen (incorporates the Richmond Agitation-Sedation Scale) and highly specific *Brief Confusion Assessment Method.*

Treatment **(Flowchart 2)**

2. Discuss evaluation and management of metabolic alkalosis.

Metabolic alkalosis may not show any symptoms. People with this type of alkalosis more often complain of the underlying conditions that are causing it. These can include—vomiting diarrhea swelling in the lower legs (peripheral edema) fatigue. Severe cases of metabolic alkalosis can cause—agitation disorientation seizures coma. The severe symptoms are most common when the alkalosis is caused by chronic liver disease. The causes of metabolic alkalosis can be summarized in **Table 1**.

Flowchart 2: Approach to management of delirium.

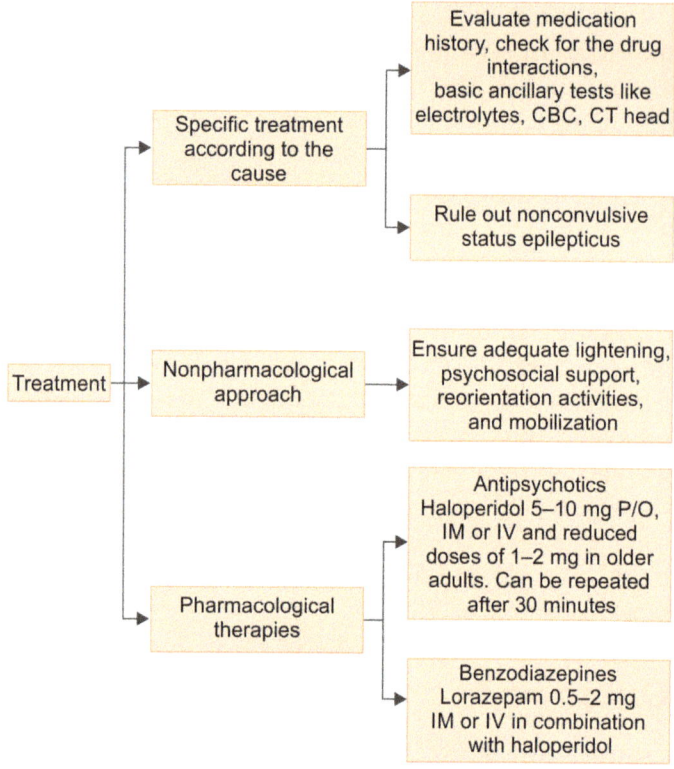

(CBC: complete blood count; CT: computed tomography; IM: intramuscular; IV: Intravenous)

TABLE 1: Causes of metabolic alkalosis.

Chloride sensitive	Chloride resistant	Miscellaneous
• Gastrointestinal—vomiting gastric drainage chloride diarrhea villous adenoma • Renal—diuretics posthypercapnic • Low chloride intake • Cystic fibrosis	• Increased mineralocorticoid activity: Primary/secondary hyperaldosteronism • Cushing's syndrome, Bartter's syndrome • Severe hypokalemia	• Massive blood transfusion • Acetate containing colloids • Alkali therapy • Hypercalcemia: Milk alkali syndrome, bone metastatic

Question 5

1. Discuss evaluation and management of hypoglycemia in ED.

Management of hypoglycemia in ED or a prehospital setup includes prompt diagnosis and per oral (PO) or IV administration of rapidly metabolized carbohydrates (glucose or dextrose).
- In patients with altered mental status, 50% dextrose in water is administered IV as a bolus dose of 50 mL, which provides 25 g of glucose.
- After 15 minutes, if hypoglycemia persists, repeat the dose.

- If the patient regains consciousness, and blood sugar is >70 mg/dL, continue carbohydrates (PO administration of long-acting carbohydrates) to prevent recurrence.
- If the blood sugars have normalized but the patient is still unconscious or drowsy, continue IV infusion of dextrose (5% dextrose in water), to maintain CBG >100 mg/dL.
- Check CBG every 30 minutes for the first 2 hours, looking for rebound hypoglycemia.
- Infusion can be reduced or eventually withdrawn, if hypoglycemia is maintained by slow administration of dextrose.

For sulfonylurea-induced hypoglycemia, *octreotide is the treatment of choice.*

Octreotide:
- Octreotide, a somatostatin analog and is able to suppress insulin secretion immediately and negates the effects of the sulfonylurea.
- *Dose:* 50–100 μg, subcutaneous for a single episode. If recurrent episodes 50–100 μg subcutaneous once every 6–8 hours or constant infusion of 125 μg/h.
- Octreotide is given after the initial glucose therapy is inadequate. It is primarily given to reduce the risk of recurrent hypoglycemia.

Diazoxide:
- Also used in treatment of refractory sulfonylurea-induced hypoglycemia.
- *MOA:* Acts directly by inhibiting insulin secretion from pancreatic β-cells.
- *Dose:* 300 mg over 30 minutes every 4 hours as a slow IV infusion.
- May cause hypotension.

2. Explain the type of restrained to calm the agitated patient in ED.

Initial assessment of the agitated patient should prioritize safety, with adequate screening of the patient for weapons, interview conducted in a room that allows privacy without compromising security, easily accessible entry and exit points for the provider and readily available personnel and protocols for appropriate restraint and intervention, as necessary. The ED physician should consider the use of verbal de-escalation tactics first when the situation allows, and the patient appears to be receptive and cooperative. These include communicating with the patient in a calm, concise, respectful manner while avoiding provocative statements, threats, and condescension. If verbal techniques fail to manage the patient's agitation, the use of restraint should be considered. Typically, chemical restraint is preferable to physical restraint, but these may be used in combination as appropriate for the severely combative patient. Pharmacologic options traditionally incorporate antipsychotic agents and benzodiazepines. Classically, first-generation (typical) antipsychotics such as haloperidol (2.5–5 mg IM/IV) were used. However, second-generation (atypical) antipsychotics, such as olanzapine (10 mg IM or 5–10 mg PO) have been shown in recent studies to perform better with lower rates of adverse events compared to first-generation antipsychotics. Commonly used benzodiazepines include lorazepam (2–4 mg IM/IV) and midazolam (2.5–5 mg IM/IV). All medication used to control agitation should aim to calm, not sedate the patient, and can be titrated up to achieve the desired effect. Physical restraint, when applied, should be done so in a systematic, team-based approach with coverage of five points (four limbs and head) and avoidance of prone positioning. In any form of restraint, post-restraint monitoring and evaluation should be implemented to assess for any adverse effects from the intervention to the patient and progression of patient condition.

Question 6

1. Discuss evaluation and management of disseminated intravascular coagulation (DIC).

Disseminated intravascular coagulation is due to abnormal activation of intravascular coagulation along with fibrinolysis activation leading to disseminated intravascular coagulation with concurrent fibrinolysis. This can lead to bleeding due consumption and depletion of coagulation factors along with accelerated fibrinolysis. The activation of intravascular coagulation can also lead to thrombosis. It usually occurs due to a systemic abnormal exposure of procoagulant in conditions like sepsis, malignancy like acute promyelocytic leukemia, trauma, intrauterine uterine death of fetus, viper bite. Clinically it can present with the underlying condition along with features of bleeding from cannula sites, catheters site, mucous membranes and sometimes with organ dysfunction with renal dysfunction, liver function abnormalities. Sometimes especially in chronic DIC as in malignancies like the DIC associated with pancreatic cancer presentation can be due to thrombosis. Lab abnormalities in various permutations and combinations reflect the systemic activation of coagulation along with concurrent activation of fibrinolysis as shown by prolonged PT/APTT/low fibrinogen levels/increased d-dimer/thrombocytopenia/evidence of microangiopathic hemolysis in the peripheral smear. The treatment involves that of treating the underlying condition like antibiotics for sepsis. Prevention of bleeding includes prophylactic platelet transfusion with target platelet counts above 20,000/μL in the absence of bleeding. In the presence of bleeding or in the preparation of an invasive procedure it is important to keep platelets above 50,000/μL. In presence of bleeding fibrinogen has to be maintained above 100 mg/dL with the help of cryoprecipitate and if PT/APTT is prolonged then freash frozen plasma (FFP) should be transfused.

2. Discuss oral anticoagulants and their role in acute deep vein thrombosis (DVT).

Warfarin (Vitamin K antagonists VKAs): A hydroxycoumarin derivative, which is commonly used as oral anticoagulant. Warfarin has both antithrombotic effect by inhibiting the synthesis of factor II, VII, IX, and X and a prothrombotic effect through inhibition of protein C and S production, but during maintenance therapy, the overwhelming effect is one of the anticoagulations. It is suggested to add parenteral anticoagulant during the first 3–5 days of warfarin treatment. Its dosing is guided by desired therapeutic range if INR of 2–3 in most of cases. Drug interactions with warfarin are numerous and complex. Bleeding and skin necrosis are two major complications. The risk is clinically significant when the INR is >4.5–5. Major limitations of vitamin K antagonist lead to development of various new direct thrombin inhibitors.

Novel oral anticoagulants (NOAC)/direct thrombin inhibitors (DTI) non-vitamin K antagonist: Direct thrombin inhibitors were developed to overcome the limitations of vitamin K antagonist, used in high-risk patient including stroke and with atrial fibrillation. Currently five direct acting oral anticoagulants are available.

- *Dabigatran oral direct thrombin inhibitor,* which is used to reduce the risk of stroke and systemic embolism with nonvalvular atrial fibrillation. It has more predictable pharmacology activity than warfarin and broad therapeutic window. It is safer than warfarin, with notable exception of higher risk of major gastrointestinal (GI) bleeding. For practical purposes, a normal *thrombin clotting time* excludes a significant coagulopathy due to dabigatran.
- *Apixaban, Rivaroxaban Betrixaban, and Edoxaban*— these oral *direct factor Xa inhibitors* have predictable pharmacological properties that do not require routine laboratory monitoring. Currently used for prevention of thromboembolism in patients undergoing hip or knee replacement surgery and reduction of systemic embolism in nonvalvular atrial fibrillation. Currently available *antifactor Xa* activity assay can be used specifically for their activity.

Question 7

1. Explain the evaluation and management of blood transfusion reactions in ED.

Acute transfusion reactions occur during or shortly after (within 24 hours) the transfusion. World Health Organization (WHO) has broadly categorized acute transfusion reactions according to their severity and the appropriate clinical response—mild, moderate to severe and life-threatening transfusion reactions.

Category 1: Mild reactions
- Mild hypersensitivity—allergic, urticarial reactions

Category 2: Moderate to severe reactions
- Moderate to severe hypersensitivity (severe urticarial reactions)
- Febrile nonhemolytic reactions—antibodies to white cell or platelet antigens; antibodies to proteins, including Immunoglobulin A (IgA)

Category 3: Life-threatening reactions
- Acute intravascular hemolysis
- Bacterial contamination and septic shock
- Fluid overload
- Anaphylactic reactions
- Transfusion-associated acute lung injury (TRALI)
- Transfusion-associated circulatory overload (TACO).

Delayed complications of transfusion: Delayed transfusion reaction occurs days to month even years after transfusion. As with acute transfusion reactions, the consequence may be severe but often treatable. Delayed reactions can be classified into following types:
- Transfusion-transmitted infections
  - Alloimmunization [against red cell or human leukocyte antigen (HLA) antigens]
- Delayed hemolytic reaction
- Posttransfusion purpura
- Graft-versus-host disease
- Iron overload (in patients who receive repeated transfusions).

Management of adverse transfusion reaction: When an acute reaction first occurs, it may be difficult to decide on its type and severity as the signs and symptoms may not initially be specific or diagnostic. However, with the exception of allergic urticarial and febrile nonhemolytic reactions, adverse reactions are potentially fatal and require urgent treatment. It is essential to monitor the transfused patient closely in order to detect the earliest clinical evidence of an acute transfusion reaction. In an unconscious or anesthetized patient, hypotension and uncontrolled bleeding may be the only signs of an incompatible transfusion. In a conscious patient undergoing a severe hemolytic transfusion reaction, signs and symptoms may appear very quickly—within minutes of infusing only 5–10 mL of blood. Close observation at the start of the infusion of each unit is essential. If an acute transfusion reaction is suspected, stop the transfusion immediately. Check the blood unit labels and the patient's identity. If there is any discrepancy, consult the blood bank.

2. What is treating malignant hypertension in ED?

Hypertensive emergency (malignant hypertension): Severe hypertension with evidence of acute target organ failure. Clinical presentation of hypertensive emergencies in emergency department is associated with different diseases and they manifest in various forms such as pulmonary edema myocardial ischemia, aortic dissection, preeclampsia hypertensive encephalopathy. Controlled blood pressure (BP) reduction to target goals should be achieved in order to prevent organ damage. Care should be taken to not lower blood pressure rapidly and to normal levels. The therapeutic approach should be to refrain from a rapid reduction in BP as this approach has been found to be associated with considerable morbidity. Clinical presentation guides the choice of antihypertensive agents in hypertensive emergencies.

Question 8

1. Discuss approach to a patient with monkey bite in ED.

In India, most of the human rabies cases occur due to bite of a rabid dog. There is also possibility of contracting rabies through the bites of cats, **monkey**, horses, sheep, goat, etc. As a prerequisite to transmission, the saliva of the biting animal must contain the virus at the time of bite.

Postexposure prophylaxis (PEP) for rabies: Human rabies is essentially a fatal disease once the clinical signs develop, although 100% preventable. Rabies PEP consists of thorough wound care along with administration of modern anti-rabies vaccine and rabies immunoglobulin. This is highly effective if carried out systematically and diligently. If a person has received pre-exposure prophylaxis (PrEP), then it eliminates the need for rabies immunoglobulin (RIG) in case of an exposure. The key to survival is administration of PEP as soon as possible. A patient with category III exposure needs thorough wound cleansing and a first dose of vaccine along with rabies immunoglobulin on the day of bite or day of reporting **(Table 2)**. The vaccination is done according to one of the WHO approved schedules to achieve a serum antibody titer of >0.5 IU/mL which is considered acceptable according to WHO. In case of any confusion regarding exposure it is always better to give overtreatment rather than undertreatment for prevention of rabies.

TABLE 2: Postexposure prophylaxis in rabies.

Categories	Nature of contact	Recommended treatment — Unknown, sick, proven, wild animal	Recommended treatment — Healthy animal
I	Touching or feeding animals, licks on intact skin no mucous membrane exposure	None	None
II	Nibbling of uncovered skin, minor scratches or abrasions without bleeding	Modern tissue culture rabies vaccine	Modern tissue culture rabies vaccine
III	Single or multiple transdermal bites or scratches, contamination of mucous membrane or broken skin with saliva from animal licks, exposure due to direct contact with bats	• Modern tissue culture rabies vaccine • And rabies immunoglobulins (RIG)	• Modern tissue culture rabies vaccine • And RIG

- Start preexposure vaccination particularly in children and others likely to have repeated animal contact, and are at a risk of dog bites.
- Start full treatment on first day and discontinue vaccine if animal is alive and well on day 10, or if it has been found rabies negative on reliable laboratory examination. Encourage patient to return for another dose of vaccine on day 21, so that a full pre-exposure series has been completed.
- If there is significant delay in presentation or if the patient is immunosuppressed, it may appropriate to double the first dose of vaccine. Administration of two ampoules of vaccine, one in each arm, on day 0.

2. Enumerate the management of needle stick injury in healthcare worker in ED.

- *Immediate actions to be taken.* Do not panic, do not put cut/pricked finger.
  Post-HIV exposure management/prophylaxis (PEP): It is necessary to determine the status of the exposure and the HIV status of the exposure source before starting PEP immediate measures: Wash with soap and water, no added advantage with antiseptic/bleach.
  Next step: Prompt reporting, postexposure treatment should begin as soon as possible, preferably within 2 hours, not recommended after 72 hours. Late PEP? May be yes. Is PEP needed for all types of exposures? NO.
- *Initial base line investigations to be done:* Initial base line investigations of exposed HIV I and II hepatitis B virus

surface antigen (HbsAg) hepatitis C virus (HCV) anti-hepatitis B surface (HBS). The health care provider should be tested for HIV as per the following schedule baseline HIV test—at time of exposure repeat HIV test—at 6 weeks following exposure second repeat HIV test—at 12 weeks following exposure. On all three occasions, Pre- and post-test counseling must be provided by Health Care Worker (HCW). HIV testing should be carried out on three ERS (ELISA/Rapid/Simple) test kits or antigen preparations. The HCW should be advised to refrain from donating blood, semen or organs/tissues and abstain from sexual intercourse. In case sexual intercourse is undertaken a latex condom should be used consistently. In addition, women HCW should not breastfeed their infants during the follow-up period.

- *Which medicines/injections you would like to give him immediately?:* The decision to start PEP is made on the basis of degree of exposure to HIV and the HIV status of the source from whom the exposure/infection has occurred.
  Basic regimen: Zidovudine (AZT)—600 mg in divided doses (300 mg/twice a day or 200 mg/thrice a day for 4 weeks + Lamivudine (3TC)—150 mg twice a day for 4 weeks
  Expanded regimen: 4 weeks therapy, basic regimen (+ Indinavir—800 mg/thrice a day, or any other protease inhibitor)
- *How to follow him up?:* PEP should be started, as early as possible, after an exposure. It has been seen that PEP started after 72 hours of exposure is of no use and hence is not recommended. The optimal course of PEP is not unknown, but 4 weeks of drug therapy appears to provide protection against HIV. If the HIV test is found to be positive at any time within 12 weeks, the HCW should be referred to a physician for treatment.

TABLE 3: Toxidrome: Common toxic syndrome.

Drugs	Common syndromic features
Cholinergic: (Organophosphorus carbamates insecticides physostigmine edrophonium some mushroom)	Confusion CNS depression weakness salivation lacrimation urinary/fecal incontinence GI cram vomiting muscle fasciculation pulmonary edema miosis bradycardia/tachycardia seizure
Anticholinergics: Antihistamine antiparkinsonians, atropine scopolamine amantadine antipsychotics antidepressants antispasmodics muscle relaxants	Delirium tachycardia dry flushed skin, dilated pupil myoclonus, temperature, urinary retention diminished bowel sound, seizure
Sympathomimetics: Cocaine amphetamines methamphetamines, decongestant in cough syrup (phenylpropanolamine, ephedrine, pseudoephedrine)	Delusion, paranoia tachycardia hypertension hyperpyrexia diaphoresis mydriasis hyperreflexia seizure hypotension arrhythmias
Opioid/sedative/ethanol: Narcotics, barbiturates benzodiazepines ethchlorvynol glutethimide, ethanol clonidine meprobamate	Respiratory depression, hypotension, miosis bradycardia hypothermic, pulmonary edema diminished bowel sound hyporeflexia seizure coma
Salicylates	Fever, metabolic acidosis, respiratory alkalosis, tinnitus, and altered sensorium
Serotonins: SSRI, TCA, and MAOI	Hyperreflexia, clonus, sweating, tremor, flushing, and hypertension

(CNS: central nervous system; GI: gastrointestinal; MAOI: monoamine oxidase inhibitors; SSRI: selective serotonin reuptake inhibitors; TCA: tricyclic antidepressants)

Question 9

1. Describe various toxidromes presenting to ED.

Toxidromes-toxic syndrome: Toxidrome word is used when a specific class of toxin/chemical/poison produces a group of signs and symptoms. Toxidromes are helpful in identifying the particular toxins and narrow down the differential diagnosis when history is uncertain or inadequate. On the basis of these toxidromes (group of signs and symptoms specific to toxins) physicians incorporates appropriate diagnostic tests and treatment into their management plan. But confusing mixed syndrome picture appears in cases of polydrug overdoses. Common toxidromes are anticholinergic syndrome, sympathomimetic syndrome, opioid/sedative/ethanol syndrome, cholinergic syndrome, and serotonin syndrome. Salient features of common toxidromes are listed in **Table 3**.

2. Discuss management of cannabinoid hyperemesis syndrome.

Cannabinoid hyperemesis syndrome (CHS) is a condition in which a patient develops cyclical nausea, vomiting, and abdominal pain after long-term use of cannabis. Many studies categorize CHS into three phases—prodromal, hyperemetic, and recovery. The prodromal, or pre-emetic phase, is characterized by early morning nausea without emesis and abdominal discomfort. Management includes **(Flowchart 3)**:

- Intravenous fluid replacement for dehydration.
- Medicines to help decrease vomiting and relieve anxiety benzodiazepines.
- Pain medicine.
- Proton-pump inhibitors to treat stomach inflammation.
- Frequent hot showers.

Flowchart 3: Approach to management cannabinoid hyperemesis syndrome.

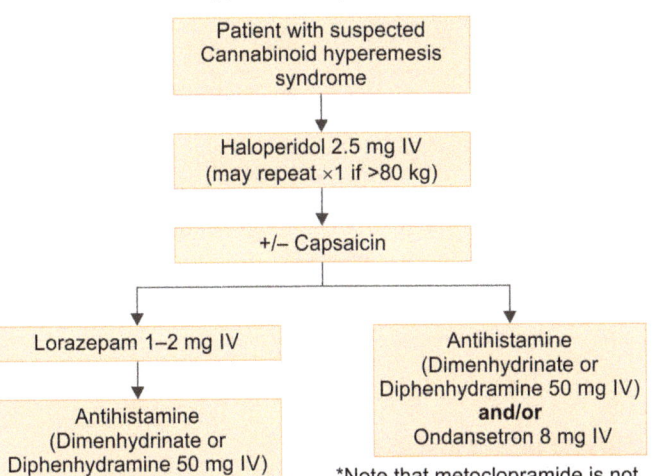

of the vagal nerve and sympathetic withdrawal. Both of this cause a slowing conduction through the AV node, thus helping in blocking re-entry. A physical examination to rule out a carotid bruit is necessary. Resuscitation equipment should be ready. Attach the monitor for continuous ECG monitoring. Pressure is applied in a firm circular manner at the level of the cricoid cartilage for about 5 seconds. Repeat the procedure on the opposite side if the tachyarrhythmia persists.

Drug therapy: Antiarrhythmic drugs which are helpful for immediate control **(Table 4)** and long-term maintenance therapy **(Table 5)** are summarized in tables below.

Catheter ablation: Catheter ablation has a very high success rate (>95%) and a low recurrence rate (<5%) in patients with accessory pathways. Complications of catheter ablation include perforation, bleeding, AV fistula, venous thrombosis, pulmonary embolism, myocardial perforation, valve damage, systemic embolism and rarely, death.

Question 10

1. Discuss management of supraventricular arrhythmias.

Vagal maneuvers: Carotid sinus massage stimulates baroreceptors triggering a reflexive increase in the activity

2. Discuss drug therapy in a COVID patient, hypoxic and nonhypoxic, at time of ED presentation.

Progression of illness due to severe acute respiratory syndrome coronavirus-2 (SARS-CoV-2) is classified in to three categories—mild, moderate, and severe. Treatment approach based on severity is shown in **Table 6**.

TABLE 4: Drugs therapy for immediate control of SVT.		
Drugs	**Doses**	**Side effects**
SVT without preexcitation		
Adenosine	Give 6 mg rapid intravenous followed by fluid bolus; if no response within 1–2 minutes, give 12 mg more	Facial flushing, chest pain, and hypotension common; transient asystole bronchospasm atrial fibrillation ventricular fibrillation
Verapamil	5 mg every 3–5 minimum, to maximum 15 mg	Hypotension, heart block, inotropic effect negative
Diltiazem	0.25 mg/kg of body weight over a 2-minutes period; if no response, additional dose of 0.35 mg/kg over a 2-minutes period; maintenance infusion of 5–15 mg/h	Hypotension, heart block, inotropic effect negative
Metoprolol	5 mg over a 2-minutes period; up to 3 doses in 15 minutes	Hypotension, heart block, bradycardia bronchospasm
SVT with preexcitation or WPW with AF		
Procainamide	30 mg/min continuous infusion to a maximal dose of 17 mg/kg (maintenance infusion of 2–4 mg/min)	Hypotension, widening of QRS complex, torsade de Pointes
Flecainide	2 mg/kg over a 10-minutes period	Negative inotropic effect conducting atrial flutter, widening of QRS
Ibutilide	If ≥60 kg: 1 mg over a 10-minutes period if <60 kg: 0.01 mg/kg over a 10-minutes period, repeat once if no response after 10 minutes	Prolongation of QT interval, torsade de Pointes

(AF: atrial fibrillation; SVT: supraventricular tachycardia; WPW: Wolff-Parkinson-White)

TABLE 5: Drugs for long term management of SVT.

Drugs	Doses	Side effects	Contraindication
SVT without preexcitation			
• Beta-blockers • Metoprolol atenolol	50–200 mg daily 80–240 mg daily	Hypotension and heart block	Asthma, CHF
• Calcium channel blockers • Diltiazem verapamil	180–360 mg daily 120–480 mg daily	Hypotension and heart block	CHF
Digoxin	0.125–0.375 mg daily	Digitalis toxicity	Preexcitation
SVT with pre-excitation			
First-line drugs: • Flecainide • Propafenone	100–300 mg daily 450–900 mg daily	VT enhanced AV nodal conduction interaction with digoxin	Ischemic and structural heart disease
Second-line drugs: • Amiodarone • Sotalol	200 mg daily 160–320 mg daily	Skin discoloration thyroid dysfunction GI pulmonary and hepatotoxicity corneal deposit tremor optic neuritis Hypotension heart block bradycardia	

(CHF: congestive heart failure; SVT: supraventricular tachycardia)

TABLE 6: COVID patient treatment nonhypoxic (mild cases) and hypoxic (moderate-severe) cases.

Mild	• No oxygen dependency • No respiratory distress • Room air SpO$_2$ >95% • No hypotension • No multiorgan involvement	• Balanced diet • Adequate sleep • Breathing exercises • Remain physically active • Hot water gargles 3 times a day • Positive mood and outlook • In case of symptoms seek medical advice • Monitor saturation with pulse oximeter • Temperature monitoring and paracetamol as needed • Multivitamins *Zinc, Vitamin C, Vitamin D*
Moderate–Severe	• Oxygen dependency/± Respiratory distress • Tachypnea RR >24 • SpO$_2$ <93% on room air • In severe disease progression— • Presence of hypotension • Shock and multiorgan involvement • Septic shock—persisting hypotension in spite of volume resuscitation requiring vasopressor to maintain MAP >65	• *Target SpO$_2$:* 92–96% (88–92% in patients with COPD) • The device for administering oxygen (nasal prongs, mask, or masks with breathing/nonrebreathing reservoir bag) depends upon the increasing requirement of oxygen therapy. If HFNC or simple nasal cannula is used, N95 mask should be applied over it. • Awake proning may be used as a rescue therapy. • Tab dexamethasone 6 mg/day orally for 10 days OR • IV dexamethasone 20 mg/day intravenous (IV) × 5 days followed by 10 mg/day IV × 5 days; titrate dose and duration to culmination of oxygen dependency • LMWH (low molecular weight heparin)

(COPD: chronic obstructive pulmonary disease; HFNC: high-flow nasal cannula)

SUGGESTED READING

1. Richhariya D, López Tapia JD, Bajan K, Sharma B. Signs and Symptoms in Clinical Practice. 1st edition. New Delhi: Jaypee Brothers Medical Publishers (P) Ltd; 2020. Chapter 40. (Question 1).
2. Richhariya D, Sharma B. Textbook of Emergency Medicine including Intensive Care and Trauma, 2nd edition. New Delhi: Jaypee Brothers Medical Publishers (P) Ltd; 2022. p. 339. (Question 1).
3. Richhariya D, Sharma B. Textbook of Emergency Medicine including Intensive Care and Trauma, 2nd edition. New Delhi: Jaypee Brothers Medical Publishers (P) Ltd; 2022. pp. 245, 1399. (Question 2).
4. Richhariya D, Sharma B. Textbook of Emergency Medicine including Intensive Care and Trauma, 2nd edition. New Delhi: Jaypee Brothers Medical Publishers (P) Ltd; 2022. pp. 435, 651. (Question 3).

5. Richhariya D, Sharma B. Textbook of Emergency Medicine including Intensive Care and Trauma, 2nd edition. New Delhi: Jaypee Brothers Medical Publishers (P) Ltd; 2022. pp. 815, 306. (Question 4).
6. Richhariya D, Sharma B. Textbook of Emergency Medicine including Intensive Care and Trauma, 2nd edition. New Delhi: Jaypee Brothers Medical Publishers (P) Ltd; 2022. pp. 867, 1050. (Question 5).
7. Richhariya D, Sharma B. Textbook of Emergency Medicine including Intensive Care and Trauma, 2nd edition. New Delhi: Jaypee Brothers Medical Publishers (P) Ltd; 2022. pp. 536, 983. (Question 6).
8. Richhariya D, Sharma B. Textbook of Emergency Medicine including Intensive Care and Trauma, 2nd edition. New Delhi: Jaypee Brothers Medical Publishers (P) Ltd; 2022. pp. 514, 990. (Question 7).
9. Richhariya D, Sharma B. Textbook of Emergency Medicine including Intensive Care and Trauma, 2nd edition. New Delhi: Jaypee Brothers Medical Publishers (P) Ltd; 2022. p. 1345. (Question 8).
10. Richhariya D, Sharma B. Textbook of Emergency Medicine including Intensive Care and Trauma, 2nd edition. New Delhi: Jaypee Brothers Medical Publishers (P) Ltd; 2022. p. 1395. (Question 9).
11. Richhariya D, Sharma B. Textbook of Emergency Medicine including Intensive Care and Trauma, 2nd edition. New Delhi: Jaypee Brothers Medical Publishers (P) Ltd; 2022. pp. 478, 626. (Question 10).

Emergency Medicine Paper 44

Jidhin Janardhanan

Question 1

1. What should be the choice of fluid for resuscitation of a trauma victim in the ER based on recent trials?

The controversy of crystalloid versus colloid for resuscitation still remains, but as per recent studies balanced crystalloids are the choice of fluids in a trauma victim in the emergency room (ER), though balanced crystalloids contain lactate and acetate, are buffered solutions, and have less chloride compared to normal saline. Common modifications of isotonic fluids include use of acetate instead of lactate in Ringer's solution.

Packed red blood cells (PRBCs) are the most commonly transfused blood product, if the patient is in hemorrhagic shock. Using only PRBCs in a patient with traumatic shock and ongoing bleeding (without plasma and platelets) will do little to promote hemostasis and may not restore tissue oxygenation. If the hemorrhage is definitively controlled, do not transfuse if the hemoglobin concentration is >10 g/dL. Consensus recommendation for transfusion is a hemoglobin concentration between 6 and 7 g/dL (60–70 g/L) for those without cardiopulmonary, cerebral, or peripheral vascular disease. For a hemoglobin concentration between 6 and 10 g/dL (60–100 g/L), use clinical judgment for transfusion.

2. Discuss the introduction of ECMO unit in the ER.

Extracorporeal membrane oxygenation (ECMO), also known as extracorporeal life support (ECLS), is a recent introduction in the management of cardiac arrest. Its use is well documented in the neonatal and pediatrics population, and in adults for refractory respiratory failure and cardiogenic shock. Use in refractory cardiac arrest is also known as extracorporeal cardiopulmonary resuscitation (ECPR). ECPR is a bridging therapy to definitive treatments, such as percutaneous coronary interventions, cardiac bypass surgery, or heart transplant. The ECMO equipment consists of a blood pump, a venous reservoir, an oxygenator for exchanging both oxygen and carbon dioxide, and a heat exchanger to warm the blood used. The whole system is monitored through pressure, oxygen saturation, and temperature monitors. Three types of ECMO circuits are available:

a. *Venoarterial ECMO (VA ECMO):* It pumps blood from the venous side to the arterial side to facilitate gas exchange and provide hemodynamic support. The blood is pumped from the venous circulation through a cannula inserted in either the inferior vena cava or the right atrium, through the oxygenator where gas exchange occurs and then warmed and returned to the patient through a cannula placed in either the aortic arch or the femoral artery into the arterial circulation. This is the modality that is used to support cardiac arrest patients.

b. *Venovenous (VV ECMO):* It removes blood from the right atrium, passes it through the gas exchanger, and returns it across the tricuspid valve into the right ventricle. It does not provide hemodynamic support. This modality is used mainly for refractory respiratory failure.

c. *Arteriovenous ECMO (AV ECMO):* It makes use of the patient's own arterial pressure to pump the blood from the arterial to the venous side and facilitates gas exchange in the process. This does not require the use of a separate blood pump.

Indications: (a) Good premorbid condition before cardiac arrest, (b) intervention to be curative and not palliative, and (c) reversible trigger event for cardiac arrest [dysrhythmia, ST-elevation myocardial infarction (STEMI), etc.]

Contraindications: Advanced age; advanced malignancy; poor baseline neurologic function; baseline inability to perform activities of daily living; preexisting "do not resuscitate" order, suspect aortic dissection, or severe aortic regurgitation; traumatic cardiac arrest, unwitnessed cardiac arrest, and no bystander cardiopulmonary resuscitation (CPR); long pre-hospital transport time; and prolonged cardiac arrest unless good perfusion and metabolic support are documented.

Medical complications: These complications include intracranial and systemic hemorrhage, initial cardiac stunning that may occur soon after initiation of ECMO, pneumothorax, acute kidney injury, gastrointestinal bleeding, sepsis, and metabolic derangement.

Question 2

1. Discuss the management of a physiologically difficult airway in the ED.

The four physiologically difficult airways described include hypoxemia, hypotension, severe metabolic acidosis, and right ventricular failure. The emergency physician should account for these physiologic derangements with airway management in critically ill patients regardless of the predicted anatomic difficulty of the intubation.

1. *Hypoxia:* Patients with hypoxemic respiratory failure are at high risk for rapid desaturation during intubation, which may result in hemodynamic instability, hypoxic brain injury, and potentially cardiopulmonary arrest. Preoxygenation is an important step in every intubation. Preoxygenation and apneic oxygenation should be performed in all critically ill patients. Supraglottic airways may be considered when higher pressures are needed or a mask seal with nasal intermittent positive pressure ventilation (NIPPV) cannot be achieved. Nasal continuous positive airway pressure with a nasal mask may be useful in maintaining alveolar recruitment during intubation in patients at high risk.

2. *Hypotension:* For patients unresponsive to volume resuscitation, a norepinephrine infusion should be initiated. Peripherally administered vasopressor boluses can be prepared quickly at the bedside and may maintain blood pressure during intubation and resuscitation. This intervention has not been studied in critically ill adults; however, diluted epinephrine (given as 10–50 µg boluses with a concentration of 1–10 µg/mL) may be preferred due to its inotropic effect. For patients without shock who have a transient drop in blood pressure after intubation due to the vasodilatory effects of induction agents or transition to positive pressure ventilation, diluted phenylephrine (given as 50–200 µg boluses with a concentration of 100 µg/mL) may be useful.

3. *Severe metabolic acidosis:* A short trial of NIPPV may adequately support the respiratory work of breathing until correction of the underlying metabolic acidosis can occur and will provide an estimate of the patient's intrinsic minute ventilation by measuring the patient's respiratory rate and tidal volume delivered with each breath. Rapid-sequence intubation should be avoided if possible, and if one is deemed necessary, a short-acting neuromuscular blocker such as succinylcholine should be used.

4. *Right ventricular (RV) failure:* Bedside echocardiographic assessment of RV function should be performed to assess RV dysfunction versus RV failure. If the patient has some contractile reserve (RV dysfunction), cautious fluid resuscitation should be performed. The goals of mechanical ventilation include maintenance of a low mean airway pressure and avoidance of hypoxemia, atelectasis, and hypercapnia, which increase RV afterload.

2. Discuss the role of newer airway aides used by an emergency physician.

Several recommendations should be considered while managing emergency airways such as adequate hemodynamic monitoring, continuous capnometry, availability of functioning high-efficiency suction devices, and the implementation of checklists. Suction-assisted laryngoscopy and airway decontamination, known as the SALAD technique, advocates the use of suction along with emergency airway management to address the problem of massive airway contamination. The SALAD technique may be considered in a clinical setting such as regurgitation of gastric contents, copious secretions, postoperative upper airway bleeding, and upper gastrointestinal hemorrhage. It has also been used outside the operating room, in cases of upper airway hemorrhage or trauma.

a. *Point-of-care ultrasound (POCUS) in airway management:* POCUS imaging is an expanding area that has been recently applied to airway management, contributing to a reduction in morbimortality related to airway interventions. The assessment consists in placing the linear ultrasound probe transversely across the suprasternal notch and identifying the endotracheal tube cuff balloon. If there is esophageal intubation, there will be a "double tract sign" with two air-filled structures with acoustic shadowing. This evaluation can be further supported by thoracic ultrasonography, which confirms bilateral lung sliding.

b. *Artificial intelligence in airway management:* Robotic endoscope-automated laryngeal imaging for tracheal intubation (REALITI) is a video-endoscopic stylet that guides endotracheal intubation.

c. *Teleguided technology for intubation:* A scoping review of teleguided technology for endotracheal intubation elucidated the feasibility, barriers, and complications inherent to its use. Teleguided-facilitated intubation appears to be as effective as in-person supervision, with no further complications. It also has educational purposes, allowing progressive autonomy for the trainees.

d. *The future of extraglottic devices:* The Baska Mask™ is an extraglottic device that allows a perilaryngeal seal with a self-energizing sealing cuff. The intubating laryngeal tube (ILTS-D™) is a second-generation extraglottic device that allows laryngeal tube suction and the possibility of secondary tracheal intubation. The Video Laryngeal Mask™ and SafeLM™ are two examples of video laryngeal masks available. Their structure includes a disposable second-generation supraglottic airway device (SAD) with a silicone cuff, anatomically curved tube, reusable videoscope, and a monitoring screen.

e. *Video laryngoscope:* It is a new videoscope for airway management that was originally designed for combat medicine owing to its ready-to-use quality.
f. *Infrared red intubation system (IRRIS):* The technique consists of a small infrared light source (wavelength between 730 and 1,000 nm), placed on the anterior cervical surface, over the cricothyroid membrane. The device emits infrared red light through the skin of the patient skin to the subglottic space.
g. *Endotracheal tube and conductor:* It is a single-lumen endotracheal tube with an integrated high-resolution camera at its tip. The integrated camera provides visual assurance during intubation, enables continuous intraoperative tube evaluation, and monitors the bronchial blockers placement. The device is available in sizes of 7.0–8.0 mm.

Question 3

1. Discuss the evaluation and management of dehydration in a child presenting with diarrhea to the emergency department (ED).

Assessment of a child with dehydration: A child with diarrhea should be assessed for (a) dehydration, (b) blood in diarrhea, (c) coexisting malnutrition, and (d) serious non-intestinal infections.

History should focus on the duration of diarrhea and number of watery stools per day; volume of water in stool; presence of blood in the stool; frequency of urination; presence of vomiting, fever, cough, or seizures; preillness feeding practices; fluids, food, and drugs taken during illness; and immunization history.

Examination should include general condition of the child, signs of dehydration, nutritional status [weight/weight for height/mid-arm circumference (MAC)], severity of malnutrition, if any, and presence of blood in stool besides general, physical, and systemic examination. Classification of dehydration **(Table 1)** is of utmost importance in the management of dehydration.

Management of dehydration **(Table 2)** consists of assessment and correction of dehydration and correction of specific etiology besides symptomatic management. Since acute vomiting is mostly seen as a part of acute gastroenteritis, our discussion here will be focused on that.

Objectives: (a) Prevent and treat dehydration, (b) drugs (antibiotics, zinc), (c) nutritional management, and (d) education.

Indications for hospital admission are: (a) Shock, (b) severe dehydration, (c) neurological abnormalities (lethargy, seizures), (d) intractable or bilious vomiting, (e) failure of oral rehydration, (f) suspected surgical condition, and (g) conditions for a safe follow-up and home management are not met.

2. Discuss the management of a child with persisting drooling in the ED.

Drooling is a common occurrence in children with central nervous system and muscular disorders, such as cerebral palsy, facial nerve palsy, myasthenia gravis, and polymyositis. Prevention of excessive mouthing of fingers or objects helps reduce the stimulus of saliva production and encourages lip closure. Treatment options for moderate and severe drooling include physiotherapy, behavioral or biofeedback modification, pharmacotherapy, and surgery **(Flowchart 1)**.

TABLE 1: Classification of dehydration.

Severe dehydration (two of the following are present)	Some dehydration (two of the following are present)	No dehydration
Lethargy/unconscious	Restless, irritable	Not enough signs to classify some or severe dehydration
Sunken eyes	Sunken eyes	
Not able to drink/drinking poorly	Drinks eagerly, thirsty	
Skin pinch goes back very slowly	Skin pinch goes back slowly	

TABLE 2: Plan of treatment for dehydration.

Severe dehydration	Some dehydration	No dehydration
Plan C	Plan B	Plan A
Urgent care in hospital	Treat dehydration with ORS/IV fluid	Home care

(IV: intravenous; ORS: oral rehydration solution)

Flowchart 1: Approach to management of drooling in a child.

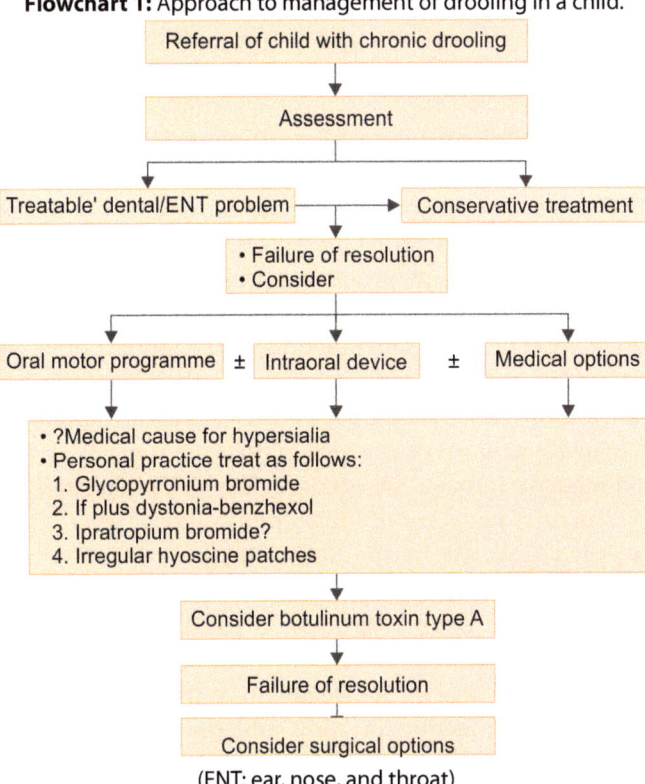

(ENT: ear, nose, and throat)

Question 4

1. Describe the pyramid of evidence-based medicine.

Figure 1 is given to help us understand how to weigh different levels of evidence in order to make health-related decisions. It helps us put the results of each study design into perspective, based on the relative strengths and weaknesses of each design. At the top of the pyramid is filtered evidence including systematic reviews, meta-analyses, and critical appraisals. These studies evaluate and synthesize the literature. The top of the pyramid represents the strongest evidence.

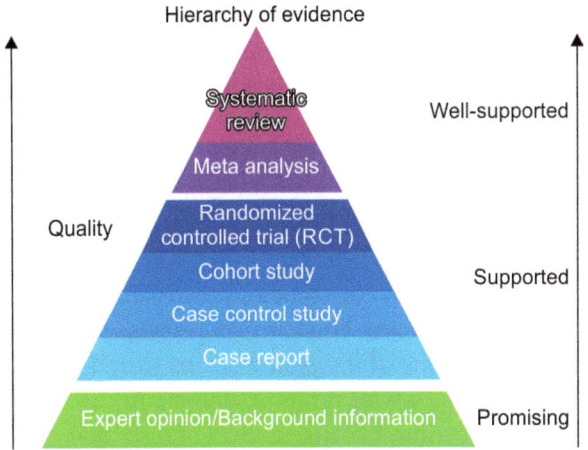

Fig. 1: Pyramid of evidence-based medicine.

2. Discuss the significance of *p* value.

The *p* value is defined as the probability under the assumption of no effect or no difference (null hypothesis), of obtaining a result equal to or more extreme than what was actually observed. *p* stands for probability and measures how likely it is that any observed difference between groups is due to chance:

p value <0.05 = Statistically significant difference

p value >0.05 = No statistically significant difference

Question 5

1. Discuss the role of an automated chest compressor device in the ED.

An automated chest compressor is a chest compression device composed of a constricting band and half backboard that is intended to be used as an adjunct to CPR during advanced cardiac life support by professional healthcare providers. The AutoPulse uses a distributing band to deliver the chest compressions **(Fig. 2)**.

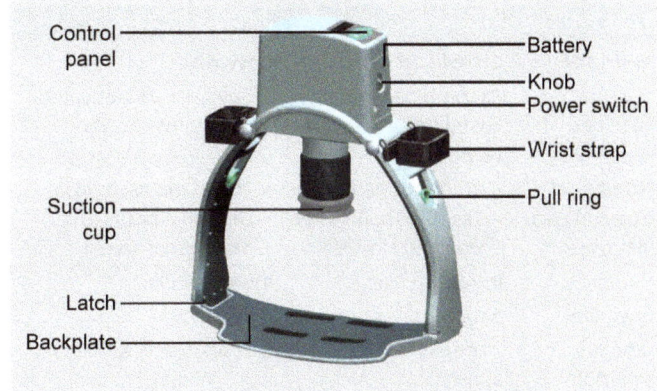

Fig. 2: Automated chest compressor device.

2. What are the interim guidelines for CPR in a COVID-19 patient in the ED?

Cardiopulmonary resuscitation in suspected or confirmed COVID-19 patients needs a modified approach as compared to the conventional approach.
a. In high-risk patients, proactively move the patient to a negative-pressure room, if available.
b. Consider "do-not-attempt CPR (DNACPR)" in patients with poor prognosis.
c. Limit the number of staff in the room.
d. Timely and clearly communicate COVID-19 status to any new providers.
e. If shockable rhythm, consider three attempts of shocks before wearing personal protective equipment (PPE) and starting chest compression.

f. Place an oxygen mask and supplement oxygen, if not done already.
g. Consider video laryngoscopy for intubation and pause chest compression during intubation.
h. Consider a mechanical compression device, if there is a need for prolonged CPR.
i. Ensure the safe removal of PPE.

Question 6

1. Write about any two COVID-19 vaccines.

Two COVID-19 vaccines (Covishield and Covaxin) were approved by India's top drug regulator for emergency and restricted use against COVID-19 on January 3, 2021. *Covishield* vaccine by Oxford University–AstraZeneca has an average efficacy of 70.4%. It is developed by the world's largest vaccine manufacturer, the Serum Institute of India. Against COVID-19, *Covaxin* is India's first home-produced vaccine developed by Bharat Biotech in collaboration with the Indian Council of Medical Research and the National Institute of Virology **(Table 3)**.

TABLE 3: Characteristics of Covishield and Covaxin vaccines.

Indicators	Covishield	Covaxin
Type of vaccines	Recombinant vaccine based on viral vector technology	Whole virion inactivated corona virus vaccine
Number of doses in each vial/dose	• 10/0.5 mL each dose • Discard 4 hours after opening of vials	• 10/0.5 mL each dose • Discard 4 hours after opening of vials
Route	Intramuscular	Intramuscular
Shelf life	6 months	6 months
Course/schedule	2 doses/6–8 weeks apart	2 doses/6–8 weeks apart
Storage and transportation	+2 to +8°C at all levels	+2 to +8°C at all levels
Adverse events following immunization (AEFI)	• Injection site tenderness, headache, fatigue, myalgias malaise, pyrexia, chills • Paracetamol may be used for symptomatic relief	• Injection site tenderness, headache, fatigue, myalgias, malaise, pyrexia, chills, nausea, vomiting, dizziness, giddiness, sweating • Paracetamol may be used for symptomatic relief

2. Discuss newer COVID variants.

Omicron: New variant of SARS CoV-2 (severe acute respiratory syndrome coronavirus-2): Mutation at spike protein region makes the variant attain the potential to develop an immune escape mechanism. The omicron variant has more than 30 mutations in the spike protein region. This variant is a major cause of concern because most of the vaccine works by forming antibodies against spike proteins, so vaccines have to be reviewed. There are possibilities of decreased efficacy of the existing COVID-19 vaccines. Structural changes have been observed in the omicron variant which is indicative of adherence to the same cellular receptors with increase in affinity and transmission.

Oxygen and steroid still remain the promising drugs. Apart from the Favipiravir, which is described earlier in this chapter, two new promising drugs Molnupiravir and Paxlovid are investigational drugs for the treatment of SARS CoV-2. Molnupiravir is an oral drug which inhibits multiple ribonucleic acid (RNA) viruses including SARS CoV-2 and is most effective when used early. Paxlovid, a protease inhibitor, is an investigational drug which inhibits the viral replication at proteolysis (a stage that occurs before viral replication).

The drug regulator of India approved two new COVID vaccines, Covovax by the Serum Institute of India and Corbevax by Biological E, for restricted use in an emergency situation. The Drug Regulator of India also approved Molnupiravir, an oral drug, which has shown promising results in early use in the treatment of mild-to-moderate SARS CoV-2 infection in adult and reduces the risk of hospitalization and death.

Questions 7

1. Discuss the ER management of testicular torsion in a 6-year-old boy with sickle cell trait.

a. Testicular torsion is a time-sensitive emergency. Manual detorsion can be attempted before surgical intervention but should not delay surgical intervention. *Trials of manual detorsion* have been found to decrease ischemia time. Even if the testicle is manually detorsed, surgery is still required. Surgical exploration is the definitive management for testicular torsion. Before performing manual detorsion, it must be explained that the procedure is painful but, if successful, it will alleviate the pain. Analgesic medication, local analgesia injection (i.e., local lidocaine), or procedural sedation should be administered.
b. Stand at the foot of the bed or to the right of the patient. Holding the testicle between the thumb and index finger, rotate it in an outward direction (like opening a book) from medial to lateral. The initial attempt should be with one and a half full rotations (540°). Relief of pain is a positive end point. You can also reassess with bedside ultrasonography. If the pain worsens with detorsion in the medial to lateral rotation, detorse in the lateral to medial direction, because a third of testicular torsions occur with medial to lateral rotation.

2. Discuss the evidence from hypothermia trials after cardiac arrest.

The TTM2 (targeted temperature management-2) trial is the largest trial conducted to date, across 14 countries with more than 1,800 subjects, and published in 2021. It compared the effect of targeted hypothermia at 33°C to targeted normothermia at 37.5°C. Therapeutic hypothermia involves use of a servo-controlled device and blanket to lower the core body temperature by 3°C for 72 hours followed by a period of rewarming in which the temperature is increased by 0.5°C/hr for 6 hours until normothermia is achieved. Studies suggest that after achieving return of spontaneous circulation (ROSC) (period of global cerebral hypoxia–ischemia), mild- induced hypothermia is used as a neuroprotective and outcome-improving measure. Mild-induced hypothermia suppresses the many pathological processes leading to delayed cell death, including apoptosis (programmed cell death). Hypothermia reduces the release of excitatory amino acids and free radicals and decreases the cerebral metabolic rate for oxygen ($CMRO_2$) by about 6% for each 1°C reduction in core temperature. Hypothermia reduces the inflammatory response associated with the post-cardiac arrest syndrome.

Question 8

1. What is MIS-C in COVID-affected children?

Multisystem inflammatory syndrome in children (MIS-C) is a new entity in children characterized by unremitting fever >38°C and epidemiological linkage with SARS CoV-2.

WHO diagnostic criteria of MIS-C: Children and adolescents 0–18 years of age with fever ≥3 days and any two of the following features:
a. Rash or bilateral nonpurulent conjunctivitis or signs of mucocutaneous inflammation (oral, hands or feet)
b. Hypotension or shock
c. Features of myocardial dysfunction, pericarditis, valvulitis, or coronary abnormalities [including echocardiogram (ECHO) findings or elevated troponin/N-terminal pro-brain natriuretic peptide(NT-pro BNP)]
d. Evidence of coagulopathy [prothrombin time (PT), partial thromboplastin time (PTT), and elevated D-dimers]
e. Acute gastrointestinal problems (diarrhea, vomiting, or abdominal pain)
   i. *And* raised inflammatory markers such as erythrocyte sedimentation rate (ESR) (>40 mm), C-reactive protein (>5 mg/L), or procalcitonin
   ii. *And* no other possible microbial cause of inflammation, e.g., bacterial sepsis, staphylococcal or streptococcal shock syndromes
   iii. *And* evidence of recent COVID-19 infection [reverse transcription-polymerase chain reaction (RT-PCR), antigen test or serology positive], or likely contact with a COVID-19-infected patient

The following conditions must be excluded before making a diagnosis of MIS-C:
a. Tropical infections (malaria, dengue, scrub typhus, enteric fever)
b. Toxic shock syndrome (staphylococcal or streptococcal)
c. Bacterial sepsis

2. Discuss the anticipated injuries and ED management in a child falling on an outstretched hand.

FOOSH is the nickname for an injury caused by having "fallen onto an outstretched hand." These injuries are among the most common injuries affecting the hands and wrists that occur when trying to break a fall. Treatment of a FOOSH injury depends on its severity. The severity of FOOSH injuries can vary greatly depending on various factors:
a. Distal radius fracture
b. Radial or ulnar styloid fracture
c. Radial head fracture
d. Scapholunate tear
e. Scaphoid fracture
f. Distal radioulnar joint fracture
g. Hamate fracture
h. Synovitis
i. Cellulitis
j. Bruise
k. Clavicle or shoulder injury

Question 9

1. Discuss the management of long COVID syndrome.

Some people, especially those who had severe COVID-19, experience multi-organ effects or autoimmune conditions with symptoms lasting weeks, months, or even years after COVID-19 illness. Multiorgan effects can involve many body systems, including the heart, lung, kidney, skin, and brain **(Fig. 3)**. Long COVID symptoms are presented heterogeneously, so patients need to be closely monitored. In order to develop effective treatment strategies, holistic assessment is necessary to consider preexisting conditions and to identify specific symptoms. Symptom-based approach is followed in managing long COVID. Comprehensive assessment through medical history and examination is essential. It is recommended to obtain a complete assessment including full blood count, renal function test, C-reactive protein, liver function test, thyroid function, glycated hemoglobin (HbA1c), vitamin D, magnesium, B₁₂, folate, and ferritin levels. Robust clinical care also requires additional assessments for appropriate referrals to specialists. Importantly, while long COVID is diagnosed, other non-COVID-19-related diagnoses should also be considered unless they could be excluded. Appropriate treatments are provided according to clinical symptoms. Dietary supplements, such as vitamins and minerals, contain anti-inflammatory and anti-oxidative components, so they have become potential treatments for long COVID. A pilot study demonstrates that multivitamin supplements improve clinical symptoms among long COVID patients. Dietary supplements may also have beneficial effect in modulating systemic inflammation and immunity. Natural flavonoids such as luteolin and quercetin are promising immunomodulatory agents which have showed inhibitory effects on mast cells.

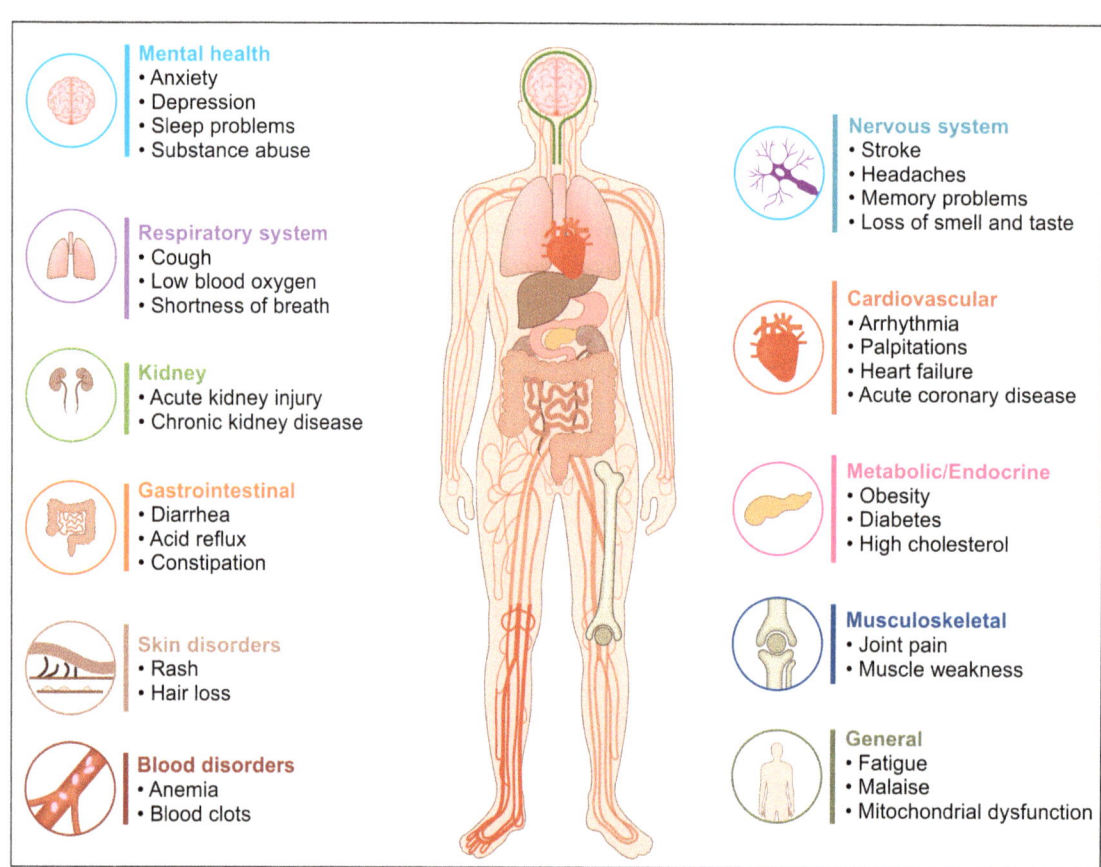

Fig. 3: Manifestation of long COVID syndrome.

2. Discuss the radiology of acute coronary syndrome.

Cardiac magnetic resonance (MR) imaging is an increasingly used technique for initial work-up of chest pain and early post-reperfusion and follow-up evaluation of acute coronary syndrome (ACS) to identify patients at high risk for further cardiac events. Coronary CT is an advanced cardiac noninvasive imaging modality with excellent diagnostic accuracy for the detection of coronary artery disease (CAD) and safe, efficient, and cost-effective tool. Coronary CT angiography (CTA) has been shown to be a highly sensitive test for the detection of CAD with negative predictive values approaching 97–99%. *Triple rule-out (TRO) CT examines coronary, pulmonary, and thoracic aorta in a single test* and is helpful in the diagnosing the fatal causes of acute chest pain such as acute pulmonary embolism and aortic dissection. *Coronary CT is an attractive modality for rapid triaging of chest pain*, reducing the hospitalization and being cost effective without compromising the safety and quality of care.

Question 10

1. Discuss the pediatric abdominal surgical emergencies.

Most of the abdominal surgical emergencies in children present with pain in abdomen, vomiting, distension, fever, and poor feeding. Due to the inherent difficulties involved in pediatric history taking and examination, the recognition of the urgency is often delayed. In 21.66% cases, the cause of acute abdomen is congenital and in 78.33% the cause is acquired. A long list of pathologies presenting with broadly the same symptoms can confuse and/or delay the physician from ordering the ideal singular diagnostic investigation and making a timely diagnosis **(Table 4)**. Morbidity and mortality in children vary with age and the condition.

TABLE 4: Nontraumatic cause of pediatric surgical abdomen.

Newborns (0–1 month)	• Duodenal obstruction • NNEC • Intestinal malrotation • Volvulus • Anorectal malformation • Hirschsprung's disease
Infants and toddlers (1 months to 2 years)	• IHPS • Intussusception • Obstructed hernia • Foreign body ingestion
Young children (2–5 years)	• Appendicitis • Meckel's causing intussusception • Foreign body ingestion • Intestinal obstruction? Band
Older children (3 years and older)	• Appendicitis • Cholecystitis • Pancreatitis • Abdominal cyst • Gonadal (ovarian/testicular torsion)

(IHPS: infantile hypertrophic pyloric stenosis; NNEC: neonatal necrotizing enterocolitis)

BOX 1: GRACE risk score for the entire spectrum of acute coronary syndromes (ACS).

Range: 1–372
Low risk: <109
Intermediate risk: 109–140
High risk: >141

Based on *eight variables at admission:*
a. Age
b. Heart rate
c. SBP
d. Serum creatinine
e. Killip class
f. Cardiac arrest
g. ST-segment deviation on ECG
h. Elevated cardiac enzymes/markers

(ECG: electrocardiogram; SBP: systolic blood pressure)

2. Discuss the GRACE guidelines for low-risk chest pain.

GRACE guidelines offer a pragmatic, evidence-based framework for shared decision-making in patients with recurrent low-risk chest pain **(Box 1)**.

SUGGESTED READING

1. Richhariya D, Sharma B. Textbook of Emergency Medicine including Intensive Care and Trauma, 2nd edition. New Delhi: Jaypee Brothers Medical Publishers (P) Ltd; 2022. pp. 347, 1535. (Question 1).
2. Richhariya D, Sharma B. Textbook of Emergency Medicine including Intensive Care and Trauma, 2nd edition. New Delhi: Jaypee Brothers Medical Publishers (P) Ltd; 2022. pp. 215-7. (Question 2).
3. Richhariya D, Sharma B. Textbook of Emergency Medicine including Intensive Care and Trauma, 2nd edition. New Delhi: Jaypee Brothers Medical Publishers (P) Ltd; 2022. pp. 1178-80. (Question 3).
4. Richhariya D, Sharma B. Textbook of Emergency Medicine including Intensive Care and Trauma, 2nd edition. New Delhi: Jaypee Brothers Medical Publishers (P) Ltd; 2022. pp. 80-90. (Question 4).
5. Richhariya D, Sharma B. Textbook of Emergency Medicine including Intensive Care and Trauma, 2nd edition. New Delhi: Jaypee Brothers Medical Publishers (P) Ltd; 2022. pp. 625-7. (Question 5).
6. Richhariya D, Sharma B. Textbook of Emergency Medicine including Intensive Care and Trauma, 2nd edition. New Delhi: Jaypee Brothers Medical Publishers (P) Ltd; 2022. pp. 629-30. (Question 6).
7. Richhariya D, Sharma B. Textbook of Emergency Medicine including Intensive Care and Trauma, 2nd edition. New Delhi: Jaypee Brothers Medical Publishers (P) Ltd; 2022. pp. 237, 789. (Question 7).
8. Richhariya D, Sharma B. Textbook of Emergency Medicine including Intensive Care and Trauma, 2nd edition. New Delhi: Jaypee Brothers Medical Publishers (P) Ltd; 2022. p. 1163. (Question 8).
9. Richhariya D, Sharma B. Textbook of Emergency Medicine including Intensive Care and Trauma, 2nd edition. New Delhi: Jaypee Brothers Medical Publishers (P) Ltd; 2022. pp. 625-7 (Question 9).
10. Richhariya D, Sharma B. Textbook of Emergency Medicine including Intensive Care and Trauma, 2nd edition. New Delhi: Jaypee Brothers Medical Publishers (P) Ltd; 2022. pp. 455, 1235. (Question 10).

Emergency Medicine Paper 45

Sreekrishnan TP

Question 1

1. Describe the pathophysiology of diabetic ketoacidosis versus hyperglycemic hyperosmolar syndrome.

Pathophysiology of diabetic ketoacidosis: Relative or absolute insulin deficiency in the presence of catabolic counterregulatory hormones (glucagon, catecholamines, growth hormones, and cortisol) is the basic underlying mechanism. This leads to hepatic overproduction of glucose, unrestrained hepatic fatty acid oxidation and release of free fatty acids into the circulation from adipose tissue (lipolysis), and production of ketone bodies [β-hydroxybutyrate (β-OHB) and acetoacetate], resulting in ketonemia and metabolic acidosis. Hyperglycemia results in osmotic diuresis leading to dehydration and loss of electrolytes.

Pathophysiology of hyperglycemic hyperosmolar syndrome (HHS): The development of HHS is attributed to three main factors: (a) Insulin resistance and/or deficiency, (b) an inflammatory state with marked elevation in pro-inflammatory cytokines (C-reactive protein, interleukins, tumor necrosis factors) and counter-regulatory hormones (growth hormone, cortisol) that cause increased hepatic gluconeogenesis and glycogenolysis, and (c) osmotic diuresis followed by impaired renal excretion of glucose. In a patient with type 2 diabetes, physiologic stresses combined with inadequate water intake in an environment of insulin resistance or deficiency lead to HHS. As serum glucose concentration increases, an osmotic gradient develops, attracting water from the intracellular space into the intravascular compartment, causing cellular dehydration.

2. Classify and describe the pathophysiology of lactic acidosis.

Cohen and Woods divided lactic acidosis into two categories: Type A and type B. Type A is lactic acidosis occurring in association with clinical evidence of poor tissue perfusion or oxygenation of blood (e.g., hypotension, cyanosis, cool and mottled extremities). Type A lactic acidosis is due to hypoxia in the setting of sepsis and poor tissue perfusion. It is a more serious diagnosis requiring blood pH <7.35 and serum lactate levels >45–54 mg/dL (>5–6 mmol/L). Type B lactic acidosis, however, happens in the absence of hypoxemia. Known causes include underlying liver disease (leading to decreased lactate clearance), thiamine deficiency, toxins (drugs), and malignancy. Avoid vasopressors when possible, for types A and B lactic acidosis because they worsen tissue ischemia.

Pathogenesis: Lactic acidosis occurs when lactic acid production exceeds lactic acid clearance. The increase in lactate production is usually caused by impaired tissue oxygenation, from either decreased oxygen delivery or a defect in mitochondrial oxygen utilization. The symptoms of lactic acidosis include abdominal or stomach discomfort, decreased appetite, diarrhea, fast and shallow breathing, a general feeling of discomfort, muscle pain or cramping, and unusual sleepiness, tiredness, or weakness. The pathway of lactate production is summarized in **Flowchart 1**.

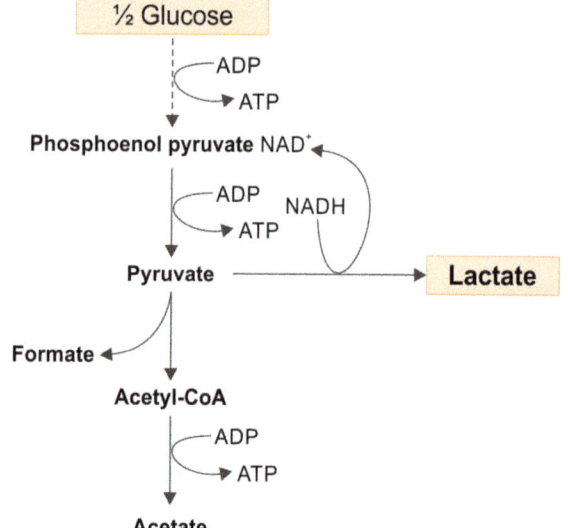

Flowchart 1: Lactate production pathways.

(ADP: adenosine diphosphate; ATP: adenosine triphosphate; CoA: coenzyme A; NAD$^+$: nicotinamide adenine dinucleotide; NADH: nicotinamide adenine dinucleotide (NAD) plus hydrogen; NADPH: nicotinamide adenine dinucleotide phosphate)

Question 2

1. Describe the anatomy and physiology of neuromuscular junction.

The neuromuscular junction (NMJ) is a synaptic connection between the terminal end of a motor nerve and a muscle (skeletal/smooth/cardiac). It is the site for the transmission of action potential from the nerve to the muscle **(Fig. 1)**. It is also a site for many diseases and a site of action for many pharmacological drugs.

2. Enumerate the differential diagnosis of acute-onset quadriparesis.

Acute-onset quadriparesis can occur in any age group and needs urgent evaluation and prompt and appropriate therapeutic intervention. Lesions at the following sites explain the muscle weakness:

a. *Muscle:* Inflammatory myopathies
b. *NMJ:* Myasthenia gravis, botulism, Lambert–Eaton syndrome
c. *Peripheral nerves:* Porphyria neuropathies, neuropathies due to heavy metal toxicity
d. *Motor nerve root:* Infectious polyradiculopathies, diabetic polyradiculopathies
e. *Anterior horn cell:* Poliomyelitis

Lower motor neurons: Antiganglioside antibody-related neuropathy

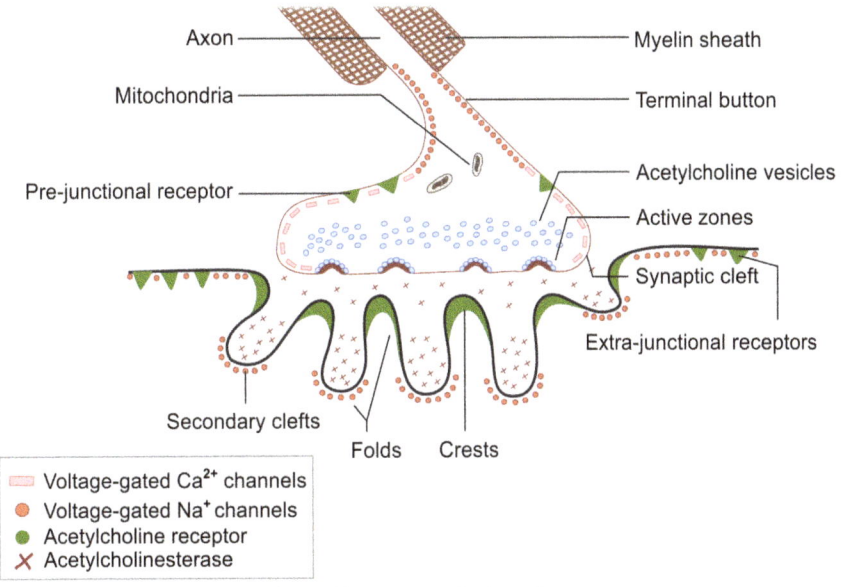

Fig. 1: Neuromuscular junction.

Question 3

1. Draw a diagram and describe the physiology of lung volumes and capacities.

There are four lung volumes and four lung capacities. Lung volumes and lung capacities are measured by a spirogram **(Fig. 2)**.

Lung volumes: Lung volume parameters are measured directly by a spirometer.

Four types are (a) tidal volume (TV), (b) inspiratory reserve volume (IRV), (c) expiratory reserve volume (ERV), and (d) residual volume (RV).

The values are small.

Lung capacities: Values are calculated by combining two or three volumes. Four types of lung capacities are (a) vital capacity (VC), (b) inspiratory capacity (IC), (c) total lung capacity (TLC), and (d) functional residual capacity (FRC). The values are large.

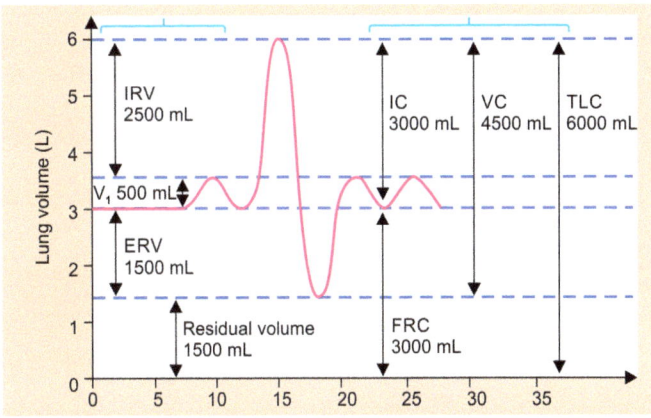

Fig. 2: Spirogram showing volume and capacity of the lungs. (ERV: expiratory reserve volume; FRC: functional residual capacity; IC: inspiratory capacity; IRV: inspiratory reserve volume; TLC: total lung capacity; VC: vital capacity)

2. Discuss the initial ventilator settings for metabolic acidosis.

Acute metabolic acidosis decreases the pH of the arterial blood and strongly stimulates the peripheral chemoreceptors to increase ventilatory drive. The increased ventilatory drive results in decreased partial pressure of arterial carbon dioxide ($PaCO_2$) and subsequent rise in plasma pH **(Table 1)**. Metabolic acidosis increases ventilatory drive. With severe metabolic acidosis, it is not uncommon to encounter patients with minute ventilations that are likely well over 40 L/min [e.g., 1–1.5 L TV at a respiratory rate (RR) of 40 breaths/min], whereas safe invasive ventilation may be difficult to achieve as the minute ventilation approaches approximately 30 L/min.

TABLE 1: Initial goals of ventilator strategy for metabolic acidosis.

Goal CO_2 (mm Hg)	Minute ventilation (L)
40	6–8
30	12–14
20	18–20

Question 4

1. Draw and label circle of Willis.

The structure of the *circle of Willis includes* left and right internal carotid arteries, left and right anterior cerebral arteries, and left and right posterior cerebral arteries **(Fig. 3)**.

2. Describe the pathophysiology of acute ischemic stroke.

According to the multicenter Trial of Acute Stroke Treatment (TOAST), there are three kinds of ischemic strokes: (a) Large vessel stroke, (b) small vessel stroke or lacunar stroke, and (c) cardioembolic stroke.

Large artery strokes could be due to thrombotic or embolic occlusion of the major arteries of the brain such as the internal carotid artery, middle cerebral artery, anterior cerebral artery, or the vertebrobasilar system. Lacunar strokes are more often due to involvement of smaller or perforating blood vessels supplying the deeper structures of the brain **(Fig. 4)**.

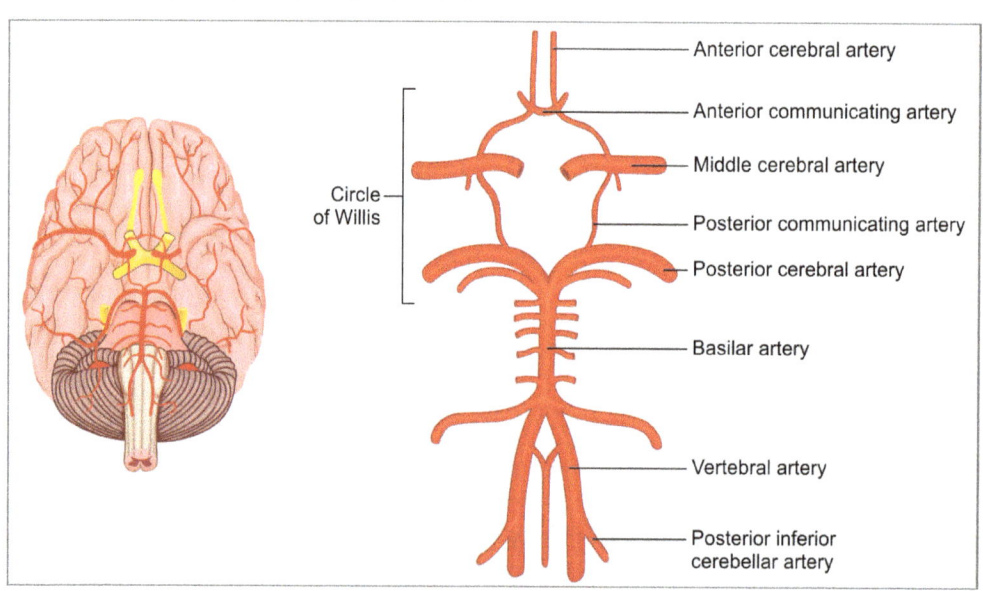

Fig. 3: Circle of Willis.

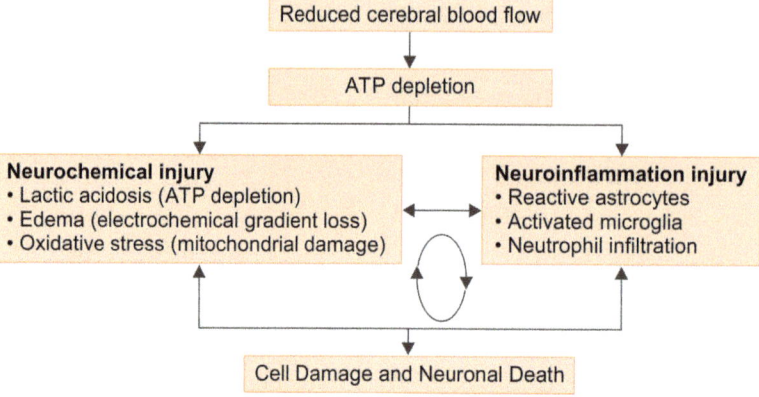

Fig. 4: Pathophysiology of acute ischemic stroke. (ATP: adenosine triphosphate)

Question 5

1. Draw, label, and describe the countercurrent mechanism.

The countercurrent mechanism is used to concentrate urine in the kidneys by the nephrons of the human excretory system. The loop of Henle utilizes the countercurrent mechanism/multiplier system to increase the concentration of solute and ions within the interstitium of the medulla. This ultimately allows the nephron to reabsorb more water and concentrate the urine while at the same time using as little energy as possible (**Fig. 5**).

2. Discuss the pathophysiology of acute kidney injury due to rhabdomyolysis.

Rhabdomyolysis is a syndrome characterized by skeletal muscle injury which is measured with myoglobin, creatine kinase (CK), and lactate dehydrogenase. Muscle injury can cause significant life-threatening electrolyte disorders; acute renal injury and muscle injury are secondary to trauma, myositis, medications, and muscle dystrophies (**Flowchart 2**).

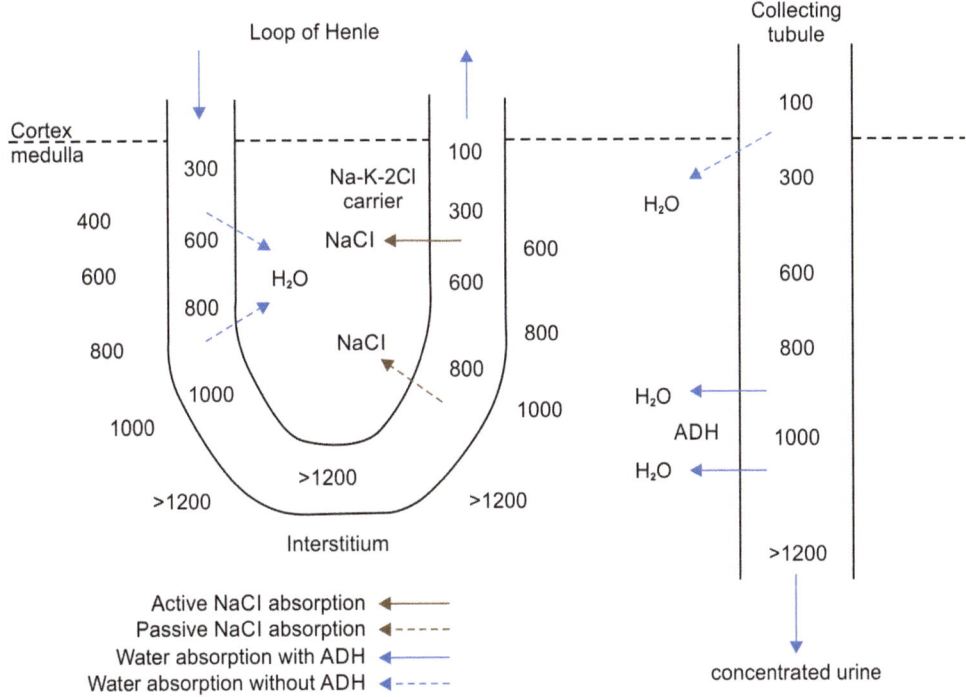

Fig. 5: Countercurrent mechanism. (ADH: antidiuretic hormone)

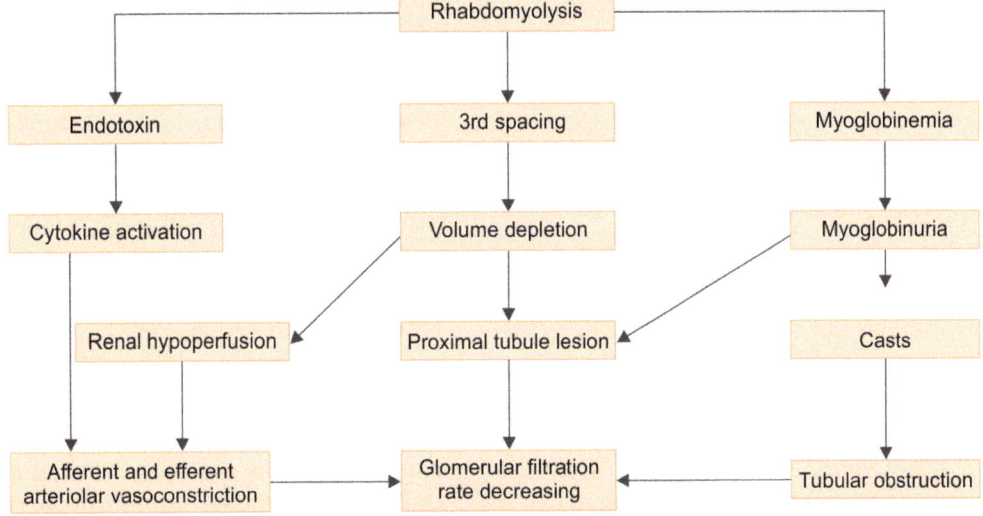

Flowchart 2: Pathophysiology of acute kidney injury due to rhabdomyolysis.

Question 6

1. Describe the buffer systems and respiratory and renal regulations of acid–base balance.

Acid-base equilibrium: It is closely tied to fluid metabolism and electrolyte balance; a pH of 7.37–7.43 is required to maintain ideal homeostasis with the help of pulmonary and renal mechanism **(Fig. 6)**.

Acid-base physiology: CO_2 produced during metabolism combines with water (H_2O) in the blood to create carbonic acid (H_2CO_3), which dissociates into hydrogen ion (H^+) and bicarbonate (HCO_3^-). The H^+ binds with hemoglobin in red blood cells and is released with oxygenation in the alveoli, at which time the reaction is reversed by another form of carbonic anhydrase, creating water (H_2O), which is excreted by the kidneys, and CO_2, which gets exhaled.

Acid-base balance: It is maintained by chemical buffering, pulmonary activity, and renal activity.

a. *Chemical buffering:* Intracellular and extracellular buffers provide an immediate response to acid–base disturbances. An ideal buffer is made up of a weak acid and its conjugate base. The conjugate base can accept H^+ and the weak acid can relinquish it. The relationship between the pH of a buffer system and the concentration of its components is described by the Henderson–Hasselbalch equation:

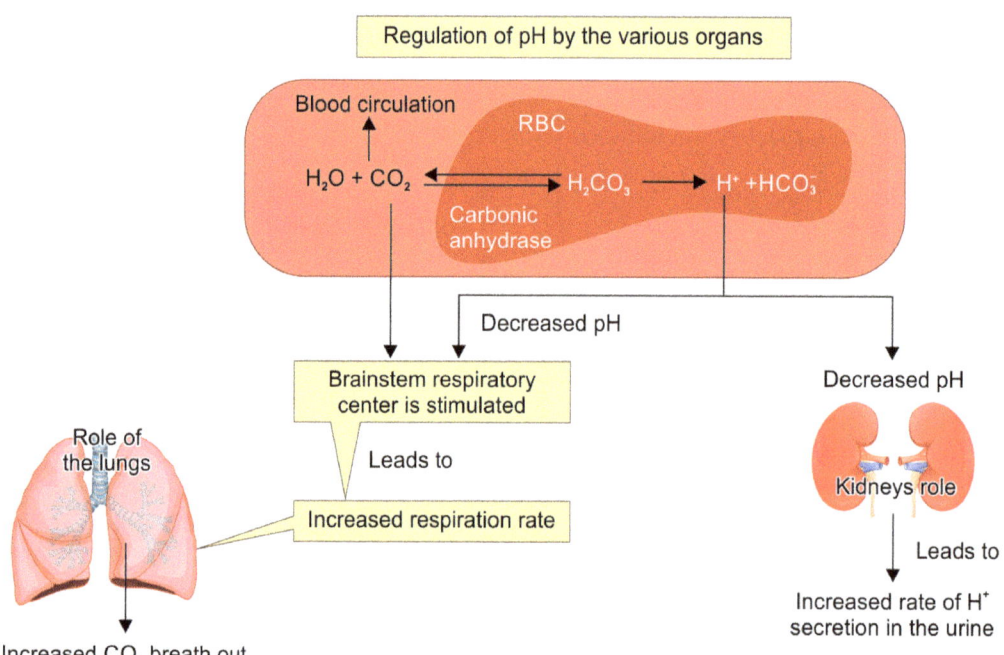

Fig. 6: Respiratory and renal regulations of acid–base balance. (RBC: red blood cells)

$pH = pKa + log\ [(anion)/(weak\ acid)]$ where pKa is the dissociation constant of the weak acid.

The most important extracellular buffer is the HCO_3/CO_2 system, described by the equation:

$H^+ + HCO_3^- \rightleftharpoons H_2CO_3 \rightleftharpoons CO_2 + H_2O$

An increase in H^+ drives the equation to the right and generates CO_2. CO_2 is controlled by alveolar ventilation while H^+ and HCO_3^- concentrations can be finely regulated by renal excretion. Other important chemical buffers include organic and inorganic phosphates and proteins such as hemoglobin and plasma proteins.

b. *Pulmonary pH regulation:* A decrease in pH leads to increase in TV or RR thus facilitating elimination of CO_2. It is about 50–75% effective and takes minutes to hours for compensation.

c. *Renal pH regulation:* The kidneys control pH by adjusting the amount of HCO_3^- that is excreted or reabsorbed. HCO_3^- reabsorption occurs mostly in the proximal tubule and collecting tubule. H_2O dissociates into H^+ and hydroxide (OH^-); in the presence of carbonic anhydrase, OH^- combines with CO_2 to form HCO_3^-, which is transported back into the circulation. Acid is actively excreted into the proximal and distal tubules where it combines with urinary buffers such as phosphate (HPO_4^{-2}), creatinine, uric acid, and ammonia to be excreted. The ammonia buffering system is especially important as the tubular cells actively regulate ammonia production in response to changes in acid load.

2. Discuss the acid–base disorders and coagulation derangement in trauma.

Common acid–base disorders and their causes are given in **Table 2**.

TABLE 2: Primary changes in acid–base disorders and compensatory responses.

Disorder	Primary disturbance	Compensatory response	Mechanism involved in compensatory response
Metabolic acidosis	Decrease in HCO_3	Decrease in PCO_2	Hyperventilation
Metabolic alkalosis	Increase in HCO_3	Increase in PCO_2	Hypoventilation
Respiratory acidosis	Increase in PCO_2	Increase in HCO_3	Increased H^+ secretion
Respiratory alkalosis	Decrease in PCO_2	Decrease in HCO_3	Decreased H^+ secretion

(PCO_2: partial pressure of carbon dioxide)

Appropriate fluid administration might help to maintain homeostasis in trauma. Inappropriate fluid administration will do just the opposite. In cases of penetrating trauma to the torso, research shows that withholding isotonic IV fluid had a mortality benefit. Hence, it is assumed that the benefit may come from decreased dilatational coagulopathy and hemostatic maintenance **(Fig. 7)**.

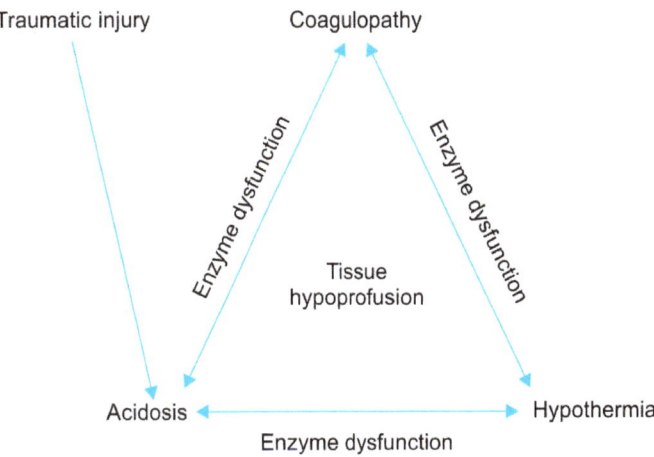

Fig. 7: Acid–base disorder and coagulopathy in trauma.

Question 7

1. Discuss the anatomical and physiological differences seen in a pregnant female.

Knowledge of physiologic and anatomic changes in pregnancy and their clinical impact on symptoms and manifestations are important in management **(Table 3)**.

TABLE 3: Anatomic and physiologic changes in pregnancy.

Anatomic changes	Clinical relevance	Physiological changes	Clinical relevance
Edematous and friable airway	Difficult airway, may require smaller ETT	Increase in oxygen consumption	Require high flow oxygen
Uterus extent beyond bony pelvis after 12 weeks, gravid uterus after 20 weeks	Direct injury to uterus, supine hypotension due to compression of inferior vena cava	• Increase in plasma volume • Increase heart rate/low blood pressure	• Delay in identification of shock • Poor marker of hemodynamic stability
Bladder moves superiorly	Direct bladder injury	Increase in bladder and uterine blood flow	Increase in bleeding risk with direct injury
Diaphragm moves upward 4 cm	Pneumothorax, tension pneumothorax tube placement 2–3 space upward	• Increase in renal plasma blood flow and GFR • Increase in bicarbonate excretion	• Precaution with drugs which excrete through the renal system • Susceptible to acidosis
Small bowel moves up	Direct blunt/penetrating bowel injury	Decrease in platelets, PT, PTT increase in fibrinogen D dimer	Precipitates DIC early
Peritoneum–abdominal wall stretches with progression of pregnancy	Poor assessment of organ injury intra-abdominal bleeding	Other hematopoietic changes in pregnancy are decrease in hemoglobin, hematocrit, and platelets, increase in white blood cell count, fibrinogens factors VIII and X	Awareness about these changes helps in resuscitation and anticipation of various complications

(DIC: disseminated intravascular coagulation; ETT: endotracheal tube; GFR: glomerular filtration rate; PTT: partial thromboplastin time; PT: prothrombin time)

2. Describe the indication and procedure of postmortem cesarean section.

Resuscitative hysterotomy: It is also called perimortem cesarean delivery (PMCD). It is usually done in patients who are >20 weeks pregnant or the uterus is above the level of umbilicus. During maternal cardiac arrest, if return of spontaneous circulation (ROSC) is not obtained within 4 minutes, it is necessary to deliver the baby as this relieves the occlusion of inferior vena cava (IVC) by the uterus and thereby improves the cardiac output. Delivery also improves the thoracic wall compliance, and this improves the cardiopulmonary resuscitation (CPR) effectiveness. It is preferred to do it in the place where the maternal resuscitation is carried out. Shifting the patient to the operating room (OR) will cause delay in all the crucial resuscitations. It can be carried out with a scalpel and scissors as waiting for the surgical equipment will cause unnecessary delay. Steps for PMCD are as follows **(Fig. 8)**:
a. While continuing maternal resuscitation and manual left uterine displacement, if antiseptic solution is available, pour over the abdomen.
b. Make an incision over the abdomen—vertical incision (preferred over Pfannenstiel) from xiphisternum to pubic symphysis as it allows more space for visualization.
c. Incision from skin to peritoneum.
d. Make a vertical incision over the uterus from the fundus to the lower segment of uterus.
e. Stretch the uterine incision through fingers to allow easy access to the delivery.
f. Deliver the baby after cutting the cord between the two umbilical clamps. Hand over the baby to neonatologist.
g. Deliver the placenta.
h. Uterus should be closed in layers followed by closure of abdomen as done in a regular manner

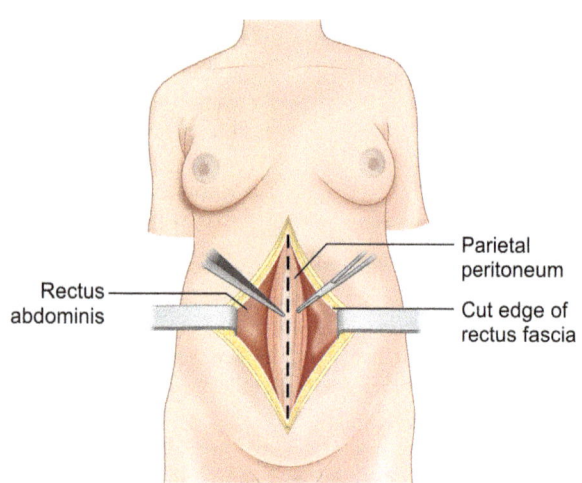

Fig. 8: Resuscitative hysterotomy.

Question 8

1. Describe pathways and mechanism for transmission of acute-onset pain.

Pain receptors are free nerve endings present in the superficial layer of skin, arterial walls, joint surfaces, and the falx and tentorium in cranial vault. Pain can be elicited by stimuli such as mechanical, thermal, and chemicals pain stimuli. Fast pain is elicited by mechanical and thermal stimuli, whereas slow pain by all three types. Chemicals that excite chemical pain are bradykinin, serotonin, histamine, potassium ions, acetylcholine, and proteolytic enzymes. Prostaglandins and substance P enhance sensitivity of pain endings. Increase in sensitivity of pain receptors is called hyperalgesia. Slow pain is carried by C fibers and fast pain by Aδ fibers. First-order neurons of slow pain synapse in substantia gelatinosa in the dorsal horn of spinal cord **(Fig. 9)**. Second-order neurons cross over to the opposite side and ascend in the anterolateral pathway. The tract carrying slow pain is called paleospinothalamic tract and that carrying fast pain is called neospinothalamic tract.

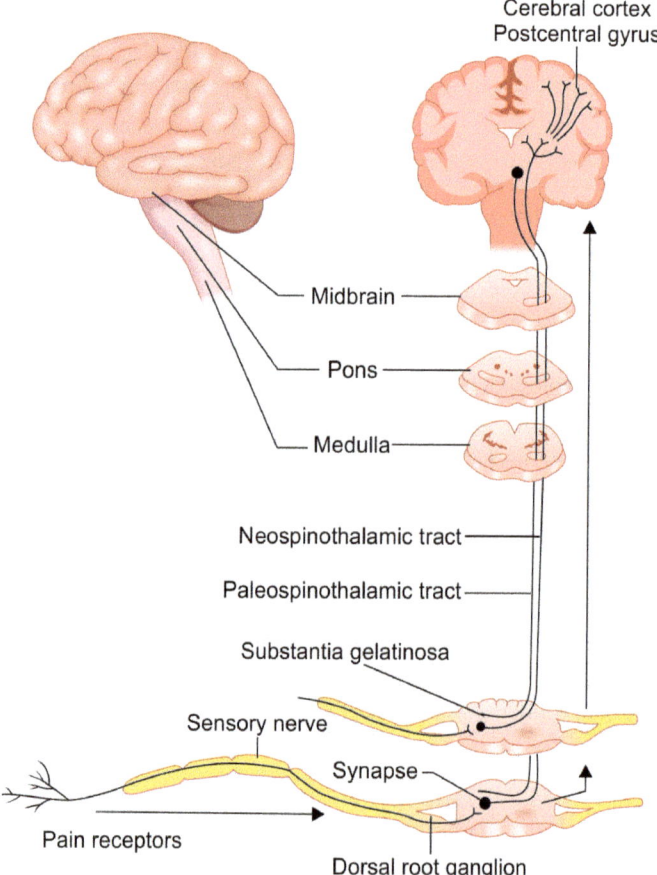

Fig. 9: Pathways of transmission of pain.

2. Discuss pain scales in the nonverbal age group.

The FLACC (face, legs, activity, cry, and consolability) scale is a measurement used to assess pain for children between the ages of 2 months and 7 years or individuals who are unable to communicate their pain **(Table 4)**. The scale is scored in a range of 0–10 with 0 representing no pain. FLACC scale is a more specific pain score for children that takes into consideration things specific to children.

TABLE 4: FLACC scale.

FLACC scale	0	1	2
Face	No particular expression or smile	Occasional grimace or frown, withdrawn, disinterested	Frequent to constant frown, clenched jaw, quivering chin
Legs	Normal position or relaxed	Uneasy, restless, tense	Kicking, or legs drawn up
Activity	Lying quietly, normal position, moves easily	Squirming, shifting back and forth, tense	Arched, rigid, or jerking
Cry	No crying (awake or asleep)	Moans or whimpers, occasional complaint	Crying steadily, screams or sobs, frequent complaints
Consolability	Content, relaxed	Reassured by occasional touching, hugging or being talked to, distractible	Difficult to console or comfort

Question 9

1. Draw a labeled diagram of knee joint and describe various tests to evaluate it clinically.

The knee joint is a synovial joint that connects three bones: femur, tibia, and patella. It is a complex hinge joint composed of two articulations: *tibiofemoral joint* and *patellofemoral joint*. The tibiofemoral joint is an articulation between the tibia and the femur, whereas the patellofemoral joint is an articulation between the patella and the femur **(Fig. 10)**.

Articular surfaces:
a. *Tibiofemoral joint*: Lateral and medial condyles of femur, tibial plateaus
b. *Patellofemoral joint*: Patellar surface of femur, posterior surface of patella

Ligaments and menisci:
a. *Extracapsular ligaments*: Patellar ligament, medial and lateral patellar retinacula, tibial (medial), collateral ligament, fibular (lateral) collateral ligament, oblique popliteal ligament, arcuate popliteal ligament, and anterolateral ligament (ALL)
b. *Intracapsular ligaments*: Anterior cruciate ligament (ACL), posterior cruciate ligament (PCL), medial meniscus, and lateral meniscus

Innervation: Femoral nerve (nerve to vastus medialis, saphenous nerve), tibial and common fibular (peroneal) nerves, posterior division of the obturator nerve

Blood supply: Genicular branches of lateral circumflex femoral artery, femoral artery, posterior tibial artery, anterior tibial artery, and popliteal artery

Movements: Extension, flexion, medial rotation, and lateral rotation.

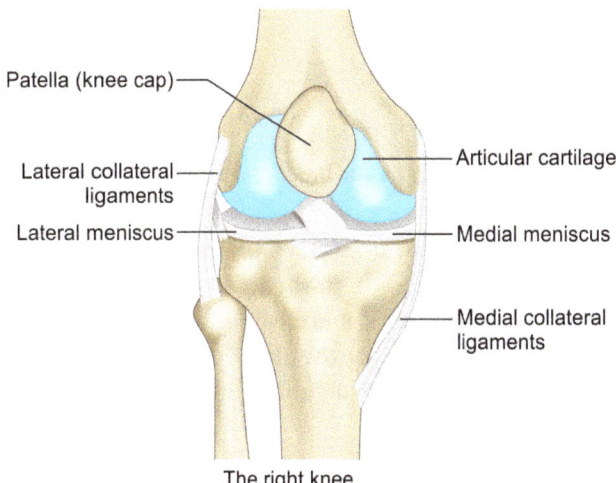

Fig. 10: Anatomy of the knee joint.

Anterior drawer test: It identifies the tears of the ACL. The test is performed with the patient in a supine position, hip flexed at 45°, and knee flexed at 90°.

While stabilizing the patient's foot, the examiner places his or her thumbs over the joint line while pulling the tibia forward. The thumbs are used to palpate for any translation of the tibia relative to the femur. A positive test result is defined as greater anterior translation of the tibia relative to the femur as compared with the other knee.

Lachman test: It is specific for ACL injury. It is done with the knee flexed at 20–30° while the examiner uses one hand to grasp and stabilize the femur. The tibia is then pulled anteriorly, and the examiner notes tibial excursion. The examiner records "firmness" or a "soft end point." The end point can be graded as 1+ (0–5 mm more displacement than on the normal side), 2+ (5–10 mm), or 3+ (>10 mm).

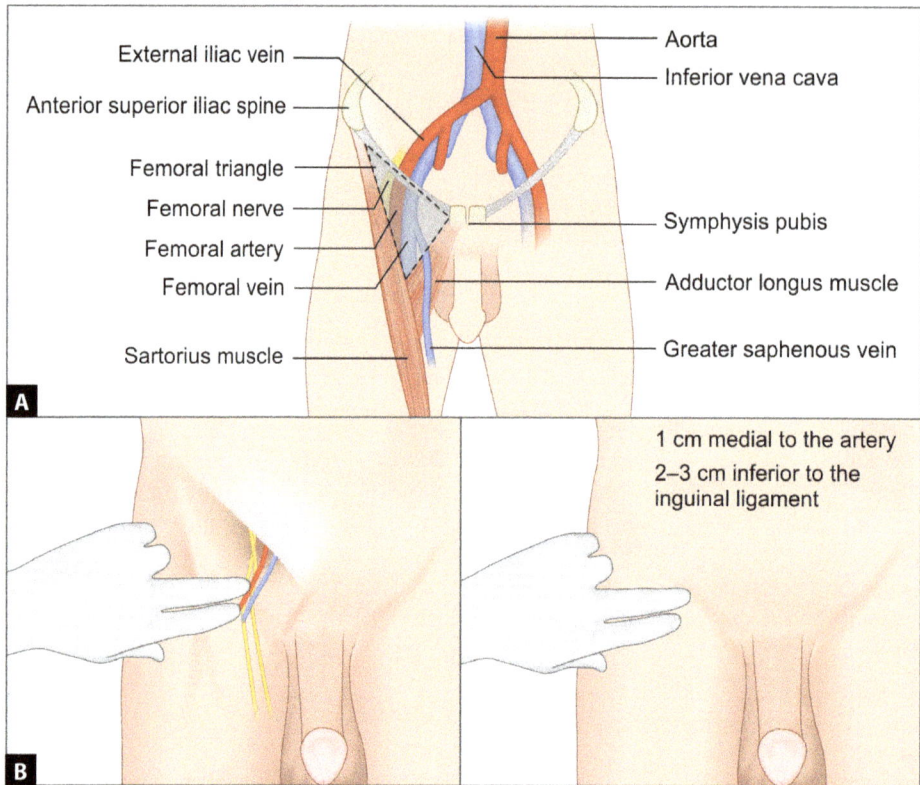

Figs. 11A and B: Landmark technique for insertion of the central venous catheter at the femoral vein site.

Posterior drawer test: It assesses CL injury. The posterior drawer test can be accomplished with the patient's knee flexed at 90° and the foot stabilized by the examiner. A smooth backward force is applied to the tibia. Posterior displacement of the tibia > 5 mm, or a soft end point, indicates injury to the PCL.

Posterior sag sign test: It also indicates PCL integrity. The patient is placed in a supine position, and a pillow is placed under the distal thigh for support, resting the heel on the stretcher. The knee is flexed to 45° or 90°. If the tibia sags backward, the test result is positive, indicating PCL insufficiency.

2. Draw a labeled diagram and describe the clinical significance of femoral triangle.

The femoral triangle in the anterior superior third of the thigh is a subfascial space that appears as a triangular depression inferior to the inguinal ligament; the depression is visible when the thigh is abducted, flexed, and laterally rotated **(Figs. 11A and B)**. The floor of the femoral triangle is comprised of the adductor longus, pectineus (medially), psoas major, and iliacus muscles (laterally). The floor is gutter-shaped since all the muscles forming the floor pass to the posterior aspect of the femur.

Since the femoral triangle provides easy access to a major artery, coronary angioplasty and peripheral angioplasty are often performed by entering the femoral artery at the femoral triangle. Heavy bleeding in the leg can be stopped by applying pressure to points in the femoral triangle.

The femoral triangle is used as a site for vascular catheterization for a number of interventional and corrective procedures. Catheterization of the femoral vessels provides access to the ipsilateral and contralateral lower limb, the vessels of the abdomen and thorax, and the cerebral vessels.

Question 10

1. Discuss spinal cord syndromes.

Incomplete spinal cord syndrome (ISCS) occurs when lesions involve specific structural and/or functional anatomic regions of the cord, with some preservation of sensory and/or motor function below the lesion **(Fig. 12)**. The clinical presentation of the incomplete spinal cord syndromes is largely determined by the involvement of the three tracts: (1) corticospinal tract, (2) spinothalamic tract, and (3) posterior column of the spinal cord. There are eight types of incomplete spinal cord syndromes based on clinical presentations: (a) Central cord syndrome, (b) Brown–Séquard syndrome (unilateral cord syndrome), (c) anterior cord syndrome, (d) posterior syndrome, (e) caudal equine syndrome, (f) conus medullaris syndrome, (g) subacute combined degeneration myelopathy, and (h) cruciate paralysis. Central cord syndrome occurs due to syringomyelia. Anterior cord syndrome occurs due to anterior spinal artery occlusion. Posterior cord syndrome occurs due to posterior spinal artery occlusion.

2. Draw, label, and locate the lesion in visual pathway in right homonymous hemianopia.

Homonymous hemianopsia (**Fig. 13**) is a condition in which a person sees only one side, right or left. The most common cause of this type of vision loss is stroke. However, any disorder that affects the brain including tumors, inflammation, and injuries can be a cause.

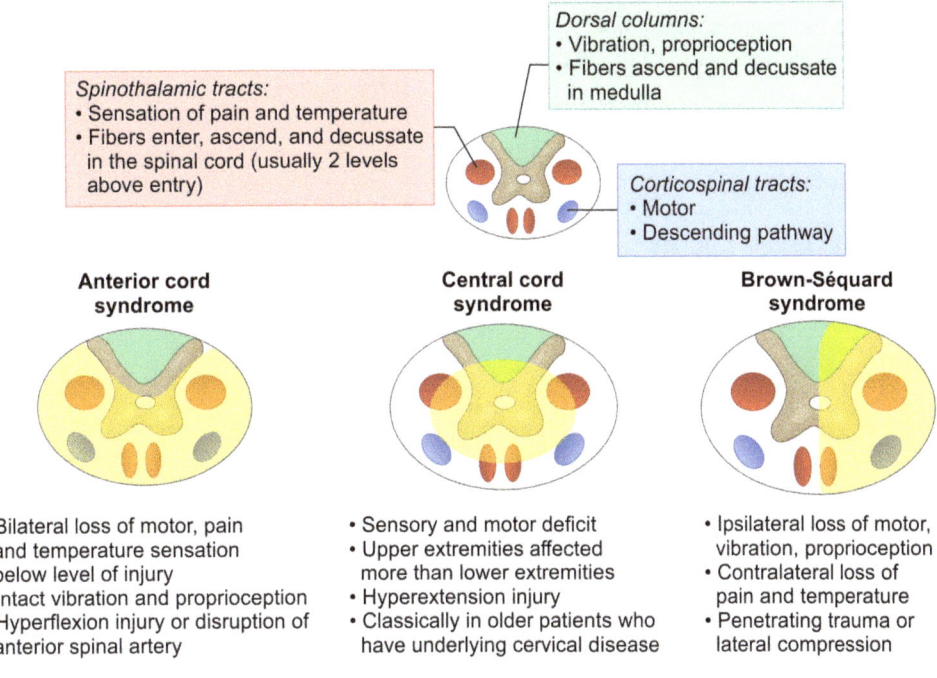

Fig. 12: Incomplete spinal cord syndrome.

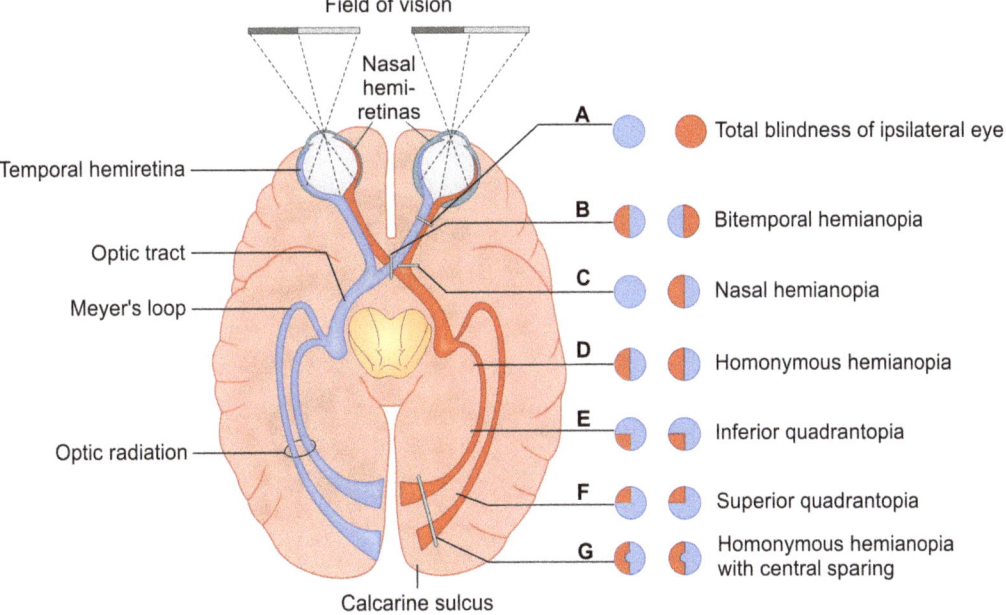

Fig. 13: Homonymous hemianopia.

SUGGESTED READING

1. Richhariya D, Sharma B. Textbook of Emergency Medicine including Intensive Care and Trauma, 2nd edition. New Delhi: Jaypee Brothers Medical Publishers (P) Ltd; 2022. pp. 871-81. (Question 1).
2. Richhariya D, Sharma B. Textbook of Emergency Medicine including Intensive Care and Trauma, 2nd edition. New Delhi: Jaypee Brothers Medical Publishers (P) Ltd; 2022. pp. 838-43. (Question 2).
3. Richhariya D, Sharma B. Textbook of Emergency Medicine including Intensive Care and Trauma, 2nd edition. New Delhi: Jaypee Brothers Medical Publishers (P) Ltd; 2022. p. 580 (Question 3).
4. Richhariya D, Sharma B. Textbook of Emergency Medicine including Intensive Care and Trauma, 2nd edition. New Delhi: Jaypee Brothers Medical Publishers (P) Ltd; 2022. pp. 820-6. (Question 4).
5. Richhariya D, Sharma B. Textbook of Emergency Medicine including Intensive Care and Trauma, 2nd edition. New Delhi: Jaypee Brothers Medical Publishers (P) Ltd; 2022. pp. 747-50. (Question 5).
6. Richhariya D, Sharma B. Textbook of Emergency Medicine including Intensive Care and Trauma, 2nd edition. New Delhi: Jaypee Brothers Medical Publishers (P) Ltd; 2022. pp. 304-5. (Question 6).
7. Richhariya D, Sharma B. Textbook of Emergency Medicine including Intensive Care and Trauma, 2nd edition. New Delhi: Jaypee Brothers Medical Publishers (P) Ltd; 2022. pp. 1114-5. (Question 7).
8. Richhariya D, Sharma B. Textbook of Emergency Medicine including Intensive Care and Trauma, 2nd edition. New Delhi: Jaypee Brothers Medical Publishers (P) Ltd; 2022. pp. 355-8. (Question 8).
9. Richhariya D, Sharma B. Textbook of Emergency Medicine including Intensive Care and Trauma, 2nd edition. New Delhi: Jaypee Brothers Medical Publishers (P) Ltd; 2022. pp. 1634-5. (Question 9).
10. Richhariya D, Sharma B. Textbook of Emergency Medicine including Intensive Care and Trauma, 2nd edition. New Delhi: Jaypee Brothers Medical Publishers (P) Ltd; 2022. p. 1571. (Question 10).

Emergency Medicine Paper 46

Sreekrishnan TP

Question 1

A 65-year-old nonhelmeted patient presents to the emergency department with history of head injury on collision with a four-wheeler. On arrival, he has noisy breathing and mouth is full of blood. His BP is 76/60 mm Hg, pulse rate 112 with saturation 76%. He is opening eyes to painful stimuli, moaning with abnormal flexion.

1. Describe the approach and management of the case.

The patient is a case of trauma. Hence as per advanced trauma life support (ATLS) we will approach the patient with airway, breathing, circulation, disability, exposure (ABCDE).

Airway: We will give supplemental oxygen to patient and look for any foreign body or secretions to be suctioned out. And put cervical collar to prevent cervical injury.

Breathing: Look for any asymmetrical chest rise to rule out pneumothorax, flail chest, etc. To call for chest X-ray imaging. Left lung can have pneumothorax or hydropneumothorax.

Circulation: Intravenous fluids given to patient, 1 liter warm isotonic fluid. And call for blood in case of transfusion required.

Disability: Level of consciousness and pupillary reflexes along with plantar reflexes. Act accordingly.

Exposure: Preserve hypothermia.

Management: To protect airway from hemorrhage and mechanical obstruction, remove avulsed teeth or foreign bodies. Bag mask ventilation requires two people due to loss of normal structure. Always plan for difficult airway and to prevent administer of paralytics unless patient can be bagged effectively or alternate airway devices kept in place.

Keeping cricothyrotomy kept as a backup if other airway securing methods fail.

Hemorrhage: Control posterior nasal epistaxis early with nasal tampon, dual balloon device or Foley's catheter placement. After intubation, oral packing might be needed with severe facial bleeding.

2. Discuss the management of hemorrhagic shock in trauma.

Hemorrhage is the most common cause of early death in trauma patients. During resuscitation of hemorrhagic shock, volume infusion in the face of continued blood loss results in dilutional coagulopathy and hypothermia, while the transient elevation in blood pressure contributes to further bleeding from wounds and vessels. Permissive hypotension, therefore, can facilitate an environment that optimizes coagulation, albeit at the potential expense of optimal tissue perfusion pressure, until repair restores the integrity of the system. Permissive hypotension is the act of maintaining a blood pressure lower than physiologic levels in a patient that has suffered from hemorrhagic blood loss. The practice is employed in order to maintain adequate vasoconstriction, organ perfusion, and prevent an undesired coagulopathy during initial fluid resuscitation. Permissive hypotension is contraindicated in patients with traumatic brain injury, because reduced perfusion pressure and oxygenation can lead to secondary brain injury. In such situations, a mean arterial pressure (MAP) of >80 mm Hg (a cerebral perfusion pressure of approximately 60 mm Hg) is required in order to maintain cerebral perfusion pressure. Hemorrhagic shock in trauma classification is given in **Table 1**.

The Assessment of Blood Consumption (ABC) score in trauma was developed to assist clinicians in deciding when massive transfusion would be required to resuscitate trauma patients. Massive transfusion protocols (MTPs) have been designed to accelerate the release of blood products but can result in waste if activated inappropriately. The ABC score **(Table 2)** has become a widely accepted score for MTP activation.

TABLE 1: Classification of hemorrhagic shock in trauma.

	Class I	Class II	Class III	Class IV
Absolute blood loss	<750 mL	750–1500 mL	1,500–2,000 mL	>2,000 mL
Relative blood loss	<15%	15–30%	30–40%	40%
Pulse rate	<100	100–120	120–140	>140
Blood pressure	Normal	Normal	Decreased	Decreased
Pulse pressure	Normal/Increased	Decreased	Decreased	Decreased
Capillary refill	Normal	Decreased	Decreased	Decreased
Respiratory rate	14–20	20–30	30–40	>35
Urine output (mL/h)	>30	20–30	5–15	Negligible
CNS (mental status)	Slightly anxious	Anxious	Anxious confused	Confused lethargic
Fluid replacement	Crystalloid	Crystalloid	Crystalloid + Blood	Crystalloid + Blood

(CNS: central nervous system)

TABLE 2: Assessment of blood consumption (ABC) score.

Components	Points
Penetrating injury	1
FAST positive	1
Heart rate >100/min	1
Systolic BP <90 mm Hg	1

Trigger for massive blood transfusion protocol ≥2 (accuracy of prediction of MTP 75%)

Question 2

1. Describe various clinical decision rules in ordering CT cervical spine in adult.

The CT cervical spine or C-spine protocol serves as an examination for the assessment of the cervical spine. It is usually performed as a non-contrast study. In certain situations, it might be combined or simultaneously acquired with a CT angiography of the cerebral arteries or a CT of the neck.

NEXUS criteria: The criteria state that a patient with suspected C-spine injury can be cleared provided the following are true: No posterior midline cervical spine tenderness. No evidence of intoxication, normal level of alertness, no focal neurological deficit, no painful distracting injury.

CANADIAN C-spine rule: Define whether any high-risk factors are present such as age (≥65 years) or dangerous mechanism (includes high speed or roll over or ejection, motorized recreation vehicle or bicycle crash). If this is the case, an X-ray of the cervical spine should be performed.

2. Describe the management of a suicidal hanging patient brought to emergency department.

Hanging is increasingly described as a method chosen by adults to self-harm. Hanging is defined as death due to external pressure on the neck when a ligature is applied to the neck of a wholly or partly suspended individual. The main pathophysiological theories described were respiratory asphyxia, interruption to cerebral blood flow because of occlusion of vessels in the neck, and cardiac inhibition secondary to nerve stimulation.

Maintenance of airway, oxygenation, measures to reduce cerebral edema and general care are the main forms of treatment. Return of brainstem reflex can be used as a prognostic factor.

Endotracheal intubation (ETI) may become necessary with appropriate measures; judicious use of fluid resuscitation, risk of ARDS, and cerebral edema. Monitor for cardiac arrhythmias, radiology X-ray soft tissue neck, CT cervical spine and brain. Consider CT angiography—head and neck/ MRA—head and neck. Start treatment like cerebral edema with elevated intracranial pressure in alterd and comatose patient. All hanging victims even if the initial presentation is clinically benign, and those with vascular compromise should be admitted for 24 hours observation in view of risk of delayed airway (tracheal stenosis) pulmonary complications (pulmonary edema and aspiration pneumonia) and carotid intimal dissection or thrombus formation.

Pulmonary Edema
- *Neurogenic:* Centrally mediated, massive sympathetic discharge; often in association with serious brain injury, poor prognostic implication.
- *Postobstructive:* Due to marked negative intrapleural pressure, generated by forceful inspiratory effort against extrathoracic obstruction; when obstruction removed, may have rapid onset pulmonary edema leading to ARDS.

Neurologic sequelae: A wide array of complications may occur in survivors of strangulations and near-hangings, including muscle spasms, transient hemiplegia, central cord syndrome, and seizures. Spinal cord injury can also cause long-term paraplegia or quadriplegia and short-term autonomic dysfunction.

Question 3

1. Describe the uses of Foley's catheter balloon tamponade.

Most Foley catheters are made of silicone, latex, or a combination, and are available in a variety of sizes. Once placed, the balloon is distended with a solution; the inflated balloon then aids retention of the catheter in the urinary bladder.

A Foley catheter is used with many disorders, procedures, or problems such as these:

- Retention of urine leading to urinary hesitancy, straining to urinate, decrease in size and force of the urinary stream, interruption of urinary stream, and sensation of incomplete emptying
- Obstruction of the urethra by an anatomical condition that makes it difficult for one to urinate—prostate hypertrophy, prostate cancer, or narrowing of the urethra
- Urine output monitoring in a critically ill or injured person
- Collection of a sterile urine specimen for diagnostic purposes
- Nerve-related bladder dysfunction, such as after spinal trauma (a catheter can be inserted regularly to assist with urination)
- Imaging study of the lower urinary tract
- After surgery

2. Describe the indication and procedure of resuscitative endovascular balloon occlusion of the aorta (REBOA).

Resuscitative endovascular balloon occlusion of the aorta (REBOA) has recently come up as a minimally invasive alternative to open aortic cross-clamping in the management of nonresponsive category of polytrauma patients. It will help in controlling noncompressible hemorrhage arising below the diaphragm. It is being used in both blunt and penetrating abdominal trauma. The use of REBOA provides for temporary hemorrhage control and improved hemodynamic until definitive surgical/endovascular control of hemorrhage achieved **(Fig. 1)**. REBOA is being used in Zone I and III of the aorta. Zone 1 of the aorta extends from the left subclavian artery to the celiac artery. Zone 2 continues from the celiac artery to the renal artery. Zone 3 extends from the origin of the lowest renal artery to the aortic bifurcation (infrarenal aorta). Zone 1 occlusion is utilized in patients in cardiac arrest or those in hemorrhagic shock with evidence of noncompressible hemorrhage arising below the diaphragm. Zone 2 is considered to be a no-occlusion zone. Zone 3 occlusion is reserved for patients without evidence of intra-abdominal hemorrhage but with evidence of a pelvic fracture.

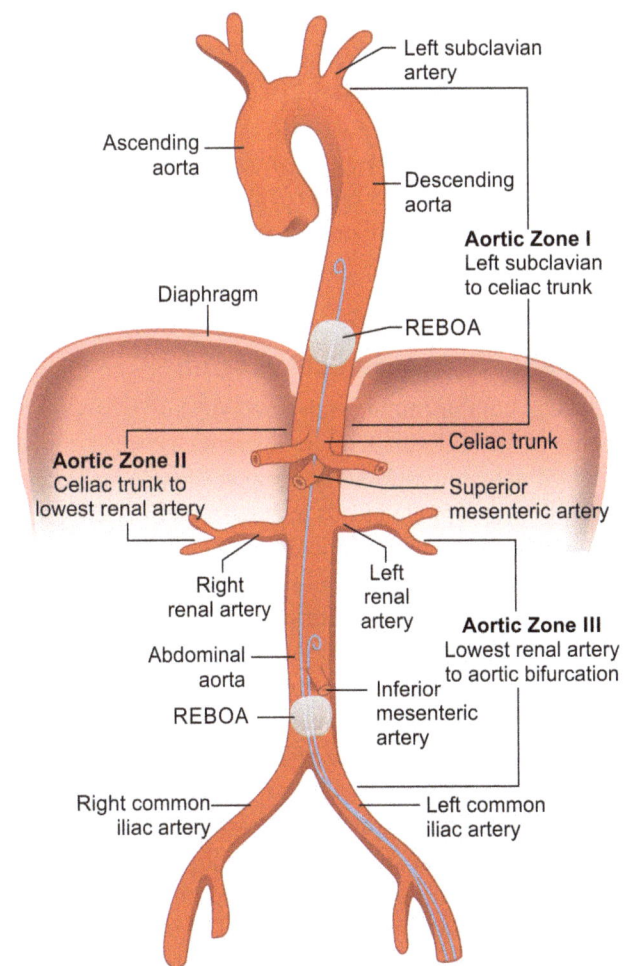

Fig. 1: Resuscitative endovascular balloon occlusion of the aorta (REBOA).

Question 4

1. Discuss the point of care ultrasound signs in chest trauma patients.

A sonographic physiologic assessment for shock, often described as the rapid ultrasound in shock (RUSH) examination, has gained popularity. This framework organizes the potential etiologies of shock into three

broad, sonographically-assessable systems that drive hemodynamics, simplified as:
1. *The Pump:* Cardiac function
2. *The Tank:* Intravascular volume status
3. *The Pipes:* Vascular emergencies in the venous and arterial system

Careful evaluation of these components can enable clinicians to quickly identify the underlying etiology of shock in patients with undifferentiated hypotension and subsequently allow early initiation of the most appropriate treatment.

a. Pericardial effusion
b. Global left ventricular (LV) contractility
c. Right ventricular (RV) strain
d. Intravascular volume status to assess the IVC
e. A FAST examination is performed to evaluate for fluid in the peritoneal and thoracic cavities
f. To assess for a tension pneumothorax
g. Aortic aneurysms and dissection

2. Describe the assessment and management of abdominal compartment syndrome.

Abdominal compartment syndrome (ACS) occurs when the pressure in the abdominal cavity elevates beyond 20 mm Hg. In abdominal compartment syndrome, the displacement of the diaphragm cephalad leads to compression of the thorax, which causes an increase in work of breathing, ventilation/perfusion inequality, and increases in both peak and plateau pressures. Abdominal compartment syndrome is most commonly due to excessive fluid resuscitation (>5 L in 24 hours) or massive blood transfusion (>10 units in 24 hours). Clinical signs are nonspecific and appear late. Classic findings are of increased airway pressure, decreased urine output, and a tense abdomen. A tense distended abdomen, respiratory distress (or high peak inspiratory pressures if mechanically ventilation is used), and oliguria constitute the classic clinical triad of abdominal compartment syndrome. This triad is often accompanied by hypotension. Diagnosis of ACS is to measure intra-abdominal pressure. Intra-abdominal pressure >20 mm Hg and evidence of organ failure support the diagnosis of abdominal compartment syndrome. The current method for measuring intra-abdominal pressure is to measure bladder pressure.

Medical management for treatment of intra-abdominal hypertension (IAH) involves an overall goal to improve the following—abdominal wall compliance with decreased muscle contraction, evacuation of luminal contents by decompression (NG tube), evacuation of abdominal fluid by drainage, and correction of positive fluid balance through goal-directed volume resuscitation. The early use of nonsurgical interventions may prevent the progression of IAH to ACS. The most effective abdominal compartment syndrome treatment is surgical decompression of abdomen. After surgical laparotomy for compartment syndrome, the abdominal fascia may be closed using temporary closure devices such as (vacs, meshes, and zippers). The fascia can be appropriately closed after 5–7 days after the compartment pressures and swelling decreased.

Question 5

1. Describe the differential diagnosis and management of massive uterine bleeding in pregnant female.

Possible causes of bleeding:
- Placenta previa
- Placental abruption
- Vasa previa
- Premature or term labor
- Genitourinary lesion or laceration
- Genitourinary infection
- Congenital or acquired bleeding disorders

Abruption of placenta: It means premature separation of placenta.

Symptoms: Abdominal pain, bleeding, severe shock

Signs: Shock spasm of uterus fetal part hard to feel, often no fetal heart sound. All emergency protocols should be considered the shift the patient to obstetric emergency unit.

Pathophysiology: Abruptio placentae, premature separation of normal implanted placenta from the uterine lining; spontaneous abruptio placentae between 24 and 28 weeks.

Clinical presentation: Mild abruption has mild uterine tenderness, no or mild vaginal bleed, normal maternal vital signs, no coagulopathy, and fetal distress.

Severe abruption has no or severe vaginal bleeding, fetal distress, coagulopathy, severe uterine pain or tenderness, continuous uterine contractions, maternal hypotension or shock, nausea, vomiting.

Emergency department management includes:
- Maternal stabilization
- Electronic fetal monitoring (cardiotocodynamometry) to identify fetal distress
- Emergency obstetrician consultation
- Place two large bore IV lines
- Obtain complete blood count (CBC), coagulation panel, fibrin degradation product, crossmatch maternal blood
- Administer anti-D Ig IM if mother is Rh-negative.

- Transvaginal scan for retroplacental clot
- Immediate delivery indicated

2. Describe McMahon score.

The McMahon score first described in 2013 used in patients ≥18 years old with rhabdomyolysis [Creatine phosphokinase (CPK) >5,000 U/L within 72 hours of admission]. The McMahon score calculated in patient with rhabdomyolysis on admission for the prediction of risk of renal failure requiring RRT or mortality, The McMahon score includes admission creatine kinase (extreme elevations in excess of 40,000, along with other indicators of severity (hypocalcemia, hyperphosphatemia and acidosis) and patient variables (gender, age, and type of injury). A McMahon score <5 indicates a 3% risk of either need for RRT or death, whereas a score >10 indicates a 52% risk of RRT or death **(Table 3)**; predicts mortality or acute kidney injury (AKI) in rhabdomyolysis patients; should not be used for patients with preexisting end-stage renal disease or with elevated CPK due to MI.

TABLE 3: McMahon risk prediction score for rhabdomyolysis patient predicting risk of renal failure and mortality.

Variable		Score
Age	>50 to <70 years	1.5
	>70 to <80 years	2.5
	>80 years	3.0
Female sex		1.0
Initial creatinine	1.4–2.2 mg/dL	1.5
	>2.2 mg/dL	3.0
Initial calcium	<7.5 mg/dL	2.0
Initial CK	>40,000 U/L	2.0
Initial phosphate	4–5.4 mg/dL	1.5
	>5.4 mg/dL	2.0
Underlying cause other than seizure syncope exercise statins or myositis		3.0
Initial serum bicarbonate	<19 mEq/L	2.0

Question 6

1. Describe the assessment and management of acute onset vertigo.

Vertigo is the illusion of movement in which the patient feels the environment around him or himself spinning when the environment is stationary. Vertigo is a symptom, not a disease.

The most common causes of this condition are benign paroxysmal positional vertigo, acute vestibular neuronitis or labyrinthitis, Ménière's disease, migraine, and anxiety disorders. Less common causes include vertebrobasilar ischemia and retrocochlear tumors. The distinction between peripheral and central vertigo usually can be made clinically and guides management decisions.

A diagnosis of the underlying disease is required for the proper management of vertigo. Vertigo may also be a component of the drowsiness or vertigo complaint expressed as dizziness. Dizziness is nonspecific and can result from a disorder in any organ system. In peripheral vertigo, the pathology is mostly in the temporal bone, especially in the labyrinth. Central pathologies are the reflection of pathologies in the area extending from the vestibular system to the brain. The most important feature in distinguishing between central and peripheral vertigo is the features of nystagmus. Centrally derived nystagmus are seen in brain and brainstem lesions. These may be in the horizontal plane, as in peripheral lesions, or in the form of vertical nystagmus. The most important point in diagnosis is history and physical examination. After a well-received history and physical examination, the diagnosis is largely approached.

Benign paroxysmal positional vertigo usually improves with a canalith repositioning procedure. Acute vestibular neuronitis or labyrinthitis improves with initial stabilizing measures and a vestibular suppressant medication, followed by vestibular rehabilitation exercises. Ménière's disease often responds to the combination of a low-salt diet and diuretics. Vertiginous migraine headaches generally improve with dietary changes, a tricyclic antidepressant, and a beta-blocker or calcium-channel blocker. Vertigo associated with anxiety usually responds to a selective serotonin reuptake inhibitor.

2. Describe the assessment and management of Ludwig's angina.

Ludwig's angina is a potentially life-threatening condition with rapid progression within hours; the cellulitis starts from the submandibular space and spreads to the connective tissues of floor of mouth and neck. Odontogenic polymicrobial cellulitis mostly caused by *viridans group streptococci (VGS), Staphylococcus aureus* and anaerobes.

Dental pathologies: Dental caries, recent dental procedures, poor oral hygiene.

Trauma: Mandibular fractures, facial fractures, piercings of tongue.

Other causes: Submandibular sialadenitis, oral malignancy, systemic illness with immunocompromised status (AIDS, diabetes mellitus, post-transplant patients). Patients mostly present with neck pain and swelling, along with dysphagia. Other symptoms include dysphonia "hot potato" muffled voice, drooling of saliva, pain over floor of mouth, tongue swelling, restricted neck movement and fever. Red flags (serious clinical features) are **Toxic general appearance, Altered mental status, Airway obstruction, Poor hydration status, Poor oral acceptance.**

Investigations: Clinical presentation forms the base of diagnosis, though no specific laboratory tests are indicated, CT scan of neck with IV contrast enhancement is the study of choice, as it gives details of airway compromise, soft-tissue swelling, and involvement of mediastinum.

Treatment: Comforting the patient's posture, maintaining airway patency and oxygenation should be the priority, wide bore IV access should be immediately secured and crystalloid fluid should be administered. Advanced airway should be placed without any delay in case of compromised airway.

Antibiotic therapy: Broad-spectrum empirical antibiotics should be administered with priority. Both aerobic and anaerobic coverage should be given. Patients with less severe symptoms and patent airway may be treated with oral antibiotics. Oral penicillin VK and amoxicillin are first-line choices while levofloxacin, cefuroxime, and amoxicillin-clavulanate are the second-line choice. While patients with suspicion of deep neck infections should be treated with IV piperacillin/tazobactam, imipenem-cilastatin, and ertapenem. Surgical drainage should be done if CT suggests abscess.

Question 7

1. Discuss acute painful loss of vision.

Painful diminution of vision, e.g., acute angle closure glaucoma, acute iridocyclitis, acute keratitis/corneal ulcer.

Unilateral painful vision loss: Corneal abrasion, acute angle closure glaucoma, inflammation, cavernous sinus thrombosis, toxic/caustic exposure, trauma.

Bilateral painful vision loss: Keratitis toxic/caustic exposure trauma.

2. Explain orbital cellulitis.

Orbital cellulitis: Extension of sinus infection into orbit or traumatic inoculation.
- *Bacteria: Streptococcus pneumoniae* (*S. pneumoniae*), *Haemophilus influenzae* (*H. influenza*), *Catarrhalis, Aureus, Streptococcus pyogenes* (*S. pyogenes*), *Bacteroides*.
- Seen as erythema and swelling around eye
- Suspect if eyelid or periorbital inflammation is accompanied by any—ptosis, impaired extra-ocular movements, pain with eye movement, chemosis, and afferent papillary defect.
- Inpatient management, possible surgical drainage.

- Oral antibiotics to complete 3 weeks' course.
- Cefuroxime (50 mg/kg IV every 8 hours)
- Ampicillin-sulbactam (50 mg/kg IV every 6 hours)
- If anaerobic infection suspected clindamycin 10 mg/kg every 6 hours.

Question 8

1. Discuss the fractured tooth management in emergency department.

Dental avulsion is described as a complete displacement of a tooth from its socket in the alveolar bone, and it is one of the most traumatic dental injuries which originate exposure of the cells of the periodontal ligament to the external environment as well as disruption of the blood supply to the pulp **(Table 4)**.

TABLE 4: Dental avulsion.	
Traumatic injuries to teeth are very common and usually associated with road-traffic accidents, contact sports such as boxing, taekwondo, karate, etc., or fights. This is very common with children than adults while playing or falling.	
Pathophysiology	Pain due to trauma can be because of exposure of pulp, avulsion, or luxation
Clinical presentation	Pain is severe-like pulpitis but associated with bleeding
Red flags	Fractured crown of tooth
History	It is very important for clinician to know cause of injury, angle of impact and object of impact to know the extent of injury.
Physical examination	• Mobility of tooth is very common, sometimes fracture can occur at the root which is very painful but show no sign clinically • Radiographs are helpful in such cases
Investigations	Radiographs OPG or IOPA are most commonly done
Treatment	• If the fracture is at crown of the tooth exposing the pulp of tooth, then root canal treatment is done followed by restoration of the tooth • If there is luxation, splinting is done • In case of avulsion, teeth can be replanted under half an hour of injury if the tooth is preserved in saliva or milk and periodontal ligament fibers are intact

2. Discuss the management of acute rib fracture pain.

Rib fractures are common injuries that occur most often following blunt thoracic trauma but can also result from severe coughing, athletic activities (e.g., rowing, swinging golf clubs, throwing), and nonaccidental trauma (i.e., child abuse). Thoracic trauma leading to multiple fractured ribs (MFR) remains very common. Good analgesia may help to improve a patient's respiratory mechanics and to avoid intubation of the trachea for ventilatory support and therefore may dramatically alter the course of recovery. Analgesia options for patients with MFR (**Fig. 2**). Thoracic epidural, thoracic paravertebral, and intercostal blocks are the top choices for patients with MFR and they are of equivalent efficacy.

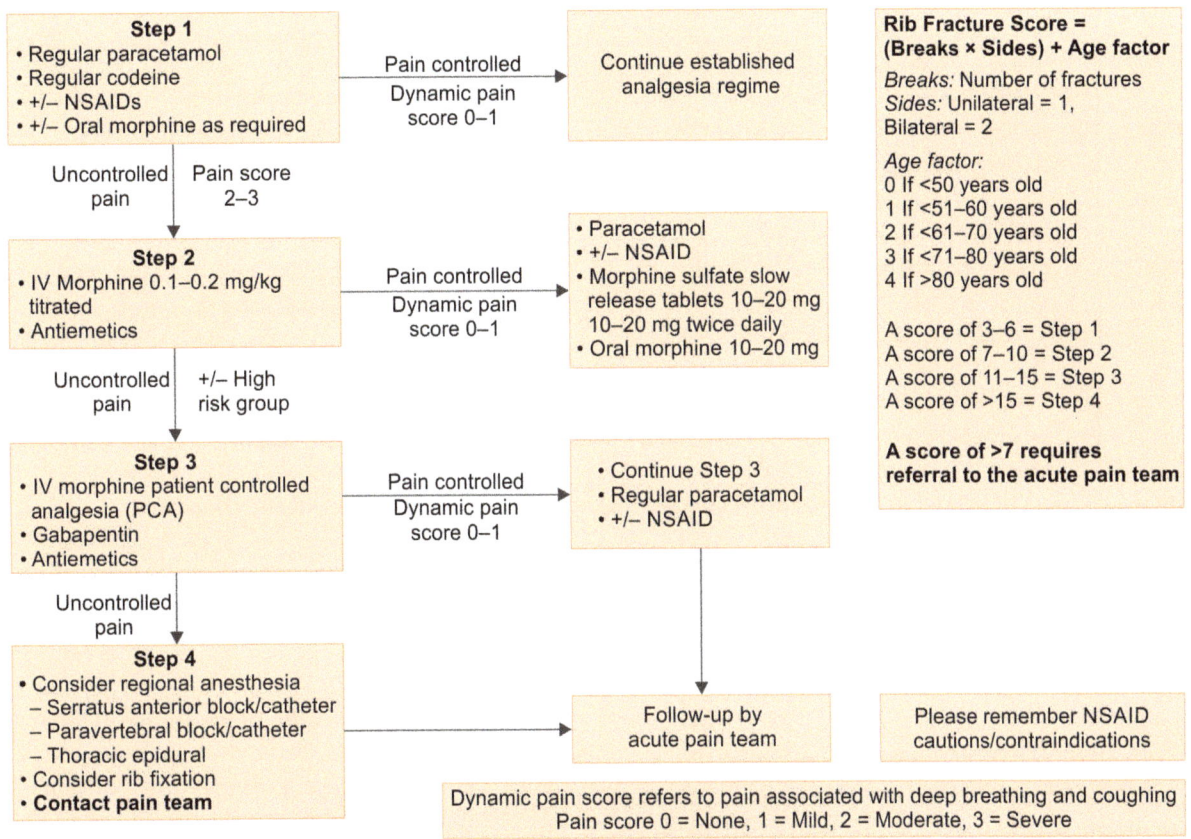

Fig. 2: Rib fracture pain management algorithm.

Question 9

1. Describe Lisfranc injury.

- A *Lisfranc injury* is a tarsometatarsal fracture dislocation characterized by traumatic disruption between the articulation of the medial cuneiform and base of the second metatarsal.
- Diagnosis is confirmed by radiographs which may show widening of the interval between the 1st and 2nd ray.
- Treatment is generally operative with either ORIF or arthrodesis.

2. Describe the clinical decision rules to evaluate knee and ankle injuries.

The Ottawa knee rules are a set of rules used to help physicians determine whether an X-ray of the knee is needed. They state that an X-ray is required only in patients who have an acute knee injury with one or more of the following:

- Aged 55 years or over.
- Tenderness at the head of the fibula.
- Isolated tenderness of the patella.
- Inability to flex knee to 90°.
- Inability to bear weight (defined as an inability to take four steps, i.e., two steps on each leg, regardless of limping) immediately and at presentation.

The Ottawa ankle rules indicate that a radiograph is indicated if any of the following is positive:

- Tenderness along the posterior medial or lateral malleoli,
- Base of the 5th metatarsal, navicular or
- If the patient is unable to bear weight for four steps following the injury.

Question 10

1. Describe the classification of liver and kidney injury.

Road traffic accident is the most common mechanism for abdominal trauma. It is the cause in up to 75% of the cases, followed by blows to the abdomen in approximately 15%, and falls in up to 9% of the cases of blunt abdominal trauma, and any such history should raise suspicion for the same. All cases of concomitant head or chest injuries must be ruled out for abdominal trauma **(Table 5)**.

TABLE 5: Liver and spleen trauma grades.		
Grade	**Liver description**	**Spleen description**
I: Hematoma	Subcapsular *nonexpanding*, <10% surface area	Subcapsular, <10% surface area (SA)
I: Laceration	Capsular tear *nonbleeding*, <1 cm depth	Capsular tear, <1 cm parenchymal depth
II: Hematoma	• Subcapsular, 10–50% SA • Intraparenchymal, <10 cm diameter	• Subcapsular, 10–50% SA • Intraparenchymal, <5 cm diameter
II: Laceration	1–3 cm parenchymal depth, <10 cm length	1–3 cm parenchymal depth, not involving vessel
III: Hematoma	• Subcapsular, >50% SA or expanding • Ruptured subcapsular/parenchymal hematoma • Intraparenchymal >10 cm or expanding	• Subcapsular, >50% SA or expanding • Ruptured subcapsular/parenchymal hematoma • Intraparenchymal >5 cm or expanding
III: Laceration	>3 cm parenchymal depth	>3 cm depth or involving trabecular vessels
IV: Laceration	25–75% of hepatic lobe parenchymal disruption or 1–3 Couinaud segments within a lobe	Laceration of segmental or hilar vessels with major devascularization (>25% of spleen)
V: Laceration	>75% of hepatic lobe parenchymal disruption or >3 Couinaud segments within a lobe	Completely shattered spleen
V: Vascular	Juxta hepatic venous injuries, i.e., retrohepatic vena cava or central major hepatic veins	Hilar vascular injury with devascularized spleen
VI	Vascular: Hepatic avulsion	–

2. Discuss classification of pelvic fractures.

Pelvic trauma is classified using Young and Burgess-mechanism of the injury **(Figs. 3A to G)**. It is commonly used to predict distant associated injuries, resuscitation needs and mortality rates.

Tile classification—based in biomechanical stability used for surgical planning. Emergency teams should be able to resuscitate, diagnose, and treat the associated injuries. Priority is given to get the hemodynamic corrected and exclude causes of bleeding from thorax, abdomen pelvis, and extremities. Simple AP view of pelvis, and inlet and outlet view radiograph gives ample information to ascertain the degree of the injury and its effect on stability of the pelvis. CT pelvis with reconstruction is needed for detailed study and planning of the surgery.

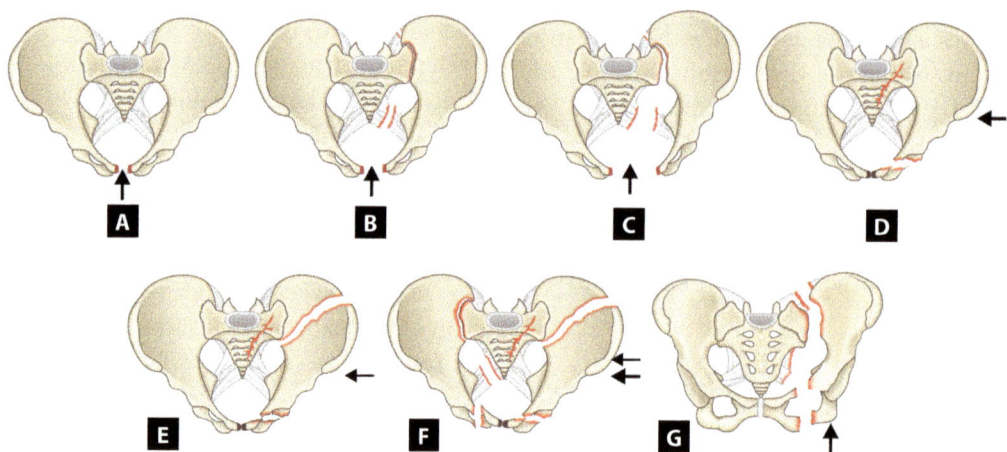

Figs. 3A to G: (A) Anteroposterior compression type I; (B) Anteroposterior compression type II; (C) Anteroposterior compression type III; (D) Lateral compression type I; (E) Lateral compression type II; (F) Lateral compression type III; (G) Vertical shear.

Stable fractures—stable are those involving only one part of the ring (pubic rami fractures), minimally displaced (<2.5 cm of diastasis) and avulsion fractures (ischial tuberosity), and transverse sacral fractures.

Unstable fractures are those involving the pelvic ring in two places with involvement of the posterior ring. These result from a combination of anteroposterior, lateral, vertical and rotational forces during the impact. Diastasis of >2.5 cm and widening of sacroiliac joint, vertical fractures of the sacrum with asymmetrical sacral foramina, avulsion fracture of the 5th lumbar transverse process with vertical displacement suggest highly unstable injury.

SUGGESTED READING

1. Richhariya D, Sharma B. Textbook of Emergency Medicine including Intensive Care and Trauma, 2nd edition. New Delhi: Jaypee Brothers Medical Publishers (P) Ltd; 2022. pp. 1557-64. (Question 1).
2. Richhariya D, Sharma B. Textbook of Emergency Medicine including Intensive Care and Trauma, 2nd edition. New Delhi: Jaypee Brothers Medical Publishers (P) Ltd; 2022. pp. 1570-8. (Question 2).
3. Richhariya D, Sharma B. Textbook of Emergency Medicine including Intensive Care and Trauma, 2nd edition. New Delhi: Jaypee Brothers Medical Publishers (P) Ltd; 2022. p. 1594. (Question 3).
4. Richhariya D, Sharma B. Textbook of Emergency Medicine including Intensive Care and Trauma, 2nd edition. New Delhi: Jaypee Brothers Medical Publishers (P) Ltd; 2022. pp. 1559-80. (Question 4).
5. Richhariya D, Sharma B. Textbook of Emergency Medicine including Intensive Care and Trauma, 2nd edition. New Delhi: Jaypee Brothers Medical Publishers (P) Ltd; 2022. pp. 750, 1095. (Question 5).
6. Richhariya D, Sharma B. Textbook of Emergency Medicine including Intensive Care and Trauma, 2nd edition. New Delhi: Jaypee Brothers Medical Publishers (P) Ltd; 2022. pp. 801, 931. (Question 6).
7. Richhariya D, Sharma B. Textbook of Emergency Medicine including Intensive Care and Trauma, 2nd edition. New Delhi: Jaypee Brothers Medical Publishers (P) Ltd; 2022. p. 900. (Question 7).
8. Richhariya D, Sharma B. Textbook of Emergency Medicine including Intensive Care and Trauma, 2nd edition. New Delhi: Jaypee Brothers Medical Publishers (P) Ltd; 2022. pp. 938, 1580. (Question 8).
9. Richhariya D, Sharma B. Textbook of Emergency Medicine including Intensive Care and Trauma, 2nd edition. New Delhi: Jaypee Brothers Medical Publishers (P) Ltd; 2022. pp. 1609-10. (Question 9).
10. Richhariya D, Sharma B. Textbook of Emergency Medicine including Intensive Care and Trauma, 2nd edition. New Delhi: Jaypee Brothers Medical Publishers (P) Ltd; 2022. pp. 1593, 1608. (Question 10).

Emergency Medicine Paper 47

Devendra Richhariya

Question 1

A 26-year-old patient presents to an emergency department (ED) with acute onset chest pain. His pulse rate is 100/minute, BP 130/90 mm Hg and oxygen saturation is 95%. His initial ECG is normal.

1. How will you assess and manage the patient?
2. Describe various risk stratification scores you will use in this case.

Patients presenting with chest pain to ED with normal ECG and cardiac markers on arrival should be observed for a period of 6–12 hours before ruling out acute coronary syndrome (acute coronary syndrome). Simultaneously other life-threatening causes of chest pain such as pulmonary embolism, tension pneumothorax, cardiac tamponade and aortic dissection should be considered high risk based on clinical presentation and managed and admitted immediately. In emergency department observation unit (EDOU) performing serial ECG/cardiac biomarkers and stress tests helps to identify ACS or patients at risk who would benefit from timely intervention to reduce their risk of *major adverse cardiac event (MACE)*. TIMI score **(Table 1)** and HEART score **(Table 2)** are used for risk stratification in chest pain.

TABLE 1: Risk stratification: Thrombolysis in Myocardial Infarction (TIMI) score - 1 point for each positive score.

History	Age >65 years
	Three or more risk factors for CAD
	Known CAD
	Aspirin use in the past 7 days
Presentation	Recent (<24 hours) severe angina
	Positive cardiac biomarkers
	ST deviation >0.5 mm

Higher TIMI scores mandate admission: Predicts risk of an adverse cardiac outcome within 14 days of presentation with unstable angina or non-STEMI.
Vancouver chest pain rule: Used to determine very low-risk chest pain patients and help in early discharge.
(CAD: coronary artery disease)

TABLE 2: Risk stratification: HEART risk score for chest pain patients in ED.

History	• Highly suspicious	2
	• Moderately suspicious	1
	• Slightly suspicious	0
ECG	• Significant ST depression	2
	• Nonspecific repolarization changes	1
	• Normal	0
Age	• >65 years	2
	• 45–65 years	1
	• <45 years	0
Risk factors	• >3 risk	2
	• 1 or 2	1
	• No risk	0
Troponins	• >3 × normal limit	2
	• 1–3 × normal limit	1
	• <normal limit	0

Heart score	Risk of MACE	Recommendations
0–3	0.9%	ED discharge
4–6	12%	Observation
>6	65%	Cardiology admission

Question 2

1. Discuss the causes, work-up, and management of nontraumatic subarachnoid hemorrhage (SAH).

Subarachnoid hemorrhage usually presents with severe thunderclap headache but may also present with syncope, decreased level of consciousness, neck pain, nuchal rigidity, seizure, and other nonspecific symptoms. The range of symptoms of spontaneous intracerebral hemorrhage (ICH) is even wider, and depending on the site of bleeding and the volume may vary from a mild headache to a deep coma with/without focal neurologic deficits. An important point is that over first hours, the symptoms may worsen or rarely improve. Taking everything into account, there is no definite finding in terms of diagnosis of hemorrhagic stroke patients, and diagnostic certainty always needs brain imaging.

Subarachnoid hemorrhage and ICH have some same and also specific management in terms of both surgical and nonsurgical interventions. All patients with SAH need neurological surgeon's consultation. Patients with ICH are generally managed medically by neurologists, though there are few indications for surgical intervention: *Airway management, blood pressure control, blood sugar control, reversal of anticoagulation, anti-fibrinolytic, seizure management, intracranial pressure control,* and *surgical interventions.*

The hematoma itself or the surrounding edema can result in increased intracranial pressure (ICP), which can precipitate secondary brain injury and neurologic deterioration. Elevation of the head of the bed and providing the patient with adequate analgesia and sedation are the mainstay of preventing ICP elevation in ICH. The patients should be treated with normal saline and hypotonic fluids should be avoided.

In case of elevated ICP, osmotic agents such as mannitol and hypertonic saline are the first-line agents.

2. Describe the utility and method of Alberta stroke program early CT (ASPECT) scoring.

The ASPECTS is a 10-point quantitative topographic CT scan score used in patients with middle cerebral artery (MCA) stroke. It has also been adapted for the posterior cerebral circulation. An ideal ASPECTs score is 10 when none of the vital structures are involved by acute ischemic changes. But patients with scores ≥8 have a higher chance for an independent outcome. An ASPECTS score less than or equal to 7 predicts a worse functional outcome at 3 months as well as symptomatic hemorrhage.

Segmental estimation of the MCA vascular territory is made, and 1 point is deducted from the initial score of 10 for every region involved:
- Caudate
- Putamen
- Internal capsule
- Insular cortex
- M1: "Anterior MCA cortex" corresponding to the frontal operculum
- M2: "MCA cortex lateral to insular ribbon" corresponding to the anterior temporal lobe
- M3: "Posterior MCA cortex" corresponding to the posterior temporal lobe
- M4: "Anterior MCA territory immediately superior to M1"
- M5: "Aateral MCA territory immediately superior to M2"
- M6: "Posterior MCA territory immediately superior to M3"

Question 3

1. Briefly discuss the management of sepsis in patients with febrile neutropenia in ED.

Febrile neutropenia (FN) is defined as "single oral temperature of >38.3°C (>101°F) or a temperature of >38.0°C (>100.4°F) sustained for >1 hour and an absolute neutrophil count (ANC) of <500 cells/mm^3 or expected to fall to <500 cells/mm^3 in next 48 hours".

Initial assessment includes targeted history, physical examination with emphasis on hydration, oral cavity, oropharynx, skin including any indwelling catheter, lungs, abdomen, perianal area, and mental status. CBC, creatinine, electrolytes, liver function test, blood culture (two set), culture and stain samples from suspected site of infection, imaging studies if any site suspected.

Outpatient management may be considered in low-risk patient who resides close to the hospital, can come for frequent clinic visits and has a 24 hours care-giver.

Inpatient management includes broad-spectrum antibiotics guided by patient's history and examination, allergies and culture data of the institution should be started within 60 minutes of presentation. Infectious Diseases Society of America (IDSA) recommends: Cefepime 2 g/8 hourly, ceftazidime 2 g/8 hourly, piperacillin tazobactam 4.5 g/6 hourly, meropenem 1 g/8 hourly and imipenem cilastatin 500 mg/6 hourly. Aminoglycoside, fluoroquinolones may be added in patients with complicated presentation.

2. Discuss Sepsis 3.0 guidelines for sepsis.

The definition further evolved and presently Sepsis-3 in 2016, defines sepsis as a *"life-threatening organ dysfunction caused by dysregulated host response to infection."* Whereas septic shock is recognized as, *"A subset of sepsis in which underlying circulatory and cellular metabolism abnormalities are profound enough to substantially increase mortality."*

In present definition of sepsis, authors emphasized that previous distinction of sepsis, severe sepsis, and septic shock is no longer relevant. An infection without organ dysfunction or hypotension or evidence of hypoperfusion does not warrant similar aggressive response, and can simply be categorized as having an infection only and not "'sepsis"; whereas previous "severe sepsis" is now termed as "sepsis". For standardization of organ dysfunction purpose, task force promotes use of quick sequential organ failure assessment (qSOFA) score **(Table 3)** in out of ICU settings and sequential organ failure assessment (SOFA) score for ICU settings. Screening tool for sepsis in ED is given in **Table 4**.

TABLE 3: qSOFA score.

H	**H**ypotension: SBP less than or equal to 100 mm Hg
A	**A**ltered mental status (any GCS <15)
T	**T**achypnea: Respiratory rate greater than or equal to 22/min

(GCS: Glasgow Coma Scale)

TABLE 4: Screening tool for rule in/out sepsis in ED.

This is a simplified tool that can be used to screen patients for sepsis in the ED or in critical care unit

1. Obtain proper history for any potential source of infection	Lung infections, kidney infections such as urinary tract infection, infection lingering in the abdomen, meningitis and endocarditis, skin and soft tissue infection, wound infection, catheter-related infections, blood-stream infections	Yes/No
2. Search for signs and symptoms that would indicate	Fever >38.3°C or temperature <36°C, altered mental status with a GCS <15, heart rate >90 bpm (tachycardia), respiratory rate >20 bpm (tachypnea), leukocytosis or leukopenia (WBC count >12,000 µ/L or <4,000 µ/L respectively)	Yes/No

If both the above are Yes, suspicion of infection is present. Laboratory investigations that should be ordered are complete blood count with differential, blood lactate and cultures, basic metabolic panel. Ultrasound abdomen, CT scan, chest X-ray, amylase, lipase, ABG, procalcitonin should be obtained according to the signs and symptoms and according to physician discretion.

3. Whether organ dysfunction criteria present?	If suspicion of infection and organ dysfunction are present, the patient's condition is labeled as *Septic Shock* and should be entered into the protocol.	Yes/No

(ABG: arterial blood gas; GCS: Glasgow Coma Scale)

Question 4

1. Describe the clinical presentation, pathophysiology, and management of scorpion bite.

Clinical presentation: Pain, erythema, induration, wheal, paresthesia and hyperesthesia are the local features.

Systemic features: Allergic—urticaria, wheeze, and angioedema.

Autonomic: Sympathetic—tachycardia, hyperthermia, hypertension, profuse sweating, and urinary retention. *Parasympathetic*—bradycardia, hypotension, urination, hypersalivation, bronchospasm and priapism; mixed dysfunction.

Cardiovascular: Hypertension, tachycardia, cardiogenic shock and arrhythmias.

Gastrointestinal: Nausea, vomiting, diarrhea, and abdominal pain.

Neurological: Cranial nerves—nystagmus, miosis/mydriasis, tongue fasciculations.

Peripheral: Spasticity, clonus, brisk reflexes, and ascending paralysis.

Central: Respiratory failure, coma, and stroke.

Rare: Disseminated intravascular coagulation (DIC), pulmonary edema, rhabdomyolysis, and renal failure.

Pathophysiology

Complex venom: Phospholipase, acetylcholinesterase, hyaluronidase, serotonin, and neurotoxins.

Mode of action: Neurotoxins—bind reversibly to voltage-gated ion channels (sodium, calcium, and potassium) and keep them in open state. Affect somatic and autonomic nervous system (autonomic storm—primary cause of morbidity and mortality). Hyperkalemia, hyperglycemia, increased secretion of renin and aldosterone—characteristic of India red scorpion.

Management: First aid—paracetamol (pain relief); airway maintenance and ventilation; anaphylaxis—adrenaline, chlorpheniramine, and hydrocortisone.

Hospital: Airway, breathing and circulation; local anesthesia for severe pain. Hourly monitoring—temperature, pulse, BP, respiratory rate, and oxygen saturation. ECG monitoring (cardiac arrhythmias). ABG and serum electrolytes (potassium, magnesium, and calcium). Scorpion antivenom—systemic envenomation; tetanus prophylaxis; fluid imbalance correction (crystalloids); benzodiazepines for delirium and agitation.

Bawaskar's protocol:
- *Stage I (0-4 hours):* Sweating salivation, mydriasis, priapism, hypertension, hypotension, cold extremities. Treatment—Antiscorpion venom (ASV) + prazosin
- *Stage II (0-6 hours):* Hypertension tachycardia cold extremities. Treatment—ASV + prazosin
- *Stage III (6-10 hours):* Tachycardia, hypotension, pulmonary edema, cold extremities Treatment ASV + prazocin + dobutamine + NIV or MV
- *Stage IV (0-6 hours):* Massive pulmonary edema treatment ASV + sodium nitroprusside/Nitroglycerine + NIV/MV
- *Stage V (>12 hours):* Warm extremities, tachycardia, hypotension, pulmonary edema. Treatment—Dobutamine.

Preventive Measures

- Clear debris and rubbish from areas of work and rest. Use insect repellants.
- Inspect shoes and clothes for scorpions. Use flashlight when walking in dark places.

2. Discuss calcium channel blocker versus beta-blocker toxicity.

Calcium channel blocker clinical features: Bradycardia, hypotension, AV conduction anomalies, idioventricular rhythms and complete heart block; altered mental status, convulsions, stroke, renal failure, noncardiogenic pulmonary edema and coma; respiratory distress.

Diagnosis: Blood level analysis

Treatment: Intravenous (IV) access, continuous ECG monitoring HR, BP, serum electrolytes, renal function test (RFT), random blood sugar (RBS), ABG.

Airway support and oxygenation GI decontamination calcium therapy for hypocalcemia 0.6–1.2 mL/kg/h of 10% calcium gluconate

- *High-dose insulin euglycemia (HIE) treatment:* 1 U/kg of regular insulin bolus along with 0.5 g/kg dextrose intravenously (IV) is administered. Watch for hypokalemia.
- *Lipid emulsion therapy:* Initial bolus of 1.5 mL/kg of 20% lipid emulsion followed by 0.25–0.5 mL/kg/min over 30 minutes.

Beta-blockers toxicity: Manifestations of overdose include hypotension, bradycardia, arrhythmias, delirium, seizures, mydriasis, coma, and respiratory failure. Hypoglycemia is common feature in children. The complications of profound hypotension may include acute renal failure, respiratory failure, and noncardiogenic pulmonary edema. Other cardiovascular effects may include atrioventricular block, intraventricular conduction delays, ventricular arrhythmias, pulmonary edema, cardiac arrest, and asystole. Central nervous system (CNS) depression is common in patients with significant cardiovascular toxicity. Beta-blockers, which are more lipid soluble are more likely to cross the blood-brain barrier causing drowsiness, confusion, seizures, hallucinations, dilated pupils and in severe cases coma. Hydrophilic beta blockers have few CNS side effects.

Beta-blocker Toxicity Management

Mild: Activated charcoal, stomach wash, whole bowel irrigation (for sustained release preparation), atropine 1 mg IV for bradycardia, fluid boluses for hypotension.

Moderate: As for mild poisoning, plus endotracheal intubation. *Glucagon:* A bolus of 5–10 mg IV in adults should be administered over 1–2 minutes (beware of the risk of vomiting and aspiration), followed by an infusion initially 50–150 µg/kg/h (e.g., 2.5 mg/h for an adult weighing 50 kg or 4 mg/h for an adult weighing 80 kg) titrated to clinical response. In children a bolus of 50–150 µg/kg IV should be administered over 1–2 minutes, followed by an infusion initially of 50 µg/kg/h, titrated to clinical response atropine up to 3 mg IV.

- *High-dose insulin euglycemia (HIE) treatment:* 1 U/kg of regular insulin bolus along with 0.5 g/kg dextrose intravenously (IV) is administered. Watch for hypokalemia.
- *Lipid emulsion therapy:* Initial bolus of 1.5 mL/kg of 20% lipid emulsion followed by 0.25–0.5 mL/kg/min over 30 minutes.

Severe: Initiate treatment as for moderate poisoning
- Intra-arterial and pulmonary pressure monitoring
- *Inotropes and vasopressors:*
  - *Isoproterenol*—start at 0.1 µg/kg/min, titrate rapidly to effect or
  - *Dobutamine*—start at 2.5 µg/kg/min, titrate rapidly to effect or
  - *Noradrenaline*—start at 0.1 µg/kg/min, titrate rapidly to effect
  - *Adrenaline*—start at 0.02 µg/kg/min, titrate rapidly to effect or
- *Phosphodiesterase inhibitors,* e.g., milrinone 50 µg/kg IV bolus over 2 minutes, then 0.25–1.0 µg/kg/min.
- Ventricular pacing
- Extracorporeal or intra-aortic balloon pump

Question 5

1. Discuss Cairo–Bishop criteria.

Tumor lysis syndrome (TLS) refers to metabolic consequences resulting from sudden release of intracellular metabolites, nucleic acids and proteins from tumor cells undergoing death spontaneously or posttreatment. It is divided into two groups, i.e., laboratory and clinical based on Cairo-Bishop definitions.

Laboratory TLS is defined as presence of ≥2 of following laboratory abnormalities, i.e., uric acid ≥8 mg/dL, potassium ≥6 mEq/L, phosphorus >4.5 mg/dL in adults (≥6.5 mg/dL in children) and calcium ≤7 mg/dL or 25% change in these laboratory values from baseline, present within 3 days before or 7 days after initiation of therapy.

Clinical TLS is defined as laboratory TLS accompanied with ≥1 of the following—serum creatinine ≥1.5 times the upper limit of normal, seizure, cardiac dysrhythmia or death.

The clinical manifestations noted are acute kidney injury, seizures and cardiac dysrhythmias or cardiac arrest. Renal failure occurs due to the precipitation of uric acid within renal tubules. Phosphorus released from cells may combine with calcium and get precipitated in renal tubules and parenchyma also. Hyperkalemia causes cardiac dysrhythmias or cardiac arrest. Hypocalcemia may cause tetany and seizures and can lead to dysrhythmias. Hypovolemia can further precipitate renal failure.

2. Briefly outline the steps in the management of thyroid storm.

Thyroid storm is unrecognized, undertreated, life-threatening form of severe thyrotoxicosis. Thyroid storm is rare and mostly acute reaction to thyroid and non-thyroid surgery, trauma infections contrast media, amiodarone, after delivery in preexisting hyperthyroidism. Other risk factors are acute coronary syndrome, pulmonary embolism, and diabetic ketoacidosis.

Prompt recognitions and treatment are warranted as mortality is almost 100%. The causes of mortality in patient of thyroid storm: Sepsis, multiorgan failure, congestive heart failure arrhythmias, disseminated intravascular, and coagulation. Clinical features of thyroid storm are typical and include hyperpyrexia, out of proportion tachycardia, altered mental status (agitation, delirium coma) along with clinical picture of hyperthyroidism. Classic features of thyroid storm include fever, marked tachycardia, heart failure, tremor, nausea and vomiting, diarrhea, dehydration, restlessness, extreme agitation, delirium or coma. Fever is typical and may be >105.8°F (41°C).

Thyroid function test: Usual findings include elevated triiodothyronine (T3), thyroxine (T4), and free T4 levels; increased T3 resin uptake; suppressed thyroid-stimulating hormone (TSH) levels; and an elevated 24-hour iodine uptake.

The management of thyroid storm is summarized in **Table 5**.

TABLE 5: Management of thyroid storm.

β-adrenergic blockers	• Propranolol 60–80 mg orally every 4 hours (IV 0.5–1.0 mg as test dose then repeat 1–2 mg every 15 minutes till desired effect then 1–2 mg every 3 hours) or • Metoprolol 25–50 mg orally every 6 hours or • Esmolol 50–100 µg/kg/min infusion
Inhibition of thyroid hormone synthesis	Propylthiouracil 500–1,000 mg loading then 250 mg every 4 hours or Methimazole 60–80 mg/day
Inhibition of thyroid hormone release	Saturated potassium iodide solution (50 mg/drops) 1–2 drops orally or per rectally or Lugol's solution 5–7 drops
Corticosteroid	Hydrocortisone 300 mg IV then 100 mg every 8 hours
Treatment of underlying precipitant	Empirical antibiotics
Supportive measures	Volume resuscitation cooling blankets, fan ice packs/lavage
Others	Lorazepam/diazepam

Question 6

1. Describe the differential diagnosis and management of acute onset vesiculobullous lesions.

Major groups of dermatologic emergencies include: Vesiculobullous disorder **(Table 6)** and drug reaction, infections, autoimmune disorders, inflammatory cutaneous disorders, environmental disorder. *Vesiculobullous disorders* are:
- Erythema multiforme major
- Stevens–Johnson syndrome (SJS)—it is considered to be a severe form of EM.
- Toxic epidermal necrolysis (TEN)—it is considered to be more severe form of SJS.
- Generalized bullous fixed drug eruption
- Pemphigus vulgaris
- Bullous pemphigoid
- DRESS syndrome

TABLE 6: Differentiation among EM, SJS/TEN, bullous fixed drug eruption.

	Erythema multiforme major	SJS/TEN	Generalized bullous fixed drug eruption
Lesion pattern	Typical target lesion present	Flat/atypical target lesion present	Absence of target lesions/bullous lesions with surrounding rim of erythema
Mucosal involvement	Yes	Yes	Yes/No
Distribution	Mainly acral involvement/limbs	Widespread	Widespread
Blister/erosions	Yes at the center of target lesions	Yes <10%—SJS; 10–30%: SJS/TEN overlap; >30%: TEN	Yes
Recurrence history	Occasional	Rare	Common
Prognosis	Excellent	Mortality depends on risk factors (SCORTEN)	Generally favorable if <20% body surface area is involved

2. Enumerate Lynch algorithm.

The Modified Lynch Algorithm provides a systematic approach to the diagnosis of rashes by providing a number of questions and branching points to narrow down the differential diagnosis of important and life-threatening rashes for the emergency physician.

Question 7

1. Describe coagulation cascade and approach to a bleeding patient on warfarin.

Physiology of hemostasis: The normal hemostatic system consists of a complex process that limits blood loss through the formation of a platelet (primary hemostasis) and the production of cross-linked fibrin (secondary hemostasis), which strengthens the platelet plug. These reactions are counter-regulated by the fibrinolytic system **(Fig. 1)**. Hemostasis is a process of balance between the coagulation and the fibrinolytic system. The coagulation system consists of two main components primary and secondary hemostasis.

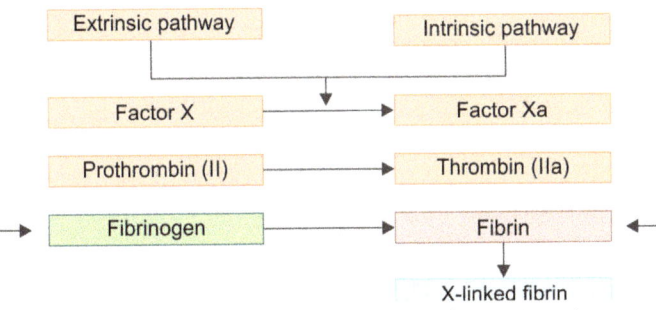

Fig. 1: Physiology of hemostasis extrinsic and intrinsic pathways.

Management of warfarin-induced bleeding: The reversal of warfarin needs immediate and sustained therapy. Immediate reversal is achieved by the therapy of prothrombin complex concentrates (PCC) and fresh frozen plasma (FFP), and sustained reversal is achieved through vitamin K administration **(Table 7)**.

2. Discuss the management of massive hematemesis in ED.

Rapid evaluation and resuscitation should be done before the diagnostic evaluation in unstable patients with acute severe bleeding. The patients should be evaluated for the immediate risk of rebleeding, complications and the cause of bleed after he is hemodynamically stabilized. Patients who are hemodynamically stable at the time of presentation with minor GI bleed can be evaluated in an outpatient setting.

Approximately 80% of GI bleed stop spontaneously and 15% of the patients continue to bleed requiring urgent intervention such as endoscopy. Patients who present with continued bleed, history of syncope, hypotension, tachycardia, low urine output, hemoglobin level <8 g, and advanced age can be categorized as high-risk patients who require urgent intervention whereas patients of younger age, without any feature of hypovolemic shock are low-risk patients. So, early categorization of patients in emergency department is important for management planning.

The emergent treatment of the patient presenting with GI bleed is very important. Initial rapid resuscitative measures should be promptly started in emergency which includes putting two large bore intravenous cannula and fluid resuscitation. Blood samples should be collected for complete blood counts, liver and renal function tests, coagulation profile, and blood grouping/crossmatching. Patients with massive upper GI bleed may need endotracheal intubation for airway protection.

TABLE 7: Management of vitamin K antagonists-induced high INRs and bleeding.

Condition	Interventions
Raised INR but <5; absent significant bleeding	Lower/Omit dose. Increase frequency of monitoring. Resume therapy at a lower dose if INR more than minimally supratherapeutic
INR ≥5.0 but ≤10.0; absent significant bleeding	Omit 1–2 doses. Increase frequency of monitoring. Resume therapy when INR therapeutic Or Omit dose. Give 1.0–2.5 mg oral vitamin K. If the patient is at increased risk of bleeding, If requires more rapid reversal for a surgical procedure, give 2–4 mg oral vitamin K; the INR should decrease within 24 h. If the INR remains elevated, additional vitamin K (1–2 mg orally) may be given
INR >10; absent significant bleeding	Hold warfarin therapy. Give 5–10 mg oral vitamin K; the INR should decrease within 24–48 h. Increase frequency of monitoring. Administer additional vitamin K if necessary. Resume therapy when INR within therapeutic range
Serious or life-threatening bleeding	Hold warfarin therapy. Give 10 mg vitamin K by slow IV infusion, in addition to 4-factor PCC or FFP. Vitamin K may be given every 12 h

(FFP: fresh frozen plasma; INR: International Normalized Ratio; PCC: prothrombin complex concentrate)

There is a controversial role of nasogastric tube placement in all GI bleeds, can be useful in upper GI bleed. Bloody nasogastric aspirate confirms the source in upper GI tract. Nasogastric tube placement should be done in patients with suspected upper GI bleed and gastric lavage should be done as it facilitates in clear view during endoscopic procedure.

Patients presenting with massive GI bleed should be given packed RBC in the ED only as rapid blood loss can result in vital organ hypoperfusion leading to multiorgan dysfunction. In euvolemic patients with upper GI hemorrhage, the packed red blood cells (PRBC) transfusion should be planned to *target hemoglobin level of 7 g%*. Overzealous PRBC transfusion should be avoided as it may increase the risk of rebleed and transfusion-related complications. Patients with acute GI bleed who are on anticoagulants, efforts should be made by emergency physician to reverse the effect of anticoagulant. Patients on warfarin or dicoumarin (vitamin K antagonists) should be given *intravenous vitamin K*.

Intravenous PPI is recommended in all patients presenting with acute upper GI bleed. Emergency physician should consider intravenous PPI in all patients with upper GI hemorrhage before the endoscopic therapy. In patients with ulcer-related upper GI bleed, *80 mg IV pantoprazole/omeprazole in the ED followed by continuous infusion @8 mg/h for at least 72 hours (preferably up to 5 days)* reduces the risk of rebleed and need for surgery. Somatostatin and its analog reduce the blood flow to portal system by causing vasoconstriction, thus decrease the variceal bleed. *The dose of somatostatin is 250 µg IV bolus followed by 250 µg/h continuous infusion for 3-5 days whereas the dose of octreotide is 50 µg IV bolus followed by 50 µg/h continuous infusion for 3-5 days.* Terlipressin causes vasoconstriction and therefore reduces portal blood flow and also increases the resistance to variceal blood. *The dose of terlipressin in variceal bleed is 1 mg IV every 6 hours for 5 days.* Cardiac and bowel ischemia are potential side effects which can limit the use of this agent.

In patients with upper GI bleed, the endoscopy is both diagnostic and therapeutic as it helps in confirming the cause of the bleed and also enables us to do measure to stop the bleed. For varices-related bleed, endoscopic band ligation of varices, glue injection (for gastric varices), endoscopic sclerotherapy can be performed to stop the bleed. For nonvariceal bleed (such as ulcer related, Mallory–Weiss tear, Cameron ulcer, esophagitis), injection therapy/hemoclip/argon plasma coagulation/hemospray or combination therapy can be used to achieve hemostasis.

Question 8

1. Discuss the assessment and management of agitated patient.

Physical or chemical restrain of patient is required whenever there is possibility of "self-harm" and agitated behavior dangerous to hospital staff. Close observation of patient is required to record changes in tone, speech, irritability, clinched jaw, and fist for intervention at the right time. Physician must record the GCS before applying any measures for agitation control. Medications used for chemical restrain are haloperidol (antipsychotic agent)/lorazepam.

Few characteristic features of commonly used haloperidol and lorazepam

Drug therapy: Haloperidol is commonly used first line medication for delirium. *Haloperidol* given in 2—5 mg intramuscular. *Olanzapine*: 2.5-5 mg orally once a day; *Risperidone* 0.5 mg orally twice daily. *Quetiapine* 12.5-25 mg orally twice daily is used for hypoactive form of delirium. *Benzodiazepine*: Lorazepam 2 mg IV is also used commonly alone or with haloperidol, diazepam is the drug of choice when delirium is suspected due to alcohol withdrawal.

2. Discuss thrombolytic therapy for stroke in ED.

Dose of tPA: As per the guidelines infuse 0.9 mg/kg (maximum dose 90 mg) over 60 minutes, with 10% of the dose given as a bolus over 1 minute.

For treatment within 3 hours of stroke onset, alteplase led to a good outcome for 33%, versus 23% for control [odds ratio (OR) 1.75, 95% CI 1.35-2.27]. The number needed to treat (NNT) for one additional patient to achieve a good outcome was 10.

For treatment from 3-4.5 hours, the proportion with a good outcome in the alteplase and control groups was 35 and 30% (OR 1.26, 95% CI 1.05-1.51, NNT 20).

The benefit of IV defibrinogenating agents and of IV fibrinolytic agents other than alteplase and tenecteplase is unproven; therefore, their administration is not recommended outside a clinical trial. Tenecteplase administered as a 0.4 mg/kg single IV bolus has not been proven to be superior or non-inferior to alteplase but might be considered as an alternative to alteplase in patients with minor neurological impairment and no major intracranial occlusion.

Question 9

1. Discuss the cause and management of sympathetic crashing acute pulmonary edema.

Pulmonary edema is often caused by *congestive heart failure*. When the heart is not able to pump efficiently, blood can back up into the veins that take blood through the lungs. As the pressure in these blood vessels increases, fluid is pushed into the air spaces (alveoli) in the lungs. Causes are acute tachy- or bradyarrhythmia, infection, fever, acute MI, severe hypertension, acute mitral or aortic regurgitation, increased circulating volumes [Na ingestion, blood transfusion, pregnancy, increased metabolic demands (exercise hyperthyroidism)], pulmonary embolism, and noncompliance [sudden discontinuation of chronic congestive heart failure (CHF) medication].

The management of acute pulmonary edema is shown in **Flowchart 1**.

Flowchart 1: Management of acute pulmonary edema.

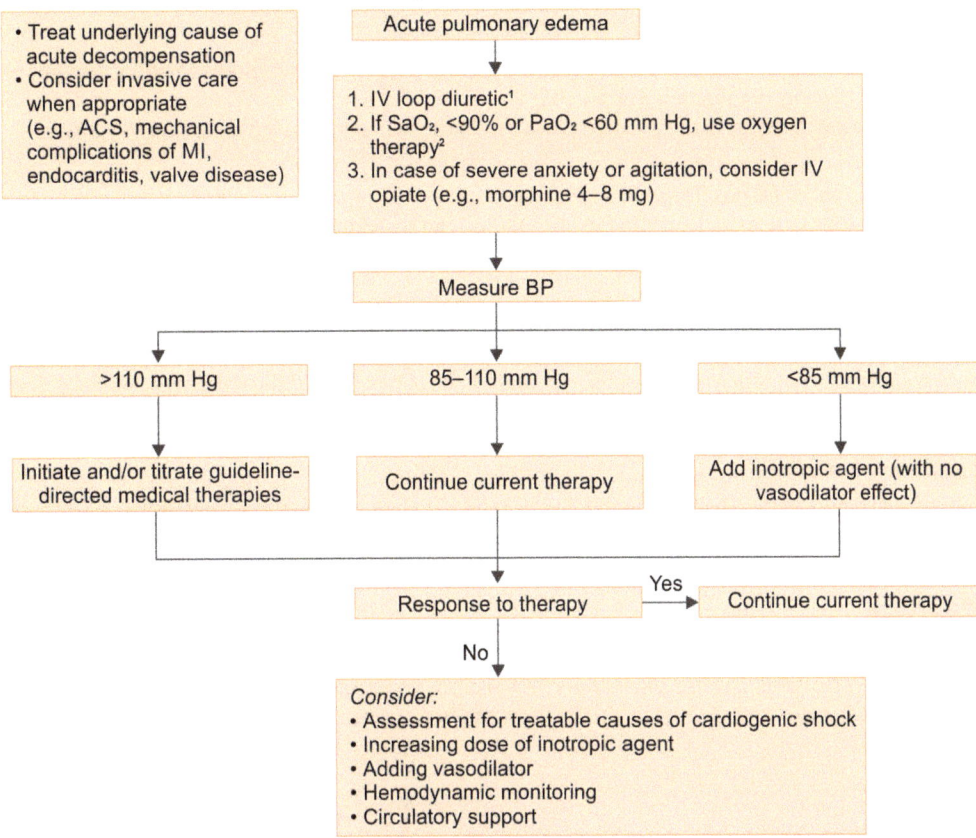

(BP: blood pressure; IV: intravenous; NIV: noninsive mechanical ventilation)
[1]At a dose 2.5 times higher than in long-term treatment; repeat when necessary.
[2]Higher-concentration oxygen (start with FIO_2 40–60%; target SaO_2 >90%) if there is no response, consider NIV or intubation and mechanical ventilation.

2. Discuss the types and management of heat-related illnesses in adults.

Heat illness is a common medical emergency in tropical areas, especially the heat stroke is cause of concern, clinically diagnosed as a core temperature >40°C with central nervous system dysfunction or multiorgan dysfunction (core temperature is at which blood perfusion of hypothalamus, and vital organ of body like heart brain are maintained, normal core body temperature is 36–37.5°C and rectal temperature being the closest approximation). Heat illness is a spectrum of disorders due to environmental exposure to heat. It ranges from minor conditions such as heat cramps, heat syncope, and heat exhaustion to the more severe condition known as heat stroke. A number of heat illnesses exist across a broad spectrum of presentations **(Table 8)**.

TABLE 8: Classification of heat illness characteristic features and treatment.	
Type	**Characteristic features and treatment**
Heat cramps	• Muscular pain which happens after exercise in hot conditions • *Heat cramp*: After heat cramps occur, the affected patient should avoid strenuous work and exercise for several hours to allow adequate recovery
Heat edema	• Cutaneous condition characterized by dependent edema from vasodilatory pooling • *Heat edema*: People visiting hot climates from colder climates may also have an increased risk of heat edema
Heat rash	• Irritation of the skin that results from excessive sweating during hot and humid weather • *Heat rash*: Medical treatment is necessary only if the area becomes infected. Heat rash can be prevented by avoiding hot, humid conditions, wearing lose fitting clothes, and using air-conditioning or fans to allow air to circulate

Contd...

Contd...

Type	Characteristic features and treatment
Heat tetany	• A result of short periods of stress in intense heat. Symptoms may include hyperventilation, respiratory problems, numbness or tingling, or muscle spasms • Treatment includes removing the affected person from the heat and slowing the breathing pattern
Heat syncope	• Dizziness as a result of excess heat • *Treatment*: The patient is positioned in a seating or supine position with legs raised. If the patient can tolerate it, oral rehydration with salt or a drink containing electrolytes, can be administered slowly, and the patient is moved to a cooler area preferably under a shade. The affected person should be advised rest; as heat syncope can lead to heat exhaustion and subsequently heat strokes
Heat exhaustion	• A precursor of a heatstroke which includes heavy sweating, rapid breathing and a fast, weak pulse • *Treatment*: Basic management includes moving the person to a cool place with removal of extra layers of clothes. Passive cooling by fanning wet towels and increase intake of oral fluids if the patient is conscious. Specific management includes following the usual airway, breathing and circulation (ABC) approach. Supplemental oxygen may be required and if the patient is confused with impaired level of consciousness and/or vomiting intravenous fluids and electrolyte replacement is needed
Heat stroke	• A core body temperature of >40°C (104°F) due to environmental heat exposure with either a lack or dysfunction of the central and peripheral thermoregulation center. Symptoms include dry skin, rapid, strong pulse and dizziness • *Treatment:* Maintain airway breathing and circulation, cardiac monitoring. Important recommended investigations are summarized – Treatment of heat stroke involves rapid mechanical cooling along with resuscitation measures. The body temperature must be lowered quickly. The patient should be moved to a cool area which is either indoor or in a shade and clothing may need to be removed to promote passive clothing. Active cooling methods include immersion in cold water, or a hyperthermia vest can be applied

Question 10

1. Discuss the management of vasopressor-resistant shock.

Management of vasopressor-resistant shock is multiphasic and various modalities of treatment used. Immediate management of shock includes fluid therapy, vasoactive therapy, and ventilator therapy along with correction of electrolyte imbalance. Along with the symptomatic treatment therapy should be directed at the underlying cause. Most cases of shock are due to myocardial infarction, prompt reperfusion therapy should be instituted. Revascularization therapy (PTCA or CABG) reduces the hospitalization, long-term mortality, and MI-related mechanical complication.

Positive pressure ventilation (PPV) support: It provides different effects for the RV and the LV. In cases of LV failure leading to cardiogenic shock, PPV may unload the LV by decreasing preload and afterload.

Pulmonary artery catheterization (PAC): PA catheter insertion may be helpful in monitoring of patient with shock. It gives information about hemodynamic parameters such as right and left ventricular filling pressures, systemic and pulmonary vascular resistance, right ventricular ejection fraction, and mixed venous oxygen (SvO_2) saturation, and thermodilution derived cardiac out.

Mechanical support is ultimate approach to improve hemodynamic parameters. Nowadays number of devices are available with different mechanism of action and effectiveness. These devices provide cardiac chambers (right left biventricular) support. Intra-aortic balloon pumps (IABP), extracorporeal membrane oxygenation (ECMO), percutaneous left ventricular assist device (LVAD) are available for mechanical support. These devices are indicated when all ICU measures fail to provide adequate tissue and organ perfusion and risk of multi organ failure develops.

2. Discuss the approach to hypercalcemia in ED.

Hypercalcemia of malignancy is characterized by rise in serum calcium levels above the upper limit of the normal laboratory reference range, related directly or indirectly to tumor. *Causes are secretion of parathyroid hormone-related peptide*: Any squamous cell carcinoma.

Osteolytic metastases: Lung cancer, breast cancer, and prostate cancer. *Production of vitamin D analogs:* Lymphomas, ectopic hyperparathyroidism.

Clinical symptoms depend on rate of development of hypercalcemia, instead of actual calcium levels (unless very high levels). A well-known mnemonic describes it—stones (kidney/biliary), bones (bone pain), groans (abdominal discomfort), moans (nonspecific symptoms), thrones (constipation, urinary frequency), muscle tone (muscle weakness, decreased reflexes), and psychiatric overtones (depression, anxiety, cognitive dysfunction). Hypercalcemic crisis can also present with life-threatening complications such as acute pancreatitis, renal failure, and coma. The approach to hypercalcemia management in ED is shown in **Flowchart 2**.

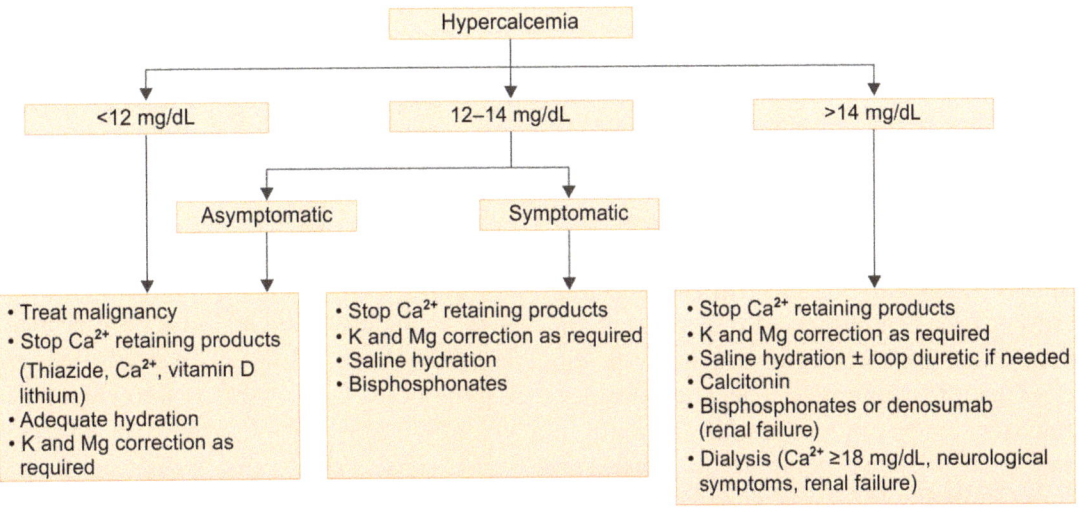

Flowchart 2: Management of hypercalcemia.

SUGGESTED READING

1. Richhariya D, Sharma B. Textbook of Emergency Medicine including Intensive Care and Trauma, 2nd edition. New Delhi: Jaypee Brothers Medical Publishers (P) Ltd; 2022. p. 19. (Question 1).
2. Richhariya D, Sharma B. Textbook of Emergency Medicine including Intensive Care and Trauma, 2nd edition. New Delhi: Jaypee Brothers Medical Publishers (P) Ltd; 2022. p. 831. (Question 2).
3. Richhariya D, Sharma B. Textbook of Emergency Medicine including Intensive Care and Trauma, 2nd edition. New Delhi: Jaypee Brothers Medical Publishers (P) Ltd; 2022. pp. 319, 973. (Question 3).
4. Richhariya D, Sharma B. Textbook of Emergency Medicine including Intensive Care and Trauma, 2nd edition. New Delhi: Jaypee Brothers Medical Publishers (P) Ltd; 2022. pp. 1455-7, 1736. (Question 4).
5. Richhariya D, Sharma B. Textbook of Emergency Medicine including Intensive Care and Trauma, 2nd edition. New Delhi: Jaypee Brothers Medical Publishers (P) Ltd; 2022. pp. 891, 971. (Question 5).
6. Richhariya D, Sharma B. Textbook of Emergency Medicine including Intensive Care and Trauma, 2nd edition. New Delhi: Jaypee Brothers Medical Publishers (P) Ltd; 2022. p. 1021. (Question 6).
7. Richhariya D, Sharma B. Textbook of Emergency Medicine including Intensive Care and Trauma, 2nd edition. New Delhi: Jaypee Brothers Medical Publishers (P) Ltd; 2022. pp. 543, 655-60. (Question 7).
8. Richhariya D, Sharma B. Textbook of Emergency Medicine including Intensive Care and Trauma, 2nd edition. New Delhi: Jaypee Brothers Medical Publishers (P) Ltd; 2022. pp. 717, 824. (Question 8).
9. Richhariya D, Sharma B. Textbook of Emergency Medicine including Intensive Care and Trauma, 2nd edition. New Delhi: Jaypee Brothers Medical Publishers (P) Ltd; 2022. pp. 465, 1691. (Question 9).
10. Richhariya D, Sharma B. Textbook of Emergency Medicine including Intensive Care and Trauma, 2nd edition. New Delhi: Jaypee Brothers Medical Publishers (P) Ltd; 2022. pp. 463, 973. (Question 10).

Emergency Medicine Paper 48

Devendra Richhariya

Question 1

1. Discuss the role of airway ultrasound during rapid sequence intubation.

Rapid sequence intubation is the cornerstone of emergency airway management and it consists of three phases—preoxygenation, endotracheal tube placement, and confirmation of tube placement. Any delay in the latter two phases leads to compromised patient outcomes. Recent studies have demonstrated the utility of point of care ultrasound (POCUS) in speeding up the process of rapid sequence intubation (RSI) and at the same time, improving the efficacy of the process. Ultrasound enables us to identify important sonoanatomy of the upper airway such as thyroid cartilage, epiglottis, cricoid cartilage, cricothyroid membrane, tracheal cartilages, and esophagus. Ultrasound has recently been used to confirm endotracheal intubation with real time images by placing a linear ultrasound probe transversely on the anterior aspect of the neck at the level of the cricothyroid membrane. The study shows that ultrasound can reliably image all the airway structures. This study suggests that hyomental distance is a more valid criterion in predicting difficult intubation.

2. Discuss push dose pressors.

Bolus administration of intravenous vasopressors and inotropes has been used by anesthesiologists in the operating room, to temporize blood pressure. However, this technique is not a standard emergency medicine or intensive care practice. These *"push-dose pressors"* are the perfect solution to short-lived hypotension, e.g., post-intubation or during procedural sedation. They also can act as a bridge to infusion vasopressors, while the latter are being mixed or while a central line is being placed.

Phenylephrine and ephedrine are the standard push-dose pressors in the anesthesia (**Table 1**). Because of short half-life and easy dosing, phenylephrine is a useful drug for the emergency department; ephedrine has a long half-life and it may not be ideal, when misdosed, has been associated with cardiac complications. Instead, epinephrine may be the ideal second push-dose pressor for the emergency department and intensive care unit. Phenylephrine is a pure vasoconstrictor, so its use makes sense in tachycardic patients, because it will not increase the heart rate and may even decrease it by reflex parasympathetic response. Epinephrine is an inopressor; in addition to vasoconstriction, it will increase heart rate and inotropy.

TABLE 1: Push dose vasopressors.

	Epinephrine	Phenylephrine
Mechanism of action	α and β1 & 2 agonist	α agonist
Onset	1 minute	1 minute
Duration	5–10 minutes	10–20 minutes
Duration	5–20 µg	50–200 µg
Dose interval	2–5 minutes	2–5 minutes
Indications	• Hypotension with bradycardia • Anaphylactic shock • Septic shock • Cardiac arrest with ROSC • Cardiogenic shock • Neurogenic shock • Hemorrhagic shock	

(ROSC: return of spontaneous circulation)

Question 2

1. Discuss approach to acute stridor in a child.

Causes of stridor: In newborn and infants, the most common cause is laryngomalacia, a condition in which tissues located in the throat above the vocal cords are too soft and flop into the airway. This causes inspiratory stridor, meaning the symptoms of noisy breathing occur when a child inhale (**Table 2**).

TABLE 2: Most common causes of stridor in infants and children.

	Nasopharyngeal	Laryngeal	Tracheal
Neonates	• Rhinitis • Choanal atresia or stenosis • Craniofacial abnormalities • Micrognathia	• Laryngomalacia • Intubation trauma • Reflux laryngitis • Laryngotracheal stenosis • Vocal cord palsy	• Tracheal bronchomalacia • Tracheal stenosis • Vascular compression
Children	• Allergic rhinitis • Adenoiditis • Adenotonsillar hypertrophy • Foreign bodies	• Croup • Hemangioma • Papillomatosis • Intubation trauma • Vocal cord palsy	• Foreign bodies • Tracheal stenosis

2. Describe the algorithmic approach in neonatal seizures.

Neonatal seizures are a commonly encountered neurologic condition in neonates. They are defined as the occurrence of sudden, paroxysmal, abnormal alteration of electrographic activity at any point from birth to the end of the neonatal period. During this period, the neonatal brain is developmentally immature. Thus, neonatal seizures have unique pathophysiology and electrographic findings resulting in clinical manifestations that can be different (and more difficult to identify) when compared to older age groups. The evaluation and treatment of neonatal seizures require algorithm-based approach **(Flowchart 1)**.

Flowchart 1: Algorithmic approach in neonatal seizures.

```
Neonate with seizures (level I–II clinical certainty)
Seen on EEG/aEEG or strong clinical suspicion
                    ↓
        Correct glucose/electrolytes          ⇐ Immediately
                    ↓
Phenobarbital      Phenobarbital 20 mg/kg IV
maintenance   ←    If seizures persist after 15 minutes give 2nd dose    ⇐ 1st line
4–6 mg/kg/day  If responsive  10–20 mg/kg (may need ventilator on 20 minutes)
                    ↓
Levetiracetam      Add/change to levetiracetam 20 mg/kg IV
maintenance, up to ←  If seizures persist after 30 minutes give 2nd dose  ⇐ If sz persist after 30 minutes
60 mg/kg/day   If responsive
                    ↓
Phenytoin          Add/change to Phenytoin 20 mg/kg IV
maintenance   ←    If seizures persist repeat dose after 30 minutes,     ⇐ If sz persist after 60 minutes
5 mg/kg/day    If responsive       consider pyridoxine
                    ↓
            Add/change Miedazolam 0.15 mg/kg bolus                       ⇐ If sz persist after 30 minutes
            followed by infusion of 0.06–0.4 mg/kg/hour
```

(aEEG: amplitude-integrated electroencephalogram; EEG: electroencephalogram; sz: seizures)

Question 3

1. Discuss approach to a cyanotic baby.

Also called as hyperpneic spells, hypoxic spells, anoxic, blue, Cyanotic or Tet spells are paroxysmal hypoxic events in a child due to decreased pulmonary blood flow and right to left shunting. They can occur in any heart condition involving ventricular septal defect (VSD) and a restriction to pulmonary blood flow. Increased contractility (due to catecholamines) and decreased right ventricular size (due to various factors) can trigger a reflex resulting in hyperventilation, some peripheral vasodilation without bradycardia, and this may initiate a spell **(Flowchart 2)**. Place infants with hypercyanotic spells in the knee-chest position and give oxygen; sometimes, opioids (morphine or fentanyl), volume expansion, sodium bicarbonate, beta-blockers (propranolol or esmolol), or phenylephrine may help. Repair surgically at 2-6 months or earlier if symptoms are severe.

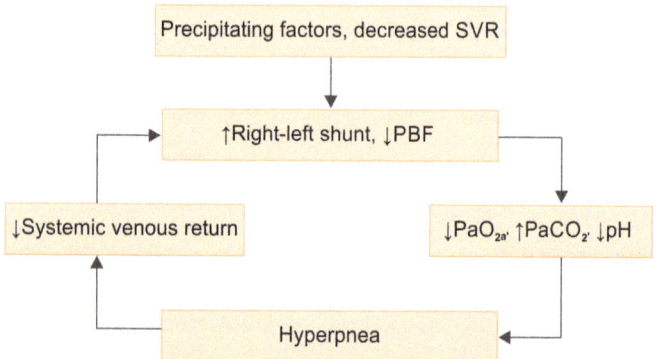

Flowchart 2: Pathophysiology of cyanotic spell.

(PBF: peripheral blood flow; SVR: systemic vascular resistance)

Approach to management of cyanotic spell: The definitive diagnosis is readily established by detailed echocardiography. Prostaglandin E1 (alprostadil) intravenous (IV) infusion to keep the patent ductus arteriosus (PDA) open (dose 10-60 ng/kg/min, if poor response saturations and acidosis not improving) the dose can be increased to maximum 300-400 ng/kg/min. Apnea is a common side effect of prostaglandin E1 (PGE1) so infusion should be started in intensive care unit (ICU) settings with ventilator support available. Flushing, diarrhea, and hypotension are other common side effects. Intravenous fluid for blood volume expansion 10 mL/kg 0.9% saline bolus, improves preload, repeat until liver edge is palpable, enhance further opening of the PDA and pulmonary blood flow through the duct; correction of metabolic abnormalities, e.g., hypoglycemia, hypocalcemia, acidosis and sepsis. Oxygenate to maintain the saturations 75-85% (do not give 100% oxygen by mask in patients with duct dependent lesions as high level of oxygen triggers closure of ductus arteriosus). Inotropes/vasopressors are required to maintain adequate systemic perfusion. If above measures are not helpful, intubation and ventilation with adequate sedation are required to improve oxygenation and minimize the metabolic demands.

Definitive management includes: For transposition of great vessels—arterial switch operation, total anomalous pulmonary venous connection, surgical rerouting of pulmonary veins, severe valvular pulmonary stenosis, balloon valvotomy and ductal stenting/Blalock-Taussig (BT) shunt for duct dependent pulmonary circulation.

2. Discuss approach to an inconsolable crying child with crush injury to foot.

Etiologic Mnemonic for Crying Infant "IT CRIES"

"IT CRIES": I-infection, T-trauma, C-cardiac disease, R-reflux, reaction to medicines, I-intussusception, E-eyes (corneal abrasion), S-surgical emergency (strangulation, torsion, hernia).

Considering the heightened parental concern, appropriate assessment of airway, breathing, circulation and necessary basic interventions such as oxygen administration, intravenous access, fluid administration, bedside glucose testing should be initiated.

Reassurance: Inform the parents the benign nature of the disease and its natural course. Red flag signs should be sought after and managed accordingly.

Question 4

1. Discuss the key differences between pediatric Glasgow Coma Scale (GCS) versus adult GCS.

The GCS is used to objectively describe the extent of impaired consciousness in all types of acute medical and trauma patients. The scale assesses patients according to three aspects of responsiveness—eye-opening, motor, and verbal responses **(Table 3)**.

2. Describe injuries related to mechanism with fall on outstretched hand.

FOOSH is the nickname for an injury caused by having "fallen onto an outstretched hand." These injuries are among the most common injuries affecting the hands and wrists that occur when trying to break a fall. Treatment of a FOOSH injury depends on its severity. The severity of FOOSH injuries can vary greatly depending on various factors.
a. Distal radius fracture
b. Radial or ulnar styloid fracture
c. Radial head fracture
d. Scapholunate tear
e. Scaphoid fracture
f. Distal radioulnar joint fracture
g. Hamate fracture
h. Synovitis
i. Cellulitis
j. Bruise
k. Clavicle or shoulder injury.

TABLE 3: Adult Glasgow Coma Scale (GCS) versus pediatric GCS.

Adult Glasgow coma score	Score	Pediatric coma score	Score
Eye opening response			
Spontaneously	4	Spontaneously	4
To verbal stimuli	3	To verbal stimuli	3
To pain	2	To pain	2
No response to pain	1	No response to pain	1
Best motor response			
Obeys verbal command	6	Spontaneous or obeys verbal command	6
Localizes to pain	5	Localizes to pain or withdraws to touch	5
Withdraws from pain	4	Withdraws from pain	4
Abnormal flexion to pain (decorticate)	3	Abnormal flexion to pain (decorticate)	3
Abnormal extension to pain (decerebrate)	2	Abnormal extension to pain (decerebrate)	2
No response to pain	1	No response to pain	1
Best verbal response			
Orientated + converses	5	Alert, babbles, coos, words to usual ability	5
Disorientated + converses	4	Less than usual words, spontaneous irritable cry	4
Inappropriate words	3	Cries only to pain	3
Incomprehensible sounds	2	Moans to pain	2
No response to pain	1	No response to pain	1
Maximum score	15	*Maximum score*	15

Question 5

1. Describe the key salient features of forest plot.

A forest plot is a graphical display of estimated results from a number of scientific studies addressing the same question. A forest plot is an essential tool to summarize information on individual studies, give a visual suggestion of the amount of study heterogeneity, and show the estimated common effect, all in one figure **(Fig. 1)**.

2. Describe the critical appraisal points of a research article.

Critical appraisal is the systematic examination of the research evidence reported in the scientific articles to assess their validity, reliability, and applicability before using their findings to inform decision-making. It should be considered as the first step to grade the quality of evidence **(Fig. 1)**. Critical appraisal of an article is a literary and scientific systematic dissection in an attempt to assign merit to the conclusions of an article. Ideally, an article will be able to undergo scrutiny and retain its findings as valid. Key points in critical appraisal are internal validity—the degree to which the study truly answers the question it poses; external validity—the study results can be generalized to other populations.

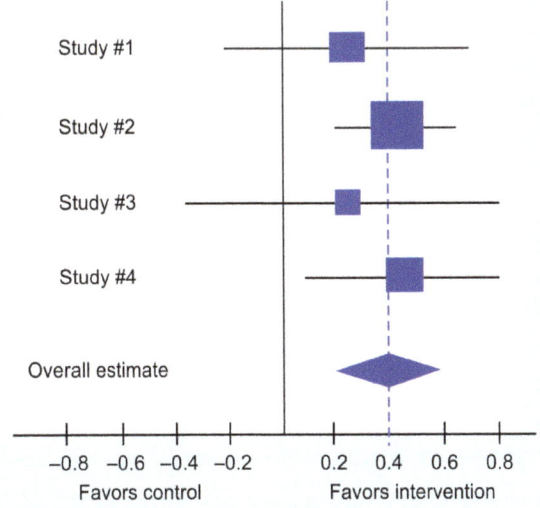

Fig. 1: Example of forest plot.

How to Critically Appraise a Paper?

a. Is the study question relevant?
b. Does the study add anything new to the evidence?
c. What type of research question is being asked?
d. Was the study design appropriate for the research question?
e. Did the methodology address important potential sources of bias?

Question 6

1. Discuss the opportunities and challenges of emergency care research.

Conducting research in emergency care settings poses unique *methodological and operational challenges*. Therefore, new approaches and strategies that address these challenges need to be developed and will require increased attention from scientists, academic institutions, and the global health research funding community. Relatively *low research investments and lack of expertise* in emergency care research have resulted in considerable disparities between the burden of emergency diseases and research output. Emergency care is a critical entryway into the healthcare system and a key determinant of individual and population health. Experts anticipate research gaps, needs and opportunities, and presenting some innovative solutions.

Research challenges in emergency care:
a. *Defining and capturing the population of interest:* At least initially, patients present with symptoms and not diagnoses; it is often difficult to consistently capture all patients presenting with diseases or symptoms of interest to the researchers.
b. *Defining interventions and outcomes:* Interventions are relatively easy to define in emergency care, while outcomes are often difficult to set.
c. *Study design and data collection:* There are clear challenges in data collection, data analysis, and comparability of research findings.
d. *Ethical issues:* Privacy, community engagement, fair participant selection and the ability to give and obtain quality informed consent in emergency care settings can be difficult.
e. *Research capacity and research environment:* Emergency department remains largely a hospital service with very few academic activities in medical colleges.

2. Discuss various grief counselling methods.

Grief counselling refers to a specific form of therapy, which focuses on general counselling with the goal of helping the individual grieve and addresses personal loss in a healthy manner. Grief counselling is offered by psychologist, counsellor or by social worker. Specific task of grief counselling includes emotional expression about the loss, accepting the loss, adjusting the life after loss, coping with changes within oneself and the world after the loss. Typical feeling experienced by individual and addressed in grief counselling include sadness, anxiety, anger, loneliness, guilt, isolation, confusion or numbness.

Purpose of grief counselling is to help individual work through the feelings, thoughts, and memories associated with the loss of loved ones. Grief counselling generally directed toward positive adjustment following loss after the death of loved ones. Grief counselling helps individual cope with the pain associated with the loss, feel supported through the anxiety surrounding life changes that may follow the loss and develop strategies for seeking support and self-care.

Question 7

1. Discuss various triage protocols used during disaster for pediatric population.

Triaging in pediatric age group: Children are usually uncooperative during examination and give poor history so it is very important to recognize markers of serious illness; useful signs are drowsiness, hypotonia, respiratory grunt, wheeze, crepitation, stridor tachypnea, pallor, fever, signs of dehydration, abnormal posture, cold periphery, vomit or less urination, convulsion, and tender abdomen. Use Jump-START **(Flowchart 3)** triaging methods in pediatric age group mass casualty.

2. Discuss ultrasound-guided triage during disaster.

Lung ultrasound (US) is proven a reliable tool in diagnosing lung inflammatory processes—the results are immediate and the examination is safe, repeatable, and cheap. Lung parenchymal alterations can be observed at the onset, and a disposable probe cover can ensure a clean procedure. Severe acute respiratory syndrome coronavirus 2 (SARS-CoV-2) infections, symptoms from fever, dry cough, fatigue, and lymphopenia to viral pneumonia with acute respiratory distress syndrome (ARDS). US examinations are easily performed at the point of care, which can be the patient's bedside or even outside the hospital. All these qualities make it a precious tool in clinical practice, optimal to assist clinicians even in initial patient triage. Early literature suggests that patients with confirmed coronavirus disease-2019 (COVID-19) pneumonia demonstrate typical lung imaging features, including pleural line irregularities, B lines, and multifocal consolidations. Early use of lung US is used in Italy in COVID-19 patients, for early diagnoses and appropriate management. Every "field hospitals" (tent) equipped with US scanner to avoid contact between infected patients and noninfected ones, permit early diagnosis outside the hospital, effectively implementing a "US triage." Limitations for the implementation of US triage are the lack of specific protocols and operator experience, which influences the validity of test results.

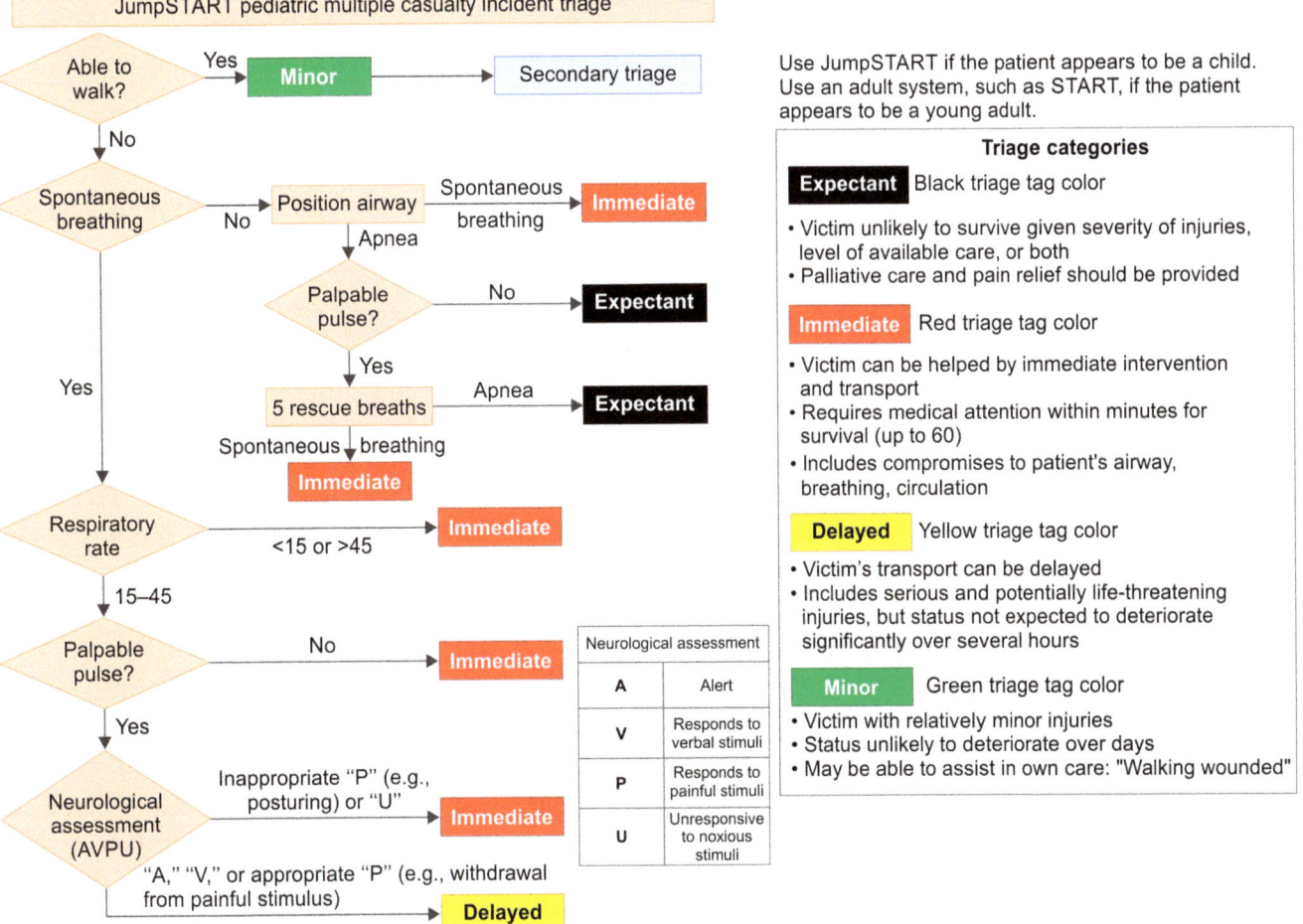

Flowchart 3: JumpSTART triaging methods in pediatric age group mass casualty.

Question 8

1. Discuss the important critical appraisal findings of targeted temperature management-2 (TTM-2) trial.

The TTM-2 trial was the largest trial conducted to date, across 14 countries with >1,800 subjects, and published in 2021. It compared the effect of targeted hypothermia at 33°C to targeted normothermia at 37.5°C. Therapeutic hypothermia involves use of a servo-controlled device and blanket to lower the core body temperature by 3°C for 72 hours followed by a period of rewarming in which the temperature is increased by 0.5°C per hour for 6 hours until normothermia is achieved. Studies suggest that after achieving ROSC (period of global cerebral hypoxia-ischemia), mild-induced hypothermia is used as a neuroprotective and outcome improving measures. Mild-induced hypothermia suppresses the many pathological process leading to delayed cell death, including apoptosis (programmed cell death). Hypothermia reduces the release of excitatory amino acids, free radicals and decreases the cerebral metabolic rate for oxygen ($CMRO_2$) by about 6% for each 1°C reduction in core temperature. Hypothermia reduces the inflammatory response associated with the postcardiac arrest syndrome.

2. Discuss the critical appraisal points of COACT trial.

The COACT trial demonstrated that in unconscious, hemodynamically stable patients surviving a VT/ VF OOHCA (out of hospital cardiac arrest), a strategy of immediate angiography (IA) did not improve survival. While time to reperfusion is critical to prognosis in ST-elevation myocardial infarction (STEMI), these data suggest that this is not the case for most VT/VF OOHCA survivors with reduced GCS and no STEMI. This study had low prevalence of unstable coronary lesions and so there is uncertainty as to whether IA may be of benefit in these patients but even if it was shown to be beneficial, the challenge is in identifying them on presentation. The COACT trial showed that immediate angiography with an intent to revascularize is not superior to delayed angiography among patients presenting with out-of-hospital cardiac arrest secondary to a shockable rhythm and with no ECG evidence of ST-segment elevations post-ROSC.

Question 9

Discuss the method of conducting and reporting of studies.

1. Explain randomized control trial.

Randomized controlled trials (RCT) are prospective studies that measure the effectiveness of a new intervention or treatment. Although no study is likely on its own to prove causality, randomization reduces bias and provides a rigorous tool to examine cause-effect relationships between an intervention and outcome. Randomization is a scientific method of allocation of subjects between the treatment and control groups. This method ensures that there is no bias or preference in selecting specific treatment for any subjects. Further, randomization provides equal chance/probability to subjects for allocation into different groups. Importantly a prerequisite, all statistical tests of significance assume that the sample drawn is random, which is met through randomization.

Randomization techniques used in RCTs are simple randomization or stratified randomization. In simple randomization, subjects are allocated to different groups without any matching. On the other hand, in stratified randomization technique, subjects are classified in groups, i.e., strata and then within a group they are randomized to various treatment groups. This ensures matching of subjects for confounding factors that might influence the outcome and thus helps in drawing the valid conclusions netting out the effects of confounders.

2. What are case reports?

A case report is a detailed report of the symptoms, signs, diagnosis, treatment, and follow-up of an individual patient. Case reports usually describe an unusual or novel occurrence and as such, remain one of the cornerstones of medical progress and provide many new ideas in medicine. Unique cases that cannot be explained by known diseases or syndromes. Cases that show an important variation of a disease or condition. Cases that show unexpected events that may contain new or useful information. Cases in which one patient has two or more unexpected diseases or disorders. Case reports should consist of five sections—an abstract, an introduction with a literature review, a description of the case report, a discussion that includes a detailed explanation of the literature review, and a brief summary of the case and a conclusion.

Question 10

A 25-year-old man presents with fracture of right hip joint with a pain score of 9/10.

1. Discuss the concept of block on arrival.

"On Arrival Block," a brachial block is given to a severely injured upper extremity as the first step of the management protocol. A short "hospital arrival-to-surgery interval" time, rapid pain relief, and early and efficient resuscitation are key factors in obtaining good outcomes after a major trauma to the upper limb. "On Arrival Block" has many advantages:

a. Immediate pain relief, delivering a humane touch, and one which improves patient confidence in the healthcare system.
b. Avoids administration of major opioids for pain, which can create difficulties during the assessment phase of the injury.
c. A tourniquet can be applied without causing pain before the initial dressing is removed in anticipation of massive bleeding.
d. Permits a pain-free detailed clinical evaluation of the injury.
e. Facilitates taking radiographs in the main operating room, with no overlap of fractured bones, as often occurs when X-rays of major injuries are taken with bandages being intact.
f. This block anesthetic is used for the definitive surgery, avoiding a need for general anesthesia or major sedation.
g. Using the "On Arrival Block" system, emergency room assessment and resuscitation is bypassed. The patient is only resuscitated once, instead of twice. This avoids much duplication of effort, wasted time, patient suffering, unnecessary costs, and mistakes generated by miscommunication between two resuscitation teams. The anesthesiologist and the surgeon work together as key members of the first assessment and management team in the main operating room.

The following are mandatory requirements to the practice of "On Arrival Block":

a. The place where "On Arrival Block" is done must have all the resuscitative equipment and drugs.

b. A senior anesthesiologist and a senior plastic/hand surgeon must be on call 24 × 7 and be available to receive the emergency patient.
c. If need be, it must be possible to carry out surgery immediately. This means availability of an operating room at all times for such cases.

2. Discuss pericapsular nerve group (PNEG) block versus fascia iliaca compartment block.

The PENG block is a novel regional analgesia technique that can be used to reduce pain after hip surgery and hip fractures and demonstrated better analgesia compared to other peripheral blocks administered for this type of surgery. The PENG block has recently been proposed as a novel method to treat pain due to hip or pelvis fracture by targeting the terminal sensory articular nerve branches of the femoral nerve (FN), obturator nerve (ON), and accessory obturator nerve (AON) **(Figs. 2A and B)**.

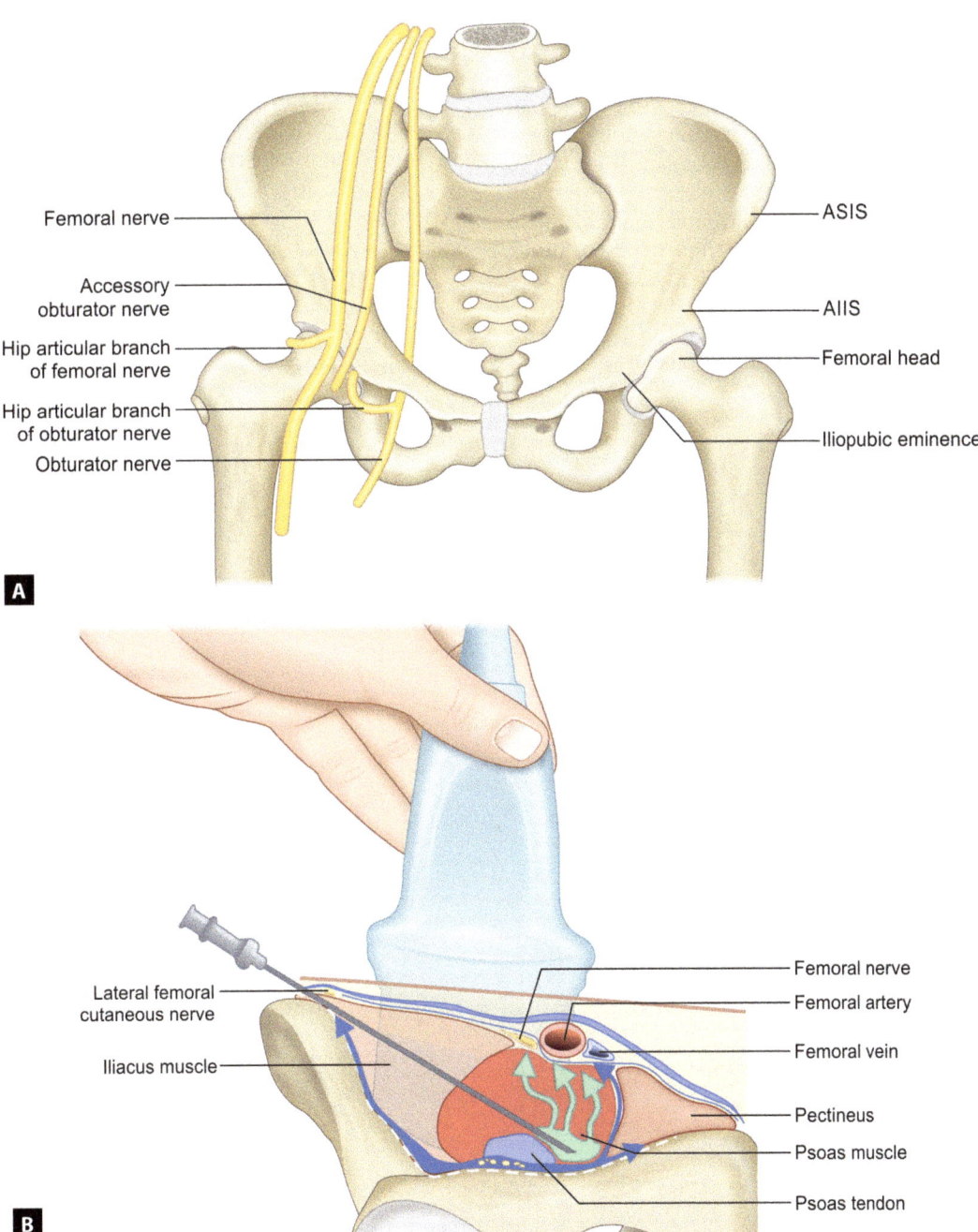

Figs. 2A and B: (A) Innervation and anatomical landmark of anterior aspect of hip joint; (B) PNEG block. (AIIS: anterior inferior illiac spine; ASIS: anterior superior illiac spine; PNEG: pericapsular nerve group)

SUGGESTED READING

1. Richhariya D, Sharma B. Textbook of Emergency Medicine including Intensive Care and Trauma, 2nd edition. New Delhi: Jaypee Brothers Medical Publishers (P) Ltd; 2022. pp. 212, 335. (Question 1).
2. Richhariya D, Sharma B. Textbook of Emergency Medicine including Intensive Care and Trauma, 2nd edition. New Delhi: Jaypee Brothers Medical Publishers (P) Ltd; 2022. pp. 1159, 1214. (Question 2).
3. Richhariya D, Sharma B. Textbook of Emergency Medicine including Intensive Care and Trauma, 2nd edition. New Delhi: Jaypee Brothers Medical Publishers (P) Ltd; 2022. pp. 1144, 1195. (Question 3).
4. Richhariya D, Sharma B. Textbook of Emergency Medicine including Intensive Care and Trauma, 2nd edition. New Delhi: Jaypee Brothers Medical Publishers (P) Ltd; 2022. pp. 1115, 1127. (Question 4).
5. Richhariya D, Sharma B. Textbook of Emergency Medicine including Intensive Care and Trauma, 2nd edition. New Delhi: Jaypee Brothers Medical Publishers (P) Ltd; 2022. p. 89. (Question 5).
6. Richhariya D, Sharma B. Textbook of Emergency Medicine including Intensive Care and Trauma, 2nd edition. New Delhi: Jaypee Brothers Medical Publishers (P) Ltd; 2022. pp. 80, 136. (Question 6).
7. Richhariya D, Sharma B. Textbook of Emergency Medicine including Intensive Care and Trauma, 2nd edition. New Delhi: Jaypee Brothers Medical Publishers (P) Ltd; 2022. pp. 172-5. (Question 7).
8. Richhariya D, Sharma B. Textbook of Emergency Medicine including Intensive Care and Trauma, 2nd edition. New Delhi: Jaypee Brothers Medical Publishers (P) Ltd; 2022. p. 237. (Question 8).
9. Richhariya D, Sharma B. Textbook of Emergency Medicine including Intensive Care and Trauma, 2nd edition. New Delhi: Jaypee Brothers Medical Publishers (P) Ltd; 2022. pp. 80-90. (Question 9).
10. Richhariya D, Sharma B. Textbook of Emergency Medicine including Intensive Care and Trauma, 2nd edition. New Delhi: Jaypee Brothers Medical Publishers (P) Ltd; 2022. pp. 386-92. (Question 10).
11. Sabapathy SR, Venkateswaran G, Boopathi V, Subramanian JB. "On Arrival Block"—management of upper extremity trauma with resuscitation in the operating room. Plast Reconstr Surg Glob Open. 2020;8(10):e3191. (Question 10).

Emergency Medicine Paper 49

Devendra Richhariya

Question 1

1. Define brain death.

Brain death: It is a legal term (in most countries), defined as the irreversible cessation of the entire brain function, which includes the brainstem.

Medical and legal definitions: No standard definition exists internationally for the term "brain death." Medicolegal guidelines and the definition of brain death are internationally inconsistent. Healthcare providers should know the local laws, institutional regulations, and guidelines before the declaration of brain death.

In 2014, a summary was published outlining the development of international guidelines for the diagnosis of brain death with the phrase—cessation of neurologic function being used in lieu of brain death or brainstem death.

2. Discuss clinical evaluation of a patient to confirm brain death.

Diagnosis of brain death by neurologic criteria based on current medical guidelines is done through clinical examination, laboratory values, and radiological findings. The examination shows that the patient's eyes are not held open voluntarily and that no movements are made to verbal or noxious stimuli. Standard points of noxious stimulation include nailbed and supraorbital or temporomandibular pressure.

a. *Confounders of brain death:*
   i. Severe hypothermia, core temperature ≤32°C
   ii. Severe hypotension, systolic blood pressure (SBP) <100 mm Hg
   iii. *Drugs:* Alcohol, poisons, recent sedation, and neuromuscular blocking (NMB) agents
   iv. Severe dyselectrolytemia
   v. Hypoglycemia
   vi. Acid–base abnormalities
b. *Documentation of coma:*
   i. Absence of motor response to a standardized painful stimulus
   ii. Beware of local spinal reflexes causing spontaneous or stimulus-related motor movements
c. *Documentation of absence of brainstem reflexes:*
   i. Brainstem reflexes are lost in a rostral to caudal direction
   ii. Reflexes in medulla oblongata are the last to cease
d. *Documented tests:*
   i. *Absent pupillary reflexes* (nerves—optic and oculomotor)
   ii. *Absent oculocephalic movement:* Doll's eye reflex (nerves—vestibular parts of vestibulocochlear, oculomotor, and abducens)
   iii. *Absent oculovestibular reflex:* Cold calorie test (nerves—vestibular parts of vestibulocochlear, trochlear, and abducens)
   iv. *Absent corneal reflex* (nerves—trigeminal and facial)
   v. *Absent cough reflex* (nerves—glossopharyngeal and vagus)

3. Discuss the pathophysiology of acute blood transfusion hemolytic reaction.

Acute transfusion reactions occur during or shortly after (within 24 hours) the transfusion. The World Health Organization has broadly categorized acute transfusion reactions according to their severity and the appropriate clinical response: mild, moderate-to-severe, and life-threatening transfusion reactions. When the antibodies present in the blood of the recipient bind with the red blood cells of the donor, complement activation takes place. As a result of complement activation, red cells are lysed releasing hemoglobin into the circulation (**Flowchart 1**).

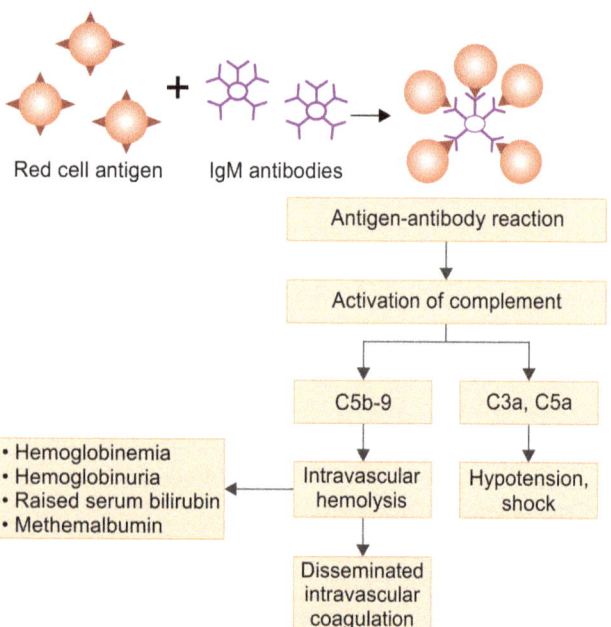

Flowchart 1: Pathophysiology of an acute blood transfusion hemolytic reaction.

Question 2

1. Discuss the physical status classification system of assessment of airway by the American Society of Anesthesiologists (ASA).

The ASA physical status classification is used at the time of the surgical procedure procedure and physical status of a patient includes its airway anatomy. The disease process which presents at the time of the surgical procedure should be graded because it predisposes to risk stratification **(Table 1)**.

TABLE 1: American Society of Anesthesiologists (ASA) physical status classification of airway assessment.

ASA physical status classification	Definition of patient status
ASA I	Normal healthy
ASA II	Mild systemic disease
ASA III	Severe systemic disease
ASA IV	Severe systemic disease with constant threat of life
ASA V	Moribund; not expected to survive without operation
ASA VI	Declared brain dead

2. Discuss LEMON mnemonic for evaluation of difficult direct laryngoscopy.

LEMON evaluation is used to assess the difficulty in intubation and direct laryngoscopy.

L—Look externally: A quick external examination of the patient should be conducted for potential signs of airway problems and their management. First, external markers of difficult intubation should be examined which are based on the specialist's clinical impression. For example, a severely combative trauma patient with facial fracture, immobilized by a cervical collar on a spine board, gives immediate impression of anticipated difficult intubation.

E—Evaluate: 3-3-2 rule: Examine the airway for structural and anatomic factors that may make intubation difficult. Normally, a mouth opening should accommodate three of the patient's fingers, a distance/measurement of three fingers from the mentum to the hyoid bone, and a distance of two fingers from the hyoid bone to the thyroid notch. When present, these factors predict sufficient spatial relationships between the mouth, the mandible, temporomandibular joint mobility, and the larynx to allow for successful direct laryngoscopy and eventual endotracheal intubation **(Figs. 1A to C)**.

- Interincisor distance less than three fingers means inadequate mouth opening which leads to difficulty in inserting a laryngoscope.
- Thyromental distance less than three fingers means that the larynx is anterior and leads to difficulty in visualization of vocal cord.
- Thyrohyoid distance less than two fingers means high larynx which makes vocal cord visualization more difficult.

M—Mallampati score: It is assessment of the posterior oropharyngeal structures visualized when the mouth is open and the tongue is fully protruded **(Fig. 2)**. Visibility of the oral pharynx ranges from complete visualization, including the tonsillar pillars (class I) to no visualization at all, with the tongue pressed against the hard palate (class IV). Classes I and II signify adequate oral access, class III signifies moderate difficulty, and class IV signifies a high degree of difficulty.

O—Obstruction: Obstruction of upper airway by foreign bodies, local edema, stridor, or soft-tissue masses makes intubation difficult or impossible. Examine the patient for any airway obstruction and assess the patient's voice to confirm the evaluation. Conditions which make the definitive airway placement difficult are epiglottitis, cancer of head and neck, Ludwig's angina, hematoma of neck, glottis swelling, or glottic polyps. Obese patients generally are more difficult to intubate than their nonobese counterparts; they desaturate quickly and cause increased difficulty with ventilation using bag mask ventilation (BMV) or an esophagogastroduodenoscopy (EGD).

N—Neck mobility: Neck positioning is maintained to achieve optimum angles for visualization of the glottis to facilitate definitive airway. Neck movement is restricted in conditions such as cervical spine injuries, rheumatoid arthritis, or degenerative arthritis. Neck mobility is assessed by flexion and extension of the patient's head and neck through a full range of motion. Neck extension is the most important motion, but placing the patient in the full sniffing position provides the optimal laryngeal view by direct laryngoscopy. The "S" in *LEMONS* refers to the patient's *oxygen saturation*.

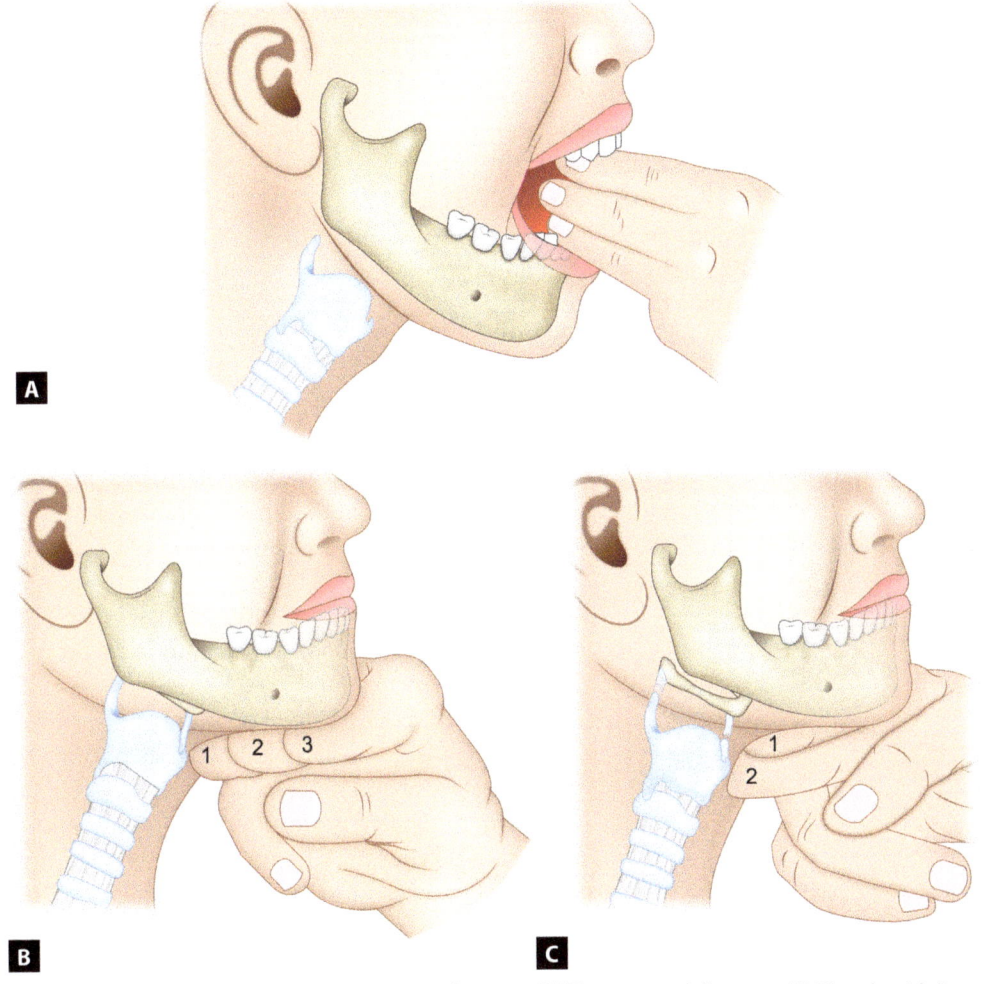

Figs. 1A to C: *3-3-2 rule assessment:* (A) Interincisor distance; (B) Thyromental distance; (C) Thyrohyoid distance.

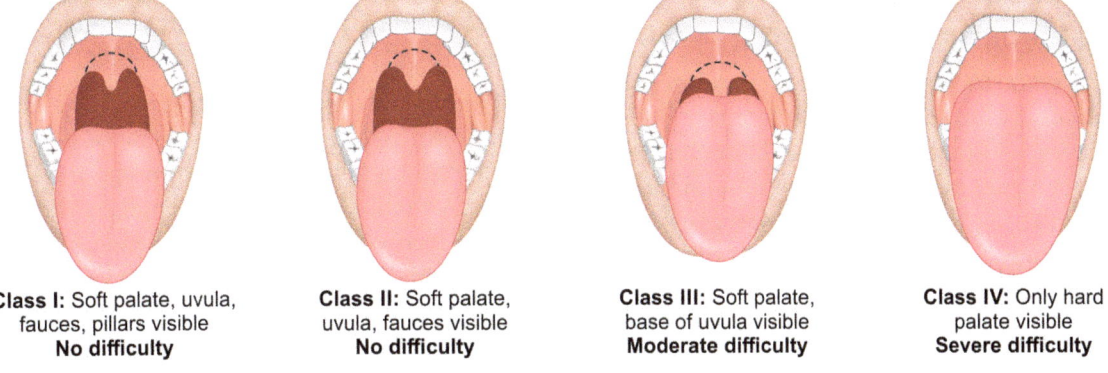

Class I: Soft palate, uvula, fauces, pillars visible
No difficulty

Class II: Soft palate, uvula, fauces visible
No difficulty

Class III: Soft palate, base of uvula visible
Moderate difficulty

Class IV: Only hard palate visible
Severe difficulty

Fig. 2: Mallampati classification.

Question 3

1. Discuss the pathophysiology of anaphylaxis.

Anaphylaxis is a severe systemic hypersensitivity reaction that is rapid in onset; characterized by life-threatening airway, breathing, and/or circulatory problems; and usually associated with skin and mucosal changes. Because it can be triggered in some people by minute amounts of antigen (e.g., certain foods or single insect stings), anaphylaxis can be considered the most aberrant example of an imbalance between the cost and benefit of an immune response. The current understanding of the immunopathogenesis and pathophysiology of anaphylaxis (**Flowcharts 2 and 3**) focuses on the roles of IgE and IgG antibodies, immune effector cells, and chemical mediators thought to contribute to examples of the disorder. Anaphylaxis causes the immune system to release a flood of chemicals (**Table 2**) that can cause you to go into shock—blood pressure drops suddenly and the airways narrow, blocking breathing. Signs and symptoms include a rapid, weak pulse; a skin rash; and nausea and vomiting.

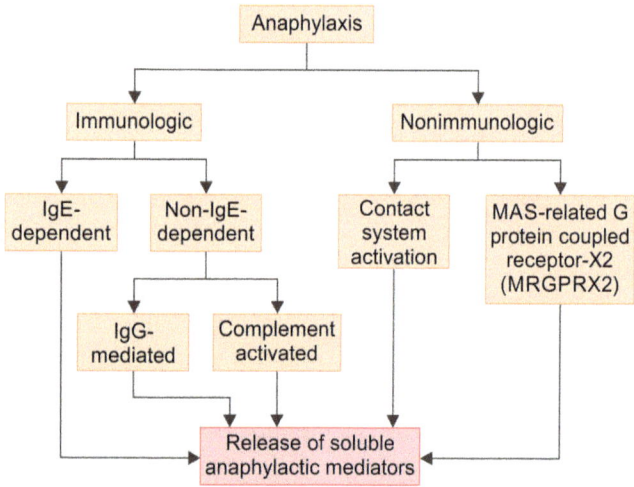

Flowchart 2: Immunopathogenesis of anaphylactic shock.

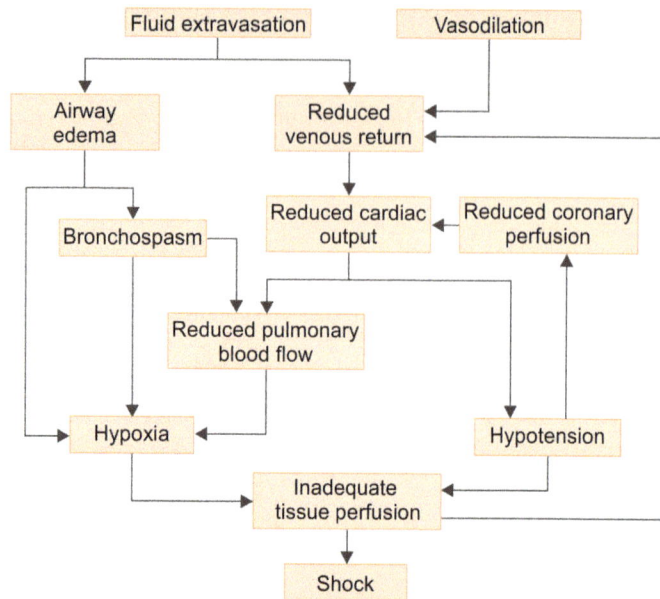

Flowchart 3: Pathophysiologic mechanism of anaphylactic shock.

Criteria 1: Acute onset of an illness (minutes to several hours) with simultaneous involvement of the skin, mucosal tissue, or both (e.g., generalized hives, pruritus or flushing, or swollen lips–tongue–uvula), and at least one of the following:
a. Respiratory compromise (e.g., dyspnea, wheeze-bronchospasm, stridor, reduced peak expiratory flow, hypoxemia)
b. Reduced blood pressure or associated symptoms of end-organ dysfunction [e.g., hypotonia (collapse), syncope, incontinence].
c. Severe gastrointestinal symptoms (e.g., severe crampy abdominal pain, repetitive vomiting), especially after exposure to nonfood allergens.

Criteria 2: Acute onset of hypotension or bronchospasm or laryngeal involvement after exposure to a known or highly probable allergen for that patient (minutes to several hours), even in the absence of typical skin involvement.

2. Discuss the diagnostic criteria for anaphylaxis.

The Australasian Society of Clinical Immunology and Allergy defines anaphylaxis as any acute-onset illness with typical skin features (urticarial rash or erythema/flushing, and/or angioedema) plus involvement of respiratory and/or cardiovascular, and/or persistent severe gastrointestinal symptoms; or any acute onset of hypotension, bronchospasm, or upper airway obstruction where anaphylaxis is considered possible, even if typical skin features are not present. *Anaphylaxis is highly likely when any one of the following two criteria are fulfilled:*

3. Discuss the physiological changes in elderly person relevant to emergencies.

Older people often present to the emergency department (ED) with atypical clinical presentations, physical findings, and investigation results due to age-related physiologic and anatomic changes. These changes can result in vague or delayed complaints with absence of typical findings, confounded by polymorbidity, and polypharmacy with drugs that may cause or mask disease symptoms.

Vital signs: Due to age-associated changes, interpreting vital signs in older patients requires enhanced knowledge and skills of physicians. These changes lead to loss of regulatory and adaptive mechanisms.

Neurologic system: A complete neurologic examination may sometimes be difficult because of cognitive or sensory impairment.

Cardiovascular system: With age, a weakening cardiovascular system leads to increased risk of disease processes including coronary artery disease, dissection, heart failure, valvopathies, and other comorbidities.

TABLE 2: Release of chemical mediators by activation of the immune system.

	Chemical mediator	Action
Arachidonic acid metabolites	• Cysteinyl Leukotrienes • Prostaglandins • Platelet activating factor	• Bronchoconstriction, coronary vasoconstriction • Increased vascular permeability, mucus hypersecretion • Eosinophil activation and recruitment
Chemokines	• IL-8 • MIP-1α • Eosinophil chemotactic factors	Neutrophil and eosinophil chemotaxis, inflammatory cell recruitment, activation of NADPH oxidase
Cytokines	• GM-CSF • IL-3, -4, -5, -6, -10, and -13 • TNF-α	Eosinophil chemotaxis and activation, inflammatory cell activation and recruitment, induction of IgE-receptor expression, induction of apoptosis
Proteases	• Chymase • Tryptase • Carboxypeptidase A	Cleavage of complement proteins and neuropeptides, inflammatory-cell chemoattractant, conversion of angiotensin I to angiotensin II, activation of protease-activated receptor-2
Proteoglycans	• Chondroitin sulfate • Heparin	Anticoagulation, complement inhibition, eosinophil chemoattractant, kinin activation
Others	• Histamine • Nitric oxide	• Vasodilation, bronchial and gastrointestinal • Smooth muscle contraction, mucus hypersecretion • Vasodilation, increased vascular permeability

(GM-CSF: granulocyte-macrophage colony-stimulating factor; Ig: immunoglobulin; IL: interleukin; MIP-1α: macrophage inflammatory protein-1 alpha; NADPH: nicotinamide adenine dinucleotide phosphate; TNF-α: tumor necrosis factor-alpha)

Respiratory system: Pulmonary functions decrease with age and cardiopulmonary diseases can further decrease respiratory reserve.

Gastrointestinal system: Compared to younger patients, older patients with intra-abdominal infections tend to present atypically or delayed, which is associated with increased likelihood of surgical intervention, morbidity, and mortality.

Genitourinary system: Urinary tract infections (UTIs) are commonly overdiagnosed, largely due to the high prevalence of asymptomatic bacteriuria in older people (up to 19% in community-dwelling older people).

Musculoskeletal system: Given the increased prevalence of osteoporosis in older patients, even minor trauma such as a fall from standing height can lead to fractures.

Integumentary examination: Aging skin loses elastin and collagen, the epidermis becomes thin, and there is decreased subcutaneous support. As such, older adults have fragile skin and are more prone to soft-tissue injuries. With immobilization, pressure ulcers may develop in as little as 4–6 hours and become a potential source of infection.

Medications: Polypharmacy increases with advanced age. Due to physiologic changes with aging, pharmacokinetics (what the body does to a drug) and pharmacodynamics (what a drug does to the body) are different in older patients.

Question 4

1. Discuss the physiology of potassium homeostasis.

Potassium homeostasis means the maintenance of the total body potassium content and plasma potassium level within narrow limits in the face of potentially wide variations in dietary potassium intake. It involves two concurrent processes: *Internal balance (intra- and extracellular fluid K^+ distribution) and external balance (renal excretion of K^+)* **(Fig. 3)**. Potassium is the major intracellular cation, predominantly in the cell. About 98% of the potassium in the body is contained in the cell. While the serum potassium level is 3.5–5 mEq/L, it is found in the cell at 140 mEq/L level.

The Na–K-ATPase pump provides sodium and potassium passage through the cell membrane. Potassium regulates excitability in all muscles including myocardium and nerves. Changes in serum potassium levels above or below normal levels can cause fatal rhythm problems, cardiac arrest, paralysis of the muscles, and respiratory arrest. The serum potassium level is determined by exogenous potassium intake, absorption, potassium exchange between extracellular fluid and cells, and the balance between sodium and potassium excretion through urine.

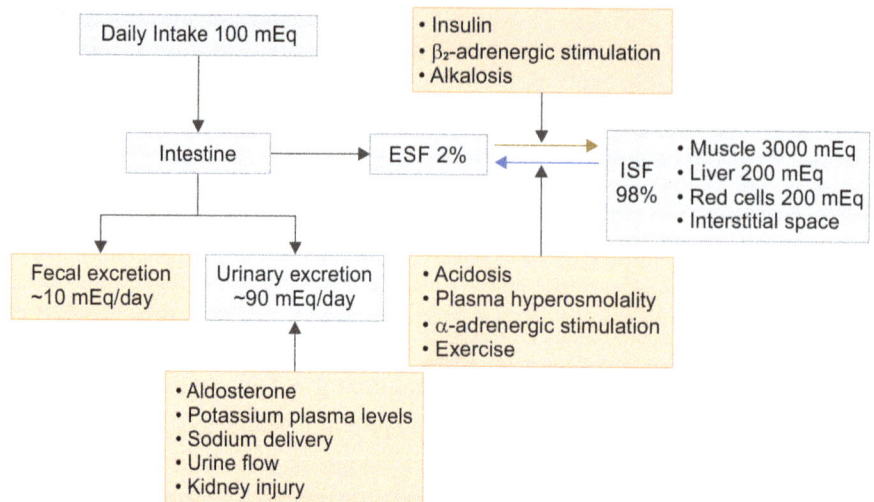

Fig. 3: Potassium homeostasis. (ECF: extracellular fluid; ICF: intracellular fluid)

2. Discuss the etiology of hyperkalemia.

Hyperkalemia occurs when potassium intake (diet containing high potassium and low sodium) increases; supportive tablets containing potassium and IV fluids containing high potassium or nutritional solutions are taken; and in cases such as saved (2–3-week-old) bank blood transfusion, cardioplegic solutions, metabolic acidosis, hypoaldosteronism, pseudo-hypoaldosteronism, rhabdomyolysis, electrical trauma, hemolysis, hyperkalemic periodic paralysis, decreased potassium excretion; kidney failure [glomerular filtration rate (GFR): If the GFR falls below 15–20 mL/kg, even if a high amount of potassium is not taken, the potassium level may increase], renal tubular acidosis, drugs [potassium-sparing diuretics, angiotensin-converting-enzyme (ACE) inhibitors, nonsteroidal anti-inflammatory drugs (NSAIDs), penicillin G potassium, heparin, β-blockers antifungals, succinylcholine], and pseudohyperkalemia.

3. Discuss about end-tidal capnogram and its utility in the ED.

Capnography is a mandatory tool in airway management in ED and ambulances. It is essential to confirm tube placement after intubation, monitoring of intubated patients in ED, and also during medical transport. Capnometry is the continuous measurement of carbon dioxide (CO_2) in a sample of gas and is represented in a graphic form (time on the x-axis and expired partial pressure of CO_2 on the y-axis). The end-tidal CO_2 ($ETCO_2$) is the maximal partial pressure or concentration of CO_2 in the respiratory gases at the end of an exhaled breath. A capnometry monitor displays the $ETCO_2$ value alone, whereas a capnography monitor displays the $ETCO_2$ value plus a continuous capnography waveform. *Capnography wave has four phases* of normal capnography wave morphology **(Fig. 4)**:

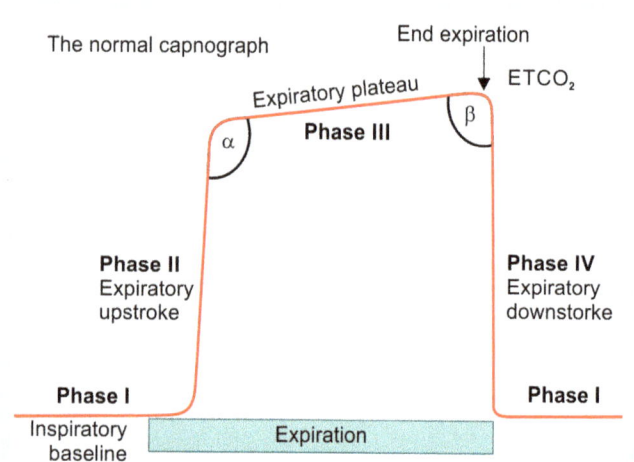

Fig. 4: Morphology of a normal capnography wave.

Phase I (inspiratory phase) represents inspiratory phase, so no CO_2 is detected. The end of phase I represents the beginning of expiration, but because the initial gases expired originate from unventilated dead space, the capnography trace remains at zero.

Phase II (expiratory upstroke) represents expiration of both dead space gas and alveolar gas from the respiratory bronchioles and alveoli.

Phase III (alveolar plateau) represents phase of expiration of alveolar gases. At the end of phase III, the maximal value of CO_2 measured is equivalent to the $ETCO_2$. Note that if the alveoli all contained exactly the same partial pressure of CO_2, phase III would be completely horizontal.

Phase IV (expiratory downstroke) represents the beginning of the next breath, with the CO_2 content returning rapidly to zero. Healthy patients with normal respiratory function will produce a capnography trace with this form. Lung pathologies will change the appearance of the capnograph due to a number of different factors: bronchoconstriction and obstruction to airflow, destruction of alveoli, an increase in the range of alveolar time constants (alveoli that empty at different rates), and an increase in ventilation (V)/perfusion (Q) spread (variation in the CO_2 content of each alveolus). As a result, the slope of phase III is often markedly increased in respiratory disease.

Question 5

1. Discuss two triage systems for adults and one triage system for children in mass casualty incidents in the field settings.

In a mass casualty situation, the number of patients and their severity are much more than the existing capability for management. Triage is the most important part of any disaster response. The main objective of mass casualty/disaster triage is to do the maximum help to the maximum number of people. Major incidents which cause mass casualties are road traffic accident, building collapse, earthquake, flood, major fire, train derailment, explosion, air crash, terrorist attack, and hazardous material release. The main objectives of triaging in disaster and mass casualty are to decompress the disaster area, most critical casualty should get the best care, and special care should be provided for burn and crush injuries. In this critical situation, a simple triaging format [START **(Flowchart 4)** and SALT **(Flowchart 5)**] should be used. Use START (simple triage and rapid treatment)/SALT (sort, assess, lifesaving interventions, and treatment/transport) triaging methods in adult age group mass casualty.

Triaging in the pediatric age group: Children are usually uncooperative during examination and give poor history so it is very important to recognize markers of serious illness. Useful signs are drowsiness, hypotonia, respiratory grunt, wheeze, crepitation, stridor, tachypnea, pallor, fever, signs of dehydration, abnormal posture, cold periphery, vomit or less urination, convulsion, and tender abdomen. Use JumpSTART **(Flowchart 6)** triaging methods in pediatric age group mass casualty.

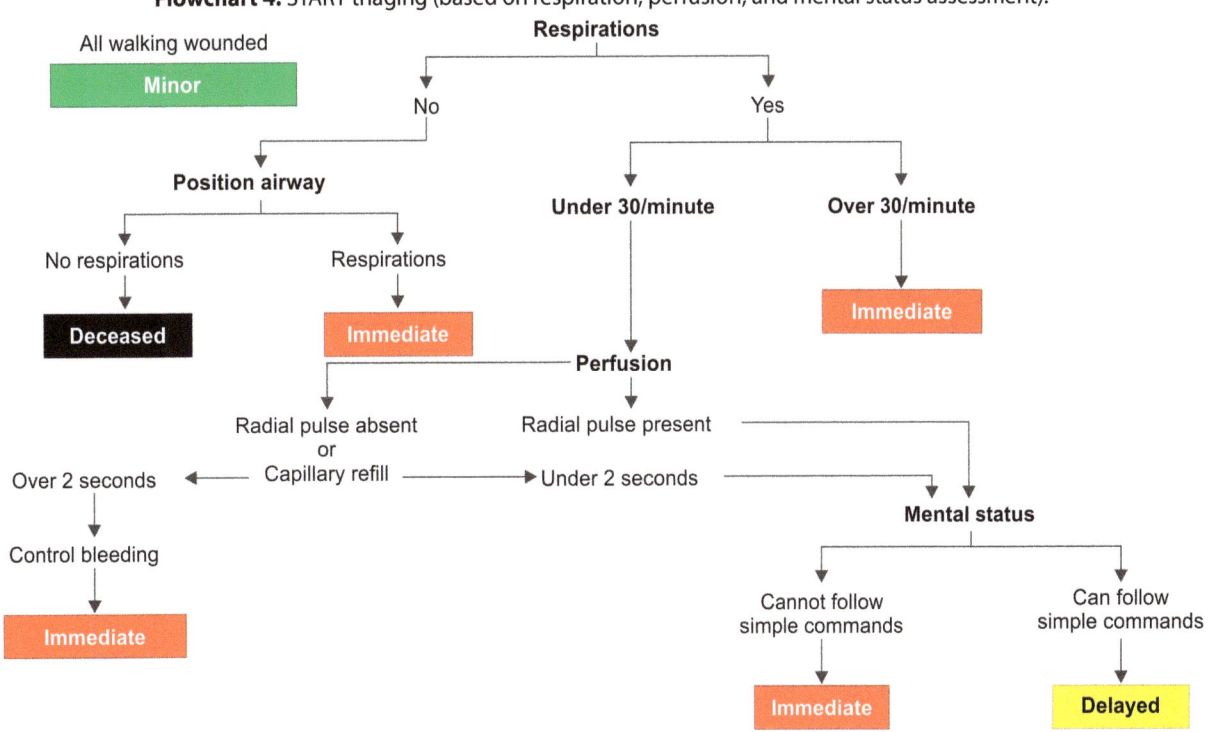

Flowchart 4: START triaging (based on respiration, perfusion, and mental status assessment).

(START: simple triage and rapid treatment)

Flowchart 5: SALT Triage Scheme.

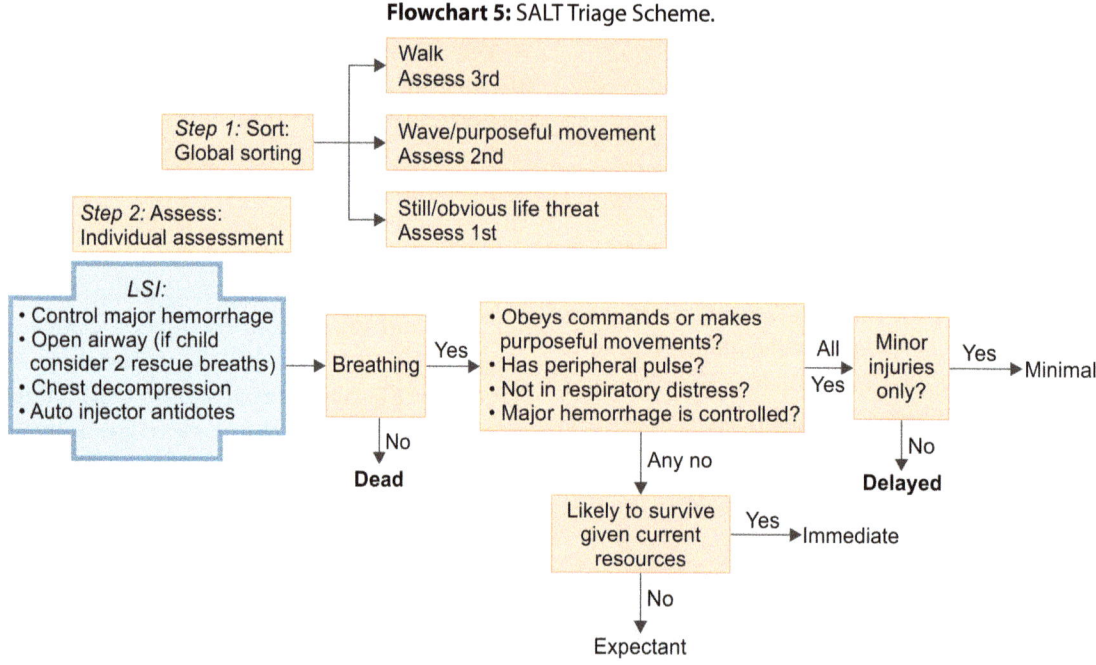

(LSI: lifesaving interventions; SALT: sort, assess, life-saving interventions, and treatment/transport)

Flowchart 6: JumpSTART triaging methods in pediatric age group mass casualty.

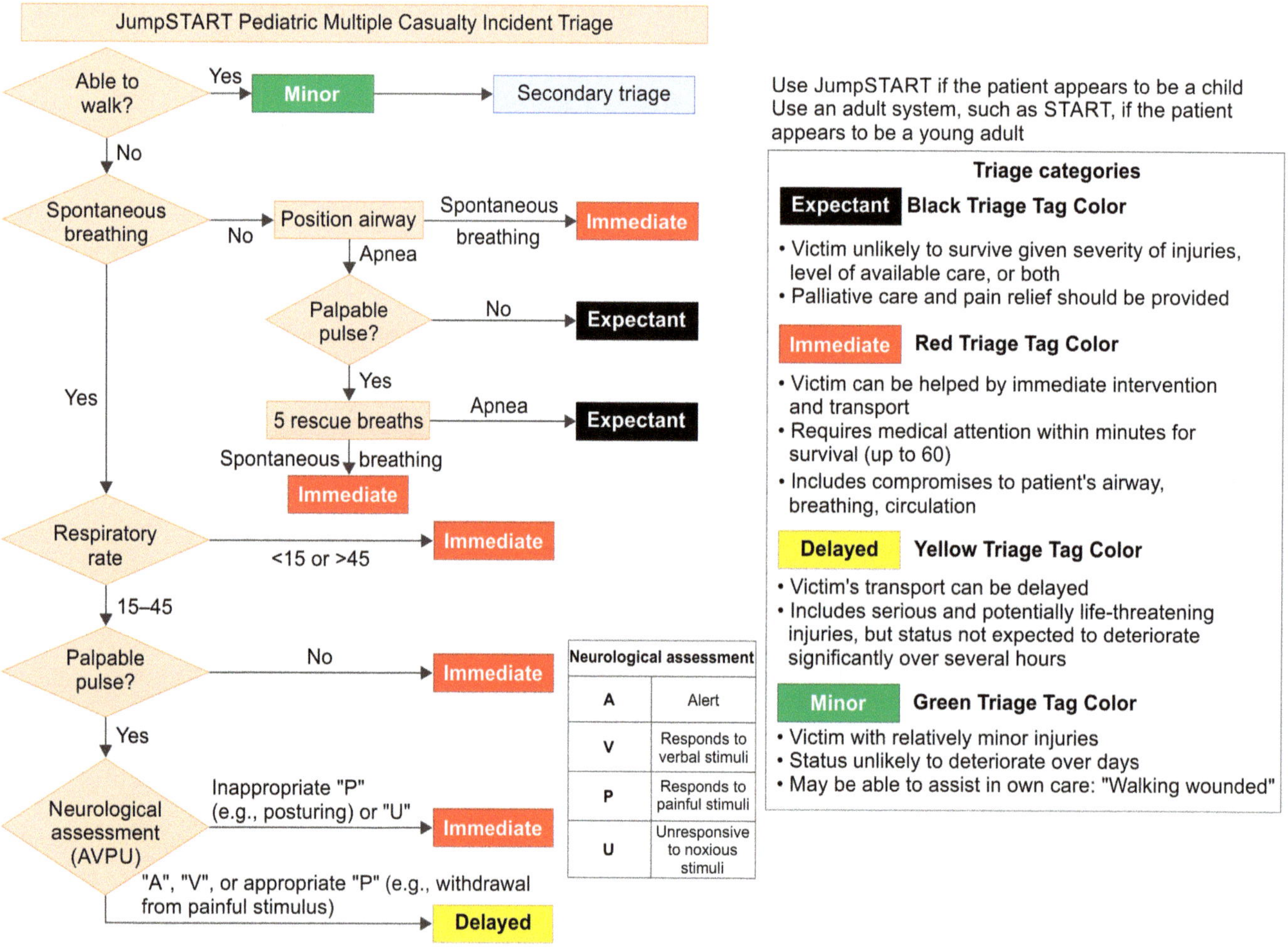

Question 6

1. Discuss and draw the life cycle of *Plasmodium vivax*.

The life cycle of *Plasmodium* includes two hosts (mosquito and human) and various sequences of stages. *Infective:* The uninucleate, lancet-shaped sporozoite (approximately 1 × 7 μm). Sporozoites are produced as a result of sexual reproduction in the midgut of vector *Anopheles* mosquitoes and migrate to the salivary gland. During a blood meal of infected *Anopheles* mosquito, there is transmission of sporozoites from the saliva of vector into the small blood vessels in the human. On entering the systemic circulation of human (second host), there is uptake of protozoans into the liver parenchymal cells. This occurs within 30 minutes of inoculation. After the uptake, the parasite develops into a multinucleate spherical schizont within the liver, comprising 2,000–40,000 uninucleate merozoites. This process is called exoerythrocytic schizogony (liver phase). This period takes 5–21 days and is dependent of the type of *Plasmodium*. In *P. vivax* and *P. ovale*, the maturation phase can take up to 1–2 years and at this time dormant parasites are called hypnozoites. The life cycle of *Plasmodium* is summarized in **Flowchart 7**.

Flowchart 7: Life cycle of *Plasmodium*.

```
Mosquito side                    Human cycle
                                      ↓
Sporozoite ←──────────────────── Sporozoites
   ↑      When mosquito              ↓
   │      bites infect man       Liver cells
   │                                 ↓
   │                             Merozoites
   │                                 ↓
   │                       Erythrocytic schizogony
   │                                 ↓
Oocyst                      Immature─┐
   ↑                                 ├→ Trophozoites
   │  Stomach               Mature ──┘
   │  of mosquito                    ↓
Ookinete                            ─── Mature
   ↑                        Schizont ╱
   │                                 ╲── Immature
   │                                 ↓
                                 Merozoite
                         Male and female gametocytes
                                     ↓
                         When mosquito bites, it takes
                         male and female gametocytes
                                     ↓
                                In mosquito
Zygotes ←──────────── Macro- and microgametes
```

2. How will you diagnose malaria caused by *P. vivax* and *P. falciparum*?

Diagnosis of malaria is based on clinical suspicion and laboratory confirmation of parasitemia and microscopic examination of peripheral blood smear (PBS). Confirmation is done by thin and thick film (more reliable when parasitemia is very low). Nothing can be found better than direct examination of smear, but it is time consuming, needs infrastructure, and single negative PBS cannot rule out malaria. Microscopic features of early trophoblast (*vivax* and *falciparum*) and mature stages of *vivax* and *falciparum* are shown in **Figures 5A and B.** To improve the measures for diagnosing malaria, various rapid diagnostic testing is available **(Table 3)**.

TABLE 3: Rapid diagnostic testing for malaria.

Microscopic methods	• Acridine orange staining • QBC testing
Molecular methods	• DNA and rRNA probes • PCR
Antigen detection	• HRP-2 antigen detection • ParaSight-F test • Parasite LDH detection
Other methods	Immunochromatographic test

(DNA: deoxyribonucleic acid; HRP: histidine-rich protein; LDH: lactate dehydrogenase; PCR: polymerase chain reaction; QBC: quantitative buffy coat; rRNA: ribosomal ribonucleic acid)

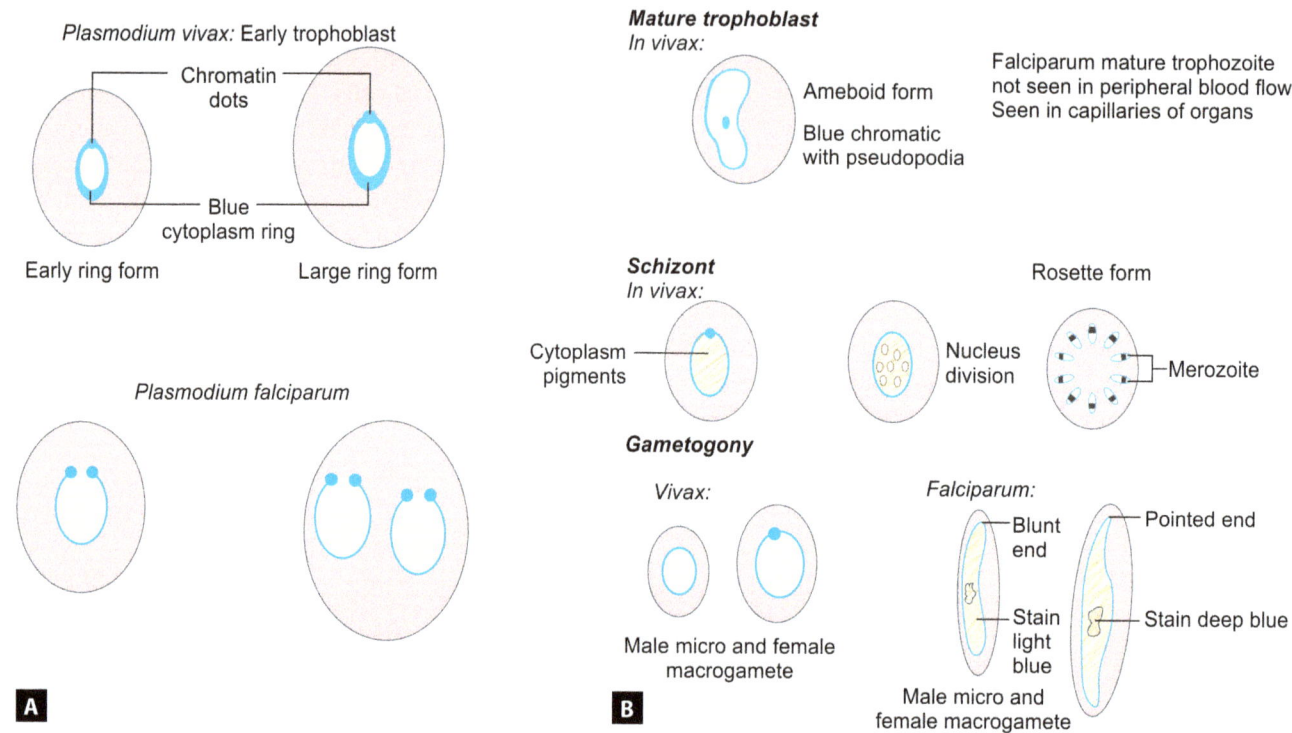

Figs. 5A and B: (A) Microscopic features of early trophoblast (*vivax* and *falciparum*); (B) Mature stages of *vivax* and *falciparum*.

Question 7

1. Discuss incident command system for an external disaster.

The incident command system (ICS) is an emergency management system that helps the primary responders and responding agencies to unify services. Medical disaster can quickly lead to chaos and confusion and ICS provides medical facilities with an organized management structure that promotes immediate, focused direction of activities during a disaster and allows for prompt resumption of normal operations. ICS is headed by the incident commander whose responsibilities are administration, planning, finance, and arranging logistics (**Table 4**). It is helpful in defining the roles and responsibilities, prioritizing duties, and providing predictable management structure (**Box 1**). Public information officer, safety officer, and liaison officer are the other important members of the ICS, and their roles are clearly defined. Incident command organization chart is shown in **Flowchart 8**.

TABLE 4: Overall responsibilities of the head of incident command center.

Logistic (Provide support)	Planning (Prepare action plan)	Finance (Cost accounting and procurement)	Operations (Direct tactical action)
Responsible for acquisition and maintenance of facilities, services, personnel equipment, materials	• Collect, analyze, display information • Prepare incident action plan • Maintain situation and resource status • Maintain incident documentation • Prepare demobilization • Promote continuity of operations	• Monitors incident costs • Maintains financial records • Administers procurement contracts	Carry out the medical objective to the best of their ability
Other important command staff			
Public information officer		*Safety officer*	*Liaison officer*
Provides information to the news media, serves as the one central point for information dissemination		Monitors the facility and anticipates, detects, and corrects unsafe situations	Functions as incident contact person for representatives from other assisting and cooperating agencies

BOX 1: Responsibilities and advantages of the incident command system (ICS).

Responsibilities of ICS:
- Create an emergency operation center
- Prepare department kits
- Plan how and when to activate ICS
- Implementation and training

Advantages of ICS:
- A logical predictable management structure
- Clearly defined roles and responsibilities
- Distribution of work
- Lessens liability
- Prioritization of duties
- Facilitation of communication via common language
- Thorough documentation of actions taken
- Flexibility and adaptability
- Position-driven system not person-driven
- Promotes financial recovery

2. Discuss the physics of radiation.

Radiation is energy that comes from a source and travels through space at the speed of light. This energy has an electric field and a magnetic field associated with it and has wave-like properties. Events associated with the exposure of humans and the environment to dangerous levels of radiation are rare. However, their destructive potential for harm to exposed humans and the environment, coupled with their long-term implications in exposed populations and infrastructures, makes them genuinely formidable threats. Radioactive material exposes responders to various health risks depending on several factors such as the amount of radiation received, and the length of time over which the dose is received. Radiation that was dispersed with or without an associated explosive component results in either direct (blast injury) or indirect (projectiles) trauma, flash, and/or thermal burns, with subsequent radiation sickness. Upon confirming the initial fatalities after an explosion, the future radiation can be determined. This will be dependent upon the grade of radioactive material and the amount that has been released.

Flowchart 8: Incident command organization chart.

```
                        Incident command
                              |
                    Information safety
                         liason
                              |
    ┌─────────────────┬───────┴────────┬─────────────────────┐
Operation section  Planning section  Logistic section   Finance/administration
                                                              section
    │                   │                 │                    │
• Staging areas    • Resource unit   • Communication unit   • Time unit
• Task force       • Situation unit  • Medical unit         • Procurement unit
• Air operation    • Documentation   • Food unit            • Claim unit
  branch           • Demobilization  • Supply unit          • Cost unit
                     unit            • Facilities unit
                                     • Ground support unit
```

First responders to the scene are prompted to utilize time, distance, and shielding (TDS) to reduce or eliminate radiation exposure. Initial triage of patients should attempt to ascertain the extent of exposure, associated injuries, and the degree of internal and external contamination. Symptoms of exposure are influenced by factors such as the type of radiation, total dose, amount and rate, individual susceptibility, and surface area irradiated. Clinical signs may include nausea, vomiting, and erythema within the first 48 hours of exposure, a latent phase with no apparent symptoms, followed by the manifestation of disease days to weeks post-exposure in the form of various hematopoietic, gastrointestinal, cutaneous, and neurovascular syndromes. Management involves decontamination measures such as removal of contaminated debris, washing of skin and nasal passage, wound debridement and irrigation, internal decontamination with chelating agents, and antibiotic coverage as well as appropriate surveillance, testing, and supportive therapy as needed.

Question 8

1. Discuss the anatomy of neck relevant to trauma.

Anatomy: Neck is divided into three zones: Zone I, zone II, and zone III **(Table 5)**. In penetrating trauma, zone designations have anatomic, diagnostic, and management implications. Since the zone system is helpful in guiding management decisions, it is preferable to employ the zone system when describing traumatic injuries. An understanding of the anatomy of the neck, especially the location of important structures, is essential to providing optimal care **(Fig. 6)**.

a. *Zone I:* This is the area between the clavicles and the cricoid cartilage. This zone contains vital structures which include the innominate vessels, the origin of the common carotid artery, subclavian vessels and vertebral artery, brachial plexus, trachea, esophagus, the apex of the lung, and thoracic duct. Furthermore, surgical exposure and access can be difficult in this zone, because of the presence of the clavicle and bony structures of the thoracic inlet.

b. *Zone II:* This is the area between the cricoid cartilage and the angle of mandible. The following structures are located here: the carotid and vertebral arteries, the internal jugular veins, trachea, and the esophagus. This zone has comparatively easy access for clinical examination and surgical exploration. It is the largest zone and the most commonly injured part in the neck.

c. *Zone III:* This is the area between the angle of the mandible and the base of the skull. This area contains the distal carotid and vertebral arteries and the pharynx. Since it is very close to the base of the skull, this area is less amenable to physical examination and difficult to explore during surgical evaluation.

Other important anatomic features are as follows:

a. There is anatomic continuity in the fascial layers between the neck and the anterior mediastinum.
b. The platysma muscle sits between the superficial and deep cervical fascia—violation of the platysma increases the likelihood of deep structure injury and should be explored in the operating room immediately.

Anatomically, the neck is also described in triangles. The sternocleidomastoid muscle separates the neck into two triangles. The anterior triangle contains most of the major anatomic structures of the neck including larynx, trachea, pharynx, esophagus, and major vascular structures. The posterior triangle contains muscles, the spinal accessory nerve, and the spinal column.

TABLE 5: Anatomical zones of the neck and their structures.

	Zone I	Zone II	Zone III
Anatomic landmarks	Clavicle/sternum to cricoid cartilage	Cricoid cartilage to the mandible	Superior angle of the mandible
Anatomic structures in zone	• Proximal common carotid artery • Subclavian artery • Vertebral artery • Lung apices • Trachea • Thyroid • Esophagus • Thoracic duct • Spinal cord	• Carotid artery • Vertebral artery • Jugular vein • Pharynx • Trachea • Esophagus • Larynx • Vagus nerve • Recurrent laryngeal nerve • Spinal cord	• Vertebral artery • Distal carotid artery • Distal jugular vein • Salivary and parotid glands • Cranial nerves IX–XII • Spinal cord

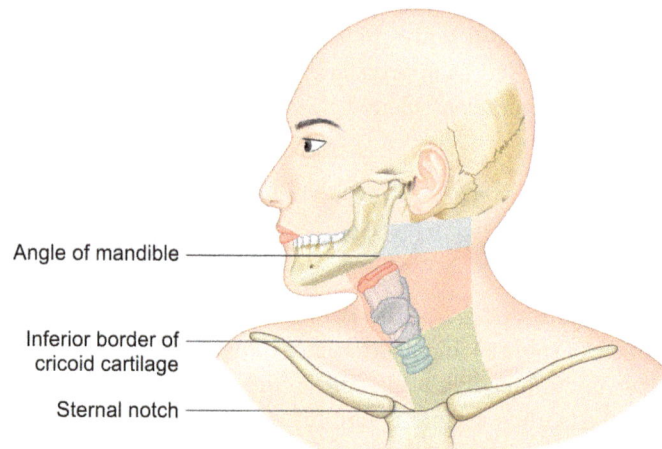

Fig. 6: Anatomical zones of the neck.

2. Discuss the classification and pathophysiology of hemorrhagic shock.

Classification of hemorrhagic shock is given in **Table 6**.

TABLE 6: Classification of hemorrhagic shock.

	Class I	Class II	Class III	Class IV
Blood loss (%)	<15%	15–30%	31–40%	>40%
Heart rate	60–100	101–120	121–140	>140
Blood pressure	Normal	Normal	Decreased	Decreased
Mental status	Slightly anxious	Mildly anxious	Anxious, confused	Confused, lethargic
Fluid requirements	Crystalloid	Crystalloid	Crystalloid, blood products	Crystalloid, blood products

Pathophysiology of hemorrhagic shock: The pathophysiology of hemorrhagic shock involves a decrease in systemic DO_2 to a level less than what is needed to maintain cellular function VO_2 **(Fig. 7)**.

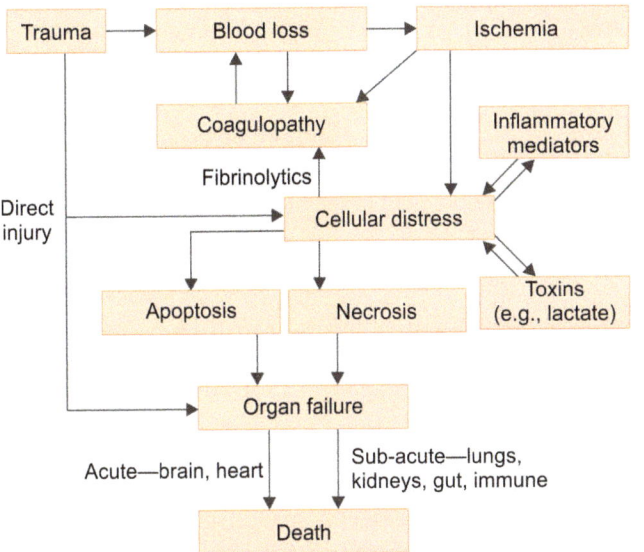

Fig. 7: Pathophysiology of hemorrhagic shock.

Question 9

1. Discuss imaging modalities for foreign bodies in soft tissue.

Identifying and removing foreign bodies are important because retained foreign bodies increase the risk of delayed wound healing and infection. Any foreign body that can be easily seen should be removed. If the object can be reliably palpated, the wound should be explored to make an attempt to remove it, provided there is no risk to the underlying critical structures. A nonirritant foreign body, such as glass or metal that is not in a critical area (e.g., a joint space) or adjacent to a vital structure (e.g., major blood vessel) and not causing any ongoing irritation, may be left in place if unable to be removed, and the wound sutured. Irritant material, such as wooden splinters, can be a source of later infection and should be removed even if it requires exploration of the base of the wound. Direct wound inspection may fail to detect all foreign bodies, particularly if the base of the wound cannot be seen. Deep wounds, wounds on the head or foot, and wounds due to trauma in a motor vehicle accident or due to glass cut injuries are more likely to contain retained glass. Radiologic evaluation by a plain X-ray is helpful if the foreign body is radiopaque and should be considered as an adjunct to visual inspection if history indicates a possibility of a foreign body or debris.

2. Discuss the various nonabsorbable sutures along with their usage in the ED.

Sutures may be monofilamentous (Prolene or Ethilon) or multifilamentous (silk). The designation for suture strength is the number of zeros **(Table 7)**. The higher the number of zeros (1-0 to 10-0), the smaller the size and the lower the strength. They can also be defined as absorbable (dissolve within 14–180 days) or nonabsorbable. Types of suture material used in laceration are summarized in **Table 8**.

TABLE 7: Choosing appropriate suture material for body regions and their removal.				
Body part	**Suture material (skin)**	**Suture material (deep)**	**Closure**	**Suture removal**
Scalp	3-0 or 4-0 NA	4-0 SA	Single tight layer	7–12 days
Ear	6-0 NA	5-0 SA	Interrupted	4–6 days
Eyebrow	6-0 NA	4-0 or 5-0 SA	Layered closure	4–6 days
Eyelid	6-0 NA	–	Single-layer horizontal mattress	4–6 days
Lip	6-0 NA	4-0 silk/SA (mucosa)	Three-layer closure	4–6 days
Oral cavity	–	4-0 SA	Layered closure if tongue muscles are involved	7–8 days
Face	6-0 NA	4-0 or 5-0 SA	Layered closure if full thickness laceration	4–6 days
Neck	5-0 NA	4-0 SA (subcutaneous)	Two-layer closure for best cosmetic results	4–6 days
Trunk	4-0 or 5-0 NA	4-0 SA (subcutaneous)	Single or layered closure	7–12 days
Extremities	4-0 or 5-0 NA	3-0 or 4-0	Splint if wound over the joint	7–12 days
Hand and feet	4-0 or 5-0 NA	–	Only skin closure	7–12 days
Nailbed	5-0 SA	–	Replace nail until cuticle	Allow to dissolve

[NA: nonabsorbable suture (nylon, polypropylene); SA: synthetic absorbable suture]

TABLE 8: Sutures and suturing methods for advanced laceration.

Laceration parameters	Type of needle	Type of suture material	Special suturing techniques
Superficial facial lacerations	Reverse cutting	Prolene or Ethilon (6-0)	Simple interrupted skin sutures
Deep facial lacerations (layered closure)	Reverse cutting	• 5-0 polydioxanone suture (PDS) or Monocryl • Prolene or Ethilon (6-0)	• Subdermal interrupted sutures • Simple interrupted skin suture
Tongue	Taper cut	4-0 or 5-0 Vicryl	Vertical mattress sutures
Oral mucosa	Taper cut	4-0 or 5-0 Vicryl	Vertical mattress sutures
Eyelid	Taper cut	6-0 silk or Prolene	Simple interrupted skin sutures
Nailbed	Reverse cutting/taper cut	6-0 or 7-0 plain catgut	Simple interrupted sutures
Limbs and torso	Reverse cutting	4-0 or 5-0 Ethilon or Prolene	Simple interrupted sutures or vertical mattress sutures

Note: Suture removal: The timing of suture removal varies with the anatomic site. (a) *Eyelids:* 2–3 days; (b) *Neck:* 3–4 days; (c) *Face:* 5 days; (d) *Scalp:* 7–14 days; (e) *Trunk and upper extremities:* 8–10 days; (f) *Lower extremities:* 8–10 days.

Question 10

1. Discuss the classification of anti-arrhythmic agents.

There are four main classes of anti-arrhythmic drugs as given in **Table 9**.

2. Discuss the classification of vasopressors and ionotropic agents.

Adrenergic agents such as phenylephrine, norepinephrine, dopamine, and dobutamine are the most commonly used vasopressor and ionotropic agents in critically ill patients **(Table 10)**.

TABLE 9: Classification of anti-arrhythmic drugs.

	IA	IB	IC
Class I Membrane stabilizing (Na channel blockers) Class I A—moderately prolong conduction Class I B—minimal effect on conduction Class I C—marked prolongation of conduction	Quinidine Procainamide Disopyramide	Lidocaine Mexiletine	Propafenone Flecainide
Class II (blockade of β-adrenergic receptors)	Propranolol Esmolol Sotalol (class III properties also)		
Class III (prolongation of repolarization)	Amiodarone Dronedarone Dofetilide Ibutilide		
Class IV (calcium channel blockers)	Verapamil Diltiazem		
Drugs for paroxysmal supraventricular tachycardia	Adenosine Digoxin		

TABLE 10: Common vasopressors and inotropes.

Agent	Initial dose	Maintenance dose	Maximum dose	Characteristics and role
Vasopressors (α-1 adrenergic)				
Norepinephrine	8–12 µg/min (0.1–0.15 µg/kg/min) A lower initial dose of 5 µg/min may be used, e.g., in older adults	2–4 µg/min (0.025–0.05 µg/kg/min)	35–100 µg/min (0.5–0.75 µg/kg/min; up to 3.3 µg/kg/min has been needed rarely)	Initial vasopressor of choice in septic, cardiogenic, and hypovolemic shock. Must be diluted, e.g., usual concentration is 4 mg in 250 mL of D5W or NS (16 µg/mL)

Contd...

Contd…

Agent	Initial dose	Maintenance dose	Maximum dose	Characteristics and role
Epinephrine (adrenaline)	1 µg/min (0.014 µg/kg/min)	1–10 µg/min (0.014–0.14 µg/kg/min)	10–35 µg/min (0.14–0.5 µg/kg/min)	• Initial vasopressor of choice in anaphylactic shock • Typically an add-on agent to norepinephrine in septic shock • Increases heart rate; may induce tachyarrhythmias and ischemia • Must be diluted; e.g., usual concentration is 1 mg in 250 mL D5W (4 µg/mL)
Phenylephrine	100–180 µg/min (0.5–2 µg/kg/min)	20–80 µg/min (0.25–1.1 µg/kg/min)	80–360 µg/min (1.1–6 µg/kg/min)	• Pure α-adrenergic vasoconstrictor: • Initial vasopressor when tachyarrhythmias preclude use of norepinephrine • May decrease stroke volume and cardiac output in patients with cardiac dysfunction • May be given as bolus dose of 50–100 µg to support blood pressure during rapid-sequence intubation • Must be diluted; e.g., usual concentration is 10 mg in 250 mL D5W OR NS (40 µg/mL)
Dopamine	2–5 µg/kg/min	5–20 µg/kg/min	20 to >50 µg/kg/min	• An alternative to norepinephrine in septic shock in highly selected patients (e.g., with compromised systolic function or absolute or relative bradycardia and low risk of tachyarrhythmias) • More adverse effects (e.g., tachycardia, arrhythmias particularly at doses >20 µg/kg/min) and less effective than norepinephrine for reversing hypotension in septic shock • Lower doses (e.g., 1–3 µg/kg/min) should not be used for renal protective effect and can cause hypotension during weaning • Must be diluted; e.g., usual concentration is 400 mg in 250 mL D5W (1.6 mg/mL)
Antidiuretic hormone				
Vasopressin	0.01–0.03 units/min	0.03–0.04 units/min	0.04–0.07 units/min (dose >0.04 units/min can cause cardiac ischemia and should be reserved for salvage therapy)	• Add-on to norepinephrine to raise blood pressure. Not to be used as first-line vasopressor • Pure vasoconstrictor; may decrease stroke volume and cardiac output in myocardial dysfunction or precipitate ischemia in coronary artery disease • Must be diluted; e.g., usual concentration is 25 units in 250 mL D5W or NS (0.1 units/mL)
Inotrope (β-1 adrenergic)				
Dobutamine	0.5–1 µg/kg/min	2–20 µg/kg/min	20–40 µg/kg/min; doses >20 µg/kg/min are not recommended in heart failure and should be reserved for salvage therapy	• Initial agent of choice in cardiogenic shock with low cardiac output and maintained blood pressure • Add-on to norepinephrine for cardiac output augmentation in septic shock with myocardial dysfunction • Increases cardiac contractility and rate; may cause hypotension and tachyarrhythmias • Must be diluted; a usual concentration is 250 mg in 500 mL D5W or NS (0.5 mg/mL)
Inotrope (nonadrenergic, PDE3 inhibitor)				
Milrinone		0.125–0.75 µg/kg/min		• Alternative for short-term cardiac output augmentation to maintain organ perfusion in cardiogenic shock refractory to other agents • Increases cardiac contractility and heart rate at high doses; may cause peripheral vasodilation, hypotension and/or ventricular arrhythmias • Renally cleared; dose adjustment in renal impairment needed • Must be diluted; e.g., a usual concentration is 40 mg in 200 mL D5W (200 µg/mL)

[D5W: (5%) dextrose water; MAP: mean arterial pressure; NS: (0.9%) normal saline; PDE3: phosphodiesterase 3]

SUGGESTED READING

1. Australasian Society of Clinical Immunology and Allergy. (2023). ASCIA Guidelines: Acute Management of Anaphylaxis. [online] Available from: https://www.allergy.org.au/hp/papers/acute-management-of-anaphylaxis-guidelines. [Last accessed May, 2023]. (Question 3).
2. Richhariya D, Sharma B. Textbook of Emergency Medicine including Intensive Care and Trauma, 2nd edition. New Delhi: Jaypee Brothers Medical Publishers (P) Ltd; 2022. p. 216. (Question 4).
3. Richhariya D, Sharma B. Textbook of Emergency Medicine including Intensive Care and Trauma, 2nd edition. New Delhi: Jaypee Brothers Medical Publishers (P) Ltd; 2022. p. 480. (Question 10).
4. Richhariya D, Sharma B. Textbook of Emergency Medicine including Intensive Care and Trauma, 2nd edition. New Delhi: Jaypee Brothers Medical Publishers (P) Ltd; 2022. pp. 1247-50. (Question 3).
5. Richhariya D, Sharma B. Textbook of Emergency Medicine including Intensive Care and Trauma, 2nd edition. New Delhi: Jaypee Brothers Medical Publishers (P) Ltd; 2022. pp. 1328-40. (Question 6).
6. Richhariya D, Sharma B. Textbook of Emergency Medicine including Intensive Care and Trauma, 2nd edition. New Delhi: Jaypee Brothers Medical Publishers (P) Ltd; 2022. pp. 152-8, 990-2. (Question 1).
7. Richhariya D, Sharma B. Textbook of Emergency Medicine including Intensive Care and Trauma, 2nd edition. New Delhi: Jaypee Brothers Medical Publishers (P) Ltd; 2022. pp. 1565-6. (Question 8).
8. Richhariya D, Sharma B. Textbook of Emergency Medicine including Intensive Care and Trauma, 2nd edition. New Delhi: Jaypee Brothers Medical Publishers (P) Ltd; 2022. pp. 1658, 1664. (Question 9).
9. Richhariya D, Sharma B. Textbook of Emergency Medicine including Intensive Care and Trauma, 2nd edition. New Delhi: Jaypee Brothers Medical Publishers (P) Ltd; 2022. pp. 174-6. (Question 7).
10. Richhariya D, Sharma B. Textbook of Emergency Medicine including Intensive Care and Trauma, 2nd edition. New Delhi: Jaypee Brothers Medical Publishers (P) Ltd; 2022. pp. 191-2. (Question 7).
11. Richhariya D, Sharma B. Textbook of Emergency Medicine including Intensive Care and Trauma, 2nd edition. New Delhi: Jaypee Brothers Medical Publishers (P) Ltd; 2022. pp. 208-11. (Question 2).
12. Richhariya D, Sharma B. Textbook of Emergency Medicine including Intensive Care and Trauma, 2nd edition. New Delhi: Jaypee Brothers Medical Publishers (P) Ltd; 2022. pp. 314-5. (Question 4).
13. Richhariya D, Sharma B. Textbook of Emergency Medicine including Intensive Care and Trauma, 2nd edition. New Delhi: Jaypee Brothers Medical Publishers (P) Ltd; 2022. pp. 328-33. (Question 8).
14. Richhariya D, Sharma B. Textbook of Emergency Medicine including Intensive Care and Trauma, 2nd edition. New Delhi: Jaypee Brothers Medical Publishers (P) Ltd; 2022. pp. 335-40. (Question 10).
15. Richhariya D, Sharma B. Textbook of Emergency Medicine including Intensive Care and Trauma, 2nd edition. New Delhi: Jaypee Brothers Medical Publishers (P) Ltd; 2022. pp. 42-3. (Question 5).
16. Whyte AF, Soar J, Dodd A, Hughes A, Sargant N, Turner PJ. Emergency treatment of anaphylaxis: concise clinical guidance. Clin Med (Lond). 2022;22(4):332-9. (Question 3).

Emergency Medicine Paper 50

Devendra Richhariya

Question 1

1. Compare and contrast anterior versus posterior shoulder dislocation with regard to history, physical findings, and X-ray findings.

Anterior shoulder dislocation most commonly describes a forward dislocation of the humerus. The arm is slightly abducted and externally rotated. There is a loss of the rounded shape of the normal shoulder (more obvious in thin patients). The acromion is prominent, where the top of the bone is toward the front of the body. Patient holds the arm away from the body. The humeral head can often be palpated in the front of the shoulder. Internal rotation and adduction are limited. Movement is usually very painful as a result of muscle spasms.

Posterior shoulder dislocations are characterized by the bone being forced behind the shoulder joint. Signs and symptoms of a dislocation include: Joint is visibly deformed or out of place, numbness or tingling at the joint, swollen or discolored. Check for range of movements, palpable fullness below the coracoid process and toward the axilla, possible damage to rotator cuff musculature and bone. Vascular injuries may result from traction of the axillary blood vessels, resulting in a reduced pulse pressure or a transient coolness in the hands. Look for peripheral nerve injuries.

X-ray of shoulder joint:
- *Anterior dislocation*—the humeral head lies below the coracoid on the anterior-posterior (AP) view, the Y-view shows the humeral head anterior to the glenoid.
- In the axial view a lesion is often seen in dislocation, known as a Hill–Sachs deformity. This always occurs in recurrent dislocations.
- The tear that occurs to the lower part of anterior labrum, is called as *Bankart lesion.* Sometimes a tear develops in the upper labrum, often referred to as superior labral anteroposterior tear (or SLAP lesion), this occurs often due to sports injury and not dislocation.
- *Posterior dislocation*—the humeral head may appear to have the contour of a "light bulb" rather than a "walking stick". The Y-view shows the humeral head lying posteriorly.

2. Discuss classification and management of proximal humerus fractures.

Classification based on four fracture segments **(Fig. 1)**:
1. The articular segment
2. The greater tuberosity
3. The lesser tuberosity
4. The humeral shaft classification describes only displaced segments which are defined as 1.0 cm displacement or 45° angulation. Multiple fracture configurations are possible. A total of 80% of proximal humeral fracture are minimally displaced.

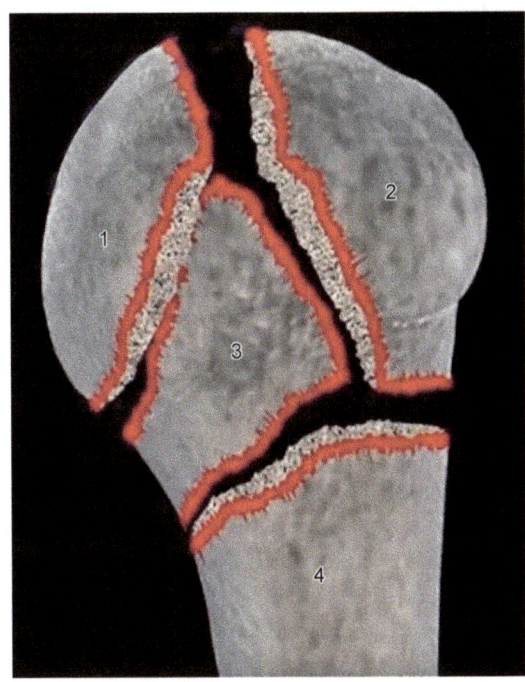

Fig. 1: Proximal humerus fracture.

Fixation with percutaneous techniques, intramedullary nails, locking plates, and arthroplasty are all acceptable treatment options. With internal fixation, special attention should be paid to medial comminution, varus angulation, and restoration of the calcar **(Flowchart 1)**.

Flowchart 1: Approach to management of proximal humerus fracture.

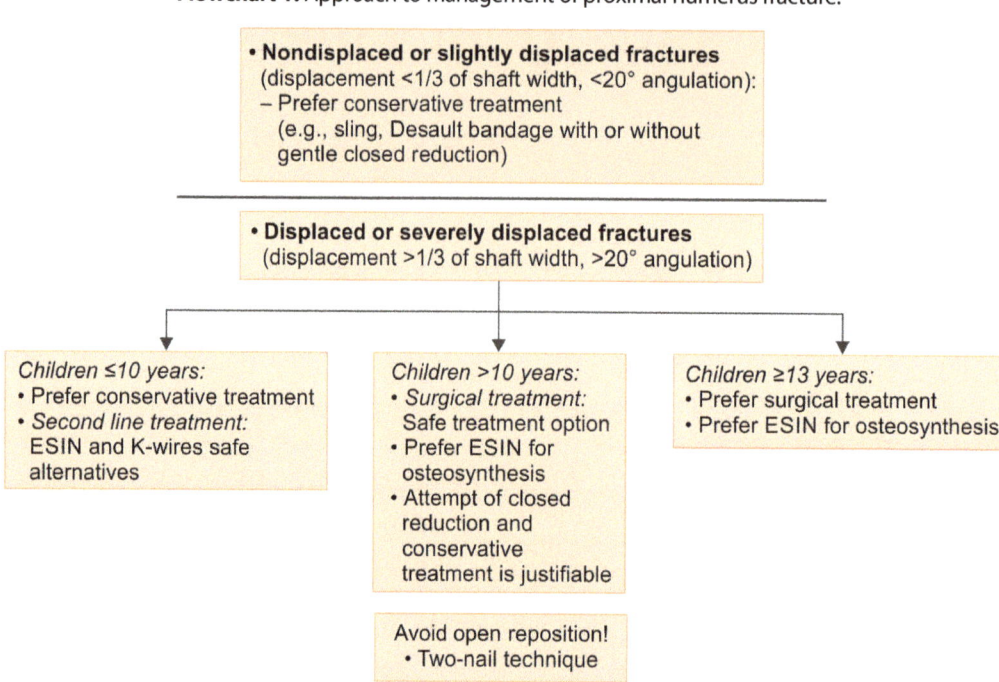

(ESIN: elastic stable intramedullary nailing)

Question 2

A 67-year-old patient presents to the emergency department with acute onset of upper abdominal pain for the past 4 hours. The pain was non-colicky and radiated to the back. On examination, his pulse was 120/min and blood pressure was 96/60 mm Hg.

1. **Discuss differential diagnosis of abdominal pain in this patient.**
2. **How will you investigate him?**
3. **How will you manage him in the emergency department?**

Differential diagnosis: Many intra-abdominal disorders cause abdominal pain and also several extra abdominal diseases can present with abdominal pain. Some of these are immediately life-threatening, requiring rapid diagnosis and surgery. The knowledge of abdominal anatomy and its innervation helps for differential diagnosis; however a systematic and logic approach, with a careful medical history and clinical evaluation, is fundamental. Focused clinical history and physical examination are able to place a right diagnostic hypothesis in 80% of patients with abdominal pain. There are some alert signs and symptoms that must always be taken into careful consideration, because they probably underlie a serious condition. Often a definitive diagnosis is impossible in the emergency department but the emergency physician has always to identify and rule out life-threatening clinical conditions. These include ruptured abdominal aorta aneurism (AAA), perforated viscus, mesenteric ischemia, and ruptured ectopic pregnancy. Other diseases (e.g., acute appendicitis, acute diverticulitis, severe acute pancreatitis, intestinal obstruction) are also serious and nearly as urgent. Emergency physician must correlate between anatomical site of abdominal pain and the differential diagnosis.

Cardiac: Acute myocardial infarction, angina, pericarditis.

Pancreatic: Pancreatitis or tumors.

Vascular: Aortic dissection, mesenteric ischemia.

Management: A thorough history usually suggests the diagnosis. It is necessary to promptly investigate the symptomatology in particular with regard to onset, quality, duration, intensity, irradiation, relationship with meals, and trigger or relieving factors. Of particular importance are characteristics and pain location, associated symptoms and duration. Vital signs must be evaluated in all patients as well as level of consciousness. General appearance is important—a sick patient is anxious, pale, diaphoretic, or in obvious pain. The abdomen must be evaluated starting with inspection to evaluate skin color, palpation to check distention of obvious masses and auscultation of bowel sounds. Blood tests in abdominal pain should be focused according to clinical evaluation, keeping in mind that specificity and diagnostic accuracy are low. Abdominal, contrast enhancement CT scan is the examination with the highest specificity and sensitivity, but bedside ultrasound is now considered the first diagnostic approach in the emergency department. It is also the fundamental in the diagnosis of aortic syndrome, also in diagnosing perforation. **Flowchart 2** summarizes the management of abdominal pain.

Flowchart 2: Management of abdominal pain.

Question 3

1. How will you assess an adult patient with thermal burns in the emergency department?

Superficial or epidermal burns involve only the epidermal layer of skin. Partial-thickness burns involve the epidermis and portions of the dermis. Full-thickness burns extend through and destroy all layers of the dermis **(Table 1)**.

Rule of nine in adults: It is used for estimation of adult burn size. The front and back of each arm and hand equal 9% of the body's surface area. The chest equals 9% and the stomach equals 9% of the body's surface area. The upper back equals 9% and the lower back equals 9% of the body's surface area. The front and back of each leg and foot equal 18% of the body's surface area **(Fig. 2)**.

Burn depth	Histology/anatomy	Example	Healing
Superficial (1 degree)	• Epidermis • No blisters, painful	Sunburn	7 days
Superficial partial thickness (2nd degree)	Epidermis and superficial dermis blisters and very painful	Hot water scald	14–21 days, no scar
Deep partial thickness (deep 2nd degree)	• Epidermis, and deep dermis, sweat glands, hair follicle • Blister and very painful	Hot liquid steam, flame	3–8 weeks, permanent scar
Full thickness (3rd degree)	Entire epidermis and dermis charred, pale, leathery, no pain	Flame	Months, severe scarring
Fourth degree	Entire epidermis and dermis, as well as bone, fat	Flame	Months

TABLE 1: Classification of thermal burn based on depth.

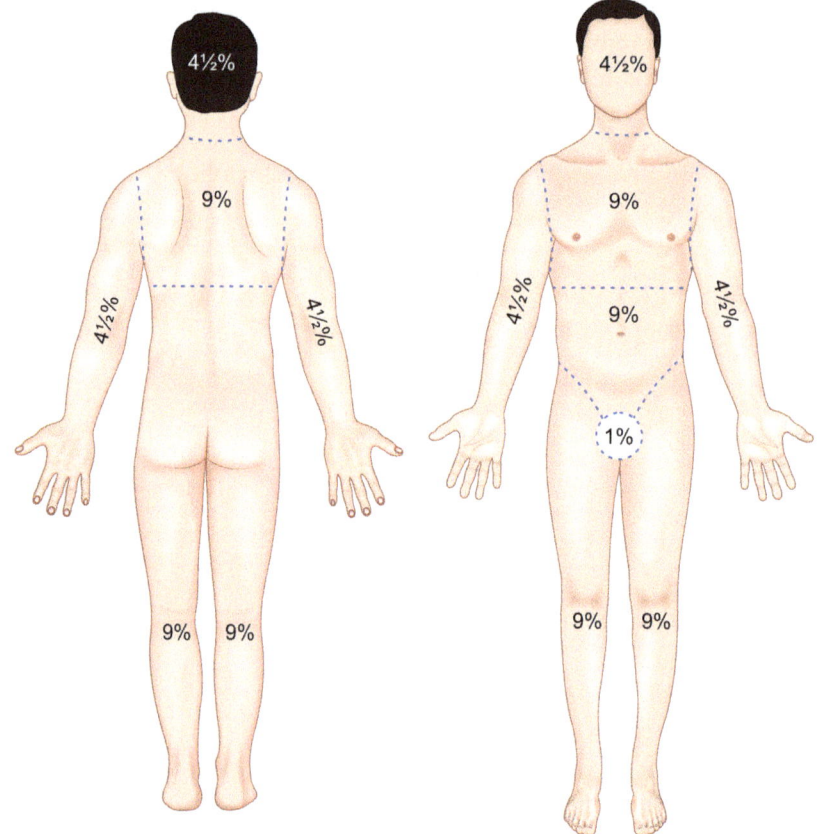

Fig. 2: Rule of nine—estimation of adult burn.

2. Mention hard and soft signs of neck injuries.

Emergency medicine clinician must be familiar with hard and soft sign related to neck trauma **(Table 2)**. In pediatrics it is prudent to consider **stridor** as an additional **"hard"** sign as it may indicate impending airway loss secondary to bleeding into the airway or from swelling encroaching on the patency of the airway. A patient with an apparently stable airway, in the first few hours, may deteriorate quickly due to edema even minor signs should still lead to very careful observation.

TABLE 2: Clinical features of concern in neck trauma.

Hard signs	Soft signs
• Airway compromise • Expanding and pulsatile hematoma • Active, brisk bleeding • Hemorrhagic shock • Hematemesis • Neurologic deficit • Massive subcutaneous emphysema • Air bubbling through wound	• Hemoptysis • Oropharyngeal blood • Dyspnea • Dysphagia • Dysphonia • Nonexpanding hematoma • Chest tube air leak • Subcutaneous or mediastinal air • Vascular bruit or thrill • Crepitus

Question 4

1. Discuss secondary brain injury following traumatic head injury. How will you reduce chances of secondary brain injury?

Head trauma leads to brain parenchymal injury which is termed as traumatic brain injury (TBI). It is defined as any disruption in function of brain due to external force. TBIs are due to falls, road traffic accident, blunt head injury, assault, blast injury, and sometime child abuse. Ability of autoregulation and maintenance of cerebral blood flow is disrupted when any traumatic brain injury occurs. Cerebral vasoconstriction occurs due to hypertension, alkalosis, and hypocarbia and cerebral vasodilation occurs due to hypotension, acidosis, and hypercarbia. After TBI increase in intracranial blood volume (due to vasodilatation) causes brain swelling, this is the compensatory mechanism of brain to maintain optimal cerebral blood flow in view of damaging brain tissue. Secondary to traumatic brain injury various devastating intracranial and extracranial events occurs such as severe intracranial hypertension, seizures and cerebral edema, hypotension, hypoxia, anemia, and hyper- and hypocapnia. These devastating events determine the final outcome in the patient after traumatic brain injury. Hypotension and hypoxia clearly worsen the patient outcome. In short pathophysiology of TBI involves alteration in: Cerebral blood flow, parenchymal injury, cerebral edema, intracranial pressure, and herniation. Main objective in the management of patients with head trauma is the prevention of secondary injury such as ischemia and hypoxia.

Measures to maintain intracranial pressure: It is important to maintain equal volume of each compartment [brain blood cerebrospinal fluid (CSF)] of skull. If volume of one component is increased [due to space-occupying lesions (SOL), intracranial hemorrhage, edema] then volume of other component should decrease as a compensatory mechanism. Mismatch in compensatory mechanism leads to rise in intracranial pressure decrease in cerebral perfusion pressure ultimately causes cerebral ischemia. Intracranial pressure monitoring is preferred in severe traumatic injury by placing external ventricular drain which is helpful in measuring the global intracranial pressure (ICP) and controlling it by CSF drainage.

2. Explain the classification and management of splenic injury.

Computed tomography (CT) is useful in deciding for *operative versus conservative non-operative management* (NOM) of abdominal trauma by providing a detailed anatomy and a severity-based solid viscera injury grading. High-resolution helical CT helps identifying vascular injuries, aneurysms, and arteriovenous fistulae. Percutaneous transcatheter coiling and temporary endovascular balloon occlusion are other examples of upcoming treatment modalities. Angioembolization is useful in evidence of active contrast extravasation on CT scan and in retroperitoneal arterial bleeding. A large vessel injury should not be missed. Both *hepatic and splenic injuries* are graded according to the American Association of Surgery for Trauma (AAST) liver and spleen injury scales (I–V) respectively. The AAST Liver and Spleen Injury Scale (1994 Revision) is summarized in **Table 3**. Vast majority of patients with blunt hepatic and splenic injury require conservative NOM.

TABLE 3: Liver and spleen trauma grades.

Grade	Liver description	Spleen description
I: Hematoma	Subcapsular *non-expanding*, <10% surface area	Subcapsular, <10% surface area (SA)
I: Laceration	Capsular tear *non-bleeding*, <1 cm depth	Capsular tear, <1 cm parenchymal depth
II: Hematoma	• Subcapsular, 10–50% SA • Intraparenchymal, <10 cm diameter	• Subcapsular, 10–50% SA • Intraparenchymal, <5 cm diameter
II: Laceration	1–3 cm parenchymal depth, <10 cm length	1–3 cm parenchymal depth, not involving vessel
III: Hematoma	• Subcapsular, >50% SA or expanding • Ruptured subcapsular/parenchymal hematoma • Intraparenchymal >10 cm or expanding	• Subcapsular, >50% SA or expanding • Ruptured subcapsular/parenchymal hematoma • Intraparenchymal >5 cm or expanding
III: Laceration	>3 cm parenchymal depth	>3 cm depth or involving trabecular vessels
IV: Laceration	• 25–75% of hepatic lobe parenchymal disruption or 1–3 • Couinaud segments within a lobe	Laceration of segmental or hilar vessels with major devascularization (>25% of spleen)
V: Laceration	• >75% of hepatic lobe parenchymal disruption or >3 • Couinaud segments within a lobe	Completely shattered spleen
V: Vascular	Juxta hepatic venous injuries, i.e., retro-hepatic vena cava or central major hepatic veins	Hilar vascular injury with devascularized spleen
VI	*Vascular:* Hepatic avulsion	—

Question 5

1. Discuss etiology and clinical features of brachial plexus injuries.

Brachial plexus injuries (also known as Erb's palsy and Dejerine–Klumpke palsy) are caused by damage to nerves, typically from trauma, tumors, inflammation, pressure, athletic injuries, or being stretched too far. Some brachial plexus injuries can happen to babies during birth. Clinical features are numbness or loss of feeling in the hand or arm; inability to control or move the shoulder, arm, wrist or hand; burning, stinging or severe and sudden pain in the shoulder or arm **(Fig. 3)**.

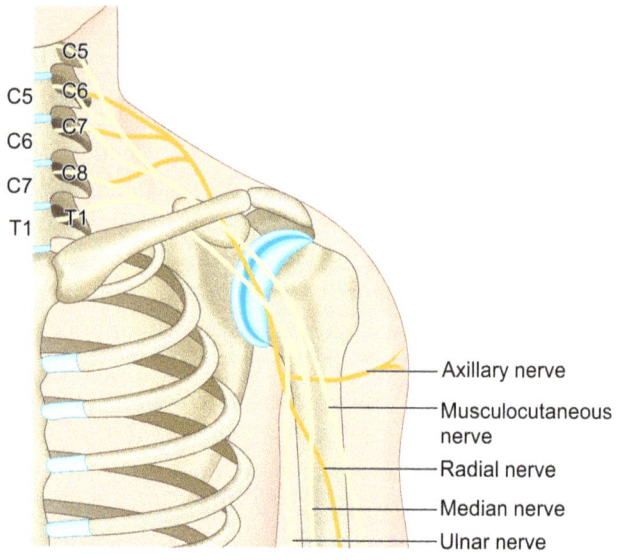

Fig. 3: Brachial plexus.

2. Discuss differential diagnosis of acute, painful, and unilateral scrotal swelling.

The presentation of an acute scrotum can be broken down into four subcategories—*the painful swollen testicle, the painless swollen testicle, the erythematous testicle, and the traumatic testicle.* Within each of these groups there is a diagnosis that cannot be missed. However, not all scrotal emergencies present with pain in the genital area. It is important to rule out scrotal emergencies in patients presenting with acute painful scrotal swelling **(Table 4)**.

TABLE 4: Differential diagnoses for acute scrotal pain.

Ischemic	Testicular torsion, torsion of the testicular appendage
Infectious	Epididymitis, epididymo-orchitis, orchitis, scrotal cellulitis, scrotal abscess, Fournier gangrene, Hansen disease, filariasis
Traumatic	*Blunt:* Testicular contusion, testicular rupture, penetrating testicular rupture, hematocele, scrotal degloving
Inflammatory	Henoch–Schönlein purpura
Idiopathic	Idiopathic scrotal swelling
Oncologic	Testicular tumors
Other	Strangulated/incarcerated inguinal hernia, Referred pain from abdominal pathology, e.g., ruptured abdominal aortic aneurysm or nephrolithiasis

Question 6

1. Discuss Le Fort injury patterns of face.

Le Fort facial fractures are classified as below **(Fig. 4)**:

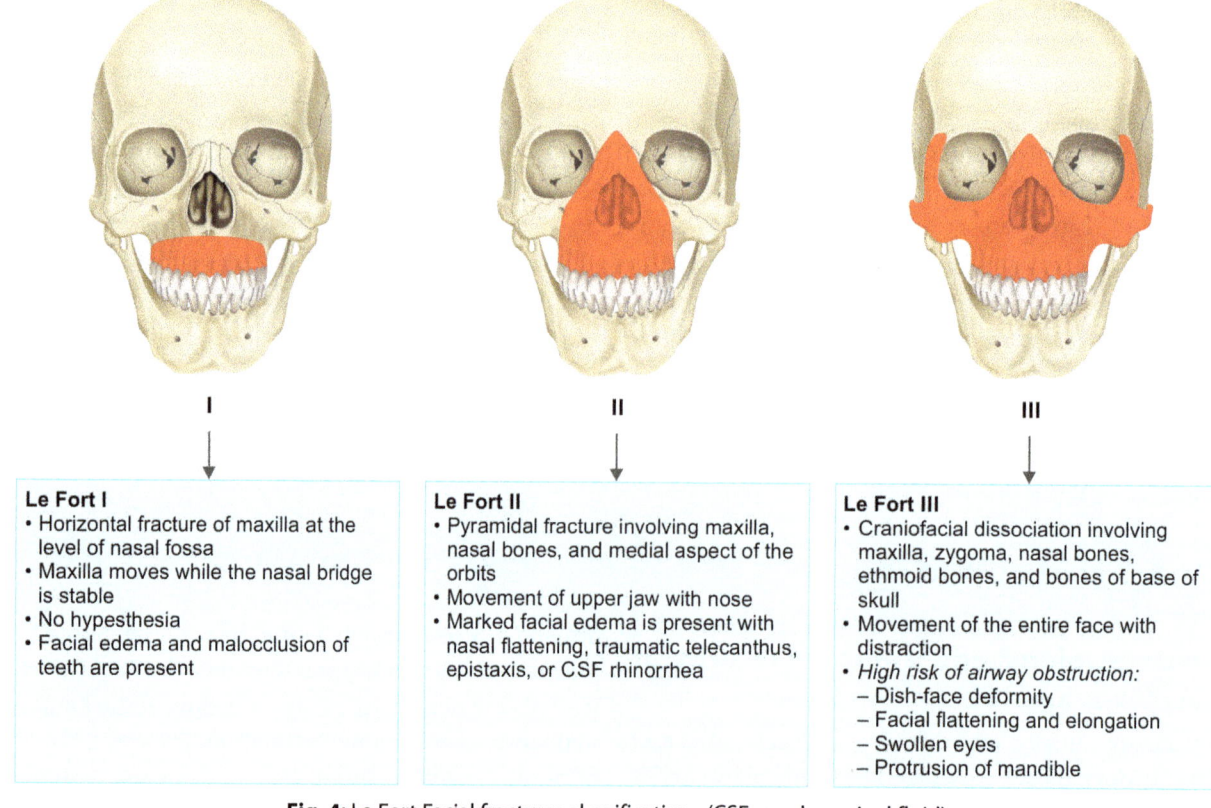

Fig. 4: Le Fort Facial fractures classification. (CSF: cerebrospinal fluid)

Le Fort I: Body of maxilla separated from pterygoid plate and nasal septum. Teeth and hard palate move.

Le Fort II: Pyramidal fracture across central maxilla and hard palate.

Le Fort III: Entire face is separated from skull from fractures of zygomatic suture line, across orbits and base of nose and ethmoids.

Le Fort IV: It includes Le Forte III and frontal bone.

2. Discuss clinical features, diagnosis, and treatment of urethral injuries in a male.

Clinical features of urethral injury: Blood at the urethral meatus is the most important sign of a urethral injury. The most common symptoms of urethral injuries include blood at the tip of the penis in men or the urethral opening in women, blood in the urine, an inability to urinate, and pain during urination. Bruising may be visible between the legs or in the genitals. Other symptoms may arise when complications develop. The symptoms of urethral injuries include pain with voiding or inability to void. Additional signs include perineal, scrotal, penile, and labial ecchymosis, edema, or both.

Diagnosis of urethral injury: Retrograde urethrogram remains the preferred initial diagnostic modality to evaluate a suspected urethral injury. Retrograde urethrography (RUG) or ascending urethrography is used to image male anterior urethra in cases of blunt perineal trauma to assess for urethral disruption, suspected urethral stricture, and fistulas. The patient is positioned in a 45° oblique position and water-soluble iodinated contrast media is gently instilled into a stretched penis through a 12–16 gauge Foley catheter positioned with its balloon in the fossa navicularis and spot films are taken. Many cases of anterior urethral injury need surgery. Minor of these injuries can be treated with a catheter through the urethra; catheter is often left in place for 14–21 days.

Treatment of urethral injury: Anterior urethral injury—initial management by suprapubic cystostomy later stricture can be managed by endoscopy (for short stricture) and urethroplasty (for long stricture). Posterior urethral injury—a suprapubic catheter is placed and delayed repair is done (urethroplasty) at 3 months.

Question 7

1. Discuss medical management of a patient with ectopic pregnancy.

Rapid fluid resuscitation: Ectopic pregnancy is a time-specific emergency. Immediate airway breathing circulation assessment should be done and volume status should be supported by intravenous fluid and blood and blood products. Further management decision should be taken on the basis of ultrasonography (USG) and beta-human chorionic gonadotropin (β-hCG).

Medical management with methotrexate: If minimal symptoms patient is stable, normal baseline LFT and RFT, tubal mass <3.5 cm in diameter, no fetal heart, no evidence of rupture and future fertility is desirable.

Methotrexate acts as an anti-mitotic, folic acid (FA) antagonist, inhibits dihydrofolate reductase (DHFR) enzyme, interferes with fetal DNA synthesis, destroys rapidly dividing cells, and causes involution of pregnancy. Monitoring of doses is done according to serial HCG levels. *Success Rate is*—85–98%, not much difference between single/multiple dose regimen but depends upon pretreatment hCG levels. Prognostic factors which can lead to higher failure rate are: (1) Larger tubal diameter; (2) Fetal cardiac activity present; 3. Higher pretreatment beta-hCG; (4) Severe abdominal pain. *Failure rate* is 14.3% (if pretreatment hCG >5000 IU) in such cases multiple doses are recommended, 3.7% (if pretreatment hCG <5000 IU). Contraindications of methotrexate use are presented in **Table 5**. Dose: 50 mg/m² single IM dose. *Patient need rescue surgery in 5% cases of* methotrexate (MTX) failure—if unstable vital signs, decreasing hemoglobin, intolerable pain, and evidence of rupture on USG.

TABLE 5: Contraindications to methotrexate (MTX) administration.

Absolute contraindications	Relative contraindications
Intrauterine pregnancy	Embryonic cardiac activity detected by transvaginal ultrasound scan (TVS)
Evidence of immunodeficiency	hCG >5000 mIU/mL
Moderate-to-severe anemia, leukopenia, thrombocytopenia	Ectopic pregnancy >4 cm in size (TVS)
Insensitivity to MTX	Refusal to accept blood transfusion
Acute pulmonary disease	Inability for patient to return for follow-up
Active peptic ulcer disease	
Hepatic/renal dysfunction	
Breastfeeding	
Hemodynamic instability	

Follow-up is done with β-hCG on (D4, D7) initial rise in beta-hCG till D4, then between D4-7, 15% decrease from pre-therapy level—if not, repeat MTX dose. After D7, weekly β-hCG till it comes to zero; this might take 2–3 months. If weekly reports do not show a fall of 15% or more, repeat dose of MTX can be given (maximum 3 doses).

Side effects—abdominal pain (75%), flatulence, stomatitis, vaginal bleeding, weakness, dizziness, syncope, hair loss. *"Separation pain"* happens 3–7 days after MTX treatment due to tubal abortion/distension due to hematoma formation. It is a lower abdominal pain, self-limited and responds to non-steroidal anti-inflammatory drugs (NSAIDs). It is suggested to perform complete blood count (CBC) and USG to differentiate such pain from ruptured tube pain. Unwanted outcomes are—long resolution period, increased waiting time for future fertility.

2. Discuss differential diagnosis and management of acute onset of dyspnea in a 40-week-pregnant patient.

Hypoxia: Acute myocardial infarction (MI), cardiomyopathy, anaphylaxis, aortic dissection, aspiration.

Thromboembolism: Amniotic fluid embolism, pulmonary embolism, acute MI air embolism.

Trauma: Tension pneumothorax tamponade.

Amniotic fluid embolism (AFE) is one of the rare causes of cardiac arrest in pregnancy. Amniotic fluid embolism (AFE) is an obstetric condition characterized by the triad of cardiovascular collapse, hypoxic respiratory failure, and coagulopathy. It is also commonly associated with neurologic symptoms (encephalopathy/coma/seizures) with persistent neurologic deficits in survivors. Low incidence of syndrome is may be due underestimation and diagnosis by exclusion and also due to underreporting. Significant mortality and morbidity is associated with AFE, and emergency physician should be aware about this clinical situation and resuscitation considerations differ slightly from other causes of cardiopulmonary collapse.

Risk factors associated with increased risk of AFE include advanced maternal age (35 years or older), placental abnormalities (previa, accreta, abruption, rupture), medical induction of labor, operative deliveries (cesarean delivery, forceps-assisted delivery, vacuum-assisted delivery, termination of pregnancy), amniocentesis, trauma, eclampsia, cervical lacerations, prolonged gestation, male fetus, and multiple gestations.

More than 90% of patient may present as hypoxia which is an early finding. Severe ventilation and perfusion mismatch from the initial embolism and cardiogenic pulmonary edema causes early hypoxia. Later hypoxia may be due to non-cardiogenic pulmonary edema from alveolar capillary leakage of a proteinaceous exudative edema containing amniotic fluid debris, consistent with acute respiratory distress syndrome. Encephalopathy and neurologic injuries can also be observed due to hypoxia in survivors. Bradycardia may be observed on fetal monitoring due to hypoxia.

Chest radiographs reveal nonspecific findings such as diffuse bilateral opacities. Evidence of right ventricular (RV) strain and leftward deviation of the intraventricular septum can be noted on echocardiogram examination. Differential diagnoses to consider include puerperal sepsis, thromboembolic pulmonary embolism, air embolism, aspiration pneumonitis, myocardial infarction, and eclampsia.

Management: Patient should be treated in intensive care unit; treatment is supportive and should include multidisciplinary team including maternal-fetal medicine, critical care, anesthesia, and respiratory therapy. Critical care management is focused on hemodynamic support (mechanical ventilation, vasopressors, and inotropes). Avoid excessive crystalloid fluid administration. In the case of cardiac arrest, a presumptive diagnosis of AFE standard high-quality cardiopulmonary resuscitation (CPR) with advanced cardiovascular life support (ACLS) protocols should continue.

Question 8

1. Discuss etiology and management of epistaxis.

Pathology behind epistaxis is erosion of mucosa and rupture of superficial arteries or veins. Nearly 90% of patients present with anterior epistaxis from Little's area. Rest 10% patients present with posterior epistaxis that is more serious than anterior and more commonly seen in old age patients with comorbidities. *Blood investigations* are not routinely indicated in single infrequent cases. For recurrent bleeding or patient with other comorbidities, few routing blood tests can be done, i.e., CBC, PT-INR, aPTT, liver function tests, etc. CT scan or MRI is indicated to evaluate surgical anatomy or local pathology. Angiography is rarely required.

Treatment: First stage of treatment is to maintain hemodynamic instability. Hypotension or hypertension should be managed accordingly. Local treatment of epistaxis is divided into *surgical or nonsurgical management*. Aim of management is to identify and control source of bleeding. There are various methods to control bleeding:
- *Manual hemostasis*
- *Cauterization*

- *Nasal packing*—anterior nasal packing Posterior nasal packing
- *Surgical treatment.*

2. Discuss evaluation and management of retropharyngeal and peritonsillar abscess.

Retropharyngeal abscess (RPA) is a polymicrobial abscess of posterior pharyngeal wall involving the deep tissues of neck mostly seen in children with peak incidence between 3 and 5 years of age.

It is a multifactorial and polymicrobial infection caused by Group A β-hemolytic streptococci, *Staphylococcus aureus* (*S. aureus*) (including methicillin-resistant *S. aureus*), *Haemophilus influenzae* (*H. influenza*), *Bacteroides*, *Peptostreptococcus*, and *Fusobacterium* species.

Evaluation history: Poor oral hygiene and lack of regular brushing, cleaning of oral cavity in children. Any penetrating neck injuries in adults along with the above-mentioned complaints should lead to suspicion of RPA.

Physical examination: Though physical examination alone is not sufficient to make the diagnosis, one should look for cervical lymphadenopathy and restricted neck movement or torticollis. Also look for trismus, stridor, and drooling as these may indicate further worsening of the condition. There may be tenderness on moving larynx and trachea side to side referred to as tracheal "rock" sign.

Red flags (serious clinical presentation): Airway compromise, drooling neck tenderness, and rigidity stridor respiratory distress trismus.

Investigations: There are no specific laboratory tests for confirmation, however contrast-enhanced CT scan of neck is the preferred modality of choice for diagnosis of this condition. The abscess appears as a hypodense lesion with peripheral ring enhancement in retropharyngeal space.

Treatment: Assessing and securing the airway, breathing and circulation is the key to save patients life. Early endotracheal intubation or tracheostomy should be performed on patient with impending obstruction and respiratory distress. Empirical IV antibiotic therapy should be started early; penicillin G with metronidazole or piperacillin/tazobactam is the first line antibiotics to be given. In case patient does not respond well or there is risk for methicillin-resistant *Staphylococcus aureus* (MRSA), patients should be given vancomycin or linezolid. IV fluids should be started if patient has dehydration or signs of inadequate perfusion. Supportive care including painkillers should be administered as per symptoms of patients. Urgent otolaryngologic consultation should be taken for any surgical intervention.

Peritonsillar abscess (PTA): Also known as *Quincy*, it is the collection of pus in peritonsillar space. It is a complication of tonsillitis which leads to spread of infection to tonsillar crypts further invading peritonsillar tissues causing cellulitis and abscess formation.

Etiology: It occurs due to complication of tonsillitis; various bacterial species are responsible for this condition.

Aerobic bacteria: *Group A beta-hemolytic Streptococci (GABHS), Corynebacterium diphtheria, Staphylococcus aureus, Streptococcus milleri* group.

Anaerobic bacteria: *Fusobacterium necrophorum, Bacteroides, Peptostreptococcus, Prevotella.* Patients usually have prior symptoms of sore throat, fever. The symptoms progress once there is spread of pus through the neck structures. There is worsening of sore throat, dysphagia, odynophagia, otalgia (ipsilateral), high-grade fever, drooling, and trismus. Most patients have a characteristic muffled, "hot potato" voice with halitosis.

Red flags (serious clinical features): **T**oxic general appearance, **A**ltered mental status, **A**irway obstruction, **P**oor hydration status, **P**oor oral acceptance.

Treatment: The main surgical intervention includes needle aspiration, incision and drainage, and tonsillectomy. Needle aspiration of abscess acts as a diagnostic aid, is easy to perform and provides immediate symptom relief. Antibiotic treatment should not be delayed, oral antibiotics may not be suitable due to poor oral compliance thus intravenous antibiotics are preferred. Intravenous (IV) penicillin G along with metronidazole or third generation cephalosporins with metronidazole are drugs of choice. In case one is allergic to penicillin group IV piperacillin/tazobactam may be used. If the patient is stable with no complications they may be started on oral antibiotics, amoxicillin/clavulanate is the preferred oral drug.

Disposition: Patients with signs of toxemia, poor hydration status, airway compromise should be hospitalized and surgical intervention should be performed without delay.

Question 9

1. Explain the management of a foreign body in the nose.

Patients presenting with a foreign body in the nose are not an uncommon occurrence in the emergency department. This population of patients comprises mainly of children <4 years of age, but it may also present in patients with psychiatric disease or intellectual disabilities. Culprit objects found in the nasal cavities are often divided into organic (e.g., seeds, peanuts, insects, worms) and inorganic (e.g., jewelry, toys, pens/pencils, button, batteries, coins, paper) substances, with inorganic items being more commonly encountered.

Nasal foreign bodies are more likely to be found in the right side of the nose. Children who insert these objects into their nose are often brought by caregivers or parents who witnessed the insertion. Therefore, a significant number of nasal foreign bodies are brought due to an observed or suspected history of insertion, within 24 hours of the incident, and with no clinical symptoms secondary to the foreign body. However, as time passes, patients are more likely to manifest with nasal pain, unilateral nasal discharge, epistaxis and, less frequently, with features of surrounding cellulitis or even meningitis.

Radiography is seldom useful in the evaluation of nasal foreign bodies since substances such as wood or plastic are unlikely to be easily visualized. A head lamp or stand lamp, with or without adjuncts such as nasal speculums, can be used to enhance the visual field.

Since impacted nasal foreign bodies have a tendency to trigger inflammatory reactions in surrounding tissue or mucosa, it is often advisable to apply topical analgesia (e.g., lidocaine nasal drops) or topical decongestant (e.g., phenylephrine or oxymetazoline) prior to initiation of removal techniques.

Positive pressure methods: This method generally employs the concept of introduction of positive pressure through an alternate orifice such as the mouth or nostril opposite to the affected side in order to push the foreign body outward from its impacted region.

Mechanical extraction: Similar to aural foreign bodies, various instruments can be used to grasp or anchor behind the nasal foreign body under direct visualization, including alligator forceps, Katz extractors, wax curettes and right-angle hooks, with care taken not to push the foreign object further into the nasal cavity during manipulation.

2. Discuss prehospital care for an avulsed tooth.

Traumatic injuries to teeth are very common and usually associated with road traffic accidents, contact sports such as boxing, taekwondo, karate, etc., or fights. This is very common with children than adults while playing or falling. Dental avulsion is described as a complete displacement of a tooth from its socket in the alveolar bone, and it is one of the most traumatic dental injuries which originate exposure of the cells of the periodontal ligament to the external environment as well as disruption of the blood supply to the pulp. Pain is severe like pulpitis but associated with bleeding. Management of pain and bleeding is important. Rinse avulsed tooth gently in milk, saline, or saliva; use care not to touch root with fingers. If possible, replant avulsed tooth. Seek immediate dental treatment. The golden time for replantation is 20–30 minutes; if it is not possible, the tooth should be kept in an appropriate storage media for preserving the viability of the periodontal ligament cells.

3. Discuss acute red eye without loss of vision.

The causes of red eye range from a minor irritation to a more serious condition or infection. Conditions that involve red eye include conjunctivitis, corneal ulcers, dry eye syndrome, and blepharitis **(Flowchart 3)**.

4. Explain the acute otitis media in adults.

Otitis media (OM) primarily affects infants and children with incidences peaking in the preschool years (6–18 months of age) and declining with advancing age. Acute OM is much less common in adults than children. The most common bacterial pathogens recovered in adults with *acute OM* are *Streptococcus pneumoniae*, *H. influenzae*, methicillin-sensitive *S. aureus*, *Pseudomonas aeruginosa* (*P. aeruginosa*). Young adults remain protected from all *Haemophilus* strains as they have received the *H. influenzae* type b vaccine. The predominant organisms involved in *chronic OM* are *S. aureus*, *P. aeruginosa*, *Aspergillus*, Anaerobic bacteria (less common). *Viral OM* caused predominantly by respiratory syncytial virus and rhinovirus occur in those under the age of 10.

Clinical features: Otalgia, otorrhea, hearing loss, deafness (older children), and nonspecific symptoms such as fever, lethargy, irritability and poor feeding (younger children). Prodrome of an upper respiratory infection (younger children), bulging or retracted tympanic membrane which may be red in color, with associated loss of light reflex may be present on otoscopic examination. Pneumatic otoscopy almost uniformly demonstrates impaired mobility. Assess facial nerve function in view of its proximity to the middle ear.

Treatment measures include analgesia, oral antibiotics, urgent specialist consultation for patients appearing septic or for those who present with complications of acute otitis media. Strongly consider IV antibiotics in such cases. The preferred initial antibiotic treatment:

- Amoxicillin 250–500 mg PO three times daily for 7–10 days
- Azithromycin 500 mg PO daily for 1 day then 250 mg PO daily for 4 days
- Cefuroxime 500 mg PO two times daily for 10 days.

Flowchart 3: Causes of red eye.

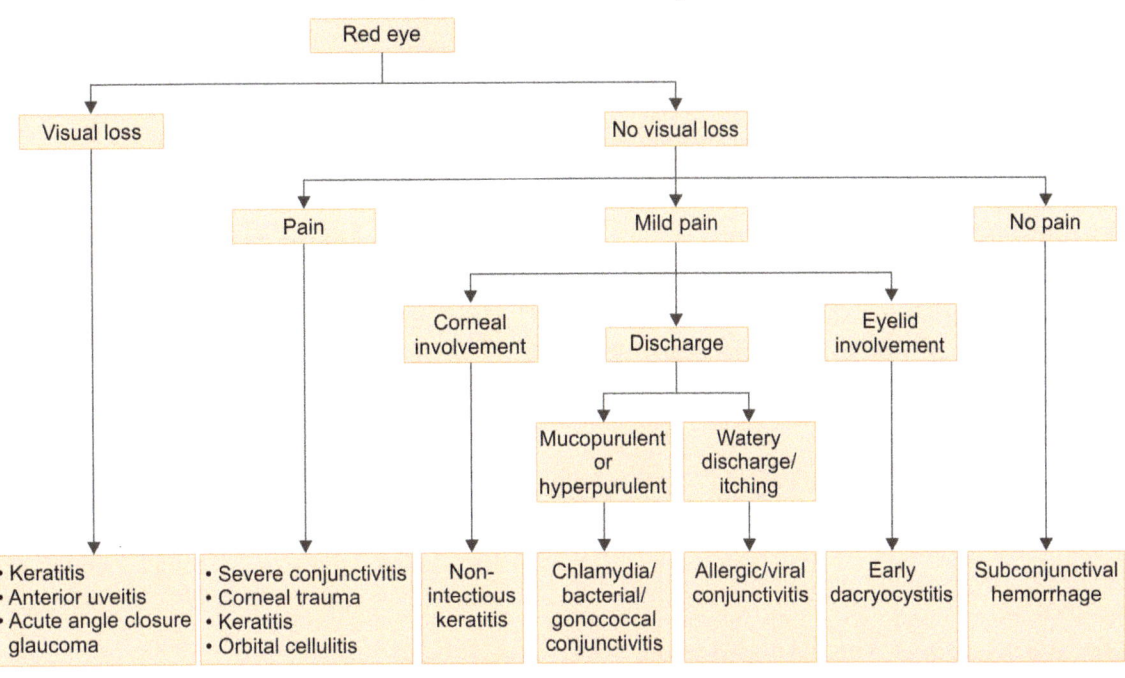

Complications of otitis media are: Tympanic membrane perforation, hearing loss, acute serous labyrinthitis, facial nerve paralysis, acute mastoiditis, lateral sinus thrombosis, cholesteatoma, intracranial complications (meningitis and brain abscess).

Question 10

1. Discuss rotator cuff injuries.

Rotator cuff muscles surround the proximal humerus and move the arm in different directions.

Four muscles formed the rotator cuff **(Fig. 5)**:

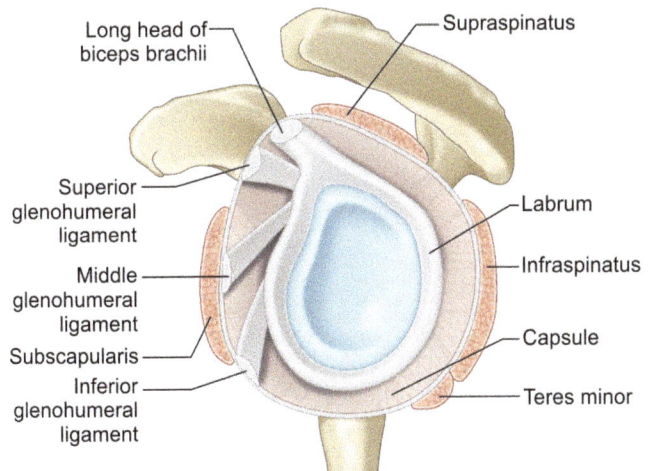

Fig. 5: Anatomy of rotator cuff around shoulder.

1. *Supraspinatus muscle:* Arises from supraspinatus fossa on dorsal scapula/attach to superior facet on greater tuberosity of humerus/abduct the arm.
2. *Infraspinatus muscle:* Arises from infraspinous fossa on dorsal aspect of scapula/attach to middle facet of greater tuberosity of humerus/externally rotates the arm.
3. *Teres minor:* Arises from superior part of lateral border of scapula/attach to inferior facet of greater tuberosity of humerus/externally rotating of arm.
4. *Subscapularis:* Arises from ventral surface of scapula/attach to lesser tuberosity of humerus/internally rotate the arm.

Examination findings in rotator cuff injuries
Drop arm test (supraspinatus muscle): Ask the patient to lower the arm slowly from abduction Positive test result—immediate drop of the arm accompanied by pain.

External rotation lag test (infraspinatus and supraspinatus) Examiner passively rotates the patient arm in external rotation.

Positive result—patient unable to maintain a position of full external rotation.

Internal rotation lag test (subscapularis): Hand of affected arm is lifted off of back by examiner, and ask to maintain position.

Positive result—unable to maintain position.

2. How will you investigate a patient with suspected rotator cuff injury?

X-ray: It does not show rotator cuff tear but to visualize the bone spurs or other potential cause of pain like arthritis.

Ultrasound: This test helps to produce images of structures particularly soft tissue such as muscle and tendons. It helps to assess the structure during movement.

MRI: It helps to display all structures in great detail.

Conservative treatments—such as *rest, ice, and physical therapy*—sometimes are all that is needed to recover from a rotator cuff injury. If injury is severe, patient need surgery.

3. Discuss flexor and extensor tendon injuries of hand.

Flexor tendon injuries typically occur from a cut on the palm side of fingers, hand, wrist, or forearm. Flexor tendons can also be injured when a finger or thumb is violently pulled away from you while you are attempting to grasp something, such as the jersey of an opposing player in sports. Flexor tendon injuries are traumatic injuries to the flexor digitorum superficialis and flexor digitorum profundus tendons that can be caused by laceration or trauma. Diagnosis is made clinically by observing the resting posture of the hand to assess the digital cascade and the absence of the tenodesis effect. Treatment is usually direct end-to-end tendon repair.

An extensor tendon injury is a cut or tear to one of the extensor tendons. Due to this injury, there is an inability to fully and forcefully extend the wrist. It is common when a ball or other object strikes the tip of the finger or thumb and forcibly bends it. Boutonnière deformity describes the bent-down (flexed) position of the middle joint of the finger.

SUGGESTED READING

1. Richhariya D, Sharma B. Textbook of Emergency Medicine including Intensive Care and Trauma, 2nd edition. New Delhi: Jaypee Brothers Medical Publishers (P) Ltd; 2022. pp. 1615-20. (Question 1).
2. Richhariya D, Sharma B. Textbook of Emergency Medicine including Intensive Care and Trauma, 2nd edition. New Delhi: Jaypee Brothers Medical Publishers (P) Ltd; 2022. pp. 633-9. (Question 2).
3. Richhariya D, Sharma B. Textbook of Emergency Medicine including Intensive Care and Trauma, 2nd edition. New Delhi: Jaypee Brothers Medical Publishers (P) Ltd; 2022. pp. 1566, 1676. (Question 3).
4. Richhariya D, Sharma B. Textbook of Emergency Medicine including Intensive Care and Trauma, 2nd edition. New Delhi: Jaypee Brothers Medical Publishers (P) Ltd; 2022. pp. 1558, 1593. (Question 4).
5. Richhariya D, Sharma B. Textbook of Emergency Medicine including Intensive Care and Trauma, 2nd edition. New Delhi: Jaypee Brothers Medical Publishers (P) Ltd; 2022. p. 785. (Question 5).
6. Richhariya D, Sharma B. Textbook of Emergency Medicine including Intensive Care and Trauma, 2nd edition. New Delhi: Jaypee Brothers Medical Publishers (P) Ltd; 2022. pp. 1551, 1599. (Question 6).
7. Richhariya D, Sharma B. Textbook of Emergency Medicine including Intensive Care and Trauma, 2nd edition. New Delhi: Jaypee Brothers Medical Publishers (P) Ltd; 2022. pp. 1075, 1119. (Question 7).
8. Richhariya D, Sharma B. Textbook of Emergency Medicine including Intensive Care and Trauma, 2nd edition. New Delhi: Jaypee Brothers Medical Publishers (P) Ltd; 2022. pp. 915, 930-2. (Question 8).
9. Richhariya D, Sharma B. Textbook of Emergency Medicine including Intensive Care and Trauma, 2nd edition. New Delhi: Jaypee Brothers Medical Publishers (P) Ltd; 2022. pp. 901, 910, 938, 945. (Question 9).
10. Richhariya D, Sharma B. Textbook of Emergency Medicine including Intensive Care and Trauma, 2nd edition. New Delhi: Jaypee Brothers Medical Publishers (P) Ltd; 2022. p. 1617. (Question 10).

Emergency Medicine Paper 51

Devendra Richhariya

Question 1

1. Enumerate the common pathogens of community-acquired pneumonia based on age-group and describe CURB-65 rule.

The common pathogens of community-acquired pneumonia (CAP) based on age-group **(Table 1)** are described under CURB-65 rule **(Table 2)**.

TABLE 1: Community-acquired pneumonia age-specific etiology.

Age	Etiology
<1 month	Group B, *Streptococcus*, *E. coli*, *L. monocytogenes*, CMV, HSV
1–3 month	Virus *S. pneumoniae*, *S. aureus*
3 month–5 years	Virus *S. pneumoniae*, *S aureus*
School age	Virus *M. pneumoniae*, *S. pneumoniae*, *C. pneumoniae*

(CMV: cytomegalovirus; HSV: herpes simplex virus)

TABLE 2: CURB-65 rule.

CURB-65	
Confusion + 1 • Blood urea nitrogen >7 mmol/L + 1 • Respiratory rate >30 + 1 • Systolic blood pressure <90 mm Hg or diastolic blood pressure <60 mm Hg + 1 • Age >65 + 1	Assessment of the severity of illness is important for diagnostic and treatment decisions for pneumonia. These assessments of illness by scoring system affect the decision between inpatient and outpatient treatment and ICU admission versus admission to a general ward. CURB-65 is a severity of illness score. This score is helpful in decreasing the admission rates and health care costs. However, the scoring system does not consider dynamic observation of patients over time, the ability to take oral medications, home supports, and access to follow-up. CURB-65 is a more simplified tool that uses five criteria to determine patients at lower risk for adverse events. These criteria are confusion; uremia [blood urea nitrogen (BUN) >7 mmol/L]; respiratory rate (>30); blood pressure (60 diastolic); age 65 years or greater.

2. Discuss investigations and management of community-acquired pneumonia in an adult in the emergency department.

Radiology: Chest X-ray is always advisable for patients with clinical suspicion of pneumonia. We most commonly see the patchy consolidation mainly confined to the lobes with air bronchogram or interstitial infiltrates as nonhomogeneous opacity and or cavity. If chest X-ray is not informative, then we may have to ask for chest CT to rule out mass, effusion, cavity, etc. Ultrasound of chest is also useful for detection of pleural effusion or pneumonia with parapneumonic effusion.

Microbiology: Sputum Gram stain and cultures are advised for all admitted patients. The sputum Gram stain is very useful for directing the choice of initial therapy but needs to be performed on a good quality sample and by a skilled microbiologist. Infectious Diseases Society of America (IDSA) now recommends sputum and blood culture in patients with severe disease as well as in all inpatients who is on empirically treatment for methicillin-resistant *Staphylococcus aureus* (MRSA) or *Pseudomonas aeruginosa*.

Hematological: Total and differential leukocyte count (TLC and DLC) is of great value in dealing with pneumonia patients. In bacterial pneumonia it is usually raised with neutrophilic predominance. It is also used for monitoring treatment response. Other important hematological tests apart from routine liver and renal function test are CRP, ESR and serum procalcitonin. CRP and ESR has good prognostic role and serum procalcitonin is of diagnostic value for bacterial pneumonia.

Serologic testing: In the emergency department serologic testing for CAP, e.g., for *Chlamydia* sp., *Legionella*, and some fungi are useful only from a retrospective perspective because they usually require both acute and convalescent serum titters. For influenza and respiratory syncytial virus (RSV) rapid antigen tests are also available. These serological tests may be useful as an adjunctive ED test for infection control purposes for hospital inpatients and as an aid in decision making regarding family and contact prophylaxis.

For *Streptococcus pneumoniae* and *Legionella pneumophilia* UATs (urinary antigen tests) are commercially available in patients with more severe illness these tests have the highest diagnostic yield. These antigen tests are rapid, simple to use, have high specificity in adults.

The management of CAP is described in **Table 3**.

TABLE 3: Initial empiric antimicrobial therapy for CAP.

Outpatient	*No comorbidities or risk factors for MRSA or Pseudomonas aeruginosa:* Amoxicillin or doxycycline or macrolide (if local pneumococcal resistance is 25%)
	With comorbidities: Combination therapy with amoxicillin/clavulanate or cephalosporin and macrolide or doxycycline OR monotherapy with respiratory fluoroquinolone
Inpatient	*Non-ICU (non-severe):* A beta-lactam + macrolide OR respiratory fluoroquinolone
	ICU (severe) Pseudomonas not suspected: A beta-lactam plus either azithromycin or a fluoroquinolone
	Pseudomonas not suspected but patient allergic to beta-lactam: A fluoroquinolone and aztreonam
	Pseudomonas suspected: An antipneumococcal, antipseudomonal beta-lactam (piperacillin–tazobactam, cefepime, imipenem, or meropenem plus ciprofloxacin or levofloxacin 750 mg; or the above beta-lactam plus aminoglycoside and azithromycin. Or the above beta-lactam plus an aminoglycoside and an antipneumococcal fluoroquinolone (in penicillin-allergic patients use aztreonam instead of the beta-lactam)
	If MRSA is suspected add vancomycin, or linezolid
	India being a TB prevalent country fluoroquinolone are not recommended for empiric treatment
	Add MRSA or *P. aeruginosa* coverage and obtain cultures/nasal PCR to allow de-escalation or confirmation of need for continued therapy (if prior respiratory isolation of same).

(CAP: community-acquired pneumonia; MRSA: methicillin-resistant *Staphylococcus aureus*)

After empiric therapy we must follow up the patients and if there is no response to the therapy within after 48–72 hours they should be re-evaluated. Once the culture report is available, the pathogen-targeted therapy, if not started earlier can be started. To chase the culture report is very important for escalation or de-escalation of antibiotics. The first and foremost treatment of pneumonia is antibiotic but other supportive care also needs to be addressed such as:
- Antipyretics
- Clear the airway
- Oxygen therapy if needed
- Adequate hydration and nutrition
- Evaluate for ICU care
- Need to be seen for requirement of ventilator (noninvasive or invasive).

In emergency, oxygen supplement has very important role when respiratory failure is there. Respiratory failure (RF) may range from mild to severe and is of different types. It is very important to understand and diagnose (on basis of ABG, SpO$_2$, etc.) the type of respiratory failure that would help in management.

Question 2

1. Discuss differential diagnosis of acute intravascular hemolysis.

Hemolytic anemia: Whenever suspicion of hemolytic anemia—*low Hb* (with no another obvious cause), *high reticulocyte count* (with no recent bleed, no repletion of iron, vitamin B$_{12}$, folate or erythropoietin).

Features of *RBC destruction:* High LDH and indirect bilirubin, low haptoglobin, it is important to localize site of hemolysis **(Fig. 1)**. It tells the:

a. By-products of hemolysis will route through reticuloendothelial system (RES) *(extravascular)* or directly into blood circulation *(intravascular)*.
b. Cause **(Flowchart 1)**
c. Need for more aggressive treatment.

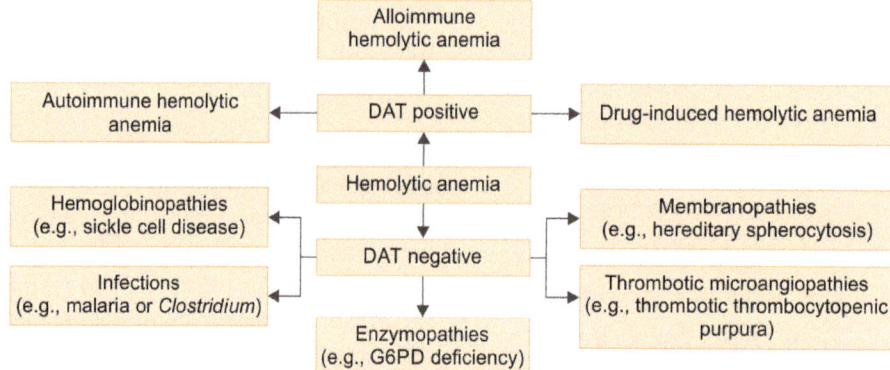

Fig. 1: Differential diagnosis of acute *intravascular hemolysis*. (AIHA: autoimmune hemolytic anemia; DAT: direct antiglobulin test; G6PD: glucose-6-phosphate dehydrogenase; HTR: hemolytic transfusion reaction)

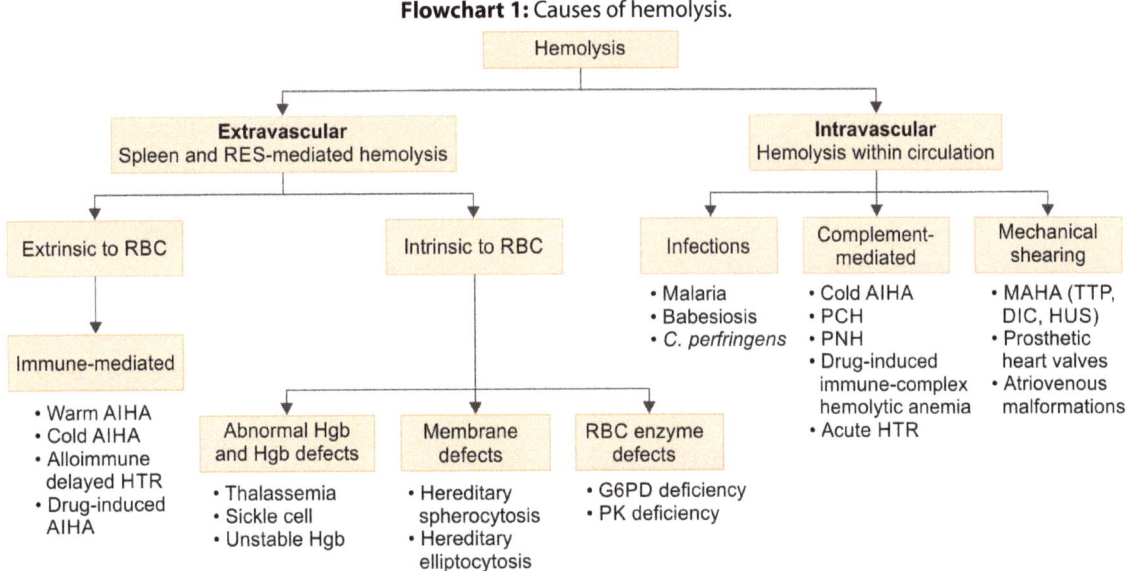

Flowchart 1: Causes of hemolysis.

(AIHA: autoimmune hemolytic anemia; DIC: disseminated intravascular coagulation; G6PD: glucose-6-phosphate dehydrogenase; HTR: hemolytic transfusion reaction; MAHA: microangiopathic hemolystic anemia; PCH: paroxysmal cold hemoglobinuria; PK: pyruvate kinase; PNH: paroxysmal nocturnal hemoglobinuria; TTP: thrombotic thrombocytopenic purpura)

TABLE 4: Drug therapy for migraine in emergency department.

Preventive medications for migraine	Abortive medication for migraine		
	Analgesics	Nonsteroidal anti-inflammatory drugs	Antiemetics
Propranolol: 40–120 mg BD	Aspirin 500–650 mg	Ibuprofen 200–300 mg	Metoclopramide 5–10 mg
Metoprolol: 100–200 mg/day	Paracetamol 500 mg	Diclofenac 50–100 mg	Chlorpromazine 10–25 mg
Amitriptyline: 25–75 mg HS	Propoxyphene 65 mg	Naproxen 500–700 mg	Promethazine 50–100 mg
Valproate: 400–600 mg BD	Codeine 60 mg	Flurbiprofen 50–100 mg	Diphenhydramine 50 mg
Flunarizine: 5–15 mg/day	Ergot derivatives are low-cost medications with vasoconstriction effect. Main adverse effects are nausea, vomiting, angina, cramps, numbness, and tingling. Contraindicated in hepatic renal failure, coronary artery disease, peripheral vascular disease, and pregnancy hypertension. Triptans: Efficacy and safety is established by well-designed trials. Triptans are 5HT 1B/1D receptor antagonist. Adverse effects are skin reaction, dizziness, hypertension, and chest discomfort. Contraindicated in angina and coronary artery disease. Sumatriptan, naratriptan, rizatriptan, and zolmitriptan are in use. Parenteral sumatriptan: A total of 6 mg of subcutaneous sumatriptan are highly effective in acute attack.		
Serotonin antagonists Pizotifen: 0.3–3 mg/day			
Methyleserzide: 1–6 mg/day			

2. Explain the clinical features and emergency department treatment of an acute attack of migraine.

Migraine: It is a common headache disorder after tension headache. Migraine is typically unilateral recurrent throbbing associated with nausea, photophobia, and phonophobia either associated with aura or without aura. Medications used to treat in ED are summarized in **Table 4**.

Question 3

1. Describe the pathogenesis of paracetamol toxicity.

At therapeutic dose, around 90% of acetaminophen is metabolized in the liver and around 2–3% is excreted unchanged in urine. Rest of the metabolism takes place via cytochrome P450 oxidase pathway and gets converted to a toxic metabolite N-acetyl-p-benzo quinonimine (NAPQI). This NAPQI gets conjugated with glutathione to form nontoxic metabolites which are excreted in urine. In case of overdosage, the glucuronide and sulfate get saturated and more of NAPQI is produced. With depletion of glutathione stores in liver due to excess of NAPQI, the concentration of toxic metabolite NAPQI increases leading to liver damage and hepatic necrosis. Patients taking substances or medications that induce the cytochrome P450 system (alcohol, anticonvulsant or antituberculous drugs) or those with glutathione depletion (poor nutrition, alcoholics and acquired immunodeficiency syndrome patients) are at increased risk of hepatic toxicity **(Fig. 2)**.

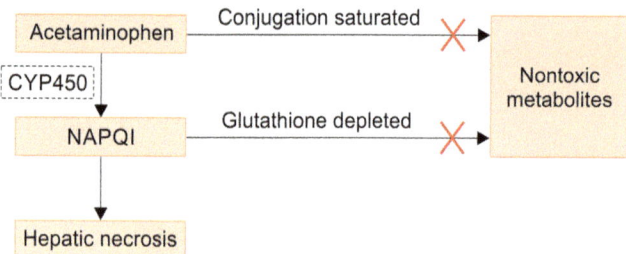

Fig. 2: Pathogenesis of paracetamol toxicity. (NAPQI: N-acetyl-p-benzo quinonimine)

2. How will you assess the risk of hepatotoxicity after an acute ingestion of paracetamol?

The clinical features of acetaminophen toxicity have been divided into four stages **(Table 5)**.

Investigations

a. Serum acetaminophen concentration—should be obtained 4 hours after ingestion.
b. Liver function tests (LFT)—may not be abnormal until >18 hours after the overdose. Alanine aminotransferase (ALT) and aspartate aminotransferase (AST) are the most sensitive markers of liver damage.
c. International normalized ratio (INR)—is a very sensitive marker of liver damage and the best prognostic parameter.
d. Renal function—creatinine is a useful prognostic marker and a low urea may suggest malnutrition and therefore glutathione depletion.
e. Blood sugar levels—to look for hypoglycemia.
f. Blood gas analysis—to check for acid–base disturbances. Metabolic acidosis, if present, is a poor prognostic sign.

TABLE 5: Clinical features of acetaminophen toxicity.			
Stages	**Time course**	**Clinical manifestations**	**Laboratory abnormalities**
Stage 1	<24 hours	Asymptomatic or anorexia, nausea, vomiting.	Hypokalemia
Stage 2	2–3 days	• Improvement in anorexia, nausea, and vomiting • Abdominal pain, hepatic tenderness, jaundice	Elevated serum transaminases, elevated bilirubin and prolonged prothrombin time if severe
Stage 3	3–4 days	• Recurrence of anorexia, nausea, and vomiting • Encephalopathy, anuria, jaundice	Hepatic failure, metabolic acidosis, coagulopathy, renal failure, pancreatitis
Stage 4	> 4 days	Clinical improvement and recovery (7–8 days) or deterioration to multiorgan failure and death	Improvement and resolution or continued deterioration

3. Discuss the management of paracetamol toxicity in the emergency department.

Management: Treatment objectives include supportive care, prevent drug absorption, and administration of antidote.

a. Rapid assessment and stabilization of airway, breathing, and circulation.
b. Gastric decontamination—gastric lavage is useful if done within 1–2 hours of ingestion. To reduce the absorption activated charcoal should be given within 4 hours of ingestion if no contraindications are present.
c. Antiemetics should be given to control nausea and vomiting.
d. Antidote—*N-acetylcysteine (NAC) is the antidote for acetaminophen toxicity*. It binds to the toxic metabolite NAPQI and prevents hepatic damage.

    The intravenous (IV) dosing schedule is as follows:
    i. 150 mg/kg in 200 mL of 5% dextrose over 1 hour, followed by
    ii. 50 mg/kg in 500 mL 5% dextrose over 4 hours, followed by
    iii. 100 mg/kg in 1,000 mL 5% dextrose over 16 hours.

    The oral dosing schedule is as follows:
    i. 140 mg/kg PO as loading dose, followed by
    ii. 70 mg/kg PO every 4 hours for a total of 17 doses.

    N-acetylcysteine can cause side effects ranging from local erythema and urticaria around the infusion site to angioedema or life-threatening anaphylaxis. If anaphylaxis occurs, the infusion should be stopped immediately and anaphylaxis should be treated. Once anaphylaxis settles, the entire dose of acetylcysteine may then be administered, possibly at a slower rate of infusion (e.g., at a rate of 50 mg/kg/hour) or by oral route regimen.

    The timing of the overdose decides the treatment to be followed in case of acetaminophen toxicity **(Table 6)**. Paracetamol treatment nomogram **(Rumack–Matthew nomogram)** should be used to interpret the measured serum paracetamol levels. NAC should be continued if (any one of the following).
    i. Paracetamol level is on or above treatment line between 4 and 15 hours after single ingestion.
    ii. Serum paracetamol is still detectable 15 hours after single ingestion.
    iii. Serum paracetamol is detectable 4 hours after uncertain time of ingestion.
    iv. INR >1.3
    v. ALT >53 IU/L

TABLE 6: Management of acetaminophen poisoning according to timing.

Timing	Total dose	Investigations	Management
Single ingestion <1 h	>150 mg/kg	Delay blood sampling until 4 h post ingestion	Activated charcoal (50 g orally), IV antiemetic, admit for observation while sampling awaited at 4 h
Single ingestion >1 h but <4 h	>150 mg/kg	Delay blood sampling until 4 h post ingestion	Activated charcoal (50 g orally), IV antiemetic, admit for observation while sampling awaited at 4 h
Single ingestion >4 h but <8 h	<150 mg/kg	Blood sampling for serum paracetamol level	If the result is expected to be available before 8 h of ingestion, treatment should be guided by the result
	>150 mg/kg	Blood sampling for serum paracetamol level	If the result is not expected to be available before 8 h, NAC should be started immediately without waiting for result
Single ingestion 8–24 h	<150 mg/kg	Blood sampling for serum paracetamol level	Treatment should be guided by the result
	>150 mg/kg	Blood sampling for serum paracetamol level	NAC should be started immediately without waiting for result
Single ingestion >24 h	>150 mg/kg	Blood sampling for serum paracetamol level	NAC should be started immediately without waiting for result
Timing unclear or ingestion is staggered		Blood sampling for serum paracetamol level	Treatment should be started immediately without waiting for result

e. Liver transplantation—it is needed in patients with severe acetaminophen-induced liver injury not improving by NAC and supportive care. The Modified Kings College Criteria for paracetamol toxicity are used to identify patients that may require transplantation.
   i. pH <7.3 or
   ii. Arterial lactate >3.5 mmol/L after 4 hours of early fluid resuscitation or arterial lactate >3.0 mmol/L after 12 hours of fluid resuscitation, or
   iii. PT >100 seconds (INR >6.5), and
   iv. Creatinine >300 µmol/L, and
   v. Grade 3 or 4 hepatic encephalopathy.

Question 4

1. Discuss the precipitating causes, clinical features, and management of myxedema coma.

Severe hypothyroidism untreated for a prolonged duration may lead to a rare fatal disease, myxedema coma, in which the body's homeostasis goes haywire due *to precipitating factors*. These factors include infection, certain medications (amiodarone, anesthesia, barbiturates, β-blockers, diuretics, lithium, narcotics, phenothiazines, phenytoin, rifampin, and tranquilizers), and failure to reinstate thyroid replacement therapy during hospitalization, stroke, surgery, burns, hypoglycemia, hypothermia, gastrointestinal hemorrhage or trauma among others. Most (95%) of the myxedema coma cases occur due to primary hypothyroidism while hypothalamic or pituitary causes account for the remaining (5%) cases.

Clinical Presentation of Myxedema Coma

Patients with myxedema coma generally present with altered sensorium, lethargy, confusion, and possibly obtundation rather than coma. Other characteristics include hypoglycemia, bradycardia, hypoventilation, hypotension, hypothermia, (usually <95.9°F), hyponatremia, increased levels of serum creatinine and creatinine kinase **(Table 7)**.

Treatment of Myxedema Coma

Myxedema coma is a metabolic thyroid emergency condition, and the suspected patients should be administrated intensive care therapy for vital pulmonary, respiratory, and cardiovascular support. The mortality rate could be from 25–60% in myxedema coma patients despite the best treatment. Hence, the treatment for suspected myxedema coma should be initiated immediately rather than waiting for laboratory confirmation. Due to lack of studies comparing the efficacy of different treatment regimens, deciding the optimal treatment is challenging. Successful treatment depends upon the timely diagnosis, prompt treatment with thyroid hormones (intravenous levothyroxine is preferred over oral), supportive therapy (appropriate fluid management and correction of hypotension and dyselectrolytemia), administration of steroid supplement (hydrocortisone) until coexisting adrenal insufficiency is ruled out, along with the aggressive treatment of precipitating factors. The treatment of myxedema coma is detailed in **Flowchart 2**.

TABLE 7: Clinical presentation of myxedema coma.

System	Clinical presentation
Central nervous system (CNS)	• Decreased mental status—may be due to decreased cerebral blood flow and cerebral glucose metabolism • Confusion, apathy, lethargy, obtundation, and coma • Cognitive impairment and psychiatric disorders can also be seen • Hyponatremia • Hypoglycemia (~25% patients)
Respiratory system	• Respiratory depression • Fluid accumulation—pleural effusion • Obstructive sleep apnea—obesity and weight gain • Myxedematous infiltration of the pharynx and tongue requiring mechanical ventilation
Cardiovascular system (CVS)	• Bradycardia, low cardiac output, and decreased blood volume • Increased systemic peripheral resistance and pericardial effusion
Renal system	• Severe renal impairment—reduced blood flow and low glomerular filtration rate (GFR) • Elevated creatinine • Decreased sodium reabsorption leading to hyponatremia
Gastrointestinal tract (GIT)	Decreased intestinal mobility—constipation, anorexia, nausea, abdominal pain, and distension
Skin and hair	• Myxedematous facies—generalized puffiness, ptosis, macroglossia, coarse and sparse hair, and periorbital edema • Dry, pale, and thickened skin with non-pitting edema (myxedema) • Dry and brittle hair • Hoarseness in voice
Metabolic	• Hypothermia (up to 75°F)
Laboratory and others	• Reduced T4 and T3 • Elevated TSH—primary hypothyroidism; normal/low TSH—central/secondary hypothyroidism • Respiratory acidosis • ECG—bradycardia, decreased voltage, prolonged QT interval, nonspecific ST-T changes and Osborn waves in cases of hypothermia • Chest radiograph—pleural effusions and cardiomegaly

Flowchart 2: Treatment of myxedema coma.

Thyroid replacement therapy		Supportive therapy		Precipitating event
Large initial IV dose T4 (200–400 μg); *Maintenance dose:* 1.6 μg/kg/day IV/PO	*Alternative:* Initial IV T4 (200–300 μg) in combination with T3 (10–25 μg)	Hypocortisolemia	IV hydrocortisone (100 mg q8h) until the possibility of co-existing adrenal insufficiency is excluded	Identification and elimination by specific treatment, use of empirical antibiotics
			Follow-up steroid therapy: Discontinue if cortisol level >25 μg/dL or corticotropin-stimulating testing if <25 μg/dL	
T3 loading dose: 5–20 μg IV/NG once *Maintenance dose:* 2.5–10 q8h IV/PO		Hypoventilation	Intubation and mechanical ventilation	Selected cases
		Hypothermia	Passive rewarming with a blanket	Respiratory acidosis Assisted mechanical ventilation
		Hyponatremia	Free-water restriction and normal saline	
		Hypotension	Fluids and vasopressor drugs	Pulmonary edema IV furosemide
		Hypoglycemia	IV dextrose or glucose	

2. Discuss the clinical features and management of a patient with adrenal crisis.

Acute adrenal crisis is usually triggered by a stressful episode (e.g., infection, physiological stress, surgery, or trauma). Customarily a patient with adrenal crisis presents with nausea, vomiting, abdominal pain, severe hypotension, and hypovolemic shock. Fever is usual as most of the cases are triggered by an infection. This being a life-threatening medical emergency requires immediate management, and in cases of undiagnosed crisis treatment comes first rather than going for biochemical confirmation of disease. It is imperative to differentiate between Addison disease and acute adrenal crisis in which the latter presents as vomiting, abdominal pain, and hypovolemic shock. This is a rare disease but can be life-threatening when overlooked. Clinical and laboratory features of the adrenal insufficiency (AI) and acute adrenal crisis are summarized in **Table 8**.

TABLE 8: Clinical and laboratory features of adrenal insufficiency.

	Primary adrenal insufficiency	*Secondary adrenal insufficiency*
Clinical features	• Hyperpigmentation, vitiligo, weight loss, hypotension, postural dizziness, and syncope shock. • Weakness fatigue, myalgia, arthralgia, anorexia, vomiting, constipation, abdominal pain, diarrhea. • Amenorrhea, infertility, salt craving. • Depression psychosis	• Weight gain, thin axillary and pubic hair, decrease in libido, infertility, and amenorrhea. • Weakness, fatigue. • Headache, visual disturbances, anorexia, vomiting, constipation, abdominal pain, diarrhea, myalgia, arthralgia. • Depression psychosis
Laboratory features	Hyponatremia, hyperkalemia, hypochloremia, and acidosis mildly elevated BUN, mild hypoglycemia, anemia, B_{12} deficiency, type I diabetes	Hypernatremia or hyponatremia, hypokalemia or normal potassium, normal serum chloride, normal BUN, marked hypoglycemia
Risk of acute adrenal crisis	Very high	Low

- Clinical features of acute adrenal crisis
- Circulatory shock is the hallmark of acute adrenal crisis (hypotension shock tachycardia)
- Fever, fatigue, dehydration, arthralgia, myalgia, nausea, anorexia, vomiting, poor concentration, depression, disorientation. Abdominal pain (rebound tenderness rigidity), flank pain, back pain, and lower chest pain.

Management of Adrenal Crisis

Empiric treatment for adrenal crisis before confirm laboratory results:

a. Hydrocortisone is drug of choice it has both glucocorticoid and mineralocorticoid properties.
b. Empiric antibiotics can be started depending on underlying conditions.
c. Fresh frozen plasma to reverse coagulopathy.
d. Hyperkalemia should be corrected.
e. Thyroxine supplementation requirement in primary HPA axis failure (clinical hypothyroidism).
f. Correction of dehydration and hypoglycemia.
g. Vasopressors.

Treatment of adrenal crisis condition is straight forward with parenteral administration of 100 mg of hydrocortisone intravenously as bolus along with correction of hypovolemia with 1,000 mL of isotonic saline within first 1 hour, followed by 50–100 mg hydrocortisone in 5% dextrose every 6 hourly intravenously or intramuscularly depending on age and body surface area. In case hydrocortisone is not at disposal, then any other synthetic glucocorticoid, such as prednisolone can be used in proportionate doses. Baseline blood samples such as cortisol, adrenocorticotropic hormone (ACTH), blood cultures should be drawn before initiation of therapy. In addition to this aggressive fluid and vasopressor support should be started under continuous cardiac monitoring. Basis the intercurrent condition which triggered the crisis antibiotics and antithrombotic are initiated. Depending upon severity of condition patient should be admitted then to intensive care setting for further work up and management. Serum electrolytes and blood glucose levels should be watchfully checked every 4-6 hours until stabilized. Once patient is stable intravenous glucocorticoid can be tapered and oral maintenance dose started.

Long-term hormone replacement therapy should be initiated once patient is recovered from crisis, intravenous steroid should be changed to oral preparation and prednisolone with longer half-life is required only once daily. Fludrocortisone (mineralocorticoid) is usually given in patient with primary adrenal failure. Androgen transdermal dehydroepiandrosterone (DHEA) 25–50 mg is also added for primary adrenal failure.

This treatment regimen to treat hypotension with correction of electrolyte and cortisol imbalance is essentially constant leading to improvement in symptoms within 24 hours. In case recovery in not as progressive as anticipated then other causes of illness (severe sepsis with shock) should be reconsidered. The treatment guidelines for acute adrenal crisis are summarized in **Table 9**.

TABLE 9: Treatment guidelines for acute adrenal crisis.

Fluid resuscitation	At least 2–3 L of normal saline to restore volume and normal sodium balance
Intravenous steroids	Intravenous hydrocortisone 100 mg bolus followed by 100 mg two or three times per day (300–400 mg daily is initial regimen)
Antibiotics	Broad spectrum antibiotics for febrile patient
Vasopressors	In case of refractory shock
Glucose	50% dextrose may be used if required
In stabilized patient	Oral prednisolone fludrocortisone and androgen replacement
	Patient education regarding steroid management during acute febrile illness (double the dose of steroid for 3 days) regular follow-up with physician

Question 5

1. Define delirium. What are its various causes?

Delirium is defined as acute onset fluctuating changes in cognition, attention, and awareness, the changes are rapid in onset within hours or day and usually reversible **(Fig. 3)**. Patients of delirium typically present as inattention, disorganized thinking, perception disturbance, and altered conscious level (somnolent or agitated). Elderly group is at increased risk **(Box 1)** of mortality if delirium is missed in emergency department.

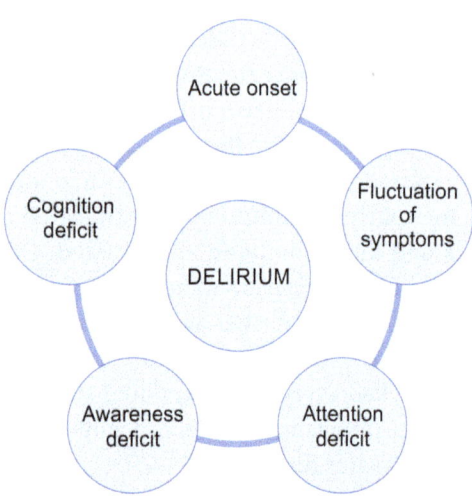

Fig. 3: Components of delirium.

2. Describe the components of Confusion Assessment Method (CAM).

Confusion Assessment Methods (CAM): First described by Inouye and colleagues in 1990 based on the *Diagnostic and Statistical Manual of Mental Disorders Revised 3rd edition* (DSMIIIR) criteria, helpful for nonpsychiatric trained physician to diagnose delirium quickly and accurately. CAM consists of four components: (1) Acute onset mental status changes fluctuating course, (2) Inattention, (3) Disorganized thinking, and (4) Altered level of consciousness. First two components are mandatory and either of two from rest of two necessary for diagnosis of delirium.

BOX 1: Risk factors for acute confusional state.

- Elderly male
- Multiple comorbidities
- Advance form of comorbidities
- Previous episode of delirium
- Advance dementia
- Chronic kidney disease
- End-stage liver disease
- Postoperative status such as recent hip fracture
- Conditions such as burn, hypoalbuminemia, dehydration
- Malnutrition, infection, acquired immunodeficiency syndrome (AIDS)
- Multiple medications and dependence such as benzodiazepine
- Alcohol abuse or withdrawal
- Socially neglected, stressful people, visual or hearing problem
- Poor mobility, terminally ill
- Prolong intensive care unit admission

3. Describe Richmond Agitation-Sedation Scale.

Target therapy to a desired sedation score—like any therapeutic intervention, we need an endpoint so that we know that we have administered the correct "dose" of whatever it is we are giving. For most patients an RASS of 0 to −2 is desirable. RASS = 0 means the patient is alert and calm. RASS = −2 means they awaken to voice (eyes open for <10 seconds) **(Table 10)**.

TABLE 10: Richmond Agitation-Sedation scale.

Richmond Agitation-Sedation scale			CAM-ICU
Score	Description		
+4	Combative	Violent, immediate danger to staff	RASS ≥ –2 Proceed to CAM-ICU assessment
+3	Very agitated	Pulls at or removes tubes, aggressive	
+2	Agitated	Frequent no-purposeful movements, fights ventilator	
+1	Restless	Anxious, apprehensive but movements not aggressive or vigorous	
0	Alert and calm		
–1	Drowsy	Not fully alert, sustained awakening to voice (eye opening and contact >10 s)	
–2	Light sedation	Briefly awakens to voice (eye opening and contact <10 s)	
–3	Moderate sedation	Movement or eye-opening to voice (no eye contact)	RASS < –2 STOP Recheck later
–4	Deep sedation	No response to voice, but movement or eye opening to physical stimulation	
–5	Unrousable	No response to voice or physical stimulation	

Question 6

1. Discuss acute vaso-occlusive crisis in sickle cell disease.

Acute painful episodes: Acute pain in back and extremities is classical presentation due to vaso-occlusive crisis of sickle cell disease (SCD). Bone pain is quite common during sickle cell crisis usually involving the back and extremities. This pain would be diffuse without local signs of inflammation. Hence, if there are local signs they suggest infection. The humeral or femoral heads are most commonly affected. Managing the pain in priority basis is utmost important.

Children may present with acute abdomen with acute splenic enlargement due to intrasplenic sickling and vascular obstruction. The children may be in shock. These children have increased susceptibility to infection. Most of these patients with SCD coming to ED are having a defined pain pattern. Enquiry into family history, previous pain episodes and history of chronic anemia are very important. Adult patients commonly have a youthful appearance with long, thin extremities.

The emergency physician needs to be vigilant in differentiating uncomplicated crises from other more serious pathologic conditions. Investigations may be required to rule out other causes of acute abdomen or acute chest pains or neurological complications. The use of t-PA for thrombolysis in acute non-hemorrhagic strokes is similar to acute strokes without SCD. Chronic organ system damage is common in these patients. Hence, quick review of these conditions is necessary during every ED visit. The common causes of mortality in patients with SCD are cardiopulmonary disease, chronic renal failure, acute stroke, and recurrent infections. The management of acute painful episode in Sickle cell disease is summarized in **Box 2**.

> **BOX 2:** Management of acute painful episode in sickle cell disease.
>
> *Types of pain in sickle cell disease:*
> - Usually symmetric back pain and extremities pain
> - Acute flare up of chronic pain—of bone and joints (chronic ulcer, osteomyelitis, avascular necrosis of joints bone infarction)
> - Neuropathic pain—burning paresthesia, hyperalgesias
>
> *Management of acute painful episodes:*
> - Triage the patient according to pain
> - Opioid analgesics within 30 minutes Morphine 0.1 mg/kg by intravenous/oral routes avoid intramuscular route
> - Adjuvant agents such as acetaminophen, nonsteroidal anti-inflammatory agents
> - Other therapy—intravenous fluids, oxygen (in hypoxic patient if saturation <92%)
> - Laboratory—complete blood count, reticulocyte liver function test, lactate levels, electrolytes
> - Experimental therapy—steroids, nitric oxide, possible future role of ketamine

2. Explain acute mesenteric ischemia.

Mesenteric ischemia is categorized as occlusive or non-occlusive in origin. Occlusive mesenteric ischemia either involves the superior mesenteric artery (SMA) or the superior mesenteric vein (SMV). Arterial occlusion may be embolic or thrombotic in origin. Mesenteric ischemia and ischemic colitis are different clinical entities. Patients with mesenteric ischemia typically present with abdominal pain. Patients with ischemic colitis present with lower gastrointestinal bleeding and are less likely to report abdominal pain as the primary complaint. Angiography is not indicated in cases of ischemic colitis. Predisposing cardiac conditions include arrhythmia (most commonly atrial fibrillation), myocardial infarction, cardiomyopathy, recent angiography, valvular disorder (e.g., rheumatic valve disease), or ventricular aneurysm. Following surgical embolectomy, the mortality from analyzed results from four decades is 54%.

Treatment: All patients require hemodynamic monitoring, resuscitation, intravenous fluid, broad-spectrum antibiotic administration, and pain management. Emergent surgical consultation and emergent laparotomy is required if peritoneal sign in acute ischemia, and the patient should not be given anything to eat or drink by mouth. Heparin therapy should be initiated if no contraindication, and vasopressors should be avoided. A patient with mesenteric ischemia caused by embolic phenomena would require surgical intervention for embolectomy, excision of infarcted bowel, and consideration of intraarterial papaverine. The patient with an arterial thrombus is a candidate for similar interventions—thrombectomy and revascularization. Similarly, if the patient has mesenteric venous thrombosis, thrombectomy and excision of gangrenous bowel may be indicated, and heparin therapy should be initiated. Patients with non-occlusive mesenteric ischemia (NOMI) should have the underlying cause treated as well as resection of the affected segment of bowel.

Question 7

1. Discuss pathogenesis and management of cardiogenic shock.

Cardiogenic shock occurs when about 40% of left ventricle is damaged predominantly due to ischemia. Right ventricular infarction is also recognized as the cause of cardiogenic shock in few cases. Thrombotic occlusion of artery supplying the major part of the heart is underlying pathology of the cardiogenic shock. Coronary occlusion induces depression of myocardial contractility. Reduction in myocardial contractility produces the low cardiac index and hypotension. Low cardiac index and hypotension causes severe tissue hypoperfusion which is measured by the raised serum lactate. Initially compensatory vasoconstriction occurs in which normotensive state is maintained. If this preshock stage is not recognized early and not treated well, this condition progresses to severe or refractory cardiogenic shock **(Flowchart 3)**. Inflammatory derangement capillary leakage and microcirculatory derangement also contribute to development of severe/refractory shock. According to various studies older age group, low left ventricular ejection fraction (LVEF), low cardiac index, low systolic BP, requirement of vasopressor and mechanical support, high serum lactate level are associated with high mortality rates in cardiogenic shock.

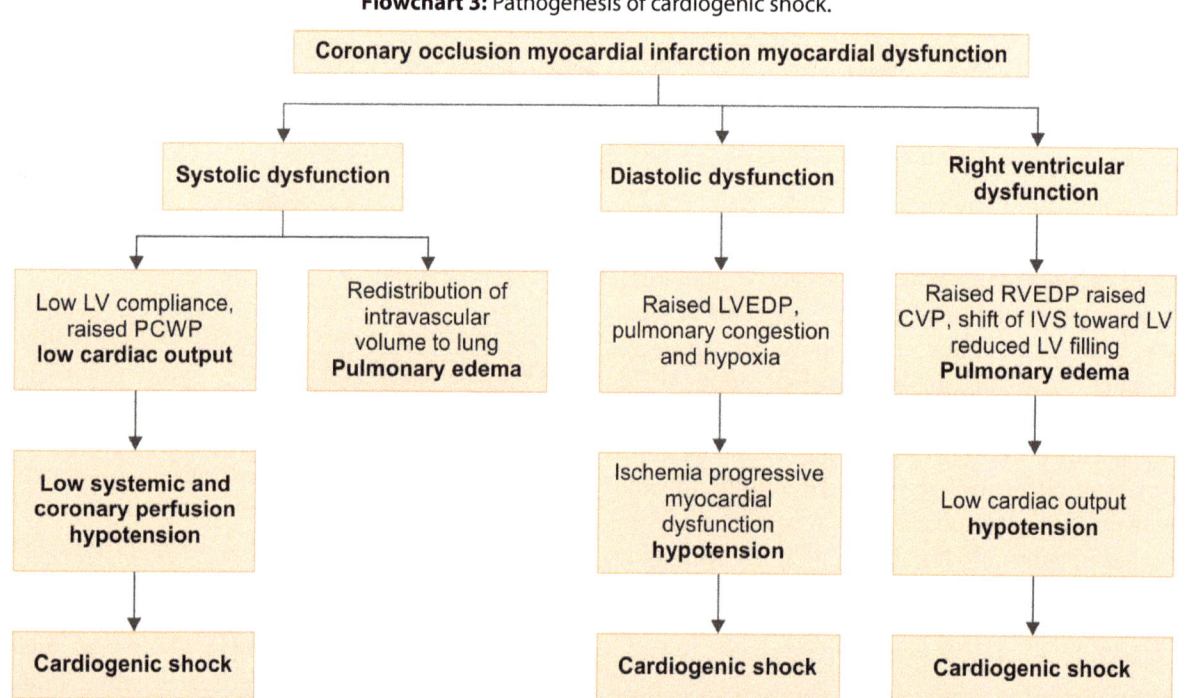

Flowchart 3: Pathogenesis of cardiogenic shock.

(CVP: central venous pressure; IVS: interventrical septum; LVEDP: left ventricular ejection diastolic pressure; PCWP: pulmonary capillary wedge pressure; REDP: right ventricula ejection pressure)

Management of cardiogenic shock should be started as early as possible to normalize hemodynamic parameter and to prevent the further damage of organ and deterioration of the patient. Management of the cardiogenic shock should target to maintain hemodynamic parameter within therapeutic range **(Fig. 4)**; maintaining the hemodynamic parameters within therapeutic range suggestive of adequate management strategies and positive outcome.

Mean arterial pressure >60 mm Hg	Pulmonary wedge pressure <18 mm Hg	Central venous pressure 8–12 mm Hg
Urine output >0.5 mL/h/kg	Arterial blood pH 7.3–7.5	Central venous O_2 saturation SvO_2 >70%

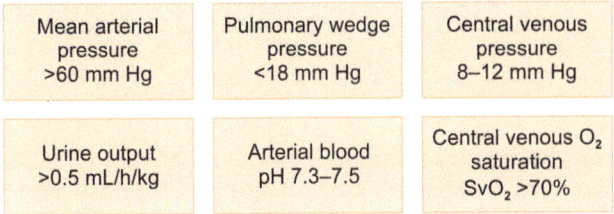

Fig. 4: Therapeutic target for hemodynamic parameters.

Management of cardiogenic shock is multiphasic, and various modalities of treatment used in cardiogenic shock are summarized in **Figure 5**. Immediate management of shock includes fluid therapy, vasoactive therapy, and ventilator therapy along with correction of electrolyte imbalance. Along with the symptomatic treatment therapy should be directed at the underlying cause. Most cases of cardiogenic shock are due to myocardial infarction, prompt reperfusion therapy should be instituted. Revascularization therapy [percutaneous transluminal coronary angioplasty (PTCA) or coronary-artery bypass grafting (CABG)] reduces the hospitalization, long-term mortality and MI-related mechanical complication.

Critical care support	Revascularization support	Mechanical support	Special situation
• Fluid administration • Vasoactive agents (vasopressor and inotrope) • Ventilator support • PA catheter	• Thrombolysis • PCI • CABG	• IABP • ECMO • Percutaneous left ventricular assist device (LVAD) e.g., Tandem heart, impella	• RVMI with shock • Surgical repair of mechanical complication (acute MR, free wall rupture)

Fig. 5: Modalities of treatment in cardiogenic shock. (CABG: coronary-artery bypass grafting; IABP: intra-aortic ballon pump; ECMO: extracarporial membrane oxygenation; PCI: percutaneous intervention; RVMI: right ventricular myocardial Infarction)

2. Discuss etiology, clinical features, investigations, and management of acute pericarditis.

Acute pericarditis, inflammation of the pericardium, is found in approximately 5% of patients admitted to the emergency department for chest pain unrelated to acute myocardial infarction. It occurs most often in men 20–50 years of age. Acute pericarditis has a number of potential etiologies including infection, acute myocardial infarction, medication use, trauma to the thoracic cavity, and systemic diseases, such as rheumatoid arthritis. However, most etiologic evaluations are inconclusive. Patients with acute pericarditis commonly present with acute, sharp, retrosternal chest pain that is relieved by sitting or leaning forward. A pericardial friction rub is found in up to 85% of patients. Classic electrocardiographic changes include widespread concave upward ST-segment elevation without reciprocal T-wave inversions or Q waves. First-line treatment includes nonsteroidal anti-inflammatory drugs and colchicine. Glucocorticoids are traditionally reserved for severe or refractory cases, or in cases when the cause of pericarditis is likely connective tissue disease, autoreactivity, or uremia. Cardiology consultation is recommended for patients with severe disease, those with pericarditis refractory to empiric treatment, and those with unclear etiologies. The management of acute pericarditis is summarized in **Table 11**.

TABLE 11: Treatment of acute and recurrent pericarditis.

Medication	***Doses***	***Duration of treatment***
Acetyle salycylic acid	500–750 mg 3–4times/day	7–10 days followed by gradual reduction 500 mg/week over 3 weeks
Ibuprofen	400–800 mg/day 3–4 times/day	14 days
Indomethacin (avoid after acute myocardial infarction)	50 mg 3 times/ day	1–2 weeks
Colchicine	0.5 mg 1–2 times/ day (patient weight <70 kg)	3 months for 1st event and 6 months for recurrence
Prednisolone	0.25–0.5 mg/kg/ day	2 weeks and 2–4 weeks for recurrence

Question 8

1. What are the clinical features of monkeypox?

Signs and symptoms:

- A new, maculopapular rash that develops into vesicles and then pustules. Lesions may be deep-seated, firm, well-circumscribed and umbilicated. The rash may:
  - Appear anywhere on the body, including palms, soles, and anogenital region
  - Be localized to a specific body site or diffuse
  - Be the only symptom people experience
  - Be painful, painless, or itchy
- Fever, headache, malaise, chills, and lymphadenopathy may occur.
- Patients may present with anorectal pain, rectal bleeding, or tenesmus in association with visible perianal skin lesions and proctitis.

2. Discuss differential diagnosis and management of genital ulcers.

Differential diagnosis and management of sexually transmitted and non-sexually transmitted genital ulcer are given in **Table 12**.

TABLE 12: Differential diagnosis and management of genital ulcers.

		STDs ulcers	
Condition	**Organism**	**Description**	**Management**

Syphilis (chancre)	Treponema pallidum
	IP: 9–90 days
		Genital ulcer:
		• Button-like papule that develops into a painless erosion and then ulcerates with raised border and scanty serous exudate. Surface may be crusted
		  – Site: Genital (95%) and extragenital (5%)
		  – Shape: Rounded or oval, regular, and well-defined
		  – Surface: Dull red, clean, oozing (scanty serous exudate)
		  – Edge: Sloping
		  – Base: Indurated.
		  – Palpation: Firm
		  – Number:
		    - Single (common)
		    - Few multiple, or kissing lesions (less commonly)
		  – Pain: Painless (unless superinfected with S. aureus)
		• Regional LNs: Regional lymphadenopathy appears within 7 days
		Nodes are:
		• Discrete
		• Firm, rubbery
		• Non-tender
		• Unilateral (more commonly)
			Not allergic to penicillin: Penicillin G Benzathine (single dose of 2.4 million units, IM)
			In allergy to penicillin: Doxycycline (100 mg, PO, twice a day/for 2 weeks)

Chancroid (soft chancre)	Hemophilus ducreyi
	IP: 4–7 days
		Genital ulcer:
		• Tender papule with erythematous halo that evolves to pustule erosion, ulcer
		  – Site: Genital and extragenital
		  – Shape: Oval, well-defined
		  – Surface: Floor—covered with gray to yellow exudate
		  – Edge: Undermined
		  – Base: It is friable with granulation tissue not indurated
		  – Margin: Surrounded by erythematous halo
		  – Palpation: Soft
		  – Number:
		    - Multiple (common), merging to form large or giant ulcers (>2 cm) with serpiginous shape
		    - Singular
		    - Pain: Painful
		• Regional LNs: The genital ulcer is followed by: Painful inguinal lymphadenitis appears 7–21 days after primary lesion:
		• Matted
		• Firm at first
		• Tender
		• Unilateral (more commonly)
		• Adherent to the overlying skin which is red, hot, edematous, and tender
			Azithromycin (1 g, PO, single dose)
			Ceftriaxone (250 mg, IM, single dose)
			Ciprofloxacin (500 mg, PO, twice for 3 days)

Granuloma inguinale	Calymmatobacterium granulomatis
	Incubation period: 2–6 weeks
		Genital ulcer:
		• Painless, granulating, progressive, ulcerative lesions of the genital and perianal areas
		• Highly vascular (i.e., a beefy red appearance) and bleed easily on contact
		• Spreads by:
		  – Direct extension or
		  – Autoinoculation of approximated skin surfaces
		• Regional LNs: No regional lymphadenopathy
		  – Large subcutaneous nodule may mimic a lymph node, i.e., pseudobubo
			Trimethoprim-Sulfamethoxazole (one double-strength tablet twice)
			Doxycycline (100 mg, PO, twice a day)
			Both for 3 weeks

Contd...

Contd...

Condition	Organism	Description	Management

Lymphogranuloma Venerum	Invasive Chlamydia trachomatis (Serotype: L1, L2, L3) IP: Primary stage: 3–12 days Secondary stage: 10–30 days	Genital ulcer:
		• *Transient primary genital ulcer:*
		– Small, painless, papule/or vesicle which breaks into non-indurated ulcer
		– Single, or grouped small ulcers (herpetiform)
		– Heals within few days
		• *In heterosexual males:*
		– Cordlike lymphangitis of dorsal penis may follow.
		– Lymphangial abscess (bubonulus) may rupture, resulting in
		– Sinuses and fistulas of urethra and deforming scars of penis
		• *Females:* Cervicitis, perimetritis, salpingitis may occur.
		• *Receptive anal intercourse (women or men): Primary anal rectal infection:* Hemorrhagic proctitis + with regional lymphadenitis
		• *Regional LNs:* The genital ulcer is followed by:
		• *Inguinal syndrome (Inguinal lymphadenitis):* Painful inguinal lymphadenopathy appearing 2–6 weeks, after presumed exposure.
		– *Initially*, nodes are discrete,
		– *BUT with progressive periadenitis* results in—a matted mass of nodes which become fluctuant and suppurative.
		– *"Groove" sign:* Extensive enlargement of inguinal nodes above and below the inguinal ligament (nonspecific)
		– *Overlying skin becomes:* Fixed–inflamed–thin–eventually develops multiple draining fistulas.
		  - Usually unilateral
		  - Palpable iliac/femoral nodes often present on same side.
			Recommended:
			Azithromycin:
			(1 g, PO, single dose)
			Doxycycline:
			(100 mg, PO, twice/for 7 days)
			Alternative:
			Erythromycin base:
			500 mg PO four times/for 7 days

Genital herpes (Herpes progentalis)	HSV-2, ≥90% of cases HSV-1, 10% of cases IP: 2–20 days	*Transmission:*
		• Usually skin-to-skin contac
		• Transmission occurs during times of asymptomatic HSV shedding (70%)
		• Transmission in discordant couples (one partner infected, the other not) (10%)
		Symptoms
		• *Primary GH*
		– Asymptomatic (most common)
		– *Symptomatic:* Constitutional symptoms fever, headache, malaise, myalgia (occurs only in 1 hourly)
		– Depending on location, pain, itching, dysuria, lumbar radiculitis, vaginal or urethral discharge are common symptoms.
		– Deep pelvic pain associated with pelvic lymphadenopathy
		
		• *Recurrent GH*
		– *Common symptoms:* Itching, burning, fissure, redness, irritation prior to eruption of vesicles
		– Dysuria, sciatica, rectal discomfort
		Genital ulcer:
		• Burning sensation precedes appearance of:
		– Initially, an *erythematous plaque* is noted, followed soon by *grouped vesicles* may evolve to *pustules*, as the overlying epidermis sloughs, they become *eroded*
		– Erosions may enlarge to *ulcerations*
		– They heal in *2–4 weeks,* (but followed by recurrence)
		  - Often with postinflammatory hypo- or hyperpigmentation
		  - Uncommonly with scarring
			Oral acyclovir (400 mg, three times/for 7–10 days)

Contd...

Contd...

Condition	Organism	Description	Management

		• Regional LNs: Inguinal/femoral lymphadenopathy:
		  – Nodes enlarged
		  – Firm, nonfluctuant
		  – Tender
		  – Usually unilateral	

		Non-STDs ulcers	
Traumatic ulcer		The ulcer appears immediately after the trauma. Soft, tender	
Fixed drug eruption		• Recurrent, superficial, soft *erosion* with surrounding violaceous margin • Lymph nodes are not enlarged	
Scabies		• The causative organism is *Sarcoptes scabiei*, which could be demonstrated in scrapings the lesion • Itching, which is more severe at night • Other lesions of scabies present in characteristic sites	
Pyogenic ulcer		History of pyogenic abscess preceding the ulcer. Soft, purulent floor	
Malignant ulcer		Old age patient, everted edges, hard, friable, and bleed easily	
Behçet's ulcer		Recurrent, multiple, superficial, tender ulcers on the scrotum or genitals. The ulcer is accompanied by aphthous ulcers in mouth and iritis.	

Question 9

1. Discuss local injuries due to exposure to cold temperature.

Frostnip and Chilblain (Erythema Pernio)

Frostnip is a temporary and mild form of cold-induced injury causing local paresthesia of the involved area that completely resolves with passive external rewarming. Chilblain (erythema pernio) is inflammatory skin changes caused by exposure to cold without actual freezing of the tissues. These skin lesions may be purple or red papular lesions which are painful or pruritic with burning or paresthesia.

Treatment: Affected part is kept elevated and passively external rewarming is used. Rubbing and massaging injured tissue is avoided. Applying ice and heat is also avoided. Protect the affected area from trauma, secondary infection, and further cold exposure.

Immersion Foot or Trench Foot

Immersion foot (or hand) is caused by prolonged immersion in cold water or mud usually below 10°C; it has three stages:

Pre-hyperemic stage: Characterized by symptoms of cold and anesthesia.

Hyperemic stage: Hot sensation, severe burning, and shooting pain

Post-hyperemic stage: With ongoing cold exposure the affected part becomes pale or cyanotic with diminished pulsation due to venospasms. This may result in blistering, swelling, redness, ecchymoses, hemorrhage, necrosis, peripheral nerve injury, and gangrene.

Treatment consists of air drying, protecting extremities from trauma and secondary infection and gradual rewarming by exposure to room temperature. Avoid using ice or heat. Avoid massaging, moistening the skin. Affected parts are elevated, cushions can be used to protect the pressure sites.

Frostbite

Frostbite is an injury from tissue freezing and formation of ice crystals in the tissue. With reperfusion of the frozen tissue, destruction occurs with damaged endothelial cell and progressive microvascular thrombosis causing further tissue damage. Only skin and subcutaneous tissue are involved in mild cases. Symptoms are prickling, numbness, itching, and pallor. Deeper structures are involved with increasing severity. The skin appears white or yellow, elasticity is lost and becomes immobile. Edema, hemorrhage, blister, necrosis, gangrene, paresthesia, and stiffness may occur.

Treatment: Secondary exposure to cold is avoided. Associated systemic hypothermia, concurrent condition and injury are evaluated and treated. Fluid is given to avoid hypovolemia and to improve perfusion.

2. Describe the pathophysiology and management of accidental hypothermia.

Pathophysiology: Resting metabolism and neurological functions are decreased as a result of cooling. Even when the core temperature is normal, skin cooling induces shivering which directly increases metabolism by increased muscle activity and indirectly by increased ventilation and cardiac output. As core temperature decreases shivering increases and reaches at maximum level when core temperature is about 32°C and stops by about 30°C. With decreasing temperature metabolism generally decreases below 32°C.

Management of Accidental Hypothermia

Out of hospital management: Before evaluating the patient and starting treatment, the patient should be moved to a safer place. Safety of the rescuers is the first priority during the rescue. Rescuers should not enter the scene if a hypothermic patient has an obvious fatal injury. After ensuring their safety, rescuers should determine whether the patient is in cardiac arrest. If there is an indication, rescuers should start resuscitation if the patient is in cardiac arrest. If vital signs are present in a patient but not alert then rescuers are advised to avoid causing cardiovascular collapse handling gently and by keeping the horizontal as much as possible. After removing the patient from the scene, encourage the victim to stay alert and focus on survival to minimize the chance of circum-rescue collapse. Rewarming and movement of extremities should be avoided to prevent increased blood flow to cool peripheral tissue with resultant increase in return of cooled blood to central circulation. Carefully check signs of life and pulse for 60 seconds as it may be difficult to detect pulse in a hypothermic patient. All patients should be provided full body insulation and rewarming unless it does not impede cardiopulmonary resuscitation or delay transport. Only electrical, chemical or forced air heating packs or blankets should be used as they provide substantial amount of heat transfer. Accidental hypothermia can be managed as per staging of the condition as described in **Table 13**.

TABLE 13: Staging and management of accidental hypothermia.

Stage	Clinical symptoms	Typical core temperature	Treatment
HT I	Conscious, shivering	35–32°C	Warm environment and clothing, warm sweet drinks, and active movement (if possible)
HT II	Impaired consciousness, not shivering	<32–28°C	Cardiac monitoring, minimal and cautious movements to avoid arrhythmias, horizontal position and immobilization, full-body insulation, active external and minimally invasive rewarming techniques (warm environment; chemical, electrical, or forced-air heating packs or blankets; warm parenteral fluids)
HT III	Unconscious, not shivering vital signs present	<28–24°C	HT II management plus airway management as required; ECMO in cases with extracorporeal membrane oxygenation with cardiac instability that is refractory to medical management
HT IV	No vital signs	<24°C	HT II and III management plus cardiopulmonary resuscitation and up to three doses of epinephrine (at an intravenous or intraosseous dose of 1 mg) and defibrillation, with further dosing guided by clinical response; rewarming with ECMO or CPB (if available) or CPR with active external and alternative internal rewarming

- Hypothermia may be determined clinically on the basis of vital signs with the use of the Swiss staging system. CPB denotes cardiopulmonary bypass, CPR cardiopulmonary resuscitation, and ECMO extracorporeal membrane oxygenation.
- Measurement of body core temperature is helpful but not mandatory. The risk of cardiac arrest increases as the core temperature drops below 32°C and increases substantially if the temperature is <28°C. To convert values for temperature to degrees Fahrenheit, multiply by 9/5 and add 32.

Question 10

Discuss the pathogenesis, clinical features, differential diagnosis, and treatment of tetanus in adults.

The tetanus is characterized by muscular rigidity and spasms caused by tetanus toxin (tetanospasmin), which is produced by *Clostridium tetani*, an anaerobic bacillus, whose spores survive in soil and cause infection by contaminating wounds.

Pathophysiology of tetanus: Tetanus toxins act by similar mechanism such as botulinum toxin. Tetanus toxin is taken up into nerve terminals of lower motor neurons, the nerve cells that activate voluntary muscles. It is a zinc-dependent metalloproteinase that targets a protein (synaptobrevin/vesicle-associated membrane protein—VAMP) that is necessary for the release of neurotransmitter from nerve endings through fusion of synaptic vesicles with the neuronal plasma membrane. Flaccid paralysis may be the initial symptom of local tetanus infection, caused by interference with vesicular release of acetylcholine at the neuromuscular junction, as occurs with botulinum toxin. Extensive retrograde transport of tetanus toxin occurs in the axons of lower motor neurons and tetanus toxin reaches the spinal

TABLE 14: Tetanus treatment.

Steps	Interventions
Wound	Identify wound and wound debridement
Antibiotic therapy	Metronidazole 500 mg IV 6 hourly, theoretically penicillin can enhance the effect of tetanospasm
Immunization	• Tetanus toxoid 0.5 mL IM at presentation then after 6 weeks and then after 6 months • Tetanus immunoglobulin 3,000–6,000 units IM (opposite arm of TT and some amount around the wound site)
Muscle relaxation	Diazepam
Respiratory distress management	Sedation neuromuscular blockade (succinylcholine/vecuronium for intubation) mechanical ventilation
Autonomic dysfunction management	Magnesium sulfate loading dose 40 mg/kg IV then continuous infusion 2 g/hour or Labetalol 0.25–1 mg/minutes IV infusion Morphine sulfate 0.5–1 mg/kg/hour Clonidine 300 μg every 8 hourly

cord or brainstem. Tetanus toxin crosses the synapses and is taken up by nerve endings of inhibitory GABAergic and/or glycinergic neurons that control the activity of the lower motor neurons. Once tetanus toxins inside the inhibitory nerve terminals, it cleaves vesicle-associated membrane protein (VAMP), thereby inhibiting the release of gamma-aminobutyric acid (GABA) and glycine, resulting functional denervation of the lower motor neurons, which leads to rigidity and spasms due to hyperactivity and to increased muscle activity.

Clinical features: Tetanus toxin causes rigidity and spasms due to hyperactivity of voluntary muscles. Rigidity is the tonic, involuntary contraction of muscles, while spasms are short lasting muscle contractions that can be elicited by sensory stimulation or by stretching of the muscles; they are termed reflex spasms. A highly reduced ability to open the mouth as rigidity of the temporal and masseter muscles leads to trismus (lockjaw). During physical examination, attempts at opening the mouth may induce spasms that cause the complete clenching of the jaws.

Differential diagnosis of tetanus: Tetanus must be differentiated from other diseases that present with fever and rigidity such as strychnine poisoning, dental infections, drug reactions, hypocalcemia, meningitis, stroke, and stiff-man syndrome. The treatment of tetanus is described in **Table 14**.

■ SUGGESTED READING

1. Richhariya D, Sharma B. Textbook of Emergency Medicine including Intensive Care and Trauma, 2nd edition. New Delhi: Jaypee Brothers Medical Publishers (P) Ltd; 2022. pp. 596-600. (Question 1).
2. Richhariya D, Sharma B. Textbook of Emergency Medicine including Intensive Care and Trauma, 2nd edition. New Delhi: Jaypee Brothers Medical Publishers (P) Ltd; 2022. pp. 796-9. (Question 2).
3. Richhariya D, Sharma B. Textbook of Emergency Medicine including Intensive Care and Trauma, 2nd edition. New Delhi: Jaypee Brothers Medical Publishers (P) Ltd; 2022. pp. 1466-71. (Question 3).
4. Richhariya D, Sharma B. Textbook of Emergency Medicine including Intensive Care and Trauma, 2nd edition. New Delhi: Jaypee Brothers Medical Publishers (P) Ltd; 2022. pp. 883, 893. (Question 4).
5. Richhariya D, Sharma B. Textbook of Emergency Medicine including Intensive Care and Trauma, 2nd edition. New Delhi: Jaypee Brothers Medical Publishers (P) Ltd; 2022. p. 815. (Question 5).
6. Richhariya D, Sharma B. Textbook of Emergency Medicine including Intensive Care and Trauma, 2nd edition. New Delhi: Jaypee Brothers Medical Publishers (P) Ltd; 2022. pp. 719, 998. (Question 6).
7. Richhariya D, Sharma B. Textbook of Emergency Medicine including Intensive Care and Trauma, 2nd edition. New Delhi: Jaypee Brothers Medical Publishers (P) Ltd; 2022. pp. 460-7. (Question 7).
8. Richhariya D, Sharma B. Textbook of Emergency Medicine including Intensive Care and Trauma, 2nd edition. New Delhi: Jaypee Brothers Medical Publishers (P) Ltd; 2022. p. 1363. (Question 8).
9. Richhariya D, Sharma B. Textbook of Emergency Medicine including Intensive Care and Trauma, 2nd edition. New Delhi: Jaypee Brothers Medical Publishers (P) Ltd; 2022. pp. 1686-91. (Question 9).
10. Richhariya D, Sharma B. Textbook of Emergency Medicine including Intensive Care and Trauma, 2nd edition. New Delhi: Jaypee Brothers Medical Publishers (P) Ltd; 2022. pp. 1314-6. (Question 10).

Emergency Medicine Paper 52

Devendra Richhariya

Question 1

1. Discuss clinical features and management of paraphimosis in a 7-year-old child.

Paraphimosis is a urological emergency in which foreskin is left retracted due to its entrapment behind the glans penis. This leads to strangulation of glans and lymphovascular compromise of the prepuce leading to venous engorgement, inflammation, pain and even necrosis, further impending the reduction of foreskin.

The patient presents with a swelling in foreskin, usually with pain. The diagnosis is often confirmed on physical examination of prepuce and the glans, both of which are markedly edematous and congested. The proximal penile shaft usually remains unremarkable. The reduction of prepucial skin becomes difficult and painful due to the swollen prepuce and constricted band of edematous tissues behind the glans.

Manual reduction: Manual reduction method may be tried in mild, early, and uncomplicated cases. Because of the pain which gets further aggravated during manipulation, it may require some form of anesthesia such as topical lignocaine gel, oral narcotics, penile nerve block or sedation.

Pharmacological therapy: Another way of reducing the preputial edema is application of mannitol (20%) soaked gauze around prepuce for a period of 30–45 minutes, with or without intermittent compression.

Minimally invasive therapy: This includes the most widely practiced method of multiple puncture technique, also known as Perth-Dundee technique.

Surgical treatment: Surgical intervention is required when above-described methods have failed to reduce the paraphimosis. This involves longitudinal dorsal slit cutting of prepuce at 12 o'clock till constricting band site and reduction of trapped prepuce back over the glans.

2. Explain the supracondylar fracture of humerus in a 6-year-old boy.

A patient in humerus supracondylar fractures presents to the emergency department with the symptoms of swelling, pain, inability to move and crepitation in the elbow. Vascular and nerve examination must be done in detail and recorded. The color and temperature of the fingers and the presence of peripheral circulation should be carefully evaluated.

Gartland Classification

Type I: Undifferentiated fractures (Type I-a if there is no medial impact here, crush in the coronal plane, slight hyperextension in the sagittal plane classified as Type I-b if any).

Type II: Dissociated fractures; but posterior cortexit is solid.

Type III: Dissociated fractures in which both the anterior and posterior cortex are not intact.

Type IV: Both anterior and posterior cortex.

They are dissociated fractures that are not intact and completely unstable.

Question 2

1. Discuss local anesthetic systemic toxicity.

Local anesthesia systemic toxicity: Dose-related clinical progression of sodium channel blockade in nontarget tissues, primary in brain and heart.

- Toxicity can be subtle neurologic symptoms to refractory seizures, cardiovascular collapse.
- Risk reduced by reducing dose limitation and techniques to minimize systemic absorption.
- Seizures treated by benzodiazepines.
- Vasopressin, tachyarrhythmias agents (beta blockers, calcium channel agonists) should be avoided in such toxicity.
- Intravenous (IV) 20% lipid emulsion 1.5 mL/kg infused over 1 minute with continuous infusion or repeat dose (maximum 10 mL/kg over initial 30 minutes) is effective treatment from local anesthesia toxicity as bupivacaine has high lipid solubility.
- Prilocaine and benzocaine cause oxidation of ferrous form, creating methemoglobin that becomes visible as cyanosis if methemoglobin concentration exceeds 1.5 g/dL.

2. Define food poisoning.

"Food poisoning" means illness specifically from a toxin in food. Food poisoning is a type of foodborne illness caused by *Salmonella* or *Escherichia (E.) coli*. Most common symptoms of food poisoning are: Diarrhea abdominal pain or cramps, nausea, vomiting, and fever.

3. Explain the clinical features and management of acute diarrhea due to *Clostridioides (C.) difficile* infection.

Clostridioides (formerly *Clostridium*) *difficile* infection (CDI) is one of the most common hospital-acquired (nosocomial) infections. *C. difficile* colonizes the human intestinal tract after the normal gut flora has been disrupted (frequently in association with antibiotic therapy) and is the causative organism of antibiotic-associated diarrhea and pseudomembranous colitis. Almost all antibiotics have a potential to cause diarrhea but it is more often seen with clindamycin and cephalosporins. Additional risk factors for CDI include age >65, recent hospitalization, and use of proton pump inhibitors. Watery diarrhea (≥3 loose stools in 24 hours) is the cardinal symptom of CDI. Other manifestations include lower abdominal pain and cramping, low-grade fever, nausea, and anorexia.

An important initial step in the treatment of CDI is discontinuation of the inciting antibiotic agent(s) as soon as possible. Further treatment depends upon stratifying the patient as per severity and follow the antibiotic protocol **(Table 1)**.

Nonsevere CDI—white blood cell count ≤15,000 cells/mL and serum creatinine <1.5 mg/dL.

Severe CDI—white blood cell count >15,000 cells/mL and/or serum creatinine ≥1.5 mg/dL.

Fulminant colitis (previously referred to as severe, complicated CDI)—hypotension or shock, ileus, or megacolon.

TABLE 1: Antibiotic regimens for treatment of *Clostridioides difficile* infections in adult.

Nonsevere disease (white blood cells ≤15,000 cells/mL and creatinine <1.5 mg/dL)	• Vancomycin 125 mg orally 4 times daily for 10 days or fidaxomicin 200 mg orally twice daily for 10 days or if both drugs are not available • Metronidazole 500 mg orally thrice daily for 10 days
Severe disease (white blood cells ≥15,000 cells/mL and creatinine >1.5 mg/dL)	Vancomycin 125 mg orally 4 times daily for 10 days or fidaxomicin 200 mg orally twice daily for 10 day
Fulminant disease (hypotension or shock, Ileus megacolon)	• Enteric vancomycin plus parenteral metronidazole • Vancomycin 500 mg orally via nasogastric tube 4 times daily • Metronidazole 500 mg intravenously thrice daily for 10 days • If Ileus presents rectal vancomycin as retention enema every 6 hours (500 mg in 100 mL normal saline per rectally, retain as long as possible)

Question 3

1. Discuss phases of clinical trials of a new drug.

New drug/vaccine development follows the stringent robust scientific protocols before introducing for mass usage by the community **(Flowchart 1)**. Many international agencies and countries are having their own regulatory authorities to approve the introduction of particular vaccine for their nationals. Development of the vaccines including after introduction for human use needs to follow more stringent protocols for their usages particularly for infants, elderly, pregnant women, and even for healthy ones.

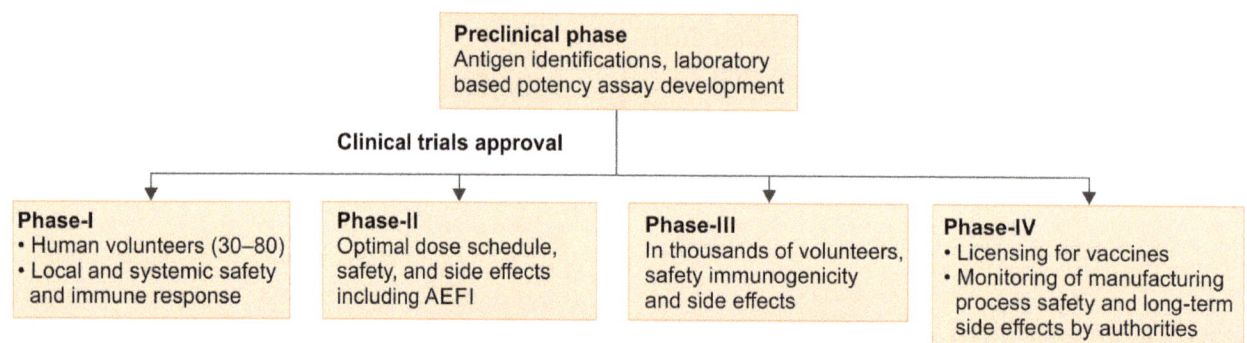

Flowchart 1: Stages of vaccine development.

(AEFI: adverse events following immunization)

2. Discuss management of a patient with suspected COVID-19 having a respiratory rate of 32/minute and oxygen saturation of 88% on room air.

Moderate-to-severe infection (increasing oxygen dependency): Severe lower respiratory infection, severe pneumonia, dyspnea, worsening nausea, vomiting, fever, confusion, and drowsiness; unusual symptoms—febrile encephalopathy, CVA, MI, oxygen dependency/± respiratory distress, tachypnea RR >30 SpO_2 <95% on supplemental oxygen on 10 L/minute, HFNC (FiO_2 50%), NIV (FiO_2 50% and EPAP 6), presence of hypotension, shock and multiorgan involvement, septic shock-persisting hypotension in spite of volume resuscitation requiring vasopressor to maintain MAP >65.

Management target SpO_2: 92–96% (88–92% in patients with COPD)—the device for administering oxygen (nasal prongs, mask, or masks with breathing/ non-rebreathing reservoir bag) depends upon the increasing requirement of oxygen therapy. If HFNC or simple nasal cannula is used, N95 mask should be applied over it. Awake proning may be used as a rescue therapy. Strongly recommended therapy (steroid)—tab dexamethasone 6 mg/day orally for 10 days OR IV dexamethasone 20 mg/day IV × 5 days followed by 10 mg/day IV × 5 days; titrate dose and duration to culmination of oxygen dependency; low molecular weight heparin (LMWH).

All patients should have daily 12-lead ECG follow CRP, D-dimer and ferritin every 48–72 hourly (if available); CBC with differential count, absolute lymphocyte count, KFT/LFT daily add antacid Zn, vitamin C, vitamin D, and antibiotic as per local guidelines.

Question 4

Define the following:

1. Positive predictive value.
2. Negative predictive value.

Positive predictive value is the probability that subjects with a positive screening test truly have the disease. *Negative predictive value* is the probability that subjects with a negative screening test truly do not has the disease.

3. Confidence interval.

A confidence interval is the mean of estimate plus and minus the variation in that estimate. This is the range of values we expect our estimate to fall between if we redo our test, within a certain level of confidence. Confidence, in statistics, is another way to describe probability. In frequentist statistics, a confidence interval is a range of estimates for an unknown parameter. A confidence interval is computed at a designated confidence level; the 95% confidence level is most common, but other levels, such as 90% or 99%, are sometimes used:

$$CI = \bar{x} \pm z \frac{s}{\sqrt{n}}$$

CI = confidence interval
$\bar{x}$ = sample mean
z = confidence level value
s = sample standard deviation
n = sample size

4. Odds ratio.

The odds ratio is a statistical measure used to quantify the association between two binary variables. It is the ratio of the odds of an event occurring in one group to the odds of the same event occurring in another group. In other words, it tells us how much more or less likely it is for an outcome to occur in one group compared to another group.

5. Likelihood ratio.

In statistics, the likelihood ratio is a measure of the strength of evidence provided by the data in favor of one statistical hypothesis over another. It is defined as the ratio of the likelihoods of two different hypotheses, given the same observed data. The likelihood ratio is often used in hypothesis testing, model selection, and parameter estimation.

Question 5

1. Discuss etiology, investigations, and treatment of acute meningitis in children.

Clinical features: Fever, irritability, headache, projectile vomiting, shrill cry, bulging, fontanelle, seizures, altered sensorium, photophobia, neck rigidity, generalized hypertonia, diplopia, ptosis, squint, poor feeding, and refusal to suck.

Kernig's sign: Extension of knee is restricted to <135° when the hip is 90° flexed position

Brudzinski's sign: On flexing the neck there is flexion of hips and knees.

Management investigations: Complete blood count—total leukocyte count may be increased in bacterial meningitis. However, a normal total leukocyte count does not rule out meningitis. Measure blood sugar levels frequently. Coagulation profile will be required before performing lumbar puncture. Chest X-ray—50% of patient with pneumococcal meningitis have evidence of chests infection in initial X-ray. Blood cultures are to be collected as soon as possible in a patient suspected with meningitis. Blood cultures are positive in 50–80% cases of bacterial meningitis. Other ancillary tests—liver function tests, renal function test. Blood biomarkers of inflammation such as procalcitonin, CRP can be used to guide treatment.

Neuroimaging: It is not mandatory to perform neuroimaging before initiating treatment in clinically suspected meningitis. Urgent CT brain should be performed in patients with signs of increased intracranial tension before performing lumbar puncture.

Treatment: Priority of treatment is prompt administration of antibiotics

Bacterial meningitis: After stabilization of airway, breathing and circulation appropriate empirical antibiotics must be administered. If the clinical suspicion is high, empirical antibiotics should be started before performing lumbar puncture. Choice of empirical antibiotics will depend on the infection suspected based on patient's age and premorbid condition **(Table 2)**. Dexamethasone may attenuate the inflammatory response and its consequences such as vasculitis, cerebral edema, etc. and shown to reduce overall mortality and neurological sequelae. First dose of dexamethasone should be administered at least 10–20 minutes before administration of antibiotics. Dose is 0.15 mg/kg. It is continued every 6 hours for next 4 days. Other corticosteroids have poor CNS penetrations, hence not to be used. All patients with meningitis have to be hospitalized and started on IV antibiotic therapy.

TABLE 2: Empirical antibiotic therapy for meningitis.

Age group	Empirical antibiotic therapy
Neonates	Ampicillin (150 mg/kg/day) + 3rd generation cephalosporin, e.g., cefotaxime (100–150 mg/kg/day)
Infant and children	Cefotaxime or ceftriaxone (80–100 mg/kg/day) + vancomycin (60 mg/kg/day)
Adults	Ceftriaxone (80–100 mg/kg/day) + vancomycin (30–60 mg/kg/day)
Immunocompromised patient	Cefotaxime (8–12 g/day) or ceftriaxone (4 g/day) + ampicillin (12 g/day) + vancomycin (30–60 mg/kg/day)
Suspected nosocomial infection	Vancomycin (30–60 mg/kg/day) + ceftazidime (6 g/day) or cefepime (6 g/day) or meropenem (6 g/day)

Viral meningitis: There is no specific treatment for viral meningitis and the treatment is largely supportive. Acyclovir 10 mg/kg 8 hourly can be given in HSV meningitis/encephalitis. Other aspects which may need emergent management in meningitis are septic shock, metabolic complications such as hypoglycemia, acidosis, hypokalemia, raised intracranial tension, seizure, and coagulopathy.

2. Explain the role of ultrasound in a patient with acute shortness of breath.

Bedside lung ultrasound in emergency (BLUE): Basic point-of-care ultrasound (POCUS) examination performed for identifying undifferentiated respiratory failure at the bedside, immediately after the physical examination, and before any radiography.

- The protocol is simple and takes only a few minutes to perform.
- It analyzes three standardized points on each hemithorax in patients with acute respiratory failure, by establishing the presence or absence of:
  - Lung sliding
  - Anterior lung rockets
  - Posterior and/or lateral alveolar and/or pleural syndrome (PLAPS)
  - A noncompressible deep vein.
- Lung ultrasonography is becoming a standard tool in critical care, due to its very high sensitivity and specificity to diagnose common chest pathologies.
  - *Left panel:* The A profile is defined as predominant A lines plus lung sliding at the anterior surface in supine or half-sitting patients (stage 1/1).
    - This profile suggests COPD, embolism, and some posterior pneumonia. Pulmonary edema is nearly ruled out.
  - *Middle:* The B profile is defined as predominant B lines in stage 1.
    - This profile suggests cardiogenic pulmonary edema, and nearly rules out COPD, pulmonary embolism, and pneumothorax.
  - *Right panel:* An A/B profile, massive B lines at the left lung, A lines at the right lung.
    - This profile is usually associated with pneumonia.

Question 6

1. Discuss physiologic monitoring during cardiopulmonary resuscitation.

The American Heart Association (AHA) recommends monitoring cardiopulmonary resuscitation (CPR) quality using end tidal carbon dioxide ($ETCO_2$) or invasive hemodynamic data.

Clinician-reported use of either $ETCO_2$ or DBP to monitor CPR quality associated with improved ROSC.

An ETCO$_2$ >10 mm Hg during CPR associated with a higher rate of survival (ETCO$_2$ 35–40 indicator of ROSC) compared to events with ETCO$_2$ ≤10 mm Hg (ROSC unlikely).

2. List the steps of high-quality cardiopulmonary resuscitation.

Five components of high-quality cardiopulmonary resuscitation (CPR):
1. Achieving a rate of 100–120 compressions per minute.
2. Compressing the chest to a depth of 2–2.4 inches (5–6 cm)
3. Avoiding leaning on the chest to allow for full chest wall recoil after each compression.
4. Minimizing pauses in compressions (chest compression fraction >60%)
5. Push hard/push fast

3. How will you assess and manage an adult patient with bradycardia?

- Call for help.
- Establish IV access.
- Bring crash cart to bedside and attach pads.
- Begin continuous cardiac and respiratory monitoring.
- *Unstable bradycardia:* Begin stabilization according to the adult unstable bradycardia algorithm.
- Evaluate underlying rhythm **(Flowchart 2)**.

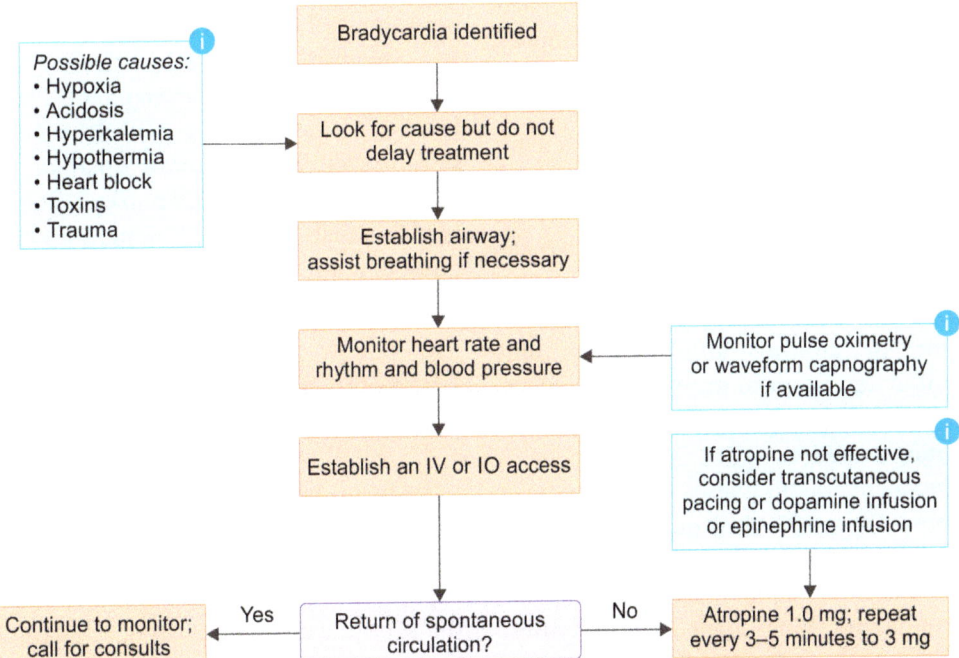

Flowchart 2: Approach to adult patient with bradycardia.

Question 7

1. Discuss recent trials carried out for determining targets of oxygen saturation and blood pressure after achieving return of spontaneous circulation.

The current AHA guidelines remain supported by the best available evidence. An oxygenation strategy of maintaining the oxyhemoglobin saturation in the range 94–99% after return of spontaneous circulation (ROSC) and down titrating the inspired oxygen while the saturation remains 100% appears appropriate; following ROSC, aim to maintain a mean arterial blood pressure of >65 mm Hg.

2. What is CRASH-3 trial?

CRASH-3 trial: According to CRASH-3 Trial, tranexamic acid is safe in patients with traumatic brain injury and that treatment within 3 hours of injury reduces head injury-related death.

Role of tranexamic acid: Tranexamic acid is an antifibrinolytic agent that reduces blood loss after surgery and may reduce blood loss after traumatic injury. It prevents cleavage of plasmin and degradation of fibrin. As early as possible after injury, with administration of tranexamic acid, within 1 hour of injury decreases relative risk from bleeding by 32% and within 1–3 hours by 21%; administration of tranexamic acid >3 hours after injury is less effective and potentially harmful. Tranexamic acid must be given before transfer/arrival to a trauma center in order to meet the time requirement of early administration. The dose is 1 g IV bolus over 10 minutes, followed by 1 g IV over 8 hours.

Question 8

1. Describe rapid sequence intubation and mention key modification to the classic RSI based on recent evidence.

Seven Ps of rapid sequence intubation (RSI):

- *Preparation:* In the initial phase, the patient is assessed for intubation difficulty, unless this has already been done, and the intubation is planned, including determining dosages and sequence of drugs, tube size, and laryngoscope type, blade, and size. Drugs are drawn up and labelled. All patients require continuous cardiac and pulse oximetry monitoring.
- *Preoxygenation:* Administration of 100% oxygen for 3 minutes of normal tidal volume breathing in a normal healthy adult establishes an adequate oxygen reservoir to permit 6–8 minutes of safe apnea before oxygen desaturation to <90% occurs.
- *Pretreatment:* During this phase, drugs are administered 3 minutes before the administration of a paralytic agent and an induction agent to mitigate the adverse physiologic effects of laryngoscopy and intubation on the patient's presenting condition.
- *Paralysis with induction:* In this phase, a potent sedative agent is administered by rapid IV push in a dose capable of producing unconsciousness rapidly. This is immediately followed by rapid administration of an intubating dose of a neuromuscular blocking agent (NMBA), either succinylcholine at a dose of 1.5 mg/kg IV or rocuronium, 1 mg/kg.
- *Positioning:* The patient should be positioned for intubation as consciousness is lost. Usually, positioning involves head extension, often with flexion of the neck on the body.
- *Placement of the tube:* Approximately 45–60 seconds after administration of the NMBA, the patient is relaxed sufficiently to permit laryngoscopy. This is assessed most easily by moving the mandible to test for mobility and absence of muscle tone.
- *Postintubation management:* After confirmation of tube placement by $ETCO_2$, obtain a chest radiograph to confirm that mainstem intubation has not occurred and to assess the lungs. If available, place the patient on continuous capnography.

2. Discuss delayed sequence intubation.

Delayed sequence intubation (DSI) is considered as "procedural sedation" using IV. Ketamine 1 mg/kg, in certain cases where preoxygenation with conventional methods like face mask is difficult due to agitation, delirium, and confusion.

3. How will you reduce chances of peri-intubation cardiac arrest in a patient who is in shock?

Confirm tube position by $ETCO_2$ and continue $ETCO_2$ monitoring if available. Take an X-ray chest to rule out endobronchial intubation. Fix endotracheal tube (ETT) appropriately and note the lip mark and document it. Plan and administer post intubation sedation and analgesia. Generally, avoid paralysis with non-depolarizing neuromuscular blockers (NDNMB) such as vecuronium and pancuronium. Make sure that no tube bite, tube block, coughing and fighting with ventilator. Manage post induction hemodynamic instability with IV fluids and vasopressors if required. An adequate dose of a benzodiazepine (e.g., midazolam, 0.1–0.2 mg/kg IV) and opioid analgesic (e.g., fentanyl, 3–5 µg/kg IV, or morphine, 0.2–0.3 mg/kg IV) is given to improve patient comfort and decrease sympathetic response to the ETT.

Question 9

1. Discuss acute radiation syndrome.

It has been stated that whole body or partial body exposure should be at least 1 Gy for the development of acute radiation syndrome. Acute radiation syndrome is not expected for exposures <0.5 Gy. After exposure, 0–2 days is defined as the prodromal phase, 2–20 days as the latent phase, and 21–60 days as the disease phase. Early symptoms are nausea, vomiting, anorexia, apathy, diarrhea, fever, headache, and tachycardia. If these symptoms started within about 2 hours, it is considered that the patient was most likely exposed to high doses, and if they started within minutes, doses exceeding 10 Gy are considered. At such high-dose exposure, in patient develops cerebrovascular syndrome and possibly dying within a few days. If cerebrovascular syndrome does not develop and only gastrointestinal syndrome develops, then the patient may recover with appropriate medical intervention. Four different syndromes that may develop related to acute radiation syndrome have been defined as cerebrovascular, gastrointestinal, hematopoietic, and cutaneous syndromes. Cerebrovascular syndrome is usually seen in doses of 10 Gy and above. It is thought that this syndrome develops due to radiation-induced deterioration in cellular permeability and CSF content, interstitial edema, and petechial hemorrhages. It has been reported that severe nausea and vomiting, confusion, disorientation, seizure, ataxia, and papilledema can be seen in cerebrovascular syndrome.

2. Discuss control zones in case of a suspected chemical release.

Control zones of a chemical release event at a scene **(Fig. 1)**.

Hot zone: It is the contaminated area or site of release. The immediate area where the suspected chemicals and victims of exposure are located is designated the hot zone. Only trained personnel in fully encapsulated protective gear should be allowed to enter. Their primary role is rescue of victims by removing them from further exposure.

Warm zone: A surrounding corridor through which each victim is washed off and decontaminated is created outside the hot zone and is designated the warm zone. This is located uphill and upwind of the hot zone.

Cold zone: A clean area where the victims who are free of external liquid contamination are received. Here, a lower level of protective equipment is necessary and a very low risk of secondary contamination exists.

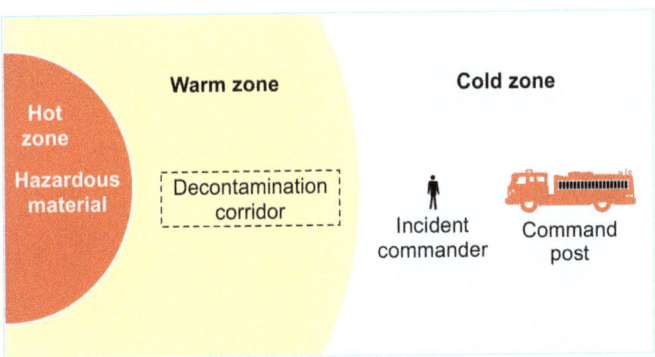

Fig. 1: Control zones of a chemical release event at a scene.

Question 10

1. Discuss the ICMR guidelines on "Do Not Attempt Resuscitation"?

Do Not Attempt Resuscitation (DNAR) is an option that may be exercised by treating physician in such a situation in the best interest of the patient. DNAR relates to CPR only and its limited value in certain situation and not to other form of treatment. ICMR (Indian Council of Medical Research) guidelines aim to guide treating physician and patient/surrogate in preserving dignity in death and avoid prolonged suffering to patient through nonbeneficial CPR while continuing to provide other potentially curative and supportive care. Open communication and decision-making would enhance mutual trust and respect between treating physician and patient/surrogate.

- DNAR would apply to a patient with a progressive debilitating, incurable, terminal illness where CPR would be inappropriate, nonbeneficial and likely to prolong the suffering of patient in the best judgment of treating physician. DNAR should be discussed with sensitivity. Compassionate care is important while applying this principle.
- DNAR is distinct from withdrawal or withholding of other life support treatment and advance directives do not come under the purview of this document.
- There should be adequate opportunity, time, and space to discuss with the patient and family in private and facilitate clear understanding of DNAR and its implication. This should be done in anticipation of an impending cardiac arrest during current hospitalization.
- Team work and good communication are of crucial importance in decision-making. Combined decision may be taken with the help of another physician, psychologist or social worker, counsellor or hospital administration.
- DNAR form should be available in the language understood by patient/surrogate and treating physician. In case the patient/surrogates does/do not sign the DNAR form, same should be recorded.
- Hospital administration should make effort to sensitize their health care professional on all issues related to DNAR.

2. Discuss the role of palliative care in the emergency department.

The World Health Organization (WHO) defines palliative care as *"an approach that improves the quality of life of patients and their families facing the problems associated with life-threatening illness, through the prevention and relief of suffering by means of early identification and impeccable assessment and treatment of pain and other problems, physical, psychosocial, and spiritual."*

■ SUGGESTED READING

1. Richhariya D, Sharma B. Textbook of Emergency Medicine including Intensive Care and Trauma, 2nd edition. New Delhi: Jaypee Brothers Medical Publishers (P) Ltd; 2022. pp. 779, 1625. (Question 1).
2. Richhariya D, Sharma B. Textbook of Emergency Medicine including Intensive Care and Trauma, 2nd edition. New Delhi: Jaypee Brothers Medical Publishers (P) Ltd; 2022. p. 650. (Question 2).

3. Richhariya D, Sharma B. Textbook of Emergency Medicine including Intensive Care and Trauma, 2nd edition. New Delhi: Jaypee Brothers Medical Publishers (P) Ltd; 2022. pp. 625, 1288. (Question 3).
4. Richhariya D, Sharma B. Textbook of Emergency Medicine including Intensive Care and Trauma, 2nd edition. New Delhi: Jaypee Brothers Medical Publishers (P) Ltd; 2022. pp. 81-90. (Question 4).
5. Richhariya D, Sharma B. Textbook of Emergency Medicine including Intensive Care and Trauma, 2nd edition. New Delhi: Jaypee Brothers Medical Publishers (P) Ltd; 2022. pp. 365, 845. (Question 5).
6. Richhariya D, Sharma B. Textbook of Emergency Medicine including Intensive Care and Trauma, 2nd edition. New Delhi: Jaypee Brothers Medical Publishers (P) Ltd; 2022. p. 222. (Question 6, 7).
7. Richhariya D, Sharma B. Textbook of Emergency Medicine including Intensive Care and Trauma, 2nd edition. New Delhi: Jaypee Brothers Medical Publishers (P) Ltd; 2022. pp. 212-5. (Question 8).
8. Richhariya D, Sharma B. Textbook of Emergency Medicine including Intensive Care and Trauma, 2nd edition. New Delhi: Jaypee Brothers Medical Publishers (P) Ltd; 2022. pp. 185-93. (Question 9).
9. Richhariya D, Sharma B. Textbook of Emergency Medicine including Intensive Care and Trauma, 2nd edition. New Delhi: Jaypee Brothers Medical Publishers (P) Ltd; 2022. pp. 134, 143-6. (Question 10).

Index

Page numbers followed by *b* refer to box, *f* refer to figure, *fc* refer to flowchart, and *t* refer to table.

A

Abdomen 196
   pain, causes of 157
   right lower quadrant of 134, 221
Abdominal aortic aneurysm 17, 196, 339
Abdominal compartment syndrome 500
   management of 500
Abdominal pain 18, 389*fc*
   acute 422
      severe 15*t*
   causes of acute-onset 264
   differential diagnosis of 15*t*, 52*t*, 542
   evaluation 53*t*
   life-threatening causes of 157
   management of 53*fc*, 543*fc*
      acute severe lower 53
   severe acute 15
Abductor digiti minimi 3
Abductor pollicis brevis 3
Abortion induction 2
Abovementioned trials 110
Abrasions 75
Abruptio placenta 99, 265
Accidental hypothermia, management of 67, 67*t*, 566, 567*t*
Acclimatization
   pathophysiology of 362
   physiology of high-altitude 122
Acetaminophen
   poisoning, management of 385*t*, 557*t*
   toxicity, clinical features of 384*t*, 556*t*
Acid–base
   disorder 367, 491, 491*f*, 491*t*
      mixed 259*fc*
   maintenance 453
Acid–base balance 453*f*
   lungs regulate 46
   regulation of 81
   renal mechanism of 4*f*, 366, 490, 490*f*
   respiratory of 490*f*
Acquired clotting disorders 147
Activated partial thromboplastin
   clotting time 21
   time 70, 104, 184
Acute aortic rupture
   external signs of 17
   management of 18
Acute cerebral hemorrhage 33, 34, 110
   antihypertensive treatment of 33, 34, 110
Acute coronary syndrome 25, 98, 102, 273, 485*b*
   classify 23
   radiology of 484
   risk stratification of 25*t*, 273*t*
   types of 24*t*, 274*t*

Acute delirium 470
   etiology of 348
Acute dysentery, case of 469
Acute dyspnea 22
   differential diagnosis for 22*t*, 102*t*
Acute ischemic stroke
   pathophysiology of 488, 488*f*
   risk factors for 255, 255*t*
Acute kidney injury 28*t*, 105, 106, 136*t*, 236, 454*t*
   classification of 27
   management of 275
   pathophysiology of 105, 489, 489*fc*
   scoring system 453
   stages of 236
Acute limb ischemia 378, 378*t*
   differential diagnosis of 378
Acute myocardial infarction 23
   classification of 274
   diagnosis of 24
Acute pancreatitis 338*t*
   common causes of 90
Acute radiation syndrome 121, 574
Acute respiratory distress syndrome 22, 102, 166, 208, 257, 448*t*
   causes for 141, 141*f*
   diagnosis of 448
   pathophysiology of 257
Acute scrotal pain, differential diagnoses for 18, 18*t*, 94*t*, 175*t*, 546*t*
Addisonian crisis 64
   management of 64
   treatment of 65*f*
Adductor pollicis 3
Adenosine
   diphosphate 253, 486
   monophosphate 466
   triphosphate 253, 486, 488
Adequate fluid resuscitation 180*fc*
Adrenal crisis 559
   acute 368*t*, 560*t*
   management of 367
Adrenal enzyme inhibitors, drug-induced 64
Adrenal hormone
   functions of 367*t*
   secretion, physiology of 367
Adrenal insufficiency 559*t*
Adrenocorticotropic hormone 448
Adult airway 169*t*, 366*t*
Adult burn, estimation of 51*f*, 544*f*
Adult Glasgow Coma Scale 519*t*
Advanced cardiac life support 35, 87
   guidelines 197
   interventions 385
Advanced trauma life support 153, 198*t*
   guidelines 197

Adverse drug reaction 126
   pathophysiology of 126
Adverse events following immunization 570
Agitated patient, management of 512
Agitation, acute 391
Airway 88
   algorithm, failed 290
   assessment, classification of 526*t*
   breathing, circulation, disability, exposures, management of 72
   management
      during pregnancy 85
      of difficult 195
      treatment options for 222
   obstruction 19
   protection of 65
   ultrasound 355
Alanine transaminase 60, 115
ALARA principle 260, 260*f*
Alcohol
   use disorder 115*t*
   withdrawal syndrome 115
      treatment for 116*t*
Aldrete score 83, 83*t*
Allis maneuver 334*f*
Alteplase 25
Alvarado score 134, 134*t*
   modified 422
Amantadine 23
Aminoglycosides, adverse effects of 7
Aminophylline 9
Aminosalicylic acid 173
Amplitude-integrated electroencephalogram 517
Amylase 15
Anaphylactic shock
   immunopathogenesis of 8*fc*, 528*fc*
   pathophysiologic mechanism of 8*fc*, 211*fc*, 528*fc*
Anaphylaxis 36
   causes of 8
   clinical criteria for 211
   current treatment of 212
   diagnosis, clinical criteria for 9
   diagnostic criteria for 528
   first-line therapy of 9
   pathophysiology of 8, 211, 528
   treatment of 9
   vaccine-induced 451
Angina, unstable 23
Angiotensin converting enzyme 164
Anion gap 4
Ankle
   injuries 503
   joint, anatomy of 255, 255*f*

Anterior cord syndrome 13, 92
Anti-arrhythmic agents 86
    classification of 1, 216, 372*t*, 538, 538*t*
Anti-arrhythmic drug 1, 371
    classification 86*t*
Antibiotic 26
    use of 71
Anticipated injuries 483
Anticoagulation 62
Anticoagulation therapy
    monitor 6
    risk stratification for 248*t*
Anticonvulsants 371
    antispasmodics 23
Antidiuretic hormone 489
Antiepileptic therapy 277
Antihistamine antiparkinsonians 23
Antimicrobial agents 7
    classification of 7*fc*
Antipsychotics 23
Anti-snake venom 65
Anxiety 437*t*
    disorder 437*t*
        classify 436
        primary 436
Aorta 79, 240, 240*f*, 499*f*
Aortic aneurysm 15
Aortic arch 447*f*
    anatomical of 447
Aortic dissection 98
    advised trial in 249
Appendage torsion 175*t*
Appendicitis 15, 456
    acute 134, 221, 264
    diagnosis of acute 134
    management of acute 264
    treatment of 422*t*
        acute 265*t*
Arrhythmias 234*t*, 428*t*
Arterial blood
    gas 252, 366, 367*t*, 383, 508
    supply 418
Arterial oxygen, partial pressure of 448
Arteriovenous malformation 432
Arthritis, causes of acute 423
Articular capsule and patella 94*f*
Ascites, pathophysiology of 43
Aspartate transaminase 60, 115
Assisted ventilation, indications for 102
Asthma
    acute 102, 233
    attack 102
    exacerbation, classify severity of 233
    grading of acute severe 22
    severity of 22, 22*fc*, 102*fc*, 233*fc*
    treatment of acute 233
Ataxia 47
Atherosclerosis 56
Atria, right 383
Atrial fibrillation 56, 247, 248*t*, 432*fc*, 475
Atropine 27
    scopolamine 23
Autoimmune hemolytic anemia 344, 554, 555
    management of 345*fc*
Automated chest compression device 117*f*, 481*f*
Automaticity 1
Autonomic dysfunction, control of 106
Avulsed tooth 550
Aztreonam 7

B

Bacitracin 7
Back pain 18
    symptoms in 377
Bacteremia 79
Bacterial meningitis, treatment of 198
Balanced crystalloid 16
Baroreceptors 45
Baroreflex 45, 46*fc*
Basic hemodynamic monitoring 162
Basic life support 35, 87, 197
Bayes' theorem 44
Beta-blocker toxicity 509
Beta-lactamase 7
Bicarbonate, role of 396
Bilevel positive airway pressure 22, 23, 394
BISAP score 174*t*
Bladder 425
    rupture, treatment 220*fc*
Blast injuries, pathophysiology of 408
Bleeding 6
    causes of severe 12
    scalp wounds, management of 270
Blinding studies, type of 246*t*
Blood
    component therapy 283
    consumption assessment of 16, 252, 415*t*, 498*t*
    film
        thick 138*f*
        thin 138*f*
    flow, mechanism of 253
    gas 406
    glucose meter 22, 102, 233
    grouping system 244, 245
    urea nitrogen 29, 174, 186
Blood pressure 22, 66, 73, 83, 88, 102, 138*f*, 233, 252, 415, 428
    control 58
    sphygmomanometric measurements of 84
Blood transfusion
    hemolytic reaction, pathophysiology of acute 525, 526*fc*
    protocol initiation 16*t*
    reactions, management of 472
Bloody diarrhea, differential diagnosis of 398
Blunt eye trauma, treatment of 331
Body
    baroreceptors in 45
    temperature, regulation of 108, 108*f*
Bomb blast injuries 206
    factors affecting 206
    field triage in 206
    pathophysiology of 206
    triaging of 207*fc*
Bomb blast, pathophysiology of 206*f*, 409*f*
Bone fracture, long 130
Bordetella pertussis infection, treatment of 71
Bowel obstruction 379, 379*t*
    causes of 379
    large 328
    management of 328*f*
Brachial artery injury 456
Brachial plexus 312*f*, 546*f*
    anatomy of 312
    injuries 312, 545
Bradycardia 573*fc*
    manage with 573
Brain dead 354, 525
    confirm 525
Brain injury
    prevent 177
        deterioration in 88
    secondary 544
    traumatic 72, 450
Breath
    acute onset shortness of 63
    acute shortness of 572
    count, single 309
Breathing 65, 88
    difficulty 22
    during primary view 55
Breathlessness, causes of acute onset of 102
Bronchial asthma 102
    pathophysiology of 406
Bronchial smooth muscle 9
Broselow pediatric emergency tape 355*f*
Broselow tape 355
    use of 355*f*
Brown-Séquard syndrome 92
Brugada syndrome 101
Buerger's disease 56
Buffer systems 366, 490
Bullet wounds, forensic evaluation of 441
Bullous fixed drug eruption 436*t*
Bullous lesions, acute onset 284
Bullous pemphigoid 284*t*
Bundle of His 79
Burch-Wartofsky point scale 434, 435*t*
Burn 75, 237
    fluid resuscitation of 90
    partial-thickness 51

C

Cairo–Bishop criteria 433, 509
Caisson sickness 363
Calcium
    channel blocker 509
    hemostasis 316, 317*f*
Canadian C-spine rule 198, 334
Cannabinoid hyperemesis syndrome, management of 474
Capnography variations, role of 214
Capnography wave 5
Carbamates insecticides physostigmine 23
Carbon dioxide 80
    monitoring 4
    partial pressure of 174, 259, 491
    tension 163

Carbon monoxide 80, 102
    poisoning 232
Carcinoma 432
Cardiac arrest 87*fc*, 213, 295*f*, 400, 483
    causes of 35*t*
    management of 35
Cardiac arrhythmia
    classify 216
    mechanisms of 1*f*, 216, 216*f*, 406*f*
Cardiac biomarkers 167
Cardiac cellular electrophysiology 405, 405*f*
Cardiac conducting system 1, 1*f*, 215, 216*f*, 405*f*
Cardiac cycle 364*f*
    phases 364*t*
Cardiac enzymes 24
Cardiac index 246
Cardiac ischemia 469
Cardiac markers 24, 274*t*
Cardiac output increases 11
Cardiac source 56
Cardiac tamponade 19
Cardiac troponin 24, 274
Cardiogenic pulmonary edema 321*t*
Cardiogenic shock
    management of 562
    pathogenesis of 562*fc*
    treatment in 563*f*
Cardiomyopathy 98
Cardiopulmonary resuscitation 5, 35, 68, 68*t*,
        86, 87, 197, 213, 214, 253, 292
    during pregnancy, steps of 86
    high quality 35
    physiologic monitoring during 572
    steps of high-quality 573
Cardiovascular system 179, 464
Carotid artery, internal 357
Carpet-layer's knee 97
Catheter, trial without 425
Catheter-directed thrombolysis 62
Cauda equina syndrome 377
Cell
    membrane functions 7
    wall synthesis inhibitors 7
Central causes 294*t*
Central cord syndrome 92
Central diabetes insipidus 2
Central nervous system 23, 65, 66, 80, 179,
        208, 215, 251, 456, 464, 474, 498
Central retinal
    artery occlusion 91
    vein occlusion 91
Central venous catheter
    complications of 78
    indications of 78
    insertion of 494*f*
Central venous
    oxygen saturation, clinical applications of 81
    pressure 196, 562
Cephalosporins 7
Cerebellar ataxia 48
Cerebellar disease, features of 47
Cerebral artery, middle 357
Cerebral autoregulation 119
Cerebral blood flow 254*f*, 255*f*, 450, 450*f*

Cerebral circulation 119
    physiology of 449
Cerebral edema, high-altitude 343, 451
Cerebral herniation syndromes 119
Cerebral palsy 73
Cerebral perfusion pressure 255*f*
Cerebral stroke
    mimics 183
    thrombolysis 183
Cerebrospinal fluid 100, 199*t*, 254, 262, 263,
        404, 404*t*, 546
    flow 404*f*
    production 404, 404*f*
Cervical lymphadenopathy 116
Cervical spine 218
    injury, mechanisms of 93*t*
    trauma 93
    unstable 77
Chemical agents, classification of 207, 208*t*
Chemical ocular injury, management of 374
Chemical release, suspected 575
Chemical terrorism, suspect 207
Chest
    drains 20
    injuries 89
    trauma 376, 499
    tube 19
Chest pain 62, 63, 101, 250*t*, 258*t*, 506*t*
    acute onset 273
    causes of 98
        acute 62*t*
    heart risk score for 273*t*
    in emergency, causes of 62
    low-risk 258, 485
    management of 258
Child abuse 439
    suspect 75
Child airway 169*t*
Child maltreatment, risk factors
        for 243, 244*t*
Child with persisting drooling,
        management of 480
Chlamydial testing 15
Cholecystitis
    diagnosis of acute 221, 221*t*
    management of acute 221
Cholesterol emboli 56
Chondromalacia patellae 98
Chronic kidney disease 7
    stages of 63, 63*t*
Chronic lithium poisoning, toxic effects
        of 107
Chronic obstructive pulmonary disease 22,
        46, 102, 166, 184, 214, 257, 476
Chronic respiratory acidosis, adaptation
        of 127
Circle of Willis 119*f*, 254, 254*f*, 488, 488*f*
Cirrhosis of liver, complications of 104
Classic technique 459*f*
Clavicle 33
Clinical dehydration scale 69*t*
Clostridioides difficile infections, treatment
        of 570*t*
Clostridium, species of 8

Coagulation cascade 511
    activation of 148*f*
Coagulopathy
    pathophysiology of 209
    trauma-induced 209*fc*
Coenzyme A 253, 486
Cold exposure, temperature regulation to 409
Cold injuries 133
Cold related emergencies 66
Cold temperature 566
Cold urticaria 66
Collateral ligament injuries, lateral 95
Colloids 16, 411
Coma
    differential diagnosis 277*t*
    management of 277
Common inotropes 538*t*
Communication skills 443
    components of 297*f*
Community-acquired pneumonia 553*t*, 554
    antibiotic therapy for 347
    etiology of 346
    management of 553
    pathogens of 553
Compare crystalloids 16
Compartment syndrome 17, 181, 181*fc*
    anatomy of 379
    causes of 16
    complications of 17
    diagnosis of 17
    investigation of 380
    management of 131, 182*fc*
    pathophysiology of 379
    suspected 181
    treatment for 17*fc*, 380
Complete blood count 60, 61, 424, 425, 470
Complex regional pain syndrome 125
Computed tomography 184
Conductive deafness 49
Confusion assessment method 560
Confusional state, acute 560*b*
Congenital abnormalities 36
Congestive heart failure arrhythmias 29
Consciousness, loss of 72
Consort guidelines 292, 444
Continuous positive airway pressure 23, 448
Co-poisoning
    diagnosis of 232
    pathophysiology of 232
Corneal abrasion
    evaluate child for 74
    management of 374
Corneal injury, suspected 463
Coronary angiography, role of 68
Coronary artery
    bypass grafting 563
    bypass surgery 24, 274
    disease 23, 24, 101, 248, 274, 506
    dissection 98
Coronary circulation, anatomy of 258, 258*f*,
        452, 452*f*
Coronary embolus 98
Coronary intervention 274
Coronary vasospasm 98

Coronavirus disease-2019 309*fc*, 351, 481, 571
    airway management in 395
    drug therapy in 475
    infection 351
        pathophysiology of 307
    pandemic 309
    positive, home isolation of 356
    syndrome
        management of 483
        manifestation of 484*f*
    triage protocol for 310*fc*
    vaccines 482
    variants, newer 482
Correlation coefficient 398*t*
Cortical vein thrombosis, diagnosis of 450*fc*
Cortical venous sinus thrombosis, diagnosis of 449
Corticosteroids 2
Corticotropin 448
Counter current mechanism 299*f*, 489
Covaxin vaccines, characteristics of 482*t*
Covishield vaccines, characteristics of 482*t*
Creatine kinase-myoglobin binding 274
Creatinine
    kinase 24
    phosphokinase 62
Critical clinical conditions, diagnosis of 260
Crohn's disease 15
Croup 36, 158
    diagnosis of 158
    treatment of 159
Cruciate ligament injuries 217
    anterior 95
    posterior 96
Crush injury 237, 518
Crystalloids 16, 411
    colloids unlike 16
Curb-65
    rule 553*t*
    score 347
Cushing's reflex 264
Cyanotic baby 517
Cyanotic spell 348
    pathophysiology of 347, 347*fc*, 518*fc*
Cyclic vomiting syndrome 66
Cystitis 231
    complicated 231
Cytomegalovirus 553

D

Dalteparin 6
Damage control resuscitation 209, 211*f*
Dashboard injury 457*f*
    management of 457
Dead space 83, 84
    measurements 84
Decompression sickness 140, 141*t*
    classification of 140
    pathophysiology of 140
Deep vein thrombosis 6, 79, 196, 325
    acute 472
    management of 325*fc*
    prophylaxis for 6
    treatment for 70*t*
Dehydration 29, 200
    classification of 201*t*, 243*t*, 480*t*
    degrees of 441*t*
    evaluate degree of 68
    management of 480
    mild-to-moderate 201
    plan of treatment for 201*t*, 480*t*
    severity of 68*t*
    treatment of 243, 243*t*
Delayed sequence intubation 574
Delirious patient, manage 61
Delirium 61, 348, 560
    assessment of 348
    causes of 61, 61*t*
    components of 560*f*
    management of 470*fc*
    mixed 61
    treatment of 61*fc*
    triage screen 61
    types of 61
Dengue 257
    fever, warning signs in 63
    investigations in 386
    phases in 386
    severe 386
    shock
        severe 64
        syndrome 64, 64*fc*
Dental avulsion 227, 227*t*, 502*t*
Deoxyribonucleic acid 7, 208, 533
Deterioration, causes of 89
Develop hospital disaster plan 38
Dexamethasone, uses of 351
Diabetes insipidus 259
Diabetic ketoacidosis 10, 10*t*, 22, 49, 49*t*, 102, 112, 185, 186
    complications of 302, 396
    criteria of 10
    diagnostic criteria for 302
    management in 395
    pathophysiology of 301, 486
    suspected 10
Diagnostic test accuracy, measures of 44
Diarrhea 480
    clinical features acute 570
    management of acute 570
Diastolic blood pressure 387
Difficile infection 570
Digital rectal examination 425
Diplopia
    causes of 460*fc*
        acute onset 460
    management of 461*fc*
Direct antiglobulin test 554
Disability 88
Disaster 169
    external 534
    ultrasound-guided triage during 520
Disequilibrium syndrome 390
Disseminated intravascular coagulation 223, 431, 491, 555
    management of 471
Distal femur 33
Diuretic
    complications of 371
    drugs, mechanism of action of 370
Diverticulitis 15
Dizziness, acute-onset 429
Dog bite 346
Down syndrome 73
Drawer test 294
    anterior 96
Drooling, management of 481*fc*
Drop arm test 56
Drug 23
    antiepileptic 37, 371*t*
    antiplatelet 314
    assisted intubation, steps of 257, 257*t*
    bioavailability of 45
    first pass effect of 45
    half-life measurement of 45
    newer antiepileptic 37
    treatment 36
Duckett Jones criteria 440
Dysdiadochokinesia 48
Dysphagia
    causes of 57
    management of acute 57
Dyspnea, causes of acute onset 22, 278, 279*t*, 548
Dysrhythmia, mechanisms of 405
Dyssynergia 48

E

Ear
    acute pain in 335, 335*t*
    nose, and throat 481
Early warning score, modified 357, 357*t*
Eclampsia 60
    management of 223
    treatment 224*t*
Ectopic pregnancy 547
    diagnosis of 133
    management of 133, 180
    pathophysiology of 132
    treatment plan for 181*fc*
Edrophonium 23
Einthoven's triangle 258, 258*f*
Elapid bite
    signs of 193*t*
    symptoms of 193*t*
Elastic stable intramedullary nailing 542
Electrical injury 390
    management of 390
Electrocardiogram 24, 53, 66, 213, 250, 273, 274, 388
    changes 143*f*
    detected on 28
Electrocardiograph 258
Electroencephalogram 517
Elevated liver enzymes 60
Emergency airway management, equipment for 290
Emergency care 36
    role of telemedicine in 296, 444

Emergency department 101, 258, 443, 542
  crowding, causes of 393
  disposition 146
  initial management in 12
  manage child in 152
  management of 12, 136
  sepsis in 252t
  setting 115t
  thermal burns in 543
  treatment 555
  triage 206
  ultrasound in 154
Emergency medicine 445
Emergency physician, osmolal gap for 288
Emergency psychiatric assessment steps 186
Emergency room 220
Emergent dialysis, indications for 28
Emergent hemodialysis indications 29t
Emergent needle thoracocentesis 19
Encephalitis 405
End stage chronic kidney disease, emergency complications of 63
End tidal carbon dioxide 5
Endoscopic retrograde cholangiopancreatography 173, 265
Endotracheal intubation 168
  complications of 169t
  long-term complications of 169
Endotracheal tube 11, 214, 491
End-tidal
  capnogram 530
  carbon dioxide 22
Enghoff calculation 84
Enoxaparin 6
Epididymitis 175t
Epigastric region 264
Epiglottitis 36
Epinephrine 9
Epiploic appendages 15
Episodic generalized weakness, causes of 47
Epistaxis
  anatomy of 176
  management of 418, 548
Erythema multiforme 145, 436
  major 145f
Erythematous rash 435
  acute onset 285
Erythrocyte sedimentation rate 424
Etomidate 402
Euthanasia 352
Evidence-based medicine, pyramid of 481, 481f
Exposure and temperature control 88
Extensor tendon injuries 552
External rotation lag test 56
Extracarporial membrane oxygenation 563
Extracellular fluid 530
  osmolality 2
Extracorporeal cardiopulmonary resuscitation 117
  technique of 118f
Extracorporeal membrane oxygenation, use of 240

Extraperitoneal bladder rupture 220, 220t
  operative treatment for 220
Eye
  anatomy of 330, 330f
  chemical injury in 75

F

Face 546
  nerve blocks of 269
Facial fractures classification 13, 14f
Facial injury 14
Falciparum
  malaria 138f
  mature stages of 534f
Fascia iliaca
  anatomy of 400
  block 400f, 401
    complications of 401
  compartment block 523
Fasciotomy 17
Febrile illness, management of acute 466
Febrile neutropenia 507
  management of 282
Femoral head 54
  dislocation of 332, 334f
Femoral neck 54
Femoral nerve block 284
Femoral shaft fracture 54
Femoral triangle 494
Femoral vein site 494f
Femur fractures, types of 54
Femur,
  classify fracture of 54
  diagnose fracture neck of 54
  supracondylar areas of 94f
Fentanyl 69, 82
Fever 100fc, 117, 281
  differential diagnosis for 100
  noninfectious
    causes of 382
    etiologies of 382t
  pathophysiology of 256, 466fc
Fibrinolysis pathway 238
Fibrinolytic agents 25t
Fibrinolytic therapy 101, 103
Fine needle aspiration cytology 460
Finger-to-nose test 48
Fishbone diagram 356f
FLACC scale 283f, 493t
Flaccid paralysis
  causes of acute 65
  diagnosis of acute 27
  etiology of acute 27t
Flaccid quadriparesis, acute onset 304t
Flail chest 376f
Flavin adenine dinucleotide 253
Flexor digiti minimi 3
Flexor pollicis brevis 3
Flexor tendon injuries 552
Florali trial 394, 394t
Fluid 36
  extravasation of 79
  resuscitation 180

Focal deficit 100
Folate 7
Foley's catheter balloon tamponade, uses of 499
Fondaparinux 6
Food poisoning 570
Foot 518
Foreign body 432
  aspiration 36
  in nose, management of 418, 549
Forest plot 351, 352f, 519f
  features of 519
Fracture 271f
  classify 129
  dislocation, complications of 332, 333t
  heal 129
  shaft tibia 181
  tooth management 502
Frank–Starling law 452f
Fresh frozen plasma 16, 239, 511
Frontal bone 13
Frostbite
  injuries, classify 133
  manage victims of 133
  risk factors precipitating 133
Functional residual capacity 213, 487

G

Gabapentin 37
Gait 111
Gallbladder 221
Gas gangrene
  manage 55
  pathogenesis of 55
  producing 55
Gastric
  decontamination 171
  lavage, role of 62
Gastroesophageal reflux disease 375
Gastrointestinal symptoms, severe 9
Gastrointestinal system 2
Generalized skin disorders 144
Generalized status epilepticus, causes of 429
Genital ulcers
  differential diagnosis of 564t
  management of 563, 564t
Geriatric trauma, management of 293
Glasgow Coma Scale 34, 58, 72, 73, 176, 198, 200, 252, 264t, 417, 508
  score 264
Glasgow Coma Score 88, 449
Glaucoma, acute angle-closure 92
Glomerular filtration rate 7, 11, 28, 63, 491
Glucose control 89
Glucose-6-phosphate dehydrogenase 244, 245, 554, 555
Gonadoliberin 448
Gonadotropin releasing hormone 448
Good Samaritan law 293
Greater trochanter 54
Groin pain 97
Growth factor, insulin-like 448
Growth hormone 448
Guillain-Barré syndrome 65

H

H1N1 infection, suspected 112
Hand
　injuries, high pressure 326
　intrinsic muscles of 450, 450t
　muscles of 3
Head
　impulse 430
　injury, traumatic 544
Headache, causes of acute 58
Head-to-toe approach 241t
Healthcare workers, hospital-based 35
Heart
　blood flow in 364
　conducting system of 1, 79, 79f
　normal conduction system of 405
　pathway 249
　risk score 258t, 506t
　sound, third 432
Heart failure 29, 246
　diagnosis of 320
　left-sided 319t
　pathophysiology of 318, 319fc
　right-sided 319t
Heat cramps 30
Heat edema 30
Heat emergencies 30, 165
Heat exhaustion 30
Heat illness, classification of 30t, 165t, 513t
Heat rash 30
Heat stroke 30, 313
　complications of 109
　cooling techniques in 108
　management of 30, 361
Heat syncope 30
Heat tetany 30
Heat-related illnesses
　management of 513
　types of 513
Heel-toe-shin test 48
HELLP syndrome 223
Hematochezia
　acute 460
　management of 148, 461fc
Hematoma
　block 361
　formation 79
Hematuria 425, 425fc
Hemodialysis
　emergency complications of 63, 63b
　history of 389
Hemodilution 58
Hemodynamic instability 382
Hemodynamic parameters, therapeutic target for 563f
Hemodynamically stable patient 388
Hemolysis 60
　causes of 555fc
Hemolytic transfusion reaction 554f, 555
Hemophilia
　A 147
　　pathophysiology of 147
　pathophysiology of 148f
　symptoms of 148f

Hemoptysis 432t
　differential diagnosis of 431, 431t
Hemorrhage 14, 497
　adrenal 64
　control 14
　intracerebral 34
　intracranial 21, 110
　intraventricular 100
　signs of 153t, 463t
　symptoms of 153t, 463t
Hemorrhagic shock 15
　causes of 51
　classification of 251, 536, 536t
　common causes of 51
　in trauma
　　classification of 251t, 498t
　　management of 497
　pathophysiology of 251, 251f, 411fc, 536, 537f
　traumatic 416
Hemostasis 291
　extrinsic pathways, physiology of 238f, 369fc, 511f
　physiology of 368
　tests of
　　primary 369
　　secondary 369
Hemothorax 79
Henderson–Hasselbalch equation 3, 126
Heparin
　complications of 238
　unfractionated 6
Hepatic encephalopathy
　acute 235
　　treatment of 235
Hepatorenal syndrome 105, 408t
Hepatotoxicity, risk of 556
Hereditary 64
Hernia
　anatomical sites of 327f
　complicated 327fc
　uncomplicated 327, 327fc
Herpes simplex virus 553
Herpes zoster 15
High altitude illnesses 122
　prevention of acute 122
High anion gap metabolic acidosis 81, 82t
Hip 96
　airway, manage 54
　dislocation, reduction of 284
　fracture 455
　　garden classification of 455f
　joint 523f
Histidine-Rich protein 533
Holliday–Segar method 243t
Homonymous hemianopia 495f
　right 495
Hospital disaster plan, organization of 408
Hospital emergency operation plan, components of 169
Housemaid's knee 97
Human immunodeficiency virus 100, 173, 281, 375
　causes of 41

Humeral head 33
Humerus
　fracture, proximal 541f
　supracondylar fracture of 130, 569
Humidifier 36
Hunt and Hess scale 58
Hydralazine 61
Hydrocephalus, management of 32, 32f
Hydromediastinum 78
Hydrothorax 78
Hydroxychloroquine 351
Hyperactive delirium 61
Hyperbaric oxygen 342
　role of 232
　therapy 125
　　indications of 126
Hyperbilirubinemia, indirect 245fc
Hypercalcemia
　approach to 514
　management of 28, 287, 515fc
Hypercoagulable states 147t
Hyperemesis gravidarum 324, 457
Hyperemesis syndrome, management cannabinoid 475fc
Hyperglycemic hyperosmolar syndrome 49, 486
Hyperkalemia 28, 28t
　etiology of 530
　tendency to 81
Hypernatremia 2
　causes of 2
　clinical effects of 2
　diagnostic algorithm of 259
　evaluate 259fc
Hyperosmolar hyperglycemic state 49
　diagnostic criteria of 48
Hyperosmolar hyperglycemic syndrome 49
　pathophysiology of 48
Hypertension
　grading of 387t
　malignant 473
Hypertensive emergency 387t
Hypertensive intracerebral hemorrhage
　hypertensive, management of 34
　management of 33
Hyperthermia, malignant 281
Hyperthyroidism 29
Hypertonic saline infusion 2
Hypervolemia 58
Hyphemia 114
Hypoactive delirium 61
Hypocalcemia 317
　causes of 317, 139t
　management of 318fc
　prolonged in 80
　treatment of 318
Hypoglycemia 139, 139t
　causes for 139
　management of 470
Hypokalemia, tendency to 81
Hyponatremia
　causes of 43, 163, 453
　clinical effects of 43
　diagnose 164fc

Hypotension, significant 63
Hypotensive resuscitation 15
Hypothenar group 3
Hypothermia 66
　causes of 256
　pathophysiological aspects of 409
　pathophysiology of 256
　signs of 66*t*
　symptoms of 66*t*
　trials 483
Hypovolemic shock, management of 411

I

Iliac crest 33
Ilioinguinal nerve entrapment 97
Iliotibial band syndrome 98
Illiac spine
　anterior inferior 523
　anterior superior 523
Imipenem 7
Immobilization dressings, types of 168
Immune system, activation of 9*t*, 212*t*, 529*t*
Immunization 107
Immunoglobulin 8
Immunotherapy 107
Impact seizure 32
Impedance threshold device 117, 117*f*
Incident command
　center, head of 38*t*, 170*t*, 534*t*
　organization chart 535*fc*
　system, advantages of 535*b*
Infantile hypertrophic pyloric stenosis 485
Infection 64
　transmission of 159
Infectious causes 63*b*
Infiltrative disorders 64
Inflammatory demyelinating polyneuropathy, chronic 47
Influenza infection 113
　suspected 112
Information technology 167
Infraspinatus muscle 56
Inguinal hernia 15
Inguinal region, right 456
Inhalational injury
　management 463
　produced by smoke 90, 179
Initial empiric antimicrobial therapy 554*t*
Initial ventilator management 306, 307
Injury
　mechanisms of 93
　report 462
Inspiratory capacity 487
Inspiratory reserve volume 487
Inspired oxygen, fraction of 448
Insulin
　euglycemic therapy, high 315
　therapy 395
Intensive blood pressure reduction 33, 34
Intensive care unit 167, 394
Intercostal chest drains 19
Intercostal drain insertion, procedure for 19
Intercostal nerve block 284

Interferon 466
Interleukin 466
Internal rotation lag test 56
Interventrical septum 562
Intestinal obstruction, management of 327
Intra-aortic balloon pump 563
Intra-arterial catheter, placement of 85
Intracellular cyclic adenosine
　　　　monophosphate 9
Intracellular fluid 530
　osmolality 2
Intracellular water loss 2
Intracerebral pressure, regulation of 451
Intracranial bleed, acute nontraumatic 191
Intracranial pressure 34, 254, 254*f*, 450, 451*f*
　signs of increased 32, 32*f*
　symptoms of increased 32, 32*f*
Intraductal papillary mucinous neoplasm 173
Intramuscular human tetanus immune
　　　　globulin 8
Intraosseous access
　complications 33
　indications for 32
Intraosseous route 33
Intraperitoneal bladder rupture 220, 220*t*
Intrauterine hypertonic saline administration 2
Intravascular hemolysis, differential diagnosis
　　　　of acute 554, 554*f*
Intravenous lipid therapy 316
Intravenous TPA infusion 184*b*
Intrinsic pathways, physiology of 238*f*, 511*f*
Intubating laryngeal mask airway 77
Intubation sick acidotic patient 401
Intussusception in child, management of 271
Invasive arterial blood pressure monitoring 85
Invasive mechanical ventilator 279
Ionizing radiation, effects of 121
Ionotropic agents 538
Ischemic stroke 21

J

Jaundice 245*f*, 281
　causes of 244, 244*t*
　　acute onset of 104
　child with 245
　fever with 137, 137*t*, 281*t*
Joint pain, acute-onset 423, 423*t*
Jugular venous pulse 162, 162*f*, 162*t*

K

Kassirer–Bleich equation 3, 4, 127
Keratoconjunctivitis, causes of 267
Ketamine 9, 69, 82, 402
Ketoacidosis, diabetes-related 49
Kidney
　basic unit of 408*f*
　disease 236*t*, 454
　functional unit of 407
　injury, classification of 504
　regulate acid-base balance 4
　role of 453
　ultrasound 425

King laryngeal tube 78
Knee
　bursal syndromes of 97
　evaluate 503
　injuries to 95
　myofascial syndromes 97
　relevant to trauma, anatomy of 94
Knee joint 95, 217, 325, 493
　anatomy of 217, 217*f*, 493*f*
Knee pain
　anterior 97, 98
　　medial 97, 98
　lateral 98
Kocher's criteria 396
Krait bite, manage patient of 65

L

Labetalol 61
Laceration 75
　wound across thigh 442
Lactate dehydrogenase 533
Lactate emergency physician, pathway of 252
Lactate production pathways 253*f*, 486*fc*
Lactic acidosis, pathophysiology of 486
Lambert–Eaton myasthenic syndrome 47
Lamotrigine 37
Laryngoscopy 526
Le Fort facial fractures classification 546*f*
Le Fort fracture, types of 262*f*
Le Fort injury patterns 546
Left bundle branch block 24, 25, 273, 274
Left ventricular
　assist device 246, 246*b*
　　complications of 247*b*
　　function 246
　ejection diastolic pressure 562
　ejection fraction 246
　end diastolic pressure 163
　failure 432
　outflow tract 289
Leg, compartments of 325, 326*f*
Levetiracetam 37
　advantages of 37
Life-threatening
　cervical spine injury, management of 464
　condition 58
　hyponatremia, management of 163
Ligament injury 95
Limb ischemia 378*t*
　management of acute 378
Lip laceration, management of 269
Lipase 15
Lisfranc injury 503
　assessment of 255
Lithium 2
　dilution cardiac output 163
　poisoning, management of chronic 107
　toxicity
　　cases, management of acute 189
　　factors precipitating 107
Liver 545*t*
　cirrhosis of 43
　failure, acute-on-chronic 235

function test 15, 325
injury, classification of 504
trauma grades 504*t*
Local anesthesia-induced systemic toxicity, management of 270
Local anesthetic
agents 356*t*, 360, 360*t*
systemic toxicity 569
Low back pain, causes of acute 377
Low molecular weight heparin 325
Low osmolarity oral rehydration solutions 243*t*
Low platelets syndrome 60
Lower abdominal pain, causes of acute 15, 224
Lower gastrointestinal bleed 227
causes of 227
Lower motor neuron 47
anatomy of 47
disease 47
weakness 47*f*
Lower subscapular nerve 312
Low-frequency probes, utility of 261
Low-molecular weight heparin 6
Ludwig's angina 226, 501
management of 501
Lumbricals 3
Lung
capacity of 487*f*
normal 448*f*
parenchymal diseases, diagnosis of 154
ultrasound, role of 260
volume
and capacities 305*f*
physiology of 305, 487
Luteinizing hormone 448
Lynch algorithm 510

M

Magnesium sulfate 9
Maintenance fluid requirements 243*t*
Malaria 257
complicated 137, 137*t*
diagnosis of 137, 533
diagnostic testing for 533*t*
emergency department management of 138
severe 137*t*
Mallampati classification 527*f*
Mallory–Weiss tear 26
Mass casualty 38
field triage of 207*f*
management 170*t*
triaging during 39
Massive blood transfusion protocol 252
Massive hematemesis, management of 511
Massive hemothorax 55
Massive transfusion
complications of 52
protocol 16, 252, 415
Massive upper gastrointestinal bleeding, causes of 25
Massive uterine bleeding 500
Maternal cardiopulmonary resuscitation 265

Maxillofacial injuries 262
management of 14*fc*, 263*fc*
McMahon score 501
Mean arterial pressure 16, 41, 200, 387
Mechanical cardiopulmonary resuscitation devices 117
Mechanical dead space 83, 84
Mechanical ventilation, indications for 233
Meckel's diverticulum 15, 422
Medial collateral ligament 95
Medial plica syndrome 98
Medical advice, discharge against 353
Medical oxygen therapy 166
Medium-bore chest tubes 20
Membrane protein, vesicle-associated 8
Meningitis 405
empirical antibiotic therapy for 200*t*, 277*t*, 572*t*
etiology of 198
in children, treatment of acute 571
types of 199*t*, 404*t*
Meniscal injury 95
Mental disorders, statistical manual of 114
Mental status assessment 531
Meralgia paresthesia 97
Mesenteric ischemia, acute 337, 561
Messenger ribonucleic acid 7
Metabolic acidosis 287, 307, 307*t*
causes of 4
ventilator
settings for 488
strategy for 488*t*
Metabolic alkalosis
causes of 46, 287*t*, 413*t*, 470*t*
common causes of 46*t*
etiopathogenesis of 413
management of 470
pathophysiology of 46
Metabolites, inhibitors of essential 7
Metacarpophalangeal joints 3
Metered-dose inhaler 407, 407*f*
Methanol poisoning 341
management of 341
pathogenesis of 341
Methicillin-resistant *Staphylococcus aureus* 554
Methotrexate administration, contraindications to 547*t*
Microangiopathic hemolytic anemia 555
Microteaching techniques 292
Midazolam 69
Middle ear 49
sagittal section of 49*f*
Midpalmar group 3
Migraine
acute attack of 555
drug therapy for 555*t*
Mitral stenosis 432
Mixed acid–base disorder, diagnosis of 259
Mnemonic thrombosis 235*t*
Monkey bite 473
Monkeypox 563
Monoamine oxidase 456
inhibitors 23, 474

Monoarticular arthritis, acute-onset 423, 424*fc*
Monro–Kellie doctrine 254
Mountain sickness
acute 343, 363
management of acute 363, 363*t*
Multidetector computed tomography 328
Multiorgan failure 29
Multiple bruises 75
Multiple casualty 38
Multiple dose-activated charcoal 62
Multisystem inflammatory system 100
Muscle
relaxants 23
spasms, control of 106
Myasthenic crisis, management of 303
Myocardial infarction 24, 274
thrombolysis in 24, 101*t*, 506*t*
Myocarditis 101
Myoglobin 24, 62
Myxedema coma 188, 188*t*, 189, 558*t*
diagnosing 188*t*
management of 557
treatment of 189*fc*, 558*fc*
Myxedema crisis 109
differential diagnosis of 109
treatment of 109

N

N-acetylcysteine 385
N-acetyl-p-benzo quinonimine 556*f*
Nails, examination of 111
Narrow complex tachycardia, management of 286*fc*
Nasal anatomy 176*f*, 418*f*
Nasal cannula, high flow 22, 257, 476
Nasal oxygen therapy, high-flow 257
Nebulization 9
Neck 536*t*
anatomical zones of 222*f*, 222*t*, 536*f*
injuries
airway compromise in 222
hard signs of 544
soft signs of 544
relevant to trauma, anatomy of 535
trauma 36, 222
concern in 222*t*, 544*t*
zones, anterior 221
Necrotizing fasciitis, management of 270
Necrotizing soft tissues infections 55
Necrotizing ulcerative gingivitis, management of acute 268
Needle decompression, procedure for 19
Needle stick injury 281
management of 473
Neglect in children, types of 243
Neonatal necrotizing enterocolitis 485
Neonatal resuscitation, steps of 242
Neonatal seizures 517, 517*fc*
Neonate with fever, management of 358
Nephron 408*f*
Nephropathy
contrast-induced 236
radiocontrast-induced 106

Neurally mediated hypotension 234*t*, 428*t*
Neurogenic shock 13, 13*t*, 123, 124, 373, 373*t*
    management of 13, 92, 124, 178
    pathophysiology of 123
Neuroleptic malignant syndrome 143, 144*t*, 280, 280*t*
Neurologic complaints 116, 117
Neurologic dysfunction 63
Neurological evaluation 3
Neuromuscular junction 303*f*, 487*f*
    anatomy of 302, 487
    physiology of 302, 487
Neuromuscular weakness 388*fc*
    causes of 388
Neurovascular complications 95
Neurovascular injury 79
Newborn care, routine 241
Newer airway aides, role of 479
Nexus C-spine rule 334
Nicotinamide adenine dinucleotide 253, 253*f*, 486
    hydrogenase 208
    phosphate 486
        hydrogen 208
Nifedipine 61
Nipah virus 160
    management of 160, 202
Nonabsorbable sutures 537
Non-accidental injury 439
Noninfectious causes 63*b*
Noninvasive arterial blood pressure monitoring 84
Noninvasive cardiac output monitoring 85
Noninvasive oxygen 4
Noninvasive ventilation 279
    contraindications of 23*t*
    indications of 23*t*
    modes of 22
Noninvasive ventilatory treatment 167
Nonparametric statistical tests 444
Non-steroidal anti-inflammatory drugs 53, 456
Non-ST-segment elevation myocardial infarction 23
Nontraumatic subarachnoid hemorrhage, management of 506
Normal anion gap metabolic acidosis 81
Normal capnogram 214
Normal capnography wave, morphology of 5, 214*f*, 530*f*
Nucleic acid replications, inhibition of 7
Nun's knee 97
Nursemaid injury 229, 230*f*
Nystagmus 430

O

Obstructed hernia 328*fc*
    management of 327
Obstructive shock 289
Obturator nerve entrapment 97
Ocular decontamination 170
Ocular injuries sustained 135
Ocular trauma, ultrasonography in 374
Ocular ultrasonography, normal 114*f*
Ocular ultrasound 248
One-handed technique 267*f*
One-way valve 117*f*
Open pneumothorax 55, 375
Ophthalmologic medications 417
Opponens digiti minimi 3
Opponens pollicis 3
Optic nerve sheath
    diameter 264
    normal values of 114
Optic neuritis 92
Oral anticoagulants 472
    novel 247
Oral rehydration solution 201, 243, 480
    complication of 69
    composition of 441
Orbital cellulitis 267, 331, 502
Organic anxiety disorder 436
Organophosphorus 23
    poisoning 26
        drug therapies 280
Orthopantomogram 227, 460
Orthopedic injury, common 168*t*, 332*t*
Orthostatic hypotension, management of 46
Oscillometry 85
Osmolal gap 4
Osmotic diuresis 2
Otalgia, causes of 133
Otitis externa
    causes of 49
    malignant 337
Otitis media 134
    acute 550
    complications of 134, 174
    microbiology of 133, 174
    pathophysiology of 174
Ottawa ankle rule 295, 334
Ottawa knee rule 295, 334
Ovarian hyperstimulation syndrome 420
Overanticoagulation, management of 6
Oxcarbazepine 37
Oxygen
    consumption 246
    delivery
        devices 410*t*
        methods of 410
    dissociation curve 80
    partial pressure of 5, 80
    saturation 83, 88
    therapy
        high flow 257, 468
        indications for high-flow 257*b*
Oxygenation 9
Oxygen-hemoglobin dissociation curve 5, 5*f*, 80*f*, 409, 410*f*

P

P value, significance of 481
Pacemaker 385
    code, five letter 385
    malfunction, causes of 385
    rhythm, latent 1
    syndrome 385
Packed RBC transfusion 26
Pain
    assessment scores 283
    causes of 52
        acute 134, 221
    pathophysiology of 124
    pathways of transmission of 360, 360*f*, 492*f*
    pharmacologic management of 455*t*
    relief 401
    shock rigidity 15
Painful episode, management of acute 561*b*
Painful eye, differential diagnosis of acute 374
Painful swelling, causes of acute 456
Painful vison loss, causes of 91, 92, 180*t*
Painless vison loss 180, 180*t*
Palliative care, role of 575
Palmar interossei 3
Pancreatitis
    acute 338
    causes of 90*t*
        acute 173, 173*t*
    complications in acute 91
    severity of acute 90, 173, 174*t*, 338*t*
    suspected acute 91, 174
Panic disorder 285
Panniculitis 66
Paracetamol overdose
    signs of 384
    symptoms of 384
Paracetamol
    acute ingestion of 556
    minimal toxic doses of 384
Paracetamol toxicity
    management of 556
    pathogenesis of 555, 556*f*
    pathophysiology of 384
Parametric statistical tests 444
Paraphimosis, management of 569
Paraquat poisoning, management of 468
Parasympathetic nervous system 79
Parkland formula 90, 180
Paroxysmal cold hemoglobinuria 555
Paroxysmal nocturnal
    dyspnea 432
    hemoglobinuria 555
Partial thromboplastin time 11, 491
Passive leg raise 163
Patellofemoral syndrome 97
PECARN versus CHALICE rules 438
Pediatric abdominal surgical emergencies 484
Pediatric airway 365, 366*t*
    anatomical characteristics of 365, 365*t*
    management of difficult 365
Pediatric emergency ultrasound protocol 296
Pediatric Glasgow Coma Scale 518
Pediatric meningitis, management of 276
Pediatric population, disaster for 520
Pediatric seizure disorder 201
Pediatric surgical abdomen, cause of 485*t*
Pelvic fracture 132, 268*t*
    classifications of 132, 268, 268*t*, 504
    management of unstable 268
    patient profile for 268
    suspected 131

Pelvic inflammatory disease 224, 420
    management of 224, 226*t*
Pelvic pain, acute 225*t*, 419, 420*t*
Pemphigus vulgaris 65, 284*t*
    treatment of 66
Penetrating eye injury, management of 267
Penicillin 7
    adverse effects of 7
    mechanism of action of 7
Percutaneous coronary intervention 24, 25, 101, 274
Percutaneous cricothyroidotomy 195*f*
Percutaneous intervention 563
Percutaneous tracheostomy, methods of 195
Pericapsular nerve group 523, 523*f*
Pericarditis 101
    management of acute 563
    treatment of
        acute 563*t*
        recurrent 563*t*
Peridialytic hypotension, differential diagnosis of 390
Peri-intubation cardiac arrest 574
Perilunate dislocation 330, 330*f*
Perimortem cesarean section 265, 266*t*
Periodontal abscess 460*t*
    management of 459
Peripartum cardiomyopathy 98
Peripheral blood
    flow 518
    smear 100
        examination 344
Peripheral venous access, complications of 79
Peripheral vertigo 123, 429
Peritonsillar abscess, management of 269, 549
Permanent teeth 226, 226*t*
Permissive hypotension 16, 251
Peroneal nerve injuries 95
Personal protective equipment 208
    level 209*f*
Pes anserine bursitis 97
Pharmacological agent 387*t*
Phenytoin 2
    sodium equivalent 37
Phlebitis 79
Physical abuse, diagnosis of 244
Physical assault, female victim of 461
Physiologically difficult airway, management of 479
Piriformis syndrome 97
Pivot shift 96
Placenta, inspect 12
Plasma 81
    osmolality 2
Plasmodium
    falciparum 100
        parasites 138*f*
    life cycle of 533*fc*
    vivax, life cycle of 533
Pneumonia 249, 346
POCSO act 442
Point-of-care
    testing 167
    ultrasound 89, 295*f*

basic physics of 411
    role of 263, 432
    use of 351
Poiseuille law 452*f*
Poisoning
    acute 62, 63
    cases of 170
Poisonous snakebite 192
Polymerase chain reaction 533
Polymorphonuclear
    leukocytes 199, 404, 423
    neutrophils 326
Polypeptides 7
Popliteal artery injury 95
Portal hypertension, causes of 43, 44*t*
Portal venous system 43, 44*f*
    diagram of 43
Positive end-expiratory pressure 448
Positive predictive value 571
Positive-pressure ventilation 102
Postcardiac arrest
    phase 68
    recovery 35
Posterior cord syndrome 13
Posterolateral injury 96
Postexposure prophylaxis 281, 346
Postmortem cesarean section, procedure of 492
Postpartum hemorrhage 12
    causes of 12*t*, 377, 377*t*, 458*t*
    complications of 377
    management of 377, 458
    risk factors of 377
Potassium homeostasis 530*f*
    pathophysiology of 260, 260*t*
    physiology of 260, 529
Potential organ donor 354
Pralidoxime 27
Preeclampsia 60
    diagnose 223, 223*t*
    severe 98
Pregabalin 37
Pregnancy 132
    affecting resuscitation 86*t*
        physiologic changes in 212
    anatomic changes in 11, 85
    chronic hypertension in 60
    emergencies during 180*t*
    physiological changes in 11, 11*t*, 85, 213*t*
    third trimester of 98
    use in 324*t*
Pregnant female 491, 500
Prehn's sign 18
Prehospital antibiotic therapy 358
Prehospital care 550
Prepatellar bursitis 97
Prerenal azotemia 408*t*
Prisoner absconding 353
Procainamide 80
Procedural sedation 73, 74, 82
    and analgesia 284
    drugs for 73*t*
    indications for 73
Prophylaxis 89
Propofol 69, 82

Pros and cons of different modalities 26
Prostaglandin 466
Prostate 425
Protein 8
    synthesis inhibitors 7
Prothrombin
    complex concentrate 239, 511
    time 11
Proton-pump inhibitors 26
Proximal femur
    anatomical classification fractures of 228*f*
    classify fractures of 228
Proximal femur fracture 228
    complications of 229
    management of 228
Proximal humerus fracture
    classification of 541
    management of 541, 542*fc*
Pseudomonas aeruginosa 49
Psoas abscess 15
Psychiatric emergency, acute 187
Psychiatric patient, medical evaluation of 186
Psychogenic causes 234*t*, 428*t*
Pulmonary artery 62, 79
    catheters 163
Pulmonary capillary wedge pressure 246, 562
Pulmonary edema
    acute 322*fc*
    high-altitude 343
    management of acute 513*fc*
Pulmonary embolism 6, 70*t*, 325, 383
    diagnosis of 70
    echocardiography in 382
    patient, resuscitation of 383*b*
    right ventricle in 383*f*
    scores for 235
Pulmonary functions 406
Pulmonary gas exchange 448*f*
Pulsatile mass 18
Pulse
    contour analysis 85
    contour cardiac output 163
    pressure variation 41, 163
Pulse-echo principle 260
Purkinje fibers 79
Push dose
    pressors 516
    vasopressors 516*t*
Pyelonephritis, differentiate 231
Pyramidal fracture 13
Pyrogenic reactions 65
Pyruvate kinase 555

Q

Q wave 80
QRS complex 80
QT interval prolongation, causes of 80
Quadriparesis
    acute onset of 303
    diagnosis of acute-onset 487
Quality improvement, fishbone analysis for 356
Quantitative buffy coat 138*f*, 533

Quick sequential organ failure assessment 156
　　score 40*t*, 200, 200*t*, 252*t*, 449*t*, 508*t*
Quinidine 80
Quinolones 7

R

Rabies 345
　　pathogenesis of 345
　　postexposure in 473*t*
　　　　prophylaxis in 346*t*
　　prophylaxis in 473*t*
Radiation physics 535
　　fundamentals of 121
Radius bone, fractures of 130
Random donor platelets 16
Rape, victim of 329
Rapid sequence intubation 69, 204
　　drugs for 204*t*
　　role of 77
Rashes 285*t*
Raynaud's disease 56
Real-time audio-visual feedback, use of 35
Receiver operating characteristic curve 44, 292*f*
Recumbent technique 459*f*
Recurrent vomiting, diagnosis of 440
Red blood cells 64, 138*f*, 490
Red eye 229
　　acute 550
　　causes of 229, 551*fc*
Red skin lesions 285*t*
Regional nerve entrapment syndromes 96
Rehydrated children 243
Renal failure 81
　　risk of 501*t*
Renal function
　　evaluation of 407
　　test 15, 425
Renal mechanism 453*f*
Renal replacement therapy 299
Renal transplant 300
Respiration 531*fc*
　　physiological principles of 448
Respiratory acidosis 306
　　pathophysiology of 127
Respiratory disease 73
Respiratory failure
　　causes of 166
　　　　type 1 166*b*
　　　　type 2 166*b*
Resuscitation 16
　　colloids for 16
　　fluid for 478
Resuscitative endovascular balloon occlusion 240*f*, 499*f*
　　of aorta, procedure of 499
Resuscitative hysterotomy 492*f*
Resuscitative thoracotomy 253
Reteplase 25
Retinal detachment 91
Retropharyngeal abscess 549
　　management of 549
Rhabdomyolysis 149, 489, 489*fc*, 501*t*
　　causes of 148, 149*t*

diagnosis of 149
　　principal causes of 149*f*
　　symptoms of 149*b*, 149*f*
　　treatment of 150
Rheumatic fever
　　management of acute 440
　　pathophysiology of acute 440
Rheumatic heart disease 56, 432*fc*
Rheumatoid arthritis 423
Rib fracture 376
　　pain management 503*f*
　　　　of acute 502
Ribosomal ribonucleic acid 7, 533
Richmond agitation-sedation scale 560, 561*t*
Rifampin 7
Right knee joint, ligaments of 94*f*
Right subclavian vein, cannulation of 447
Right ventricular myocardial infarction 563
Romberg test 48
Rotator cuff
　　around shoulder, anatomy of 56, 56*f*, 551*f*
　　shoulder 311*f*
　　tears, pathophysiology of 120
Rotator cuff injury 56, 311, 426, 551
　　clinical assessment of 426
　　risk factors for 425
　　suspected 56, 552
Rule of nine 51*f*, 544*f*
Runner's knee 97
Ruptured abdominal aortic aneurysm, classic triad of 17
Ruptured eye globe 135
　　management of 135
Rush protocol 196*t*
　　shock by 196*t*
Rutherford criteria 378

S

Saddle thromboembolism 62
Saddle thrombus, management of 62
Salbutamol 9
Salt triage scheme 532*fc*
Salt triaging 39*fc*
Salter–Harris
　　classification 271, 271*f*, 421, 421*t*
　　fracture 421*f*
SARS COV-2 infection 451
Scalds 75
Scaphoid lunate dislocation 256
Scars 75
Scorpion bite, management of 508
Scrotal pain
　　acute onset of 270
　　causes of acute 93, 175
Secure airway 36
Seidel sign 267
Seizure 234*t*, 428*t*, 429, 517
　　syncope from 234
　　treatment 89
　　type of 371*t*
Seldinger technique 20
Selective serotonin reuptake inhibitors 23, 474
Sensitivity troponin, high 249

Sensorineural deafness 49
Sensorium 100*fc*
　　altered 100, 347
Sensory state 48
Sepsis 29, 79, 200, 358
　　child with 398
　　diagnosis of 448
　　endocrine changes in 448
　　guidelines, surviving 41*t*, 200, 200*t*
　　hormonal changes in 448*f*
　　identification of 252
　　shock 40, 156
　　　　pathophysiology of 252
　　suspected 358
Septic arthritis, management of 325
Septic shock 40, 156, 467
　　initial resuscitation of 71*t*
　　resuscitation of 71
　　vasopressors in 40
Sequential organ failure assessment 200
Serious cardiac rhythm disturbances 112
Serotonin syndrome 144, 144*t*, 280, 280*t*
Setting-sun sign 32
Sexual assault
　　female victim of 111
　　treatment of female victim of 111
　　victim of 111, 329
Sexually transmitted infections 420
Shock
　　fluid volume in 364, 365*t*
　　resuscitation planning in 290*fc*
　　trauma
　　　　classification of 463
　　　　hemorrhagic 291
Shoulder
　　impingement syndrome, pathophysiology of 120
　　joint, anatomy of 120, 120*f*, 255, 255*f*
　　rotator cuff muscles of 425, 425*f*
Shoulder dislocation
　　management of anterior 381
　　types of 255
Shunt, insertion of 32*f*
Sickle cell
　　crisis, management of 282
　　disease 116, 561, 561*b*
　　trait 482
Single rescuer cardiopulmonary resuscitation 68
Sinuses 450*f*
Skin
　　lesion 285*t*
　　　　classification of 285*t*
　　rashes 285*t*
Small bowel obstruction 328
Small-bore chest tube 20
Smith's fracture 130
　　complications of 130
　　X-ray of 130*f*
Smoke inhalation
　　injury 179*t*, 464*t*
　　management of 342
Snakebite
　　cases of 192
　　syndromic approach to 193*f*

Sodium
 bicarbonate therapy 2, 275
 homeostasis 2, 43
  physiology of 453
 polystyrene sulfonate 28
Soft tissue, foreign bodies in 537
Somatic motor effects 27
Somatostatin 26
Somatropin 448
Sore throat
 acute 375
 causes of 375, 375t
 noninfectious causes of 375t
 risk stratification for 375
 signs of acute 375
 symptoms of acute 375
Sphygmomanometry 84
Spinal cord
 blood supply of 217, 218f
 injury 373
 transverse section of 218, 218f
Spinal cord syndrome 464, 494
 incomplete 13, 92, 178, 465f, 495f
 types of 178f
Spinal shock 13, 13t, 124, 373, 373t
Spirometry, abnormal 407f
Spleen trauma grades 504t, 545t
Splenic injury
 classification of 545
 management of 545
Splinting, prehospital care for 168
Spontaneous bacterial peritonitis
 diagnosis of 105t
 treatment of 105t
Spontaneous circulation, return of 35, 87, 516
Staphylococcal scalded skin syndrome 29, 349, 435
Staphylococcal toxic shock syndrome 29
 diagnostic criteria of 29
 pathogenesis of 29
Staphylococcus
 aureus 29, 49
 species 29
Status epilepticus 190
 management of 37, 191
 treatment for 37t, 278t
Steeple sign 158f
ST-elevation myocardial infarction 273
Sternum 33
Steroids, use of 13
Stevens–Johnson syndrome 349, 436
Stewart–Holmes rebound sign 48
Sting 433
Streptokinase 25
Stress cardiomyopathy 101
Stridor
 acute 516
 causes of 157, 203, 203t, 517t
Stroke
 management of 293
 mimics 21, 21t, 103, 103t, 183t
 thrombolysis 183
  in acute 21
 thrombolytic therapy for 512
 volume variation 41, 163

ST-segment elevation
 causes of 101
 myocardial infarction 25
Subarachnoid hemorrhage 58, 100
 grading scales for 58t
 suspicion of 58
Subclavian vein 447f
 anatomy of 78, 78f
Suboptimal mask seal 77
Subscapularis 56
Substance-use disorder 114, 115b
 severity of 115f
Succinylcholine 70
Sudden infant death syndrome 155
 causes for 155
 risk factors for 155
Suicidal hanging, management of 498
Suicide substrate 6
Sulfonylurea-induced hypoglycemia, manage 139
Supine hypotension syndrome 11
Supracondylar fracture 131
 late complications of 131
 management of 271
Supraglottic airways 77
Suprascapular nerve 312
Supraspinatus muscle 56
Supraventricular arrhythmias, management of 475
Supraventricular tachycardia 475
 management of 476t
Surgical embolectomy 62
Sympathetic crashing acute pulmonary edema 98
 management of 321, 512
 physiology of 321fc
Sympathetic nervous system 79
Synaptobrevin 8
Syncope 233, 234
 causes of 233
 diagnostic algorithm of 427
Syndrome of inappropriate antidiuretic hormone 164
Synovial fluid 424
 analysis 326t, 423t
Systemic inflammatory response syndrome 174
Systemic lupus erythematosus 423, 431
Systemic vascular resistance 347, 518
Systolic blood pressure 25, 34, 110, 200, 246, 252, 273, 387, 449, 485
 early intensive 33

T

T wave 80
Tachyarrhythmia
 mechanisms of 1
 narrow complex 286fc
Tachycardia 29
 narrow complex 286
 wide-complex 344
Tactical casualty combat care
 guidelines 296
 phases of 297t

Takayasu arteritis 56
Tamponade 79
Target international randomized ratio 6
Temperature control 89
Temperature regulation
 pathophysiology of 409fc
 physiology of 164, 165fc, 361
Temporary teeth 226, 226t
Temporomandibular joint dislocation 269f
 causes of 458
 management of 269
Tenecteplase 25
Tension pneumothorax 19, 55
Teres minor 56
Terlipressin causes vasoconstriction 26
Testicular torsion
 management of 482
 treatment option for 94, 175
Testis, detorsion of 19
Tetanus 237
 immune globulin 8, 237
 immunization 8, 237
 pathogenesis of 8, 236
 pathophysiology of 106
 prophylaxis 8, 8t, 237t
 toxin 8
 toxoid 8
 treatment of 237, 237t, 568t
Tetanus-diphtheria toxoid 8, 237
Therapeutic hypothermia 253
Thermal burn, classification of 51, 51t, 543t
Thermoregulation, physiology of 313
Thigh pain, anterolateral 97
Thoracic trauma 19
Thoracodorsal nerve 312
Thrombin 12
Thromboangiitis proliferans 56
Thrombocytopenia, heparin-induced 6
Thromboelastography 210f, 411, 412f
 role of 209
Thromboembolic disease, treatment of 324
Thromboembolism in pregnancy, diagnosis of 324
Thrombolysis 183
 method of 21
Thrombophilia 147
Thrombotic thrombocytopenic purpura 173, 555
Thyroid function test 187, 188t
 interpretation of 188t, 434t
Thyroid hormone production, physiology of 434, 434fc
Thyroid storm 29, 238, 434
 diagnostic criteria for 29
 management of 29, 29t, 238, 238t, 435t, 510, 510t
 precipitating factors for 29, 237
Thyroid-stimulating hormone 188, 189, 434, 448
Thyroxine 188, 189, 434, 448
Tibia
 medial areas of 94f
 subcondylar areas of 94f
Tinzaparin 6
Tissue necrosis 79
Tonsillitis 36

Topical ophthalmic medication 417*t*
Topiramate 37
Torsion testis, diagnose 18
Total body
 surface area 198
 water 259
Total lung capacity 487
Total parenteral nutrition 244
Toxic epidermal necrolysis 145, 436
Toxic syndrome 23
 common 23*t*, 474*t*
Toxidrome 23, 23*t*, 474, 474*t*
Tracheal injury 79
Tranexamic acid, role of 52
Transbronchial lung biopsy 431
Transbronchial needle aspiration 431
Transient ischemic attack 248, 429
Transthoracic echocardiography 85
Trauma
 chain of survival in 291*f*
 coagulation derangement in 491
 coagulopathy in 491*f*
 management 11
  changes in 11
 nerve blocks in 355
 scale, revised 73, 73*t*
 score, revised 73
 surgery of 253*t*
 victim 209, 478
Traumatic brain injury, management of 72, 373
Traumatic ocular injury 463
Traumatic shock, pathophysiology of 411
Tricuspid regurgitation peak gradient 383
Tricyclic antidepressant 23, 474
 overdose 142, 142*t*
 poisoning 279
 toxicity 143*f*
Triggered rhythms 1
Tri-iodothyronine 188, 189, 434, 448
 reverse 448
Trimethoprim 7
Troponins 62
Tube, placement of 69
Tubercular meningitis 404
Tubo-ovarian abscess 420
Tubular necrosis, acute 408, 408*t*
Tumor
 lysis, pathophysiology of 215*fc*
 necrosis factor 212, 466
Tumor lysis syndrome
 management of 215
 pathophysiology of 215
Two-handed technique 267*f*

U

Ulnar nerve 3
 injury 229, 451, 451*f*
Ultrasound, role of 135
Ultrasound-guided triage 295
Upper endoscopy and colonoscopy 26
Upper extremity injuries 332
Upper gastrointestinal bleeding 25, 227
 management of 26*fc*

Upper subscapular nerve 312
Uremia 81
Ureter 425
Urethral injuries 220
 diagnosis of 221
 in male, treatment of 547
Urinary bladder, nerve supply of 424, 424*f*
Urinary tract infection 231, 245, 420
 complicated 231
 uncomplicated 231
Urine
 acidification, mechanism of 299
 acute retention of 424, 425*fc*
 analysis 15, 231, 276, 408*t*
 examination 325
 formation, physiology of 370, 370*f*

V

Vaccination, role of 71
Vaccine development, stages of 570*fc*
Vaginal bleeding
 causes of 222, 265
 diagnostic algorithm of 419
 differential diagnoses of 419
Vancomycin 7, 358
Vaso-occlusive crisis 116
 acute 561
Vasopressin, role of 68
Vasopressor
 classification of 538
 common 538*t*
 resistant shock, management of 514
 therapy principles 41*f*
Vaughan-William's classification 86
Vena cava
 inferior 44, 163, 196, 289, 383
  compression of 12*f*
Venoarterial extracorporeal membrane oxygenation 241
Venomous scorpion 433
 management of 434
Venous blood gas 366, 367*t*
Venous oximetry 81
Venous oxygen saturation 81
Venous thromboembolism
 diagnostic testing for 235
 risk factors for 235
 treatment of 70
Venovenous extracorporeal membrane oxygenation 241
Ventilatory abnormalities 214, 214*f*
Ventricular repolarization 80
Ventricular tachycardia 101
Vertigo 122, 123
 acute-onset 430, 430*fc*
 benign paroxysmal positional 429
 causes of 335*t*, 429*t*
 central 123, 429
 management of acute onset 335, 501
Vesiculobullous lesions, acute onset 510
Vesiculobullous skin lesions, causes of 65
Vestibulo-ocular reflex 123

Vibrio vulnificus 56
Victim's gait 111
Violence, prevention of 399
Viperid bite 192*t*
 signs of 192*t*
Viral laryngotracheobronchitis 36
Vision
 acute loss of 417
 acute painful loss of 502
 loss of 550
Visual aids guidance 35
Visual pathway 495
Vital capacity 487*f*
Vitamin K 6
 antagonists, management of 239*t*, 511*t*
Vivax, mature stages of 534*f*
Vocal cord dysfunction 36
Vomiting, causes of 200, 200*t*
von Willebrand
 disease 369
 factor 213

W

Warfarin 511
Warfarin-induced bleeding, management of 239
Water bath technique 296, 296*f*
Waveform, components of 411
Weakness
 muscular cause of 388
 non-neurologic causes of 388
Weber test 49
Westley croup score, modified 159*t*
Wheezing 22
White blood cell 105, 138, 199, 221, 252, 326, 404, 423, 424
White cerebellar sign 294
Wolff-Parkinson-White syndrome 80, 475
Wong–Baker pain rating scale 283*f*
Wound
 management, routine 8*t*
 puncture 237
Wrist
 and hand, anatomy of 3, 3*f*
 pivot method 459*f*
Wrist joint
 anatomy of 329
 normal 329
 radiology of 329*f*

X

Xenobiotic absorption 62

Z

Zika virus
 infection 113
 management of 202
Zinc-dependent metalloproteinase 8
Zipper entrapment injury, management of 271
Zonisamide 37
Zygomatic suture line, fractures of 13

EU GSPR Authorised Reprsentative
Logos Europe, 9 rue Nicolas Poussin
1700, La Rochelle, France
Phone: +33 (0) 6 67 93 73 78
E-mail: contact@logoseurope.eu

www.ingramcontent.com/pod-product-compliance
Ingram Content Group UK Ltd.
Pitfield, Milton Keynes, MK11 3LW, UK
UKHW050703160426
5217IPUK00041B/1322